Vegetarian and Plant-Based Diets in Health and Disease Prevention

Vegetarian and Plant-Based Diets in Health and Disease Prevention

Edited by

François Mariotti

 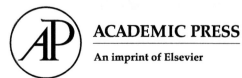

ACADEMIC PRESS
An imprint of Elsevier

Part 4: Life Events

List of Contributors

Carlo Agostoni Fondazione IRCCS Cà Granda Ospedale Maggiore Policlinico, Milan, Italy; University of Milan, Milan, Italy

Sutapa Agrawal Public Health Foundation of India, Gurgaon, India

Ute Alexy University of Bonn, Bonn, Germany

C. Alix Timko University of Pennsylvania, Philadelphia, PA, United States; Children's Hospital of Philadelphia, Philadelphia, PA, United States

Benjamin Alles Sorbonne Paris Cité Epidemiology and Statistics Research Center (CRESS), Nutritional Epidemiology Research Team (EREN), Inserm U1153, Inra U1125, Conservatoire National des Arts et Métiers (CNAM), Paris 5, 7, 13 Universities, Bobigny, France

Rossella Attini University of Torino, Torino, Italy

Yun-Jung Bae Shinhan University, Uijeongbu, Korea

Neal D. Barnard Physicians Committee for Responsible Medicine, Washington, DC, United States; George Washington University School of Medicine and Health Sciences, Washington, DC, United States

Nawel Bemrah Risk Assessment Unit – French Agency for Food, Environmental and Occupational Health & Safety (ANSES), Maisons-Alfort, France

Silvia Bettocchi Fondazione IRCCS Cà Granda Ospedale Maggiore Policlinico, Milan, Italy; Università Cattolica del Sacro Cuore, Milan, Italy

Marie-Christine Boutron-Ruault Institut Gustave Roussy, Villejuif, France; University Paris-Saclay, Villejuif, France

Patricia Burns Instituto de Lactología Industrial (CONICET-UNL), Facultad de Ingeniería Química, Universidad Nacional del Litoral, Santa Fe, Argentina

Gianfranca Cabiddu Brotzu Hospital, Cagliari, Italy

Irene Capizzi   University of Torino, Torino, Italy

Peter Clarys   Vrije Universiteit Brussel, Brussels, Belgium; Erasmus University College, Brussels, Belgium

David A. Cleveland   University of California, Santa Barbara, CA, United States

Peter Clifton   University of South Australia, Adelaide, SA, Australia; School of Health Sciences Flinders University, Adelaide, SA, Australia

Emilie Combet   University of Glasgow, Glasgow, United Kingdom

Pieter C. Dagnelie   Maastricht University, Maastricht, The Netherlands

Luc Dauchet   CHRU Lille University Medical Center, Lille, France; Lille University, Lille, France

Valentina De Cosmi   Fondazione IRCCS Cà Granda Ospedale Maggiore Policlinico, Milan, Italy; University of Milan, Milan, Italy

Peter Deriemaeker   Vrije Universiteit Brussel, Brussels, Belgium; Erasmus University College, Brussels, Belgium

Anthony Fardet   INRA, UMR 1019, UNH, CRNH Auvergne, Clermont-Ferrand, France; Clermont Université, Université d'Auvergne, Clermont-Ferrand, France

Massimo Filippi   San Raffaele Scientific Institute and Vita-Salute San Raffaele University, Milan, Italy

Ségolène Fleury   Risk Assessment Unit – French Agency for Food, Environmental and Occupational Health & Safety (ANSES), Maisons-Alfort, France

Meika Foster   University of Otago, Dunedin, New Zealand

Quentin Gee   University of California, Santa Barbara, CA, United States

Marian Glick-Bauer   City University of New York, New York, NY, United States

Daiva Gorczyca   Wroclaw Medical University, Wroclaw, Poland

Marcel Hebbelinck   Vrije Universiteit Brussel, Brussels, Belgium

Sydney Heiss University at Albany, State University of New York, Albany, NY, United States

Wolfgang Herrmann Saarland University Hospital, Homburg, Germany

Sarah R. Hoffman UNC Gillings School of Global Public Health, Chapel Hill, NC, United States

Julia M. Hormes University at Albany, State University of New York, Albany, NY, United States

Motoyasu Iikura National Center for Global Health and Medicine, Tokyo, Japan

Piia Jallinoja University of Helsinki, Helsinki, Finland

Nicole Janz University Clinic Bochum, Bochum, Germany

Carol S. Johnston Arizona State University, Phoenix, AZ, United States

Jae G. Jung Dongguk University Ilsan Hospital, Goyang, Korea; Incheon Sarang Hospital, Incheon, Korea

Sarah Jung Loma Linda University, Loma Linda, CA, United States

Hana Kahleova Institute for Clinical and Experimental Medicine, Prague, Czech Republic

Hyoun W. Kang Dongguk University Ilsan Hospital, Goyang, Korea

David L. Katz Griffin Hospital, Derby, CT, United States

Sarah H. Kehoe MRC Lifecourse Epidemiology Unit, Southampton, United Kingdom

Mathilde Kersting University Clinic Bochum, Bochum, Germany

Timothy J. Key University of Oxford, Oxford, Oxfordshire, United Kingdom

Ghattu V. Krishnaveni CSI Holdsworth Memorial Hospital, Mysore, India

Kalyanaraman Kumaran CSI Holdsworth Memorial Hospital, Mysore, India; MRC Lifecourse Epidemiology Unit, Southampton, United Kingdom

Filomena Leone   University of Torino, Torino, Italy

Valentina Loi   Brotzu Hospital, Cagliari, Italy

Kelsey M. Mangano   University of Massachusetts Lowell, Lowell, MA, United States

Jim Mann   University of Otago, Dunedin, New Zealand

François Mariotti   UMR Physiologie de la Nutrition et du Comportement Alimentaire, AgroParisTech, INRA, Université Paris-Saclay, Paris, France

Stefania Maxia   Brotzu Hospital, Cagliari, Italy

Alessandra Mazzocchi   Fondazione IRCCS Cà Granda Ospedale Maggiore Policlinico, Milan, Italy; University of Milan, Milan, Italy

Sylvie Mesrine   Institut Gustave Roussy, Villejuif, France; University Paris-Saclay, Villejuif, France

Yoshihiro Miyamoto   National Cerebral and Cardiovascular Center, Osaka, Japan

Diego Moretti   ETH Zürich, Zürich, Switzerland

Preetam Nath   S.C.B. Medical College, Cuttack, India

Kunihiro Nishimura   National Cerebral and Cardiovascular Center, Osaka, Japan

Mari Niva   University of Helsinki, Helsinki, Finland

Alexandre Nougadère   Risk Assessment Unit – French Agency for Food, Environmental and Occupational Health & Safety (ANSES), Maisons-Alfort, France

Derek Obersby   University of West London, London, United Kingdom

Michael J. Orlich   Loma Linda University, Loma Linda, CA, United States

Terezie Pelikanova   Institute for Clinical and Experimental Medicine, Prague, Czech Republic

Giorgina B. Piccoli   University of Torino, Torino, Italy; Le Mans Hospital, Le Mans, France

Fabrice Pierre   Université de Toulouse III, Toulouse, France

Jorge Reinheimer   Instituto de Lactología Industrial (CONICET-UNL), Facultad de Ingeniería Química, Universidad Nacional del Litoral, Santa Fe, Argentina

Gianna C. Riccitelli   San Raffaele Scientific Institute and Vita-Salute San Raffaele University, Milan, Italy

Gilles Rivière   Risk Assessment Unit – French Agency for Food, Environmental and Occupational Health & Safety (ANSES), Maisons-Alfort, France

Maria A. Rocca   San Raffaele Scientific Institute and Vita-Salute San Raffaele University, Milan, Italy

Hank Rothgerber   Bellarmine University, Louisville, KY, United States

Samir Samman   University of Otago, Dunedin, New Zealand; University of Sydney, Sydney, NSW, Australia

Thomas A.B. Sanders   King's College London, United Kingdom

Silvia Scaglioni   Fondazione IRCCS Cà Granda Ospedale Maggiore Policlinico, Milan, Italy

Lutz Schomburg   Charité - Universitätsmedizin Berlin, Berlin, Germany

Gina Siapco   Loma Linda University, Loma Linda, CA, United States

Shivaram Prasad Singh   S.C.B. Medical College, Cuttack, India

Frank Thies   University of Aberdeen, Aberdeen, United Kingdom

Tullia Todros   University of Torino, Torino, Italy

Serena Tonstad   Oslo University Hospital, Oslo, Norway; Loma Linda University, Loma Linda, CA, United States

Mathilde Touvier   Sorbonne Paris Cité Epidemiology and Statistics Research Center (CRESS), Nutritional Epidemiology Research Team (EREN), Inserm U1153, Inra U1125, Conservatoire National des Arts et Métiers (CNAM), Paris 5, 7, 13 Universities, Bobigny, France

Amalia Tsiami   University of West London, London, United Kingdom

Katherine L. Tucker   University of Massachusetts Lowell, Lowell, MA, United States

Laura Vacchi   San Raffaele Scientific Institute and Vita-Salute San Raffaele University, Milan, Italy

Annukka Vainio   Natural Resources Institute Finland, Helsinki, Finland

Marine van Berleere   CHRU Lille University Medical Center, Lille, France

Gabriel Vinderola   Instituto de Lactología Industrial (CONICET-UNL), Facultad de Ingeniería Química, Universidad Nacional del Litoral, Santa Fe, Argentina

Stephen Walsh   Vrije Universiteit Brussel, Brussels, Belgium

Michelle Wien   California State Polytechnic University, Pomona, Pomona, CA, United States

P. Winnie Gerbens-Leenes   University of Groningen, Groningen, The Netherlands

Ming-Chin Yeh   City University of New York, New York, NY, United States

Yoko Yokoyama   Keio University, Kanagawa, Japan

Foreword

All life must feed. For most creatures, this exigency of survival is simple, if not always easy. Sometimes, food is merely elusive. Sometimes, it runs away. Sometimes, it fights back.

Plants, rooted in the bedrock of biology on this planet, feed on sunlight itself. Herbivores feed on such plants. Carnivores, in their turn, feed on those plant-fed herbivores.

Only for omnivores are the routine difficulties of acquiring adequate sustenance compounded by the complex dilemma of choice. Uniquely, omnivores have choices to make, and we humans are constitutional omnivores. We have been omnivores since before ever our species became "*sapiens,*" let alone "*sapiens*" twice over. Our *Homo erectus* forebears were omnivores, too.

When we look over that expanse, the sweep of human history, the view of diet grows fairly dim very fast. Just consider how challenging it is to remember exactly what we ate yesterday, and we can readily forgive fairly wide error bars around breakfast in the Paleolithic. Still, there is a quite a bit we do know with confidence about the diet to which we are natively adapted. There was a great diversity of plant foods in it. Animals were wild and, in turn, nourished by their native diets and lean due to their native exertions. Water was the principal relief of thirst. Excesses of saturated fat, added sugar, or refined starch were nowhere to be found.

Where the paleoanthropologists debate, they debate the salience of meat in our native diet. Some now contend we were, as long labeled, hunter-gatherers; others contend we were more correctly gatherer-hunters. Perhaps, clans of us were both in different places at different times. Omnivores are opportunists.

The relative preponderance of plants, however, is a matter of relative consensus. Across the range of dietary patterns debated, plants predominate by volume when not by calories, and by both at the other extreme. The reasons were almost certainly the obvious: plants do not flee, and they tend not to fight back (although there are exceptions, as those who have ever picked a prickly pear know). Gathering is generally less perilous than hunting with primitive weapons, and more reliably productive.

However, we allow for debates about the Stone Age, as modern diets emphasizing animal products and processed foods are a marked departure from our adaptations.

All on its own, adaptation would make a case for a return to diets enriched with a variety of minimally processed plant foods, but we have no need to rely on only that. As laid out in the many and diverse chapters of this book, there is an enormous aggregation of modern evidence favoring plant-predominant diets for human health. The basis for plant-based diets in arguments addressing environmental impact and ethics may be stronger still, though they are the lesser emphasis here.

Across a vast expanse of studies, methods, populations, and outcomes, an emphasis on vegetables and fruits is perhaps the most consistent feature of diets associated with favorable health outcomes. This book enumerates the many particulars underlying that simple and robust assertion, addressing in turn the what, why, and how of vegetarianism and related dietary variants. The coverage is comprehensive, the evidence is presented clearly and abundantly, and the editing is methodical. The result is a source all but encyclopedic.

However strong and diverse the arguments for plant-based eating, they do not alter the omnivorous nature and legacy of *Homo sapiens*. We are, natively, omnivorous; and omnivores have choices.

This expansive, richly referenced, and meticulously edited text is dedicated to the proposition that those choices be well and fully informed.

-Fin,

David L. Katz, MD, MPH
Director, Yale University Prevention Research Center
Griffin Hospital, Derby, CT, United States
Founder, The True Health Initiative
Author (forthcoming): *The Truth About Food* (HarperOne, 2018)

Preface

The right science at the right time

"A timely initiative": that was a comment I often heard when discussing this project with my colleagues and potential contributors to this book. In a context of global population growth, particular attention is now being paid to critical transitions in subsistence modes regarding protein and energy from plant or animal sources. For a whole series of reasons grouped around the different facets of sustainability, there has been a marked change to how Western and developing countries now judge diets that are mostly contributed by plants and characterized by varied degrees and types of avoidance of animal products. This is now a burning issue and an important feature of sustainability in terms of its effects on health, a pivotal aspiration of the human condition that can help us to understand the effects of the behaviors we deploy within our environment.

Yet, this field is still only addressed in a partial and fragmentary manner, and it remains a subject of considerable controversy and clashing views. Science offers a way to overcome this problem. There is now a large body of literature that contains wide-ranging and in-depth information on the relationships between vegetarian or plant-based diets and our health. The aim of this book was therefore to assemble all these data in a single work that could offer a benchmark in the field and also provide an overview of the information available. It therefore discusses both the overall benefits of plant-based diets on health and the disease risk, and issues concerning the status in certain nutrients of the individuals consuming them, while considering the entire spectrum of vegetarian diets.

The first part of this book was designed to unravel the complex context of this issue. It thus reviews its different aspects so that readers can understand the whole picture. In particular, this section focuses on the links between our dietary choices in favor of animal or plant sources and individual social and behavioral characteristics, indicating how these may vary as a function of cultures or religions in different parts of the world and how they are articulated in terms of nutrition transitions and other aspects of sustainability. We then seek to provide a comprehensive view of the relationships between plant-based diets, health, and disease prevention by presenting different viewpoints and levels of analysis. First of all, we describe the links between health and certain important characteristics of plant-based diets, with obvious reference to the consumption of both fruits and vegetables and meat. There follow 12 chapters that analyze the relationships between plant-based or vegetarian diets and their numerous consequences with respect to health and disease outcomes. The next section explains how this issue may differ, or be highly specific, in populations of different age or physiological status. The last part of the book comprises 11 chapters that look in detail at the nutrients and substances whose intakes are related to the proportions of plant or animal products in the diet. By focusing at the nutrient/substance level, these chapters echo the section dedicated to the links between broad dietary characteristics and health, thus reflecting the different viewpoints offered by the book.

With its 45 chapters contributed by around a hundred eminent scientists from throughout the world, this book offers both students and academics an opportunity to immerse themselves in a multifaceted nutritional area that is both fascinating and highly scientific. More generally, by using science to address such a complex societal issue in an encyclopedic manner, this book could be seen as a reminiscence of our collective memory, in the same way that the Enlightenment movement tried to illuminate virtuous and sustainable pathways for humankind.

I am extremely grateful to all these contributors for their efforts. Our aim is now to grow into an international group of experts who are active in this field to sustain scientific initiatives regarding the critical and inspiring subject of plant-based diets.

Prof. François Mariotti, PhD
Professor of Nutrition
UMR PNCA, AgroParisTech, INRA
Université Paris-Saclay, Paris, France
Editor

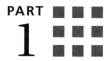

PART 1

Setting the Scene – General Features Associated With Vegetarian Diets

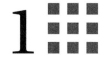

1

Vegetarian Diets: Definitions and Pitfalls in Interpreting Literature on Health Effects of Vegetarianism

Pieter C. Dagnelie[1], François Mariotti[2]

[1]MAASTRICHT UNIVERSITY, MAASTRICHT, THE NETHERLANDS; [2]UMR PHYSIOLOGIE DE LA NUTRITION ET DU COMPORTEMENT ALIMENTAIRE, AGROPARISTECH, INRA, UNIVERSITÉ PARIS-SACLAY, PARIS, FRANCE

1. Introduction

Vegetarianism refers to the practice of abstaining from the consumption of one or more types of foods from animal origin, especially flesh from animals. A brief overview of the background and history of vegetarianism is found in Wikipedia (Anonymous, 2016). The term "vegetarian" was first used in public around 1840, possibly as a combination of *vegetable* and *-arian* as a descriptor of a person's characteristics. The term was popularized in subsequent years in Western Europe by the foundation of national vegetarian societies, as well as the International Vegetarian Union. However, vegetarian tradition is much older, especially in India, where the oldest records date back to several centuries BC. In ancient Europe, vegetarianism was probably uncommon, and in the middle ages, several monk orders avoided meat, but not fish, for ascetic reasons. Eating fish instead of meat on Fridays has continued to be a very common Roman Catholic tradition in many parts of the world. In this book, "plant-based diets" refer to diets predominantly based on plant foods, including most vegetarian diets.

2. Underlying Motivation of Plant-Based and Vegetarian Diets

There is extensive literature on reasons for choosing a vegetarian diet. Some reasons for avoiding meat and/or other animal products are these:

- ethical reasons, related to killing animals and/or animal welfare;
- ecological reasons, especially the low efficiency of producing animal food (both in terms of calories and protein) from edible plant foods in relation to the world food situation and the growing world population;

Vegetarian and Plant-Based Diets in Health and Disease Prevention. http://dx.doi.org/10.1016/B978-0-12-803968-7.00001-0

- health reasons, related to the notion that consumption of large amounts of animal products high in saturated fat is associated with a wide variety of diseases in affluent societies. Another health reason may be the presence of contaminants, additives, or other unwanted substances in animal products;
- disliking certain types of animal food. This is a very common reason for avoiding one or more specific types of animal foods, e.g., certain types of fish, poultry, pork, beef, lamb, etc.

These categories may be simplified to two main reasons for being vegetarian, as applied by many authors: ethical reasons (ethical vegetarians) or health reason (health vegetarians). Of note, health effects of diet are caused by the actual foods eaten, regardless of the underlying motivation. Millions of people around the globe eat diets that are predominantly or even exclusively plant-based because animal foods are either locally unavailable or unaffordable. If we define vegetarianism as actual behavior, regardless of underlying motivation, these people would be vegetarians. Indeed, the health effects of "enforced plant-based diets" may, in some respects, resemble the health effects of "voluntary" vegetarian diets. However, the resemblance stops if unavailability of animal products due to food shortage or poverty is the cause of the enforced plant-based diets, since this will go hand in hand with otherwise suboptimal dietary composition, or even with general food shortage or famine.

Furthermore, especially in non-Western countries, vegetarianism may relate to cultural and religious adherence superimposed on other traditional determinants of vegetarian diet, as the readers can read in the first section of this book.

For the sake of consistency, in this volume, we restrict the term vegetarianism to the conscious, voluntary choice to exclude meat (poultry, beef, pork, lamb, etc.), fish, seafood (shellfish, shrimp, octopus, etc.), and possibly other animal products such as dairy and eggs from the diet.

3. Definitions

The term **vegetarian** will be used in this volume to include *all categories of vegetarian diets and vegetarians without distinction, i.e., all diets excluding meat and fish, regardless of whether other animal products such as dairy and/or eggs are also excluded.* Of note, in the literature, many authors apply the term "vegetarian" as a synonym for "ovolactovegetarian" because ovolactovegetarians are the most numerous category of vegetarians. We discourage this utilization because its meaning is ambiguous. If ovolactovegetarians are specifically meant, we will use the term "ovolactovegetarian" and not "vegetarian."

Ovolactovegetarian: Refers to a diet composed of (or people consuming) dairy and eggs, but no meat, fish, or other seafood (shellfish, shrimp, octopus, etc.). Some definitions (e.g., by the Dutch Vegetarian Society) restrict the term ovolactovegetarian to someone who avoids not only flesh from killed animals (meat and fish) but also gelatin and cheese curdled with rennet of animal origin. Here, we will not follow this definition.

Lactovegetarian: As ovolactovegetarian, consuming dairy but not eggs.

Ovovegetarian: As ovolactovegetarian, consuming eggs but not dairy.

Pescetarian/pesco-vegetarian: Refers to a diet containing (or people who eat) fish and/or seafood but no meat.

Vegan: Refers to a diet not containing (or people who do not consume) any animal foods. Also, by-products of animal husbandry, e.g., milk and honey, are excluded from the diet.

Many vegans also exclude other animal-derived products such as leather, but since the focus of this volume is on diet, we will not make a distinction regarding the use of nonedible products.

Semivegetarian, also called "flexitarian": Refers to people following a predominantly vegetarian diet of any type, but with the occasional inclusion of animal products; usually, the term "semi" refers to meat and fish. In scientific literature, it is essential to define what is meant by "occasional," since this could just as well be once per month as three times per week. In scientific studies, different definitions may be relevant depending on the context. For example, in a prospective cohort study on the etiological relation between meat consumption and cancer, a cutoff point of one time per week would be relevant; whereas in studies on nutritional adequacy of low-meat diets, a cutoff point of two to three times per week would be more relevant. Nevertheless, the fact that any cutoff point is arbitrary has contributed to the lack of congruence in the scientific literature. For the present book, we propose a cutoff point of no more than once per week.

"Low-meat eaters" or **"occasional meat eaters"** are—similar to semivegetarians—defined as people eating meat every now and then, and again in each and every publication the definition should be given. Gilsing et al. (2013) defined low-meat eaters as people eating meat once per week, which was logical in the context of the concerned study (meat in the etiology of cancer); however, as mentioned earlier, this may depend on the scientific context, similar to semivegetarians. Again, for the present book, we propose a cutoff point of no more than once per week.

Vegetarian-like diets: Many specific movements, schools, etc., exist that apply vegetarianism to a certain extent. Examples are adherents of anthroposophy and Seventh Day Adventists, some of whom avoid meat. In any such case, the food composition of such a diet (including information on variability between subjects) should be defined as precisely as possible in any study on the health effects of the concerned diet.

Macrobiotic: The macrobiotic diet does not directly fit into the aforementioned schedule, as there is no formal, strict avoidance of specific foods. In macrobiotics, the purpose is to construct a diet that is individually shaped to find a balance between two polar forces: yin and yang. The macrobiotic diet consists of cereals (especially unpolished rice), pulses, and vegetables with small additions of seaweeds, fermented food, nuts, and seeds. Most macrobiotic adherents avoid meat, dairy products, and fruits. Fish may be taken occasionally if desired, but in practice, it is eaten rarely by many adherents to the macrobiotic diet.

Strict vegetarian: Literally, this expression refers to people who strictly adhere to the type of vegetarian diet they have chosen. Strictness is the degree of perseverance or rigidity in, in this case, avoiding certain foods. Thus, in this sense, a "strict vegetarian" is someone who eats "strictly vegetarian diets," i.e., who *strictly adheres to whatever type of vegetarianism he/she applies*. So, a strict lactovegetarian is someone who never uses meat, and a strict vegan is someone who strictly avoids all animal foods.

Some authors use the term "strict vegetarian" as a synonym for people avoiding many or all animal foods, especially vegans. Since this application of "strict" does not specify which foods are avoided, it is ambiguous and should be avoided.

In this volume, strictness is used only as referring to the degree to which people adhere to their vegetarian diet, regardless of the type of vegetarianism they have chosen.

True vegetarian: This term is used for people who truly adhere to a vegetarian diet, i.e., identical to the term "strict vegetarian."

4. Methodological Pitfalls in Interpreting the Literature on Health Effects of Vegetarian Diets

4.1 Heterogeneity in Dietary Composition

No two human beings are the same, nor are their diets. Even when restricting the definition of vegetarianism to a "conscious voluntary choice", there are essential caveats in studies on health effects of vegetarian diets. Vegetarians are in no way a homogeneous or well-defined group: the diet of two vegetarians may be as different as the diet of two omnivores, or even more. Consequently, it is useless to speak about "health effects of vegetarian diets" without a further definition. For example, health effects may markedly differ between (1) someone who dislikes meat and just leaves it out of the diet without any dietary adaptations and (2) someone who replaces meat by another source of high-quality protein, such as dairy products or soy-based foods, and includes a vitamin B_{12} supplement.

Furthermore, any combinations of types of avoidance of meats such as pork, lamb, beef, herring, or trout are possible. People may avoid meat at home but not at a barbecue. Also, people may make new choices all the time. A person may decide today to stop eating all animal foods and in a month may change his/her mind to reinclude dairy products. All this is part of human life, but for science, this means that the description of health effects of vegetarianism—like any dietary behavior—is a true challenge.

For causal inference regarding health effects of vegetarianism, science has to seek for consistent dietary patterns. This is also the basis of this volume on vegetarianism; therefore we have earlier defined some types of vegetarianism. However, the reader should always keep in mind that any definition is no more than a template, and that in practice the limitation of any study on vegetarianism is that diets may not fall exactly within one category, and they may differ between participants or over time. Of course, this applies not only to the avoidance of animal products but also in other aspects of diet and lifestyle in general.

4.2 Self-Defined Vegetarianism Versus "Measured" Degree of Avoidance of Specific Animal Foods

Many publications on vegetarian diets have relied on self-defined vegetarianism. For instance, in the Continuing Survey of Food Intake (CFSII) by individuals in the United States (Haddad and Tanzman, 2003), self-defined vegetarians and nonvegetarians were defined as those who responded positively or negatively, respectively, to the question "Do you consider yourself to be a vegetarian?"

But if someone calls himself a "vegetarian," does he also fit into the "objective" definition given earlier? In a survey in Dutch families with alternative food habits, some respondents calling themselves "vegetarian" actually consumed meat several times per week (van Staveren et al., 1985). In adolescents in Finland (Vinnari et al., 2009), only 13% of self-reported vegetarians in fact followed an ovolactovegetarian diet or stricter according to the food frequency questionnaire (FFQ), but the average meat consumption per day was much lower than in their omnivorous peers (15 vs. 103 g/day).

Gilsing et al. (2013) reported that in the Netherlands Cohort Study on diet and cancer, 50% of the self-reported vegetarians consumed some meat according to the FFQ, but with a mean consumption frequency of ~1 time/week. Again, this was much lower than in the "omnivorous" participants.

Finally, in the CFSII, 64% of the self-defined vegetarians reported in the FFQ to consume ≥10 g/day of meat (Haddad and Tanzman, 2003), and the remaining group consumed <10 g/day of meat. The consumption of vegetables and fruits in the self-defined vegetarians was higher and their BMI was lower than in the self-defined nonvegetarians, regardless of whether they were true vegetarians or consumed a small amount of meat.

Although these studies clearly show that self-defined vegetarianism is quite different from actual complete avoidance of meat, they do not answer the question of whether misclassification based on self-defined vegetarianism could lead to bias in association studies with health outcomes.

Gilsing et al. (2015) studied this question by comparing the associations between vegetarianism and colorectal cancer, using the self-defined vegetarians and vegetarianism based on the FFQ. Although both methods of classification yielded statistically nonsignificant protective effects, the association was considerable stronger for confirmed vegetarians than for nonvegetarians, suggesting that some attenuation occurs when merely relying on self-definition for classification purposes.

This remains unknown for many studies that have only data on self-defined vegetarianism, which is therefore a clear limitation when interpreting the literature. In many studies in vegetarian diets, it remains unclear whether a reported association with reduced risk of chronic diseases is due to the avoidance of meat or to a better balanced diet with more vegetables, fruits, whole grain cereals, etc. Generally, the latter is more likely to be the cause of the reduction of disease than the mere avoidance of meat.

For future studies, a validated method of dietary assessment should be used as a basis to divide participants in "vegetarians" versus "nonvegetarians." Dietary studies should assess actual consumption by using a validated dietary assessment tool such as an FFQ, a dietary recall, or food diary.

Also in research reports and publications, basing the classification of participants with regard to vegetarianism on a validated dietary assessment method rather than on a "self-reported vegetarianism" is preferred. The additional major advantage of this approach is the possibility to describe the total diet (not limited to the type of animal food) in much more detail than just "vegetarian," and the same applies to studies of etiological or prognostic associations.

4.3 Confounding

The choice for a vegetarian diet may be associated with a wide range of other personal, psychological, or social characteristics. So when it comes to investigating the health effects of vegetarian diets, we have a major risk of confounding. A few examples are given here.

First, factors like gender, age, education, and income may be determinants of choosing a vegetarian diet. In a large Dutch cohort of individuals aged 55–69 years, vegetarians were more likely to be women, have higher education, less likely to be smokers, and have fewer children (Gilsing et al., 2013). Associations of vegetarianism with socioeconomic status and healthy lifestyle are a major limitation in deciphering the health effect of vegetarian diets per se.

There may also be an association between diet and personality structure. For instance, a report suggested an association between vegetarianism and dietary restraint in female students and faculty members in Colorado, USA (Curtis and Comer, 2006). The authors reported higher levels of dietary restraint in weight-motivated semivegetarians (defined as eating no red meat but occasionally chicken and/or fish) than in semivegetarians not motivated by weight. The association was absent in non-vegetarians and in "full vegetarians" (i.e., all types of true vegetarians). Thus, there remains the possibility that the choice for (semi) vegetarian diets could be associated with different psychological characteristics, and that (semi) vegetarianism could be associated with dieting and thus with generally different food choices (e.g., low-calorie foods). Likewise, vegetarianism in adolescents and young adults has been proposed to be actually an indicator of potentially harmful weight control behavior, as will be discussed in detail in Chapter 4.

Finally, it is important to consider that people may shift to vegetarian-like diets for health reasons, such as the presence of a priori disease, suboptimal health, allergic response, food intolerance, etc. This was observed for parents of macrobiotic children in The Netherlands, where in a population-based study in 173 Dutch macrobiotic families 42% of the mothers shifted to this diet for health reasons of at least one of the parents (Dagnelie, 1988; unpublished data). Vegetarianism was also more frequent in subjects with cancer than in noncancer individuals (Gilsing et al., 2013). The existence of many confounding factors associated with vegetarianism is one rationale for the many chapters in the first section of this book that intend to show the context of the utilization of plant-based and vegetarian diets.

4.4 Is the Study Sample Representative for the Concerned Base Population?

Human health research must meet basic ethical principles, including rules for recruiting subjects and informed consent. The fact that participation is voluntary means people may participate for specific reasons. In a cross-sectional study or in a cohort study comparing the health of vegetarians with nonvegetarians, especially healthy conscious people may participate. This could mean, for instance, that participating vegetarians take more vitamin B_{12} supplements than vegetarians in general would do, which leads to a better vitamin B_{12} status than in vegetarians in general.

To date, we know of only a single study that was performed in a representative sample. This study was performed in two stages. First, a comprehensive inventory of all macrobiotic families with children under 8 years of age in The Netherlands was made and the families were invited to participate in a cross-sectional study with anthropometric assessment of all these children of age less than 8 (Dagnelie et al., 1988). Out of a total of 216 eligible families, 18 families (8%) could not be traced, e.g., due to departure, 15 families (7%) were not visited and 10 families (5%) refused. Thus, overall participation was 80% of the families. In a second step, all children between 4 and 18 months old were followed in a mixed-longitudinal design, with repeated assessment of diet and growth over 6 months, with blood sampling for vitamin status and a medical examination at the end of the 6-month period. A matched group of children on omnivorous diets was used as control in this study (Dagnelie and van Staveren, 1994). Unfortunately, such population-based studies in a representative sample have remained an exception; yet, such studies are imperative if one wants to obtain a true picture of the nutritional status and health effects of vegetarian diets.

To overcome this problem, it has been suggested to simply reweight existing and future studies to correct for the proportion of diseased and healthy vegetarians in the study population relative to the estimated prevalence of disease in the full population. Although this option sounds attractive, it does not provide a solution, for two reasons. First, as already discussed in the preceding paragraphs, vegetarians are clearly a select population, i.e., there is selection bias (which cannot be controlled for in studies with selective sampling, nor in statistical analyses). Second, there is the risk of reverse causation; for example, health food stores will not only attract ethical vegetarians but also vegetarians who have stopped eating meat because of chronic disease, hypersensitivities, etc.

Therefore, as mentioned, the only true solution will be to perform population-based studies in which either a complete vegetarian population is being studied or a representative study sample is obtained from a well-defined vegetarian population. As mentioned, hardly any such studies exist to date, which severely hampers our current knowledge about health effects of vegetarian diets.

5. Conclusion

In this volume on vegetarian diets, vegetarianism is defined as the conscious, voluntary choice to exclude one or more types of animal food from the diet. Vegetarian is used to include all categories of vegetarian diets and vegetarians without distinction. Different degrees of vegetarianism include ovolactovegetarian diets, which included dairy products and eggs, and vegan diets, which exclude all animal products. A strict vegetarian is someone who strictly adheres to his/her vegetarian diet, regardless of the type of vegetarianism.

Methodological pitfalls in interpreting the literature on health effects of vegetarian diets include heterogeneity in composition of the diet, the use of "self-defined" vegetarians instead of definition based on a dietary inventory, confounding by dietary and lifestyle characteristics that are associated with taking a vegetarian diet, and lack of representativeness of the study population in the overwhelming majority of published studies. These methodological flaws make it extremely difficult to draw valid conclusions regarding the health effects of vegetarian diets.

References

Anonymous, June 9, 2016. https://en.wikipedia.org/wiki/Vegetarianism dd.

Curtis, M.J., Comer, L.K., May 2006. Vegetarianism, dietary restraint and feminist identity. Eat. Behav. 7 (2), 91–104. PubMed PMID: 16600838.

Dagnelie, P.C., van Staveren, W.A., May 1994. Macrobiotic nutrition and child health: results of a population-based, mixed-longitudinal cohort study in The Netherlands. Am. J. Clin. Nutr. 59 (Suppl. 5), 1187S–1196S. PubMed PMID: 8172122.

Dagnelie, P.C., van Staveren, W.A., van Klaveren, J.D., Burema, J., December 1988. Do children on macrobiotic diets show catch-up growth? A population-based cross-sectional study in children aged 0–8 years. Eur. J. Clin. Nutr. 42 (12), 1007–1016. PubMed PMID: 3266149.

Gilsing, A.M., Weijenberg, M.P., Goldbohm, R.A., Dagnelie, P.C., van den Brandt, P.A., Schouten, L.J., 2013. The Netherlands Cohort Study-Meat Investigation Cohort; a population-based cohort over-represented with vegetarians, pescetarians and low meat consumers. Nutr. J. 12, 156. PubMed PMID: 24289207; Pubmed Central PMCID: 4220685.

Gilsing, A.M., Schouten, L.J., Goldbohm, R.A., Dagnelie, P.C., van den Brandt, P.A., Weijenberg, M.P., 2015. Vegetarianism, low meat consumption and the risk of colorectal cancer in a population based cohort study. Sci. Rep. 5, 13484. PubMed PMID: 26316135; Pubmed Central PMCID: 4551995.

Haddad, E.H., Tanzman, J.S., September 2003. What do vegetarians in the United States eat? Am. J. Clin. Nutr. 78 (Suppl. 3), 626S–632S. PubMed PMID: 12936957.

van Staveren, W.A., Dhuyvetter, J.H., Bons, A., Zeelen, M., Hautvast, J.G., December 1985. Food consumption and height/weight status of Dutch preschool children on alternative diets. J. Am. Diet. Assoc. 85 (12), 1579–1584. PubMed PMID: 4067152.

Vinnari, M., Montonen, J., Harkanen, T., Mannisto, S., April 2009. Identifying vegetarians and their food consumption according to self-identification and operationalized definition in Finland. Public Health Nutr. 12 (4), 481–488. PubMed PMID: 18462562.

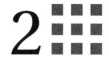

2

Attitudes Toward Meat and Plants in Vegetarians

Hank Rothgerber

BELLARMINE UNIVERSITY, LOUISVILLE, KY, UNITED STATES

…little is known about associated attitudes, behavior, and lifestyle of the 'new' vegetarians
Dwyer et al. (1974, p. 529)

1. Introduction

In some ways, much has changed since this quote from early work on the psychology of vegetarianism, but as this review will emphasize, there is much more to learn. To begin, here is a definition: an *attitude* is a psychological tendency that is expressed in evaluating a particular entity with some degree of favor or disfavor (Eagly and Chaiken, 1993). *Psychological tendency* refers to a state that is internal to the person, and *evaluating* refers to all classes of evaluative responding, whether overt or covert, cognitive, affective, or behavioral. Attitudes have been central to the study of social psychology for decades. There has been considerable interest in theories specifying when attitudes predict behavior (e.g., the theory of planned behavior, Ajzen, 1991) and in cognitive consistency theories predicting that behavior may cause attitude change (e.g., cognitive dissonance, Festinger, 1957).

This review uses attitudes as a lens to better understand the social psychology of vegetarianism. Questions asked include the following: How favorably do vegetarians evaluate meat and plant sources of diet relative to meat eaters? Do vegetarians who are less rigorous in adhering to their diet have different attitudes than those stricter in adherence? Do vegetarians who eschew all animal products (i.e., vegans) differ in attitudes than those who consume dairy and eggs? Do vegetarians motivated by ethical concerns differ in their attitudes compared to those motivated by health concerns? Before building up too much hype, a caveat is in order: Research on the psychology of vegetarianism has come a long way but is still in its youth. There are sample limitations and inconsistent definitions of what constitutes a vegetarian dispersed throughout the emerging literature. Many studies only examine attitudes toward one type of food—meat—and at that, they rarely distinguish between different types of meat. Without claiming to offer definitive answers, then, the review should assist the reader in better understanding how attitudes may predict diet choice and diet maintenance. It also considers the possibility that diet choice influences attitudes and draws upon evidence from cognitive dissonance, moralization, and social identity in doing so.

2. Studies Comparing Attitudes Among "Vegetarians" to Meat Eaters

During the last 25 years, almost a dozen studies have described attitudes that vegetarians have toward meat or directly compared these attitudes to ones held by meat eaters. For the most part, these studies have been extremely liberal in defining who constitutes a vegetarian and have also not attempted to analyze differences between vegetarian subgroups. In what may be the first work to extensively examine how vegetarians evaluate the food that they have chosen to avoid, Amato and Partridge (1989) documented a number of negative attitudes vegetarians associated with meat. The clear majority of over 300 vegetarians studied intimated that they would never consider eating meat again. Central to the reaction of many were feelings of disgust toward meat, particularly when thinking of sensory characteristics such as its sight or smell.

As far as we know, the first peer-reviewed study of vegetarian attitudes toward meat was conducted by Beardsworth and Keil (1992), who conducted an in-depth qualitative analysis of 76 vegetarians (including 5 semivegetarians, 18 pescetarians, 26 ovolactovegetarians, 9 lactovegetarians, and 18 vegans) in the United Kingdom. While noting that participants varied in their interest in food and their concern with and knowledge of health and nutrition, the researchers identified strong antimeat attitudes among vegetarians. Many vegetarians reported a strong sense of revulsion toward meat even if they were not certain whether the roots of disgust were physical or psychological. Specifically, participants singled out as distressing the sensory characteristics of meat, the appearance of red meat in particular, and blood and other factors not hiding the animal's actual appearance. A later detailed qualitative examination by Kenyon and Barker (1998) replicated many of these results in an English sample of 15 vegetarian teenage girls (i.e., no meat in their diet) relative to 15 nonvegetarian counterparts. They found, for example, that two-thirds of vegetarians made reference in some way to an animal when describing meat, indicating that they were unable and/or unwilling to use the strategy of dissociating the animal from meat that is employed by many meat eaters to justify meat consumption (see Hoogland et al., 2005; Kubberød et al., 2002; Rothgerber, 2013a, 2014a).

Relying on a convenience sample in the United Kingdom, Povey et al. (2001) moved beyond a two-group comparison and assessed attitudes toward food choices among 25 meat eaters, 26 "meat avoiders" (in fact pescetarians), 34 "vegetarians" (in fact ovolactovegetarians), and 26 vegans (to be discussed later). Meat eaters were the only respondents to report any positivity toward meat. Although unclear if degree of diet restriction was related to strength of negative attitudes and beliefs, the vegetarian groups overall expressed strong negativity toward meat. The most common beliefs about meat for pescetarians included *cruel and barbaric, fattening, unhealthy, environmentally problem-atic, and expensive*. Ovolactovegetarians most often associated meat with *unhealthy, cruel and barbaric, health scares, inhumane, and murderous*. It should be noted that although pescetarians and ovolactovegetarians generally evaluated vegetarian diets positively, it is impossible to know if this assessment resulted from positive attitudes toward plants and vegetables, negative attitudes toward meat, or some combination of the two.

Barr and Chapman (2002) focused on perceptions of red meat among a Canadian sample of current vegetarians ($n=90$; including 14 occasional meat eaters, 37 pescetarians, 22 ovolactovegetarians, 11 lactovegetarians, and 6 vegans), former vegetarians ($n=35$), and nonvegetarian women ($n=68$) recruited through notices in university and community newspapers as well as word of mouth. Vegetarians were more negative than former vegetarians and meat eaters in their evaluation of red meat on nearly every question assessed. For items involving specific prompts about nutrients, toxins, antibiotics, and unnatural hormones and those assessing more general health, a strong majority of vegetarians believed that red meat was unhealthy. A large majority of current vegetarians also reported not liking the sensory quality of meat or digesting it.

While most of the aforementioned studies have sought to understand vegetarian attitudes toward meat by comparing them to those who eat meat without restriction, several studies (Rothgerber, 2015a,b) have examined ways that vegetarians may differ from a seemingly more similar group, conscientious omnivores (COs, Singer and Mason, 2006), those who only consume animal flesh that has met certain ethical standards. Relative to mainstream eaters, vegetarians and COs share convictions that food choices matter beyond their impact on the individual consumer and that following one's conscience in food choices is appropriate. Most importantly, they both express principled opposition to factory farming, an opposition driven by a combination of health, animal, and environmental motives. It turned out that attitudes were critical in explaining how individuals practice behavioral resistance to factory farming. Across two studies recruiting participants using an Internet platform (study 1: vegetarian – $n=206$, CO – $n=143$; study 2: vegetarian – $n=70$, CO – $n=109$), numerous differences emerged in attitudes toward meat between vegetarians and COs. Vegetarians expressed greater disgust over factory-farmed meat (e.g., "eating factory-farmed meat is offensive, repulsive, and disgusting") and sensory dislike of meat, rating its taste, smell, and appearance more negatively than did COs. In one study (Rothgerber, 2015b), these beliefs about meat helped explain differences between COs and vegetarians in the perceived acceptability of killing animals for food, arguably the underlying distinction between the groups. In the other (Rothgerber, 2015a), attitudes toward meat helped account for the greater guilt vegetarians felt relative to COs when they violated their diet.

Swanson et al. (2001) conducted the only study in the review to single out white meat; they compared attitudes toward it and nonmeat protein sources (e.g., tofu, nuts, etc.) between self-identified vegetarians ($n=34$) and meat eaters ($n=66$) attending university in the northwestern United States. As expected, direct measures revealed that vegetarians preferred nonmeat protein sources to white meat and that meat eaters preferred white meat to nonmeat protein sources.

This study was also the first published article to implicitly measure vegetarian attitudes toward meat. Results of an Implicit Association Test (IAT), in which participants were presented with either pictures of white meat or nonmeat protein paired with either pleasant or unpleasant words, indicated that vegetarians implicitly preferred nonmeat protein to white meat and implicitly identified with nonmeat protein more than white meat. The opposite findings occurred for meat eaters. Implicit and explicit attitude measures were moderately correlated, and self-reported consumption of white meat and nonmeat protein were correlated in the expected direction with all measures. These results do raise an interesting question. Because the IAT involves a relative comparison and the explicit measure was calculated by subtracting nonmeat protein liking from white meat liking, it is unclear whether vegetarian attitudes reflected strong disdain for white meat, strong endorsement of nonmeat protein sources, or some combination of the two.

This issue was addressed in several subsequent studies measuring implicit and explicit meat and vegetable attitudes between vegetarians and meat eaters. In a sample of 47 Belgian university vegetarians (with one-half being pescetarian) and 49 meat eaters, participants rated the tastiness of pictured meats and vegetables, separately indicated their attitudes toward vegetables and toward meat (the latter in terms of hedonic, health, environmental, moral, and affective beliefs), and completed an IAT and Extrinsic Affective Simon Test (EAST), the latter which allowed implicit attitudes toward vegetables and meat to be individually assessed (De Houwer and De Bruycker, 2007). For the implicit tests, the meat stimuli consisted of pictures of steak, hamburger, dried sausages, pate, and bacon, while the vegetable stimuli depicted pictures of cabbages, carrots, beans, broccoli, and peas. Overall, the implicit tests revealed that relative to meat eaters, vegetarians had a stronger preference for vegetables over meat. Scores on the EAST showed that vegetarians marginally preferred vegetables more than meat eaters who in turn, marginally preferred meat more than vegetarians. These effects were even greater for the explicit measures, which strongly predicted vegetarian status without contribution from the implicit measures.

A study of 16 vegetarian (one-half were pescetarian) and 16 meat-eating Irish college students replicated many of these findings, albeit showing weaker effects for meat eaters (Barnes-Holmes et al., 2010). On explicit measures, vegetarians were again strongly provegetable and antimeat, while meat eaters favored meat more than vegetables (but only slightly). On implicit measures (IAT and the Implicit Relational Assessment Procedure), vegetarians showed provegetable and antimeat biases that differed significantly from meat eaters' provegetable and promeat biases (neither of which were statistically significant). Unlike De Houwer and De Bruycker (2007), implicit and explicit attitudes were only weakly correlated. Barnes-Holmes et al. (2010) also found that explicit attitudes were a weak (but significant) predictor of diet status and that implicit measures enhanced predictions moderately.

Thus, while these studies assessing vegetarian implicit attitudes reveal certain consistencies, they are unclear on the relative importance of more regulated and controlled attitudes associated with meat as opposed to those existing without conscious awareness. The significant correlations between implicit and explicit measures clearly indicate some overlap between these processes, but which exerts a stronger influence on behavior? The inability of explicit measures to predict vegetarian status in Barnes-Holmes et al. (2010) may support the conclusion that what best distinguishes vegetarians from meat eaters is not what they carefully reflect on and report but attitudes that they may be unaware of or unwilling to share. If so, it would be unfortunate that so few studies have measured implicit relative to explicit attitudes about meat and vegetables. However, Barnes-Holmes et al. (2010) only examined 16 participants in each diet condition and anecdotally noted that some of the meat eaters were ambivalent about meat because they perceived it as fattening, potentially underestimating explicit differences between vegetarians and meat eaters. There is also the problem that implicit measures did not predict vegetarian status in De Houwer and De Bruycker (2007). The researchers note that implicit attitudes could be important in influencing controlled processes responsible for diet choice or by shaping the likelihood of maintaining a vegetarian diet. Future research is needed to resolve the discrepancies between these two studies and to shed more light on the relative contribution of implicit and explicit attitudes to the psychological experience of vegetarianism.

2.1 Limitations to Studies Comparing Attitudes Among "Vegetarians" to Meat Eaters

While a fair number of studies have examined the way vegetarians evaluate meat and a few have extended it to beliefs about vegetables, research on attitudes toward other potential contributors to a vegetarian diet—fruit, dairy, and meat substitution products—are virtually nonexistent. One study directly assessed female vegetarian attitudes toward dairy and found these attitudes to be more negative than those held by meat eaters (Barr and Chapman, 2002). Approximately half of vegetarians believed that dairy products contain antibiotics and unnatural hormones, and that they are not needed by adults, while only 26% believed that a diet with dairy is healthier than without. These effects were not simply driven by vegans, as the most common intended dietary change among vegetarians was to use fewer dairy products. Studies on vegetarian perceptions of meat substitution products are also rare. Hoek et al. (2011) found that 84% of Dutch vegetarians and 46% of UK vegetarians were classified as heavy users of meat substitution products (>1 time per week), but attitudes of vegetarians were not specified. Heavy users, in general, were more likely to prefer meat substitution products dissimilar to meat, likely as a way to avoid disgust and reminders of sensory qualities of meat.

Because of the scarcity of studies assessing vegetarian attitudes of plant-based foods as opposed to meat, it is difficult to know how important these attitudes are in choosing a vegetarian diet and in maintaining it. One possibility is that vegetarians are attracted to and sustain their diet because of affection for fruits, vegetables, and nonmeat protein sources. Support for the position that vegetable preference is what most critically distinguishes between vegetarians and meat eaters comes from Barnes-Holmes et al. (2010), who found that vegetarians explicitly rated vegetables much higher than did meat eaters, whereas differences between the groups in their ratings of meat only approached significance. However, a logical problem with this position is that admiration of vegetables would not by itself cause an individual to abandon an omnivore diet in favor of a vegetarian diet because both allow the individual to consume as many calories from vegetables as desired. That is, what distinguishes an omnivore from a plant-based diet is the consumption of meat, not vegetables. It thus seems more likely that negative attitudes toward meat are what would most greatly motivate a change and adherence to a vegetarian diet. This fits the observations of Beardsworth and Keil (1992), who in relatively unstructured interviews found that vegetarians generated many more antimeat statements than provegetable statements. De Houwer and De Bruycker (2007) also found that attitudes toward meat more strongly differentiated between vegetarians and meat eaters than did attitudes about vegetables. For example, vegetarians and meat eaters differed in their EAST scores for vegetables only when the IAT was administered before the EAST. No such qualifications occurred for meat attitudes. In addition, both explicit measures and the IAT were correlated with the EAST for meat but not for vegetables, suggesting that the EAST score was most influenced by attitudes toward meat. Because they are thought to exert much more influence on behavior and because researchers have devoted considerably more attention to them, the remainder of this chapter will focus exclusively on attitudes toward meat. This is, of course, not to suggest that attitudes toward vegetables are unimportant to the dietary behavior of vegetarians. Even if not the underlying cause of vegetarianism, attitudes toward vegetables likely shape food choices as vegetarians show an inclination and actively search for vegetables.

Future research should also more carefully consider whether vegetarian attitudes toward meat vary depending on the particular type of meat. With few exceptions (Barr and Chapman, 2002; Swanson et al., 2001), research on vegetarians has not separated out attitudes toward specific types of meat and none have directly compared attitudes toward one type with attitudes toward another. There are strong reasons to suspect that red meat would produce more disgust and revulsion than other forms of meat. Some of this evidence comes from studies of nonvegetarians. Fessler et al. (2003) found that meat avoiders motivated by health ate less red meat. Santos and Booth (1996) found that among English college students choosing to eat a vegetarian dish, beef and lamb were the meat dishes most likely to be avoided. Similarly, an analysis of 206 Norwegian students found that most preferred white meat to red (Kubberød et al., 2002), with decreased hedonic ratings of meat as it increased in red color intensity, especially for females.

Among vegetarians, a common progression is to first eliminate red meat, then chicken, then fish, and then for vegans, dairy and eggs (Jabs et al., 1998), and others have observed that red meat is avoided earlier than white meat (Beardsworth and Keil, 1991, 1992; Maurer, 2010; Twigg, 1979, 1983). Dwyer et al. (1974) reported that all of their 100 "new vegetarians" avoided red meat, with dairy and eggs being avoided by the least. Some have speculated that the apparent revulsion for red meat may stem from its mammalian origins, but it seems more attributable to the presence of blood that is seen in red meat (Kenyon and Barker, 1998; Santos and Booth, 1996). There are fewer disgust-eliciting cues in pork, chicken, and fish because they appear white once the blood has been drained. Even among meat eaters, many are disgusted by bloody meat (Beardworth and Keil, 1992; Fiddes, 1991; Kenyon and Barker, 1998; Kubberød et al., 2002; Twigg, 1979; Santos and Booth, 1996). Given that red meat is avoided earlier than white meat when moving into vegetarianism, it seems reasonable to assume that vegetarians would hold more negative attitudes toward red meat, but this awaits more careful empirical verification.

While certainly informative, the reviewed studies leave unanswered questions. Given that vegetarians constitute a relatively small percent of the population and are not easily discernible from the general public, it may be difficult to identify them as research participants. This explains the small number of vegetarian participants in the cited studies (only Rothgerber, 2015a included more than 100 vegetarians) and sampling techniques that may not always capture the range of diversity among vegetarians. Consequently, it is unclear whether the published attitudes associated with meat and vegetables would hold for larger, more age and gender diverse samples taken from settings outside North America and the United Kingdom.

On this note, it is also uncertain whether male and female vegetarians would differ in these attitudes. Given meat's connection to masculinity and its greater consumption by men (e.g., Rothgerber, 2013a; Rozin et al., 2012), one possibility is that male vegetarians would be more favorable or less negative toward meat than would female vegetarians. Conversely, male and female vegetarians may exhibit less alignment with traditional gender roles and may evaluate meat similarly. Suggestive evidence for gender being unrelated to attitudes among vegetarians comes from Kalof et al. (1999), who found that gender differences in vegetarianism disappeared when controlling for beliefs. A similar question may be applied to age: do older vegetarians hold similar attitudes toward meat and vegetables as younger vegetarians? There is some evidence that older vegetarians may be more influenced by health motives (MacNair, 1998), but it is unclear whether age would influence attitudes independent of diet motivation.

There is also a certain lack of precision apparent in a number of these earlier studies. The qualitative studies (e.g., Beardsworth and Keil, 1992) provide the richest sources of raw data, but they also tend to be vague about reporting trends, making it difficult to estimate exactly how many vegetarians share a certain attitude. In some cases, researchers combine vegetarians and meat eaters into a single category, rendering it impossible to know how beliefs about meat and nutrition vary between the two groups (e.g., Lea and Worsley, 2001). More substantially, both qualitative and quantitative studies have suffered from a lack of precision in defining what constitutes a vegetarian (see Ruby, 2012) and in analyzing such distinctions appropriately.

One frequent problem is that studies are overinclusive in determining who constitutes a vegetarian and include as "vegetarian" participants who indeed consume animal flesh; for example, in Beardsworth and Keil (1992), one-third of the vegetarian sample ate meat or fish. In Barr and Chapman (2002), 57% of so-called vegetarians reported occasionally eating fish, and 16% occasionally eating chicken; according to a strict definition of vegetarianism, a clear majority of vegetarian participants were semivegetarian or not even vegetarian at all! In Barnes-Holmes et al. (2010) and De Houwer and De Bruycker (2007), about half of vegetarian participants consumed fish. One study stated that vegetarians ate "no meat" (Kenyon and Barker, 1998), but it is unclear if this included fish as well, and another did not specify what defined a vegetarian (Swanson et al., 2001). The powerful phenomenon of semivegetarianism (see Rothgerber, 2014b) suggests that care needs to be taken to avoid labeling participants as vegetarian when they fail to adhere to strict dietary standards. Readers can refer to Chapter 1 of the present book for further details about the spectrum of vegetarian diets.

Perhaps the larger criticism is not that studies include such participants but that they fail to distinguish between these different diet types in the analysis, a regrettable but understandable omission given the small or modest sample sizes in many of the studies. Incidentally, this practice of analyzing semivegetarians and true vegetarians as one group is common across vegetarian studies covering a variety of psychological domains (e.g., Dietz et al., 1995; Shickle et al., 1989). Whether partial or semivegetarians differ from true vegetarians in their attitudes toward meat and vegetables, then, cannot generally be known from these reviewed studies.

Moving to the more restrictive side of the vegetarian diet, there is also a problem in analyzing data related to vegans. Most studies do not indicate how many vegetarian participants were vegan, and in some cases, the dietary survey may not have been sensitive to this difference. Several studies (e.g., Barr and Chapman, 2002; Beardsworth and Keil, 1992; Santos and Booth, 1996) identified some participants as vegan, but with the exception of Povey et al. (2001) and Rothgerber (2015a), none of them directly compared vegans with other vegetarians, thus, making it difficult to discern if vegan attitudes toward meat and vegetables were comparable to those held by vegetarians. To make matters even more complicated, studies relying merely on self-identified vegetarian status may be muddying the waters, as one study comparing self-reported vegetarian status with descriptions of eating behavior found that many vegetarians, especially pescetarians and vegans, incorrectly identified themselves (Pribis et al., 2010).

2.2 Summary

In short, it is apparent that the vegetarians who have been studied in the review thus far expressed strong disdain for meat. This disdain took several forms that seemed largely consensual even across samples divergent in their demographic characteristics. Vegetarians expressed disgust at meat, finding the thought of eating it abhorrent and revolting. Sensory characteristics such as the taste and smell of meat generated negative reactions. Blood and other physical reminders of the dead animal were also singled out as particularly offensive. Vegetarians did not dissociate the animal from its meat form but conversely thought of meat as a dead animal. Meat was viewed as generally unhealthy, with some concern for its contamination potential, and that it contains toxins, hormones, and antibiotics. Vegetarian attitudes toward vegetables seemed positive and toward dairy were negative, but it is less clear how strong these attitudes were and how much they contributed to the decision to adopt and maintain a vegetarian diet. Red meat seemed to be abhorred the most, but the relative rating of other meat varieties was unclear. These conclusions should be viewed tentatively because most studies relied on small sample sizes and may not represent the full range of vegetarians. It is possible that attitude differences based on gender, age, and other demographic characteristics have been overlooked. The studies have also been exceedingly liberal in defining who constitutes a vegetarian and have not generally analyzed differences in attitudes between varying types of vegetarians.

In the next section, I will consider (mostly newer) studies that have addressed this last issue and have specifically examined differences between semivegetarians and true vegetarians, between vegans and other vegetarians, and between health and ethical vegetarians in their attitudes toward meat.

3. Differences in Attitudes Toward Meat Between Varying Types of Vegetarians

3.1 Semivegetarians Versus True Vegetarians

To borrow from Beardsworth and Keil (1992), vegetarianism may best be understood as a continuum of categories measuring the progressive degree to which animal foods are avoided. At one end are what we would term in this chapter and in the entire book (see Chapter 1) "semivegetarians" (most similar to Beardsworth and Keil's type I vegetarians), individuals defining themselves as vegetarian but still eating animals on occasion. It is worth asking: how common is this phenomenon?

In addition to the aforementioned studies in the first section that examined attitudes toward meat and vegetables, it turns out that a number of studies have documented that people will claim they are vegetarian but then simultaneously acknowledge that they eat red meat, chicken, and/or fish. These studies span geography and age, ranging from American teenage samples (Perry et al., 2001; Robinson-O'Brien et al., 2009), to Australian teenagers (Worsley and Skrzypiec, 1998), to representative American samples (Gossard and York, 2003; Time/CNN/Harris Interactive Poll, 2002), to female physicians in the United States (White et al., 1999), to Canadians (National Institute of Nutrition, 1997, 2001), to Canadian women (Barr and Chapman, 2002), to women in the southwestern United States (Kwan and Roth, 2004), to expansive and small American samples (Cooper et al., 1985; Krizmanic, 1992), to Londoners (Willetts, 1997), and to a highly educated group from the United Kingdom (Beardsworth and Keil, 1992). A majority of self-identified vegetarians in these studies admitted to eating red meat, chicken, or seafood regardless of the timeframe. In a telephone survey of well-educated and wealthy respondents in the eastern United States, 7.2% indicated that they were vegetarian, but only 2.5% said that they never ate poultry, and only 1.5% reported never eating fish or poultry (Dietz et al., 1995). Similar results were attained across several representative studies in the United States (Maurer, 2010). A team of researchers at Yale University School of Medicine concluded that less than one-tenth of 1% of Americans are true vegetarians (cited in Herzog, 2011). Semivegetarians, then, appear to greatly outnumber those strictly committed to a vegetarian diet.

For the task of analyzing vegetarian attitudes toward meat and vegetables, it is important to understand *why* individuals define themselves in one category but behave quite differently from membership criteria. It is possible that individuals are practicing self-deception to reduce the dissonance associated with eating meat (see Rothgerber, 2014a). To the extent that vegetarians are seen as a desirable group to some, this may bias the individual to generate definitions to fit their own practice (Bedford and Barr, 2005) and to sustain self-definition in the event of a lapse (Willetts, 1997). There is also the possibility that these individuals do not suffer from cognitive or motivational distortions and fully intend to abandon meat consumption but differ from true vegetarians in terms of structural (see Ruby, 2012) or psychological variables such as being unassertive or having weak impulse control. It may also be the case that semivegetarians have different attitudes toward meat and animals than true vegetarians, and these differences are responsible for differences in behavior.

To address this latter possibility, Rothgerber (2014b) surveyed 214 participants recruited through the Vegetarian Resource Group, a nonprofit organization dedicated to educating the public on vegetarianism and related issues. Based on participants' self-reported consumption of a range of animal products, 59 were labeled by the author as semivegetarian, those reluctantly or readily eating at least one animal product while still self-identifying as vegetarian, and 155 were coded as true vegetarians, those refusing to eat all animal products. The groups did not differ in their perceptions of living animals, specifically in how similarly they perceived human and animal emotional experience. This was true for all emotions studied: primary emotions, secondary emotions, and emotional states of pigs and dogs. Past research (Bilewicz et al., 2011) has argued that the reason meat eaters perceive greater human–animal difference is that it justifies meat consumption, evidently not the case for semivegetarians. Rather, the chief difference between semivegetarians and true vegetarians rested in their attitudes toward dead animals served as meat. True vegetarians reported disliking the sensory characteristics of meat—its taste, smell, texture, and appearance—more than did semivegetarians. Similarly, true vegetarians were more disgusted by meat than were semivegetarians, specifically agreeing more that emotionally they could not chew and swallow meat and that they found meat more offensive, repulsive, or disgusting. This is certainly not to suggest that semivegetarians overly enjoyed the taste or other sensory characteristics of meat, at least relative to more frequent meat eaters. In fact, Timko et al. (2012) found that the majority of semivegetarians cited sensory factors or taste as the number one reason for meat avoidance, both in terms of why they initiated it and why they maintained it.

These results suggest that there is danger in combining all vegetarians into a single category based on self-identification. They also suggest that in addition to the reasons listed earlier to explain semivegetarianism, the phenomenon may result when individuals have simultaneous congruent and incongruent attitudes with more loyal vegetarians. The findings that meat disgust, to mention one attitude, differed between semivegetarians and true vegetarians suggests that self-identification may be limited in predicting attitudes. Studies that have included semivegetarians may be underestimating how much disdain true vegetarians have toward meat, a bias potentially made larger by Rothgerber (2014b) likely oversampling more committed semivegetarians.

3.2 Vegans Versus Other Vegetarians

By the same standard, studies that have combined vegans and other vegetarians together may overestimate vegetarian disdain of meat. That is, an emerging literature has begun to demonstrate that vegans are not only behaviorally distinct from other vegetarians but also attitudinally distinct. While vegans were more likely than other vegetarians to be concerned with the impact of diet choice on the environment (Ruby, 2008) and to believe that a meatless diet was healthier (Ruby et al., 2011), most often the choice to exclude a wider range of animal products was motivated by a concern for animal welfare (Rothgerber, 2013b); relative to other vegetarians, vegans held more positive attitudes toward animals (Rothgerber, 2015a,b; Ruby, 2012; Ruby et al., 2011), were more concerned with the practices of the meat industry (Ruby et al., 2011) and the impact of their diet on animal welfare (Ruby, 2008) and animal suffering (Ruby et al., 2011), and perceived greater human–animal emotional similarity (Rothgerber, 2013c, 2015a,b). Consequently, they were more likely to believe in the wrongness of killing animals for food (Rothgerber, 2015b), a view held so strongly that vegans were more likely to experience guilt over feeding their pet an animal-based diet and were less likely to feed their pet dog a diet high in meat or fish (Rothgerber, 2013c, 2014c). Vegans also judged meat abstainers who violated their diet and ate meat more negatively, especially when the violator was a vegan ingroup member (Rothgerber, 2014d). The moral opposition to the exploitation of animals was strong enough that vegans indicated that their diet represented more of a lifestyle than a diet (Fox and Ward, 2008), and for some, these convictions were so strong they refused sexual intimacy with nonvegans (Potts and Parry, 2010).

It appears that these favorable attitudes toward living animals manifest themselves as greater disdain for meat than even vegetarians express. Povey et al. (2001) found that for vegans, the most frequent characterization of meat was *cruel and barbaric*, whereas for other vegetarians, it was *unhealthy*. In samples of 17 and 207 vegans, respectively, Rothgerber (2015a,b) found that vegans relative to other vegetarians scored higher on meat disgust and sensory dislike of meat, and that they scored lower on a meat-eating justification scale. Specifically, vegans were significantly less likely than other vegetarians to justify meat consumption by endorsing religious, health, fate, and hierarchical justifications, by denying animal suffering, by endorsing promeat attitudes, by dissociating the animal from food, and by avoiding thinking about the treatment of animals. Once again, it appears that researchers may be obfuscating vegetarian attitudes toward meat by analyzing vegetarian participants with vegans. This time, the effect is likely to make vegetarian attitudes toward meat seem more *negative* than they really may be.

3.3 Health Versus Ethical Vegetarians

The range of animal products avoided along with how religiously they are shunned is clearly associated with attitudes toward meat. However, as important as diet itself may be, the reasons for following one's diet may be equally or even more important. A number of recent studies suggest that one's motives for abstaining from meat are associated with a spectrum of social psychological perceptions. By far, the two most common motives cited in the literature involve ethics (primarily the treatment of animals and to a lesser extent the environment) and personal health. There is actually some contention about which of these motives is most prevalent: Ruby's (2012) review concluded that recent studies showed ethical vegetarianism to be the most popular type, whereas Herzog (2011) stated that most studies have found health motives to be widespread. What is agreed on is that despite behaving similarly when it comes to diet, these groups appear largely different in attitudes, beliefs, values, and personal philosophies. Jabs et al. (1998) proposed that each motivation was clearly distinct and related to a separate model for adopting a vegetarian diet. Even meat eaters were sensitive to distinctions between these groups, with exposure to an ethical but not health vegetarian setting in motion dissonance-reducing perceptions (Rothgerber, 2014a).

Ethical vegetarians resist meat largely because it increases animal suffering and because of their belief that modern-day factory farming is inhumane (Rothgerber, 2013b; Rozin et al., 1997). Hamilton (2000) argued that for ethical vegetarians, meat symbolizes not only violence and aggression, but also death; it stands as a horrific reminder of the pain and suffering of the animal. Hamilton (2000) drew parallels between these beliefs and religion, and others have noted that ethical vegetarians frame their diet within a philosophical, ideological, or spiritual context (Fox and Ward, 2008) and are motivated by humanistic values (Lindeman and Sirelius, 2001). These values include strong feelings of affinity toward animals. This affinity was reflected in the belief that animals have primary and secondary emotions similar to humans (Rothgerber, 2013c), and in the practice of feeding pet dogs a diet less derived from meat or fish, and when failing to do so, feeling greater guilt over the animals used to make pet food (Rothgerber, 2013c, 2014c). Ethical vegetarians perceived themselves as being more radical than health vegetarians (Fox and Ward, 2008). Indeed, they displayed stronger opposition to foxhunting and capital punishment and stronger support for nuclear disarmament than other vegetarians (Hamilton, 2006). Ethical vegetarians seemed aware of their unique characteristics, evaluating health vegetarians more negatively relative to judgments toward vegans (Rothgerber, 2014e). In general, ethical vegetarians shared more similarities with vegans than do other vegetarians and were more likely to transition to veganism than health vegetarians (Jabs et al., 1998).

In contrast, health vegetarians adopt an internal focus, addressing desires to sustain good health and avoid illness. Consuming dead animals was seen as a form of contamination (Hamilton, 2000). Personal health, fitness, and energy were valued rather than other living creatures (Fox and Ward, 2008). Many health vegetarians traced their diet to personal experiences rather than ideology. Lindeman and Sirelius (2001) suggested that the ideology of health vegetarians is more conservative and normative value driven, concerned with personal safety and security. This may explain why health vegetarians were less negative in their evaluation of an ingroup member who violated their diet than were ethical vegetarians (Rothgerber, 2014d). Presumably, such a vegetarian could engage in compensatory behavior aimed at well-being to offset the negative health effects of meat intake. Health vegetarians tended to gradually eliminate meat from their diet and were less likely to eliminate all animal products from their diet (Jabs et al., 1998). As such, they appear to be closer to the mainstream than ethical vegetarians and seem less concerned with animal welfare.

Rozin et al. (1997) conducted the first quantitative comparison of attitudes toward meat between ethical and health vegetarians. Recruiting an adult sample in Pennsylvania, they identified 36 participants who listed a moral reason for first being vegetarian and 26 participants who listed a health reason as motivating their vegetarianism. Relative to health vegetarians, ethical vegetarians offered a wider range of reasons for their vegetarianism and rejected a larger range of animal products. They were also more disgusted by meat (assessed in terms of mental state, contamination potency, and feeling of nausea), reported stronger emotional reaction to the consumption of meat, expressed more concern when watching others eating meat, and more strongly believed that meat causes undesirable personality changes, such as violence and aggression.

This greater sense of disgust among ethical rather than health vegetarians was corroborated by Hamilton's (2006) in-depth qualitative study of 47 vegetarians in the United Kingdom. When asked to imagine how they would feel if they learned that they had inadvertently eaten meat, ethical vegetarians displayed negative reactions including anxiety, anger, guilt, a sense of contamination, harm, unease, discomfort, queasiness, deep revulsion, and sickness. None of the health vegetarians reported such feelings from unknowingly ingesting meat; their focus was restricted to digestive concerns. Jabs et al. (1998) had earlier reported that relative to the health vegetarians ($n=8$) whom they studied, ethical vegetarians ($n=11$) were unable to dissociate meat from its animal origins and were more disgusted by meat.

Rothgerber (2014b, 2015a) also made comparisons between ethical ($n=115$ and $n=245$) and health vegetarians ($n=33$ and $n=168$) in attitudes toward meat. Consistent with Rozin et al. (1997), ethical vegetarians rated meat as more disgusting (e.g., cannot chew or swallow it, more nauseating, etc.). Sensory evaluations were inconsistent: in Rothgerber (2014b), ethical vegetarians reported disliking the taste and texture of meat more than health vegetarians, but in Rothgerber (2015a), similar to Rozin et al. (1997), there were no differences between ethical and health vegetarians in sensory ratings of meat. Clearly, researchers examining attitudes toward meat among vegetarians would be wise to measure motives and to analyze this factor appropriately.

4. The Role of Values

The fundamental difference between ethical and health vegetarians likely resides in the different value systems held by the groups. Values are important to the present work because, along with beliefs (the cognitive component of attitudes, understood to be linkages between the attitude object and various attributes, Fishbein and Ajzen, 1975), they are thought to be the building blocks of attitudes (Eagly and Chaiken, 1993). Values may be viewed as abstract cognitions or global attitudes; they serve as standards for beliefs, attitudes, and behavior (Rokeach, 1968). In terms of structure, values are more general and are at a higher level than beliefs and attitudes, which are more specific manifestations of values.

When an attitude is ambivalent or contains contrary beliefs, values help determine which beliefs will be most influential. For example, two individuals may hold simultaneous beliefs that eating meat constitutes cruelty to animals and that meat tastes good. If the first individual values nonviolence, the animal cruelty concerns would more likely influence their attitudes toward meat eating than would hedonism, whereas if the second individual values pleasure, the good taste of meat would likely exert more influence on attitudes toward meat eating than would concerns about mistreatment. All of this suggests that to more thoroughly understand attitudes and beliefs toward meat, it may be first necessary to understand values. For example, one study found that values influenced vegetarian diet choice through the mediating role played by beliefs about the benefits of vegetarianism (Kalof et al., 1999). In an examination of attitudes toward food attributes not directly related to vegetarianism, Dreezens et al. (2005) found that those valuing universalism rated genetically modified food low and organic food high, while the opposite pattern was observed for those valuing power; the value–attitude link was again modified by beliefs. That values lead to attitudes and beliefs, which in turn lead to behavior, has been supported by a number of studies outside the food domain (Bernard et al., 2003; Homer and Kahle, 1988; Maio and Olson, 1995; Thøgersen and Ölander, 2002).

Several studies have examined value differences between vegetarian subgroups. Vegans were lower in social dominance than were other vegetarians (Bilewicz et al., 2011) and higher in idealism (Rothgerber, 2015b). Ethical vegetarians were more humanistic (Lindeman and Sirelius, 2001) and more greatly valued compassion, nonviolence, and ecological preservation than health vegetarians (Jabs et al., 1998). These specific values shape beliefs and attitudes within these groups, shape how influential specific beliefs and attitudes are, and ultimately shape the behavioral differences observed in the literature. For example, valuing compassion more, ethical vegetarians may feel greater empathy toward animals and, therefore, express greater concern when witnessing others consuming meat. Vegans and other vegetarians may both believe in the difficulty in following a vegan diet, but greater idealism may cause vegans to be less influenced by this perceived difficulty when evaluating veganism and, subsequently, more likely to behave in accordance with it.

Other research has identified value differences between undifferentiated vegetarians and nonvegetarians. The most commonly identified value difference is that relative to meat eaters, vegetarians reject social power, social dominance, inequality, and authoritarianism (Allen et al., 2008, 2000; Bilewicz et al., 2011; Dietz et al., 1995; Kalof et al., 1999). This seems logical given that meat symbolizes these attributes and that plant-derived foods represent a rejection of these values (Adams, 2015; Allen and Ng, 2003; Allen et al., 2008; Fiddes, 1991; Lea and Worsley, 2001; Twigg, 1983). Indeed, according to deFrance (2009), the upsurge in meat eating is a recent phenomenon to establish social distinctions of wealth and status and to foster social unity through the symbolic manipulation of animals. As Eder (1996) observed, "Vegetarian life is the negation of social power."

Another important value difference is that vegetarians emphasize nonviolence and compassion (Jabs et al., 1998; Hamilton, 2000, 2006) more than meat eaters. They are also more likely to espouse liberal political ideology (Gale et al., 2007; White et al., 1999), to value environmental protection (Dietz et al., 1995; Jabs et al., 1998; Kalof et al., 1999), and to reject traditional values (Dietz et al., 1995; Kalof et al., 1999).

5. The Role of Attitudes Toward Meat in Becoming a Vegetarian and in Maintaining a Vegetarian Diet

At this point, I would offer the idea that *the decision to adopt a vegetarian diet is influenced by a value or set of values that lead to proanimal attitudes and beliefs, and for health vegetarians, by a value leading to antimeat attitudes and beliefs* (see Fig. 2.1). Those that value social equality and reject dominance over nature or other beings would develop a host of attitudes on a number of issues, including being favorable toward environmental protection and toward antidiscrimination policies; developing favorable attitudes toward animals and supporting their welfare would follow. This general support would be evident in more detailed beliefs about animals in the food system, such as they should not suffer to satisfy our consumption desires. Eventually, these attitudes and beliefs would cause some individuals to seek behavioral change and reduce meat intake or adopt a vegetarian diet. Valuing nonviolence and compassion would cause individuals to have positive attitudes

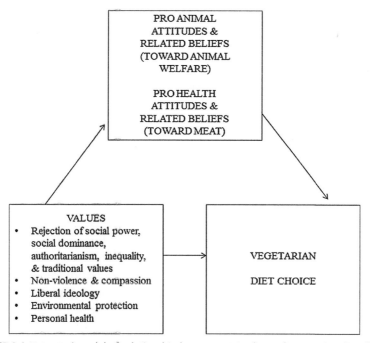

FIGURE 2.1 Proposed model of relationship between attitudes and vegetarian diet choice.

toward measures designed to reduce animal suffering and cause negative attitudes toward actions that inflicted harm on animals. These attitudes would produce a number of beliefs, including that factory farming is unjust. Embracing liberal ideology and rejecting traditional values may cause individuals to hold positive attitudes toward social change movements and to have positive attitudes toward alternative diets disavowing themselves from the traditional meal structure (e.g., meat, vegetables, and a starch). These attitudes would then affect beliefs, such as that a vegetarian diet is worth the social disruption it may cause.

The values previously identified with vegetarians are those most related to ethical vegetarians. Health vegetarians are less likely to share these values, and for them, the principal value inspiring their attitudes, beliefs, and behavior is that of personal health. A concern with one's well-being would trigger a number of positive attitudes toward behavior reflecting this: to exercise, to sleep well, and of course, to eat in a healthy way. These individuals are more likely open to alternative diets that may produce health benefits. For some, beliefs that a vegetarian diet is healthy and that meat is unhealthy would be strong enough to motivate behavioral change.

This perspective suggests that health vegetarians are not as concerned with the living animal but focus more on meat itself as a potential contaminant to the body. Even so, opposition to meat would be more practical and not have the sort of moral and emotional condemnation associated with outrage over animal welfare. Conversely, for ethical vegetarians, when it comes to the initial decision to become vegetarian, views on meat (i.e., the dead animal on the plate) are not as centrally motivating, well-elaborated, or emotionally developed as views on animals in general.

There is available evidence to support the notion that for many vegetarians, the strong disdain for meat evident in this review does not necessarily predate their decision to become vegetarian. For example, only a relatively small percent of vegetarians state that disgust with meat or a dislike of its sensory characteristics is a primary motive for their conversion to vegetarianism (Amato and Partridge, 1989; Beardsworth and Keil, 1992; Hamilton, 2006; Kalof et al., 1999; Kenyon and Barker, 1998; Rozin et al., 1997; Timko et al., 2012); rather the focus is on the living animal or one's personal health. In studies specifying the percent changing their diet because of gustatory dislike, the figure is around 10% (Amato and Partridge, 1989; Hamilton, 2006; Rozin et al., 1997) or much lower (Timko et al., 2012). Amato and Partridge (1989) reported that 48% of the vegetarians they studied experienced cravings for meat, and these cravings fade over time to the point where 82% stated that they would never consider eating meat again. That the cravings fade over time indirectly supports the premise that attitudes toward meat become more negative the longer one has followed a vegetarian diet and do not primarily motivate the initial decision to convert. In addition, the majority of vegetarians in one study reported that they had liked and enjoyed many or all types of meat before becoming vegetarian (Hamilton, 2006). Similarly, Beardsworth and Keil (1992) noted that some vegetarians had not always been disgusted and repulsed by meat. These authors also reported that many ethical vegetarians were not disgusted by cooked meat, missed not eating it, and some even craved it, especially bacon: bacon nostalgia as they term it (Beardsworth and Keil, 1992).

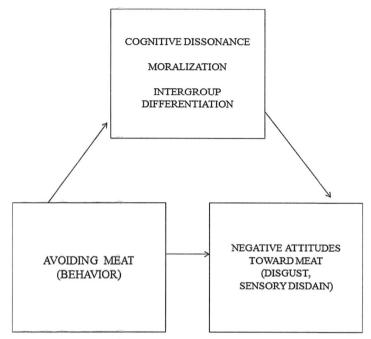

FIGURE 2.2 Proposed model of relationship between attitudes and vegetarian diet maintenance.

To explain diet maintenance and what transpires after following a vegetarian diet for some time, attitudes toward meat play a more prominent role and become intensified. That is, *I believe that negative attitudes toward meat develop more strongly and become more salient as a result of following a vegetarian diet* (see Fig. 2.2). The increasing negative attitudes toward meat occur because of at least three distinct processes: cognitive dissonance, moralization, and a desire for positive intergroup distinctiveness, each of which will be presented.

5.1 Vegetarian Diet and Dissonance Theory

The process of not eating meat produces psychological effects on the individual, above and beyond the individual's values, beliefs, and attitudes that led to the behavioral change in the first place. Although dissonance theory has more often been applied to the psychological experience of meat eaters (see Joy, 2011; Rothgerber, 2014a), it may also be relevant to the psychological experience of new vegetarians. Vegetarians may experience some or all of the following: social tension with family and friends over their diet (Jabs et al., 1998, 2000); a number of negative emotions from meat eaters (Adams, 2003); negative reactions in meat eaters anticipating moral reproach (Minson and Monin, 2012); a need to abandon familiar restaurants because of limited vegetarian options; difficulty finding appropriate food when traveling or in unfamiliar circumstances; burdening those hosting them for meals; and worrying about satisfying certain nutritional requirements.

From classical dissonance theory (Festinger, 1957), dissonance may result from the individual wanting to maintain consistency ("My diet offends others; I do not like offending people" or "My diet burdens others; I do not like being a burden"). From the "new look" dissonance (Cooper and Fazio, 1984), dissonance may result from the individual wanting to avoid aversive consequences ("I follow a vegetarian diet; this diet creates social disharmony" or "I follow a vegetarian diet; this diet makes it difficult to eat out"). In either case, the individual would experience strong motivational pressures to justify the costs of being vegetarian. While there are several ways of doing so, one approach is to condemn meat itself, to turn it from a liked or tolerated food to a disgusting, abhorrent, ill-smelling, and ill-tasting reminder of a dead animal. In essence, meat disdain becomes a consonant cognition that then reduces the dissonance brought on by being a vegetarian.

5.2 Vegetarian Diet and Moralization

Rozin and colleagues offer a separate account for how converting to vegetarianism may cause meat to be viewed as more disgusting. In a process they term moralization, Rozin et al. (1997) describe how for ethical vegetarians, meat eating changes from a neutral activity to a moral one. What may have been a preference to avoid meat becomes thought of in terms of values, which are more durable, internalized, and central to the self. Values tend to produce strong moral emotions, such as anger, shame, contempt, guilt, and disgust, with this last emotion serving as a focal point of their research. Rozin et al. (1997) argue that ethical vegetarians evaluate meat as more disgusting because having adopted an antimeat stance on ethical and philosophical grounds, they then connect meat eating with powerful emotions that provide additional motivational force for their position. Disgust occurs in vegetarians as a way of supporting and internalizing meat avoidance. That is, the shift in meat from a liked to a disliked or disgusting food occurs because once philosophically opposed to meat, a dislike for its sensory and inherent qualities motivates further avoidance of it.

Rothgerber (2015b) has offered the moralization concept as one way to explain why COs do not develop the same level of disgust for animal flesh as vegetarians. Factory-farmed animal products are probably not dissimilar enough from ethical animal products in taste, smell, texture, and appearance to cultivate in COs a disgust specific to factory-farmed foods comparable to the level of disgust that vegetarians can develop for meat. This interpretation has also received indirect support from Rothgerber (2014b), who found that self-identified vegetarians who nonetheless consumed animal flesh reported being less disgusted by meat. The possibility that diet could cause disgust (or a lack thereof) is also supported by research confirming that disgust reactions to meat are a consequence, not a cause, of meat avoidance (Fessler et al., 2003). The work of Allen et al. (2008) also sheds light on how perceptions of taste can be affected by what food is thought to represent rather than its actual physical properties. Specifically, they found that those scorning social power gave a more favorable taste evaluation when they believed they had tasted a vegetarian alternative to a sausage roll than when they believed they had tasted a sausage roll, regardless of the product they actually ate.

5.3 Vegetarian Diet and Social Identity

A third explanation for why committing to vegetarianism would cause an increase in meat disgust and other negative attitudes toward meat emphasizes that being a vegetarian becomes an important aspect of one's social identity. Like other valued social identities, the individual is motivated to feel favorable about the ingroup and to achieve positive intergroup differentiation (Tajfel and Turner, 1986). Because the defining behavior of vegetarianism is in not eating meat, it stands that vegetarians would be highly motivated to define meat abstention in a positive way. One obvious way to do so is by devaluing meat. This suggests that over time, vegetarians would become more negative toward meat because it helps them feel better about a valued ingroup. Few empirical studies have approached vegetarianism from a social identity perspective, so I will elaborate a bit more.

Meat can be seen as a social construction in that its social importance seems greater than nutritionally warranted (see Allen et al., 2000). The symbolic value associated with meat, then, lends itself to identity building. A number of scholars have discussed vegetarianism as a form of identity (Allen et al., 2000; Jabs et al., 1998; Fox and Ward, 2008; Joy, 2011; Fischler, 1988; Kremmel, 2006; Hamilton, 2000; Rothgerber, 2014a). For example, Fox and Ward (2008) noted that their vegetarian respondents did not define vegetarianism simply as a diet but a broader lifestyle tied to identity. Jabs et al. (1998) described vegetarianism in religious terms, noting that it became an identity that produced a "spiritual transformation" occupying central importance to its followers. Vegetarianism defines the self, who one is, the sort of being one is, what it is to be human, and the relationship with the other (i.e., nonhuman animals) (Hamilton, 2000).

Fischler (1988) discussed how food choices are intermeshed with self-identities. To this, I would expand: they are related to *social* identities. Many vegetarians are involved in vegetarian subcultural groups, such as message boards, animal rights groups, etc. (Kremmel, 2006). According to Back and Glasgow (1981), many vegetarians erect a strong boundary against their identity and society. They want to associate with like-minded individuals, they reject their upbringing and socially imposed inhibitions, and they espouse strong ideological preferences. Vegetarians feel isolated from society and have a strong sense of ingroup belonging. Vegetarianism may be the aspect of others' identity that is most salient to nonvegetarians (Kremmel, 2006). While meat eaters only experience diet as a form of social identity when they interact with vegetarians, vegetarians are reminded of identity every time food is eaten or discussed in the presence of meat eaters (Kremmel, 2006). Vegetarians do not define themselves simply as a set of dietary behaviors, and it seems that omnivores do not see them this way either (see Joy, 2011; Rothgerber, 2014a). This potentially creates a good deal of tension, especially within families and holiday celebrations where meat eaters may feel threatened by the rejection of tradition (Jabs et al., 1998; Rothgerber, 2014a). Indeed, negative encounters with outgroup members and lack of social support are major reasons for abandoning vegetarian diets (Jabs et al., 1998).

Several writers have commented on how vegetarian outrage and disgust at unknowingly ingesting meat products far exceeds the harm to animals that such cases may bring.

In these instances, the animal is already dead, the food is already prepared, and their refusal to eat, likely with little awareness on the part of others, would have minimal long-term effect on industrial farming. But in identity terms, such violations are so upsetting because they violate the symbolic identity of vegetarians. This relates to the concept of boundary work; that is, vegetarians consider their social identity as important, and they work to symbolically defend its boundaries. One way is to reject fake or semivegetarians, who may harm the integrity of the collective group.

Rothgerber (2014d) specifically studied how vegans and other vegetarians reacted to ingroup violators. While violators were typically devalued, the specific reaction depended on the social context. Situations that made norm violations more damaging to the ingroup intensified vulnerable groups' negativity toward disloyalty. One such situation involves mainstream salience because norms differentiating vulnerable groups from the mainstream become more important when the mainstream is salient. Another situation that impacted ingroup negativity was whether the violation was concealed because unconcealed violations may be more damaging to the group and used by outgroup members to undercut its survival. It was shown statistically that concerns that disloyal members would undermine intergroup distinctiveness and undercut the message of the group were central to the disapproval shown to norm violators. This shows that vegetarians are worried about others' reactions to their group and the impact that disloyalty has on others and the way the ingroup is perceived, rather than simply being a personal or internal matter. There is also the notion that evaluations and perceptions of vegetarian subgroups (e.g., vegan–vegetarian, and health vegetarian–ethical vegetarian) are subject to the horizontal hostility phenomenon demonstrated in other minority groups and shown to be motivated by social identity concerns (Rothgerber, 2014e; White and Langer, 1999; White et al., 2006).

In short, there is general recognition that vegetarianism is not simply a behavior but that it represents a deeper set of values and attitudes. It seems to have all the characteristics of a group typically studied in the intergroup relations literature: self-definition; differentiated behavior; ingroup pride; disgust toward outgroup behavior; hostility from the outgroup; group boundary work; devalued perceptions of ingroup violators; status differentiation within the group; smaller groups organized around the larger group; and the horizontal hostility phenomenon.

There is reason to suspect that vegetarian identity would become more important as one adheres to the diet over a longer period. To maintain status as a good ingroup member and to maintain distance from the outgroup, I would expect vegetarians to place even greater importance on and value the one dimension that most clearly defines the group: not eating meat. Meat should, therefore, be devalued, denigrated, and defamed as a way to achieve positive intergroup differentiation. In practice, this means that following a vegetarian diet for a longer time should cause an increase in meat disgust, negative sensory ratings of meat, and in general, negative attitudes and beliefs about meat. This appears to be an untested proposition.

6. Conclusion

For omnivores, attitudes toward meat and animals are "nonattitudes": they are not strongly felt and do not predict behavior (Herzog, 2011). For vegetarians, these attitudes are fundamentally important. Dietz et al. (1995) suggest that values, beliefs, and attitudes predict the decision to become vegetarian. This review generally concurs: certain attitudes differentiate vegetarians from nonvegetarians, and they also are critical in differentiating between semivegetarians and true vegetarians, vegans and other vegetarians, and health and ethical vegetarians. There are still, of course, important questions to resolve. Dietz et al. (1995) conclude that these internal social psychological processes are more important than demographic factors, but this may be a false dichotomy. Demographic factors (such as gender) may predict values, attitudes, and beliefs, and we need more research to determine if demographic factors become nonsignificant when controlling for internal processes. A critical question is why do attitudes matter: How much do they cause diet choice, and how much do they result from it? Does this answer depend on the type of attitude (meat, vegetable, or animal) or a specific type of meat at that? The answer to why attitudes matter may involve both possibilities. Some attitudes (chiefly, toward animals) may cause diet choice, and others (toward meat) may result from diet choice. But even this seems more complicated and likely depends on whether the specific vegetarian is primarily motivated by ethics or health. There is also a question about the extent to which these attitudes impact other behaviors related to health. That is, it is possible that other behaviors are as strongly attached to vegetarianism as the diet itself, but this remains unclear. Once again, motives for vegetarianism may be relevant, as the connection may be direct for health vegetarians and indirect for ethical vegetarians. In short, we have come a long way since the assessment of Dwyer et al. (1974), but there are more questions than ever to answer.

References

Adams, C.J., 2003. Living Among Meat Eaters: The Vegetarian's Survival Handbook. Bloomsbury Publishing.

Adams, C.J., 2015. The Sexual Politics of Meat: A Feminist-Vegetarian Critical Theory. Bloomsbury Publishing, USA.

Ajzen, I., 1991. The theory of planned behavior. Organ. Behav. Hum. Decis. Process. 50 (2), 179–211.

Allen, M.W., Ng, H.S., 2003. Human values, utilitarian benefits and identification: the case of meat. Eur. J. Soc. Psychol. 33 (1), 37–56.

Allen, M.W., Gupta, R., Monnier, A., 2008. The interactive effect of cultural symbols and human values on taste evaluation. J. Consum. Res. 35 (2), 294–308.

Allen, M.W., Wilson, M., Ng, S.H., Dunne, M., 2000. Values and beliefs of vegetarians and omnivores. J. Soc. Psychol. 140 (4), 405–422.

Amato, P.R., Partridge, S.A., 1989. The New Vegetarians: Promoting Health and Protecting Life. Plenum Press, New York.

Back, K.W., Glasgow, M., 1981. Social networks and psychological conditions in diet preferences: gourmets and vegetarians. Basic Appl. Soc. Psychol. 2 (1), 1–9.

Barnes-Holmes, D., Murtagh, L., Barnes-Holmes, Y., Stewart, I., 2010. Using the implicit association test and the implicit relational assessment procedure to measure attitudes toward meat and vegetables in vegetarians and meat-eaters. Psychol. Rec. 60, 6.

Barr, S.I., Chapman, G.E., 2002. Perceptions and practices of self-defined current vegetarian, former vegetarian, and nonvegetarian women. J. Am. Diet. Assoc. 102 (3), 354–360.

Beardsworth, A.D., Keil, E.T., 1991. Vegetarianism, veganism, and meat avoidance: recent trends and findings. Br. Food J. 93, 19–24.

Beardsworth, A., Keil, T., 1992. The vegetarian option: varieties, conversions, motives and careers. Sociol. Rev. 40, 253–293.

Bedford, J.L., Barr, S.I., 2005. Int. J. Behav. Nutr. Phys. Act. 2, 4.

Bernard, M.M., Maio, G.R., Olson, J.M., 2003. The vulnerability of values to attack: inoculation of values and value-relevant attitudes. Personal. Soc. Psychol. Bull. 29 (1), 63–75.

Bilewicz, M., Imhoff, R., Drogosz, M., 2011. The humanity of what we eat: conceptions of human uniqueness among vegetarians and omnivores. Eur. J. Soc. Psychol. 41, 201–209.

Cooper, C.K., Wise, T.N., Mann, L., 1985. Psychological and cognitive characteristics of vegetarians. Psychosomatics 26 (6), 521–527.

Cooper, J., Fazio, R.H., 1984. A new look at dissonance theory. Adv. Exp. Soc. Psychol. 17, 229–266.

deFrance, S.D., 2009. Zooarchaeology in complex societies: political economy, status, and ideology. J. Archaeol. Res. 17, 105–168.

De Houwer, J., De Bruycker, E., 2007. Implicit attitudes toward meat and vegetables in vegetarians and nonvegetarians. Int. J. Psychol. 42, 158–165.

Dietz, T., Frisch, A.S., Kalof, L., Stern, P.C., Guagnano, G.A., 1995. Values and vegetarianism. An exploratory analysis. Rural Sociol. 60, 533–542.

Dreezens, E., Martijn, C., Tenbült, P., Kok, G., De Vries, N.K., 2005. Food and values: an examination of values underlying attitudes toward genetically modified-and organically grown food products. Appetite 44 (1), 115–122.

Dwyer, J.T., Mayer, L.D.V.H., Dowd, K., Kandel, R.F., Mayer, J., 1974. New vegetarians: the natural high. J. Am. Diet. Assoc. 65, 529–536.

Eagly, A.H., Chaiken, S., 1993. The Psychology of Attitudes. Harcourt Brace Jovanovich College Publishers.

Eder, K., 1996. The Social Construction of Nature: A Sociology of Ecological Enlightenment. Sage Publications, Inc.

Fessler, D.M., Arguello, A.P., Mekdara, J.M., Macias, R., 2003. Disgust sensitivity and meat consumption: a test of an emotivist account of moral vegetarianism. Appetite 41 (1), 31–41.

Festinger, L., 1957. A Theory of Cognitive Dissonance, vol. 2. Stanford University Press, Palo Alto, CA.

Fiddes, N., 1991. Meat. A Natural Symbol. Routledge, London.

Fischler, C., 1988. Food, self and identity. Soc. Sci. Inf. 27 (2), 275–292.

Fishbein, M., Ajzen, I., 1975. Belief, Attitudes, Intention, and Behavior. An Introduction to Theory and Research. Addison–Wesley, Massachussets.

Fox, N., Ward, K., 2008. Health, ethics and environment: a qualitative study of vegetarian motivations. Appetite 50, 422–429.

Gale, C.R., Deary, I.J., Schoon, I., Batty, G.D., 2007. IQ in childhood and vegetarianism in adulthood: 1970 British cohort study. BMJ 334 (7587), 245.

Gossard, M., York, R., 2003. Social structural influences on meat consumption. Soc. Am. Ecol. 10, 1–9.

Hamilton, M., 2000. Eating ethically: 'spiritual' and 'quasi-religious' aspects of vegetarianism. J. Contemp. Relig. 15 (1), 65–83.

Hamilton, M., 2006. Eating death: vegetarians, meat, and violence. Food Cult. Soc. 9, 155–177.

Herzog, H., 2011. Some We Love, Some We Hate, Some We Eat: Why It's So Hard to Think Straight About Animals. HarperCollins, New York, NY.

Hoek, A.C., Luning, P.A., Weijzen, P., Engels, W., Kok, F.J., de Graaf, C., 2011. Replacement of meat by meat substitutes. A survey on person-and product-related factors in consumer acceptance. Appetite 56 (3), 662–673.

Homer, P.M., Kahle, L.R., 1988. A structural equation test of the value-attitude-behavior hierarchy. J. Personal. Soc. Psychol. 54 (4), 638.

Hoogland, C.T., de Boer, J., Boersema, J.J., 2005. Transparency of the meat chain in the light of food culture and history. Appetite 45 (1), 15–23.

Jabs, J., Devine, C.M., Sobal, J., 1998. Model of the process of adopting vegetarian diets. Health vegetarians and ethical vegetarians. J. Nutr. Educ. 30, 196–203.

Jabs, J., Sobal, J., Devine, C.M., 2000. Managing vegetarianism: identities, norms and interactions. Ecol. Food Nutr. 39 (5), 375–394.

Joy, M., 2011. Why We Love Dogs, Eat Pigs, and Wear Cows: An Introduction to Carnism. Conari Press.

Kalof, L., Dietz, T., Stern, P.C., Guagnano, G.A., 1999. Social psychological and structural influences on vegetarian beliefs. Rural Sociol. 64, 500–511.

Kenyon, P.M., Barker, M.E., 1998. Attitudes towards meat-eating in vegetarian and non-vegetarian teenage girls in England – an ethnographic approach. Appetite 30, 185–198.

Kremmel, S., 2006. Understanding Eating Boundaries: A Study of Vegetarian Identities (Graduate theses and dissertations). http://scholarcommons.usf.edu/etd/3801.

Krizmanic, J., 1992. Here's who we are. Veg. Times 182 (72–76, 78–80).

Kubberød, E., Ueland, Ø., Rødbotten, M., Westad, F., Risvik, E., 2002. Gender specific preferences and attitudes towards meat. Food Qual. Prefer. 13 (5), 285–294.

Kwan, S., Roth, L., 2004. Meat consumption and its discontents: vegetarianism as counter-hegemonic embodiment. In: Conference Papers–American Sociological Association, pp. 1–14.

Lea, E., Worsley, A., 2001. Influences on meat consumption in Australia. Appetite 36, 127–136.

Lindeman, M., Sirelius, M., 2001. Food choice ideologies: the modern manifestations of normative and humanist views of the world. Appetite 37, 175–184.

MacNair, R.M., 1998. The psychology of being a vegetarian. Veg. Nutr. Int. J. 2, 96–102.

Maurer, D., 2010. Vegetarianism: Movement or Moment. Promoting a Lifestyle for Cultural Change. Temple University Press, Philadelphia, PA.

Maio, G.R., Olson, J.M., 1995. Relations between values, attitudes, and behavioral intentions: the moderating role of attitude function. J. Exp. Soc. Psychol. 31 (3), 266–285.

Minson, J.A., Monin, B., 2012. Do-gooder derogation disparaging morally motivated minorities to defuse anticipated reproach. Soc. Psychol. Personal. Sci. 3 (2), 200–207.

National Institute of Nutrition, 1997. Tracking Nutrition Trends. Retrieved from: http://www.ccfn.ca/pdfs/canadian%20nutrition%201997.pdf.

National Institute of Nutrition, 2001. Tracking Nutrition Trends. Retrieved from: http://www.ccfn.ca/pdfs/rap-vol17-1.pdf.

Perry, C.L., Mcguire, M.T., Neumark-Sztainer, D., Story, M., 2001. Characteristics of vegetarian adolescents in a multiethnic urban population. J. Adolesc. Health 29 (6), 406–416.

Potts, A., Parry, J., 2010. Vegan sexuality. Challenging heteronormative masculinity through meat-free sex. Fem. Psychol. 20, 53–72.

Povey, R., Wellens, B., Conner, M., 2001. Attitudes towards following meat, vegetarian and vegan diets: an examination of the role of ambivalence. Appetite 37, 15–26.

Pribis, P., Pencak, R.C., Grajales, T., 2010. Beliefs and attitudes toward vegetarian lifestyle across generations. Nutrients 2, 523–531.

Robinson-O'Brien, R., Perry, C.L., Wall, M.M., Story, M., Neumark-Sztainer, D., 2009. Adolescent and young adult vegetarianism: better dietary intake and weight outcomes but increased risk of disordered eating behaviors. J. Am. Diet. Assoc. 109 (4), 648–655.

Rokeach, M., 1968. Beliefs, Attitudes and Values: A Theory of Organization and Change. Jossey-Bass Inc., Publishers, San Francisco, US.

Rothgerber, H., 2013a. Real men don't eat (vegetable) quiche: masculinity and the justification of meat consumption. Psychol. Men Masc. 14, 363–375.

Rothgerber, H., 2013b. Vegetarianism, Veganism, and the Causes of Meat Abstention. (Unpublished manuscript).

Rothgerber, H., 2013c. A meaty matter: pet diet and the vegetarian's dilemma. Appetite 68, 76–82.

Rothgerber, H., 2014a. Efforts to overcome vegetarian-induced dissonance among meat eaters. Appetite 79, 32–41.

Rothgerber, H., 2014b. A comparison of attitudes toward meat and animals among strict and semi-vegetarians. Appetite 72, 98–105.

Rothgerber, H., 2014c. Carnivorous cats, vegetarian dogs, and the resolution of the vegetarian's dilemma. Anthrozoos 27, 485–498.

Rothgerber, H., 2014d. Evaluation of ingroup disloyalty within a multi-group context. Soc. Psychol. 45, 382–390.

Rothgerber, H., 2014e. Horizontal hostility among non-meat eaters. PLoS One 9 (5), e96457.

Rothgerber, H., 2015a. Can you have your meat and eat it too? Conscientious omnivores, vegetarians, and adherence to diet. Appetite 84, 196–203.

Rothgerber, H., 2015b. Underlying differences between conscientious omnivores and vegetarians in the evaluation of meat and animals. Appetite 87, 251–258.

Rozin, P., Markwith, M., Stoess, C., 1997. Moralization and becoming a vegetarian. The transformation of preferences into values and the recruitment of disgust. Psychol. Sci. 8, 67–73.

Rozin, P., Hormes, J.M., Faith, M.S., Wansink, B., 2012. Is meat male? A quantitative multimethod framework to establish metaphoric relationships. J. Consum. Res. 39 (3), 629–643.

Ruby, M.B., 2008. Of Meat, Morals, and Masculinity: Factors Underlying the Consumption of Non-human Animals, and Inferences about Another's Character (Master's thesis) Available from cIRcle at: http://circle.ubc.ca/handle/2429/1504.

Ruby, M.B., 2012. Vegetarianism: a blossoming field of study. Appetite 58, 141–150.

Ruby, M.B., Cheng, T.K., Heine, S.J., 2011. Cultural Differences in Food Choices and Attitudes Towards Animals. (Unpublished raw data).

Santos, M.L.S., Booth, D.A., 1996. Influences on meat avoidance among British students. Appetite 27, 197–205.

Shickle, D., Lewis, P.A., Charny, M., Farrow, S., 1989. Differences in health, knowledge and attitudes between vegetarians and meat eaters in a random population sample. J. R. Soc. Med. 82 (1), 18.

Singer, P., Mason, J., 2006. The Ethics of What We Eat. Text Publishing, Melbourne.

Swanson, J.E., Rudman, L., Greenwald, A.G., 2001. Using the Implicit Association Test to investigate attitude-behaviour consistency for stigmatised behaviour. Cogn. Emot. 15 (2), 207–230.

Tajfel, H., Turner, J.C., 1986. The social identity theory of intergroup behavior. In: Worchel, S., Austin, W.G. (Eds.), The Psychology of Intergroup Relations, pp. 7–24.

Thøgersen, J., Ölander, F., 2002. Human values and the emergence of a sustainable consumption pattern: a panel study. J. Econ. Psychol. 23 (5), 605–630.

Time/CNN/Harris Interactive Poll, 2002. Do You Consider Yourself a Vegetarian? Available at: http://i.timeinc.net/time/covers/1101020715/poll/images/poll_body.gif.

Timko, C.A., Hormes, J.M., Chubski, J., 2012. Will the real vegetarian please stand up? An investigation of dietary restraint and eating disorder symptoms in vegetarians versus non-vegetarians. Appetite 58 (3), 982–990.

Twigg, J., 1979. Food for thought: purity and vegetarianism. Religion 9, 13–35.

Twigg, J., 1983. Vegetarianism and the meaning of meat. In: Murcott, A. (Ed.), The Sociology of Food and Eating. Gower, Aldershot, pp. 18–30.

White, J.B., Langer, E.J., 1999. Horizontal hostility: relations between similar minority groups. J. Soc. Issues 55, 537–559.

White, J.B., Schmitt, M.T., Langer, E.J., 2006. Horizontal hostility: multiple minority groups and differentiation from the mainstream. Group Process. Intergroup Relat. 9, 339–358.

White, R.F., Seymour, J., Frank, E., 1999. Vegetarianism among US women physicians. J. Am. Diet. Assoc. 99 (5), 595–598.

Willetts, A., 1997. Bacon sandwiches got the better of me: meat eating and vegetarianism in south-east London. In: Caplan, P. (Ed.), Food, Health, and Identity. Routledge, New York, NY.

Worsley, A., Skrzypiec, G., 1998. Teenage vegetarianism: prevalence, social and cognitive contexts. Appetite 30 (2), 151–170.

3

Nutrition Knowledge of Vegetarians

Sarah R. Hoffman

UNC GILLINGS SCHOOL OF GLOBAL PUBLIC HEALTH, CHAPEL HILL, NC, UNITED STATES

1. Introduction

1.1 Vegetarians as Unwitting Nutrition Educators

Vegetarians are defined by what they do not consume, differentiating themselves in most societies by rejecting a widespread social norm (Back and Glasgow, 2010). As a result, vegetarians are frequently confronted by curious nonvegetarians with nutrition-related questions: "But where do you get your protein?," "How do you live without meat?," "What about iron?" These interactions often require vegetarians to defend the adequacy of their diet, unwittingly becoming nutrition educators. This phenomenon is epitomized by the common inquiry "But where do you get your protein?," which has generated innumerable responses on the Internet in the form of humorous cartoons and a range of educational blogs, articles, and videos. "But where do you get your protein?" has arguably become a fixture of vegetarian culture, or the shared experience of the realities of being a vegetarian in a society of mostly nonvegetarians.

Occasionally, nonvegetarians assume that vegetarian diets are inherently *healthier* than nonvegetarian diets. In this case, vegetarians may find themselves confronted with uninformed compliments: "You're vegetarian? No wonder you're so thin and healthy!" In this case, the nutritionally savvy vegetarian might remind the nonvegetarian that "even Oreos [a popular brand of chocolate sandwich cookies] are vegan" and that nearly all cakes, cookies, pies, and other "junk" foods are suitable for vegetarian diets.

As dietary minorities, vegetarians unwittingly find themselves in the position of nutrition educator. New vegetarians who intend to interact with family members, friends, or coworkers around food may search for legitimate responses to the common misconceptions they are confronted with by nonvegetarians. As a result of nutritional interrogations by nonvegetarians, some vegetarians may become well versed in nutrition and may even find themselves educating their own healthcare providers (Castillo et al., 2015; Mulliner et al., 1995).

Some vegetarians are born into vegetarian families. In most societies, they too will find themselves confronted with questions posed by nonvegetarian classmates, friends, neighbors, coworkers, and other nonvegetarians. Do children raised in vegetarian families or cultures acquire the knowledge needed to answer these questions passively as a natural result of their upbringing? As of mid-2016, no systematic investigation of this question has been published.

Vegetarians who are not born into vegetarian families must undertake an experience of *becoming* vegetarian. Interestingly, "vegetarian" is not only a diet, but it is also something that a person can become or transform themselves into. Perhaps acquiring new knowledge is a natural consequence of this transformation.

2. Defining Nutrition Knowledge

Nutrition knowledge may be procedural, declarative (Worsley, 2002), or social (Miyazaki, 1994). **Procedural nutrition knowledge** specific to vegetarians may include where to buy and how to cook tofu and how to identify vegetarian food in a nonvegetarian restaurant. An example of **declarative nutrition knowledge** is an awareness of which vegetarian foods are good sources of protein. In the case of vegetarianism, declarative nutrition knowledge may be thought of as the "awareness of the nutritional implications of vegetarianism, and of basic nutritional concepts relating to micro- and macronutrients" (Hoffman et al., 2013). Throughout this chapter, the term "declarative-procedural nutrition knowledge" may be used to refer to declarative and procedural nutrition knowledge collectively.

Researchers measure declarative nutrition knowledge using validated instruments that are incorporated into questionnaires. Table 3.1 presents a global survey of 19 validated nutrition knowledge instruments from 1974 to 2015, and includes articles published in Italian and Korean (Alsaffar, 2012; Anderson et al., 2002; da Vico et al., 2010; Dickson-Spillmann et al., 2011; Feren et al., 2011; Freeland-Graves et al., 1982; Gower et al., 2010; Hoffman et al., 2013; Jones et al., 2015; Kim et al., 1999; Kim, 2009; Moynihan et al., 2007; Obayashi et al., 2003; Parmenter and Wardle, 1999; Rovner et al., 2012; Spendlove et al., 2012; Verrall et al., 2000; Whati et al., 2005; Zinn et al., 2005). The most widely used, previously validated nutrition knowledge instrument is the General Nutrition Knowledge Questionnaire (GNKQ) developed for adults in the United Kingdom by Parmenter and Wardle (1999). The GNKQ has been adapted and modified for use in the United States (Jones et al., 2015), Turkey (Alsaffar, 2012), elite athletes in Australia (Spendlove et al., 2012), obese adults in Norway (Feren et al., 2011), older adults in England (Moynihan et al., 2007), sports nutrition research in New Zealand (Zinn et al., 2005), and vegetarians living in the United States (Hoffman et al., 2013). Thus, much of what is currently known about nutrition knowledge is limited to studies of declarative knowledge in nonvegetarians, as measured by instruments created for use in the West (Table 3.1).

It is easy to fall into the trap of thinking about nutrition "knowledge" as limited to scientific explanations about food. To do so would typecast alternative knowledge systems as "beliefs" and would be an act of ethnocentrism (Bryant et al., 2003). Declarative-procedural nutrition knowledge need not be limited to scientific explanations, e.g., micro- and macronutrients. In some cases, declarative or procedural nutrition knowledge may even precede a biochemical understanding of its mechanism, e.g., nixtamalization of corn/maize in Mesoamerica.

Table 3.1   A global Survey of 19 Validated Nutrition Knowledge Instruments from 1974 to 2015

Author (Year)	Instrument	Intended Population
Jones et al. (2015)	Parmenter and Wardle (1999), modified for the US population, with items from Obayashi et al. (2003)	Adults in California, United States
Hoffman et al. (2013)	Parmenter and Wardle (1999), abbreviated, and modified for US vegetarians	Adult vegetarians taking an online survey, United States
Alsaffar (2012)	Parmenter and Wardle (1999), modified and translated into Turkish	Adults in Turkey
Rovner et al. (2012)	Type 1 Diabetes Nutrition Knowledge Survey (NKS)	Youth with type 1 diabetes and their parents in Boston, Massachusetts
Spendlove et al. (2012)	Parmenter and Wardle (1999), modified for the Australian population	Elite Australian athletes
Dickson-Spillmann et al. (2011)	Short, consumer-oriented nutrition knowledge questionnaire	German-speaking part of Switzerland
Feren et al. (2011)	Synthesis of existing instruments including Parmenter and Wardle (1999)	Obese adults; tested in patients waiting for a gastric bypass operation in Norway
da Vico et al. (2010)	Italian version of Moynihan et al. (2007)	Italian hospital patients
Gower et al. (2010)	A computer nutrition knowledge survey for elementary school students	First through fourth grade students from Salt Lake City, Utah, United States, area schools
Kim (2009)	Pregnancy nutrition knowledge scale	Pregnant women, Korea
Moynihan et al. (2007)	Select items from Parmenter and Wardle (1999)	Older adults (60+ years) residing in sheltered accommodation in England
Whati et al. (2005)	A nutrition knowledge questionnaire for urban South African adolescents	South African adolescents living in urban areas
Zinn et al. (2005)	Sports nutrition knowledge questionnaire with items from Parmenter and Wardle (1999)	Developed in New Zealand for use by clinicians and researchers
Anderson et al. (2002)	Knowledge of applied nutrition, food preparation, and perceived confidence in cooking skills	UK children in afterschool care in an area of high social disadvantage
Obayashi et al. (2003)	Nutrition knowledge scale(s) developed for the 1995 Diet and Health Knowledge Survey (DHKS)	US adults
Verrall et al. (2000)	Caregivers' Nutrition Knowledge, Attitudes and Beliefs	Caregivers of children with cerebral palsy
Parmenter and Wardle (1999)	General Nutrition Knowledge Questionnaire (GNKQ) for adults	UK adults
Kim et al. (1999)	The Food and Living Survey	Validated in the Boston, Massachusetts, area in 1974
Freeland-Graves et al. (1982)	A nutrition knowledge test with a vegetarian nutrition subtest	Developed for the purpose of comparing nutrition knowledge of vegetarians to that of nonvegetarians

Declarative-procedural nutrition knowledge does not exist in a vacuum; it is developed and applied in the context of social nutrition knowledge. **Social nutrition knowledge** consists of social representations, widespread beliefs, interpretative repertoires, and internalized social contingencies related to food (Miyazaki, 1994). Food-related social representations and interpretive repertoires live alongside declarative-procedural nutrition knowledge and are important yet easily overlooked motivators of dietary behavior.

Individual food items are polysemic symbols (Bryant et al., 2003). A polysemic symbol is "a symbol that carries several meanings simultaneously" (Bryant et al., 2003). These meanings may evolve over time and differ between cultures (Bryant et al., 2003). In some cases, meanings for an individual food item may even conflict. Meat, for example, represents physical strength and power, higher status, virility, cruelty, killing, disgust, and poor health (Rozin et al., 2012; Ruby et al., 2013). A firmly established example of social representation and food symbolism related to vegetarianism is the common association between meat and masculinity (Rozin et al., 2012). In classroom testing spanning at least a decade, North American students consistently classified steak as masculine and strawberries as feminine (Bryant et al., 2003).

Interpretive repertoires of a society guide its members toward a common understanding of which animals to eat or not eat (Norman, 2014). In a nonvegetarian-predominant culture, there exists an interpretative repertoire on the difficulty of maintaining a vegetarian or vegan diet (Norman, 2014). Perhaps the most important vegetarian-related interpretative repertoire of all (in the West) is that a "vegetarian" is something a person "is" or "is not" (Norman, 2014). Widespread beliefs and interpretive repertoires about food, such as the prevalent misunderstanding around protein in vegetarian diets, may be factually incorrect and yet retain a powerful influence on dietary behavior and social norms.

3. Transcultural Considerations

Vegetarians living in Western countries may experience their vegetarianism differently from vegetarians living in a context where vegetarianism is more widespread due to spiritual customs, poverty, or both. That is, **vegetarians by choice** may differ in significant ways from **vegetarians by context**. It follows that nutrition knowledge may develop and function differently in these two groups.

While vegetarians by context are steeped in procedural and social knowledge about vegetarianism from birth, vegetarians by choice are often not. Vegetarians by choice who are living in nonvegetarian societies must develop a high level of declarative nutrition knowledge to explain and defend their diet to others while developing the procedural nutrition knowledge necessary for their own survival. Social representations, widespread beliefs, interpretative repertoires, and internalized social contingencies related to vegetarianism may differ from society to society, and even differ dramatically between vegetarian-predominant cultures and nonvegetarian cultures. Furthermore, knowledge and beliefs about vegetarianism in a Buddhist or Hindu country likely differ from knowledge and beliefs about vegetarianism in a country where meat is virtually absent due to scarcity. More research is needed to understand how the experiences of vegetarians vary by context in relation to nutrition knowledge.

Deeper investigation into nutrition knowledge of vegetarians in predominantly vegetarian countries is called for. Most of what is currently known about nutrition knowledge and vegetarianism is limited to studies of declarative nutrition knowledge in white, Western vegetarians (Hoffman et al., 2013). Procedural nutrition knowledge that is embedded into the regular dietary practices of some cultures, e.g., the consumption of rice with dal and bread in India or nixtamalization of corn/maize in Mesoamerica, is not testable by declarative nutrition knowledge instruments. A global survey of transcultural procedural nutrition knowledge from vegetarian-predominant cultures could be informative to vegetarians by choice, nutritionists, and researchers.

4. Measuring Nutrition Knowledge in Vegetarians

Freeland-Graves et al. (1982) developed a test to measure general and vegetarian-specific nutrition knowledge in vegetarians and nonvegetarians. The instrument consisted of three parts: 40 questions concerning general nutrition knowledge (e.g., functions of nutrients, the Four Food Groups), 40 questions regarding vegetarian nutrition (e.g., limiting amino acids, nutritional advantages and disadvantages of vegetarianism), and three questions regarding previous nutrition training and current sources of nutrition information. The test was validated in two university nutrition classes (Freeland-Graves et al., 1982).

The "Four Food Groups" referenced by the Freeland-Graves instrument were developed by the United States Department of Agriculture (USDA) and included (1) vegetables and fruits, (2) milk, (3) meat, and (4) cereals and breads. This model was eventually replaced by the USDA's 1992 Food Guide Pyramid. In this sense, the Freeland-Graves et al. (1982) instrument is specific to a particular place and time, i.e., the United States in the 1970s or early 1980s, when it was developed. Were the test to be administered today, subjects would be unfamiliar with the "Four Food Groups" and therefore achieve lower test scores. This instrument would need to be updated and revalidated to be administered again.

It is important, when developing questions for or interpreting results from any test, to reflect on what phenomena are being measured by the instrument. Questions about the "Four Food Groups" do not necessarily measure knowledge of nutrition truths but the internalization of a framework for thinking about food as promoted by the USDA in the mid-20th century. While this type of nutrition knowledge is probably worth measuring, interpretations of test scores should incorporate the implications of the types of questions posed to the study participants and whether such questions measure knowledge of truths that will survive the test of time.

Instruments developed to measure nutrition knowledge in nonvegetarians can be modified to exclude references to meat and other animal products and to include questions specific to vegetarianism. In 2013, the widely used Parmenter and Wardle (1999) questionnaire was abbreviated and modified for use in US adult vegetarians (Hoffman et al., 2013). The GNKQ for adults (Parmenter and Wardle, 1999) is a 50-item instrument developed in the UK. Six items were borrowed from this questionnaire to create four items assessing awareness of basic nutritional concepts relating to micro- and macronutrients and energy. Nonvegan foods were eliminated and/or replaced with similar vegan options. All but one item contained several subitems, resulting in a total of 22 individual questions (Tables 3.2a and 3.2b). An eight-item section dedicated to vegetarian nutrition was also developed. Items were based upon educational material written by registered dietitians, publicly available on the Vegetarian Resource Group website. Such information is widely available through other

Table 3.2a   Items From the General Nutrition Knowledge Questionnaire (Parmenter and Wardle, 1999) Modified for Use in a Sample of US Adult Vegetarians

Parmenter and Wardle (1999)	Hoffman et al. (2013)
Do you think these are high or low in fat? (tick one box per food: high, low, not sure)	**Please select the most appropriate category for each food item: (carbohydrate, fat, protein, unsure)**
Pasta (without sauce)	Rice
Low fat spread	Nuts
Baked beans	Bananas
Luncheon meat	Olive oil
Honey	Pasta
Scotch egg	Potato
Nuts	Avocado/guacamole
Bread	Tempeh, seitan, and meat analogues
Cottage cheese	Coconut
Polyunsaturated margarine	
Do you think experts put these in the starchy foods group? (tick one box per food: yes, no, not sure)	
Cheese	
Pasta	
Butter	
Nuts	
Rice	
Porridge	
Do you think these are high or low in protein? (tick one box per food: high, low, not sure)	
Chicken	
Cheese	
Fruit	
Baked beans	
Butter	
Cream	

Table 3.2b Items From the General Nutrition Knowledge Questionnaire (Parmenter and Wardle, 1999) Modified for Use in a Sample of US Adult Vegetarians

Parmenter and Wardle (1999)	Hoffman et al. (2013)
Do you think these are high or low in fiber/roughage? (tick one box per food: high, low, not sure)	**Do you think the following are high or low in fiber? (high, low, unsure)**
Cornflakes	Cornflakes
Bananas	Bananas
Eggs	Tofu
Red meat	Apple Juice
Broccoli	Nuts
Nuts	Beans
Fish	
Baked potatoes with skins	
Chicken	
Baked beans	
Which of the following has the most calories for the same weight? (tick one)	**Which of the following has the most calories (energy) per gram (unit of weight)? Choose one.**
Sugar	Sugar
Starchy foods	Starch
Fiber/roughage	Fiber
Fat	Fat
Not sure	Protein
	Not sure
Do you think these are high or low in salt? (tick one box per food: high, low, not sure)	**Do you think the following food items are high or low in sodium (salt)? (high, low, unsure)**
Sausages	Tofurky, Boca burger, other faux meat products
Pasta	Frozen vegetables
Kippers	Cinnamon roll
Red meat	Cheese or vegan cheese analogues
Frozen vegetables	Tofu
Cheese	Olive oil

popular vegetarian organization websites. The questions were administered in a "true/false" fashion (Table 3.3). The resulting instrument consisted of 30 unique items (22 general, 8 vegetarian). Scoring was completed by calculating the percentage correct for the entire instrument ($[n/30]*100$). This modified nutrition knowledge instrument showed acceptable reliability (Cronbach's alpha = 0.74, $n = 312$) in a sample of US adult vegetarians recruited through online advertisements on heavily trafficked social media platforms.

5. Nutrition Knowledge of Vegans as Compared to Ovolactovegetarians

In a representative sample of Shanghai vegetarians (Mao et al., 2015), vegans were more likely than ovolactovegetarians (70% vs. 58%, $n = 274$) to believe that a "vegetarian diet" is

Table 3.3 Vegetarian-Specific Nutrition Knowledge Questions Developed by Hoffman et al. (2013)

Do You Agree or Disagree With the Following Statements? (Agree, Disagree, Unsure)
1. Iron found in plant foods is in a different form than iron found in animal foods.
2. Drinking a glass of orange juice with an iron-rich, vegetarian meal will enhance the iron absorption.
3. It is untrue that all essential amino acids must be eaten together at the same meal to form a complete protein.
4. Fortified foods or supplements are an important source of vitamin B_{12} for strict vegetarians and vegans.
5. The calcium in some greens (spinach, chard) is not readily absorbed, but the calcium in other greens (kale, collard) is.
6. Vegetarian sources of vitamin D include fortified foods and supplements.
7. Saturated fat occurs naturally in some plant foods.
8. It is important to eat a variety of foods, even when following a vegetarian/vegan diet.

a healthy dietary pattern that will not have any nutrient deficiencies. Hoffman et al. (2013) found that greater dietary restriction was significantly associated with increased nutrition knowledge scores: vegans who consume honey scored highest on the nutrition knowledge questionnaire (mean = 0.81), followed by vegans who never consume honey (mean = 0.79), and ovolactovegetarians (mean = 0.71) (Hoffman et al., 2013).

6. Nutrition Knowledge of Vegetarians as Compared to Nonvegetarians

Lindamood and Gunning (1977) compared nutrition knowledge between vegetarian and nonvegetarian college students at San Diego State University. Of 71 students who completed the nutrition knowledge questionnaire, 45% defined themselves as vegetarian. No significant difference in nutrition knowledge was found between vegetarians and nonvegetarians, with both groups answering 41% of the questions correctly (Lindamood and Gunning, 1977).

Freeland-Graves et al. (1982) administered a nutrition knowledge test to 106 vegetarians and 106 nonvegetarians at a large state university in the Southwest. Vegetarians were recruited by newspaper advertisements, posters in health food stores and restaurants, and "personal contact." The "vegetarian" sample included 11 vegans and 15 pescetarians. Nonvegetarians consisted of local resident and student volunteers who were matched to vegetarians (1:1 matching) by age, gender, city of residence, and amount of nutrition training. Vegetarians scored significantly higher than nonvegetarians on both the general and the vegetarian nutrition subtests. Both vegetarians and nonvegetarians scored fairly low on the test, with vegetarians earning a mean score of 59% (percentage of questions answered correctly) and nonvegetarians earning a mean score of 50%, while university-level nutrition students scored 86% on average. Both vegetarians and nonvegetarians scored significantly higher on the general nutrition subtest than on the vegetarian nutrition subtest (Freeland-Graves et al., 1982).

Kim et al. (1999) compared nutrition knowledge between vegetarians and nonvegetarians residing in the Boston, Massachusetts area in 1974 and 1997. An 88-item survey containing a nutrition knowledge questionnaire was developed and validated in 1974 and distributed to customers at health food stores and traditional supermarkets. The instrument was distributed a second time in 1997 at a vegetarian food fair. In 1974, the 23 vegetarian respondents and 366 nonvegetarian respondents achieved similar nutrition knowledge scores (0–7-point scale, mean ± SD: 4.6 ± 0.8 and 4.1 ± 1.2, respectively). In 1997, the 103 vegetarian and 81 nonvegetarian respondents recruited at a vegetarian food fair also achieved similar nutrition knowledge scores (0–7-point scale, mean ± SD: 4.8 ± 1.3 and 4.8 ± 1.1, respectively) (Kim et al., 1999).

Leonard et al. (2014) conducted a cross-sectional assessment of nutrition knowledge and iron consumption among women aged 18–35 years living in Newcastle, Australia, in 2012–13. A 30-item questionnaire was developed to measure knowledge about dietary sources of iron and iron physiology. Nine vegetarians and 22 self-described "partial vegetarians" (a term left undefined in the article) performed better on the nutrition knowledge questionnaire than 76 nonvegetarians (mean ± SD: 12.1 ± 3.7 and 10.6 ± 3.2, respectively, $P = .04$). The authors noted that "vegetarians may have a heightened interest in nutrition, resulting in their higher knowledge scores, than nonvegetarians." There was no significant difference in mean iron intake between the two groups (10.54 ± 3.31 mg/day and 11.5 ± 4.0 mg/day) (Leonard et al., 2014).

In summary, only four studies compared nutrition knowledge between vegetarians and nonvegetarians, and one focused on iron, which is highly pertinent to vegetarianism.

7. Nutrition Knowledge of Ethically Oriented as Compared to Health-Oriented Vegetarians

A typical finding of qualitative studies on vegetarianism is that there are two primary motivations for the diet: ethical concerns and health considerations. Readers can refer to Chapters 1 and 2 for details. Hoffman et al. (2013) compared nutrition knowledge scores of health and ethical vegetarians categorized by both initial and current motivation for becoming vegetarian. Subjects who became vegetarian for ethical reasons scored similarly on the nutrition knowledge instrument (mean = 0.760, standard error = 0.0087) as health vegetarians (mean = 0.745, standard error = 0.017). Results were similar when subjects were grouped by current reason for remaining vegetarian (Hoffman et al., 2013).

Perhaps, there is no difference in nutrition knowledge acquisition by health versus ethical orientation among US adult vegetarians, i.e., vegetarians living in a nonvegetarian-predominant society, who regardless of health or ethical orientation may study nutrition to defend and maintain their dietary practices. This may seem counterintuitive since it might be thought that health vegetarians would know more about health, and consequently nutrition, than other vegetarians. It is possible that ethical vegetarians, given their higher personal conviction levels (Hoffman et al., 2013), study nutrition and other aspects of their lifestyle more intensely and by way of this intensity develop just as much nutrition knowledge as their health-oriented counterparts. No correlation was found between nutrition knowledge and personal conviction regarding one's own vegetarianism, however (Hoffman et al., 2013). Further research using larger samples of vegetarians are necessary to draw any conclusion regarding whether nutrition knowledge varies by motivation, to elucidate the process of nutrition knowledge formation in vegetarians, and to understand the relationship between nutrition knowledge and health behavior among vegetarians.

8. Nutrition Knowledge and Dietary Behavior Among Vegetarians

Hoffman et al. (2013) found a significant relationship between nutrition knowledge and dietary restriction in a sample of US adult vegetarians, with dietary restriction defined as the number of animal-derived foods from a provided list that were currently "never" consumed by the subject ($r = 0.32$, $r^2 = 0.1024$). This overall association could have been driven by the presence of many ethical vegetarians in the sample (234 ethical vegetarians and 58 health vegetarians), as nutrition knowledge was significantly associated with dietary restriction in ethical vegetarians ($r = 0.36$) but not in health vegetarians. Dietary restriction was greater in ethical vegetarians than in health vegetarians when subjects were categorized by current motivation for following a vegetarian diet. While health versus ethical orientation may not be associated with differences in nutrition knowledge (Hoffman et al., 2013), orientation does seem to have implications for the relationship between nutrition knowledge and dietary restriction. Furthermore, among ethical vegetarians (but not in health vegetarians), the relationship between nutrition knowledge and number of years as vegetarian approached significance. This finding suggests that nutrition knowledge is accumulated over time, or it supports the longevity of a vegetarian lifestyle, or both.

More recently, Radnitz et al. (2015) examined differences in dietary behavior in a sample of 246 vegans located in the United States, Canada, and other (undisclosed) countries. Participants completed an online survey and were grouped according to their reason for following a vegan diet. Behaviors of health-oriented ($n = 45$) and ethically oriented ($n = 201$) vegans were compared. While ethical vegans reportedly consumed more soy-based foods, foods high in vitamin D, and beverages high in polyphenols than health-oriented vegans, ethical vegans also consumed greater quantities of sweets per day. Ethical vegans were more likely than health-oriented vegans to report taking a multivitamin (30% vs. 9%), any supplement (82% vs. 60%), a vitamin D supplement (37% vs. 20%), or a vitamin B_{12} supplement (64% vs. 47%) (Radnitz et al., 2015). In addition, Radnitz et al. (2015) found that ethical vegans reported a significantly longer duration on a vegan diet than did health-oriented vegans, a finding that is consistent with Hoffman et al. (2013). If nutrition knowledge is not substantially different between health and ethical vegetarians, then the question of what drives these behavioral differences remains open.

9. Nutrition Knowledge and the Process of Becoming a Vegetarian

Nonvegetarians can be former or future vegetarians, and vegetarians can be former nonvegetarians. It is possible that some nonvegetarians become vegetarian because of nutrition knowledge. If the "facts of life" regarding meat are considered to be nutrition knowledge, then nutrition knowledge plays a definitive role in the process of becoming vegetarian for ethical vegetarians.

In a paper entitled "Once You Know Something, You Can't Not Know It: An Empirical Look at Becoming Vegan," McDonald (2000) reports their use of a qualitative methodology to identify a psychological process of how people learn about and adopt veganism, asking "how do people learn to become vegan?" McDonald used snowball sampling to identify vegans from a small core group recruited at the June 1996 nationwide March for the Animals in Washington, DC. Only vegans who had been practicing veganism for at least 1 year were included ($n = 12$). All the individuals reported having gone through a "catalytic experience" that introduced them to animal cruelty. Upon learning these facts, some of the future vegans went into a state of repression and remained there until another catalytic experience. Upon receiving the catalytic experience, the future vegans eventually became "oriented," and they entered a learning period in which they gathered knowledge about animal cruelty and how to live as a vegetarian or specifically a vegan (e.g., acquiring nutrition knowledge). After a period of learning that could span multiple years, the participants made the choice to become vegan, adopting a new world view to guide their new lifestyle (McDonald, 2000).

Thus, for these 12 ethically oriented vegans identified and interviewed by McDonald (2000), knowledge and its acquisition formed the very foundation for their veganism. However, it was not knowledge alone that made them vegan but the decision to act upon that knowledge in such a way that all animal-derived foods and products are avoided. The question remains: when confronted with the same facts, what makes it so that some humans make this decision while others do not? The same question can be asked of health-oriented vegetarians as compared to nonvegetarians who possess the same knowledge regarding the health benefits of a vegetarian diet.

10. Discussion

10.1 Does Nutrition Knowledge Precede or Result From Vegetarianism or Both?

McDonald (2000) demonstrated that nutrition knowledge (in this case, knowledge of where animal-derived foods come from) both preceded and contributed to the transition to vegetarianism for 12 ethically oriented vegans. A parallel process may take place in health-oriented vegetarians, in which knowledge of the benefits of a vegetarian diet and potential harms of animal-derived foods precede and contribute to the transition to vegetarianism. It is clear, and perhaps intuitive, that knowledge precedes vegetarianism, but do vegetarians gain additional knowledge over time so that a vegetarian of 10 years knows twice as much as a vegetarian of 5 years?

Hoffman et al. (2013) and Freeland-Graves et al. (1982) found that nutrition knowledge was not related to the length of time a person had been vegetarian, suggesting that knowledge does not increase over time after becoming vegetarian. These studies did not set out to compare newer and older vegetarians in terms of nutrition knowledge, and they were not longitudinal studies able to establish a temporal, causal relationship between nutrition knowledge and length of time on a vegetarian diet; so it is wise to interpret their findings cautiously. An analysis of cross-sectional data might find a positive association, for instance, if comparing nutrition knowledge among vegetarians of 3 months or less to vegetarians of 1 year or more. A longitudinal study that follows new vegetarians might find that nutrition knowledge test scores in the first 3 months of becoming vegetarian are associated with whether an individual is still adhering to a vegetarian diet 10 years later.

It is possible that vegetarians do acquire additional nutrition knowledge over time, but the type of knowledge that vegetarians accumulate is not necessarily the type of knowledge tested by available instruments. Further qualitative research with larger samples of vegetarians and more extensive instrumentation is needed to understand how new knowledge arises or does not arise after a successful transition to a vegetarian diet. Additional questions to be studied might include these: (1) What drives vegetarians-by-choice to seek nutrition knowledge, after becoming vegetarian,? What types of knowledge do they seek? (2) Once acquired, how is nutrition knowledge used by vegetarians? So far, it appears that nutrition knowledge is most heavily relied upon to make the transition from a nonvegetarian lifestyle to a vegetarian lifestyle, but what happens after? (3) Is knowledge and corresponding behavior related to how long an individual remains vegetarian? Finally, (4) would educational interventions prevent nutritional deficiencies and/or cessation of vegetarianism in vegetarians?

10.2 Synthesis

Nutrition knowledge is more than an internalized system of declarative, scientific "facts." Beyond declarative knowledge, there exist other forms of knowing as it relates to nutrition, including procedural and social knowledge. Vegetarians may be vegetarian by choice or by context, with implications for the role of each type of knowledge in their lives. Numerous instruments have been developed to measure nutrition knowledge, but only one has been developed and validated specifically for vegetarians and is applicable across temporal and geographic contexts (Hoffman et al., 2013). Four studies have been completed to evaluate differences in nutrition knowledge between vegetarians and nonvegetarians and only one controlled for confounding and found a statistically significant difference in test scores (Freeland-Graves et al., 1982). Nutrition knowledge was not substantially different between health and ethical vegetarians in one small, uncontrolled analysis, and it appears that ethical motivation has more profound implications for dietary behavior than nutrition knowledge alone.

References

Alsaffar, A.A., 2012. Validation of a general nutrition knowledge questionnaire in a Turkish student sample. Public Health Nutr. 15 (11), 2074–2085. http://doi.org/10.1017/S1368980011003594.

Anderson, A.S., Bell, A., Adamson, A., Moynihan, P., 2002. A questionnaire assessment of nutrition knowledge–validity and reliability issues. Public Health Nutr. 5 (3), 497–503. http://doi.org/10.1079/PHNPHN2001307.

Back, K.W., Glasgow, M., 2010. Social networks and psychological conditions in diet preferences: gourmets and vegetarians. Basic Appl. Soc. Psychol. 2 (1), 1–9. http://doi.org/10.1207/s15324834basp0201_1.

Bryant, C., DeWalt, K., Courtney, A., Schwartz, J., 2003. The Cultural Feast: An Introduction to Food and Society, second ed. Thomson Wadsworth, Belmont, California.

Castillo, M., Feinstein, R., Tsang, J., Fisher, M., 2015. Basic nutrition knowledge of recent medical graduates entering a pediatric residency program. Int. J. Adolesc. Med. Health. 1–2. http://doi.org/10.1515/ijamh-2015-0019.

da Vico, L., Biffi, B., Agostini, S., Brazzo, S., Masini, M.L., Fattirolli, F., Mannucci, E., 2010. Validation of the Italian version of the questionnaire on nutrition knowledge by Moynihan. Monaldi Arch. Chest Dis. 74 (3), 140–146 IRCCS [and] Istituto di clinica tisiologica e malattie apparato respiratorio, Universita di Napoli, Secondo ateneo.

Dickson-Spillmann, M., Siegrist, M., Keller, C., 2011. Development and validation of a short, consumer-oriented nutrition knowledge questionnaire. Appetite. 56 (3), 617–620. http://doi.org/10.1016/j.appet.2011.01.034.

Feren, A., Torheim, L.E., Lillegaard, I.T.L., 2011. Development of a nutrition knowledge questionnaire for obese adults. Food & Nutr. Res. 55. http://doi.org/10.3402/fnr.v55i0.7271.

Freeland-Graves, J.H., Greninger, S.A., Vickers, J., Bradley, C.L., Young, R.K., 1982. Nutrition knowledge of vegetarians and nonvegetarians. J. Nutr. Educ. 14 (1), 21–26. http://doi.org/10.1016/S0022-3182(82)80058-7.

Gower, J.R., Moyer-Mileur, L.J., Wilkinson, R.D., Slater, H., Jordan, K.C., 2010. Validity and reliability of a nutrition knowledge survey for assessment in elementary school children. J. Am. Diet. Assoc. 110 (3), 452–456. http://doi.org/10.1016/j.jada.2009.11.017.

Hoffman, S.R., Stallings, S.F., Bessinger, R.C., Brooks, G.T., 2013. Differences between health and ethical vegetarians. Strength of conviction, nutrition knowledge, dietary restriction, and duration of adherence. Appetite 65, 139–144.

Jones, A.M., Lamp, C., Neelon, M., Nicholson, Y., Schneider, C., Wooten Swanson, P., Zidenberg-Cherr, S., 2015. Reliability and validity of nutrition knowledge questionnaire for adults. J. Nutr. Educ. Behav. 47 (1), 69–74. http://doi.org/10.1016/j.jneb.2014.08.003.

Kim, E., Schroeder, K., Houser, R., Dwyer, J., 1999. Two small surveys, 25 years apart, investigating motivations of dietary choice in 2 groups of vegetarians in the Boston area. J. Am. Diet. Assoc. 99 (5), 598–601.

Kim, H.W., 2009. Development of the pregnancy nutrition knowledge scale and its relationship with eating habits in pregnant women visiting community health center. J. Korean Acad. Nurs. 39 (1), 33–43. http://doi.org/10.4040/jkan.2009.39.1.33.

Leonard, A.J., Chalmers, K.A., Collins, C.E., Patterson, A.J., 2014. The effect of nutrition knowledge and dietary iron intake on iron status in young women. Appetite. 81, 225–231. http://doi.org/10.1016/j.appet.2014.06.021.

Lindamood, D.M., Gunning, B.E., 1977. College nonvegetarians vs. Vegetarians-food habits and knowledge. J. Nutr. Educ. Behav. 9 (1), 25. http://doi.org/10.1016/S0022-3182(77)80113-1.

Mao, X., Shen, X., Tang, W., Zhao, Y., Wu, F., Zhu, Z., Cai, W., 2015. Prevalence of vegetarians and vegetarian's health dietary behavior survey in Shanghai. Wei Sheng Yan Jiu 44 (2), 237–241.

McDonald, B., 2000. Once you know something, you can't not know it: an empirical look at becoming vegan. Soc. Anim. 8 (1), 1–23. http://doi.org/10.1163/156853000X00011.

Miyazaki, Y., 1994. Social Knowledge of Food: How and Why People Talk about Foods. The University of Waikato.

Moynihan, P.J., Mulvaney, C.E., Adamson, A.J., Seal, C., Steen, N., Mathers, J.C., Zohouri, F.V., 2007. The nutrition knowledge of older adults living in sheltered housing accommodation. J. Hum. Nutr. Diet.Official J. Br. Diet. Assoc. 20 (5), 446–458. http://doi.org/10.1111/j.1365-277X.2007.00808.x.

Mulliner, C.M., Spiby, H., Fraser, R.B., 1995. A study exploring midwives' education in, knowledge of and attitudes to nutrition in pregnancy. Midwifery. 11 (1), 37–41. http://doi.org/10.1016/0266-6138(95)90055-1.

Norman, A., 2014. Interpretations of Meat Consumption – a Critical Analysis of Interpretative Repertoires of Individuals Working in an Environmental NGO. Swedish University of Agricultural Sciences.

Obayashi, S., Bianchi, L.J., Song, W.O., 2003. Reliability and validity of nutrition knowledge, social-psychological factors, and food label use scales from the 1995 Diet and Health Knowledge Survey. J. Nutr. Educ. Behav. 35 (2), 83–91.

Parmenter, K., Wardle, J., 1999. Development of a general nutrition knowledge questionnaire for adults. Eur. J. Clin. Nutr. 53 (4), 298–308.

Radnitz, C., Beezhold, B., DiMatteo, J., 2015. Investigation of lifestyle choices of individuals following a vegan diet for health and ethical reasons. Appetite. 90, 31–36. http://doi.org/10.1016/j.appet.2015.02.026.

Rovner, A.J., Nansel, T.R., Mehta, S.N., Higgins, L.A., Haynie, D.L., Laffel, L.M., 2012. Development and validation of the type 1 diabetes nutrition knowledge survey. Diabetes Care. 35 (8), 1643–1647. http://doi.org/10.2337/dc11-2371.

Rozin, P., Hormes, J.M., Faith, M.S., Wansink, B., 2012. Is meat male? A quantitative multimethod framework to establish metaphoric relationships. J. Cons. Res. 39 (3), 629–643. http://doi.org/10.1086/664970.

Ruby, M.B., Heine, S.J., Kamble, S., Cheng, T.K., Waddar, M., 2013. Compassion and contamination. Cultural differences in vegetarianism. Appetite. 71, 340–348. http://doi.org/10.1016/j.appet.2013.09.004.

Spendlove, J.K., Heaney, S.E., Gifford, J.A., Prvan, T., Denyer, G.S., O'Connor, H.T., 2012. Evaluation of general nutrition knowledge in elite Australian athletes. Br. J. Nutr. 107 (12), 1871–1880. http://doi.org/10.1017/S0007114511005125.

Verrall, T.C., Berenbaum, S., Chad, K.E., Nanson, J.L., Zello, G.A., 2000. Children with Cerebral Palsy: Caregivers' Nutrition Knowledge, Attitudes and Beliefs. Can. J. Diet. Pract. Res. 61 (3), 128–134.

Whati, L.H., Senekal, M., Steyn, N.P., Nel, J.H., Lombard, C., Norris, S., 2005. Development of a reliable and valid nutritional knowledge questionnaire for urban South African adolescents. Nutrition. 21 (1), 76–85. http://doi.org/10.1016/j.nut.2004.09.011.

Worsley, A., 2002. Nutrition knowledge and food consumption-can nutrition knowledge change behaviour? Asia Pac. J. Clin. Nutr. 11, S579–S585. http://doi.org/10.1046/j.1440-6047.11.supp3.7.x.

Zinn, C., Schofield, G., Wall, C., 2005. Development of a psychometrically valid and reliable sports nutrition knowledge questionnaire. J. Sci. Med. Sport/Sports Med. Aust. 8 (3), 346–351.

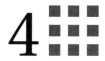

4

Vegetarianism and Eating Disorders

Sydney Heiss[1], Julia M. Hormes[1], C. Alix Timko[2,3]

*[1]UNIVERSITY AT ALBANY, STATE UNIVERSITY OF NEW YORK, ALBANY, NY, UNITED STATES;
[2]UNIVERSITY OF PENNSYLVANIA, PHILADELPHIA, PA, UNITED STATES;
[3]CHILDREN'S HOSPITAL OF PHILADELPHIA, PHILADELPHIA, PA, UNITED STATES*

It has long been speculated that there is a connection between eating disorders and vegetarianism. While this idea tends to permeate popular belief, research to support the hypothesis that the two phenomena are causally linked is limited, and the existing literature on this subject is plagued by inconsistencies in both measurement strategies and findings. Researchers have employed a number of approaches to studying the hypothesized relationship between vegetarianism and eating disorders: they have examined the rates of vegetarianism in samples of individuals with eating disorders (Zuromski et al., 2015; Bardone-Cone et al., 2012; Bas et al., 2005; O'Connor et al., 1987) and the prevalence of eating disorders in samples of vegetarians (Timko et al., 2012a; Trautmann et al., 2008; Klopp et al., 2003; Lindeman et al., 2000). Researchers have also cross-sectionally compared vegetarians to nonvegetarians on a number of other eating-related variables, including dieting and dietary restraint (e.g., Forestell et al., 2012; Timko et al., 2012a; Trautmann et al., 2008; Fisak et al., 2006).

Prior to discussing the evidence for and against a causal role of vegetarianism in the etiology and/or maintenance of eating disorders, it is useful to briefly revisit a number of topics that help set the context for such a discussion, namely definitions of vegetarianism as used in the literature, the importance of motives for avoiding meat or animal products, the assessment of eating pathology specifically in vegetarians, and common methodological difficulties in exploring the relationship between eating pathology and vegetarianism. Even though the former two topics have been explored in depth elsewhere in this volume, the issue of operational definitions and the reasons behind a vegetarian diet have slightly different implications in the context of eating pathology and therefore merit inclusion in the present discussion.

1. Defining Terminology

1.1 Defining Meat Avoidance

Understanding the relationship between eating disorders and vegetarianism is fraught with difficulties, not the least of which is the poor operational definition of "vegetarianism." There are significant inconsistencies in the way in which vegetarianism has been defined. Although the operational definition of "vegetarian" appears to be fairly clear-cut, it has been rather loosely applied in the research literature. The readers can refer to Chapter 1 for more detail. The inconsistencies in the use of the term "vegetarian" may be at least partially responsible for the common perception that vegetarianism plays a role in the development eating disorders and disordered eating. Overall, there appear to be two commonly used approaches: (1) grouping together all types of "vegetarians" (i.e., degrees of meat avoidance ranging from vegans to ovolactovegetarians, lactovegetarian, pescetarian, or semivegetarians) and comparing them to nonvegetarians or omnivores who consume all animal products (e.g., Bardone-Cone et al., 2012; Bas et al., 2005) or (2) attempting to differentiate between distinct subgroups, such as vegans, ovolactovegetarians, semivegetarians, and omnivores (e.g., Forestell et al., 2012; Timko et al., 2012a). The latter approach, which is arguably the stronger research design, tends to be the exception, likely due to the difficulty of recruiting sufficiently large numbers of the different types of vegetarians to draw meaningful between-group comparisons.

When presenting research results, we will use the terminology employed by the research referenced and, whenever possible, will provide an operational definition of the term as used by the researcher. However, in our discussions, we will use the following terminology: we define *vegans* as those who refrain from eating any animal products, including meat, fish, eggs, and dairy. The term *ovolactovegetarian* refers to individuals who refrain from eating the flesh of an animal but do consume milk and eggs. We use the term *semi-vegetarian* to describe individuals who refrain from consuming only some types of meat, for example, individuals who avoid red meat or pork but will eat fish, poultry, or both, as well as those who follow a primarily vegetarian diet but occasionally consume meat. In research on eating pathology, the frequency of meat consumption is rarely reported, including in individuals who consume a predominantly, but not exclusively, vegetarian diet. Thus, it is impossible to determine with certainty the frequency with which semivegetarians surveyed in the existing literature include meat in their diet. When speaking of a combination of any of these categories of avoidance, we will simply refer to it as *vegetarianism*. Finally, *omnivore* refers to someone who consumes and uses all types of animal products.

It may seem unnecessary to clearly differentiate these subgroups of meat avoiders beyond general vegetarianism. However, in the context of eating pathology (where elimination of specific food groups from the diet is likely to be pathological or problematic and can result in significant macro- and micronutrient deficiencies), it is essential to have a good grasp of what exactly is being excluded from the diet. A review of the literature reveals that many studies combine vegans, ovolactovegetarians, and semivegetarians into one group to have a large enough sample for meaningful statistical analyses. Thus, much research on "vegetarians" is really on a wide range of different types of meat avoiders. While combining all subgroups aids in addressing issues of statistical power, there is a serious conceptual problem with grouping all meat avoiders together: the small body of research that does clearly differentiate these subgroups indicates that semivegetarians are categorically different from vegans, vegetarians, and omnivores, specifically when it comes to symptoms of eating pathology (Timko et al., 2012a).

Compounding this problem is the common reliance on self-report of vegetarianism. Most research reports do not specify if operational definitions of different types of vegetarians (or even a definition of "vegetarian") were provided to study participants. Individuals who consume fish, for example, will frequently self-identify as "vegetarian," as opposed to "pescetarian" or "semivegetarian." For example, in a study examining disordered eating in vegetarians, we asked individuals to identify whether they adhered to a vegetarian diet and, if so, what type (Timko et al., 2012a). We provided clear operational definitions of each type of vegetarian. Later in the same survey, we asked participants to note how frequently they ate a variety of foods, including several animal products. We then confirmed self-identified vegetarian status by reviewing the food frequency questions. Approximately a dozen individuals who self-identified as some type of vegetarian endorsed at least occasional consumption of food inconsistent with that diet. As small samples are typical in research on vegetarianism and eating pathology, even a small number of individuals who misrepresent their diet could adversely impact findings.

1.2 The Motive for Meat Avoidance

Understanding the reasons for avoiding meat and animal products is arguably as important as capturing the exact nature of the avoidance. For a general review of the research on vegetarianism and attitude toward meat the readers can refer to Chapter 2. In the context of eating pathology, the reasons why meat is initially eliminated from the diet can play a key role in determining whether it is related to eating pathology and provides important information for treatment. For example, vegetarianism in someone recovering from anorexia may not be as relevant to the treatment of the disorder if that individual's family is vegetarian, has been vegetarian for the patient's lifetime, and/or is vegetarian for religious or other ideological reasons. However, if that same individual opted to adhere to a vegan diet exclusively during the course of anorexia, their veganism may be directly related to the illness and should be addressed in treatment.

Assessing the rationale for a vegetarian diet is not straightforward, as vegetarians typically endorse many motives, often simultaneously. Cited reasons for meat avoidance include moral, health, ecological concerns, religious and other personal convictions, appeal, taste, disgust, and other sensory issues, and concerns about cost (Rozin et al., 1997). Moral meat avoidance is typically associated with animal welfare concerns, such that the refrainer believes that abstinence from meat and/or other animal products is an ethical imperative: that we as humans "ought" not to exploit or allow the cruel and inhumane treatments of farmed animals. Such moral considerations are the most common reason for vegetarianism in Americans, with 59% of a combined sample of vegetarians citing morals as a beginning and continuing cause of vegetarianism (Timko et al., 2012a).

Health reasons are the second most common one given, with 20% of vegetarians adhering to the diet due to the perceived health benefits associated with meat and animal product avoidance (i.e., lowered risk of cardiovascular disease and cancer; Timko et al., 2012a, Campbell et al., 1998, Hart, 2009). Health concerns as a reason for diet adoption can, however, mask unhealthy motivations: specifically, adopting a vegetarian diet due to health and weight concerns. Individuals with eating disorders adopt a vegetarian diet for this reason more frequently than in the population at large (Bardone-Cone et al., 2012). Approximately 4% of the general population adopts a vegetarian diet for shape and weight reasons (Timko et al., 2012a). Because weight is often equated with health, unless specifically queried, weight and shape motivations may be grouped in a broader category of "health" concerns as the stated rationale for the adoption of a vegetarian diet. Without querying for this distinction, individuals who state their dietary change was motivated by health concerns may have actually done so to influence their weight and shape.

Though less frequent, individuals can adopt a vegetarian diet due to the belief that meat production has negative effects on the environment (ecological reasons), for example, increased water usage or methane gas emission from livestock. Eleven percent of the vegetarian population cites environmental concerns as a motivation for their diet. Disgust, referring to the perception of meat as being repulsive or offensive, is another commonly cited reason for meat avoidance, with approximately 20% of another sample of vegetarians citing disgust as a current reason for vegetarianism (Rozin et al., 1997). Personal, economic, and taste or other sensory reasons typically are the least frequently cited as initial reasons for meat avoidance. Personal reasons include beliefs about the adverse effects of eating meat, for example, of one's personality (e.g., making one behave more like an animal, making one more aggressive or violent). Economic avoiders do so due to a vegetarian diet being perceived as less expensive, whereas taste avoiders simply do not enjoy the flavor or other sensory properties of meat. It is important to note that many individuals will cite multiple reasons for diet adoption. For those with eating disorders, any of these reasons may provide legitimacy to their decision to eliminate meat.

Religious vegetarians avoid meat in adherence to the rules of their faith. This is a relatively uncommon motivation for the diet, with only 3.5% of a vegetarian sample reporting religious concerns (Timko et al., 2012a). At various points in the Old Testament, pork and shellfish are described as forbidden foods. Likewise, the Quran forbids the consumption of pork. Hindu texts do not explicitly forbid consumption of animal products, but the faith's tenets of nonviolence are typically interpreted as being consistent with the adoption of a ovolactovegetarian diet. It can be more difficult to determine whether vegetarianism is linked to an eating disorder in the cases of religious reasons for meat avoidance. As we noted earlier, in these cases, it is often important to look for a shift to a vegan diet.

Determining the rationale for adherence to a vegetarian diet is further complicated by dynamic changes in motives over time. A process coined "moralization" may play a role in these changes. Moralization is considered the "acquisition of moral qualities by objects or activities that previously were morally neutral" (Rozin et al., 1997, p. 67). It is possible that individuals who began their vegetarian diet due to nonmoral concerns may later assign moral value to their behavior. It is therefore important to determine both initial and current reasons for adherence, as well as length of time of meat avoidance, since motives appear to change and evolve dynamically over time. The process of moralization in vegetarianism, specifically in the context of eating pathology, is not well understood. Historically, eating disorders, particularly anorexia, have been associated with asceticism.

While the understanding of eating disorders has moved away from the ascetic interpretation commonly articulated in early psychoanalytic writing (Mogul, 1980), anecdotally, some individuals with anorexia will describe feelings of being empty, pure, and strong when restricting. It is likely that the moralization of vegetarianism can parallel some of these feelings and strengthen the desire to maintain a vegetarian diet (even if it was started for weight control or as a way to mask eating pathology).

2. Vegetarianism and Restrained Eating

When reviewing the literature on meat avoidance and eating disorders, three main categories of eating pathology emerge: restrained eating, disordered eating, and clinical eating disorders.

2.1 Defining Restrained Eating

"Dietary restraint" or "restrained eating" is frequently used as a marker of pathological eating behaviors. Restrained eating is difficult to describe, as there is no standard operational definition. In general, restraint refers to "chronic dieting" or intentional restriction of intake to influence body weight, often punctuated with episodes of overeating (or eating more than wanted) (Lowe and Thomas, 2009; Stroebe, 2008; Laessle et al., 1989). Essentially, restrained eaters are individuals who fail at restraining or restricting their eating. In experimental studies, restrained eaters will consume more after eating "forbidden" (i.e., diet rule–violating) foods (for a review, see Stroebe, 2008), undergoing a negative mood induction (Cardi et al., 2015), or being exposed to threats to their self-esteem (Wallis and Hetherington, 2004). Restraint is not associated with a reduction in overall caloric intake, but rather with a reduction in consumption of specific macronutrients (e.g., fats or carbohydrates) or types of foods (e.g., desserts) (Timko et al., 2012b, 2017).

Even though restraint and dieting are sometimes used interchangeably, they are not synonymous: while most individuals who currently identify as dieters are also restrained eaters, not all restrained eaters identify as currently dieting (Lowe and Timko, 2004). Restraint, therefore, is often considered to be a more stable or traitlike approach to eating, whereas dieting is assumed to be more state-based (Lowe, 1993). Restrained eating is different from disordered eating; however, measures used to assess restraint are often used when disordered eating is the actual behavior of interest. Thus, restraint (for better or worse) has become a marker for disordered eating and is believed to be a risk factor for the development of an eating disorder (Stice, 2002; Polivy and Herman, 2002).

There is no standard method of measuring restraint, and a number of measures currently exist that tap into the construct of restraint. A review of the literature on eating disorders and meat avoidance revealed that the most common measures of restraint used to quantify eating-related behaviors in vegetarians are the Dutch Eating Behavior Questionnaire (DEBQ) (Van Strien et al., 1986) and the Three-Factor Eating Questionnaire (TFEQ) (Stunkard and Messick, 1985). We were able to identify five articles that used the DEBQ to assess restraint in vegetarians (Fisak et al., 2006; Gilbody et al., 1998; McLean and Barr, 2003; Timko et al., 2012a; Trautmann et al., 2008) and nine articles that have used the TFEQ to assess restraint associated with a vegetarian diet (Barr et al., 1994; Curtis and Comer, 2006; Fisak et al., 2006; Forestell et al., 2012; Janelle and Barr, 1995; Martins et al., 1999; McLean and Barr, 2003; Kahleova et al., 2013; Moore et al., 2015).

2.2 Specific Findings

Within the limited studies that specifically assess the relationship between vegetarianism and restraint, the majority tend to find that vegetarians endorse higher levels of dietary restraint compared to nonvegetarians (Trautmann et al., 2008; Martins et al., 1999; Gilbody et al., 1998; McLean and Barr, 2003); however, this finding has not been consistently replicated. For example, Fisak et al. (2006) found no difference in restrained eating between vegetarians and nonvegetarians. A close examination of the research reveals that the some self-identified vegetarian participants studied are in fact semivegetarians (Trautmann et al., 2008; Gilbody et al., 1998). The failure to accurately categorize vegetarians is the likely cause of the inconsistencies within this literature. Specifically, the association between levels of restrained eating and vegetarianism varies depending on the operational definition of "vegetarian." While it is often assumed that the data is clear-cut in that vegetarians are more restrained and therefore more disordered in their eating, the reality is that the picture is much cloudier.

Studies that drew clear distinctions between different groups of vegetarians found that ovolactovegetarian and vegan women had significantly lower levels of dietary restraint compared to omnivores (Janelle and Barr, 1995; Barr et al., 1994). Other research indicated that ovolactovegetarians and pescetarians were no different than omnivores in terms of restraint, but both semivegetarians and flexitarians (defined as "cutting back on meat, rather than abstaining completely") were significantly more restrained (Forestell et al., 2012). Ultimately, individuals who restricted a variety of meats from their diet (as opposed to only eliminating one or two type of meat) had lower scores on the restraint subscale of the TFEQ (Forestell et al., 2012). Another study found that semivegetarians were significantly more restrained than a combined group of ovolactovegetarians and vegans, though semivegetarians' restraint scores were no different from nonvegetarians (Curtis and Comer, 2006). The finding that semivegetarians are the only group of meat avoiders who exhibit significantly elevated levels of restraint is fairly robust (Curtis and Comer, 2006; Timko et al., 2012a; Forestell et al., 2012). Therefore, the belief that restrained eating (and, by default, more disordered eating) is associated with vegetarianism is only true for semivegetarians. These findings seem almost paradoxical considering that full vegetarians are more restrictive in their intake, compared to semivegetarians, but nevertheless seem to endorse less restraint in formal assessments (Forestell et al., 2012). The current data suggest that a semivegetarian diet may be more of a risk or complicating factor for restrained/disordered eating than a vegetarian or vegan diet.

A caveat to this research is that most is correlational, making it difficult to draw conclusions about causality between restraint and vegetarianism. There are, however, two studies that were designed in such a way that causality could be better asserted: if the onset of the meat avoidance can be assessed, it can be determined with somewhat greater certainty whether vegetarianism causes an increase in restrained eating. In these studies, researchers assessed the relationship between dietary restraint and vegetarianism by asking individuals to change their diet for health purposes (since vegetarian diets are often adopted in response to specific medical or other health conditions) and then measured their dietary restraint using the TFEQ. In the first study, a vegetarian diet was used to increase healthy behaviors in a diabetic population. Ultimately, individuals who adhered to a low-calorie vegetarian diet as opposed to a low-calorie conventional diet endorsed lower levels of dietary restraint, suggesting that in the context of dieting, vegetarianism can lower dietary restraint (Kahleova et al., 2013). In the second study, participants were randomized to a vegetarian diet (e.g., vegan, ovolactovegetarian, pescetarian, semivegetarian) for weight loss (Moore et al., 2015); there were no significant between-group differences in restraint scores as a result of this dietary change. More research of this type needs to be conducted to fully understand the relationship between restraint and vegetarianism.

2.3 Summary

Restraint is typically used as a marker for disordered eating; but in practice, vegetarianism is restrictive by nature, regardless of any cooccurring eating pathology. Across the board, semivegetarians consistently appear to exhibit more pathological eating behaviors (as discussed later), even though in practice they are restricting fewer macronutrients than ovolactovegetarians and vegans. What is missing from many of the studies discussed here is the reason why someone chooses a vegetarian diet. It is possible that semivegetarians are more likely to eliminate some meat products for weight and shape reasons than vegans or vegetarians, who may be driven primarily by concerns about morality and ethics. Those individuals who consider the consumption of meat to be immoral or unethical may not feel as though they have to consciously restrict, as meat is not an option in their mind; whereas it takes consistent willpower to refrain from meat to control body shape. More research is certainly needed to test this specific hypothesis.

Another caveat or limitation to existing research on the relationship between restrained eating and vegetarianism is that current measures of restraint may inadequately measure restrictive behaviors in vegetarians. Some participants may score higher on measures of restraint because they restrict animal products on a daily basis, and not due to disordered eating behaviors. Additionally, restraint does not exclusively result in a reduction of overall calories consumed, but instead it is more related to the restriction of specific macronutrients, which could also translate into higher scores for vegetarians, being that "meat," "dairy," and "eggs" all fall under the macronutrient umbrella. As such, restraint scales may not be properly measuring eating pathology among vegetarians, and they could, in fact, overestimate pathological eating behavior in this group.

3. Vegetarianism and Disordered Eating

3.1 Defining Disordered Eating

The second type of eating-related pathology often described in the literature on vegetarianism is "disordered eating" or "subclinical eating disorders." These categories typically include individuals who score highly on self-report measures of disordered eating, report engaging in extreme or unhealthy dieting behaviors, binge, and/or have significantly distorted body image, but they fall shy of the criteria for a formal diagnosis of a clinical eating disorder. The primary difference between "disordered eating" and "eating disorders" is that individuals who endorse disordered eating do not reach the diagnostic threshold for a formal eating disorder diagnosis. Disordered eating behaviors are on the same spectrum and can be as clinically significant as formally diagnosable eating disorders in regards to mental health and personal well-being.

A review of the literature on eating disorders and meat avoidance revealed that the most common measures used to assess disordered eating in vegetarians are the Eating Attitudes Test (EAT) and its shortened version (EAT-26) (Garner and Garfinkel, 1979; Garner et al., 1982). The EAT-26 ostensibly assesses eating disorders; it has a "clinical cutoff," but it is most frequently used to evaluate disordered eating. Individuals who indicate a score of 20 or higher on the EAT-26 are considered high risk and should be referred for a clinical interview with a mental health professional (Garner and Garfinkel, 1979; Garner et al., 1982; Mintz, 2000). The EAT-26 is often used as a brief eating disorder screening tool. Even if an individual's score does not exceed the cutoff for clinical significance, a higher score on this questionnaire is generally considered to be a marker for the likely use of unhealthy means of weight loss. At the time of publication, seven published articles address the question of whether vegetarians endorse higher levels of eating pathology, compared to omnivores, as measured by the EAT or EAT-26 (Timko et al., 2012a; Forestell et al., 2012; Trautmann et al., 2008; Fisak et al., 2006; Bas et al., 2005; Klopp et al., 2003; Lindeman et al., 2000).

3.2 Specific Findings

Four studies found vegetarians to score higher on measures of disordered eating using the EAT-26 (Bas et al., 2005; Lindeman et al., 2000; Trautmann et al., 2008) or EAT (Klopp et al., 2003); others found no statistically significant difference between vegetarians and nonvegetarians (Fisak et al., 2006; Forestell et al., 2012; Timko et al., 2012a). Within the studies that found no significant difference between vegetarians and nonvegetarians, there nevertheless seems to be a consistent trend toward semivegetarians having the highest scores of disordered eating (Timko et al., 2012a; Forestell et al., 2012). One study examined other additional markers of disordered eating, namely skipping meals and dietary supplement use, a measurement in itself that may be biased against vegetarians, since vegetarians are often directed by health care professionals to take dietary supplements, but it found no significant group differences (Klopp et al., 2003). Another study reported that vegetarians' increased scores on the EAT-26 were not associated with an increase in self-reported importance of weight control (Lindeman et al., 2000).

As noted previously, the way in which vegetarianism is measured varies to such an extent across studies that it is difficult to make meaningful between-group comparisons in EAT scores. As is the case in the literature on restrained eating, combining subgroups of vegetarians into one group is a common trend in research on disordered eating as well. For example, of the studies employing the EAT/EAT-26, no two studies approached the definition/grouping of vegetarian in the same way. One group of researchers broke down participants into four distinct groups: vegan, ovolactovegetarian, semivegetarian, and omnivore (Timko et al., 2012a), whereas another split participants into seven different categories based on their diet: vegan, lactovegetarian (refrains from meat and egg, consumes dairy), ovovegetarian (refrains from meat and dairy, eats egg), pescetarian, semivegetarian, flexitarian (generally tries to consume less meat), and omnivore (Forestell et al., 2012). The latter study ultimately combined the first three groups to run statistical analyses. One study combined semivegetarians and ovolactovegetarians, with a majority of participants in that joint group actually identifying as semivegetarian (77% vs. 23% who followed a ovolactovegetarian diet; Klopp et al., 2003). Similarly, in another study, of the 30 vegetarians in the group, none were vegan and a "majority" were semivegetarians, though a detailed breakdown was not included. Importantly, these authors report that even in the nonvegetarian group, 14% reported refraining from beef, and 23% reported refraining from pork (Trautmann et al., 2008). Yet another group stated that while they found the vegetarian group to be "relatively heterogeneous in their dietary practices," with vegetarian participants being vegan, ovolactovegetarian, lactovegetarian, and semivegetarian, all meat refrainers were combined into one group for analysis (Fisak et al., 2006). One group of researchers asked participants to respond yes or no to the question, "Are you a vegetarian?" but specific type of vegetarianism was not assessed (Bas et al., 2005). Finally, Lindeman et al. (2000) chose to exclude semivegetarians from their study. They defined vegetarianism classically: as the avoidance of red meat, white meat, and fish; this group, though, did not break vegans into a separate category.

3.3 Summary

The data on whether vegetarianism is associated with more disordered eating is equivocal. The lack of a standard operational definition for different types of vegetarians and the lack of a standardized method of categorizing individuals as vegetarian makes it difficult to interpret the literature on disordered eating and vegetarianism. As with the literature on restrained eating and vegetarianism, it appears as if semivegetarians may be the most disordered in their eating. Again, the reason for adopting a vegetarian diet may be more important than the diet itself in assessing the relationship with disordered eating. Finally, the existing research on disordered eating and vegetarianism is exclusively cross-sectional in nature, so causality cannot be determined. Overall, more research is needed in this area. Future work should include a clear differentiation of different types of meat avoiders, should query the rationale for adopting a vegetarian diet, and should track eating behaviors in vegetarians longitudinally to determine cause and effect.

4. Vegetarianism and Clinical Eating Disorders

4.1 Defining Clinical Eating Disorders

The final area of research focuses on vegetarian diets in individuals with clinical eating disorders, specifically those with either anorexia nervosa or bulimia nervosa. Anorexia nervosa is defined by a clinically significant restriction of dietary intake in comparison to biological needs that results in a weight lower than what is expected given the person's age and developmental trajectory (APA, 2013). In addition, individuals with anorexia express a significant fear of gaining weight or being fat, experience disturbances in their experience of weight or shape, and/or engage in behaviors to avoid gaining weight despite the extent of their illness (APA, 2013). The majority of studies assessing the relationship between vegetarianism and eating disorders focus specifically on anorexia nervosa.

Individuals with bulimia nervosa often try to restrict their dietary intake, but this restriction is interrupted by frequent periods of overeating, known as bingeing. During a binge, individuals with bulimia will objectively eat more in one sitting than other individuals would eat in a similar period, and they will also experience a subjective feeling of loss of control while eating (APA, 2013). Bingeing is followed by one or more compensatory behaviors (e.g., vomiting, use of diuretics, excessive exercise, fasting, or extreme dieting) to prevent weight gain. Very little research on vegetarianism and eating disorders has focused specifically on bulimia. Finally, binge eating disorder is also characterized by recurring binges, but in the absence of compensatory behaviors (APA, 2013). To our knowledge, there are no studies assessing a relationship between binge eating disorder and vegetarianism.

Research on clinical eating disorders and vegetarianism takes two forms: assessing for eating pathology and vegetarianism in nonclinical samples or assessing for vegetarianism in clinical populations. In the former, eating pathology is quantified in a variety of ways. In terms of questionnaires, the Eating Disorder Examination-Questionnaire (EDE-Q) (Fairburn and Beglin, 1994; Fairburn et al., 1999) is perhaps the most commonly used in research on eating disorders. It can be used to generate clinical diagnoses and has a total (global) score as well as four subscales capturing "restraint," "shape concern," "weight concern," and "eating concern" (Fairburn and Beglin, 1994). Surprisingly, this questionnaire has been used relatively infrequently in studying vegetarianism; at the time of publication we could only identify three articles and one conference proceeding citing the EDE-Q as a measure (Timko et al., 2012a; Bardone-Cone et al., 2012; Zuromski et al., 2015; Sieke et al., 2013). In a large sample of undergraduate males and females, vegetarians scored significantly higher than nonvegetarians on the eating, shape, and weight concern subscales of the EDE-Q (Sieke et al., 2013). Interestingly, in this study, there were no differences between groups on the restraint subscale of the EDE. It is important to note that the restraint scale of the EDE-Q does not measure restrained eating as measured in the preceding but rather caloric restriction. Vegetarians who adopted the diet for health or shape/weight concerns on average had a higher EDE-Q score than those who chose to be a vegetarian for other (such as religious or ethical) reasons (Sieke et al., 2013). This finding highlights the key role that the rationale for a vegetarian diet plays when trying to understand its relationship to eating pathology. Finally, in a sample of both college students and the general population, semivegetarians scored higher than omnivores only on the Eating Concern subscale of the EDE-Q (Timko et al., 2012a,b).

Nonstandardized assessments designed to detect disorder pathology appear to be more common in research on vegetarians. When asking five "yes" or "no" questions aimed at quantifying binge eating, compensatory behaviors (including use of laxatives, diuretics, and self-induced vomiting), and following a strict diet, researchers found that vegetarians (determined by a "yes" or "no" response to the question "are you vegetarian now") were no different from omnivores in their response to eating disorder–related questions (Estima et al., 2012). Similarly, another group of researchers asked general questions of participants about binge eating and weight control behaviors and found that vegetarian status (determined by a "yes" or "no" answer to the question "are you a vegetarian now") was associated with significantly greater binge eating and use of unhealthy weight control measures (Robinson-O'Brien et al., 2009). A study of young women self-identifying as vegetarians found that they were healthier than nonvegetarians in terms of body mass index and level of physical activity, but they were at increased risk for worse mental health (Baines et al., 2007).

4.2 Anorexia Nervosa and Vegetarianism

Vegetarianism is often believed to play a causal role in the development of eating disorders, as the restrictive nature of the diet can easily hide restriction characteristic of eating disorders. The research on clinical eating disorders and vegetarianism is primarily cross-sectional or conducted via retrospective chart reviews, making it nearly impossible to assess causality. When comparing the level of eating pathology in clinical groups to other groups (even those with subclinical eating pathology), those with a clinical diagnosis were found to score highest in both self-reported vegetarianism and all subscales of the EDE-Q (Zuromski et al., 2015). In this study, vegetarianism was assessed via self-report on a continuum from vegan to ovolactovegetarian to semivegetarian to omnivore. The authors found that vegetarianism (defined as a combined group of self-reported vegans, ovolactovegetarians, or semivegetarians) was most common within the clinical group. They also noted that the subclinical group reported higher lifetime rates of vegetarianism than the nonclinical group, lending at least preliminary support to the idea that vegetarianism may be related to either the facilitation or maintenance of eating disorders.

Retrospective chart reviews are typically used to determine the rates of vegetarianism in samples of individuals with an eating disorder and to compare those with an eating disorder who are vegetarian to those with an eating disorder who do not adhere to a vegetarian diet. In three retrospective chart reviews (Hadigan et al., 2000; O'Connor et al., 1987; Kadambari et al., 1986), approximately half of all patients who were diagnosed with anorexia reported adhering to a vegetarian diet. In all three studies, the subtype of vegetarianism was not specified (i.e., we do not know if the individuals self-identified as vegans, vegetarians, or semivegetarians): the most recent study did not specify the way in which they determined vegetarian status, aside from observing food intake and comparing to a 1-month self-report history (Hadigan et al., 2000). One study defined vegetarianism as the avoidance of red meat (O'Connor et al., 1987), suggesting that many of the "vegetarians" surveyed were likely semivegetarians. The third study defined vegetarianism as being either "absent," "occasional," "usual," or "severe" and failed to describe the operational definition for these categories and the way in which an individual received the label (Kadambari et al., 1986). In retrospective chart reviews, Kadambari et al. found inpatient anorectic vegetarians to be more "weight phobic," as indicated by a greater fear of gaining weight, and more likely to indicate greater restriction to avoid weight gain. These patients were also more likely to consume large portions of noncaloric foods and exhibited a greater fear of fatness than their nonvegetarian counterparts (Kadambari et al., 1986). Interestingly, the majority of vegetarians would not classify themselves as "occasional," "usual," or "severe," begging the question as to whether the assigned label correctly reflected actual eating behavior or if the label accurately reflected vegetarianism.

4.3 Bulimia Nervosa and Vegetarianism

In addition to the relationship with anorexia, there may be an association between vegetarianism and bulimia nervosa (bulimia). There have been relatively fewer studies focusing specifically on bulimia and vegetarianism; therefore, it is difficult to determine the exact nature of the relationship between these two phenomena. Within the existing literature, there have been reports that adolescent and young adult vegetarians, in general, are more likely to report binge eating and a subjective sense of loss of control in respect to their eating (Robinson-O'Brien et al., 2009). Adolescent vegetarians have been found to be four times as likely as nonvegetarians to vomit for weight control and eight times as likely to use laxatives for weight control purposes (Perry et al., 2001). These findings suggest a need to further assess bingeing behavior in vegetarians, specifically in the context of both bulimia and binge eating disorder.

4.4 Summary

Many of the studies described failed to draw a clear distinction between subgroups of vegetarians, not only because all types of meat avoiders were grouped together, but because the definition of vegetarian in querying participants used was very vague. Because of this, it is almost impossible to truly understand the relationship between vegetarianism and eating disorders. It is also unclear if we should focus on the rates and level of eating pathology in vegetarian samples or, conversely, on rates of vegetarianism in samples of individuals with eating disorders. Regardless, the limited data we have indicates that vegetarianism of some sort occurs at a higher rate in patients with eating disorders than in subclinical or nonclinical groups. As with other research, literature on eating pathology lacks standardized methods of assessment. The dearth of studies that include the EDE-Q to assess type and prevalence of vegetarianism in relation to eating disorders highlights the need to be very specific in both the measurement of eating pathology and the sample surveyed. A review of the items of the EDE-Q reveals that very few are likely to be biased against vegetarians (such that they would unfairly pathologize behaviors that are normative in individuals avoiding some or all animal products). Items from the weight and shape concerns scales specifically highlight issues related to dietary restriction. Thus, the EDE-Q, perhaps better than any other measure, may tap into those who chose a vegetarian diet for these reasons and may, in fact, be at greater risk for eating pathology. Furthermore, we need to be specific in the reasons for adopting a vegetarian diet and when, in the course of the development of an eating disorder, the adoption of a vegetarian diet occurred.

5. Is Vegetarianism a (Causal) Risk Factor for Eating Pathology?

Of the eating disorders, anorexia is commonly considered to be most strongly related to vegetarianism. Vegetarianism is believed to be a socially acceptable way in which one can refrain from eating specific foods, and it may thus allow individuals with an eating disorder to significantly restrict their intake without causing alarm or concern. In fact, two-thirds of individuals with a history of an eating disorder believed that their vegetarianism was related to their eating disorder by giving them another way to restrict caloric intake and increase the feeling of control over diet, but the majority (60%) also indicated that the adherence to the vegetarian diet emerged at least one year *after* the onset of their illness (Bardone-Cone et al., 2012). Thus, vegetarianism may not be causal in the development of an eating disorder, but it may be a symptom of the illness or even a maintaining factor.

In one attempt to assess the directionality of the association between anorexia and adherence to a vegetarian diet, researchers described three distinct groups of red meat refrainers: true vegetarians (who engaged in meat avoidance before the onset of illness), pseudovegetarians (meat avoidance began after the onset of illness), and nonvegetarians (i.e., omnivores) (O'Connor et al., 1987). It is important to note that in this study, vegetarianism was operationally defined as refraining from red meat; thus a portion of these vegetarians were actually what we would consider semivegetarians or (depending on the frequency of fish and poultry consumption) not vegetarians at all. The researchers found that of the clinical population, 54% of their participants refrained from red meat, but only 6% had refrained from meat consumption before the onset of their illness. Interestingly, it has been suggested that individuals with other mental disorders, including depression, anxiety, and somatoform disorders, are also disproportionately likely to self-identify as vegetarian, and in most cases, the mental disorder preceded the onset of the diet (Michalak et al., 2012).

There is also some evidence that a vegetarian diet may maintain the illness and/or impede recovery from eating disorders. Women who had previously been diagnosed with anorexia and were not in remission (defined as the absence of "normal eating, normal weight, and regular menses for the past 12 months") were significantly more likely to identify as vegetarian, compared to respondents in remission (Yackobovitch-Gavan et al., 2009).

In another study examining recovery in anorexia, 6 out of 12 patients who were consuming insufficient calories identified as vegetarian or semivegetarian (Windauer et al., 1993).

When assessing the association between vegetarianism and eating disorders, the timing of the start of adherence to the vegetarian diet seems to be of particular importance. There are significant differences between rates of vegetarianism in individuals with an active eating disorder compared to those in partial recovery, or in full recovery, such that those with an active eating disorder are most likely to be vegetarian, and those in full recovery are the least likely to be vegetarian (Bardone-Cone et al., 2012). Additionally, there seem to be important demographic and clinical differences between anorexic patients who started their vegetarian diet before versus after the onset of illness. Typically, vegetarians have similar demographic and clinical characteristics (e.g., age, mean duration of anorexia, mean BMI), compared to nonvegetarians, whereas the semivegetarians (or "pseudovegetarians" referred to by the authors) reported longer duration of illness and a lower BMI throughout the course of illness (O'Connor et al., 1987).

We currently do not have the data to unequivocally indicate that meat avoidance in itself is a risk factor or causally related to eating pathology. It appears most likely that adherence to a vegetarian diet does not cause eating disorders; rather, vegetarianism is used to "camouflage" existing eating disorders (Bas et al., 2005). It is also likely that it maintains eating pathology and may contribute to difficulties in recovery. Although we posit that vegetarianism is more likely to play a maintenance role in the eating pathology than to be causally linked to the development of eating disorder, research designed to definitively address this issue is needed.

5.1 Clinical Implications

Regardless of whether vegetarianism is etiological in the development of eating disorders, or anorexia specifically, it may hinder recovery. Generally, maintaining a vegetarian or vegan diet while trying to recover from an eating disorder (particularly anorexia) is difficult and frequently not recommended. The reintroduction of meat to eating disordered vegetarians has been suggested for three specific reasons: (1) to decrease rule-driven eating behavior, (2) to decrease familial conflicts, and (3) to ensure adequate iron intake (O'Connor et al., 1987). The likelihood of successful meat reintroduction was found to be inversely correlated with length of vegetarianism: the shorter the time the individual had refrained from red meat, the more likely they were to successfully reincorporate red meat into their diet when they were able to choose their own meals toward end of treatment. True vegetarianism was associated with a longer amount of time of meat avoidance (7.8 years as opposed to 3.3 years in semivegetarians) (O'Connor et al., 1987). This suggests that those who reported vegetarianism before the onset of illness may be more likely to want to continue to refrain from meat when responsibility over their own intake. It also highlights the need to understand the rationale for the adoption of a vegetarian diet.

Practically, the first step of eating disorder treatment is typically to work toward increasing body weight and stabilizing eating patterns. Individuals at the start of recovery from anorexia nervosa tend to be hypermetabolic, meaning that when attempting to gain weight, they must increase their daily intake of calories beyond that of an individual without this diagnosis (Weltzin et al., 1991). Much research has been done on refeeding for weight restoration in general, but there has been relatively little research conducted on refeeding in the context of a vegetarian diet (Marzola et al., 2013). Generally, vegetarian diets are not recommended during the renourishment process for a number of reasons. Vegetarianism can be associated with lower calorie foods, and many meat substitutes (such as tofu) are relatively lower in calories, compared to animal-derived proteins. Thus, individuals in a hypermetabolic state will have to eat a much larger volume of vegetarian food to ingest the 3500–4500 daily calories typically needed for successful weight restoration.

It is also easier to ensure adequate intake of several micronutrients, including iron, calcium, and fatty acids, when a diet includes meat (Marzola et al., 2013). For example, anorexia patients tend to consistently avoid fatty foods. As such, when entering treatment, they have often inadequate intake of some fatty acids (Holman et al., 1995). Eicosapentaenoic acid (EPA) and docosahexaenoic acid (DHA) are two omega-3 fatty acids that are important for proper bodily functioning (Marzola et al., 2013). EPA is the precursor to eicosanoids, which are vital in a number of different bodily functions. DHA is one of the building blocks for brain gray matter. Both EPA and DHA are most commonly found in the highest concentrations in eggs, meat, and especially fish (Marzola et al., 2013), the very foods that are typically rejected by vegetarian and vegan patients, so it is of particular importance to ensure a diet used in refeeding meets the dietary needs of patients. While vegetarians do tend to reject the foods with the highest concentration of fatty acids, it has been suggested that supplementing EPA in pill form can have a beneficial effect on mood and general functioning while in weight restoration treatment (Ayton et al., 2004).

In addition to, and perhaps more importantly than, concerns about nutritional deficits, the rigidity of the vegetarian diet may interfere with successful eating disorder recovery. Typically, individuals with eating disorders, particularly anorexia, have inflexible dietary rules. When an individual with an eating disorder adopts a vegetarian diet, feared or "unhealthy" foods can often be avoided, and a rigid meal plan can be followed under the guise of being "vegetarian." Not only can this facilitate reduced macronutrient and caloric intake, but the diet itself may become negatively reinforced. Adhering to a vegetarian diet can aid in anxiety reduction by allowing for the avoidance of feared foods; and the reintroduction of meat into the diet as part of treatment, in turn, may cause elevated anxiety and fear, a significant contributor to nonremission (Yackobovitch-Gavan et al., 2009). Ultimately this means that anorexia patients may have a more difficult time with remission if they continue to adhere to a vegetarian diet. This is of particular importance due to the finding that anorexia patients are more likely to return to restrictive eating behaviors, including vegetarianism, as well as dieting after treatment (Hasson et al., 2011).

5.2 Areas of Future Study

5.2.1 Cultural Variation

Most of the studies discussed here were conducted in the United States. One study based in Turkey, though, found that 58% of vegetarians chose diet due to taste preferences, 19% chose the diet to be healthier, and 10% adhered for weight control (Bas et al., 2005). This is a noticeable difference from American-based populations, who cite personal ethics or morals as their primary motivation for abstention a majority of the time (Timko et al., 2012a). A rare cross-cultural study of eating behaviors in vegetarian Hindus in India found evidence for elevated scores on the EAT-26 oral control subscale compared to Omani and European participants but no significant correlation between BMI and body dissatisfaction or abnormal eating behaviors that is normally observed specifically in female respondents (Kayano et al., 2008). Due to this difference between populations, a better understanding of motives for vegetarianism and its association with eating behaviors across cultures is necessary.

5.2.2 Gender

As is typical in eating disorder research, much of the existing research on eating disorders and vegetarianism has been done in female participants. Those studies that included male participants found that nearly all vegetarian men were underweight, whereas not all of their female vegetarian counterparts were similarly underweight (Bas et al., 2005). Additionally, male vegetarians appear to be at a much higher risk for extreme weight loss behaviors, such as using supplements, laxatives, or vomiting (Perry et al., 2001). Vegetarianism thus appears to be a marker of potential eating-related pathology specifically in men (Perry et al., 2001), though further research in this population is needed.

6. Final Summary

Vegetarianism appears to be disproportionately associated with disordered eating or eating pathology. However, the relationship is complex and requires further study before definitive conclusions can be made. Across studies comparing subgroups of vegetarians, consistent trends have emerged that indicate a definitive need for distinguishing between different types of meat avoiders. Even among nonclinical samples, subgroups of vegetarians look markedly different in measures of pathological eating behaviors. When compared to true vegetarians, vegans, and omnivores, it appears the semivegetarians are the "most pathological." Not only are they more likely to restrict their diet, but they also more susceptible to overeating. Semivegetarians are also more likely to restrict their food intake due to dietary concerns (Timko et al., 2012a), whereas ovolactovegetarians and vegans adhere to a vegetarian diet primarily due ethical and animal welfare concerns (Forestell et al., 2012; Curtis and Comer, 2006). Adolescent vegetarians are more likely to frequently weigh themselves, experience body dissatisfaction, practice both healthy and unhealthy weight control measures, and to have been diagnosed with an eating disorder (Perry et al., 2001).

In contrast, vegans and vegetarians typically endorse significantly lower levels of restraint and external eating, and greater levels of food acceptance, in comparison to semivegetarians. These findings suggest that semivegetarians are categorically different from ovolactovegetarians and vegans, and this distinction should be considered when assessing diet type and pathological eating (Robinson-O'Brien et al., 2009).

In clinical samples, not only is the type of vegetarianism important to assess but also the reason and timing of vegetarian diet. The latter is particularly important in determining whether vegetarianism played a causal role in the development of the eating disorder. While the question of causality has certainly been at the forefront of researchers' minds, we interpret the existing evidence to indicate less of a causal role of vegetarianism in the development of eating disorders. Rather, we hypothesize that vegetarianism may occur early in the disorder as a way to restrict intake in a socially acceptable fashion, and it may maintain the illness by facilitating a restrictive or rigid diet. This hypothesis requires further study.

References

APA, 2013. Diagnostic and Statistical Manual of Mental Disorders (DSM-5). American Psychiatric Association, Washington, DC.

Ayton, A.K., Azaz, A., Horrobin, D.F., 2004. A pilot open case series of ethyl-EPA supplementation in the treatment of anorexia nervosa. Prostagl. Leukot. Essent. Fat. Acids 71, 205–209.

Baines, S., Powers, J., Brown, W.J., 2007. How does the health and well-being of young Australian vegetarians and semi-vegetarian women compare with nonvegetarians. Public Health Nutr. 10, 436–442.

Bardone-Cone, A.M., Fitzsimmons-Craft, E.E., Harney, M.B., Maldonado, C.R., Lawson, M.A., Smith, R., Robinson, D.P., 2012. The inter-relationships between vegetarianism and eating disorders among females. J. Acad. Nutr. Diet. 112, 1247–1252.

Barr, S.I., Janelle, K.C., Prior, J.C., 1994. Vegetarian versus nonvegetarian diets, dietary restraint, and subclinical ovulatory disturbances: prospective 6-month study. Am. J. Clin. Nutr. 60, 887–894.

Bas, M., Karabudak, E., Kiziltan, G., 2005. Vegetarianism and eating disorders: associations between eating attitudes and other psychological factors among Turkish adolescents. Appetite 44, 309–315.

Campbell, T.C., Parpia, B., Chen, J., 1998. Diet, lifestyle, and the etiology of coronary artery disease: the Cornell China study. Am. J. Cardiol. 82, 18T–21T.

Cardi, V., Leppanen, J., Treasure, J., 2015. The effects of negative and positive mood induction on eating behaviour: a meta-analysis of laboratory studies in the healthy population and eating and weight disorders. Neurosci. Biobehav. Rev. 57, 299–309.

Curtis, M.J., Comer, L.K., 2006. Vegetarianism, dietary restraint, and feminist identity. Eat. Behav. 7, 91–104.

Estima, C.C.P., Philippie, S.T., Leal, G.V.S., Pimentel, C.V.M.B., Alvarenga, M.S., 2012. Vegetarianism and eating disorder risk behavior in adolescents from Sao Paulo, Brazil. Rev. Esp. Nutr. Hum. Diet. 16, 94–99.

Fairburn, C.G., Beglin, S.J., 1994. Assessment of eating disorders: interview or self-report questionnaire? Int. J. Eat. Disord. 16, 363–370.

Fairburn, C.G., Cooper, Z., O'connor, M., 1999. Eating disorder examination. Int. J. Eat. Disord. 6, 1–8.

Fisak, B., Peterson, R.D., Tantleff-Dunn, S., Molnar, J.M., 2006. Challenging previous conceptions of vegetarianism and eating disorders. Eat. Weight Disord. 11, 195–200.

Forestell, C.A., Spaeth, A.M., Kane, S.A., 2012. To eat or not to eat red meat. A closer look at the relationship between restrained eating and vegetarianism in college females. Appetite 58.

Garner, D.M., Garfinkel, P.E., 1979. The eating attitudes test: an index of the symptoms of anorexia nervosa. Psychol. Med. 9, 273–279.

Garner, D.M., Olmsted, M.P., Bohr, Y., Garfinkel, P.E., 1982. The eating attitudes test: psychometric features and clinical correlates. Psychol. Med. 12, 871–878.

Gilbody, S.M., Kirk, S.F.L., Hill, A.J., 1998. Vegetarianism in young women: another means of weight control? Int. J. Eat. Disord. 26, 87–90.

Hadigan, C.M., Anderson, E.J., Miller, K.K., Hubbard, J.L., Herzog, D.B., Klibanski, A., Grinspoon, S.K., 2000. Assessment of macronutrient and micronutrient intake in women with anorexia nervosa. Int. J. Eat. Disord. 26 (3), 284–292.

Hart, J., 2009. The health benefits of a vegetarian diet. Altern. Complement. Ther. 15, 64–68.

Hasson, L.M., Bjorck, C., Bigegard, A., Clinton, D., 2011. How do eating disorder patients eat after treatment? Dietary habits and eating behaviour three years after entering treatment. Eat. Weight Disord. 16.

Holman, R.T., Adams, C.E., Nelson, R.A., Grater, S.J.E., Jaskiewicz, J.A., Johnson, S.B., Erdman, J.W., 1995. Patients with anorexia nervosa demonstrate deficiencies of selected essential fatty acids, compensatory changes in nonessential fatty acids and decreased fluidity of plasma lipids. J. Nutr. 125, 901–907.

Janelle, K.C., Barr, S.I., 1995. Nutrient intakes and eating behaviors scores of vegetarian and nonvegetarian women. J. Am. Diet. Assoc. 95, 180–189.

Kadambari, R., Gowers, S., Crisp, A., 1986. Some correlates of vegetarianism and anorexia nervosa. Int. J. Eat. Disord. 5, 539–544.

Kayano, M., Yoshiuchi, K., Al-Adawi, S., Viernes, N., Dorlov, A.S.S., Kumano, H., Kuboki, T., 2008. Eating attitudes and body dissatisfaction in adolescents: cross-cultural study. Psychiatry Clin. Neurosci. 62, 17–25.

Kahleova, H., Hrachovinova, T., Hill, M., Pelikanova, T., 2013. Vegetarian diet in type 2 diabetes–improvement in quality of life, mood and eating behaviour. Diabet. Med. 30 (1), 127–129.

Klopp, S.A., Heiss, C.J., Smith, H.S., 2003. Self-reported vegetarianism may be a marker for college women at risk for disordered eating. J. Am. Diet. Assoc. 103, 745–747.

Laessle, R.G., Tuschl, R.J., Kotthaus, B.C., Prike, K.M., 1989. A comparison of the validity of three scales for the assessment of dietary restraint. J. Abnorm. Psychol. 98, 504.

Lindeman, M., Stark, K., Latvala, K., 2000. Vegetarianism and eating-disordered thinking. Eat. Disord. 8 (2), 157–165.

Lowe, M.R., 1993. The effects of dieting on eating behavior: a three-factor model. Psychol. Bull. 114, 100.

Lowe, M.R., Thomas, J.G., 2009. Measures of restrained eating: conceptual evolution and psychometric update. In: Handbook of Assessment Methods for Obesity and Eating Behaviors, pp. 137–185.

Lowe, M.R., Timko, C.A., 2004. What a difference a diet makes: towards an understanding of differences between restrained dieters and restrained nondieters. Eat. Behav. 5, 199–208.

Martins, Y., Pliner, P., O'connor, R., 1999. Restrained eating among vegetarians: does a vegetarian eating style mask concerns about weight? Appetite 32, 145–154.

Marzola, E., Nasser, J.A., Hashim, S.A., Shish, P.B., Kaye, W.H., 2013. Nutritional rehabilitation in anorexia nervosa: review of literature and implications for treatment. BMC Psychiatry 13.

Mclean, J.A., Barr, S.I., 2003. Cognitive dietary restraint is associated with eating behaviors, lifestyle practices, personality characteristics and menstrual irregularity in college women. Appetite 40, 185–192.

Michalak, J., Zhang, X.C., Jacobi, F., 2012. Vegetarian diet and mental disorders: results from a representative community survey. Int. J. Behav. Nutr. Phys. Act. 9.

Mintz, L.B., 2000. The eating attitudes test: validation with DSM-IV eating disorder criteria. J. Personal. Assess. 74, 489–503.

Mogul, S.L., 1980. Asceticism in adolescence and anorexia nervosa. Psychoanal. Study Child 35, 155–175.

Moore, W.J., Mcgrievy, M.E., Turner-Mcgrievy, G.M., 2015. Dietary adherence and acceptability of five different diets, including vegan and vegetarian diets, for weight loss: the new DIETs study. Eat. Behav. 19, 33–38.

O'connor, M.A., Touyz, S.W., Dunn, S.M., Beumont, P.J.V., 1987. Vegetarianism in anorexia nervosa? A review of 116 consecutive cases. Med. J. Aust. 147, 540–542.

Perry, C., Mcguire, M., Neumark-Sztainer, D., Story, M., 2001. Characteristics of vegetarian adolescents in a multiethnic urban population. J. Adolesc. Health 29, 406–416.

Polivy, J., Herman, C.P., 2002. Causes of eating disorders. Annu. Rev. Psychol. 53, 187–213.

Robinson-O'brien, R., Perry, C.L., Wall, M.M., Story, M., Neumark-Sztainer, D., 2009. Adolescent and young adult vegetarianism: better dietary intake and weight outcomes but increased risk of disordered eating behaviors. J. Am. Diet. Assoc. 104, 648–655.

Rozin, P., Markwith, M., Stoess, C., 1997. Moralization and becoming a vegetarian: the transformation of preferences into values and the recruitment of disgust. Psychol. Sci. 8, 67–73.

Sieke, E.H., Carlson, J.L., Lock, J., Timko, C.A., Peebles, R., February 2013. Drivers of disordered eating in University students reporting a vegetarian diet. Soc. Adolesc. Med. J. Adolesc. Health 52 (2).

Stice, E., 2002. Risk and maintenance factors for eating pathology: a meta-analytic review. Psychol. Bull. 128, 825.

Stroebe, W., 2008. Restrained Eating and the Breakdown of Self-regulation.

Stunkard, A.J., Messick, S., 1985. The three-factor eating questionnaire to measure dietary restraint, disinhibition and hunger. J. Psychosom. Res. 29, 71–83.

Timko, C.A., Anohkina, A., Serpell, L., Dakanalis, A., 2017. Restraint ≠ Restriction. (in preparation).

Timko, C.A., Hormes, J.M., Chubski, J., 2012a. Will the real vegetarian please stand up? An investigation of dietary restraint and eating disorder symptoms in vegetarians versus non-vegetarians. Appetite 58, 982–990.

Timko, C.A., Juarascio, A., Chowansky, A., 2012b. The effect of a pre-load experiment on subsequent food consumption. Caloric and macronutrient intake in the days following a pre-load manipulation. Appetite 58, 747–753.

Trautmann, J., Rau, S.I., Wilson, M.A., Walters, C., 2008. Vegetarian students in their first year of college: are they at risk for restrictive or disordered eating behaviors? Coll. Stud. J. 42, 340–347.

Van Strien, T., Frijters, J.E., Bergers, G., Defares, P.B., 1986. The Dutch eating behavior questionnaire (DEBQ) for assessment of restrained, emotional, and external eating behavior. Int. J. Eat. Disord. 5, 295–315.

Wallis, D.J., Hetherington, M.M., 2004. Stress and eating: the effects of ego-threat and cognitive demand on food intake in restrained and emotional eaters. Appetite 43, 39–46.

Weltzin, T.E., Fernstrom, M.H., Hansen, D., Mcconaha, C., Kaye, W.H., 1991. Abnormal caloric requirements for weight maintenance in patients with anorexia and bulimia nervosa. Am. J. Psychiatry 148, 1675–1682.

Windauer, U., Lennerts, W., Talbot, P., Touyz, S.W., Beumont, P.J.V., 1993. How well are 'cured' anorexia nervosa patients? An investigation of 16 weight-recovered anorexic patients. Br. J. Psychiatry 163, 195–200.

Yackobovitch-Gavan, M., Golan, M., Valevski, A., Kreitler, S., Bachar, E., Lieblich, A., Mitrani, E., Weizman, A., Stein, D., 2009. An integrative quantitative model of factors influencing the course of anorexia nervosa over time. Int. J. Eat. Disord. 42, 306–317.

Zuromski, K.L., Witte, T.K., Smith, A.R., Goodwin, N., Bodell, L.P., Bartlett, M., Siegried, N., 2015. Increased prevalence of vegetarianism among women with eating pathology. Eat. Behav. 19, 24–27.

Cognitive Processes Underlying Vegetarianism as Assessed by Brain Imaging

Massimo Filippi, Gianna C. Riccitelli, Laura Vacchi, Maria A. Rocca

SAN RAFFAELE SCIENTIFIC INSTITUTE AND VITA-SALUTE SAN RAFFAELE UNIVERSITY, MILAN, ITALY

1. Introduction

The term "neuroscience" was first introduced in 1962 by Francis O. Schmitt in his Neuroscience Research Program with the goal of bringing together different disciplines to stimulate their interaction in the study of the nervous system. Today, it is an interdisciplinary science field that is mainly centered around biology, chemistry, medicine, cognitive science, psychology, physics, and statistics to investigate the nervous system from different perspectives (e.g., developmental, structural, and functional).

Social cognitive neuroscience (SCN) investigates the neural mechanisms of social cognition and interactions. It is also concerned with deficits of sociocognitive processes in humans such as depression, schizophrenia, sociopathy, and autism. This part of cognitive neuroscience is directed toward a better understanding of the complex aspects of social behavior, such as empathy, attractiveness, self-awareness, moral reasoning, intentionality, and imitation. Traditionally, social brain science has been focused on specific cognitive domains. Most studies emphasize emotional and motivational features rather than other aspects of cognition such as language. Social cognition includes the study of mental processes necessary to the understanding and storing of information about the self and other persons, as well as interpersonal norms and procedures to navigate efficiently in the social world (Van Overwalle, 2009). Basic abilities underlying human social cognition include the perception and evaluation of social stimuli, the integration of perceptions with contextual knowledge, and the representation of possible responses to the situation. One of the hallmarks of social cognition in humans is the ability to understand conspecifics as beings like oneself, with intentional and mental lives like one's own (Decety and Chaminade, 2003). Accordingly, human beings tend to identify with conspecifics and attribute mental states to them. Such abilities rely on the activity of several brain regions located in the frontal lobes (the orbitofrontal cortex, medial prefrontal cortex, and cingulate cortex), the temporal lobes (including the amygdala), the fusiform gyrus, and the somatosensory cortices (Decety and Jackson, 2004; Hein and

Singer, 2008; Singer and Lamm, 2009). The majority of these regions seem to be critically involved in the "empathy network" as well as in the processing of emotions (Adolphs, 2002). This suggests that the merging between emotions and feelings experienced by oneself and those perceived in other individuals may be a key ingredient of social understanding, and it may play a major role in promoting empathy, prosocial behaviors, and moral norms (Decety and Jackson, 2004; Van Overwalle, 2009).

2. Quantitative Methods in Neuroscience

From the beginning of SCN studies, to collect a significant amount of data, researchers have made use of instruments such as surveys, questionnaires, and interviews. All these instruments are based on the request of pieces of information of different natures, such as demographic variables, facts, perceptions or feelings about oneself, others, or external events. Generally, surveys and questionnaires are self-administered and self-compiled, using structured and predetermined questions; conversely, interviews are administered by a trained interviewer who can ask more or less structured questions in a more dynamic environment and exchange.

In SCN, more standardized measures are tests or scales, which are usually aimed at assessing the individual's performance on a task or about a variable of investigation. They are usually composed of a series of items. Performance on these items produces a test score, which is usually normalized with respect to a reference population. This score reflects a more general construct, such as emotional functioning, personality, cognitive ability, or aptitude. Differences in test or scale scores/performance should reflect individual differences in the construct that the test or the scale is supposed to measure.

In the last decades, there has been a growing interest to understand the neural mechanisms of cognitive processes, such as thought, perception, and language, and it has been mainly driven by significant advances in the development of technology to observe the activity of the human brain. Techniques such as event-related potentials (ERPs), positron emission tomography (PET), and functional magnetic resonance imaging (fMRI) have improved our understanding of how the human brain processes sensory information and movement control, improves language abilities, and experiences emotions.

Briefly, ERPs are thought to reflect the summed activity of postsynaptic potentials produced when a large number of similarly oriented cortical pyramidal neurons (in the order of thousands or millions) fire in synchrony while processing information (Peterson et al., 1995). They are time locked to sensory, motor, or cognitive events that provide a safe and noninvasive approach to study psychophysiological correlates of mental processes. ERPs in humans can be divided into two categories: early waves, or components, peaking roughly within the first 100 ms after stimulus, are termed "sensory" or "exogenous," as they depend largely on the physical parameters of the stimulus; in contrast, ERPs generated later reflect the manner in which the subject evaluates the stimulus and are termed "cognitive" or "endogenous" ERPs, as they examine information processing. The waveforms are described according to latency and amplitude.

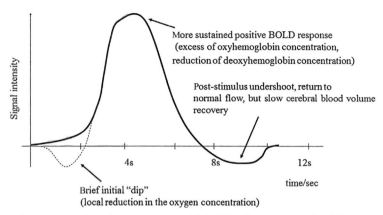

FIGURE 5.1 Schematic representation of the time course of the blood oxygenation level dependent (BOLD) response to an increase in neuronal activity. The *dotted line* indicates that the brief initial dip of the BOLD response can be variable.

The advent of radionucleotide methods, such as PET, have seen an increasing interest in the evaluation of cerebral blood flow in healthy volunteers. This technique has a good reproducibility, but it is invasive since it requires the administration of radionucleotide agents and in general has a poorer spatial and anatomical resolution compared to MRI methodologies.

fMRI is a relatively new technique that is being widely used to study the neuronal mechanisms of central nervous system (CNS) functioning since it is noninvasive, safe, and provides a high spatial resolution, despite a relatively low temporal resolution (particularly when compared to neurophysiologic techniques). The signal changes seen during fMRI studies are determined by the blood oxygenation level dependent (BOLD) mechanism (Ogawa et al., 1993). The activation of a cerebral tissue determines an increase in local synaptic activity, which results in a rise of blood flow and oxygen consumption; because the increase of blood flow is greater than that of oxygen consumption, an increase of the ratio between oxygenated and deoxygenated hemoglobin is produced, which enhances the MRI signal (Ogawa et al., 1993, 1998) (Fig. 5.1). As these signal changes are very modest (usually ranging from 0.5% to 1.5%), it is necessary to obtain a large amount of brain images acquired during alternated periods of activations (motor, sensorial, and cognitive) and rest (Vanzetta and Grinvald, 1999). By analyzing these data with appropriate statistical methods, it is possible to obtain information about the location and extent of specific areas involved in the performance of a given task in healthy subjects and in patients suffering from a given condition (Bandettini et al., 1993; Worsley and Friston, 1995). Currently, fMRI methods of analysis allow making inferences at group levels, whereas improvements are still needed to achieve a more robust comparison of interindividual profiles. Many caveats need to be considered when planning or analyzing fMRI experiments, including standardization and repeatability of the experiments, ability of the subjects to understand and perform the tasks, and interindividual variability in task performance. Other confounders include hemispheric dominance, age, and gender.

3. Vegetarianism and Social Cognitive Neuroscience

Alternative diets characterized, to a greater or lesser degree, by the avoidance of animal products have recently gained increasing popularity in the general population (about 2% of the UK population in 2012). Within vegetarianism, the extent to which the individual may avoid animal products may vary, from the avoidance of red meat only to that of meat, fish, and eggs (lactovegetarian), or to that of all products derived from animals (vegan), as fully described in Chapter 1 of this book.

During the past decade, there has been growing interest from SCN to observe brain profiles and behavioral characteristics of vegetarians. Cooper et al. (1985) performed the first study in the field and described the psychological characteristics of vegetarians. The study group consisted of 20 well-educated, young adults of normal weight who had been vegetarians for an average of 9 years. All of them filled out a questionnaire pertaining to demographic characteristics, the rationale for their dietary habits, attitudes about health beliefs, and the utilization of various nontraditional health providers. Moreover, participants completed a battery of psychometric inventories to assess both psychological and cognitive variables. Despite that vegetarians scored higher than the normal population, but lower than a psychiatric population, at Hopkins Symptom Checklist (HSCL-90) (a test that aims to assess psychological distress), globally, the psychometric findings of the study showed no significant differences between vegetarians and normal controls, suggesting that vegetarian dietary style does not coexist with psychological or cognitive alterations.

3.1 Vegetarianism and Motivation

The term "motivation" refers to the reasons for people's actions, desires, and needs (Elliot and Covington, 2001) or the reason that prompts a person to act in a certain way or to develop an inclination for specific behaviors (Pardee, 1990). Behavior can be driven by internal or external motivations. Internal motivations include self-desires to seek out new things and new challenges, to analyze one's capacity, to observe, and to gain knowledge (Ryan and Deci, 2000a,b). External motivation comes from influences outside the individual. Common external motivations are competition or rewards for showing the desired behavior and the threat of punishment following misbehavior.

Another important distinction is that between push and pull motivations (Uysal and Jurowski, 1994). The first occurs when people push themselves toward their goals or to achieve something (e.g., escape, adventure, social interaction, prestige, and health); in pull motivations, it seems that it is the goal that is pulling us toward it. This latter motivation can be influenced by novelty, attractiveness of the destination, benefit expectation, and marketing image (with an essential role of media and social networks) but also by moralization.

Maslow's theory (Maslow, 1943) is one of the most widely discussed theories of motivation: individuals possess a constantly growing inner drive, organized in a hierarchy system from basic (lowest-earliest) to most complex (highest-latest) motives (Pardee, 1990): physiological (hunger, thirst), safety (personal, financial), love/belonging (family, friendship), esteem (self-esteem, confidence, respect of others), self-actualization (ethics, morality), and self-transcendence (altruism, spirituality). According to Maslow, people are motivated by unsatisfied needs that influence their behavior. Only after the lower level needs are at least minimally satisfied can people advance to the next level of needs, arranged in order of importance to human life. Interestingly, one of the highest level of motivation is driven by ethical and moral needs.

There are many possible reasons why people choose to follow meat avoidance, with different vegetarian diets (including vegan diets) over and above the traditional meat-centered diet. Cooper et al. (1985) investigated the reason for dietary preferences in 20 vegetarians and found that 65% mentioned health, 60% noted the desire to avoid cruelty to animals, and 50% disliked the eating of animal flesh; 40% spoke of fear of a world food shortage as a reason for their vegetarianism, while only 15% said that meat tasted bad to them. Ten percent had adopted a vegetarian diet owing to the influence of their spouses. None had adopted vegetarianism for religious reasons. Personal health and animal cruelty are the most reported motivations by vegetarians (Lea and Worsley, 2001; Hoek et al., 2004), although disgust or repugnance with eating flesh (Santos and Booth, 1996; Rozin et al., 1997; Kenyon and Barker, 1998) and food beliefs influences from peers or family (Lea and Worsley, 2001) do also occur. While health vegetarians choose to avoid meat to derive certain health benefits or lose weight (Kim et al., 1999; Wilson et al., 2004; Key et al., 2006), ethical vegetarians consider meat avoidance as a moral imperative (Whorton, 1994; Fessler et al., 2003). Health vegetarians tended to make gradual "trial adoptions" of food choices, while "ethical vegetarians" made more sudden changes in their diet to support beliefs, such as animal welfare/rights, and create consistency in their lives (Hamilton, 1993). Health concerns are also the major reason motivating individuals who are "partial vegetarians," who choose not to eat red meat, limit their consumption of flesh to fish, or select only organic products (Hoek et al., 2004; Bedford and Barr, 2005).

Vegetarianism has been linked to concerns with the environmental and ecological impact of meat (Lindeman and Sirelius, 2001; Gaard, 2002; Hoek et al., 2004). Kalof et al. (1999) found that the belief that a vegetarian diet is less harmful to the environment was the only factor significantly differentiating vegetarians and nonvegetarians. Fox (1999) suggests that a vegetarian economy contributes to "ecosystem health" by reducing the impact of pollution on environment and economies, affecting both developed and less developed countries. Beyond health and ethical reasons, the incorporation into practice and beliefs of a broader number of environmental commitments was another essential element of the vegetarian trajectory (Jabs et al., 1998). These commitments ranged from the use of organic food to a variety of behaviors that contribute to an "environmentally friendly" lifestyle. While initial motivation to adopt a vegetarian diet may be divergent (Fox and Ward, 2008a,b), there may also be convergence among those who have adopted a vegetarian diet. Fox and Ward (2008a,b) explored this convergence and specifically examined vegetarians' own perspectives to investigate the interactions between beliefs over health, animal cruelty, and the environment and how these may contribute to food choice trajectory. The authors identified two distinct initial motivations for vegetarianism: personal health and animal welfare/rights. Health was a significant motivator, both in terms of reducing symptoms of illness or discomfort, and as a preventive measure to avoid a range of minor and major illnesses; while ethical reasons concerning animal welfare/rights were based both upon affective and philosophical reasons. No respondent cited environmental concerns as a primary motivation for vegetarianism, suggesting that convictions on the environmental benefits of vegetarianism may be subsequent to, or a consequence of, a decision to avoid meat, rather than the cause of this dietary choice (Fox and Ward, 2008a,b). Taken together, these studies provide evidence that the motivations for vegetarianism are complex, following trajectories that developed in new lifestyles or outlooks. Convergence between different motivations for vegetarianism may be more common than indicated in previous investigations, and this suggests that not only do values and beliefs affect behavior (Jabs et al., 1998; Kenyon and Barker, 1998; Lindeman and Sirelius, 2001) but that behavior may subsequently influence attitudes and beliefs, in turn leading to further behavioral changes. This aspect is described in full by Prof. Rothberger in Chapter 2 of this book.

3.2 Vegetarianism and Empathy

Empathy refers to the ability to experience and understand the feelings of others. In other words, it designates an attitude toward others characterized by a commitment to understand the other, excluding any personal emotional attitude (sympathy, antipathy) and any moral judgment. Empathy is the process by which one infers the affective state of another person and experiences a similar state, being aware that the origin of that experience is the other and not oneself (Singer et al., 2009).

Two main forms of empathy can be distinguished:

- affective empathy (or emotional empathy) (Shamay-Tsoory et al., 2009): the capacity to respond with an appropriate emotion to another's mental states (Rogers et al., 2007). Being affected by another's emotional or arousal state (emotional contagion) (de Waal, 2008) exerts an effect on the ability to empathize emotionally;
- cognitive empathy: the capacity to understand another's perspective or mental state (Rogers et al., 2007; Gerace et al., 2013).

The ability to attribute internal mental states, either feeling, desires, intentions, or emotions, to others requires high-level brain functions such as language and metacognition (Stone and Gerrans, 2006). Such abilities rely on the activity of many brain regions.

Several fMRI studies have shown that observing the emotional state of another individual activates a neuronal network involved in processing the same state in oneself, whether it is pain, disgust, or touch (Decety and Jackson, 2004; Hein and Singer, 2008; Singer and Lamm, 2009). Affective empathy has been related to recruitment of the somatosensory cortices, limbic regions, anterior insula, dorsal anterior cingulate cortex (ACC), anterior midcingulate cortex (MCC), supplementary motor area, and amygdala (Jackson et al., 2005; Lamm et al., 2011). Cognitive empathy network includes the ventromedial prefrontal cortex (vmPFC), superior temporal sulcus, temporo-parietal junction, temporal poles/amygdala, and posterior cingulate cortex (PCC)/precuneus (Frith and Frith, 2006). The ability to integrate cognition and emotion requires the enrollment of prefrontal regions such as the vmPFC, orbitofrontal cortex (OBF), and ACC (Decety and Svetlova, 2012). The mirror neuron system (MNS) has a central role in social cognition, especially for emotional empathy (Shamay-Tsoory et al., 2009).

The majority of studies attempting to characterize empathy-related responses did not separate empathy toward humans from that toward animals. In some of the available studies, scenes showing animals were treated as a neutral condition. However, a study (Rae Westbury and Neumann, 2008) that compared stimuli depicting human and nonhuman animal targets, demonstrated an increased subjective empathy as the "stimuli" became closer in phylogenetic relatedness to humans (mammalian vs. bird stimuli), thus indicating that empathic response toward humans may generalize to other species.

We postulated that the neural representation of conditions of abuse and suffering might be different among subjects who made different eating choices due to ethical reasons, resulting in the engagement of different components of the brain networks associated with empathy and social cognition (Filippi et al., 2010). Specifically, we hypothesized that the neural processes underlying empathy in ovolactovegetarians and vegans may operate for representations not only about humans but also animals. Vegetarians who decided to avoid the use of animal products for ethical reasons have a moral philosophy of life based on a set of basic values and attitudes toward life, nature, and society that extends well beyond food choice. The central ethical question related to vegetarianism is whether it is right for humans to use and kill animals. We also hypothesized that, in addition to a common shared pattern of cortical processing of human and animal suffering, ovolactovegetarians and vegans might also experience a different functional brain architecture reflecting their different motivational factors and believes. We recruited 20 meat eaters, 19 ovolactovegetarians, and 21 vegans, matched for sex and age. A questionnaire was filled in by all the subjects before fMRI acquisition to investigate eating habits, reasons/motivations of the eating choices, and the time elapsed from such a choice. All ovolactovegetarians and vegans reported to have made their eating choice for ethical reasons. They had a stable eating habit for 3.8 years and were recruited among vegetarian associations. Meat eaters were recruited by advertisement and none of them had been vegetarian before the study. Eight vegans had been ovolactovegetarians before becoming vegans. All the subjects were naïve about the goal of the study. None of the subjects had any history of neurological, major medical, or psychiatric disorders (including depression), nor either alcohol or drug abuse. In addition, none of the subjects were taking any medical treatment at the time of fMRI assessment, and all of them had a normal neurological examination.

Brain activations were investigated using fMRI and an event-related design. A series of 150 pictures was presented in a random order: 40 showed negative valence scenes related to humans, 40 showed negative valence scenes related to animals, and the remaining 70 showed "neutral" natural landscapes. Pictures were pseudorandomized so that no more than two pictures of the same category were presented consecutively. Negative valence scenes were taken from the International Affective Picture System (IAPS), newspapers, books, or magazines. Human and animal pictures were comparable in terms of valence and arousal rating. Non-IAPS pictures were validated in a group of 50 healthy subjects that did not participate in the fMRI experiment. Participants also completed the empathy quotient, a self-report questionnaire (Baron-Cohen and Wheelwright, 2004) developed to measure the cognitive and affective aspects of empathy.

Ovolactovegetarians and vegans showed a common functional architecture of emotional processing characterized by an increased engagement of empathy-related areas while observing negative scenes, independently of the species involved, including the ACC and inferior frontal gyrus (IFG) (Fig. 5.2). This pattern of activations in ovolactovegetarians and vegans is likely to reflect a stronger empathic response compared to meat eaters;

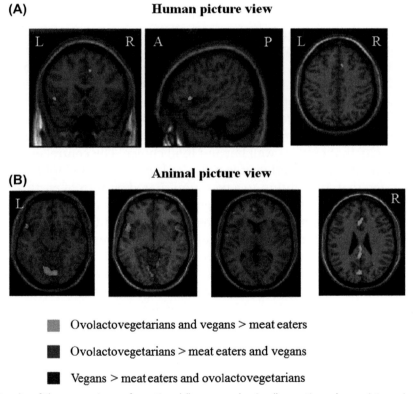

(A)   **Human picture view**

(B)   **Animal picture view**

◼ Ovolactovegetarians and vegans > meat eaters

◼ Ovolactovegetarians > meat eaters and vegans

◼ Vegans > meat eaters and ovolactovegetarians

FIGURE 5.2 Results of the comparisons of emotional (human and animal) negative valence picture views (showing mutilations, murdered people, human/animal threat, tortures, wounds, etc.) between meat eaters, ovolactovegetarians and vegans. Results are superimposed on a high-resolution T1-weighted image in the standard Montreal Neurological Institute space, at a threshold of $P < .05$ corrected for multiple comparisons. Areas activated during human picture view in ovolactovegetarians and vegans versus meat eaters are shown in yellow (white in print versions). Activations specific for ovolactovegetarians are shown in blue (dark gray in print versions). Activations specific for vegans are shown in red (light gray in print versions). (A) Human picture view and (B) animal picture view. Images are in neurological convention. *With permission from Filippi, M., Riccitelli, G., Falini, A., Di Salle, F., Vuilleumier, P., Comi, G., Rocca, M.A., 2010. The brain functional networks associated to human and animal suffering differ among omnivores, vegetarians and vegans. PLoS One 5 (5), e10847.*

indeed, ACC has been associated with alert states, self-awareness, and pain processing (Mottaghy et al., 2006). Remarkably, ovolactovegetarians and vegans also had an increased recruitment of empathy-related areas while observing negative scenes regarding animals rather than humans, with the additional activation of the middle prefrontal cortex (mPFC), PCC, and some visual areas (Fig. 5.2). Recruitment of mPFC and PCC is frequently observed in conditions involving representation of the self and self-values (D'Argembeau et al., 2010). The PCC is also thought to be involved in memory and visuospatial processing (Maddock, 1999), particularly in relation to emotions and social behavior (D'Argembeau et al., 2010), as well as when subjects have to judge the valence of emotionally salient words or episodic memories, with the strongest responses seen when unpleasant stimuli are presented (Maddock, 1999). During the animal suffering view, ovolactovegetarians and vegans also experienced a reduced activation of the right amygdala in comparison to meat eaters. The amygdala responds to various kinds of aversive stimuli, most strongly to fearful and threatening scenes (Hariri et al., 2002) and, to a lesser extent, to those associated with disgust (Phillips et al., 1997).

In addition to the previous shared pattern of functional activations, we also detected a significantly different functional architecture between ovolactovegetarians and vegans during observation of negative scenes. During human suffering viewing, activations specific to ovolactovegetarians were located along the inferior parietal lobule (IPL), which is involved in bodily representations that distinguish the self from the other (Decety and Jackson, 2004), and it was found to be more activated when pictures of mutilations were presented than when contamination or neutral pictures were shown (Schienle et al., 2006). More critically, for animal pictures, activations specific to ovolactovegetarians were found in the ACC and the lingual gyrus, whereas activations specific to vegans were found in the bilateral IFG and the left middle frontal gyrus (MFG). ACC is a region highly interconnected with limbic and prefrontal structures, and it is thought to play a key role in normal and dysfunctional emotional self-control as well as social behavior (Devinsky et al., 1995). A meta-analysis study (Phan et al., 2002) found that emotional tasks with explicit cognitive components (e.g., recognition or evaluation of emotional stimuli and biographic material) engaged specifically the ACC as compared to passive emotional conditions. The recruitment of this region in ovolactovegetarians might therefore correspond to their distinctive behavioral response to pictures of animal suffering, e.g., enhanced attention and empathic pain (Singer et al., 2004), or increased self-control and monitoring (Botvinick, 2007). On the other hand, the activation of the IFG seen in vegans during animal suffering might be related to aspects of cognitive control during emotion processing. The IFG is also considered to be part of the MNS. Increased activation of MNS areas has been shown during social interaction, as well as during observation and imitation of emotional faces (Iacoboni, 2009) (Fig. 5.3).

This study was the first to assess the neural correlates of empathy toward nonconspecifics in people with different social norms, as reflected by their eating habits. Our results converge with theories that consider empathy as accommodating a shared representation of emotions and sensations between individuals, allowing to understand

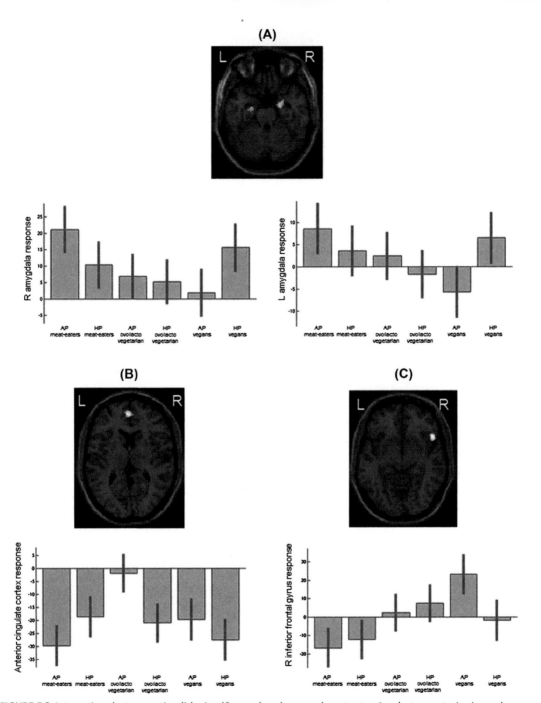

FIGURE 5.3 Interactions between stimuli (animal/human) and groups (meat eaters/ovolactovegetarian/vegan). An interaction was found in the right amygdala (A) indicating greater increase to animal negative valence picture view in meat eaters and to human negative valence picture view in vegans. An interaction between "human pictures" and "vegan group" was also found in the left amygdala (A). An interaction was found in anterior cingulate cortex (ACC) (B) between the "meat-eater group" and "human pictures," as well as between "ovolactovegetarian group" and "animal pictures," and in the right inferior frontal gyrus (IFG) between "animal pictures" and "vegan group" (C). Foci of activations are shown on a high-resolution T1-weighted image in the standard Montreal Neurological Institute space. Plots indicate activation changes detected in the three groups during the two experimental conditions in each of these regions. Images are in neurological convention. *With permission from Filippi, M., Riccitelli, G., Falini, A., Di Salle, F., Vuilleumier, P., Comi, G., Rocca, M.A., 2010. The brain functional networks associated to human and animal suffering differ among omnivores, vegetarians and vegans. PLoS One 5 (5), e10847.*

others (Decety and Jackson, 2004). They also support the hypothesis that the neuronal bases of empathy involve several distinct components including mirroring mechanisms (Iacoboni, 2009), as well as emotion contagion and representations of connectedness with the self (Singer, 2006). Brain areas similar to those showing different emotional responses between groups in our study (such as the IFG and the mPFC) have also been found to be modulated by religiosity (Kapogiannis et al., 2009), further supporting a key role of affect and empathy in moral reasoning and social values.

Inference on other people's emotional states and intentions is facilitated by processing and understanding actions performed with the mouth by other individuals. Functional imaging studies have identified a set of brain areas, located mainly in the parietal and frontal lobes, that are involved in processing of observation of mouth actions performed not only by humans but also by other species (i.e., monkeys and dogs) (Buccino et al., 2004). While actions belonging to the observer's repertoire (e.g., speech reading) are mapped in areas of the motor system located in the IFG, actions that are not part of such a repertoire (e.g., barking) are processed on the basis of their visual properties and mapped to visual areas (Buccino et al., 2004). As previously discussed, the neuronal network that involves the IFG and IPL, which form part of the MNS, is also at work for emotion recognition and contagion, which contribute to emotional empathy (Shamay-Tsoory et al., 2009; Shamay-Tsoory, 2011). Several factors modulate empathic response, including the subjective attitude toward the observed individual (Singer, 2006) and personal experience (Cheng et al., 2007).

Based on such a background, we hypothesized that brain representation of mouth actions performed by other humans and other species might differ among individuals with different dietary habits and ethical beliefs (Filippi et al., 2013). We assumed that, due to their propensity to identify nonconspecifics as being like themselves and their increased empathic response toward animal actions, when compared to meat eaters, ovolactovegetarians and vegans would exhibit a different pattern of recruitment of regions involved in the processing of mouth actions, including those located in the fronto-parietal lobes. We also supposed that, since different motivational factors and beliefs characterize ovolactovegetarianism and veganism, in addition to a common shared pattern of cortical processing of mouth actions, ovolactovegetarians and vegans might also experience a different functional architecture. Finally, we postulated that the recruitment of the previous regions might differ according to the species involved and their phylogenetic proximity to humans. Using a block design fMRI, 20 meat eaters, 19 ovolactovegetarians, and 21 vegans were scanned while watching a series of silent videos that presented a single mouth action performed by a human, a monkey, and a pig in each block. The inclusion/exclusion criteria and subjects' characteristics were identical to those of the previous experiment (Filippi et al., 2010). The mouth actions observed were (1) biting and (2) oral communicative actions (OCAs). Monkey scenes were recorded in a free environment. Participants were instructed to look at the scenes and focus their attention on mouth movements, without providing any specific response during the fMRI acquisition. Each block consisted of 12 s of video, followed by a 12 s resting period. During each block, the same action (i.e., biting or OCA) was presented four times. During the resting phase of a given block, the subjects had to observe a static frame of the same action for 12 s. Each of the six blocks of the experiment was performed four times within a run. The order of videos in the various blocks was counter-balanced across subjects. To assess whether processing of mouth actions performed by distinct species differs between ovolactovegetarians and vegans versus meat eaters, since speech processing is a key aspect of social interactions, we compared observation of OCAs and biting by the human, monkey, and pig within and between the three study groups (Fig. 5.4). In contrast to OCAs, biting was associated with an increased activation of several regions in the temporo-occipital lobes, the parietal lobes, and the cerebellum. Conversely, in contrast to biting, OCAs resulted in increased activity of several regions along the middle and superior temporal cortices and the IFG, with a different expression in the three study groups. The STS is involved in several functions, including theory of mind, audio–visual integration, motion perception, speech processing, and perception of faces (Hein and Knight, 2008). A review of foci of activations in this region reported in several previous fMRI studies has led to the identification of an anterior portion, mainly involved in speech processing, and a posterior one, mainly recruited by cognitive demands (Hein and Knight, 2008). The left pars opercularis of the IFG contains a representation of mouth actions performed by humans (Buccino et al., 2001). Recruitment of this region, together with regions located in the parietal and temporal lobes, contributes to the understanding of actions performed by others by transcoding the observed action into a corresponding motor plan (Rizzolatti et al., 2001). During "human scenes," the comparison of OCA versus biting showed an increased activity of the right amygdala in ovolactovegetarians and vegans versus meat eaters. The amygdala contributes to the analysis of body movements for perception of actions through its connections with the STS and the frontal cortex (Allison et al., 2000), thus adding emotional salience to sensory inputs.

To verify the existence of brain functional architectural differences between ovolactovegetarians and vegans, regions of activations specific to each group were further investigated. Compared with the other two groups, ovolactovegetarians showed a selective increased recruitment of the right MFG and right posterior insula, whereas vegans recruited selectively the left MFG, IFG (pars opercularis), and MTG (posterior portion). The MFG contributes to social cognitive processes (such as making inferences of others and social perception) (Murty et al., 2010). Recent meta-analysis studies have shown that the insula can be parcellated in an anterior and a posterior portion (Cauda et al., 2012; Chang et al., 2013): the first being mostly activated by cognition and the latter by interoception, perception, and emotion (Cauda et al., 2012). The insula also modulates connections between the MNS and the limbic system in social mirroring and in the ability to empathize with others (Iacoboni, 2009). The left IFG and posterior portion of the MTG are part of the MNS. Collectively, these results indicate that different portions of the empathy-related networks contribute to the modulation of social interactions with other individuals in ovolactovegetarians and vegans compared to meat eaters.

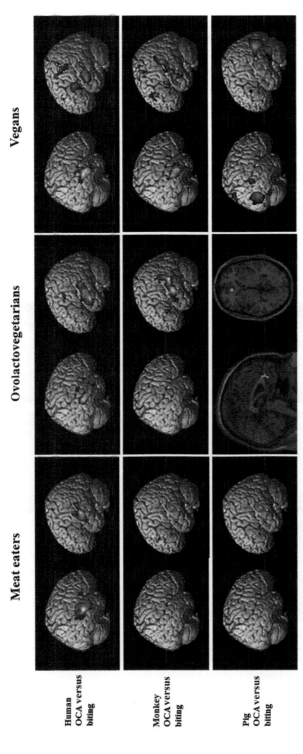

FIGURE 5.4 Cortical activations on a rendered brain from meat-eater, ovolactovegetarian, and vegan subjects during the comparison of oral communicative actions (OCAs) versus biting by a human, a monkey, and a pig (within-group analysis, two-sample t tests, *P* < .05 corrected for multiple comparisons). Images are in neurological convention. *With permission from Filippi, M., Riccitelli, G., Meani, A., Falini, A., Comi, G., Rocca, M.A., 2013. The "vegetarian brain": chatting with monkeys and pigs? Brain Struct. Funct. 218 (5), 1211–1227.*

The analysis of "animal scenes" provided some additional interesting results (Fig. 5.5). During "monkey scenes," compared to meat eaters, ovolactovegetarians and vegans experienced an increased activity of the bilateral cuneus and left MTG, in a region that roughly corresponds to the location of the Wernicke's area. Ovolactovegetarians selectively activated the left MTG and IFG, and vegans the right MTG and middle occipital gyrus. All these areas are recruited consistently in healthy individuals during lipreading (Paulesu et al., 2003). The increased recruitment of Wernicke's area and cuneus in ovolactovegetarians and vegans might be secondary to their attempt to decode monkey mouth gesture. Ovolactovegetarians had a preferential recruitment of the left IFG, which suggests an additional process of matching mouth action of the monkey with that of the viewer, whereas vegans engaged associative temporo-occipital areas in the right hemisphere, suggesting a role of higher cognitive processes involved in sentence comprehension (Just et al., 1996).

During the comparison of OCA versus biting in "pig scenes," ovolactovegetarians showed a selective increased activity of the anterior cingulum, which likely reflects a

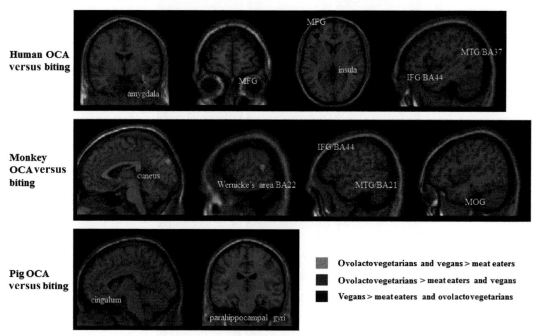

FIGURE 5.5 Results of the between-group comparisons of oral communicative actions (OCAs) versus biting during "human/monkey/pig scenes" superimposed on a T1-weighted image in the Montreal Neurological Institute space. Yellow (white in print versions) indicates areas activated in ovolactovegetarians and vegans versus meat eaters. Blue (dark gray in print versions) indicates activations specific to ovolactovegetarians. Red (light gray in print versions) indicates activations specific to vegans. Images are presented in neurological convention. *BA*, Brodmann area; *IFG*, inferior frontal gyrus; *MFG*, middle frontal gyrus; *MOG*, middle occipital gyrus; *MTG*, middle temporal gyrus. *With permission from Filippi, M., Riccitelli, G., Meani, A., Falini, A., Comi, G., Rocca, M.A., 2013. The "vegetarian brain": chatting with monkeys and pigs? Brain Struct. Funct. 218 (5), 1211–1227.*

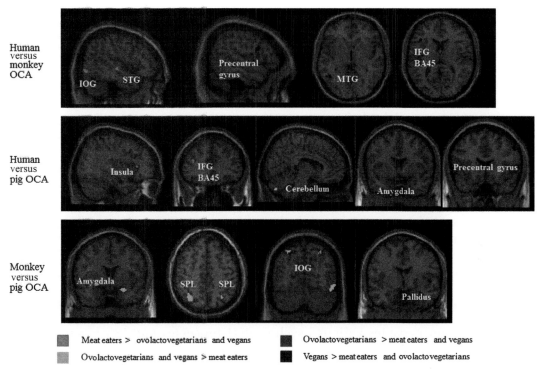

FIGURE 5.6 Results of the between-species comparisons of oral communicative actions (OCAs) among meat eaters, ovolactovegetarians, and vegans, superimposed on a T1-weighted image in the Montreal Neurological Institute space (between-group analysis, ANOVA, p<0.05 corrected for multiple comparisons). Green (lighter gray in print versions) indicates areas activated in meat eaters versus ovolactovegetarians and vegans. Yellow (lightest gray in print versions) indicates areas activated in ovolactovegetarians and vegans versus meat eaters. Blue (dark gray in print versions) indicates activations specific to ovolactovegetarians. Red (light gray in print versions) indicates activations specific to vegans. Images are in neurological convention. *BA*, Brodmann area; *IFG*, inferior frontal gyrus; *IOG*, inferior occipital gyrus; *MTG*, middle temporal gyrus; *SPL*, superior parietal lobule; *STG*, superior temporal gyrus. *With permission from Filippi, M., Riccitelli, G., Meani, A., Falini, A., Comi, G., Rocca, M.A., 2013. The "vegetarian brain": chatting with monkeys and pigs? Brain Struct. Funct. 218 (5), 1211–1227.*

strong empathic response (Devinsky et al., 1995; Phan et al., 2002) or simply an enhanced attention (Singer et al., 2004), whereas vegans activated the bilateral parahippocampal gyrus, which has a role in auditory-verbal memory functions (Grasby et al., 1993) and, through its connections with the amygdala, contributes to emotion-driven learning (Murty et al., 2010).

To address the hypothesis that processing of mouth actions differs according to the species involved and their phylogenetic proximity to humans, we limited the analysis to OCAs, since they represent the basis of intra- and intergroup relationships in humans (Fig. 5.6). During human versus monkey OCA, compared to ovolactovegetarians and vegans, meat eaters had an increased activity of part of the visual areas of the observation–execution matching system. Vegans experienced a selective increased activity of the left MTG and the frontal portion of the system, further supporting the notion of an increased recruitment of regions of the MNS in these subjects. Consistent with its role in interpersonal interactions, the anterior portion of the insula was more active, in combination with the left IFG, in meat eaters compared to ovolactovegetarians and vegans during human versus pig OCA. Additional between-group differences in processing human versus pig actions were found in areas involved in empathy processing, including the amygdala and the anterior lobe of the cerebellum. This latter region plays a crucial role in motor learning and language processing as demonstrated by a recent meta-analysis (Jirak et al., 2010). Overall, these findings support the notion that despite ovolactovegetarians and vegans showing a characteristic pattern of recruitment of regions that are part of the MNS during processing mouth actions executed by other animals, the activity of this system is higher when they are dealing with actions performed by their conspecifics, probably as a consequence of the matching of the observed human action with their motor repertoire, as part of a common representational format. Additionally, species proximity with humans can modulate MNS recruitment in these subjects, as suggested by the between-group differences observed for monkey but not pig OCAs.

3.3 Vegetarianism, Affect System, and Cognition

The affect system pervades various psychological processes and has a primary role also in the food domain. According to nutritional needs of the organism, food stimuli could be associated to different affective responding (e.g., sweet for preference, taste for aversion; Rozin and Vollmecke, 1986). In humans, ideational reasoning provides further means determining affective responding, potentially overriding the pleasure based on the flavor of selected food items (Rozin et al., 1997; Martins and Pliner, 2005). Thus, vegetarianism is a good model to explore the effects of a hedonic shift from liking to dislike toward specific food items based on ideational reasoning. One study focused on the affective guidance of selective attention processes. Through EEG registration, the late positive potential (LPP), occurring between 300 and 700 ms after stimulus onset, has shown an enlarged amplitude when viewing pleasant or unpleasant stimuli rather than neutral pictures (Cuthbert et al., 2000; Schupp et al., 2006). Consequently, the authors expected a greater LLP response when meat stimuli were presented to vegetarians. Participants performed also an explicit attention task in which target stimuli were defined by an additional food category (desserts) to verify the hypothesis that enlarged LPP amplitudes to significant stimuli reflects an implicit process. They recruited 24 participants without eating disorders who were asked to first passively view the pictures (passive viewing), then to see the same picture set and silently count the dessert pictures (explicit task), and finally to rate each of the depicted food on a 3-point hedonic rating scale with "do like it a lot" [1], "neither/nor" [0], or "do not like it at all" [−1]. The passive viewing and the explicit task were performed during an EEG recording. The LPP measurement showed a heightened state of selective attention when viewing affective pictures (Nieuwenhuis et al., 2005; Schupp et al., 2006). Meat pictures elicited enlarged

LPP amplitudes in vegetarians compared to meat eaters. Brain potentials to comparable pictures of vegetable dishes did not differ significantly between vegetarians and meat eaters; thus the increased LPP amplitude was thought to be meat related. These findings support the notion that the attention capture of food is not only related to biological processes of food consumption but also shaped by the affective salience associated with ideational reasoning and symbolic meaning (Rozin, 1996).

4. Conclusions

Several studies have investigated the relationship between vegetarianism and motivation, empathy, and cognitive features. Combined with the use of fMRI techniques, such an effort has allowed to characterize the psycho-cognitive profile of vegetarians versus meat eaters. Current evidences suggest that vegetarians have a different functional recruitment of networks belonging to social mirroring, emotional contagion, and self-representation. These data may open new fields of research, contributing to improve our understanding of the dynamics at the basis of our social interactions, which are especially important in a world that has growing interest for its cultural diversity.

References

Adolphs, R., 2002. Neural systems for recognizing emotion. Curr. Opin. Neurobiol. 12 (2), 169–177.

Allison, T., Puce, A., McCarthy, G., 2000. Social perception from visual cues: role of the STS region. Trends Cogn. Sci. 4 (7), 267–278.

Bandettini, P.A., Jesmanowicz, A., Wong, E.C., Hyde, J.S., 1993. Processing strategies for time-course data sets in functional MRI of the human brain. Magn. Reson. Med. 30 (2), 161–173.

Baron-Cohen, S., Wheelwright, S., 2004. The empathy quotient: an investigation of adults with Asperger syndrome or high functioning autism, and normal sex differences. J. Autism Dev. Disord. 34 (2), 163–175.

Bedford, J.L., Barr, S.I., 2005. Diets and selected lifestyle practices of self-defined adult vegetarians from a population-based sample suggest they are more 'health conscious'. Int. J. Behav. Nutr. Phys. Act. 2 (1), 4.

Botvinick, M.M., 2007. Conflict monitoring and decision making: reconciling two perspectives on anterior cingulate function. Cogn. Affect. Behav. Neurosci. 7 (4), 356–366.

Buccino, G., Binkofski, F., Fink, G.R., Fadiga, L., Fogassi, L., Gallese, V., Seitz, R.J., Zilles, K., Rizzolatti, G., Freund, H.J., 2001. Action observation activates premotor and parietal areas in a somatotopic manner: an fMRI study. Eur. J. Neurosci. 13 (2), 400–404.

Buccino, G., Lui, F., Canessa, N., Patteri, I., Lagravinese, G., Benuzzi, F., Porro, C.A., Rizzolatti, G., 2004. Neural circuits involved in the recognition of actions performed by nonconspecifics: an FMRI study. J. Cogn. Neurosci. 16 (1), 114–126.

Cauda, F., Costa, T., Torta, D.M., Sacco, K., D'Agata, F., Duca, S., Geminiani, G., Fox, P.T., Vercelli, A., 2012. Meta-analytic clustering of the insular cortex: characterizing the meta-analytic connectivity of the insula when involved in active tasks. NeuroImage 62 (1), 343–355.

Chang, L.J., Yarkoni, T., Khaw, M.W., Sanfey, A.G., 2013. Decoding the role of the insula in human cognition: functional parcellation and large-scale reverse inference. Cereb. Cortex 23 (3), 739–749.

Cheng, Y., Lin, C.P., Liu, H.L., Hsu, Y.Y., Lim, K.E., Hung, D., Decety, J., 2007. Expertise modulates the perception of pain in others. Curr. Biol. 17 (19), 1708–1713.

Cooper, C., Wise, T.N., Mann, L.S., 1985. Psychological and cognitive characteristics of vegetarians. Psychosomatics 26 (6), 521–523 526–527.

Cuthbert, B.N., Schupp, H.T., Bradley, M.M., Birbaumer, N., Lang, P.J., 2000. Brain potentials in affective picture processing: covariation with autonomic arousal and affective report. Biol. Psychol. 52 (2), 95–111.

D'Argembeau, A., Stawarczyk, D., Majerus, S., Collette, F., Van der Linden, M., Feyers, D., Maquet, P., Salmon, E., 2010. The neural basis of personal goal processing when envisioning future events. J. Cogn. Neurosci. 22 (8), 1701–1713.

de Waal, F.B., 2008. Putting the altruism back into altruism: the evolution of empathy. Annu. Rev. Psychol. 59, 279–300.

Decety, J., Chaminade, T., 2003. When the self represents the other: a new cognitive neuroscience view on psychological identification. Conscious. Cogn. 12 (4), 577–596.

Decety, J., Jackson, P.L., 2004. The functional architecture of human empathy. Behav. Cogn. Neurosci. Rev. 3 (2), 71–100.

Decety, J., Svetlova, M., 2012. Putting together phylogenetic and ontogenetic perspectives on empathy. Dev. Cogn. Neurosci. 2 (1), 1–24.

Devinsky, O., Morrell, M.J., Vogt, B.A., 1995. Contributions of anterior cingulate cortex to behaviour. Brain 118 (Pt. 1), 279–306.

Elliot, A.J., Covington, M.V., 2001. Approach and avoidance motivation. Educ. Psychol. Rev. 13 (2), 73–92.

Fessler, D.M., Arguello, A.P., Mekdara, J.M., Macias, R., 2003. Disgust sensitivity and meat consumption: a test of an emotivist account of moral vegetarianism. Appetite 41 (1), 31–41.

Filippi, M., Riccitelli, G., Falini, A., Di Salle, F., Vuilleumier, P., Comi, G., Rocca, M.A., 2010. The brain functional networks associated to human and animal suffering differ among omnivores, vegetarians and vegans. PLoS One 5 (5), e10847.

Filippi, M., Riccitelli, G., Meani, A., Falini, A., Comi, G., Rocca, M.A., 2013. The "vegetarian brain": chatting with monkeys and pigs? Brain Struct. Funct. 218 (5), 1211–1227.

Fox, M.A., 1999. The contribution of vegetarianism to ecosystem health. Ecosyst. Health 5, 70–74.

Fox, N., Ward, K., 2008a. Health, ethics and environment: a qualitative study of vegetarian motivations. Appetite 50 (2–3), 422–429.

Fox, N., Ward, K.J., 2008b. You are what you eat? Vegetarianism, health and identity. Soc. Sci. Med. 66 (12), 2585–2595.

Frith, C.D., Frith, U., 2006. The neural basis of mentalizing. Neuron 50 (4), 531–534.

Gaard, G., 2002. Vegetarian eco-feminism: a review essay. Frontiers 23, 117–146.

Gerace, A., Day, A., Casey, S., Mohr, P., 2013. An exploratory investigation of the process of perspective taking in interpersonal situations. J. Relatsh. Res. 4 (e6), 1–12.

Grasby, P.M., Frith, C.D., Friston, K.J., Bench, C., Frackowiak, R.S., Dolan, R.J., 1993. Functional mapping of brain areas implicated in auditory–verbal memory function. Brain 116 (Pt. 1), 1–20.

Hamilton, M.B., 1993. Wholefoods and healthfoods: beliefs and attitudes. Appetite 20 (3), 223–228.

Hariri, A.R., Tessitore, A., Mattay, V.S., Fera, F., Weinberger, D.R., 2002. The amygdala response to emotional stimuli: a comparison of faces and scenes. NeuroImage 17 (1), 317–323.

Hein, G., Knight, R.T., 2008. Superior temporal sulcus–it's my area: or is it? J. Cogn. Neurosci. 20 (12), 2125–2136.

Hein, G., Singer, T., 2008. I feel how you feel but not always: the empathic brain and its modulation. Curr. Opin. Neurobiol. 18, 153–158.

Hoek, A.C., Luning, P.A., Stafleu, A., de Graaf, C., 2004. Food-related lifestyle and health attitudes of Dutch vegetarians, non-vegetarian consumers of meat substitutes, and meat consumers. Appetite 42 (3), 265–272.

Iacoboni, M., 2009. Imitation, empathy, and mirror neurons. Annu. Rev. Psychol. 60, 653–670.

Jabs, J., Devine, C., Sobal, J., 1998. Model of the process of adopting diets: health vegetarians and Ethical vegetarians. J. Nutr. Educ. 30, 196–202.

Jackson, P.L., Meltzoff, A.N., Decety, J., 2005. How do we perceive the pain of others? A window into the neural processes involved in empathy. NeuroImage 24 (3), 771–779.

Jirak, D., Menz, M.M., Buccino, G., Borghi, A.M., Binkofski, F., 2010. Grasping language–a short story on embodiment. Conscious. Cogn. 19 (3), 711–720.

Just, M.A., Carpenter, P.A., Keller, T.A., Eddy, W.F., Thulborn, K.R., 1996. Brain activation modulated by sentence comprehension. Science 274 (5284), 114–116.

Kalof, L., Dietz, T., Stern, P.C., Guagnano, G.A., 1999. Social psychological and structural influences on vegetarian beliefs. Rural Sociol. 64, 500–511.

Kapogiannis, D., Barbey, A.K., Su, M., Zamboni, G., Krueger, F., Grafman, J., 2009. Cognitive and neural foundations of religious belief. Proc. Natl. Acad. Sci. U.S.A. 106 (12), 4876–4881.

Kenyon, P.M., Barker, M.E., 1998. Attitudes towards meat-eating in vegetarian and non-vegetarian teenage girls in England–an ethnographic approach. Appetite 30 (2), 185–198.

Key, T.J., Appleby, P.N., Rosell, M.S., 2006. Health effects of vegetarian and vegan diets. Proc. Nutr. Soc. 65 (1), 35–41.

Kim, E.H., Schroeder, K.M., Houser Jr., R.F., Dwyer, J.T., 1999. Two small surveys, 25 years apart, investigating motivations of dietary choice in 2 groups of vegetarians in the Boston area. J. Am. Diet. Assoc. 99 (5), 598–601.

Lamm, C., Decety, J., Singer, T., 2011. Meta-analytic evidence for common and distinct neural networks associated with directly experienced pain and empathy for pain. NeuroImage 54 (3), 2492–2502.

Lea, E., Worsley, A., 2001. Influences on meat consumption in Australia. Appetite 36 (2), 127–136.

Lindeman, M., Sirelius, M., 2001. Food choice ideologies: the modern manifestations of normative and humanist views of the world. Appetite 37 (3), 175–184.

Maddock, R.J., 1999. The retrosplenial cortex and emotion: new insights from functional neuroimaging of the human brain. Trends Neurosci. 22 (7), 310–316.

Martins, Y., Pliner, P., 2005. Human food choices: an examination of the factors underlying acceptance/rejection of novel and familiar animal and nonanimal foods. Appetite 45 (3), 214–224.

Maslow, A.H., 1943. A theory of human motivation. Psychol. Rev. 50 (4), 370–396.

Mottaghy, F.M., Willmes, K., Horwitz, B., Muller, H.W., Krause, B.J., Sturm, W., 2006. Systems level modeling of a neuronal network subserving intrinsic alertness. NeuroImage 29 (1), 225–233.

Murty, V.P., Ritchey, M., Adcock, R.A., LaBar, K.S., 2010. fMRI studies of successful emotional memory encoding: a quantitative meta-analysis. Neuropsychologia 48 (12), 3459–3469.

Nieuwenhuis, S., Aston-Jones, G., Cohen, J.D., 2005. Decision making, the P3, and the locus coeruleus-norepinephrine system. Psychol. Bull. 131 (4), 510–532.

Ogawa, S., Menon, R.S., Kim, S.G., Ugurbil, K., 1998. On the characteristics of functional magnetic resonance imaging of the brain. Annu. Rev. Biophys. Biomol. Struct. 27, 447–474.

Ogawa, S., Menon, R.S., Tank, D.W., Kim, S.G., Merkle, H., Ellermann, J.M., Ugurbil, K., 1993. Functional brain mapping by blood oxygenation level-dependent contrast magnetic resonance imaging. A comparison of signal characteristics with a biophysical model. Biophys. J. 64 (3), 803–812.

Pardee, R.L., 1990. Motivation Theories of Maslow, Herzberg, McGregor and McClelland. A Literature Review of Selected Theories Dealing with Job Satisfaction and Motivation. US Department of Education, Educational Resources Information Center (ERIC).

Paulesu, E., Perani, D., Blasi, V., Silani, G., Borghese, N.A., De Giovanni, U., Sensolo, S., Fazio, F., 2003. A functional-anatomical model for lipreading. J. Neurophysiol. 90 (3), 2005–2013.

Peterson, N.N., Schroeder, C.E., Arezzo, J.C., 1995. Neural generators of early cortical somatosensory evoked potentials in the awake monkey. Electroencephalogr. Clin. Neurophysiol. 96 (3), 248–260.

Phan, K.L., Wager, T., Taylor, S.F., Liberzon, I., 2002. Functional neuroanatomy of emotion: a meta-analysis of emotion activation studies in PET and fMRI. NeuroImage 16 (2), 331–348.

Phillips, M.L., Young, A.W., Senior, C., Brammer, M., Andrew, C., Calder, A.J., Bullmore, E.T., Perrett, D.I., Rowland, D., Williams, S.C., Gray, J.A., David, A.S., 1997. A specific neural substrate for perceiving facial expressions of disgust. Nature 389 (6650), 495–498.

Rae Westbury, H., Neumann, D.L., 2008. Empathy-related responses to moving film stimuli depicting human and non-human animal targets in negative circumstances. Biol. Psychol. 78 (1), 66–74.

Rizzolatti, G., Fogassi, L., Gallese, V., 2001. Neurophysiological mechanisms underlying the understanding and imitation of action. Nat. Rev. Neurosci. 2 (9), 661–670.

Rogers, K., Dziobek, I., Hassenstab, J., Wolf, O.T., Convit, A., 2007. Who cares? Revisiting empathy in Asperger syndrome. J. Autism Dev. Disord. 37 (4), 709–715.

Rozin, P., 1996. Towards a psychology of food and eating: from motivation to module to model to marker, morality, meaning, and metaphor. Curr. Dir. Psychol. Sci. 5, 18–24.

Rozin, P., Markwith, M., Stoess, C., 1997. Moralization and becoming a vegetarian: the transformation of preferences into values and the recruitment of disgust. Psychol. Sci. 8, 67–73.

Rozin, P., Vollmecke, T.A., 1986. Food likes and dislikes. Annu. Rev. Nutr. 6, 433–456.

Ryan, R.M., Deci, E.L., 2000a. Intrinsic and extrinsic motivations: classic definitions and new directions. Contemp. Educ. Psychol. 25 (1), 54–67.

Ryan, R.M., Deci, E.L., 2000b. Self-determination theory and the facilitation of intrinsic motivation, social development, and well-being. Am. Psychol. 55 (1), 68–78.

Santos, M.L., Booth, D.A., 1996. Influences on meat avoidance among British students. Appetite 27 (3), 197–205.

Schienle, A., Schafer, A., Hermann, A., Walter, B., Stark, R., Vaitl, D., 2006. fMRI responses to pictures of mutilation and contamination. Neurosci. Lett. 393 (2–3), 174–178.

Schupp, H.T., Flaisch, T., Stockburger, J., Junghofer, M., 2006. Emotion and attention: event-related brain potential studies. Prog. Brain Res. 156, 31–51.

Shamay-Tsoory, S.G., 2011. The neural bases for empathy. Neuroscientist 17 (1), 18–24.

Shamay-Tsoory, S.G., Aharon-Peretz, J., Perry, D., 2009. Two systems for empathy: a double dissociation between emotional and cognitive empathy in inferior frontal gyrus versus ventromedial prefrontal lesions. Brain 132 (Pt. 3), 617–627.

Singer, T., 2006. The neuronal basis and ontogeny of empathy and mind reading: review of literature and implications for future research. Neurosci. Biobehav. Rev. 30 (6), 855–863.

Singer, T., Critchley, H.D., Preuschoff, K., 2009. A common role of insula in feelings, empathy and uncertainty. Trends Cogn. Sci. 13 (8), 334–340.

Singer, T., Lamm, C., 2009. The social neuroscience of empathy. Ann. N. Y. Acad. Sci. 1156, 81–96.

Singer, T., Seymour, B., O'Doherty, J., Kaube, H., Dolan, R.J., Frith, C.D., 2004. Empathy for pain involves the affective but not sensory components of pain. Science 303 (5661), 1157–1162.

Stone, V.E., Gerrans, P., 2006. What's domain-specific about theory of mind? Soc. Neurosci. 1 (3–4), 309–319.

Uysal, M., Jurowski, C., 1994. Testing the push and pull factors. Ann. Tour. Res. 21 (4), 844–846.

Van Overwalle, F., 2009. Social cognition and the brain: a meta-analysis. Hum. Brain Mapp. 30 (3), 829–858.

Vanzetta, I., Grinvald, A., 1999. Increased cortical oxidative metabolism due to sensory stimulation: implications for functional brain imaging. Science 286 (5444), 1555–1558.

Whorton, J.C., 1994. Historical development of vegetarianism. Am. J. Clin. Nutr. 59 (5 Suppl.), 1103S–1109S.

Wilson, M.S., Weatherall, A., Butler, C., 2004. A rhetorical approach to discussions about health and vegetarianism. J. Health Psychol. 9 (4), 567–581.

Worsley, K.J., Friston, K.J., 1995. Analysis of fMRI time-series revisited–again. NeuroImage 2 (3), 173–181.

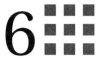

6

Geographic Aspects of Vegetarianism: Vegetarians in India

Sutapa Agrawal

PUBLIC HEALTH FOUNDATION OF INDIA, GURGAON, INDIA

1. Introduction

Readers may also refer to Chapter 1 of this book for the definition of vegetarianism and vegetarian diets. For the sake of consistency, in this volume, the term vegetarianism refers to the conscious, voluntary choice to exclude meat, fish, seafood, and possibly other animal products such as dairy and eggs from the diet. Vegetarianism encompasses a spectrum of eating patterns: from diets that leave out all animal meats and products (vegan) to diets that include eggs, milk, and milk products (ovolactovegetarian). Plant-based diets refer to diets predominantly based on plant foods, including most vegetarian diets and other diets in the spectrum, such as those including fish (pescetarian) (Tonstad et al., 2009). In general, vegetarian diets provide relatively large amounts of cereals, pulses, nuts, fruits, and vegetables. In terms of nutrients, vegetarian diets are usually rich in carbohydrates, n-6 fatty acids, dietary fiber, carotenoids, folic acid, vitamin C, vitamin E, and Mg and relatively low in protein, saturated fat, long-chain n-3 fatty acids, retinol, vitamin B(12), and Zn (Key et al., 2006). In recent years, the vegetarian dietary pattern has been adopted by an increasing number of people in Western countries (Fraser, 2009), where it is usually an adopted lifestyle by choice during adulthood (Fraser, 2009). Moreover, vegetarianism is not common in the West (<5% of the population) (Key et al., 2006), which limits the power of studies examining the macro- and micronutrient value of vegetarian diets (Fraser, 2009; Key et al., 2006; Obersby et al., 2013; Baines et al., 2007).

By contrast, a substantial proportion of the Indian population (35%) are vegetarians (Key et al., 2006) (10%–62% for different regions) (Arnold et al., 2009). The history of vegetarianism has its roots in the civilization of ancient India, and the origin of vegetarianism in India has often been linked to the cow protectionism and veneration associated with Hindu culture (Narayan, 2008). The earliest records of vegetarianism as a concept and practice among a significant number of people concerns ancient India (Spencer, 1993), where the diet was closely connected with the idea of nonviolence toward animals (called ahimsa in India) and was promoted by religious groups and philosophers (Walters and Portmess, 2001). Vegetarianism in India has unique attributes, which make it scientifically relevant to analyze the relation between vegetarian diet and disease risk: (1) it is generally a lifelong pattern and less susceptible to change, making it easier to measure at any etiologic window in the process of disease formation; (2) it is often transmitted through multiple generations, and hence easier to measure for in utero exposure, and even for the mother's in utero experience; and (3) it is associated with high consumption of whole grains, legumes, nuts and seeds, and dairy with spices and seasonings unique to the Indian diet; the combination/pattern could yield different findings than similar studies conducted in the West. Dietary patterns in India are bound by religious, cultural, and family values (Arnold et al., 2009) and are often maintained for generations. The vegetarian diet in India includes a wide range of vegetables, fruits, cereals, pulses, spices, seasonings, and cooking practices (Mudambi and Rajagopal, 2001) and hence can have different levels of bioavailability and absorption for many nutrients. Thus, information on the geographic aspects of vegetarianism across various regions of India is a valuable addition to the existing body of evidence.

1.1 Vegetarianism and Nutrition Transition in India

When considering the role of a "nutrition transition" in this trend, it is important to note that the Indian population has a long tradition of faith-based vegetarianism and remains ~40% vegetarian (FAOSTAT), a rate that ranks India as the nation with the largest population of vegetarians (estimated at 300–400 million) in the world. Moreover, data from the FAO indicate that during the past 25 years, the annual per capita consumption of meats in India has only slightly increased (by ~1 kg) to 5 kg (FAOSTAT, FAO. World Agriculture: Towards 2015/2030), primarily attributable to poultry consumption. In India, vegetarianism is mainly guided by religion, caste, and traditional values, which rule the roost. Most vegetarians abstain from eating meat, fish, or eggs because, in India, vegetarianism is not a matter of choice. (However, while strongly linked to religion and caste, some may argue that there is increasingly a choice involved. Many younger people in northern Indian cities, for example, are choosing to consume meat.) It is a traditional way of living, inherited by birth with caste and religious considerations (Narayan, 2008). Being born a vegetarian, when eating out, one may tend to eat meat occasionally due to social considerations and still call himself or herself a vegetarian. However, the fast-growing Indian middle class now consists of around 300 million people, who model their new consumer lifestyle on the West, and as a result, vegetarianism is falling out of favor (Esselborn, 2013). Over the past 10 years the amount of meat eaten in India has more than doubled: in 2009, it reached around 5.5 kg (12 pounds) per head, according to the World Food Program. Though, this is still very little in comparison with developed countries such as Germany, where 61 kg of beef, pork, and poultry are consumed per person per year (Esselborn, 2013).

India, which is home to one-seventh of the world's population, a rapidly growing economy, and the majority of the world's vegetarians, offers an ideal setting to study dynamics of the nutrition transition that may play out in a context that already has a long tradition of plant-based eating or vegetarian diet (DeLessio-Parson, 2016). With the surge in India's population, India is gradually becoming one of the largest meat-eating population in the world (Jishnu, 2014). Data compiled by the National Sample Survey Organisation (NSSO) of the government has been showing a clear increase in meat consumption in recent years.

Although NSSO covers just 100,000 people in its surveys, these provide the largest official data on consumption and expenditure. The latest Household Consumption survey (Round 558) conducted during 2011–12 and released in July 2014 shows both rural and urban India are spending more on milk, meat, and eggs as consumption of these items is rising much faster than that of cereals (NSSO, 2012–13). Animal products have also contributed to 33% of the incremental food inflation over the past 5 years, a figure that is expected to be higher in the future (Jishnu, 2014). Milk and other dairy products, derived from cows and buffalo, are widely consumed across India, and India is the largest producer of milk globally (FAOSTAT, 2016). Dairy consumption per capita is greatest in the Punjab region and is associated with socioeconomic status with greater consumption among wealthier and urban communities (Adhya et al., 2017). Other recent trends show meat production and consumption patterns are changing: wealthier Indians shop more in large supermarkets, and meat is portrayed as a symbol of status, wealth, and participation in global culture (Jishnu, 2014; Roy, 2015). These recent developments come into conflict with the country's vegetarian roots dating back to the premodern era, as presented in the Vedas and as practiced by early Brahmins. As such, religious and cultural proscriptions shape meat-eating, which varies by caste and across places (Stuart, 2008). Most practicing vegetarians were raised exclusively on plant-based diets and, while longitudinal data to produce population-level estimates of nutritional intake are scarce, there appears to be high adherence across generations (Agrawal et al., 2014). In many places, institutionalized support of vegetarianism, including state-level criminalization of cattle slaughter, remains strong just as specific policies and practices are hotly contested (DeLessio-Parson, 2016).

1.2 Types of Vegetarian Diet Consumption in India and States

An analysis of the cross-sectional data states by Agrawal et al. (2014) on 156,317 adult men and women aged 20–49 years who participated in India's third National Family Health Survey (2005–06) in India and its states shows that, overall, a majority (two-thirds, 64%) of the sample population eat a nonvegetarian diet (persons consuming fruits, vegetables, pulses or beans, animal products such as chicken or meat, fish, eggs, milk, or curd either daily, weekly, or at least occasionally), whereas one-fourth is lacto-vegetarian (persons consuming fruits, vegetables, pulses or beans, milk, or curd, either daily, weekly, or occasionally but no fish, eggs, chicken, or other meat) (see Table 6.1). Other dietary patterns are followed by a relatively smaller percentage of Indian population: semivegetarian (persons consuming fruits, vegetables, pulses, or beans either daily, weekly, or occasionally and animal products such as chicken or meat, eggs, milk, or curd, only weekly or occasionally, but no fish) constitutes 5.2%; ovolactovegetarian (persons consuming fruits, vegetables, pulses or beans, milk or curd, and or eggs either daily, weekly, or occasionally, but no fish or chicken or meat) constitutes 3.2%; pescetarian (persons consuming fruits, vegetables, pulses or beans, milk or curd either daily, weekly, or occasionally, and or eggs or fish only weekly or occasionally, but no chicken or meat) constitutes 2.2%; and vegan (no consumption of animal products such as chicken

Table 6.1 Percentage Consumption of Different Types of Diet Among Adult Population Age 20–49 Years in India and States, National Family Health Survey-3, 2005–06

India/States	Vegan N[%]	Lactovegetarian N[%]	Ovolactovegetarian N[%]	Pescetarian N[%]	Semivegetarian N[%]	Nonvegetarian N[%]	Total N
India	2,560[1.6]	37,797[24.2]	5,002[3.2]	3,446[2.2]	8,140[5.2]	99,372[63.6]	156,317
Northern Region							
Jammu and Kashmir	9[0.6]	276[18.4]	18[1.2]	9[0.6]	297[19.8]	891[59.4]	1,500
Himachal Pradesh	17[1.8]	429[45.6]	76[8.1]	13[1.4]	137[14.6]	269[28.6]	941
Punjab	138[3.4]	2,149[52.3]	275[6.7]	13[0.3]	420[10.2]	1,112[27.1]	4,107
Uttaranchal	20[1.6]	324[26.6]	84[6.9]	15[1.2]	108[8.9]	669[54.8]	1,220
Haryana	107[3.5]	2,099[68.9]	205[6.7]	6[0.2]	148[4.9]	482[15.8]	3,047
Delhi	43[2.1]	645[30.9]	222[10.6]	25[1.2]	192[9.2]	963[46.1]	2,090
Rajasthan	236[2.9]	5,060[62.1]	393[4.8]	62[0.8]	869[10.7]	1,528[18.8]	8,148
Central Region							
Uttar Pradesh	264[1.2]	8,458[37.7]	1,227[5.5]	336[1.5]	835[3.7]	11,343[50.5]	22,463
Chhattisgarh	69[2.1]	484[14.5]	101[3.0]	60[1.8]	57[1.7]	2,574[77.0]	3,345
Madhya Pradesh	294[3.1]	3,975[42.2]	479[5.1]	223[2.4]	463[4.9]	3,980[42.3]	9,414
Eastern Region							
Bihar	50[0.5]	1,812[17.3]	66[0.6]	382[3.6]	120[1.1]	8,037[76.8]	10,467
West Bengal	43[0.3]	183[1.4]	16[0.1]	554[4.1]	94[0.7]	12,548[93.4]	13,438
Jharkhand	49[1.3]	214[5.5]	37[1.0]	80[2.1]	81[2.1]	3,395[88.0]	3,856
Orissa	50[0.8]	225[3.8]	19[0.3]	432[7.2]	66[1.1]	5,168[86.7]	5,960
Northeastern Region							
Sikkim	0[0.0]	9[9.6]	1[1.1]	1[1.1]	6[6.4]	77[81.9]	94
Arunachal Pradesh	0[0.0]	2[1.3]	1[0.6]	2[1.3]	2[1.3]	152[95.6]	159
Nagaland	0[0.0]	1[0.5]	0[0.0]	1[0.5]	2[1.0]	204[98.1]	208
Manipur	1[0.3]	1[0.3]	0[0.0]	31[9.0]	3[0.9]	307[89.5]	343
Mizoram	0[0.0]	0[0.0]	1[0.7]	1[0.7]	6[4.3]	131[94.2]	139
Tripura	1[0.2]	4[0.7]	1[0.2]	46[7.8]	2[0.3]	536[90.8]	590
Meghalaya	0[0.0]	3[0.8]	1[0.3]	9[2.3]	5[1.3]	371[95.4]	389
Assam	5[0.1]	72[1.6]	13[0.3]	132[3.0]	12[0.3]	4,135[94.6]	4,369

Western Region							
Gujarat	400[4.9]	4,546[55.6]	342[4.2]	159[1.9]	399[4.9]	2,330[28.5]	8,176
Maharashtra	643[4.0]	3,614[22.7]	529[3.3]	1,35[0.8]	912[5.7]	10,068[63.3]	15,901
Goa	3[1.2]	10[3.9]	2[0.8]	30[11.8]	2[0.8]	207[81.5]	254
Southern Region							
Andhra Pradesh	45[0.4]	579[4.7]	222[1.8]	78[0.6]	1,129[9.1]	10,299[83.4]	12,352
Karnataka	41[0.4]	2,126[22.2]	385[4.0]	134[1.4]	979[10.2]	5,932[61.8]	9,597
Kerala	11[0.2]	81[1.8]	37[0.8]	234[5.2]	541[1.2]	4,045[90.7]	4,462
Tamil Nadu	21[0.2]	416[4.5]	249[2.7]	243[2.6]	740[8.0]	7,619[82.0]	9,288

or meat, fish, eggs, milk, or curd) constitutes 1.6%. More than 80% of the population consume a nonvegetarian diet in northeastern region, in southern region (except the state of Karnataka), most of the states in eastern region (except Bihar), and the western state of Goa. More than half the population in the northern states of Punjab, Haryana, Rajasthan, and in the western state of Gujarat follow a lactovegetarian diet. One in five people in Jammu and Kashmir follow a semivegetarian diet (without fish), whereas one in 10 people in Goa (11.8%) and Manipur (9.0%), 7.8% in Tripura, 7.2% in Orissa, 5.2% in Kerala, and 4.1% in West Bengal consume a pescetarian diet (dominated by fish). In the state of Delhi, 1 out of 10 people is an ovolactovegetarian, whereas the western states of Gujarat (4.9%) and Maharashtra (4.0%) have the highest percentages of vegans.

1.3 Nutritional Profile of Vegetarian Diets in India

The nutritional profile of vegetarian and nonvegetarian diet across various regions of India is not well documented (Farmer et al., 2011), although studies have shown greater amounts of antioxidants (vitamins C, A, and E) in Indian vegetarians that may make them less prone to oxidative stress and noncommunicable diseases (Manjari et al., 2001; Somannavar and Kodliwadmath, 2012). However, some studies on the nutritional profile of Indian vegetarian diet demonstrate micronutrient deficiencies of zinc and iron that are primarily attributable to reduced absorption (Agte et al., 1994, 2005) and vitamin B_{12} deficiency in rural and urban vegetarians due to low dietary intake (Yajnik et al., 2006; Misra et al., 2002). A recent study (Shridhar et al., 2014) assessing the nutrition profile of the vegetarians from four different geographic regions, representing 20 states of India, with energy, socioeconomic status, and multivariate adjusted analyses of nutritional intake found that, overall, Indian vegetarian diets were found to have a greater percentage meeting recommended daily allowance (RDA) levels of macro- and micronutrients with less fat and lower calories than nonvegetarian diets.

2. Health Implications of Vegetarianism in India

Extensive research has documented the protective effects of plant-based eating against noncommunicable diseases in wealthy countries such as the United States (Fraser, 2009; Orlich et al., 2013). In these settings, a plant-based diet is increasingly viewed as a cost-effective intervention to treat medical conditions, especially chronic ones, and reduce reliance on medicines (Tuso et al., 2013). At the aggregate level, it has been posited that plant-based eating brings more people closer to optimal health, whereas meat eaters as a group are more vulnerable to the extremes of disease-related noncommunicable diseases, i.e., both malnutrition/underweight status and excess calories/overweight (Sabaté, 2003). Yet population-level studies are often difficult to carry out given the still relatively low adherence to vegetarianism and veganism in most places. Therefore, although the health-protective effects of vegetarianism are well documented in the wealthy country context (see Section 3 in this book), less is known across the Global South, even as India is home to most of the world's vegetarians. A hospital-based survey in a district of Karnataka, a state in southwest India, documented a linear relationship between BMI and vegetarian status. BMI was lowest in vegans (23.9 kg/m^2), slightly higher among ovolactovegetarians (25.9 kg/m^2), and highest in nonvegetarians (29.2 kg/m^2) (Zaman et al., 2010). Another recent study leverages population-level data and finds that Indian vegetarians are more protected against type 2 diabetes, even after controlling for wealth; the analysis also controlled for BMI (Agrawal et al., 2014; Zaman et al., 2010). Yet unhealthy BMI itself is also a risk factor for many diseases and chronic conditions, and estimates of BMI by vegetarian status after controlling for wealth are needed. Vegetarianism generally appears to be protective against obesity globally, but estimates in India are confounded by socioeconomic status given the historical connections between vegetarianism and certain higher caste groups (DeLessio-Parson, 2016) and are thus inconclusive. However, a recent study by Jaacks et al. (2016) found that after adjustment for confounders (age, sex, education, tobacco, alcohol, and place of residence), South Asian (including India) vegetarians were only slightly less frequently overweight/obese compared with nonvegetarians: 49% [95% confidence interval (CI), 45%–53%] versus 53% (95% CI, 51%–56%), respectively.

Diet is a key culprit in perpetuating noncommunicable disease, but it can also be health promoting (DeLessio-Parson, 2016). This is particularly true when it comes to vegetarianism, which have been associated with increased longevity; reduced risk of heart disease, diabetes, and cancer; weight maintenance; and diminished need for medications (Farmer et al., 2011; Fraser, 2003, 2009; Orlich et al., 2013; Singh et al., 2003; Tuso et al., 2013). Yet societal-level dietary dynamics generally push toward greater animal protein consumption. Meat is often viewed as a high-status food globally and also in India (Twigg, 1983; York et al., 2003; Kapur, 2014). Economic development typically involves the expansion of the middle class, thereby increasing their purchasing power and generating more demand for meat, dairy, and processed foods, with a concomitant increase in noncommunicable disease (DeLessio-Parson, 2016). On the other hand, growing awareness of the negative health outcomes for people and for the planet associated with meat-heavy diets can prompt others–both individuals and policy makers–to adopt more sustainable plant-centered eating practices.

In India, the shift toward greater consumption of animal proteins has been quite limited. Nearly one in three Indians are vegetarians (36% in NFHS 2005–06) and less than 10% of the daily food supply per capita derives from animal sources (FAOSTAT, see Fig. 6.1). Even so, when examining the diet in historical context, dietary changes of the past five decades are substantial. Fig. 6.1 shows trends in the share of different foods and food groups in the diet of the average Indian (percent of food measured in kcal of daily food supply per capita). The proportion of calories from traditional grains, pulses, and unprocessed sugar has declined sharply, just as the contribution of oils, wheat, and refined sugar to the average diet has increased dramatically (DeLessio-Parson, 2016). Calories from dairy and eggs have doubled in importance, and the pace of increase appears to be picking up. The consumption of chicken has risen in recent years, but together with red meat consumption, it remains a very small proportion

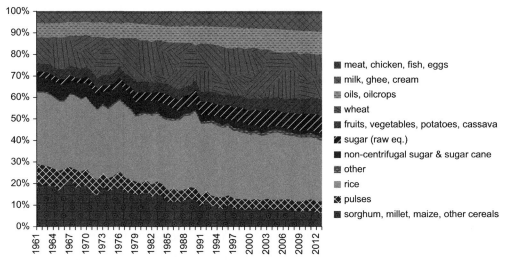

FIGURE 6.1 The unfolding nutrition transition in India. Contribution of items to daily per capita food supply (% of kcal), 1961–2013. *Created by DeLessio-Parson, A., 2016. A protective effect of plant-based diets in urbanizing India. Poster presented at the annual meeting of the Population Association of America (PAA) (Unpublished); DeLessio-Parson, A., 2016. The Protective Effect of Plant-Based Diets in Urbanizing India using food supply estimates (kcal/capita/day) of the Food and Agriculture Organization of the United Nations, FAOSTAT.*

of the average diet. However in India, the increase in red meat consumption is proportionate to the increase in population, whereas real increase is found in chicken consumption (NSSO, 2012–13). Taken together, these changes indicate the onset of the fourth stage of the nutrition transition in India, which is characterized by changes in diet and activity pattern leading to the emergence of new disease problems and increased disability (Popkin and Gordon-Larsen, 2004; Popkin, 1994). At the same time, these country-level trends mask substantial within-country variation. Moreover, they offer little in terms of understanding how Indian vegetarians may be more or less susceptible to negative health outcomes, especially obesity, in the context of changing diets (DeLessio-Parson, 2016).

In India, studies have documented notable increases in obesity, diabetes, and coronary heart disease (Misra et al., 2011). As Fig. 6.2 reveals, the absolute increase is particularly telling: the number of overweight (BMI >25) Indians tripled from around 25 million in 1980 to 75 million in 2013, with the numbers swelling among young and middle-age adults with both men and women affected. The proportion of adolescents and children with unhealthy body weights increased as well. Across much of the Global South, the BMI–wealth gradient differs sometimes quite dramatically across countries and neighborhoods (Corsi et al., 2011, 2012). The relationship is, however, clearly reversed in India: the wealthiest are the first to experience expanding waistlines, even as malnutrition, stunting, and underweight status persist in poorer segments of societies (Gouda and Prusty, 2014; Griffiths and Bentley, 2001; Patel, 2012). This positive relationship between wealth/socioeconomic status and overweight/obesity exists at

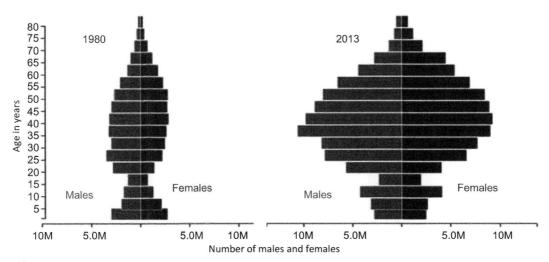

FIGURE 6.2 Burden of overweight/obesity in India. Number of males and females aged 20 years and above with BMI >25 kg/m², 1980 and 2013. *Courtesy Agrawal, S., Millett, C.J., Dhillon, P.K., Subramanian, S.V., Ebrahim, S., 2014. Type of vegetarian diet, obesity and diabetes in adult Indian population. Nutr. J. 13 (1), 89.*

both the individual and state level, underscoring the key role of economic development in health outcomes and the disease burden (Subramanian and Smith, 2006). These trends, understood within the context of population growth, draw attention to the "urgent need" for an integrated, multisector public health response (Kapil and Sachdev, 2012).

2.1 Prevalence of Diabetes and Obesity According to Types of Vegetarian Diet Consumption

An analysis of the cross-sectional data states by Agrawal et al. (2014) on 156,317 adult men and women aged 20–49 years who participated in India's third National Family Health Survey (2005–06) in India and its states shows the unadjusted prevalence of diabetes and obesity by types of diet consumption (Table 6.2). An increasing trend in diabetes prevalence based on types of diet was found (P for trend <.01). Prevalence of diabetes varied from 0.9% (95% CI: 0.8–1.1) in lactovegetarian, ovolactovegetarian (0.9%; 95% CI: 0.6–1.3), and semivegetarian (0.9%; 95% CI: 0.7–1.1) to 1.0% in vegan (95% CI: 0.6–1.7), 1.2% (95% CI: 1.1–1.3) in nonvegetarian and the highest in pescetarian diets (1.4%; 95% CI: 1.0–2.0). The range between the lowest and highest BMIs for all groups were reasonably low (less than 1 kg/m²). Mean BMI was 20.3 kg/m² in pescetarians and 20.5 kg/m² in vegans, 20.6 kg/m² in semivegetarians, 20.7 kg/m² in nonvegetarians, 21.0 kg/m² in ovolactovegetarians, and 21.2 kg/m² in lactovegetarians. For BMIs ≥23 kg/m², the prevalence of diabetes was 1.7% in ovolactovegetarians, 2.0% in semivegetarians, 2.1% in lactovegetarians, 2.6% in pescetarians, 2.8% in vegans, and 2.9% in nonvegetarians (data not shown). For BMIs ≥30 kg/m², the prevalence of diabetes was 2.1% in ovolactovegetarians, 3.7% in lactovegetarians, 3.8%

Table 6.2 Unadjusted Prevalence (% With CI) of Diabetes and Obesity According to Types of Vegetarian Diet Consumption in Adult Indian Population (n = 156,317) Aged 20–49 Years, NFHS 2005–06

Characteristics	Vegan	Lactovegetarian	Ovolactovegetarian	Pescetarian	Semivegetarian	Nonvegetarian	P for Trend Values[a]
			Type of Diets				
Diabetes							
N[%], 95% CI	26[1.0]	356[0.9]	46[0.9]	48[1.4]	71[0.9]	1,223[1.2]	<.01
	0.6–1.7	0.8–1.1	0.6–1.3	1.0–2.0	0.7–1.1	1.1–1.3	
BMI ≥23 kg/m²							
N[%], 95% CI	534[21.5]	9,722[26.9]	1,163[24.9]	650[19.5]	1,690[21.8]	21,380[22.6]	<.001
	19.5–23.7	26.3–27.5	23.4–26.5	17.8–21.3	20.7–23.0	22.3–23.0	
BMI ≥25 kg/m²							
N[%], 95% CI	286[11.5]	5,861[16.2]	697[14.9]	334[10.0]	877[11.3]	11,996[12.7]	<.001
	10.0–13.2	15.7–16.7	13.7–16.3	8.0–11.3	10.5–12.2	12.4–13.0	
BMI ≥30 kg/m²							
N[%], 95% CI	58[2.3]	1,311[3.6]	140[3.0]	56[1.7]	156[1.6]	2,269[2.4]	<.001
	1.7–3.2	3.4–3.9	2.5–3.7	1.2–2.4	1.2–2.4	2.3–2.5	
BMI, mean [±SD]	20.5[±4.2]	21.2[±4.5]	21.0[±4.1]	20.3[±3.8]	20.6[±4.0]	20.7[±4.1]	

[a]The P for trend values has been obtained from a likelihood ratio test for showing no difference between the groups for types of vegetarian diet, ignoring the correlated data. As the nonvegetarian group was expected to have the highest and the rural group the lowest levels of diabetes and BMI, trend tests were carried out scoring the groups 1 to 5 and using likelihood ratio tests.

in semivegetarians, 5.2% in vegans, 5.3% in pescetarians, and 5.4% in nonvegetarians (data not shown).

3. Conclusions

Vegetarian diets and vegetarianism are an important consideration for nutrition and the environment. This chapter provided an overview of food and diets in India and discussed the geographic aspects of vegetarianism in India. Vegetarian dietary patterns are diverse in India and are typically characterized by low consumption of animal-source foods, in particular red meat. However, diets are changing rapidly in India, with particularly pronounced increases in egg and dairy consumption.

Future decades will likely bring more fast food establishments, supermarkets, and other elements of a globalized food system that promote the consumption of more processed foods, refined sugars, and animal proteins (DeLessio-Parson, 2016). Many still rely on agriculture-based livelihoods, but population growth in urban areas—primarily metropolitan suburbs—is projected to increase (Lozano-Gracia et al., 2013). Given India's size, even a small shift away from vegetarianism percentage-wise could have a substantial impact on the resources required to feed the still-growing population. Research has found that those living in urban settings are most likely to be overweight (Gouda and Prusty, 2014), but it is not clear which neighborhood characteristics (e.g., wealth or uniquely urban environmental traits) matter most: sedentary lifestyle or the food habits. Supermarkets, fast food outlets, and Westernized eating patterns are likely to expand unevenly into communities across India, growing most rapidly in wealthier, urban neighborhoods that are most distanced from agricultural production. Interestingly, in the past 25 years, overall per capita calorie consumption has declined in rural places, while average consumption in urban areas stayed constant (Deaton and Drèze, 2009). The mechanisms of such place-based divergence are poorly understood, yet understanding these dynamics is an essential piece of the planetary health puzzle (DeLessio-Parson, 2016).

Due to the institutionalized nature of vegetarianism across some of India, the nutrition transition could unfold without a concomitant significant increase in meat consumption (DeLessio-Parson, 2016). Yet to the extent that the consumption of dairy and processed/refined foods replaces traditional eating habits, diet-related noncommunicable disease will likely rise nonetheless. A better understanding of how this protective effect of vegetarianism operates in towns and smaller cities and other geographic regions of India could thus be key to preventing future growth in obesity rates and other disease-related noncommunicable diseases. Further, Vitamin B_{12} bioavailability remains a concern and should be addressed by exploring various dietary patterns associated with deficiency across various regions of India and identifying people who need supplementation.

References

Adhya, T., Joy, E.J.M., Agrawal, S., Tak, M., 2017. Dietary patterns and implications for reactive N flows in India. In: Abrol, Y.P., Adhya, T.K., Aneja, V.P., Raghuram, N., Pathak, H., Kulshrestha, U., Sharma, C., Singh, B. (Eds.), The Indian Nitrogen Assessment: Sources of Reactive Nitrogen, Environmental and Climate Effects, Management Options, and Policies, 1st Edition. Elsevier, p. 461. 2017. https://www.elsevier.com/books/the-indian-nitrogen-assessment/abrol/978-0-12-811836-8 (forthcoming).

Agrawal, S., Millett, C.J., Dhillon, P.K., Subramanian, S.V., Ebrahim, S., 2014. Type of vegetarian diet, obesity and diabetes in adult indian population. Nutr. J. 13 (1), 1–18.

Agte, V., Chiplonkar, S., Joshi, N., Paknikar, K., 1994. Apparent absorption of copper and zinc from composite vegetarian diets in young Indian men. Ann. Nutr. Metab. 38 (1), 13–19.

Agte, V., Jahagirdar, M., Chiplonkar, S., 2005. Apparent absorption of eight micronutrients and phytic acid from vegetarian meals in ileostomized human volunteers. Nutr. J. 21 (6), 678–685.

Arnold, F., Parasuraman, S., Arokiasamy, P., Kothari, M., 2009. Nutrition in India national family health survey. In: NFHS 3. 2005–06 Mumbai: International Institute for Population Sciences, Vol. I. ICF Macro, Calverton, Maryland, USA.

Baines, S., Powers, J., Brown, W.J., 2007. How does the health and well-being of young Australian vegetarian and semi-vegetarian women compare with non-vegetarians? Public Health Nutr. 10 (5), 436–442.

Corsi, D.J., Kyu, H.H., Subramanian, S.V., 2011. Socioeconomic and geographic patterning of under- and overnutrition among women in Bangladesh. J. Nutr. 141 (4), 631–638.

Corsi, D.J., Finlay, J.E., Subramanian, S.V., 2012. Weight of communities: a multilevel analysis of body mass index in 32,814 neighborhoods in 57 low- to middle-income countries (LMICs). Soc. Sci. Med. 75 (2), 311–322.

Deaton, A., Drèze, J., 2009. Food and nutrition in India: facts and interpretations. Econ. Political Wkly. 44 (7), 42–65.

DeLessio-Parson, A., 2016. The Protective Effect of Plant-Based Diets in Urbanizing India.

Esselborn, P., January 2, 2013. Vegetarians Developing a Taste for Meat. http://www.dw.com/en/vegetarians-developing-a-taste-for-meat/a-16490496.

FAO, 2016. World Agriculture: Towards 2015/2030. An FAO Perspective. Available from: http://www.fao.org/docrep/005/y4252e/y4252e05c.htm.

FAOSTAT, 2016. Food and Agriculture Organization of the United Nations, Statistical Database. Available from: http://faostat.fao.org/.

Farmer, B., Larson, B.T., Fulgoni 3rd, V.L., Rainville, A.J., Liepa, G.U., 2011. A vegetarian dietary pattern as a nutrient-dense approach to weight management: an analysis of the national health and nutrition examination survey 1999–2004. J. Am. Diet. Assoc. 111 (6), 819–827.

Fraser, G.E., 2003. Risk factors for cardiovascular disease and cancer among vegetarians. In: Diet, Life Expectancy, and Chronic Disease: Studies of Seventh-Day Adventists and Other Vegetarians. Oxford University Press, pp. 203–230 (Chapter 12).

Fraser, G.E., May 2009. Vegetarian diets: what do we know of their effects on common chronic diseases? Am. J. Clin. Nutr. 89 (5), 1607S–1612S. http://dx.doi.org/10.3945/ajcn.2009.26736K. Epub 2009 Mar 25.

Gouda, J., Prusty, R.K., 2014. Overweight and obesity among women by economic stratum in urban India. J. Health Popul. Nutr. 32 (1), 79–88.

Griffiths, P.L., Bentley, M.E., 2001. The nutrition transition is underway in India. J. Nutr. 131 (10), 2692–2700.

Jaacks, L.M., Kapoor, D., Singh, K., Narayan, K.M.V., Ali, M.K., Kadir, M.M., Mohan, V., Tandon, N., Prabhakaran, D., September 4, 2016. Vegetarianism and cardiometabolic disease risk factors: differences between South Asian and American adults. Nutrition 32 (9), 975–984. Epub 2016 Dec 4.

Jishnu, L., December 31, 2014. Meaty Tales of Vegetarian India. Down to Earth. Available at http://www.downtoearth.org.in/coverage/meaty-tales-of-vegetarian-india-47830.

Kapil, U., Sachdev, H.P.S., 2012. Urgent need to orient public health response to rapid nutrition transition. Indian J. Community Med. 37 (4), 207–210.

Kapur, M., August 28, 2014. Many Indians Turning to Meat as Their Wallets Grow Fatter. http://edition.cnn.com/2014/08/28/world/asia/india-meat-eating/.

Key, T.J., Appleby, P.N., Rosell, M.S., February 2006. Health effects of vegetarian and vegan diets. Proc. Nutr. Soc. 65 (1), 35–41.

Lozano-Gracia, N., Young, C., Lall, S.V., Vishwanath, T., January 2013. Leveraging Land to Enable Urban Transformation: Lessons from Global Experience. The World Bank Policy Research Working Paper No. 6312. The World Bank Sustainable Development Network, Urban and Disaster Risk Management Department.

Manjari, V., Suresh, Y., Sailaja Devi, M.M., Das, U.N., 2001. Oxidant stress, anti-oxidants and essential fatty acids in South Indian vegetarians and non-vegetarians. Prostaglandins Leukot. Essent. Fatty Acids 64 (1), 53–59.

Misra, A., Vikram, N.K., Pandey, R.M., Dwivedi, M., Ahmad, F.U., Luthra, K., Jain, K., Khanna, N., Devi, J.R., Sharma, R., Guleria, R., 2002. Hyperhomocysteinemia, and low intakes of folic acid and vitamin B12 in urban North India. Eur. J. Nutr. 41 (2), 68–77.

Misra, A., Singhal, N., Sivakumar, B., Bhagat, N., Jaiswal, A., Khurana, L., December 2011. Nutrition transition in India: secular trends in dietary intake and their relationship to diet-related non-communicable diseases. J. Diabetes 3 (4), 278–292.

Mudambi, S., Rajagopal, M. (Eds.), 2001. Fundamentals of Food and Nutrition, fourth ed. New Age International, Madras.

NSSO, 2012–13. Situation Assessment Survey of Agricultural Households Conducted by the National Sample Survey Office (NSSO) for the 2012–13 Crop Year from July to June.

Obersby, D., Chappell, D.C., Dunnett, A., Tsiami, A.A., March 14, 2013. Plasma total homocysteine status of vegetarians compared with omnivores: a systematic review and meta-analysis. Br. J. Nutr. 109 (5), 785–794.

Orlich, M.J., et al., 2013. Vegetarian dietary patterns and mortality in adventist health study 2. JAMA Intern. Med. 173 (13), 1230–1238.

Patel, R., 2012. Stuffed and Starved: The Hidden Battle for the World Food System. 2 Rev Exp Edition. Melville House.

Popkin, B.M., Gordon-Larsen, P., 2004. The nutrition transition: worldwide obesity dynamics and their determinants. Int. J. Obes. 28, S2–S9. http://dx.doi.org/10.1038/sj.ijo.0802804.

Popkin, B.M., September 1994. The nutrition transition in low-income countries: an emerging crisis. Nutr. Rev. 52 (9), 285–298. http://dx.doi.org/10.1111/j.1753-4887.1994.tb01460.x.

Roy, S., 2015. The New Indian Pariahs: Vegetarians. NPR.org.. http://www.npr.org/2012/02/28/147038163/the-new-indian-pariahs-vegetarians.

Sabaté, J., 2003. The contribution of vegetarian diets to health and disease: a paradigm shift? Am. J. Clin. Nutr. 78 (3), 502S–507S.

Shankar Narayan, V. Text of speech delivered by, President of Indian Vegan Society and the Regional Coordinator for India, South & West Asia for the International Vegetarian Union (IVU), UK, on Friday, the First of August, 2008 at 04.45 pm on the occasion of 38th IVU World Vegetarian Congress (Centenary Congress) at the Festsaal, Kulturpalast, Dresden, Germany.

Singh, P.N., Sabaté, J., Fraser, G.E., 2003. Does low meat consumption increase life expectancy in humans? Am. J. Clin. Nutr. 78 (3), 526S–532S.

Somannavar, M.S., Kodliwadmath, M.V., 2012. Correlation between oxidative stress andantioxidant defence in South Indian urban vegetarians and non-vegetarians. Eur. Rev. Med. Pharmacol. Sci. 16 (3), 351–354.

Spencer, C., 1993. The Heretic's Feast. A History of Vegetarianism, pp. 33–68 London.

Shridhar, K., Dhillon, P.K., Bowen, L., Kinra, S., Bharathi, A.V., Prabhakaran, D., Reddy, K.S., Ebrahim, S., June 4, 2014. Nutritional profile of Indian vegetarian diets – the Indian Migration Study (IMS). Nutr. J. 13, 55. http://dx.doi.org/10.1186/1475-2891-13-55.

Stuart, T., 2008. The Bloodless Revolution: A Cultural History of Vegetarianism: From 1600 to Modern Times. Reprint Edition. W.W. Norton & Company, New York.

Subramanian, S.V., Smith, G.D., 2006. Patterns, distribution, and determinants of under and over nutrition: a population-based study of women in India. Am. J. Clin. Nutr. 84 (3), 633–640.

Tonstad, S., Butler, T., Yan, R., Fraser, G.E., 2009. Type of vegetarian diet, body weight, and prevalence of type 2 diabetes. Diabetes Care 32, 791–796.

Tuso, P.J., Ismail, M.H., Ha, B.P., Bartolotto, C., 2013. Nutritional update for physicians: plant-based diets. Perm. J. 17 (2), 61–66.

Twigg, J., 1983. Vegetarianism and the meanings of meat. In: Murcott, A. (Ed.), Sociology of Food and Eating: Essays on the Sociological Significance of Food. Gower Pub Co, Aldershot, Hants, England, pp. 18–30.

Walters, K.S., Portmess, L. (Eds.), 2001. Religious Vegetarianism: From Hesiod to the Dalai Lama. State University of New York Press, Albany, pp. 13–46.

Yajnik, C.S., Deshpande, S.S., Lubree, H.G., Naik, S.S., Bhat, D.S., Uradey, B.S., Deshpande, J.A., Rege, S.S., Refsum, H., Yudkin, J.S., 2006. Vitamin B12 deficiency and hyperhomocysteinemia in rural and urban Indians. J. Assoc. Physicians India 54, 775–782.

York, R., Rosa, E.A., Dietz, T., 2003. Footprints on the earth: the environmental consequences of modernity. Am. Sociol. Rev. 68 (2), 279–300.

Zaman, G.S., Akhtar Zaman, F., Arifullah, M., 2010. Comparative risk of type 2 diabetes mellitus among vegetarians and nonvegetarians. Indian J. Community Med. 35 (3), 441–442.

Further Reading

Heinrich Boll Foundation, 2014. Meat Atlas-Facts and Figures about the Animals We Eat. Heinrich Böll Foundation, Friends of the Earth, Europe.

Jenkins, D.J.A., Kendall, C.W.C., Marchie, A., Jenkins, A.L., Augustin, L.S.A., Ludwig, D.S., Barnard, N.D., Anderson, J.W., September 2003. Type 2 diabetes and the vegetarian diet. Am. J. Clin. Nutr. 78 (3), 610S–616S.

Kaveeshwar, S.A., Cornwall, J., 2014. The current state of diabetes mellitus in India. Australas. Med. J. 7 (1), 45–48.

Shetty, P.S., 2002. Nutrition transition in India. Public Health Nutr. 5 (1A), 175–182.

Singh, R.B., Pella, D., Mechirova, V., Kartikey, K., Demeester, F., Tomar, R.S., Beegom, R., Mehta, A.S., Gupta, S.B., De Amit, K., et al., 2007a. Prevalence of obesity, physical inactivity and undernutrition, a triple burden of diseases during transition in a developing economy. The Five City Study Group. Acta Cardiol. 62, 119–127.

Singh, R.B., Singh, S., Chattopadhya, P., Singh, K., Singhz, V., Kulshrestha, S.K., Tomar, R.S., Kumar, R., Singh, G., Mechirova, V., et al., 2007b. Tobacco consumption in relation to causes of death in an urban population of north India. Int. J. Chron. Obstruct. Pulmon. Dis. 2, 177–185.

Vishwanath, T., Lall, S.V., Dowall, D., Lozano-Gracia, N., Sharma, S., Wang, H.G., 2013. Urbanization beyond Municipal Boundaries: Nurturing Metropolitan Economies and Connecting Peri-urban Areas in India. Directions in Development; Countries and Regions. The World Bank, Washington, DC. Available at: http://documents.worldbank.org/curated/en/373731468268485378/Urbanization-beyond-municipal-boundaries-nurturing-metropolitan-economies-and-connecting-peri-urban-areas-in-India.

Wagner, K.H., Brath, H., 2012. A global view on the development of non communicable diseases. Prev. Med. 54 (Suppl.), S38–S41.

7 ░░░

Religious Variations in Vegetarian Diets and Impact on Health Status of Children: Perspectives From Traditional Vegetarian Societies

Ghattu V. Krishnaveni[1], Sarah H. Kehoe[2], Kalyanaraman Kumaran[1,2]

[1]CSI HOLDSWORTH MEMORIAL HOSPITAL, MYSORE, INDIA; [2]MRC LIFECOURSE EPIDEMIOLOGY UNIT, SOUTHAMPTON, UNITED KINGDOM

1. Religion and Diet

Annapurna (goddess of food), you who are eternally complete, you, the very life of Lord Shiva;

Give me food (in alms) so I can sustain my body to achieve supreme knowledge.

From Hindu scriptures

From time immemorial, food has been an integral part of a religion's spiritual identity. All the world religions promote dietary norms as a means of promoting purification of body, mind, and soul. Religion-based beliefs drive practices related to restrictions on, and prescription of, type of food, seasonal changes in dietary norms, temporary or permanent abstinence of certain foods, and fasting (Davidson, 2003). Many a time, these practices are consistent with the core premise of a religion's teaching. Vegetarianism is strongly associated with a number of religions that originated in ancient India (Hinduism, Buddhism, Jainism) that advocate "ahimsa" (nonviolence). For example, Jainism, which abhors violence of all kinds, prescribes strict vegetarianism. Moreover, the foods that have symbolic importance with a religion are either condemned or recommended. Cows are symbolic of prosperity and sacredness among Hindus, and thus beef eating is prohibited. Milk and other dairy products are preferred, perhaps for the same reason. In Islam, pigs are considered unclean, and therefore eating of pork is prohibited. Some religions instruct partaking of food prepared in a specific manner (e.g., Halal in Islam and Kosher in Judaism). Considering the great impact that diet and nutrition has on health in humans, it is not surprising that religion also plays an important contributory role in determining population health (Diaz, www.leads.ac.uk).

2. The Relationship Between Religion and Diet

The diets of followers of various religions differ depending on the extent to which they practice their religion and their socioeconomic class. The attitude toward diet and vegetarianism in Hinduism today differs from the practices of the past. In historic times, meat eating and animal sacrifices were relatively common among many Hindu castes. However, there were restrictions on meat eating, and slaughter of domestic animals was usually performed for ritual sacrifice. Moderation in diet was recommended; ancient Hindu texts suggest that diets should be just sufficient to sustain the body and soul (e.g., Bhagavad-Gita and Tirukkural). The Bhagavad-Gita recommends that food and water be taken only when hungry and satisfy 75% of the hunger with 25% remaining unfilled (http://www.gita-society.com). Over time, vegetarianism gradually propagated through the Brahmin (priestly) castes. There was a belief that meat promoted an undesirable mental state, while vegetarianism promoted a positive and healthy mental state, which was considered essential for spiritual progress (Bhagavad-Gita). A big fillip to vegetarianism in India was provided during the reign of King Ashoka (c.268 to 232 BC), who converted from Hinduism to Buddhism and advocated nonslaughter of animals. The Krishna schools, which propagate lactovegetarianism, ban not just meat and eggs but also onions, garlic, and mushrooms, which they consider to be associated with baser instincts (www.iscon.org). Most vegetarian Hindus today are ovolactovegetarians or lactovegetarians. Of nonvegetarian Hindus, chicken and fish are commonly consumed followed by lamb and goat; cows or beef are not consumed. Also nonvegetarian Hindus have many religious days on which they do not consume any meat; various groups do not eat meat on Mondays, Tuesdays, Thursdays, Fridays, and Saturdays, leaving Wednesdays and Sundays as the most common days for eating meat (anecdotal cultural beliefs). Thus, even nonvegetarian Hindus have a diet that is predominantly plant-based and not very dissimilar from that of vegetarians. Hindus also observe a number of "fasting" days for religious reasons; these could be marked by intake of just water, or milk and fruits, or avoidance of certain foods such as rice, wheat, and certain vegetables and spices. The number of religious and fasting days can vary depending on the caste and community within Hindus.

Buddhism prohibits killing humans and animals. However, this does not completely preclude followers of Buddhism from eating meat. The original Buddhist monks were not allowed to grow their own food and were dependent on alms for food; they were bound to eat whatever was put in their begging bowls, including meat, provided it had not been killed specifically for them (Davidson, 2003). The division of Buddhism into two major sects has resulted in differences in their dietary practices. The Theravada sect, which follows the original practice of begging for food, allows meat eating as they are bound to accept whatever is put in their bowls. The followers of Mahayana sect are allowed to grow their own food or use money to buy food, and thus they avoid all kinds of meat. The Jains follow a practice of total ahimsa (nonviolence) toward all living beings. Vegetarianism is mandatory, and Jains are either lactovegetarians or vegans. The practice of ahimsa extends to all living beings, including small animals and insects. This results in Jains even avoiding root plants such as onion or garlic, which are uprooted from the ground and therefore liable to cause harm to small insects (Jain, http://www.ivu.org). There are also restrictions on eating times; for example, cooking and eating after sunset was avoided in the past where there was a possibility of small insects being unknowingly ingested in the dark.

The Islam religion does not forbid a nonvegetarian diet (Hossain, 2014). However Islam advocates that all meat/food consumed is prepared in "halal" manner. Halal signifies the manner in which an animal is slaughtered or killed. Food not prepared in the halal manner is not considered fit for consumption. Similarly, Judaism also does not advocate vegetarianism, although some small groups have supported it; again all food/meat must be "kosher," referring to the manner of preparing the food/meat (Davidson, 2003).

Christianity does not promote vegetarianism, although some sects such as the Seventh-day Adventists and Eastern Orthodox Christians follow vegetarianism (Davidson, 2003). Vegetarianism and fasting is also followed by a number of Christians during the period of Lent. Taoism is similar in its approach to Chinese Buddhism. While meat eating is not banned, only the Taoist monks are probably vegetarian, but there are days of fasting and meat restriction, similar to the Christian tradition of Lent.

Sikhism does not recommend vegetarianism, although it does prohibit the ritual slaughter of animals for food. Some Sikhs avoid beef and pork, following the traditions of both Hinduism and Islam. Only a few Sikhs, such as those belonging to the Namdhari sect, are vegetarian (Singh). The Baha'i Faith does not make any preference for vegetarianism, while Zoroastrianism and Shintoism also have some vegetarian sects.

Thus, it is not surprising that all these differing practices impact diet and, consequently, nutrition status.

3. Vegetarian Diet and Health: Evidence From Religion-Based Studies

There is a huge difference in the definition of vegetarianism, not only among different religions, but among different sects and regions within an individual religion. In south India among "upper-caste" Hindus, a vegetarian diet includes consumption of dairy products, apart from plant-based food products (lactovegetarian). Although egg is not considered a part of a vegetarian diet by the majority of traditional followers of the religion, some caste Hindus do consume eggs. Eastern Orthodox Christians are permitted to eat fish, mollusks, and crustaceans during meat-less fasting seasons. Similarly, some vegetarian Hindus in coastal India also accept fish as part of an overall vegetarian diet.

Despite the various different definitions of vegetarianism, evidence from a few studies within specific religious groups shows that following a vegetarian life style has several health benefits in terms of associated lower obesity, cardiovascular disease risk factors, and cancers, and reduction in all cause mortality (Le and Sabaté, 2014). In particular, studies in Seventh-day Adventist (Le and Sabaté, 2014; Sabaté and Wien, 2010) and Eastern Orthodox Christians (Lazarou and Matalas, 2010; Sarri et al., 2003) have shown improvement in health indicators among those who follow vegetarian practices during specific religious periods compared to those who do not. Though these studies are mainly conducted among adults, some have also shown these benefits to be apparent in children and adolescents (Sabaté and Wien, 2010). However, health benefits are less apparent among South Asian vegetarians. A study comparing vegetarian and nonvegetarian adults in the United States and in South Asia (India and Pakistan) observed that South Asian vegetarians ate a less healthy diet than vegetarians in the United States, and they had relatively lower health benefits over nonvegetarians than their US counterparts (Jaacks et al., 2016). The vegetarian lifestyle was more likely to be driven by religious reasons among these individuals.

A significant issue is the quality of dietary proteins in those who are vegetarian for religious reasons. Protein in eggs is highly bioavailable and has higher biological value (Hoffman and Falvo, 2004). However, most Indian vegetarians do not consume eggs. The protein in their diet is therefore mostly derived from pulses/lentils, cereals, and dairy products (Gopalan et al., 1989). While protein in milk and milk products such as curd or cheese are of good quality, plant-based protein sources are generally of poorer quality. Specifically, cereals such as rice and wheat, which form a major source of protein due to the bulk of consumption in Indian lactovegetarians, are deficient in the essential amino acid lysine (Gopalan et al., 1989). Lentils and other pulses have lower levels of sulfur-containing amino acids, methionine, and cysteine. Thus a judicious mixture of various food groups is necessary to provide a balanced protein intake. However, lentils and dairy products are relatively expensive and not always available. Therefore, their consumption also depends on socioeconomic status and availability.

South Asian studies have consistently shown several nutritional deficiencies in adults following religions that promote vegetarianism. From a Hindu perspective, even those who eat nonvegetarian foods follow a predominantly plant-based diet. This is linked to religious practices. Among Hindus who eat animal foods, meat, fish, and eggs are usually consumed only a couple of times every week. The quantity and frequency are therefore considerably lower compared with Western meat eating populations. Some households may cook a sauce with some pieces of meat in it; the sauce is mainly consumed along with a staple such as rice, while the quantity of meat is small. There may be also gender issues: the women in the household tend to fast more frequently and eat last after feeding the men and children (Barker et al., 2006), so they may not get any pieces of meat.

During fasting days, the Hindu diet ranges from fruit, to fruit and milk, to carbohydrate-rich food such as potato and sago. In some instances, a fasting diet with high starch content and binge eating following the break of the fast (Kalra et al., 2015) may lead to greater carbohydrate and calorie intake than their normal diets. Therefore, there are significant differences in those who choose to remain vegetarian for health reasons in Western countries as opposed to those who are vegetarian for religious reasons in low- and middle-income countries.

Growing children and adolescents who have greater nutrient demands are likely to bear the brunt of unsupplemented vegetarian lifestyles. Understanding the deleterious effects of vegetarianism on the health of children, and the need for providing optimum nutritional environment for their growth, right from before birth, within the ambit of religious dictums is important in these populations.

4. Vegetarianism and Child Health: Impact of Fetal Nutritional Environment

The Developmental Origins of Health and Disease hypothesis proposes that nutrition during fetal development has a long-term impact on an individual's health (Hanson and Gluckman, 2011). Indeed, several studies from different parts of the world have shown that both intrauterine growth restriction marked by low birthweight and accelerated fetal growth caused by maternal gestational diabetes (GDM) are associated with adiposity, insulin resistance, increased blood pressure, and other disease risk indicators in children and adolescents (Barker, 1998; Dabelea, 2007; Krishnaveni et al., 2010). These findings highlight the importance of nutrition during formative years in the long-term health of children. A well-balanced maternal diet, with adequate supply of a broad range of nutrients, is essential for optimum fetal growth and development. Studies in low- and middle-income countries such as India have shown that pregnant women are likely to be undernourished, with several micronutrient deficiencies, thus compromising fetal growth (Bhutta and Haider, 2008). At the same time, increasing prevalence of maternal obesity and GDM in these populations has also been exposing the growing fetus to nutritional overload (Seshiah et al., 2004), thus causing a double burden of under- and overnutrition, and thereby increasing the disease risk in children. Some researchers argue that the practice of vegetarianism over generations, which is the main premise of major Indian religions such as Hinduism, may be one of the factors giving rise to the aforementioned associations (Yajnik et al., 2008).

In India, nutritional derangements are common in seemingly healthy pregnant women. Our collaborative group has been engaged in prospective studies examining the influence of maternal nutrition on the health of their offspring for ~20 years. The Pune Maternal Nutrition Study (PMNS) and the Mysore Parthenon study have shown that vital nutrients such as maternal vitamin B_{12} and vitamin D are likely to be deficient in the majority of pregnant women in these regions (Farrant et al., 2009; Krishnaveni et al., 2009; Yajnik et al., 2008). The PMNS mothers were also energy deficient (Rao et al., 2001). Folate, which is supplied abundantly in plant-based diets, was in surplus among pregnant women in both studies. The researchers of these studies proposed that vegetarianism driven by religion was one of the contributing factors for their findings. While in the PMNS rural mothers, thinness, and thus an undernourished status was common, in our study of urban women in Mysore, offspring were exposed to a hyperglycemic intrauterine environment (Krishnaveni et al., 2010). These studies showed that maternal nutritional imbalances as reported were associated with altered fetal growth and childhood risk factors for noncommunicable disease in the offspring (Krishnaveni et al., 2010, 2011, 2014; Yajnik et al., 2008).

The Pune study showed for the first time that offspring of mothers with B_{12} deficiency during pregnancy had higher levels of risk markers for type 2 diabetes such as higher adiposity and insulin resistance as early as 6 years of age, especially in the presence of higher maternal folate status. Subsequently, the Parthenon study in Mysore also observed higher insulin resistance among children of mothers with higher folate concentrations. In Mysore, maternal B_{12} deficiency and high folate status were also associated with a higher incidence of GDM in the mothers themselves (Krishnaveni et al., 2009). Maternal GDM was a strong predictor of increased adiposity at birth in the offspring (Hill et al., 2005). Offspring of diabetic mothers also exhibited cardiometabolic disease risk factors such as higher adiposity, glucose intolerance, insulin resistance, higher blood pressure, and increased stress reactivity even during childhood and adolescence (Krishnaveni et al., 2005, 2015, 2010). Lower vitamin B_{12} status during pregnancy has also been shown to be associated with fetal growth retardation in another cohort study in Bangalore, India (Muthayya et al., 2006); children born to B_{12}-deficient mothers had cardiac function abnormalities that may have implications for their future cardiovascular disease risk (Sucharita et al., 2014).

The Mysore Parthenon study also explored the associations of maternal vitamin D status on children's health indicators (Krishnaveni et al., 2011). The deficiency of this vitamin is common among pregnant women in the Indian subcontinent despite the abundant supply of sunlight (Sachan et al., 2005). Low dietary vitamin intake due to vegetarian lifestyle may be one of the factors causing this. The Mysore studies observed that lower maternal 25(OH)D status during pregnancy was associated with smaller muscle size, lower insulin secretion, and higher insulin resistance in the offspring during early to mid-childhood. India also has a high prevalence of anemia, especially in pregnant women (Sharma, 2003). Dietary factors could be one of the predictors of this. Iron deficiency has been shown to be particularly high in lactovegetarian populations (Rammohan et al., 2012; Mahajani and Bhatnagar, 2015). Maternal anemia has been shown to have significant associations with fetal growth and neonatal health (Rahman et al., 2016). These various studies on different nutrient components associated with vegetarianism in India give an indication of the relevance of cultural dietary practices for the fetal growth, thereby influencing their childhood and subsequent health status.

5. Vegetarian Diet During Childhood

It is well-known that diet plays a crucial role in the growth and development of an individual during early life. Childhood malnutrition is one of the major global public health problems currently, and it has been linked to increased morbidity and mortality among children under 5 years of age (Victora et al., 2008; UNICEF-WHO-World Bank Group, 2015). Both childhood undernutrition and overnutrition have adverse implications not only for the immediate health of the child, but they may also have long-term effects on the development of noncommunicable diseases in adult life. Since children are dependent on their guardians for food, their dietary habits reflect those of their providers. It has been suggested that a well-balanced vegetarian or vegan diet with appropriate micronutrient supplements may provide an optimum nutritional environment for a healthy childhood, and it may even be beneficial in terms of reducing the prevalence of obesity and cardiovascular risk markers in the long run (Di Genova and Guyda, 2007). In Western populations, vegetarian lifestyle is usually by choice, and mostly for nonreligious reasons such as health, environmental, and ethical considerations (Pribis et al., 2010). In these scenarios, a child's nutrient needs are generally met by way of supplements. However, even in these populations, a few individual case studies have reported severe adverse manifestations of vegetarianism in children such as severe vitamin B_{12} deficiency (Di Genova and Guyda, 2007). In India, vegetarianism, in particular lactovegetarian lifestyle, during childhood is universally driven by religious beliefs of the parents. Although the majority of modern families do not expect children to observe extreme dietary practices related to fasting and abstinence, it is likely that a shared cultural environment encourages children to observe some of these practices. This may further exacerbate dietary deficits.

Children in the Indian subcontinent are some of the most stunted and undernourished in the world (UNICEF-WHO-World Bank Group, 2015). In addition to energy and protein deficiency, these children have also been shown to be deficient in several essential nutrients such as vitamin D, iron, and zinc that are not available in plant-based diets (Kawade, 2012; Trilok Kumar et al., 2015; Sachdev and Gera, 2013). These deficiencies are likely manifest in those following lactovegetarian diets. While the intake of some of these nutrients is low in vegetarian diets, the bioavailability of some nutrients such as zinc and iron will be reduced in plant-based diets (Sharma, 2003). India has a high prevalence of iron deficiency anemia, especially among children below 5 years of age (Sachdev and Gera, 2013). Zinc deficiency is also high among Indian children and adolescents, and it has been shown to be associated with developmental and cognitive impairments (Kawade, 2012). Deficiency of vitamin B_{12} has also been shown to be associated with developmental delays in young children in India (Jain et al., 2015). In our study of 9- to 10-year-old children in Mysore India, we have previously observed that a lactovegetarian diet pattern was predominantly found in Hindus, and it was negatively associated with plasma vitamin B_{12} concentrations but positively with folate concentrations (Kehoe et al., 2014). These dietary imbalances may have long-term implications; a combination of low vitamin B_{12} and high folate status has been associated with neuropsychiatric and cardiometabolic risks even in adults (Morris et al., 2007).

Paradoxical to these situations, the prevalence of obesity is also on the rise among Indian children (Ranjani et al., 2016), despite widespread vegetarianism. Researchers propose that growing urbanization and the accompanying nutritional transition in India has led to increased consumption of energy-dense foods and a reduction in diet quality among vegetarians (Singh et al., 2014). In particular, whole plant-based foods such as fruits, vegetables, and nuts are being replaced by refined carbohydrates and fried foods. Thus, Indian vegetarian children are being increasingly exposed to high-calorie junk foods, especially in urban, higher socioeconomic populations. This factor, combined with prevalent micronutrient deficiencies, may be leading to the development of early risk factors for noncommunicable diseases in Indian children.

Some studies have shown general associations of vegetarian-based religions with childhood health adversities, without reference to specific nutritional parameters. A study among adolescent girls showed that the development of secondary sexual characteristics was delayed in Jain girls, who are likely to be vegans or lactovegetarians, compared to a general sample of girls (Chatterjee et al., 2009). In another study comparing childhood mortality rates between Muslims and Hindus in India using the nationally representative NFHS data, it was shown that the rates were higher among Hindus, though they were better off in terms of socioeconomic status and maternal education (Bhalotra, 2010). The mortality rates were particularly high if the mothers were vegetarian.

6. Conclusion

In conclusion, though it is generally believed that a vegetarian lifestyle has several health benefits for cardiometabolic health in adults, religion-induced vegetarianism may confer long-term adverse effects on children's health through several mechanisms. Though the studies described in this chapter do not suggest a definitive role of a vegetarian diet in development of adverse outcomes, the consistency of these associations provide circumstantial evidence for its role. However, confounding effects of other sociocultural and biological characteristics specific to these different religions cannot be ruled out. Future studies should focus on novel methods for identifying these associations more conclusively. More importantly, the focus should be on devising religion- and culture-appropriate intervention methods to prevent the adverse effects of vegetarian diets on health, at the same time as promoting the beneficial properties.

References

Barker, D.J.P., 1998. Mothers, Babies and Health in Later Life, second ed. Churchill Livingstone.

Barker, M., Chorghade, G., Crozier, S., Leary, S., Fall, C., 2006. Gender differences in body mass index in rural India are determined by socio-economic factors and lifestyle. J. Nutr. 136 (12), 3062–3068.

Bhalotra, S., 2010. Religion and Childhood Death in India: Full Research Report ESRC End of Award Report. RES-167-25-0236 ESRC, Swindon, UK. https://assets.publishing.service.gov.uk/media/57a08b16e527 4a27b2000957/60430_Full_Research_Report.pdf.

Bhutta, Z.A., Haider, B.A., 2008. Maternal micronutrient deficiencies in developing countries. Lancet 371 (9608), 186–187.

Chatterjee, M., Chakrabarty, S., Dutta, N., Mukherji, D., Bharati, P., 2009. Sexual maturation and physical status among the adolescent Jain girls of Jabalpur, Madhya Pradesh, India. Anthropol. Anz. 67 (1), 65–76.

Dabelea, D., 2007. The predisposition to obesity and diabetes in offspring of diabetic mothers. Diabetes Care 30 (Suppl. 2), S169–S174.

Davidson, J., 2003. World religions and the vegetarian diet. J. Advent. Theol. Soc. 14 (2), 114–130.

Di Genova, T., Guyda, H., 2007. Infants and children consuming atypical diets: vegetarianism and macrobiotics. Paediatr. Child Health 12 (3), 185–188.

Diaz, S.G. Religion and Food. http://www.leeds.ac.uk/yawya/science-and-nutrition/Religion%20and%20 food.html.

Farrant, H.J., Krishnaveni, G.V., Hill, J.C., Boucher, B.J., Fisher, D.J., Noonan, K., et al., 2009. Vitamin D insufficiency is common in Indian mothers but is not associated with gestational diabetes or variation in newborn size. Eur. J. Clin. Nutr. 63 (5), 646–652.

Gopalan, C., Rama Sastri, B.V., Balasubramanian, S.C., Revised and updated by Narasinga Rao, B.S., Deosthale, Y.G., Pant, K.C., 1989. Nutritive Value of Indian Foods. National Institution of Nutrition, Indian Council of Medical Research, Hyderabad.

Hanson, M., Gluckman, P., 2011. Developmental origins of noncommunicable disease: population and public health implications. Am. J. Clin. Nutr. 94 (Suppl. 6), 1754S–1758S.

Hill, J.C., Krishnaveni, G.V., Annamma, I., Leary, S.D., Fall, C.H.D., 2005. Glucose tolerance in pregnancy in South India: relationships to neonatal anthropometry. Acta Obstet. Gynecol. Scand. 84 (2), 159–165.

Hoffman, J.R., Falvo, M.J., 2004. Protein-which is best? J. Sports Sci. Med. 3 (3), 118–130.

Hossain, M.Z., 2014. What does Islam say about dieting? J. Relig. Health 53 (4), 1003–1012.

Jaacks, L.M., Kapoor, D., Singh, K., Narayan, K.M., Ali, M.K., Kadir, M.M., et al., 2016. Vegetarianism and cardiometabolic disease risk factors: differences between South Asian and US adults. Nutrition 32 (9), 975–984.

Jain, P.K. Dietary code of practice amongst Jains. http://www.ivu.org/congress/2000/jainism.html.

Jain, R., Singh, A., Mittal, M., Talukdar, B., 2015. Vitamin B_{12} deficiency in children: a treatable cause of neurodevelopmental delay. J. Child Neurol. 30 (5), 641–643.

Kalra, S., Bajaj, S., Gupta, Y., Agarwal, P., Singh, S.K., Julka, S., et al., 2015. Fasts, feasts and festivals in diabetes-1: glycemic management during Hindu fasts. Indian J. Endocrinol. 19 (2), 198–203.

Kawade, R., 2012. Zinc status and its association with the health of adolescents: a review of studies in India. Glob. Health Action 5, 7353. http://dx.doi.org/10.3402/gha.v5i0.7353.

Kehoe, S.H., Krishnaveni, G.V., Veena, S.R., Guntupalli, A.M., Margetts, B.M., Fall, C.H., et al., 2014. Diet patterns are associated with demographic factors and nutritional status in South Indian children. Matern. Child Nutr. 10 (1), 145–158.

Krishnaveni, G.V., Hill, J.C., Leary, S.D., Veena, S.R., Saperia, J., Saroja, A., et al., 2005. Anthropometry, glucose tolerance and insulin concentrations in Indian children: relationships to maternal glucose and insulin concentrations during pregnancy. Diabetes Care 28 (12), 2919–2925.

Krishnaveni, G.V., Hill, J.C., Veena, S.R., Bhat, D.S., Wills, A.K., Karat, C.L.S., et al., 2009. Low plasma vitamin B_{12} in pregnancy is associated with gestational 'diabesity' and later diabetes. Diabetologia 52 (11), 2350–2358.

Krishnaveni, G.V., Veena, S.R., Hill, J.C., Kehoe, S., Karat, S.C., Fall, C.H., 2010. Intra-uterine exposure to maternal diabetes is associated with higher adiposity and insulin resistance and clustering of cardiovascular risk markers in Indian children. Diabetes Care 33 (2), 402–404.

Krishnaveni, G.V., Veena, S.R., Winder, N.R., Hill, J.C., Noonan, K., Boucher, B.J., Karat, S.C., Fall, C.H., 2011. Maternal vitamin D status during pregnancy and body composition and cardiovascular risk markers in Indian children: the Mysore Parthenon Study. Am. J. Clin. Nutr. 93 (3), 628–635.

Krishnaveni, G.V., Veena, S.R., Karat, S.C., Yajnik, C.S., Fall, C.H., 2014. Association between maternal folate concentrations during pregnancy and insulin resistance in Indian children. Diabetologia 57 (1), 110–121.

Krishnaveni, G.V., Veena, S.R., Jones, A., Srinivasan, K., Osmond, C., Karat, S.C., et al., 2015. Exposure to maternal gestational diabetes is associated with higher cardiovascular responses to stress in adolescent Indians. J. Clin. Endocrinol. Metab. 100 (3), 986–993.

Lazarou, C., Matalas, A., 2010. A critical review of current evidence, perspectives and research implications of diet-related traditions of the Eastern Christian Orthodox Church on dietary intakes and health consequences. Int. J. Food Sci. Nutr. http://dx.doi.org/10.3109/09637481003769782.

Le, L.T., Sabaté, J., 2014. Beyond meatless, the health effects of vegan diets: findings from the adventist cohorts. Nutrients 6 (6), 2131–2147.

Levels and trends in child malnutrition, 2015. UNICEF-WHO-World Bank Group Joint Malnutrition Estimates. http://www.unicef.org/media/files/JME_2015_edition_Sept_2015.pdf.

Mahajani, K., Bhatnagar, V., 2015. Comparative study of prevalence of anaemia in vegetarian and non vegetarian women of Udaipur city, Rajasthan. J. Nutr. Food Sci. http://dx.doi.org/10.4172/2155-9600. S3-001.

Morris, M.S., Jacques, P.F., Rosenberg, I.H., Selhub, J., 2007. Folate and vitamin B-12 status in relation to anemia, macrocytosis, and cognitive impairment in older Americans in the age of folic acid fortification. Am. J. Clin. Nutr. 85 (1), 193–200.

Muthayya, S., Kurpad, A.V., Duggan, C.P., Bosch, R.J., Dwarkanath, P., Mhaskar, A., et al., 2006. Low maternal vitamin B_{12} status is associated with intrauterine growth retardation in urban South Indians. Eur. J. Clin. Nutr. 60 (6), 791–801.

Pribis, P., Pencak, R.C., Grajales, T., 2010. Beliefs and attitudes toward vegetarian lifestyle across generations. Nutrients 2 (5), 523–531.

Rahman, M.M., Abe, S.K., Rahman, M.S., Kanda, M., Narita, S., Bilano, V., et al., 2016. Maternal anemia and risk of adverse birth and health outcomes in low-and middle-income countries: systematic review and meta-analysis. Am. J. Clin. Nutr. 103 (2), 495–504.

Rammohan, A., Awofeso, N., Robitaille1, M., 2012. Addressing female iron-deficiency anaemia in India: is vegetarianism the major obstacle? Int. Sch. Res. Netw. http://dx.doi.org/10.5402/2012/765476.

Ranjani, H., Mehreen, T.S., Pradeepa, R., Anjana, R.M., Garg, R., Anand, K., et al., 2016. Epidemiology of childhood overweight & obesity in India: a systematic review. Indian J. Med. Res. 143 (2), 160–174.

Rao, S.R., Yajnik, C.S., Kanade, A.S., Fall, C.H.D., Margetts, B.M., Jackson, A.A., et al., 2001. Intake of micronutrient-rich foods in rural Indian mothers is associated with the size of their babies at birth: Pune Maternal Nutrition Study. J. Nutr. 131 (4), 1217–1224.

Sabaté, J., Wien, M., 2010. Vegetarian diets and childhood obesity prevention. Am. J. Clin. Nutr. 91 (5), 1525S–1529S.

Sachan, A., Gupta, R., Das, V., Agarwal, A., Awasthi, P.K., Bhatia, V., 2005. High prevalence of vitamin D deficiency among pregnant women and their newborns in northern India. Am. J. Clin. Nutr. 81 (5), 1060–1064.

Sachdev, H.P., Gera, T., 2013. Preventing childhood anemia in India: iron supplementation and beyond. Eur. J. Clin. Nutr. 67 (5), 475–480.

Sarri, K.O., Tzanakis, N.E., Linardakis, M.K., Mamalakis, G.D., Kafatos, A.G., 2003. Effects of Greek Orthodox Christian Church fasting on serum lipids and obesity. BMC Public Health 3, 16. http://dx.doi.org/10.1186/1471-2458-3-16.

Seshiah, V., Balaji, V., Balaji, M.S., Sanjeevi, C.B., Green, A., 2004. Gestational diabetes mellitus in India. J. Assoc. Physicians India 52, 707–711.

Sharma, K.K., 2003. Improving Bioavailability of Iron in Indian Diets Through Food-Based Approaches for the Control of Iron Deficiency Anaemia. ftp://ftp.fao.org/docrep/fao/005/y8346m/y8346m06.pdf.

Singh, J. http://www.global.ucsb.edu.

Singh, P.N., Arthur, K.N., Orlich, M.J., James, W., Purty, A., Job, J.S., et al., 2014. Global epidemiology of obesity, vegetarian dietary patterns, and noncommunicable disease in Asian Indians. Am. J. Clin. Nutr. 100 (Suppl. 1), 359S–364S.

Sucharita, S., Dwarkanath, P., Thomas, T., Srinivasan, K., Kurpad, A.V., Vaz, M., 2014. Low maternal vitamin B_{12} status during pregnancy is associated with reduced heart rate variability indices in young children. Matern. Child Nutr. 10 (2), 226–233.

Trilok Kumar, G., Chugh, R., Eggersdorfer, M., 2015. Poor vitamin D status in healthy populations in India: a review of current evidence. Int. J. Vitam. Nutr. Res. 85 (3–4), 185–201.

Victora, C.G., Adair, L., Fall, C., Hallal, P.C., Martorell, R., Richter, L., et al., 2008. Maternal and child undernutrition: consequences for adult health and human capital. Lancet 371 (9609), 340–357.

Yajnik, C.S., Deshpande, S.S., Jackson, A.A., Refsum, H., Rao, S., Fisher, D.J., et al., 2008. Vitamin B_{12} and folate concentrations during pregnancy and insulin resistance in the offspring: the Pune Maternal Nutrition Study. Diabetologia 51 (1), 29–38.

Further Reading

Bhaktivedanta Swami Prabhupad, A.C., 2015. Bhagavad Gita as It Is, English, first ed. Bhaktivedanta Book Trust, Mumbai, India.

Vegetarianism. http://www.iskcon.org/vegetarianism.

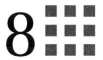

8

Dietary Transition: Longterm Trends, Animal Versus Plant Energy Intake, and Sustainability Issues

P. Winnie Gerbens-Leenes

UNIVERSITY OF GRONINGEN, GRONINGEN, THE NETHERLANDS

1. Introduction

At present, a dietary transition is taking place, in which people shift from plant energy intake toward a larger share of dietary energy from animal sources (Grigg, 1995a; Popkin, 2002; FAO, 2003; Kearney, 2010; Vranken et al., 2014). Globalization of diets includes shifts from local markets toward global trade in commodities, such as animal feed, and processes in which people and ideas spread throughout the world (Lang, 2002) and thereby change consumption. In Europe and the United States, since the 18th century, the dietary transition that accompanied economic development has caused changes in food consumption patterns (Fogel and Helmchen, 2002). In the European Union, for example, consumption patterns tend to converge toward a common diet (Gil et al., 1995). The recent economic growth in developing countries, for example in China (International Monetary Fund (IMF), 2010), has caused dietary changes, especially an increase in the consumption of meat and other foods of animal origin. It has been shown that economic factors, such as income and prices of protein, are important factors for the spatial variation in the consumption of total protein, animal protein, and animal protein as a percentage of all protein (Grigg, 1995b). At present, the increasing demand for protein from animal sources gives additional pressure on limited natural resources needed to produce the food.

Today, there are great challenges to produce food for an increasing global population (FAO, IFAD and WFP, 2015), which puts pressure on natural resources like arable land, freshwater, and biodiversity (FAO, 2003; WWF, 2007; Hoekstra and Chapagain, 2008). Climate change might worsen this situation (Fischer et al., 2002). Globally, food production has a large impact on land use (Penning de Vries et al., 1995; FAO, 2003), freshwater use (Falkenmark, 1989; Rosegrant and Ringler, 1998; Rockstrom, 1999; FAO, 2003; Hoekstra and Chapagain, 2008), and is related to greenhouse gas emissions (Kramer, 2000; Carlsson-Kanyama et al., 2005; Hedenus et al., 2014). Population growth requires the production of more food, while economic development first causes a demand for more food (Latham, 2000) and later also for different food, e.g., more foods of animal origin.

The use of natural resources for food is the combined effect of a specific consumption pattern and production system. There are links between sustainable consumption and the limited availability of natural resources (e.g., Hertwich, 2005). For example, Duchin (2005) shows that a shift from affluent consumption patterns, with large meat consumption, toward a Mediterranean-type pattern, characteristic of Greece in the 1960s, has favorable impacts on the environment.

Today, food consumption patterns show large differences, especially between developed and developing countries. In the world's poorest countries, average food consumption is often small, causing malnutrition and hunger (Azoulay, 1998). Studies on food security show that agriculture can secure physiological requirements, but an affluent diet including meat might not be possible for the whole world population (Penning de Vries et al., 1995; Schonfeldt and Hall, 2012). In the coming decades, social and cultural food aspects might become crucial for satisfying global food demand.

With respect to food, there is a difference between physical consumption and consumption in the form of expenditure because there is a physiological limit to consumption. To provide energy for the human body, requirements are the same as they were in the Stone Age, about 10 MJ per capita per day (Voedingscentrum, 1998). Economic consumption, expenditure on food, however, can rise almost infinitely. Many studies have shown that the overall composition of people's diets corresponds to their income (e.g., Braun von, 1988; Vringer and Blok, 1995; Rivers Cole and McCoskey, 2013; Vranken et al., 2014). In general, when standards of living are low, increasing incomes favor more food and especially more foods of animal origin, while the consumption of staple foods drops (Grigg, 1995a). Beyond basic constraints, larger incomes do not favor more food anymore, but more expensive foods, for example, more meat. Increasing affluence in the Netherlands, for example, resulted in a substantial rise in meat consumption over the last decades, with per capita consumption rising from 36 kg in 1950 to 76 kg in 2014 (Verhoog et al., 2015).

Meat consumption does not rise infinitely, however. In the OECD countries, already in the 1980s, the share of animal products in the diet had stabilized, so the historical trend of rapid and regular increases of meat consumption did not continue (Blandford, 1984). Vranken et al. (2014) have shown that at a certain level of income, average meat consumption will stagnate or even decline. Agricultural studies on food security (Penning de Vries et al., 1995; Bouma et al., 1998) have estimated that a shift from a vegetarian diet to an affluent diet with meat leads to a threefold increase in the land use. Gerbens-Leenes and Nonhebel (2002) have shown that the difference between an affluent consumption pattern and a vegetarian one is even larger than a factor of three. However, this is not only caused by larger consumption of meat, but shifts occur in all food categories. The so-called nonmeat changes in the diet, partly also of animal origin (more oils, beverages, fruits, cheese, ice cream, cakes, and so on), seem to have a large impact on land requirements because, in general, more affluent foods require more land. For example, the land requirement (m^2/kg) for beef, which is relatively expensive, is more than twice the requirement for pork (Gerbens-Leenes and Nonhebel, 2002).

Ehrlich and Holdren (1971) have shown that there are three factors that determine natural resource use: (1) the size of the population; (2) the level of affluence; and (3) the level of technology. Today, especially the Western countries, the United States, Canada, and most countries of the European Union, have reached a high living standard. In these affluent countries, the high living standard goes along with low population growth, high technology levels, large claims on natural resources, and huge carbon dioxide emissions. Developing countries, on the other hand, show a low standard of living that goes along with high population growth, low technology levels, and insecure food availability of inadequate quality.

The specific aims of this chapter are to show trends of the dietary transition, with a focus on animal foods, that go along with economic development and to give an impression of the consequences of this transition for sustainability issues like natural resource use. The research questions are these: (1) What is the relationship between per capita food supply and economic changes? (2) In which regions will large changes in food supply and consumption occur in the next 10 years? (3) What is the impact of dietary changes on natural resource use?

The chapter is based on earlier studies by the same author, especially on a study into "Food consumption and economic growth. Increasing affluence and the use of natural resources" (Gerbens-Leenes et al., 2010) and a study into "The water footprint of poultry, pork and beef: a comparative study in different countries and production systems" (Gerbens-Leenes et al., 2013).

2. Food Systems

Agriculture provides crops, e.g., rice, sugar cane, or wheat, and produces animal commodities, e.g., meat and raw milk. The number of agricultural commodities important for global food supply is limited to about 21 (FAO, 2010). The agricultural commodities provide ingredients for food items, such as bread, pasta, or pizza. Basically, foods consist of only four components: water, carbohydrates, fats, and proteins (Voedingscentrum, 1998; Whitney and Rolfes, 1999; FAO, 2010).

2.1 Production

The 15 main categories of crop commodities, expressed as global production (tons per year), are sugar cane, root crops, vegetables, maize, paddy rice, wheat, fruits, potato, sugar beet, cassava, soybean, barley, pulses, oil seed rape, and sorghum; the 6 main animal commodities are raw milk, pork, poultry, beef, mutton, and goat's meat (FAO, 2010). Starting in the 1960s, FAO food balance sheets (FAO, 2010) give information for almost all countries in the world on annual commodity market supply. The food industry uses agricultural commodities to manufacture foods, e.g., pizzas (Catsberg and Kempen-Dommelen van, 1997). Industry often splits commodities into fractions based on composition characteristics. The fractions form the ingredients for further production, when industry joins in and processes ingredients into food items. Soybeans, for example, are split into an oil and an oil cake fraction (Kramer and Moll, 1995). Oil is used to produce margarines and oil cake for feed. At the end of the 19th century, technological developments in agriculture, transportation, and food conservation stimulated an expansion of the food industry, shifting food preparation away from households to the food industry (Jobse-Putten van, 1995). This has been one of the causes of the dietary transition. Agricultural production determines the availability of commodities for consumer supply. Sometimes wastes are produced that are reused, for example, manure from cows or pigs are used as fertilizer, or food industry wastes are applied as ingredients for livestock feed (Nonhebel, 2004).

The production of meat and milk requires the preceding agricultural production of animal feed. With larger demand for foods of animal origin, especially in developing countries, more feed is needed. In 2020, the share of developing countries in total world meat consumption will expand from 52% in 2003 to 63% (Delgado, 2003). By 2020, developing countries will consume 107 million metric tons (mmt) more meat and 177 mmt more milk than they did in 1996/1998, dwarfing developed country increases of 19 mmt for meat and 32 mmt for milk. The projected increase in livestock production will require annual feed consumption of cereals to rise by nearly 300 mmt by 2020 (Delgado, 2003). This development will put large pressure on agricultural production systems.

2.2 Consumption

Consumer supply provides foods for consumption in a country. Foods are sold in shops or produced in home gardens (Fernandes and Nair, 1986; Pallot and Nefedova, 2003). The repeated arrangements of consumption, characterized by types and quantities of food items and their combination in dishes and meals, are termed food consumption patterns (Gerbens-Leenes and Nonhebel, 2002). Factors such as preferences (Herrmann and Röder, 1995), habits, availability, tradition, culture, and income influence these patterns (Wijn de and Weits, 1971; Ivens et al., 1992; Whitney and Rolfes, 1999; Boom-Binkhorst van der et al., 1997; Vringer and Blok, 1995; Braun von and Paulino, 1990; Musaiger, 1989; Wandel, 1988; Braun von, 1988). For instance, when income increases, people spend more money on food (Vringer and Blok, 1995; Pindyck and Rubinfeld, 2005). Food consumption patterns change over time, although sometimes this is difficult (Ivens et al., 1992). Consumption patterns can differ enormously between communities (Jobse-Putten van, 1995). In the Western societies during the 20th century, food consumption patterns have shifted away from traditional food, mainly harvested from the local environment, toward a diet of market food. Gradually a more varied consumption pattern has developed (Landbouw-Economisch Instituut/Centraal Bureau voor de Statistiek, 2002).

Throughout the world, major shifts in consumption patterns are occurring, even in the consumption of basic staple foods, toward more diversified patterns (Kearney, 2010). The transition is diverse as a result of differences in sociodemographic factors and consumer characteristics, urbanization, food industry marketing, and policies of trade liberalization. Along with the "nutrition transition," there is a process with rising rates of obesity and chronic diseases such as cardiovascular disease and cancer that might be caused by changes in food consumption. Future food policies must consider both agricultural and health sectors, thereby enabling the development of coherent and sustainable policies that will ultimately benefit agriculture, human health, and the environment (Kearney, 2010).

Hundreds of detailed studies from the dietary, social, and agricultural sciences, as well as food security studies, are available. Dietary and social studies express consumption in terms of specific food items (e.g., Mennell et al., 1992; Receveur et al., 1997; Whitney and Rolfes, 1999); agricultural studies on global food security simplify consumption to basic and affluent diets and show them in grain equivalents (GE) (e.g., Penning de Vries et al., 1995), while other studies address food security as the average per capita availability of commodities (FAO, 2003). The agricultural and food security studies often show time trends, emphasizing the need to increase agricultural production. The effect of income on food consumption patterns is recognized as one of the factors that determine food choice (e.g., De Wijn and Weits, 1971; Braun von, 1988; Wandel, 1988; Musaiger, 1989; Braun von and Paulino, 1990; Ivens et al., 1992; Vringer and Blok, 1995; Whitney and Rolfes, 1999; Boom-Binkhorst van der et al., 1997; Regmi et al., 2008; Kearney, 2010). Among the poorest people, be they individuals or nations, diets tend to be composed principally of cheap, starchy, staple foods: wheat, rice, potatoes, cassava, and the like (Jobse-Putten van, 1995; Poleman and Thomas, 1995). Regmi et al. (2008) have shown that food purchasing patterns in middle-income countries shift to the patterns in high-income countries. Convergence in consumption patterns occurs for total food, cereals, meats, seafood, dairy, sugar and confectionery, caffeinated beverages, and soft drinks. Convergence reflects consumption growth in middle-income countries due to rapid modernization of their food delivery systems, as well as to global income growth (Regmi et al., 2008). With respect to meat, the convergence can go in two directions. In developing countries in 2003, people consumed on average one-third the meat and one-quarter of the milk products per capita compared to the richer developed countries, but this is changing rapidly. The per capita amount of meat consumed in developing countries over the past has grown three times as much as it did in the developed countries (Delgado, 2003). Poor people everywhere are eating more animal products as their incomes rise above poverty level and as they become urbanized. Meat consumption does not increase infinitely though. At a certain level of income, average meat consumption will stagnate or even decline (Vranken et al., 2014). An example of declining meat consumption comes from the western Canadian Arctic. Increasing affluence in the Dene/Metis communities of indigenous peoples caused a shift in traditional diets based on animal foods harvested from the local environment, to market foods containing more items of vegetable origin, such as flour and sugar (Receveur et al., 1997).

Existing research often focuses on health issues and changes in time. General relationships between economic change and the rate of change in food consumption patterns are also important to be explored. The dietary transition began in developed countries 300 years ago. It coincided with great economic growth (Maddison, 2003). If developing countries follow the same route, it would mean a major shift in the balance between global food demand and supply, with considerable consequences for natural resources. Especially in countries with large and fast changes in food consumption patterns in combination with a large population, such as China, the impact on global natural resources would be large. In China between 1991 and 2011, food consumption patterns and eating and cooking behaviors changed dramatically (Zhai et al., 2014). The dietary shifts were affected greatly by the country's urbanization. The composition of consumption shifted toward more fats and animal protein. First there was a rapid decline of coarse grains consumption, followed by a decline of refined grains consumption and increases of edible oils and meat consumption. These changes were accompanied by major eating and cooking behavior shifts resulting in unhealthy Western types of food consumption patterns. These patterns are often based on traditional recipes with major additions and changes. The most popular meat type is pork, and consumption of poultry and eggs is increasing. The changes in food consumption patterns include an increase in snacking and eating away from home. Prior to the last decade, there was essentially no snacking in China except for hot water or green tea. Most recently, the intake of foods high in added sugar has also increased. The study of Zhai et al. (2014) has also shown that in the near future, as exemplified by the food consumption of the three largest Chinese cities, major growth in consumption of processed foods and beverages can be expected.

The trend toward larger meat consumption does not change by itself, and interventions are needed. Rivers Cole and McCoskey (2013) have shown that effectively decelerating global meat consumption requires aggressive policy interventions, which, while leaving individuals with less choice, would address the otherwise detrimental environmental impacts of increasing meat consumption. In many developing countries, such as China, the agricultural development policy focuses on livestock promotion, neglecting the potential adverse consequences for human health, which should be taken into account (Popkin and Du, 2003).

2.3 The Composition of Food Commodities

Based on the composition, food commodities form four categories: (1) *starchy staples*, crops that mainly provide carbohydrates with few proteins; (2) *protein-rich crops*, which provide proteins as well as carbohydrates; (3) *oil crops*, providing plant-based fats for the production of oil and carbohydrates and proteins for feed (Penning de Vries et al., 1989); and (4) *animal commodities*, which provide high-quality proteins and fats (Whitney and Rolfes, 1999). The composition of a specific commodity determines the suitability for food and the function in human diets (Whitney and Rolfes, 1999). For example, starchy staple crops, such as maize and potatoes, provide carbohydrates, pulses provide proteins and carbohydrates, and oil crops, such as soybean, provide plant-based oil. Shifts in the macronutrient composition of food consumption patterns also cause a demand for different commodities. With respect to protein, there are slight differences between the protein quality from animal versus plant sources and the reader can refer to Chapter 35 for a detailed review. Briefly, it is important to consider the amount of protein and the amino acid composition of the protein source that make up the diet, together with the energy intake in the developing world. Although many diets in developing countries are deficient in protein quantity compared to recommendations, the protein quality can also be important (Schonfeldt and Hall, 2012).

2.4 The Food System and Natural Resources

The requirements for natural resources for a specific food item, such as meat, are determined by the production system. In general, food items show large differences in the requirement for land (Gerbens-Leenes and Nonhebel, 2005), energy (Kramer, 2000), and freshwater (Hoekstra and Chapagain, 2007), and they differ in carbon dioxide emissions (Hedenus et al., 2014). This results in substantial variations in natural resource requirements and carbon dioxide emissions among food consumption patterns. Several studies have shown that natural resource use varies among food items and food consumption patterns (e.g., Engelenburg van et al., 1994; Kok et al., 1993; Kramer and Moll, 1995; Gerbens-Leenes and Nonhebel, 2002; Tukker and Jansen, 2006; Hoekstra and Chapagain, 2008; Gerbens-Leenes et al., 2013). As a rule, affluent Western-style food consumption patterns need more natural resources than those of poor developing countries (e.g., Gerbens-Leenes and Nonhebel, 2002; Duchin, 2005; Hoekstra and Chapagain, 2007). Hedenus et al. (2014) have shown the importance of reduced meat consumption, especially ruminant meat like beef, and dairy consumption for meeting stringent climate change targets. Tukker et al. (2011) have shown that moderate dietary shifts that include reduced meat consumption give impact reductions of up to 8%. The slightly changed food costs did not lead to significant first-order rebound effects. However, Tukker et al. (2011) have also shown that the European meat production sector will most likely compensate for losses on the domestic meat market and increase its exports. Higher impact reductions probably would need more drastic dietary changes. Westhoek et al. (2014) performed a study into the consequences in the European Union of replacing 25%–50% of animal foods with foods of vegetal origin on a dietary energy basis, assuming corresponding changes in production. Halving the consumption of meat, dairy, and eggs in the European Union would achieve a 40% reduction in nitrogen emissions, 25%–40% reduction in greenhouse gas emissions, and 23% per capita less use of cropland. The readers can refer to Chapter 9 for an analysis of plant-based diet and the mitigation of climate changes. In general, not only foods of animal origin, such as meat and milk, but also fats and beverages have relatively large energy, land, and freshwater requirements (MJ/kg, m^2/kg, m^3/kg). Therefore, all food consumption changes toward more affluent patterns have impacts on natural resource use. For example, there are large differences among water footprints (WFs) of different types of meat that also depend on how the meat was produced. This is shown in the following example.

2.5 Efficiency of Meat Production: the Example of Water Footprints of Meat

The WF is an indicator of freshwater appropriation that includes the water consumption and pollution along product supply chains (Hoekstra et al., 2011). The *green* WF refers to rainwater consumed (evaporated). The *blue* WF refers to surface water and groundwater volumes consumed (evaporated). The *gray* WF refers to the volume of freshwater required to assimilate a load of pollutants based on ambient water quality standards. The WF of meat, for example, poultry, pork, or beef, is mainly determined by the animal feed (Gerbens-Leenes et al., 2013).

Fig. 8.1 shows that, basically, three factors explain the WFs of meat. An important underlying factor is the type of production system, i.e., grazing, mixed, or industrial, since the type of production system influences the feed conversion efficiency, the feed composition, and the origin of the feed. Sometimes feed is produced in an organic way; sometimes it is produced in a conventional way. A factor that is included in Fig. 8.1, but which is quantitatively small, is the drinking water of the animals and other on-farm activities, such as cleaning.

The first factor is the feed conversion efficiency (how much feed dry mass is required to produce meat, irrespective of whether it is grazing forage or concentrates). Fig. 8.2 shows that there is an efficiency increase from grazing to mixed to industrial systems because less feed is needed to produce a unit of meat as the animals in industrial systems are fed more concentrated feed stuffs, move less, are bred to grow faster, and are slaughtered at a younger age. The feed conversion efficiency causes a general decrease of the WF of meat from grazing to mixed to industrial systems. The second factor is the feed composition (what the animals eat), more particularly the ratio of concentrates to roughages. There is an increase in the fraction of concentrates in animal feed from grazing to mixed to industrial systems. In general, concentrates

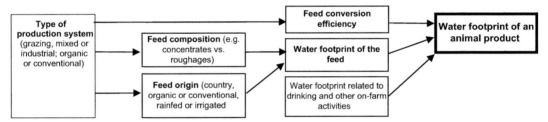

FIGURE 8.1 Factors determining the water footprint of an animal product, such as meat and milk. Three important factors are feed conversion efficiency, feed composition, and feed origin, which are all partly influenced by the type of production system. *Source: From Gerbens-Leenes, P.W., Mekonnen, M.M., Hoekstra, A.Y., 2013. The water footprint of poultry, pork and beef: a comparative study in different countries and production systems. Water Resour. Ind. 1–2, 25–36.*

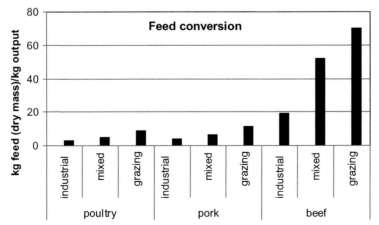

FIGURE 8.2 Average feed conversion for three types of meat for three types of production systems. *Source: Adapted from Gerbens-Leenes, P.W., Mekonnen, M.M., Hoekstra, A.Y., 2013. The water footprint of poultry, pork and beef: a comparative study in different countries and production systems. Water Resour. Ind. 1–2, 25–36.*

have a larger WF than roughage. The second factor contributes to an increase of the WF, especially the blue and gray WF, from grazing and mixed to industrial systems. The third factor is the origin of the feed. There are differences in WFs for feed among countries. The overall effect of the three factors depends on the relative importance of the separate factors, which varies case by case. A specific focus on the blue WF is needed because in the case of blue water use, groundwater, and surface water, agricultural water demand competes with other human demands for water, such as water demands for households and industries.

In general, feed conversion efficiencies are largest for broilers and pigs and smallest for cattle. This explains the general finding that beef has a much larger WF than poultry and pork. However, the large use of concentrates in the broilers feed in all systems and of pigs in industrial systems causes a relatively large blue and gray WF for poultry and pork, in several cases larger than for beef.

In general, the WFs of meat are dominated by the green portion of the WFs. The blue and gray WFs are proportionately much smaller (Table 8.1).

2.6 Food Supply and Income

Per capita food supply depends on a countries' annual per capita income (GDP). Fig. 8.3 shows that supply varies between 1600 kcal per capita per day for low GDPs and 3800 kcal for high GDPs, a difference of a factor of almost two and a half (Gerbens-Leenes et al., 2010). The figure shows that especially for low GDPs, differences per unit of GDP are large, while for high GDPs, differences are negligible, and saturation occurs.

Fig. 8.4 shows the relationship between the macronutrient composition of human diets and annual, per capita GDP.

Table 8.1   Green, Blue, and Gray Water Footprint (L/kg) of Poultry, Pork, and Beef for the World on Average, Specified by Production System

	Global Average		
	Graz.	**Mix.**	**Ind.**
Poultry			
Green WF	7,919	4,065	2,337
Blue WF	734	348	210
Gray WF	718	574	325
Pork			
Green WF	7,660	5,210	4,050
Blue WF	431	435	487
Gray WF	632	582	687
Beef			
Green WF	21,121	14,803	8,849
Blue WF	465	508	683
Gray WF	243	401	712

Graz., grazing; *Mix.*, mixed; *Ind.*, industrial.
Source: Adapted from Gerbens-Leenes, P.W., Mekonnen, M.M., Hoekstra, A.Y., 2013. The water footprint of poultry, pork and beef: a comparative study in different countries and production systems. Water Resour. Ind. 1–2, 25–36.

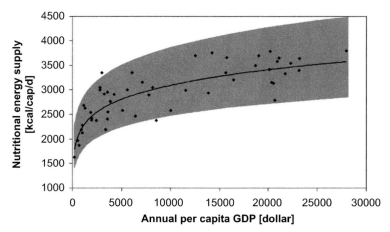

FIGURE 8.3 Relationship between annual per capita GDP (dollars) and dietary energy supply (kilocalories per capita per day). The relationship is based on data from 57 countries in different stages of development in 2001. The *solid line* shows the power-law regression (income elasticity 0.14, $R^2 = 0.71$); the shaded zone is the 90% confidence band. *Source: From Gerbens-Leenes, P.W., Nonhebel, S., Krol, M.S., 2010. Food consumption patterns and economic growth. Increasing affluence and the use of natural resources. Appetite 55, 597–608.*

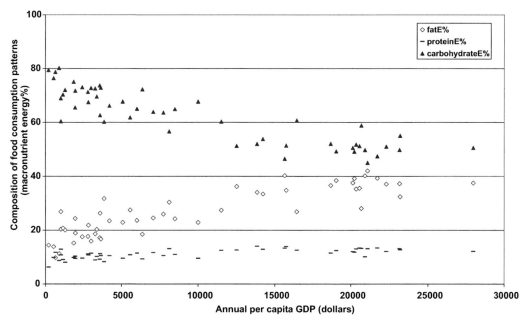

FIGURE 8.4 Relationship between annual per capita GDP and the composition of human diets in terms of the fraction of dietary energy derived from fat (fat E%), protein (protein E%), and carbohydrate (carbohydrate E%). The relationship was based on data from 57 countries in different stages of development in 2001. *Source: From Gerbens-Leenes, P.W., Nonhebel, S., Krol, M.S., 2010. Food consumption patterns and economic growth. Increasing affluence and the use of natural resources. Appetite 55, 597–608.*

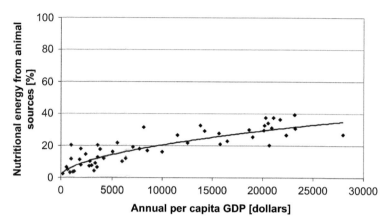

FIGURE 8.5 Relationship between annual per capita GDP and the composition of human diets in terms of the fraction of dietary energy from animal sources; the *solid line* denotes the power-law function with income elasticity 0.52, $R^2 = 0.73$. The relationship was based on data from 57 countries in different stages of development in 2001. *Source: From Gerbens-Leenes, P.W., Nonhebel, S., Krol, M.S., 2010. Food consumption patterns and economic growth. Increasing affluence and the use of natural resources. Appetite 55, 597–608.*

The figure shows that the fraction of dietary energy (E%) provided by proteins is stable, between 9 and 13 E%. The carbohydrate and fat E% show a relationship with GDP. In countries with small GDPs, people derived dietary energy mainly from carbohydrates and a small fraction from fats. In countries with large GDPs, more energy is provided by fats. Fig. 8.5 shows the relationship between the fraction of dietary energy derived from animal sources and annual per capita GDP.

When GDPs are small, the fraction of dietary energy derived from animal sources is almost negligible; when GDPs are relatively large, the fraction is about 25%–40%. The figure also shows that for small GDPs, differences per unit of GDP are large; for large GDPs, differences per unit GDP are smaller. It is important to notice that the fraction of energy from animal sources in the human diet does not increase infinitely. This is in line with the findings of Jobse-Putten van (1995), who has shown that in Western societies, high-income groups consume less meat than low-income groups. However, rich people often buy more expensive meat, e.g., more beef rather than pork.

In general, animal protein has a better quality than vegetal protein (Whitney and Rolfes, 1999). For all countries, the protein E% of per capita consumption was about the same. An increase of the fraction of dietary energy derived from animal foods, therefore, does not imply an increase of the fraction of protein but rather an improvement of protein quality. Especially for developing countries, this improves the quality of consumption. Fig. 8.5 gives the fraction of energy derived from animal foods, not the consumed amount.

2.7 Trends

Below income levels of $5000 per capita per year, large changes in food supply and dietary composition occur for relatively small annual per capita GDP changes. For a GDP between

$5000 and $12,500, changes are relatively small. When annual per capita incomes are above $12,500, food supply and the dietary composition stabilize. This is in line with studies of specific consumer groups that show that increasing affluence causes shifts of specific food consumption, e.g., the study from Rivers Cole and McCoskey (2013). Low-income countries have an increase of supply first, next a change in dietary composition. This is relevant for environmental studies. An increase of a low income initially means that people buy more of the same foods. In this situation, natural resource use is linear to supply. Next, people shift toward larger fat and animal food consumption, and this change continues for longer. This situation requires the production of food commodities with larger natural resource use, such as land and water.

Table 8.2 gives an example of differences in the per capita supply of food items (kilograms per capita per year) for three different countries with different income levels: Nigeria, Portugal, and Denmark. In 2001, the annual per capita income in Nigeria was $1200, in

Table 8.2 Per Capita Supply of Food Items in Kilograms per Capita per Year for Three Different Countries With Different Income Levels: Nigeria, Portugal, and Denmark

Food Item	Supply (Kilograms per Capita per Year)		
	Nigeria[a]	Portugal[b]	Denmark[b]
Beverages			
Beer	8.0	67.4	121.5
Wine	0	58.4	25.0
Coffee	0	3.3	8.6
Tea	0.2	0.0	0.4
Fats			
Vegetable oil and fats	14.2	30.0	43.6
Meat			
Beef	2.7	17.6	17.6
Pork	1.4	34.7	64.2
Poultry	1.7	23.0	15.3
Other meat	2.8	3.6	1.2
Dairy and Eggs			
Milk products	13.5	100.5	141.7
Butter	0.1	1.5	9.6
Cheese	0	7.2	15.9
Eggs	3.5	8.6	15.9
Cereals, Sugar, Potatoes, Vegetables, and Fruits			
Cereals	150.8	82.4	74.6
Sugar	8.8	29.2	40.5
Starchy roots and tubers (e.g., potatoes)	227	138.7	57.1
Vegetables	52.8	123.7	80.0
Fruits	70.3	103.4	64.0

[a]FAO, 2010.
[b]Gerbens-Leenes, 2006.

Portugal $14,000, and in Denmark $23,000 (Maddison, 2003). In Nigeria, the annual meat consumption is small, in Portugal, annual consumption is 79 kg, and in Denmark, it is 98 kg. In Nigeria, the consumption of cereals and starchy roots is relatively large. The table also shows that cultural differences are important. For example, there is a large difference between Portugal and Denmark regarding the consumption of wine, coffee, tea, and beer.

2.8 Future Changes

The main changes in dietary patterns occur in the category of per capita annual incomes below $12,500 (Gerbens-Leenes et al., 2010). If this trend continues, there are important consequences in the coming decade, not only for food security but also for the use of natural resources, such as arable land and freshwater. Currently, about 85% of the world population lives in six regions: (1) the OECD countries, (2) Latin America, (3) Africa, (4) China, (5) India, and (6) the rest of Asia. Especially China, India, and the rest of Asia combine relatively small GDPs with large economic growth rates. In the next 10 years, changes are likely to occur in Asia with per capita food supply increasing and dietary composition becoming more affluent, like the patterns of Western countries, with increasing consumption of animal foods and limited consumption of starchy staples. The case study of Zhai et al. (2014) of changing food consumption patterns in China confirms this trend. Although still based on traditional recipes, China's food consumption patterns and eating and cooking behaviors changed dramatically between 1991 and 2011. Macronutrient composition shifted toward more fats and protein, first caused by a decline in coarse grain consumption and, later, of refined grains in combination with increased oil consumption and larger consumption of foods of animal origin, e.g., pork, poultry, and eggs. Most recently, the intake of foods high in added sugar, such as beverages, has also increased. Zhai et al. (2014) show that the dietary shifts in China are affected greatly by the country's urbanization. The future, as exemplified by the diet of the three mega cities, promises major growth in consumption of processed foods and beverages.

2.9 The Impact on Natural Resources

Increased supply in combination with a dietary shift toward foods with greater requirements for natural resources, such as meat, results in a larger pressure on these natural resources. The European transition toward affluent dietary patterns was a gradual process, taking place over centuries. The economies developed step by step, and agriculture could keep pace with demand growth. Today, economic growth occurs relatively fast (Maddison, 2003).

At present, 38% of the global land area is used for food production (FAO, 2003), and sustainable options to increase land areas are few. Moreover, a global deceleration of yield growth has occurred (FAO, 2003). The pressure on freshwater is also large. Humans already use 86% of the available freshwater, mainly for agriculture. This water can for a large part be attributed to the consumption of animal foods, such as meat (Hoekstra and Chapagain, 2007). The expected global increase in consumption of meat, therefore, will put additional pressure on the availability of freshwater. While land and freshwater are mainly needed in agriculture, energy requirements occur in all links of a food chain. In the past decades, energy requirements for food increased not only due to consumption of different foods but also due to the use of other production and transportation methods (Gerbens-Leenes, 2006). It can therefore be expected that the general trends of consumption also have impact on energy use. Knowledge on the impact of different foods and food categories on resource use provides a tool to indicate pathways toward more sustainable diets, for example, by increased efficiency, prevention, or substitution. Dagevos and Voordouw (2013), for example, have shown that in The Netherlands, a country with an affluent Western consumption pattern, many people are meat reducers that eat no meat at least 1 day per week. Dagevos and Voordouw (2013) especially emphasize the role of politicians and policy makers who have little interest in strategies to reduce meat consumption and to encourage more sustainable food consumption patterns. Given the important environmental impact of animal food consumption and consumer awareness to reduce the consumption of meat, more interest in sustainable food consumption patterns could reduce the environmental impact. Boer de et al. (2006) have indicated that the East Mediterranean diet of the early 1960s, characterized by a relatively small consumption of animal energy intake in combination with large consumption of foods of vegetal origin, has interesting qualities for the development of options to create more sustainable, healthy food consumption patterns. Boer de et al. (2014) promote four options to improve the sustainability of food consumption patterns: (1) smaller portions of meat ("less"), (2) smaller portions using meat raised in a more sustainable manner ("less but better"), (3) smaller portions and eating more vegetable protein ("less and more varied"), and (4) meatless meals with or without meat substitutes ("veggie-days").

3. Conclusions

This chapter shows that throughout the world a dietary transition is taking place, in which people shift toward more affluent dietary consumption patterns with more meat. For small income groups, an increase in per capita GDP goes along with changes toward the Western lifestyle food consumption patterns. A second characteristic of changes in consumption is the switch in the fraction of dietary energy from carbohydrates to fats and to animal foods, while the protein fraction remains stable. People with low incomes derive dietary energy mainly from carbohydrates; the contribution of fats to dietary energy is small, that of protein the same as for high incomes, and that of animal sources negligible. People with high incomes derive dietary energy mainly from carbohydrates and fats, and the contribution of animal sources is substantial.

The importance for environmental studies is that results show that the largest changes in food consumption patterns, and thus the largest increase in the use of natural resources, occurs in the range of incomes below $5000 per year, i.e., in developing countries. With an income of above $12,500, saturation has occurred, and per capita use of natural resources for food does not necessarily increase any further.

The chapter has also shown that it is important how food, and especially meat, is produced. There are large differences in natural resource use per unit of meat, as has been shown for water. The most expensive meat type, beef, has a much larger WF than poultry or pork. However, the cheaper poultry and pork have relatively large blue and gray WFs, which are less favorable from a sustainability perspective.

In the coming 10 years, large changes in dietary patterns are likely to occur in Asia, especially in China and India. These two countries combine economic growth, low income levels, and poor nutritional patterns. Applying traditional recipes, China's food consumption patterns shift toward the affluent Western patterns characterized by large fat and animal energy intake and relatively small plant energy consumption. The European transition occurred gradually, enabling agriculture and trade to keep pace with demand growth. Changes in economic circumstances change the demand for food. A continuation of present economic trends might cause a considerable pressure on the food system because changes are occurring much faster than they did in Europe, causing additional pressure on finite natural resources. Although meat consumption decreases in some countries, the average trend toward larger meat consumption is a process that occurs globally in the world. To decrease the environmental impacts of animal energy intake, important interventions need to be made through policy.

Abbreviations

E%	Energy percentage
FAO	Food and Agriculture Organization of the United Nations
GDP	Gross domestic product
GE	Grain equivalents
WF	Water footprint

References

Azoulay, G., 1998. Enjeux de la sécurité alimentaire mondiale. Cah. Agric. 7, 433–439.

Blandford, D., 1984. Changes in food consumption patterns in the OECD area. Eur. Rev. Agric. Econ. 11 (1), 43–65.

Boer de, J., Helms, M., Aiking, H., 2006. Protein consumption and sustainability: diet diversity in EU-15. Ecol. Econ. 59 (3), 267–274. http://dx.doi.org/10.1016/j.ecolecon.2005.10.011.

Boer de, J., Schosler, H., Aiking, H., 2014. "Meatless days" or "less but better"? Exploring strategies to adapt Western meat consumption to health and sustainability challenges. Appetite 76, 120–128. http://dx.doi.org/10.1016/j.appet.2014.02.002.

Boom-Binkhorst van der, F.H., Winkelman, M.L.J., Lith van, A., von Lossonczy von Losoncz, T.O., Amesz, M.F., Schure-Remijn, P.J.M., 1997. Voedingsmiddelen en dranken in het Nederlandse voedingspatroon (Food items and beverages in the Dutch food package). In: Stafleu, A., Veen, J.M., Vredebregt-Lagas, W.H. (Eds.), Mens en Voeding (People and Food). Nijgh en van Ditmar, Baarn, The Netherlands, pp. 233–234.

Bouma, J., Varallyay, G., Batjes, N.H., 1998. Principal land use changes anticipated in Europe. Agric. Ecosyst. Environ. 67, 103–119.

Braun von, J., Paulino, L., 1990. Food in sub-Saharan Africa, trends and policy challenges for the 1990s. Food Policy 505–517.

Braun von, J., 1988. Effects of technological change in agriculture on food consumption and nutrition: rice in a West African setting. World Dev. 9, 1083–1098.

Carlsson-Kanyama, A., Engström, R., Kok, R., 2005. Indirect and direct energy requirements of city households in Sweden: options for reduction, lessons for modeling. J. Ind. Ecol. 9 (1–2), 221–235.

Catsberg, C.M.E., Kempen-Dommelen van, G.J.M., 1997. Levensmiddelenleer. Uitgeverij Intro, Baarn, The Netherlands.

Dagevos, H., Voordouw, J., 2013. Sustainability and meat consumption: is reduction realistic? Sustain. Sci. Pract. Policy 9 (2), 60–69.

Delgado, C.L., 2003. Rising consumption of meat and milk in developing countries has created a new food revolution. J. Nutr. 133 (11), 3907S–3910S.

De Wijn, J.F., Weits, J., 1971. Steensma's Voedingsleer. Steensma's Food Science. Scheltema en Holkema, Amsterdam/Haarlem, The Netherlands.

Duchin, F., 2005. Sustainable consumption of food: a framework for analyzing scenarios about changes in diets. J. Ind. Ecol. 9 (1–2), 99–114.

Ehrlich, P.R., Holdren, J.P., 1971. Impact of population growth. Science 171 (3977), 1212–1217.

Engelenburg van, B.C.W., Rossum van, T.F.M., Blok, K., Vringer, K., 1994. Calculating the energy requirements of household purchases, a practical step by step method. Energy Policy 22, 648–656.

Falkenmark, M., 1989. Water scarcity and food production. In: Pimentel, D., Hall, C.W. (Eds.), Food and Natural Resources. Academic Press, San Diego, CA, pp. 164–191.

FAO, IFAD, WFP, 2015. The State of Food Insecurity in the World 2015. Meeting the 2015 International Hunger Targets: Taking Stock of Uneven Progress. FAO, Rome.

FAO, 2003. In: Bruinsma, J. (Ed.), World Agriculture: Towards 2015/2030. An FAO Perspective. Earthscan, London.

FAO, 2010. Food Balance Sheets. http://www.fao.org.

Fernandes, E.C.M., Nair, P.K.R., 1986. An evaluation of the structure and function of tropical homegardens. Agric. Syst. 21, 279–310.

Fischer, G., Van Velthuizen, H., Shah, M., Nachtergaele, F.O., 2002. Global Agroecological Assessment for Agriculture in the 21st century: Methodology and Results. International Institute for Applied Systems Analysis, Laxenburg, Austria/Food and Agriculture Organization of the United Nations, Rome, Italy.

Fogel, R.W., Helmchen, L.A., 2002. Economic and technological development and their relationships to body size and productivity. In: Caballero, B., Popkin, B.M. (Eds.), The Nutrition Transition, Diet and Disease in the Developing World. Food Science and Technology International Series. Academic Press, London, San Diego, pp. 9–24.

Gerbens-Leenes, P.W., Nonhebel, S., 2002. Consumption patterns and their effects on land required for food. Ecol. Econ. 42, 185–199.

Gerbens-Leenes, P.W., Nonhebel, S., 2005. Food and land use. The influence of consumption patterns on the use of agricultural resources. Appetite 45, 21–31.

Gerbens-Leenes, P.W., Nonhebel, S., Krol, M.S., 2010. Food consumption and economic growth. Increasing affluence and the use of natural resources. Appetite 55, 597–608.

Gerbens-Leenes, P.W., Mekonnen, M.M., Hoekstra, A.Y., 2013. The water footprint of poultry, pork and beef: a comparative study in different countries and production systems. Water Resour. Ind. 1-2, 25–36.

Gerbens-Leenes, P.W., 2006. Natural Resource Use for Food: Land, Water and Energy in Production and Consumption Systems (thesis). University of Groningen, Groningen, The Netherlands.

Gil, J.M., Gracia, A., Perez y Perez, L., 1995. Food consumption and economic development in the European Union. Eur. Rev. Agric. Econ. 22, 385–399.

Grigg, D., 1995a. The nutrition transition in Western Europe. J. Hist. Geogr. 22 (1), 247–261.

Grigg, D., 1995b. The pattern of world protein consumption. Geoforum 26 (1), 1–17.

Hedenus, F., Wirsenius, S., Johansson, D.J.A., 2014. The importance of reduced meat and dairy consumption for meeting stringent climate change targets. Clim. Change 124 (1–2), 79–91. http://dx.doi.org/10.1007/s10584-014-1104-5.

Herrmann, R., Röder, C., 1995. Does food consumption converge internationally? Measurement, empirical tests and determinants. Eur. Rev. Agric. Econ. 22 (3), 400–414.

Hertwich, E.G., 2005. Consumption and industrial ecology. J. Ind. Ecol. 9 (1–2), 1–6.

Hoekstra, A.Y., Chapagain, A.K., 2007. Water footprints of nations: water use by people as a function of their consumption pattern. Water Resour. Manag. 21, 35–48.

Hoekstra, A.Y., Chapagain, A.K., 2008. Globalization of Water: Sharing the Planet's Freshwater Resources. Blackwell Publishing, London.

Hoekstra, A.Y., Chapagain, A.K., Aldaya, M.M., Mekonnen, M.M., 2011. The Water Footprint Assessment Manual: Setting the Global Standard. Earthscan, London.

Ivens, W.P.M.F., Dankert, G., Eng van der, P.J., Faber, D.C., van Keulen, H., Klaver, W., Lövenstein, H.M., Makken, F., Rabbinge, R., Schoffelen, E.P.L.M., Drijver-Haas de, J.S., 1992. World Food Production. Open Universiteit, Heerlen, the Netherlands.

International Monetary Fund (IMF), 2010. World Economic Database, September 2004. http://www.imf.org/external/pubs/ft/weo/2004/02/data/.

Jobse-Putten van, J., 1995. Eenvoudig Maar Voedzaam (Simple but Nutritious). SUN/P.J. Meertens-Instituut, Nijmegen/Amsterdam, The Netherlands.

Kearney, J., 2010. Food consumption trends and drivers. Philos. Trans. R. Soc. B Biol. Sci. 365 (1554), 2793–2807. http://dx.doi.org/10.1098/rstb.2010.0149.

Kok, R., Biesiot, W., Wilting, H.C., 1993. Energie-intensiteiten van voedingsmiddelen (Energy Intensities of Food Items). IVEM-report 59. Center for Energy and Environmental Studies (IVEM), Groningen, The Netherlands.

Kramer, K.J., Moll, H.C., 1995. Energie voedt, nadere analyses van het indirecte energieverbruik van voedingsmiddelen (Energy Feeds, Analysis of Indirect Energy Use of Food Items). IVEM-report 77. Center for Energy and Environmental Studies (IVEM), Groningen, The Netherlands.

Kramer, K.J., 2000. Food Matters (thesis). University of Groningen, The Netherlands.

Landbouw-Economisch Instituut (LEI-DLO) (Agricultural Economic Institute), Centraal Bureau voor de Statistiek (CBS) (Central Bureau of Statistics), 2002. Landbouwcijfers 2002 (Agricultural Data 2002). LEI/CBS, 's-Gravenhage, The Netherlands.

Lang, T., 2002. Can the challenges of poverty, sustainable consumption and good health governance be addressed in an era of globalization? In: Caballero, B., Popkin, B.M. (Eds.), The Nutrition Transition. Diet and Disease in the Developing World. In: Taylor, S.L. (Ed.), Food Science and Technology International Series. Academic Press, London, pp. 51–71.

Latham, J.R., 2000. There's enough food for everyone, but the poor can't afford to buy it. Nature 404, 222. http://dx.doi.org/10.1038/35005264.

Maddison, S., 2003. The World Economy. Historical Statistics. OECD, Paris, France.

Mennell, S., Murcott, A., Otterloo van, H.A., 1992. Sociology of Food, Eating Diet and Culture. International Sociological Association. SAGE Publications, London.

Musaiger, A.O., 1989. Changes in food consumption patterns in Bahrein. Nutr. Health 6, 183–188.

Nonhebel, S., 2004. On resource use in food production systems: the value of livestock as a 'rest-stream upgrading system'. Ecol. Econ. 48, 221–230.

Pallot, J., Nefedova, T., 2003. Trajectories in people's farming in Moscow oblast during the post-socialist transformation. J. Rural Stud. 19, 345–362.

Penning de Vries, F.W.T., Jansen, D.M., Ten Berge, H.F.M., Bakema, A.I, 1989. Simulation of Ecophysiological Processes of Growth in Several Annual Crops. Centre for Agricultural Publishing and Documentation (Pudoc), Wageningen, The Netherlands, pp. 63–64.

Penning de Vries, F.W.T., Keulen van, H., Rabbinge, R., 1995. Natural resources and limits of food production in 2040. In: Bouma, J. (Ed.), Eco-regional Approaches for Sustainable Land Use and Food Production. Kluwer Academic Publishers, The Netherlands.

Pindyck, R.S., Rubinfeld, D.L., 2005. Microeconomics, sixth ed. Pearson Education, Inc., Upper Saddle River, New Jersey 07458, USA.

Poleman, ThT., Thomas, L.T., 1995. Income and dietary change. Food Policy 20 (2), 149–159.

Popkin, B.M., Du, S., 2003. Dynamics of the nutrition transition toward the animal foods sector in China and its implications: a worried perspective. J. Nutr. 133 (11), 3898S–3906S.

Popkin, B.M., 2002. The dynamics of the dietary transition in the developing world. In: Caballero, B., Popkin, B.M. (Eds.), The Nutrition Transition. Diet and Disease in the Developing World. In: Taylor, S.L. (Ed.), Food Science and Technology International Series. Academic Press, London, pp. 111–129.

Receveur, O., Boulay, M., Kuhnlein, H.V., 1997. Decreasing traditional food use affects diet quality for adult Dene/Métis in 16 communities of the Canadian Northwest Territories. J. Nutr. 127, 2179–2186.

Regmi, A., Takeshima, H., Unnevehr, L., 2008. Convergence in food demand and delivery: do middle-income countries follow high-income trends? J. Food Distrib. Res. 39 (1), 116–122.

Rivers Cole, J., McCoskey, S., 2013. Does global meat consumption follow an environmental Kuznets curve? Sustain. Sci. Pract. Policy 9 (2), 26–36.

Rockstrom, J., 1999. On-farm green water estimates as a tool for increased food production in water scarce regions. Phys. Chem. Earth (B) 24 (4), 375–383.

Rosegrant, M.W., Ringler, C., 1998. Impact of food security and rural development of transferring water out of agriculture. Water Policy 1, 567–586.

Schonfeldt, H.C., Hall, N.G., 2012. Dietary protein quality and malnutrition in Africa. Br. J. Nutr. 108, S69–S76. http://dx.doi.org/10.1017/s0007114512002553.

Tukker, A., Jansen, B., 2006. Environmental impacts of products: a detailed review of studies. J. Ind. Ecol. 10 (3), 159–182.

Tukker, A., Goldbohm, R.A., Koning de, A., Verheijden, M., Kleijn, R., Wolf, O., Rueda-Cantuche, J.M., 2011. Environmental impacts of changes to healthier diets in Europe. Ecol. Econ. 70 (10), 1776–1788. http://dx.doi.org/10.1016/j.ecolecon.2011.05.001.

Verhoog, D., Wijsman, H., Terluin, I., 2015. Vleesconsumptie per hoofd van de bevolking in Nederland, 2005–2014. LEI 2015-120. LEI Wageningen UR, Den Haag, The Netherlands.

Voedingscentrum, 1998. Nederlandse Voedingsmiddelentabel (Dutch Food Items). In: Breedveld, B.C., Hammink, J., van Oosten, H.M. (Eds.), Voedingscentrum (Food Center), Den Haag, The Netherlands.

Vranken, L., Avermaete, T., Petalios, D., Mathijs, E., 2014. Curbing global meat consumption: emerging evidence of a second nutrition transition. Environ. Sci. Policy 39 (0), 95–106. http://dx.doi.org/10.1016/j.envsci.2014.02.009.

Vringer, K., Blok, K., 1995. The direct and indirect energy requirements of households in the Netherlands. Energy Policy 23 (10), 893–910.

Wandel, M., 1988. Household food consumption and seasonal variations in food availability in Sri Lanka. Ecol. Food Nutr. 22, 169–182.

Westhoek, H., Lesschen, J.P., Rood, T., Wagner, S., De Marco, A., Murphy-Bokern, D., Oenema, O., 2014. Food choices, health and environment: effects of cutting Europe's meat and dairy intake. Glob. Environ. Chang. Hum. Policy Dimens. 26, 196–205. http://dx.doi.org/10.1016/j.gloenvcha.2014.02.004.

Whitney, E.N., Rolfes, S.R., 1999. Understanding Nutrition, eighth ed. Wadsworth Publishing Company, Belmont, USA, pp. 3–40.

Wijn de, J.F., Weits, J., 1971. Steensma's Voedingsleer (Steensma's Food Science). Scheltema en Holkema, Amsterdam/Haarlem, The Netherlands.

WWF, 2007. Allocating Scarce Water. A WWF Primer on Water Allocation, Water Rights and Water Markets. WWF-UK, Godalming, UK.

Zhai, F.Y., Du, S.F., Wang, Z.H., Zhang, J.G., Du, W.W., Popkin, B.M., 2014. Dynamics of the Chinese diet and the role of urbanicity, 1991–2011. Obes. Rev. 15, 16–26. http://dx.doi.org/10.1111/obr.12124.

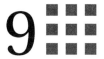

9

Plant-Based Diets for Mitigating Climate Change

David A. Cleveland, Quentin Gee

UNIVERSITY OF CALIFORNIA, SANTA BARBARA, CA, UNITED STATES

1. What Is the Diet–Climate Connection?

The large human impact on the biophysical environment has been acknowledged by the proposal for defining a new geological epoch, the Anthropocene, and the term is already widely used informally (Ruddiman et al., 2015). This impact is unsustainable (Hoekstra and Wiedmann, 2014; Steffen et al., 2015), and a large part of it is from the food system (Foley et al., 2011; Garnett, 2011). This means that the supply-side solutions to increasing demand due to growing population and increasing consumption that have defined the history of agriculture are no longer an option, and the focus needs to be on demand-side solutions (Cleveland, 2014).

Many environmental impacts of diets via resource consumption and waste emissions have been documented, including on water quality, water supply, air quality, soil quality, land use, and biodiversity. Along with animal welfare and human health, environmental benefits have long been one of the major advantages of plant-based diets (PBDs, comprising vegan and ovolactovegetarian) promoted by proponents, such as Thomas Tryon in 17th-century England (Stuart, 2008, pp. 72–73). For example, water is a critical resource, and agriculture production alone (not including the rest of the food system) uses the great majority of fresh water globally: 92% of our water footprint (Hoekstra and Mekonnen, 2012), but with large variations within and between crops (Mekonnen and Hoekstra, 2014). Animal production consumes 12% of groundwater and surface water for irrigation, and the total water footprint of animal production is 29% of the total for agricultural production (Mekonnen and Hoekstra, 2012, p. 408). Changing diets by reducing animal foods in countries worldwide could reduce global water consumption, with vegan diets having the greatest reduction: 14.4% of blue (irrigation) and 20.8% of green (precipitation held in soil) water (Jalava et al., 2014).

In this chapter, we focus on the diet–climate connection, that is, on the relative contribution of PBDs to anthropogenic climate change (hereafter simply "climate change") and its mitigation, since climate change is the major environmental threat to our species and our planet. Increasing concentration of greenhouse gases (GHG) in the atmosphere, which drives global climate change, is a prominent part of human impact in the Anthropocene, and current growth in concentration must be stabilized or even reversed to avoid a greater than 2°C or less increase in average global temperature, which would be catastrophic (Hansen and Sato, 2016; Pfister and Stocker, 2016). While estimates vary depending on methods, data, and assumptions, it is clear that the food system is responsible for a major portion of all anthropogenic GHG emissions (GHGE) into the atmosphere. Vermeulen et al. (2012, p. 198) estimated that global food systems contribute 19%–29% of total GHGE, including land use change and food waste, with production accounting for 80%–86% of this. However, Bellarby et al. (2008, p. 5) estimated that agricultural production alone accounted for 17%–32% of the global total. For the United Kingdom, Garnett (2011, p. 524) estimated that agricultural production was only 40% of the total food system GHGE, while Gerber et al. (2013, p. 15) estimated that livestock alone accounted for 14.5% of the global total, including land use change. Taken together, these and other estimates suggest that the food system contributes at least one-third or more of global GHGE.

Fortunately, there is a high correlation between foods that are good for our health and foods that are good for the climate and the environment in general, as popularized by the Barilla double pyramid (BCFN, 2015). This correlation is slowly beginning to find its way into official dietary recommendations, with one (Sweden) of four nations that have included environmental sustainability in their guidelines mentioning climate change mitigation as a reason (Gonzalez Fischer and Garnett, 2016). However, such recommendations can be very controversial, as in the United States, where the recommendation of the Dietary Guidelines Advisory Committee (DGAC) (USDA and HHS, 2015b) to make this link in the new edition of the Dietary Guidelines for Americans (DGA) (USDA and HHS, 2015a) was not taken by the government, most likely because of the pressure from the food industry, especially the meat industry (Goldman, 2015; Gonzalez Fischer and Garnett, 2016, pp. 37–38).

Research on the diet–climate connection is growing rapidly (Heller et al., 2013), and since 2005, the Food Climate Research Network at the University of Oxford has become a major source of information and discussion (http://www.fcrn.org.uk). Because the scientific study of the diet–climate relationship is in its infancy and methods and data sources are actively being developed and debated, our goal in this chapter is to provide a guide to the key issues that need to be addressed for an informed discussion of the climate impact of PBDs, and to the general conclusions that are supported, and not to comprehensively review the existing data. To do this we address three main questions: *How can diets be measured to assess their climate impact? How can climate impact be measured and attributed to diet? What do we know about the relative climate impact of different PBDs?*

2. How Can Diets Be Measured to Assess Their Climate Impact?

Climate impact is commonly measured by using the metric global warming potential (GWP) of GHGs, in units of the equivalent mass of carbon dioxide (CO_2e), with the GWP of $CO_2 = 1$ (Section 3). There are two basic methods of estimating this impact. A bottom-up, process-based life cycle assessment (LCA) assembles GHGE data from the processes comprising the life cycle of foods in a diet. A top-down, economic input–output LCA (EIO-LCA) begins with data at an aggregate system level, like a national food system, and partitions impacts to the components of the system (e.g., http://www.eiolca.net/). Hybrid approaches attempt to combine the best of these two (Matthews et al., 2016, pp. 257–264), and have been proposed and tested for assessing the GHGE of foods comprising diets. A study of the French diet found general agreement between process-based LCA and hybrid LCA results, but it found hybrid data to be more reliable (Bertoluci et al., 2016).

LCAs of foods and diets in terms of their climate impact require many decisions, which are inevitably influenced by values (Goldstein et al., 2016), much of the data required is subject to varying levels of uncertainty, and methods are not fully standardized (Hallström et al., 2015; Heller et al., 2013; Röös et al., 2014). For example, defining system boundaries, structurally, temporally, and spatially, is a key aspect of LCA, requires some subjective judgments, and is subject to debate. Another important choice in LCA is the unit of the food to be measured and allocated an environmental impact, referred to in LCA as the functional unit. Functional units based on mass (e.g., kg), energy (e.g., kcal), serving, single nutrient, or nutritional index can have very different results (Section 4.1). Therefore, we need to keep asking questions about how all of these decisions are made, what an LCA does and does not include, how impacts are defined and measured, and quality of the data used, but also about their effect on moving toward greater human and environmental health (Cleveland et al., 2015).

The impact of a diet on climate is the product of individual foods' impacts, their quantities in the diet, and the number of people following the diet. The actual diets of different segments of a population, or different populations, can be compared (Section 4.2), model diets can be constructed to highlight different impacts, or interactions and tradeoffs between them, and compared with each other or with actual diets (Section 4.3). A third way is to focus on the individual foods that differentiate diets (Section 4.4). As Katz and Meller (2014, p. 94) note, because "food selection is a discrete choice that can be made at a given time," there is also a practical advantage in making information on the climate impact of foods available as a guide to food choice. However, foods and diets can also be conflated in ways that lead to misleading results (Section 4.1).

The climate effects of foods can be evaluated in two basic ways. *First*, we can compare the emissions of different life cycles of the same food, e.g., broccoli that is grown at a nearby farm that you purchase, cook, and eat within 24 h, and is never refrigerated, versus broccoli grown at a distant farm, frozen, packaged, transported in a refrigerated truck, stored in a retail store's freezer, then in your home freezer, before cooking 6 months after it is harvested. *Second*, we can compare the emissions of different foods that serve the same or similar roles in the diet, e.g., in terms of the nutrients they supply. An example of this is the comparison of two types of milk, cow versus plant-based, which can serve the role of "milk" in diets in the Global North both in terms of their place in foods and meals and in terms of the nutrients supplied (Röös et al., 2016). Major challenges for both of these approaches are idiosyncratic differences, the need to balance the huge resource demands of determining the impact of each specific food choice, and the resulting necessity of making decisions based on incomplete information.

Finally, there are two different pathways by which foods and diets affect the environment, the food system on which most research to date has been done, and the healthcare system, which is receiving increasing attention. The *first* is the process of getting food to the eater, from the production and transport of inputs (e.g., irrigation water, fertilizers), through in-field production (e.g., fertilizer application, machinery, labor use), transportation, processing, storage, and retailing, to preparation of food in the household or institution (Sections 4.2–4.4). To this is added the impact of waste throughout the life cycle, including postconsumer plate waste and human and animal waste. The *second* is the impact of food on the environment after it is eaten, which includes its effect on the health of eaters, which drives the GHGE of the healthcare system, and the productivity of eaters, which affects the efficiency of resource use (Section 4.5).

Having considered how the diet component of the diet–climate relationship can be measured, in the next section, we discuss how the climate component can be measured.

3. How Can Climate Impact Be Measured and Attributed to Diet?

We focus in this section on GHGs because they are the most important drivers of climate change and the most commonly measured climate impact of diet. GHGs in the Earth's atmosphere absorb infrared radiation that would otherwise radiate directly into space, resulting in the greenhouse effect. While the greenhouse effect has been recognized for centuries as a beneficial factor for making the Earth much warmer on average than it would otherwise be (Weart, 2008), the additional GHG in the atmosphere due to human activity during the Anthropocene has changed the radiation balance of the Earth's climate system and increased the amount of heat retained, increasing global average temperatures and precipitation extremes (Stocker et al., 2013). The heat-retention effect of a GHG is commonly measured in terms of its net radiative forcing (RF), with a positive RF leading to an increase in heat energy gain in the Earth system, which contributes to global warming. Current rates of increasing RF are predicted to have major and even devastating consequences for humans and the Earth's climate system (Hansen and Sato, 2016; IPCC, 2014; Pfister and Stocker, 2016; Stocker, 2013; Pfister and Stocker 2016; Stocker 2013). Different GHGs have different values of RF based on their heat radiation absorption properties, their concentration in the atmosphere, and their lifetime in the atmosphere. We begin this section with the question of how the climate impact of dietary GHG can be measured.

3.1 How Can We Measure the Climate Impact of GHGs from Diets?

The GWP, the most commonly used metric for measuring the climate impact of GHG, is "An index, based on radiative properties of greenhouse gases, measuring the radiative forcing following a pulse emission of a unit mass of a given greenhouse gas in the present-day atmosphere integrated over a chosen time horizon, relative to that of carbon dioxide" (IPCC, 2013a). For example, releasing 1 kg of methane, which has a 100-year GWP of 34, has the same RF effect of 34 kg of CO_2 on the climate system over 100 years.

Because of the various properties of different GHGs, it can be quite challenging to estimate the climate impact of individual foods or diets, including PBDs. For example, methane is a powerful greenhouse gas, but it has a relatively short lifetime in the atmosphere of only 12.4 years, producing water, CO_2, and ozone (O_3) as feedbacks (Section 3.2). CO_2 is a weaker greenhouse gas, but it lasts much longer in the atmosphere. So, choosing the time periods to use as the basis for the GWP of the different GHGs is arbitrary (Section 3.2). The major world climate science and policy body has stated that there is "no scientific argument" for the 100-year versus other time periods and that it is therefore "a value judgment" (IPCC, 2013b, pp. 711–712).

There are other metrics for comparing GHGs, but they each have problems. For instance, global temperature potential (GTP) is a metric that considers the net change in temperature at a given time in the future, from a pulse of a GHG, and compares it to the temperature change from CO_2. As with the GWP, the assigned time in the future is a highly subjective decision. In the very near term, GTP can be very high for gases such as methane, but less so for times far into the future (Persson et al., 2015), so that using the very low 100-year GTP may lead to claims that do not accurately capture the climate impact of continual release of methane, or the important potential of rapid emissions reduction.

3.2 Why is Methane So Important for Understanding the Climate Impact of Diets?

Methane from the food system comes primarily from enteric fermentation of ruminant animals and anaerobic decomposition of organic waste including manure and food waste. Production of most plant foods has relatively low CH_4 emissions, with the exception of rice, which has relatively high emissions compared with other crops due to anaerobic conditions in flooded paddies. About 31% of methane in the United States comes from enteric fermentation (primarily cows) and manure management (EPA, 2016), with the largest source from ruminant production, dominated by beef, and globally, about 44% of total methane emissions are from livestock (Gerber et al., 2013, p. 15). For example, incorporating beef carcass GHGE (Pelletier et al., 2010), carcass-to-bone-free weight (Hallström and Börjesson, 2013), and a 100-year GWP of 34 for methane, yields a total GHGE impact of 43 kg CO_2e per kg of beef, with methane comprising at least half (22 kg CO_2e).

However, even though the data currently show a large contribution of methane from animal foods, top-down methods often used in national assessments may underestimate this. For example, EPA estimates of the contribution of beef and dairy production to US emissions may underestimate methane emissions by almost 50% (Turner et al., 2015), yet livestock is the only major economic sector not required to report GHGE (Halverson, 2015).

Because methane's lifetime in the atmosphere is only 12.4 years, using a shorter time frame leads to a higher GWP: the 20-year GWP for methane is 86 (including climate-carbon feedbacks), while it is 34 for a 100-year time frame (Myhre et al., 2013, p. 714, Table 8.7). The effects are less pronounced for other food system GHGs with longer lifetimes, such as N_2O with a 121-year lifetime. Most LCAs that include the climate impact of methane from the diet use the 100-year GWP, and many used outdated estimates as low as 21. The 100-year GWP detracts attention from the potential of reductions in short-lived GHGs like methane to mitigate climate change in the short-term (Scovronick et al., 2015), and because of the large proportion of methane emissions are from animal foods, a realistic estimate of the potential of PBDs to mitigate climate change may require using the 20-year GWP.

While experts may debate the relative merits of GWP versus GTP, the overall implication of either metric is clear: reducing methane, including a move to more PBDs, has the potential to contribute to rapid climate change mitigation. Immediate or rapid reductions in methane release will have a substantial impact in the critical short-term, although sustaining these reductions would mean that the benefits would bottom out in the long run as methane concentrations in the atmosphere drop. Thus, methane reductions cannot eliminate the need for CO_2 emission reductions, but they can make important contributions in the near term for rapid reductions in RF.

3.3 Is CO_2 from Respiration a Greenhouse Gas?

Biogenic CO_2 from animal respiration is usually considered climate neutral, i.e., not a GHG (Herrero et al., 2011), because the CO_2 that animals exhale is from the oxidation of the carbon compounds in the plants they eat, which were only recently created by photosynthesis by incorporating carbon in CO_2 removed from the atmosphere. However, Goodland and Anhang's (2009, 2012) much cited research asserted that 51% of the global anthropogenic GHGE is attributable to animal agriculture, including a large proportion due to respiration. Their estimate of 51% has also been widely cited and featured in the recent popular documentary *Cowspiracy* (http://www.cowspiracy.com/). As a result of criticisms of their work (Herrero et al., 2011), Goodland and Anhang (2012) proposed respiration as a "proxy" for past land use change that has resulted in less carbon uptake via photosynthesis than would have otherwise happened. But their methods are not clear, and the result could be double counting CO_2 from respiration and land use change. The impact of land use change for animal food production may be better analyzed on its own, without respiration CO_2 being included.

However, it is important to recognize that there can be longer term imbalances in the amount of CO_2 going into the atmosphere via oxidation from respiration (or burning) of organic matter and the amount of CO_2 leaving the atmosphere via photosynthesis. For example, release of CO_2 via oxidation of carbon compounds in aboveground biomass and soil organic matter as a result of changes in land use, such as clearing native vegetation for pasture or crop production, may exceed the CO_2 removed by photosynthesis during reforestation or crop growth. Omnivorous diets contribute a large proportion of these CO_2 emissions since animal agriculture occupies 80% of land used for food production globally, mostly as pasture, but including 35% of all cropland (Foley et al., 2011). Castanheira and Freire (2013) have pointed out that the large differences in net CO_2 emissions from soybean production (often used as animal feed) are correlated with differences in the amount of preexisting vegetation and soil organic matter removed and the type of tillage practiced (Section 4.4). An imbalance can also have major impacts over the long-term. There is evidence that deforestation and cultivation beginning as long as 7000 years ago, due to the increase in crop and animal agriculture, led to an imbalance that caused net release of CO_2 into the atmosphere, contributing to global warming (Kaplan et al., 2011; Ruddiman, 2013).

3.4 How Does Diet Contribute to Nitrous Oxide Emissions?

Nitrogen plays a significant role in climate change, in large part due to nitrous oxide (N_2O) emissions from the use of organic and synthetic nitrogen fertilizers in crop production (Galloway et al., 2008). N_2O has a very high GWP both short-term and long-term: 298 for a 100-year time frame and 268 for a 20-year time frame (including climate-carbon feedbacks) (Myhre et al., 2013, p. 714, Table 8.7). While it is released at a rate much lower than methane, its higher GWP makes it a significant contributor to climate change. Since ~35% of crop land is used to grow animal feed (Foley et al., 2011), it is not surprising that N_2O from feed production comprises about one-quarter of livestock total emissions of 53% of global N_2O emissions, while manure is the source of the remaining three quarters (Gerber et al., 2013, p. 15). In countries with highly industrialized agricultural systems, such as the United States, agriculture can represent 80% or more of the domestic N_2O sources (EPA, 2014), where animal feed accounts for about 45% of corn and 47% of soy production in the United States (http://www.ers.usda.gov/topics/crops/corn/background.aspx) (Olson, 2006). Even small reductions in animal foods in the diet can have important climate benefits from N_2O emission reductions. For example, reducing poultry meat consumption in most industrial countries by about 50% by 2020, the current level in Japan, would result in a reduction in global N_2O emissions from poultry of about 19% (Reay et al., 2012).

4. What Do We Know About the Relative Climate Impact of Different PBDs?

A number of studies have examined the diet–climate relationship for diets with a range of proportion of plant foods, and they are in general agreement that increasing the proportion of plant foods and decreasing the proportion of animal foods in diets results in reductions in GHGE per capita. Many of these studies have also documented reductions in mortality and morbidity with increasing proportion of plant foods as well. In one of the first systematic reviews of the environmental impact of dietary scenarios, Hallström et al. (2015) analyzed 12 studies published since 2009, and they found that vegan diets provided the largest reduction in GHGE of up to >50%, followed by ovolactovegetarian diets, although there was variation as a result of the type and amount of meat in the diet and the food substituting for meat in the scenarios. Those studies with results that have not supported this general conclusion are likely to have made questionable methodological or empirical assumptions (e.g., Tom et al., 2015) (Section 4.1).

However, while healthy PBDs generally have a much lower environmental impact than omnivorous diets, their impact will vary depending on the proportion of plant foods with different impacts (Section 4.4). Our understanding of the details of the impact of different diets is also limited due to uncertainty, lack of data, and methodological differences. Another complication is that, although climate impact is often positively correlated with other forms of dietary environmental impact, e.g., on water, soil, and biodiversity, in some cases, it may be negatively correlated. This means that PBDs could result in environmental burden shifting; e.g., PBDs or plant foods that have less GHGE than other diets and animal foods may be more water intensive (Goldstein et al., 2016). There is also the risk of burden shifting within climate impact; e.g., increasing carbon sequestration by adding reactive nitrogen (N) from fertilizers to grazing land could result in higher GHGE due to increased N_2O emissions (Henderson et al., 2015).

As discussed in Section 2, diet–climate studies have used two basic approaches: analyzing data for actual diets and estimating their current or projected climate impacts, and modeling changes in current diets following official national or international recommendations to create counterfactual diets, and then estimating the effects of these diets on health and GHGE. Other studies evaluate the climate impact of specific foods as components of diets. To estimate the total impact of diets, the kg CO_2e per kg of food can be multiplied by the food intake per person and the number of people following a diet. Many of the references cited in this section, and throughout this chapter, provide examples of kg CO_2e per kg estimates for different foods and diets and kg CO_2e per person for different populations.

4.1 What Functional Unit Can Be Used to Compare GHGE of Different Diets?

The most frequent metric used for measuring GHGE related to diets is kg CO_2e per some functional unit, for example, kg CO_2e per kg mass, per kcal, or per gram of protein. Using LCA, researchers can determine the GHGE per functional unit associated with different foods. The most comprehensive review of LCAs of climate impact of food and diets found that plant foods such as grains, soy, and other legumes, refined sugars, oils, and fruits, and vegetables generally had relatively low GHGE per kcal, per gram of protein, and per serving, while animal foods such as red meat, fish, and dairy had much higher GHGE per each of these units (Tilman and Clark, 2014). One exception was that due to their relatively low caloric content, vegetables had slightly higher emissions than dairy and eggs per kilocalorie.

A main reason for the higher GHGE intensity of animal foods is their lower efficiency in terms of resources required, and therefore more emissions, per unit of food output compared with plant foods. In other words, eating plants, which convert solar energy to food energy, is more efficient than eating animals that eat the plants since the animals consume primary production before humans consume the animals. While the degree of relatively greater efficiency varies according to the data and methods used, all studies support this conclusion. For example, one estimate for the United States is that per kcal consumed by humans, beef requires 163 times more land, 18 times more water, and 19 times more nitrogen, and produces 11 times more CO_2e than the average for three staple plant foods (wheat, potatoes, rice); and per gram of protein consumed, beef requires 42, 2, and 4 times these resources, and it produces 3 times the CO_2e than the three plant foods (calculations based on Eshel et al., 2014:SI). A study of the Swedish food system compared high-protein plant foods such as soybean, with beef, and found that per gram of protein, beef required 18 times the amount of energy, and it emitted 71 times the CO_2e as soybean (calculations based on Gonzalez et al., 2011). At the global level, an analysis of 120 LCA publications found that ruminant meat had the highest GHGE per serving, per gram of protein, and per kcal, mostly due to methane emissions; for example, per gram of protein, ruminant meat produces over 250 times as much GHGE as legumes (Tilman and Clark, 2014).

GHGE per functional unit is useful to get a sense of the impact of a given food. However, problems can arise when comparing diets based on a single functional unit, for example, energy (kcal), because the types of foods used to satisfy the energy requirement of alternative dietary scenarios can vary significantly in other ways. For instance, two studies (Tom et al., 2015; Vieux et al., 2012) analyzed dietary scenarios that included reduction in meat intake replaced by an increase in fruit and vegetable intake on a calorie for calorie basis and found that this resulted in equal or increased GHGE compared with current diets. The promotional material for Tom et al. (Rea, 2016), and subsequent popular media reports, emphasized the claim that lettuce has higher GHGE than bacon per kcal. However, replacing animal foods with plant foods on a caloric basis is a category error because these foods provide different nutrients; plant foods with high vitamin and mineral densities can have low energy density, leading to high CO_2e per kg.

One alternative to using individual functional units is to estimate the GHGE using a nutritional profile of a diet or food, but this can also be misleading. For example, Smedman et al. (2010) developed a Nutrient Density to Climate Impact (NDCI) index to evaluate different beverages in the Swedish diet, and they found cow milk more GHGE efficient than soy or oat milks, even though its CO_2e emissions per kg were over three times higher. However, Röös et al. observed that though it is important to include nutritional aspects of a beverage in the functional unit for populations with protein and micronutrient deficiency, for populations like that of Sweden that over consume most nutrients, the function of milk as a beverage may be to "wash down food and provide water." So, a more appropriate functional unit than the NDCI would be 1 kg or 1 L of beverage (Röös et al., 2014, p. 89). Three of the four authors of the Smedman paper were also employed by the Swedish Dairy Association.

Therefore, while functional units are the necessary basis for comparing the GHGE of foods, and thus of diets, for meaningful results they need to be used in ways that reflect the overall goal of improving nutrition and health, while reducing GHGE, and be relevant to the context in which they are applied. This implies that, as Hamm pointed out in reference to the misinterpretation of their results by the authors of the Tom et al. paper, diet–climate studies require a broad interdisciplinary perspective (Hamm, 2016). In the following sections, we look at how this has been accomplished in some important studies relevant to PBDs.

4.2   How Do the GHGE of Existing Diets Compare?

Studies of existing diets show that those that are more plant based have lower GHGE. Scarborough et al.'s analysis of the self-reported dietary patterns of 65,000 participants in the United Kingdom found that high meat eaters had 1.9 times and medium meat eaters about 1.5 times the GHGE as a ovolactovegetarian, and an average meat eater had about 2 times and a high meat eater 2.5 times the GHGE as a vegan eater (Scarborough et al., 2014).

The future impact of existing diets can also be compared. In one of the most exhaustive analyses of the diet–climate connection globally, Tilman and Clark (2014) defined global regions and examined the environmental effects projected to 2050 of current dietary patterns: Mediterranean, pescetarian, ovolactovegetarian, and income-dependent projection of current conventional omnivorous diets. To forecast 2050 diets assuming continuation of past trends, they used about 50 years of data for 100 of the world's more populous nations, and to estimate the GHGE of foods from cradle to farm gate, they used data from 120 LCA publications. They found that an omnivorous diet had about 4 times the GHGE per kcal as a ovolactovegetarian diet, and animal foods had much higher GHGE per kcal, per protein, and per serving than plant foods. Although they did not examine vegan diets separately, dairy accounted for about 40% of GHGE in the ovolactovegetarian diet. In terms of land required to supply the diets, the income-dependent diet required more than two times the additional cropland as the alternative diets. They also estimated the effects of the three alternative diets on mortality, type II diabetes, cancer, and chronic coronary heart disease, based on 10 million person-years of observations on diet and health, which showed reductions in relative risk for these diseases of ~5%–40% for the more PBDs compared their regional conventional omnivorous diets.

Because of the difficulty of having participants follow assigned diets, intervention studies are less common. One intervention study assigned 63 adults randomly to one of five diets— vegan, ovolactovegetarian, pescetarian, semivegetarian (reduced meat omnivorous), and omnivorous—and evaluated their N-footprint (reactive nitrogen released into the environment) at 2 and 6 months (Turner-McGrievy et al., 2016). It found that the vegan diet had significantly lower N-footprint than the other diets, which would mean lower N_2O emissions.

4.3   What Can Model Diets Tell Us?

Most studies of the diet–climate connection look at the relative effects of different model diets, including comparisons with existing diets. Heller et al. looked at the effect of changing the US diet qualitatively, based on the USDA recommended food pattern diet (USDA and HHS, 2010), and quantitatively, by reducing energy intake from the current average of 2534 kcal per day to the recommended 2000 (Heller and Keoleian, 2015). They found that the qualitative change alone actually increased CO_2e per capita per day by 12% from 3.6 to 4.0, while also adding the reduction in energy intake resulted in an overall emissions reduction of only 1%. The main reason for these results is that GHGE reduction due to a reduction in meat consumption was balanced by an increase in GHGE from an increase in dairy consumption, and to a lesser extent by an increase in seafood, fruit, oils, and vegetables. However, 2000 kcal per day USDA recommended ovolactovegetarian and vegan diets reduced emissions from the current diet by 33% and 53%, respectively, which suggests that reducing or eliminating dairy may be critical for reducing the climate impact of PBDs, and that increases in beans/peas, nuts, and soy are also highly beneficial.

Bajželj et al. (2014) created a model relating global land use and agricultural biomass flow, and six scenarios of future impacts based on predictions of future food consumption and required production to 2050. Three of the scenarios were based on current yield trends, and three on the difference between actual and potential yield via sustainable intensification to the point of yield-gap closure, which included improved irrigation efficiency and elimination of overfertilization. Food waste reduction of 50% and dietary change (reduction in sugars, saturated fats, livestock products) were the two demand-side measures that further defined two each of the yield scenarios. For each scenario they estimated forest losses, carbon emissions (from land use change and agricultural production), fertilizer use, and irrigation.

They then compared the annual GHGE of the six scenarios in relation to the estimated GHGE target for 2050 required to stay under a 2°C increase in average global temperature, and they found that the business as usual (BAU) scenario (current yield trends with no food waste reduction or diet change) would almost reach this target, meaning that all sources of GHGE other than food would have to reduce emissions to almost zero to avoid >2°C increase. Even the scenario with yield-gap closure and 50% reduction in food waste reached half of the target GHGE by 2050, but adding diet change reduced this to one-quarter. This implied to the authors that avoiding catastrophic climate change requires changing diets by reducing animal foods. They concluded that when mitigation strategies include significant demand-side measures (food waste reductions and diet change), it is possible to prevent increased agricultural expansion and to decrease GHGE, and that the implementation of healthy diets would greatly benefit both the environment and the general health of the population in regions where excessive consumption of energy-rich food occurs, or may develop.

Springmann et al. (2016) modeled the regional and global effects on GHGE, morbidity, and the economy by 2050 of three model diets—a healthy global diet, ovolactovegetarian diet (VGT), and a vegan diet (VGN)—in comparison with a BAU reference diet (REF) based on FAO projections. They used a risk assessment model to assess the effects on mortality of exposure to dietary changes in red meat and fruits and vegetables, and they linked model diets for different regions to GHGE using a previously published analysis of LCAs (Tilman and Clark, 2014).

They found that with the REF diet, CO_2e would increase >50% by 2050 to >11 Gt per year, whereas the VGT and VGN diets resulted in CO_2e emissions in 2050 that were

45%–55% lower than in 2005–07, and 63%–70% less than REF emissions in 2050 (Springmann et al., 2016). Their estimates for reduced GHGE were conservative because they did not include GHGE from land use change or better health outcomes. They found that the largest absolute reduction in emissions occurred in the Global South, while the largest per capita reduction in emissions occurred in the Global North (which would contribute to food and climate justice). Their most important result was that for a GHGE reduction pathway that would limit global temperature increase to 2°C, the ratio of food-related CO_2e emissions to all emissions increased from 16% in 2005–07 to 52% by 2050 for the REF diet, but it decreased by 1% for the VGN diet. In other words, supporting the conclusion of Bajželj et al. (2014), for the food system to make a pro rata contribution to GHGE reductions to keep global warming <2°C, the vegan (VGN) diet would be necessary.

While most estimates of GHGE from foods or diets do not include LUC because of difficulty in measuring it, it likely accounts for a large portion of diet GHGEs, especially if historical LUC is included (Ruddiman, 2013; Ruddiman et al., 2015) (Section 3.3). Erb et al. (2016) created scenarios based on assumptions about future yields, agricultural areas, livestock feed, and human diets, and they evaluated them in terms of their potential to avoid deforestation. They found that diets were the strongest determinants, and that vegan diets had the largest number of feasible scenarios. "A vegan or [lacto-ovo-]vegetarian diet is associated with only half the cropland demand, grazing intensity and overall biomass harvest of comparable meat-based human diets," and it would also have health benefits. They concluded that this reinforced the importance of demand-side measures for sustainability.

4.4 What Are the GHGE of Different Foods?

As we have seen, PBDs in general are clearly more climate friendly than omnivorous diets; however, the specific food choices can have a large effect on the magnitude of this difference. A number of studies have compared the climate impact of plant and animal foods in terms of different functional units, and we summarized some of these in Section 4.1. Also important for understanding the relative climate impact of PBDs are differences in GHGE among animal foods and among plant foods, and differences for the same foods depending on their life cycles, e.g., how they were grown, transported, processed, stored, or cooked. Extensive data bases of GHGE of different foods in Excel format are available online for the Barilla double pyramid (BCFN, 2015) and Tilman and Clark's analysis of global diets (Tilman and Clark, 2014), and one company makes their database on food carbon footprint available to researchers (http://www.cleanmetrics.com/).

As PBDs increase in popularity, so have plant-based substitutes for animal foods and studies of their comparative climate impacts. For example, a study comparing oat and dairy milk on two model Swedish farms compared the environmental impact of producing oat drink with cow milk in terms of biodiversity conservation, requirements for beef and protein, the opportunity cost of land, and the different protein content of oat and cow milk (Röös et al., 2016). They found "great potential for reduced climate impact" with oat milk, even while keeping some cow milk production.

The relative climate impact of PBDs will depend on the animal foods in the omnivorous diets they are compared with, and there is variability in GHGE between animal foods. Eshel et al.'s 2014 top-down EIO-LCA found that for the United States, beef had much higher GHGE than other animal foods. However, there can also be high variability within categories of animal foods, depending primarily on different production methods, as found in a study of meat consumed in Sweden, where the CO_2e per kg of beef varied from 20 to 41 kg (Hallström et al., 2014). Land use change can make large contributions to animal food emissions, and thus it is important to include if possible when comparing PBDs with standard omnivorous diets. For example, Nijdam et al. (2012) found an upper bound of 129 kg CO_2e per kg beef for extensive systems in Brazil, which involve a significant amount of land use change.

There can also be high variability within plant food categories due to differences in land use change. Soy is a common component of PBDs, valued for its high protein content (~8 g protein per cup, similar to cow milk), and it is often assumed to have a smaller climate impact than animal foods. Castanheira and Freire (2013) compared the GHGE of soybean grown in different ecozones, on different types of land, and using different tillage methods, and they found a very high degree of variability due to LUC, with the highest for conversion of tropical rainforest (17.8 kg CO_2e per kg of soybean) and the lowest for degraded grassland (0.1 kg CO_2e per kg of soybean). When land use change is not considered, the GHGE intensity only varied between 0.3 and 0.6 kg CO_2e per kg of soybean. In addition, all tillage systems had higher GHGE than the corresponding no-till system.

Fruits and vegetables are a major component of PBDs, and increasing their consumption in most diets for their nutritional benefits is commonly recommended (Katz and Meller, 2014), yet there can be a great deal of variation in their GHGE. For example, a study in Switzerland found large differences in CO_2e per kg for different fruits and vegetables, and for individual fruits and vegetables, depending on origin and mode of transport, and on whether they were produced in heated greenhouses (Stoessel et al., 2012). Another study found the kg CO_2e per kg for Swedish tomatoes was approximately 3–4 times that of Swedish carrots, due to the emissions from building and heating greenhouses (Röös and Karlsson, 2013).

Local foods, especially fruits and vegetables, are often assumed to be more climate friendly than imported foods, primarily because of less GHGE from transport (Cleveland et al., 2015). However, regardless of the many other benefits of local food systems, local fruits and vegetables may not have significantly lower GHGE than imported ones. A study of one county in California found that completely localizing fruit and vegetable consumption from the current level of 94% of fruits and vegetables imported from outside of the county to zero imported would reduce GHGE by less than 1% of a household's total emissions for food (Cleveland et al., 2011), in part because direct transport (farm gate to retail, or food miles) only accounts for 11% of GHGE for fruits and vegetables in the United States (Weber and Matthews, 2008). Similarly, a study in the United Kingdom found that if consumers drove more than 7.4 km to purchase organic produce at a farm stand, the GHGE would be more than from a large-scale delivery system that included imported produce, cold storage, packing, and transport to the consumer (Coley et al., 2009).

Food waste is a major contributor to climate impact because a large proportion of food produced is never eaten, and every kilogram of food wasted adds to GHGE and increases the amount of food that needs to be produced to replace it. However, the level of waste differs between foods and combined with different emissions rates, results in different total effects, and here again, PBDs appear more climate friendly than omnivorous ones. One study that modeled the effect of reducing food waste in the United States found that animal foods contributed to GHGE from waste disproportionately, accounting for 74% of CO_2e emissions, but only 33% of waste by mass, with ruminant meat (beef, veal, lamb) having the largest disparity, accounting for 31% of emissions from waste but only 3% by mass (Heller and Keoleian, 2015). Fruits and vegetables by contrast accounted for 33% of waste by mass but only 8% of CO_2e emissions.

4.5 What Are the Climate Impacts of the Effect of PBDs via the Healthcare System?

The food we eat also affects the climate after we eat it, through its influence on health and the healthcare system, and standard diets today have a high burden of disease. For example, the current US health system contributes upward of 16% or more of the US gross domestic product, healthcare GHGE is 8% of the domestic GHGE (Chung and Meltzer, 2009), and diet is a major contributor to the healthcare costs of noncommunicable diseases (Frazão, 1999). As we have seen, PBD's not only have lower GHGE than omnivorous diets, but they are generally healthier.

Hallström et al. (2017) modeled healthier alternative diets (HADs) and analyzed the associated reductions in relative risk of three noncommunicable diseases (type 2 diabetes, coronary heart diseases, and colorectal cancer) strongly linked to diet. They calculated the healthcare costs of each disease and the GHGE of those costs. They found that diets with reduced red and processed meat and refined grains, and increased fruits, vegetables, whole grains, beans, and peas, had 20%–45% lower relative risk for the three diseases and, therefore, lower healthcare costs and associated GHGE. Differences in healthcare costs contributed to differences in GHGE. For example, hospital services and pharmaceutical manufacturing have higher GHGE per dollar of economic activity than physician office services, and different diseases, such as coronary heart disease and type II diabetes, utilize such medical services in different proportions and magnitudes. More specifically, pharmaceuticals make up about 30% of economic activity for diabetes but only about 9.7% for coronary heart disease.

While the study did not consider a complete PBD, the HAD that eliminated red and processed meat resulted in 84 kg CO_2e savings per capita per year from reduced health care costs. Although this is a small portion of a typical American's total carbon footprint (about 0.5%), it likely greatly underestimates the potential because many diseases (e.g., hypertension, stroke, and forms of cancer other than colorectal cancer) associated with the foods changed in the HADs were not included due to lack of adequate documentation of relative risk. In addition, there are also potential diet–disease links for animal foods not changed in the HADs, e.g., dairy.

A less direct diet–climate link is via the effect of diet on body weight. Overweight and obesity have been increasing dramatically worldwide (Ng et al., 2014); they accounted for 6.2% of total human biomass in 2005 (Walpole et al., 2012), and they are associated with dietary change including higher intake of animal foods (Tilman and Clark, 2014), as well as with lower levels of physical activity. Overweight and obesity can increase GHGE via several pathways: increased healthcare system emissions due to association with increased incidence and prevalence of diseases such as diabetes and cancer (Hua et al., 2016) discussed earlier; increased consumption leading to increased food production, which increases emissions throughout the food chain, including from increased human waste; and increased body weight leading to increased transportation burden (Michaelowa and Dransfeld, 2008). Because healthy PBDs compared with standard diets are associated with weight loss (Barnard et al., 2015), and overweight and obesity lead to higher GHGE, a move to more PBDs has the potential to contribute to climate change mitigation, as well as improved health.

A survey of 3463 people in Australia found that both overweight and obesity were independently associated with higher CO_2 emissions from transport, which was mostly explained by greater use of motorized travel, while active transport (walking or cycling) was associated with lower CO_2 emissions (Goodman et al., 2012). The increase in food system GHGE is also evident as increased metabolic rate and respiration CO_2 emissions: based on changes in resting metabolic rate in a 6-month weight loss study, Gryka et al. (2012) estimated that if all obese and overweight adults over 20 years worldwide reduced their weight by 10 kg and maintained it over one year, it would result in a reduction in CO_2 emissions equal to 0.2% of CO_2 from fossil fuel burning and cement manufacture. However, it is important not to double count respiration CO_2 due to obesity and overweight and the life cycle CO_2 emissions from the extra food consumed (Section 3.3).

In addition, the reduction in GHGE and resulting climate change mitigation from a change to more PBDs would also reduce the negative health impacts of climate change itself, which are both direct due to increased temperatures, air and water pollution, extreme weather events, and vector borne diseases (e.g., in the United States USGCRP 2016), and indirectly as the result of disruptions to food production and distribution (Porter et al., 2014). This would, in turn, contribute to reduced GHGE from the healthcare system.

5. Conclusion

While there are many uncertainties, data gaps, and methodological issues that make discerning the detailed effects of PBDs on the climate in comparison with omnivorous diets difficult, the broad picture is clear: most PBDs have much lower GHGE than omnivorous diets, and they can make an important contribution to the urgent task of avoiding catastrophic climate change. Thus, the potential of PBDs to mitigate climate change, as well to increase human health and benefit the environment in general, strongly suggests the need for increasing adoption of PBDs. One of the biggest challenges may be the food industry, which, as mentioned in the introduction, has challenged the inclusion of environmental criteria in dietary guidelines and has actively opposed plant-based food alternatives to animal foods, like mayonnaise, in the market place (Charles, 2015). Meeting this challenge will likely require strong government positions to counter animal food industry resistance (Gonzalez Fischer and Garnett, 2016, p. 63). Another related major challenge is motivating diet change. To support change to more PBDs to mitigate climate change, we will need more action-oriented research on the determinants of diet change by individuals and communities, on the policies that can best support them in that change, and how to motivate the policy makers (Garnett et al., 2015).

Acknowledgments

We thank Elinor Hallström and Daniela Soleri for discussions of topics in this chapter.

References

Bajželj, B., Richards, K.S., Allwood, J.M., Smith, P., Dennis, J.S., Curmi, E., Gilligan, C.A., 2014. Importance of food-demand management for climate mitigation. Nat. Clim. Change 4, 924–929. http://dx.doi.org/10.1038/nclimate2353.

Barnard, N.D., Levin, S.M., Yokoyama, Y., 2015. A systematic review and meta-analysis of changes in body weight in clinical trials of vegetarian diets. J. Acad. Nutr. Diet. 115 (6), 954–969. http://dx.doi.org/10.1016/j.jand.2014.11.016.

BCFN (Barilla Center for Food & Nutrition), 2015. Double Pyramid 2015: Recommendations for a Sustainable Diet. Barilla Center for Food & Nutrition, Parma, Italy. http://www.barillacfn.com/en/publications/double-pyramid-2015-recommendations-for-a-sustainable-diet.

Bellarby, J., Foereid, B., Hastings, A., Smith, P., 2008. Cool Farming: Climate Impacts of Agriculture and Mitigation Potential. Greenpeace, Amsterdam. http://www.greenpeace.org/international/en/publications/reports/cool-farming-full-report/.

Bertoluci, G., Masset, G., Gomy, C., Mottet, J., Darmon, N., 2016. How to build a standardized country-specific environmental food database for nutritional epidemiology studies. PLoS One 11 (4), e0150617. http://dx.doi.org/10.1371/journal.pone.0150617.

Castanheira, É.G., Freire, F., 2013. Greenhouse gas assessment of soybean production: implications of land use change and different cultivation systems. J. Clean. Prod. 54, 49–60. http://dx.doi.org/10.1016/j.jclepro.2013.05.026.

Charles, D., 2015. How Big Egg Tried to Bring Down Little 'Mayo' (And Failed). The Salt: NPR. http://www.npr.org/sections/thesalt/2015/09/03/437213511/how-big-egg-tried-to-bring-down-little-mayo-and-failed.

Chung, J.W., Meltzer, D.O., 2009. Estimate of the carbon footprint of the US health care sector. JAMA 302 (18), 1970–1972. http://dx.doi.org/10.1001/jama.2009.1610.

Cleveland, D.A., 2014. Balancing on a Planet: The Future of Food and Agriculture. University of California Press, Berkeley.

Cleveland, D.A., Carruth, A., Mazaroli, D.N., 2015. Operationalizing local food: goals, actions, and indicators for alternative food systems. Agric. Hum. Values 32, 281–297. http://dx.doi.org/10.1007/s10460-014-9556-9.

Cleveland, D.A., Radka, C.N., Müller, N.M., Watson, T.D., Rekstein, N.J., Wright, H.v.M., Hollingshead, S.E., 2011. The effect of localizing fruit and vegetable consumption on greenhouse gas emissions and nutrition, Santa Barbara County. Environ. Sci. Technol. 45, 4555–4562.

Coley, D., Howard, M., Winter, M., 2009. Local food, food miles and carbon emissions: a comparison of farm shop and mass distribution approaches. Food Policy 34 (2), 150–155. http://dx.doi.org/10.1016/j.foodpol.2008.11.001.

EPA (US Environmental Protection Agency), 2014. Inventory of U.S. Greenhouse Gas Emissions and Sinks: 1990–2012. EPA, Washington, D.C. http://www.epa.gov/climatechange/ghgemissions/usinventoryreport.html.

EPA (US Environmental Protection Agency), 2016. Inventory of U.S. Greenhouse Gas Emissions and Sinks: 1990–2014. EPA, Washington, D.C. https://www3.epa.gov/climatechange/ghgemissions/usinventoryreport.html.

Erb, K.-H., Lauk, C., Kastner, T., Mayer, A., Theurl, M.C., Haberl, H., 2016. Exploring the biophysical option space for feeding the world without deforestation. Nat. Commun. 7. http://dx.doi.org/10.1038/ncomms11382.

Eshel, G., Shepon, A., Makov, T., Milo, R., 2014. Land, irrigation water, greenhouse gas, and reactive nitrogen burdens of meat, eggs, and dairy production in the United States. Proc. Natl. Acad. Sci. U.S.A. 111 (33), 11996–12001. http://dx.doi.org/10.1073/pnas.1402183111.

Foley, J.A., Ramankutty, N., Brauman, K.A., Cassidy, E.S., Gerber, J.S., Johnston, M., Mueller, N.D., O'Connell, C., Ray, D.K., West, P.C., Balzer, C., Bennett, E.M., Carpenter, S.R., Hill, J., Monfreda, C., Polasky, S., Rockstrom, J., Sheehan, J., Siebert, S., Tilman, D., Zaks, D.P.M., 2011. Solutions for a cultivated planet. Nature. 478 (7369), 337–342. http://www.nature.com/nature/journal/v478/n7369/abs/nature10452.html - supplementary-information.

Frazão, E., 1999. America's Eating Habits: Changes and Consequences, Agriculture Information Bulletin No. AIB-750. Agriculture Information Bulletin U.S. Department of Agriculture, Economic Research Service, Food and Rural Economics Division, Washington, D.C. http://www.ers.usda.gov/publications/aib-agricultural-information-bulletin/aib750.aspx.

Galloway, J.N., Townsend, A.R., Erisman, J.W., Bekunda, M., Cai, Z.C., Freney, J.R., Martinelli, L.A., Seitzinger, S.P., Sutton, M.A., 2008. Transformation of the nitrogen cycle: recent trends, questions, and potential solutions. Science 320 (5878), 889–892.

Garnett, T., 2011. Where are the best opportunities for reducing greenhouse gas emissions in the food system (including the food chain)? Food Policy 36, S23–S32. http://dx.doi.org/10.1016/j.foodpol.2010.10.010.

Garnett, T., Mathewson, S., Angelides, P., Borthwick, F., 2015. Policies and Actions to Shift Eating Patterns: What Works? FCRN; Catham House, Oxford; London. http://www.fcrn.org.uk/fcrn-publications/reports/policies-and-actions-shift-eating-patterns-what-works.

Gerber, P.J., Steinfeld, H., Henderson, B., Mottet, A., Opio, C., Dijkman, J., Falcucci, A., Tempio, G., 2013. Tackling Climate Change through Livestock – a Global Assessment of Emissions and Mitigation Opportunities. Food and Agriculture Organization of the United Nations (FAO), Rome. http://www.fao.org/ag/againfo/resources/en/publications/tackling_climate_change/index.htm.

Goldman, T.R., 2015. Health Policy Brief: Dietary Guidelines for Americans. Health Affairs. Project HOPE http://www.healthaffairs.org/healthpolicybriefs/brief.php?brief_id=149.

Goldstein, B., Hansen, S.F., Gjerris, M., Laurent, A., Birkved, M., 2016. Ethical aspects of life cycle assessments of diets. Food Policy. 59, 139–151. http://dx.doi.org/10.1016/j.foodpol.2016.01.006.

Gonzalez, A.D., Frostell, B., Carlsson-Kanyama, A., 2011. Protein efficiency per unit energy and per unit greenhouse gas emissions: potential contribution of diet choices to climate change mitigation. Food Policy 36 (5), 562–570. http://dx.doi.org/10.1016/j.foodpol.2011.07.003.

Gonzalez Fischer, C., Garnett, T., 2016. Plates, Pyramids and Planet – Developments in National Healthy and Sustainable Dietary Guidelines: A State of Play Assessment. http://www.fcrn.org.uk/fcrn-publications/reports/plates-pyramids-and-planet-%E2%80%93-developments-national-healthy-and-sustainable.

Goodland, R., Anhang, J., 2009. Livestock and Climate Change. WorldWatch, pp. 10–19.

Goodland, R., Anhang, J., 2012. Comment to the Editor on: livestock and greenhouse gas emissions: the importance of getting the numbers right, by Herrero et al. Anim. Feed Sci. Technol. 166–167, 779–782. Animal Feed Sci. Technol. 172 (3–4), 252–256. http://dx.doi.org/10.1016/j.anifeedsci.2011.12.028.

Goodman, A., Brand, C., Ogilvie, D., 2012. Associations of health, physical activity and weight status with motorised travel and transport carbon dioxide emissions: a cross-sectional, observational study. Environ. Health 11 (1), 1–10. http://dx.doi.org/10.1186/1476-069x-11-52.

Gryka, A., Broom, J., Rolland, C., 2012. Global warming: is weight loss a solution? Int. J. Obes. 36 (3), 474–476. http://dx.doi.org/10.1038/ijo.2011.151.

Hallström, E., Börjesson, P., 2013. Meat-consumption statistics: reliability and discrepancy. Sustain. Sci. Pract. Policy 9 (2), 37.

Hallström, E., C-Kanyama, A., Börjesson, P., 2015. Environmental impact of dietary change: a systematic review. J Clean. Prod. 91, 1–11.

Hallström, E., Gee, Q., Scarborough, P., Cleveland, D.A., 2017. A healthier US diet could reduce greenhouse gas emissions from both the food and health care systems. Climatic Change, (in press). http://dx.doi.org/10.1007/s10584-017-1912-5.

Hallström, E., Röös, E., Börjesson, P., 2014. Sustainable meat consumption: a quantitative analysis of nutritional intake, greenhouse gas emissions and land use from a Swedish perspective. Food Policy. 47 (0), 81–90. http://dx.doi.org/10.1016/j.foodpol.2014.04.002.

Halverson, N., 2015. US Gives Meat Producers a Pass on Climate Change Emissions. Reveal, from the Center for Investigative Reporting http://www.revealnews.org/article/us-gives-meat-producers-a-pass-on-climate-change-emissions/.

Hamm, M.W., 2016. Energy Use, GHG and Blue Water Impacts of Scenarios where US Diet Aligns with New USDA Dietary Recommendations. Food Climate Research Network. http://www.fcrn.org.uk/fcrn-blogs/michaelwhamm/new-commentary-tom-et-al-paper-energy-use-ghg-and-blue-water-impacts.

Hansen, J., Sato, M., 2016. Regional climate change and national responsibilities. Environ. Res. Lett. 11 (3), 034009.

Heller, M.C., Keoleian, G.A., 2015. Greenhouse gas emission estimates of U.S. Dietary choices and food loss. J. Ind. Ecol. 19 (3), 391–401. http://dx.doi.org/10.1111/jiec.12174.

Heller, M.C., Keoleian, G.A., Willett, W.C., 2013. Toward a life cycle-based, diet-level framework for food environmental impact and nutritional quality assessment: a critical review. Environ. Sci. Technol. 47 (22), 12632–12647. http://dx.doi.org/10.1021/es4025113.

Henderson, B.B., Gerber, P.J., Hilinski, T.E., Falcucci, A., Ojima, D.S., Salvatore, M., Conant, R.T., 2015. Greenhouse gas mitigation potential of the world's grazing lands: modeling soil carbon and nitrogen fluxes of mitigation practices. Agriculture. Ecosyst. Environ. 207, 91–100. http://dx.doi.org/10.1016/j.agee.2015.03.029.

Herrero, M., Gerber, P., Vellinga, T., Garnett, T., Leip, A., Opio, C., Westhoek, H.J., Thornton, P.K., Olesen, J., Hutchings, N., Montgomery, H., Soussana, J.F., Steinfeld, H., McAllister, T.A., 2011. Livestock and greenhouse gas emissions: the importance of getting the numbers right. Animal Feed Sci. Technol. 166–167. http://dx.doi.org/10.1016/j.anifeedsci.2011.04.083. 779–782.

Hoekstra, A.Y., Mekonnen, M.M., 2012. The water footprint of humanity. Proc. Natl. Acad. Sci. U.S.A. 109 (9), 3232–3237. http://dx.doi.org/10.1073/pnas.1109936109.

Hoekstra, A.Y., Wiedmann, T.O., 2014. Humanity's unsustainable environmental footprint. Science 344 (6188), 1114–1117. http://dx.doi.org/10.1126/science.1248365.

Hua, F., Yu, J.-J., Hu, Z.-W., 2016. Diabetes and cancer, common threads and missing links. Cancer Lett. 374 (1), 54–61. http://dx.doi.org/10.1016/j.canlet.2016.02.006.

IPCC (Intergovernmental Panel on Climate Change), 2013a. Annex III: Glossary. In: Stocker, T.F., Qin, D., Plattner, G.-K., Tignor, M., Allen, S.K., Boschung, J., Nauels, A., Xia, Y., Bex, V., Midgley, P.M. (Eds.), Climate Change 2013: The Physical Science Basis. Contribution of Working Group I to the Fifth Assessment Report of the Intergovernmental Panel on Climate Change. Cambridge, United Kingdom and New York, NY, USA. Cambridge University Press, pp. 1447–1466. http://www.climatechange2013.org.

IPCC (Intergovernmental Panel on Climate Change), 2013b. Climate change 2013: the physical science basis. In: Working Group I Contribution to the Fifth Assessment Report of the Intergovernmental Panel on Climate Change. IPCC, Geneva. http://www.climatechange2013.org/images/report/WG1AR5_SPM_FINAL.pdf.

IPCC (Intergovernmental Panel on Climate Change), 2014. Climate change 2014: impacts, adaptation, and vulnerability. In: Field, C.B., Barros, V.R., Dokken, D.J., Mach, K.J., Mastrandrea, M.D., Bilir, T.E., Chatterjee, M., Ebi, K.L., Estrada, Y.O., Genova, R.C., Girma, B., Kissel, E.S., Levy, A.N., MacCracken, S., Mastrandrea, P.R., White, L.L. (Eds.), Part A: Global and Sectoral Aspects. Contribution of Working Group II to the Fifth Assessment Report of the Intergovernmental Panel on Climate Change. Cambridge University Press, Cambridge, United Kingdom and New York, NY, USA.

Jalava, M., Kummu, M., Porkka, M., Siebert, S., Varis, O., 2014. Diet change—a solution to reduce water use? Environ. Res. Lett. 9 (7), 074016.

Kaplan, J.O., Krumhardt, K.M., Ellis, E.C., Ruddiman, W.F., Lemmen, C., Goldewijk, K.K., 2011. Holocene carbon emissions as a result of anthropogenic land cover change. Holocene 21 (5), 775–791. http://dx.doi.org/10.1177/0959683610386983.

Katz, D.L., Meller, S., 2014. Can we say what diet is best for health? Annu. Rev. Public Health 35 (1), 83–103. http://dx.doi.org/10.1146/annurev-publhealth-032013-182351.

Matthews, H.S., Hendrickson, C.T., Matthews, D.H., 2016. Life Cycle Assessment: Quantitative Approaches for Decisions that Matter. Green Design Institute, Carnegie Mellon University, Pittsburgh, PA. http://www.lcatextbook.com/.

Mekonnen, M.M., Hoekstra, A.Y., 2012. A global assessment of the water footprint of farm animal products. Ecosystems 15 (3), 401–415. http://dx.doi.org/10.1007/s10021-011-9517-8.

Mekonnen, M.M., Hoekstra, A.Y., 2014. Water footprint benchmarks for crop production: a first global assessment. Ecol. Indic. 46, 214–223. http://dx.doi.org/10.1016/j.ecolind.2014.06.013.

Michaelowa, A., Dransfeld, B., 2008. Greenhouse gas benefits of fighting obesity. Ecol. Econ. 66 (2–3), 298–308. http://dx.doi.org/10.1016/j.ecolecon.2007.09.004.

Myhre, G., Shindell, D., Bréon, F.-M., Collins, W., Fuglestvedt, J., Huang, J., Koch, D., Lamarque, J.-F., Lee, D., Mendoza, B., Nakajima, T., Robock, A., Stephens, G., Takemura, T., Zhang, H., 2013. Anthropogenic and Natural Radiative Forcing. In: Stocker, T.F., Qin, D., Plattner, G.-K., Tignor, M., Allen, S.K., Boschung, J., Nauels, A., Xia, Y., Bex, V., Midgley, P.M. (Eds.), Climate Change 2013: The Physical Science Basis. Contribution of Working Group I to the Fifth Assessment Report of the Intergovernmental Panel on Climate Change. Cambridge, United Kingdom and New York. Cambridge University Press, NY, USA, pp. 659–740. http://www.climatechange2013.org.

Ng, M., Fleming, T., Robinson, M., Thomson, B., Graetz, N., Margono, C., Mullany, E.C., Biryukov, S., Abbafati, C., Abera, S.F., Abraham, J.P., Abu-Rmeileh, N.M.E., Achoki, T., AlBuhairan, F.S., Alemu, Z.A., Alfonso, R., Ali, M.K., Ali, R., Guzman, N.A., Ammar, W., Anwari, P., Banerjee, A., Barquera, S., Basu, S., Bennett, D.A., Bhutta, Z., Blore, J., Cabral, N., Nonato, I.C., Chang, J.-C., Chowdhury, R., Courville, K.J., Criqui, M.H., Cundiff, D.K., Dabhadkar, K.C., Dandona, L., Davis, A., Dayama, A., Dharmaratne, S.D., Ding, E.L., Durrani, A.M., Esteghamati, A., Farzadfar, F., Fay, D.F.J., Feigin, V.L., Flaxman, A., Forouzanfar, M.H., Goto, A., Green, M.A., Gupta, R., Hafezi-Nejad, N., Hankey, G.J., Harewood, H.C., Havmoeller, R., Hay, S., Hernandez, L., Husseini, A., Idrisov, B.T., Ikeda, N., Islami, F., Jahangir, E., Jassal, S.K., Jee, S.H., Jeffreys, M., Jonas, J.B., Kabagambe, E.K., Khalifa, S.E.A.H., Kengne, A.P., Khader, Y.S., Khang, Y.-H., Kim, D., Kimokoti, R.W., Kinge, J.M., Kokubo, Y., Kosen, S., Kwan, G., Lai, T., Leinsalu, M., Li, Y., Liang, X., Liu, S., Logroscino, G., Lotufo, P.A., Lu, Y., Ma, J., Mainoo, N.K., Mensah, G.A., Merriman, T.R., Mokdad, A.H., Moschandreas, J., Naghavi, M., Naheed, A., Nand, D., Narayan, K.M.V., Nelson, E.L., Neuhouser, M.L., Nisar, M.I., Ohkubo, T., Oti, S.O., Pedroza, A., Prabhakaran, D., Roy, N., Sampson, U., Seo, H., Sepanlou, S.G., Shibuya, K., Shiri, R., Shiue, I., Singh, G.M., Singh, J.A., Skirbekk, V., Stapelberg, N.J.C., Sturua, L., Sykes, B.L., Tobias, M., Tran, B.X., Trasande, L., Toyoshima, H., van de Vijver, S., Vasankari, T.J., Veerman, J.L., Velasquez-Melendez, G., Vlassov, V.V., Vollset, S.E., Vos, T., Wang, C., Wang, X., Weiderpass, E., Werdecker, A., Wright, J.L., Yang, Y.C., Yatsuya, H., Yoon, J., Yoon, S.-J.,

Zhao, Y., Zhou, M., Zhu, S., Lopez, A.D., Murray, C.J.L., Gakidou, E., 2014. Global, regional, and national prevalence of overweight and obesity in children and adults during 1980-2013: a systematic analysis for the Global Burden of Disease Study 2013. Lancet 384 (9945), 766–781. http://dx.doi.org/10.1016/S0140-6736(14)60460-8.

Nijdam, D., Rood, T., Westhoek, H., 2012. The price of protein: review of land use and carbon footprints from life cycle assessments of animal food products and their substitutes. Food Policy. 37 (6), 760–770. http://dx.doi.org/10.1016/j.foodpol.2012.08.002.

Olson, R.D., 2006. Below-cost Feed Crops. An Indirect Subsidy for Industrial Animal Factories. IATP Trade and Global Governance Program. http://www.nffc.net/Learn/Reports/BelowCost6_06.pdf.

Pelletier, N., Pirog, R., Rasmussen, R., 2010. Comparative life cycle environmental impacts of three beef production strategies in the Upper Midwestern United States. Agric. Syst. 103 (6), 380–389.

Persson, U.M., Daniel, J.A.J., Christel, C., Fredrik, H., David, B., 2015. Climate metrics and the carbon footprint of livestock products: where's the beef? Environ. Res. Lett. 10 (3), 034005.

Pfister, P.L., Stocker, T.F., 2016. Earth system commitments due to delayed mitigation. Environ. Res. Lett. 11 (1), 014010.

Porter, J.R., Xie, L., Challinor, A.J., Cochrane, K., Howden, S.M., Iqbal, M.M., Lobell, D.B., Travasso, M.I., 2014. Food security and food production systems. In: Field, C.B., Barros, V.R., Dokken, D.J., Mach, K.J., Mastrandrea, M.D., Bilir, T.E., Chatterjee, M., Ebi, K.L., Estrada, Y.O., Genova, R.C., Girma, B., Kissel, E.S., Levy, A.N., MacCracken, S., Mastrandrea, P.R., White, L.L. (Eds.), Climate Change 2014: Impacts, Adaptation, and Vulnerability. Part a: Global and Sectoral Aspects. Contribution of Working Group II to the Fifth Assessment Report of the Intergovernmental Panel of Climate Change. Cambridge, United Kingdom and New York, NY, USA. Cambridge University Press, pp. 485–533.

Rea, S., 2016. Vegetarian and "healthy" Diets Could Be More Harmful to the Environment. Carnegie Mellon University News, Pittsburgh, PA. http://www.cmu.edu/news/stories/archives/2015/december/diet-and-environment.html.

Reay, D.S., Davidson, E.A., Smith, K.A., Smith, P., Melillo, J.M., Dentener, F., Crutzen, P.J., 2012. Global agriculture and nitrous oxide emissions. Nat. Clim. Change. 2 (6), 410–416. http://www.nature.com/nclimate/journal/v2/n6/abs/nclimate1458.html - supplementary-information.

Röös, E., Karlsson, H., 2013. Effect of eating seasonal on the carbon footprint of Swedish vegetable consumption. J. Clean. Prod. 59, 63–72. http://dx.doi.org/10.1016/j.jclepro.2013.06.035.

Röös, E., Patel, M., Spångberg, J., 2016. Producing oat drink or cow's milk on a Swedish farm — environmental impacts considering the service of grazing, the opportunity cost of land and the demand for beef and protein. Agric. Syst. 142, 23–32. http://dx.doi.org/10.1016/j.agsy.2015.11.002.

Röös, E., Sundberg, C., Hansson, P.-A., 2014. Carbon footprint of food products. In: Muthu, S.S. (Ed.). Muthu, S.S. (Ed.), Assessment of Carbon Footprint in Different Industrial Sectors. , vol. 1. Springer Singapore, Singapore, pp. 85–112. http://dx.doi.org/10.1007/978-981-4560-41-2_4.

Ruddiman, W.F., 2013. The Anthropocene. In: Jeanloz, R. (Ed.). Jeanloz, R. (Ed.), Annual Review of Earth and Planetary Sciences, vol. 41. Annual Reviews, Palo Alto, pp. 45–68. http://www.annualreviews.org/doi/abs/10.1146/annurev-earth-050212-123944.

Ruddiman, W.F., Ellis, E.C., Kaplan, J.O., Fuller, D.Q., 2015. Defining the epoch we live in. Science 348 (6230), 38–39. http://dx.doi.org/10.1126/science.aaa7297.

Scarborough, P., Appleby, P., Mizdrak, A., Briggs, A.M., Travis, R., Bradbury, K., Key, T., 2014. Dietary greenhouse gas emissions of meat-eaters, fish-eaters, vegetarians and vegans in the UK. Clim. Change 125 (2), 179–192. http://dx.doi.org/10.1007/s10584-014-1169-1.

Scovronick, N., Dora, C., Fletcher, E., Haines, A., Shindell, D., 2015. Reduce short-lived climate pollutants for multiple benefits. Lancet 386 (10006), e28–e31. http://dx.doi.org/10.1016/S0140-6736(15)61043-1.

Smedman, A., Lindmark-Månsson, H., Drewnowski, A., Edman, A., 2010. Nutrient density of beverages in relation to climate impact. Food Nutr. Res. 54.

Springmann, M., Godfray, H.C.J., Rayner, M., Scarborough, P., 2016. Analysis and valuation of the health and climate change cobenefits of dietary change. Proc. Natl. Acad. Sci. U.S.A. http://dx.doi.org/10.1073/pnas.1523119113.

Steffen, W., Richardson, K., Rockström, J., Cornell, S.E., Fetzer, I., Bennett, E.M., Biggs, R., Carpenter, S.R., de Vries, W., de Wit, C.A., Folke, C., Gerten, D., Heinke, J., Mace, G.M., Persson, L.M., Ramanathan, V., Reyers, B., Sörlin, S., 2015. Planetary boundaries: guiding human development on a changing planet. Science 347 (6223). http://dx.doi.org/10.1126/science.1259855.

Stocker, D.Q., 2013. Climate change 2013: the physical science basis. In: Working Group I Contribution to the Fifth Assessment Report of the Intergovernmental Panel on Climate Change, Summary for Policymakers. IPCC.

Stocker, T.F., Dahe, Q., Plattner, G.-K., 2013. Climate change 2013: the physical science basis. In: Working Group I Contribution to the Fifth Assessment Report of the Intergovernmental Panel on Climate Change. Summary for Policymakers. IPCC.

Stoessel, F., Juraske, R., Pfister, S., Hellweg, S., 2012. Life cycle inventory and carbon and water food print of fruits and vegetables: application to a Swiss retailer. Environ. Sci. Technol. 46 (6), 3253–3262. http://dx.doi.org/10.1021/es2030577.

Stuart, T., 2008. The Bloodless Revolution: A Cultural History of Vegetarianism: From 1600 to Modern Times. W. W. Norton & Company.

Tilman, D., Clark, M., 2014. Global diets link environmental sustainability and human health. Nature 515 (7528), 518–522. http://dx.doi.org/10.1038/nature13959.

Tom, M., Fischbeck, P., Hendrickson, C., 2015. Energy use, blue water footprint, and greenhouse gas emissions for current food consumption patterns and dietary recommendations in the US. Environ. Syst. Decis. 1–12. http://dx.doi.org/10.1007/s10669-015-9577-y.

Turner, A., Jacob, D.J., Wecht, K., Maasakkers, J., Lundgren, E., Andrews, A., Biraud, S., Boesch, H., Bowman, K., Deutscher, N.M., 2015. Estimating global and North American methane emissions with high spatial resolution using GOSAT satellite data. Atmos. Chem. Phys.

Turner-McGrievy, G.M., Leach, A.M., Wilcox, S., Frongillo, E.A., 2016. Differences in environmental impact and food expenditures of four different plant-based diets and an omnivorous diet: results of a randomized, controlled intervention. J. Hunger Environ. Nutr. 1–14. http://dx.doi.org/10.1080/19320248.2015.1066734.

USDA, and HHS, 2010. Dietary Guidelines for Americans, 2010, seventh ed. Washington, DC, U.S.

USDA, and HHS (Department of Agriculture and U.S. Department of Health and Human Services), 2015a. 2015 – 2020 Dietary Guidelines for Americans, eighth ed. USDA, HHS, Washington, D.C. http://health.gov/dietaryguidelines/2015/guidelines/.

USDA, and HHS (US Departments of Agriculture and Health and Human Services), 2015b. Scientific Report of the 2015 Dietary Guidelines Advisory Committee. USDA, HHS, Washington, D.C. http://www.health.gov/dietaryguidelines/2015-scientific-report/.

USGCRP (U.S. Global Change Research Program), 2016. The Impacts of Climate Change on Human Health in the United States: A Scientific Assessment. U.S. Global Change Research Program, Washington, D.C. https://health2016.globalchange.gov/.

Vermeulen, S.J., Campbell, B.M., Ingram, J.S.I., 2012. Climate change and food systems. In: Gadgil, A., Liverman, D.M. (Eds.), Gadgil, A., Liverman, D.M. (Eds.), Annual Review of Environment and Resources, vol. 37, p. 1905.

Vieux, F., Darmon, N., Touazi, D., Soler, L.G., 2012. Greenhouse gas emissions of self-selected individual diets in France: changing the diet structure or consuming less? Ecol. Econ. 75 (0), 91–101. http://dx.doi.org/10.1016/j.ecolecon.2012.01.003.

Walpole, S.C., Prieto-Merino, D., Edwards, P., Cleland, J., Stevens, G., Roberts, I., 2012. The weight of nations: an estimation of adult human biomass. BMC Public Health 12 (1), 1–6. http://dx.doi.org/10.1186/1471-2458-12-439.

Weart, S.R., 2008. The Discovery of Global Warming, Revised Edition. Harvard University Press.

Weber, C.L., Matthews, H.S., 2008. Quantifying the global and distributional aspects of American household carbon footprint. Ecol. Econ. 66 (2–3), 379–391. http://dx.doi.org/10.1016/j.ecolecon.2007.09.021.

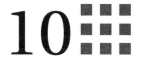

10

Barriers to Increasing Plant Protein Consumption in Western Populations

Mari Niva[1], Annukka Vainio[2], Piia Jallinoja[1]

*[1]UNIVERSITY OF HELSINKI, HELSINKI, FINLAND; [2]NATURAL RESOURCES INSTITUTE
FINLAND, HELSINKI, FINLAND*

1. Introduction

Products based on red meat and dairy are the main sources of protein in the Western countries. However, there has been a growing concern about the negative impact of the herding, slaughtering, and eating of animals on the environment, animal welfare, and human health. A high level of consumption of red meat and processed meat has been associated with increased cancer risk (Cross et al., 2007). In comparison, pulses as a source of vegetable protein are known to have several positive health effects, such as reducing the risk of diabetes and cardiovascular diseases (Rizkalla et al., 2002), as well as cancers (Finley et al., 2007; World Cancer Research Fund, 2013). In addition, it has been shown that beans, nuts, and seeds contain higher nutrient value and lower cost per 100 kcal than meat and meat products, making them more affordable in a nutritional sense (Drewnowski, 2010). From the environmental point of view, the production and consumption of red meat and dairy contribute significantly to the global greenhouse gas emissions, which accelerate anthropogenic climate change. Compared to meat-based meals, vegetable-based meals generate lower amounts of greenhouse gas emissions (Virtanen et al., 2011). It has been calculated that only a global transition to a low-meat diet, such as is commonly recommended also for health reasons, would significantly reduce mitigation costs of climate change (Stehfest et al., 2009). The cultivation of legumes also contributes to a more efficient use of nitrogen (N) that would significantly improve the environmental impacts of food production and consumption (Steffen et al., 2015).

The consumption of meat has steadily increased among the Western populations during the past decades, whereas the consumption of plant protein has been stable (de Boer et al., 2016; Vinnari and Tapio, 2009; Natural Resources Institute Finland, 2013). To better understand the conditions for increasing plant protein consumption globally and in particular in those food cultures in which plant proteins are a less culturally embedded part of the cuisine, attention needs to be paid to those factors that act as barriers to transition

Vegetarian and Plant-Based Diets in Health and Disease Prevention. http://dx.doi.org/10.1016/B978-0-12-803968-7.00010-1

to more plant-based diets. By barriers we mean both individual and structural issues that make it difficult to or prevent people from increasing their use of pulses and decreasing that of meat and dairy products. In the following sections, we first review the current consumption trends of pulses in the Western countries and the intentions that people already have for changing their diets to include less meat. After that, we examine different kinds of barriers to increasing the use of plant proteins. In the final section, we discuss potential solutions and outline some future directions for food research and policies that aim at enhancing plant protein consumption in the Western food cultures.

2. The Consumption and Cultural Place of Plant Proteins in Western Food Cultures

Despite growing public discussion of the environmental, health, and ethical problems related to meat production and consumption, in Europe the consumption of pulses as an alternative protein source is relatively low compared to many African, Asian, Middle Eastern, and South American countries, where pulses are a central part of the diet (Schneider, 2002; FAOstat, 2013). Akibode and Maredia (2011) note that whereas statistics on the production and trade volumes of legumes are readily available, consumption statistics are more difficult to find. Their approximate calculations based on FAO's food security statistics suggest that in the developing countries, the legume consumption per capita is almost twice as high as in the developed countries, and that in the early 2000s, the growth rate in consumption (0.8%) in the former countries was double the growth rate in the latter countries (0.4%) (Akibode and Maredia, 2011, p. 39). In sub-Saharan Africa and Latin America and the Caribbean the total consumption of major pulse crops (dry bean, chickpea, cowpea, fava bean, pigeon pea, and lentils) exceeds 10 kg/capita/year, whereas in the developed countries, it is below 3 kg/capita/year, and in some Asian regions, even less (Akibode and Maredia, 2011, p. 43). It is noteworthy, however, that Akibode's and Maredia's statistics do not include soybean, which tofu—a highly significant part of the food culture in many East Asian countries—is made of.

Although the current consumption volumes of beans are relatively low in Western countries, beans have by no means been unheard of by Europeans either. In fact, pulses have been a more or less visible part of European diets for centuries (Cubero, 2011). Particularly in Southern Europe, many kinds of beans are cultivated and form an established part of the food culture. In Northern Europe, the variety of cultivated beans is more limited, but broad beans and peas have been grown for a long time. In contrast, processed forms of beans such as tofu had been largely unfamiliar in Western diets until the mid-1970s (Shurtleff and Aoyagi, 2013). To take an example, in a survey conducted in 2013, only 3%–6% of Finns reported eating lentils, beans, or tofu on a weekly basis (Jallinoja et al., 2016), reflecting the vegetarian population of 2%–4% among Finns since the mid-1980s (Vinnari, 2008; Paturi et al., 2008). In the same study, especially tofu and soy products were unfamiliar: half of the population never ate tofu, and more than half never ate soy products such as soy chunks, textured soy protein, or soy sausages (Jallinoja et al., 2016).

Recently, public and media interest in cuisines and dishes from other parts of the world (Johnston and Baumann, 2015) have started to play a role in the cultural meanings of plant proteins in Western countries. More than before, European and North American meals both at home and in restaurants may now include beans in various forms, either as the main protein source or as a trimming. There are several indicators of an increased interest and acceptance of plant proteins. For example, although plant-based diets can hardly be seen as an established part of gourmet or foodie cultures, many popular and award-winning food blogs are specialized in meat-free recipes (Johnston and Baumann, 2015, p. 136), and mainstream food magazines and cookbooks increasingly include recipes for vegetarian and vegan dishes.

3. Are Consumers Trying to Change Their Use of Meat and Pulses?

During recent years an increasing amount of social scientific research has analyzed consumers' perspectives on the societal demands to diminish the consumption of animal protein, particularly that of red meat. This research has contributed to providing a better understanding of the personal, cultural, and social conditions for eating less meat and suggests that there are signs of increasing awareness of the need to reduce meat consumption and also willingness to do so among consumers (e.g., Latvala et al., 2012; Leitzmann, 2014; Niva et al., 2014). A study on the reasons for reducing meat consumption suggested that they were mostly based on health and weight concerns and taste preferences, but particularly the most active meat limiters were also motivated by animal welfare and environmental issues (Latvala et al., 2012).

The reasons for reducing meat consumption resonate with those associated with vegetarianism: health concerns and compassion toward animals and their ethical treatment have been found to be strong motivations for engaging in vegetarianism (Hoek et al., 2004; Potts and White, 2008), as fully described in other chapters of this book. In a study by Smith et al. (2000), adopting a meat-free diet was associated with these factors but also a sense of disgust related to meat. Pollard et al. (1998) found that individuals who reported a low level of red meat consumption attributed their food choices to health, natural content, weight control, and ethical concerns more likely than those who described their diets as conventional; however, vegetarians differed significantly from those describing their diets as conventional only with regard to ethical concerns. Fox and Ward (2008) suggest that vegetarians often follow a trajectory in which the initial reasons for becoming a vegetarian, such as health concerns, are over time supplemented with other considerations, such as ecological or ethical ones. It has also been noted that health-oriented and ethically oriented (self-identified) vegetarians differ from each other in their attitudes and practices. The former seem to be more flexible and may occasionally eat meat, whereas the latter are more committed to their diet and try to refrain from eating animal products (Hoffman et al., 2013). Similarly, it has been found that "semivegetarians," who identify themselves as vegetarians but who sometimes consume meat, are more motivated by health concerns than those people who more strictly adhere to the definition of vegetarianism (Rothberger, 2014). These results suggest that when people reduce their meat eating, irrespective of whether they remain omnivores or become vegetarians, the reasons for doing so are related to a variety of concerns ranging from personal health to the wider ecological impacts and ethical aspects of meat.

Interestingly, despite increasing research interest in consumers' awareness of the environmental effects of meat and in their willingness to reduce their meat eating, less research has been conducted on whether and to what extent consumers are ready to replace meat with plant proteins. Studies conducted on the acceptability of meat substitutes, such as Quorn, tofu, and other products based on soy protein, indicate that acceptance is quite low and partly influenced by consumers' evaluations of how well the substitute fits in with the whole meal (Elzerman et al., 2011). It is also evident that meat substitutes are consumed not only by vegetarians but also meat-eaters, and that consumers' categorizations of meat substitutes are strongly influenced by their categorizations of meat products and the perceived dissimilarity between substitutes and meat (Hoek et al., 2011). There is some evidence, however, that the consumption of vegetable-based proteins is most likely to first increase among those groups who already consume them. In the study by Jallinoja et al. (2016), a fifth of all respondents estimated that they would increase their consumption of beans during the following few years. Half of those who consumed beans on a weekly basis planned to further increase their bean consumption, whereas only 5% of those who never ate beans intended to do the same. It is thus evident that some familiarity with pulses is needed before people can imagine to start using them on a more frequent basis, but once such familiarity is established, an additional increase is easy to conceive.

4. Barriers to Increasing Plant-Based Protein Consumption

Barriers to increasing plant-based protein consumption in Western countries are complex and operate at multiple levels, ranging from psychological attributes and everyday life routines to wider-scale barriers associated with identity, culture, supply, environment, and economy. Moreover, sensory characteristics of food are among the most important factors affecting acceptability for consumers. This is why the taste, texture, appearance, and odor of pulses and pulse-based foods—which differ from the sensory characteristics of meat—may function as barriers to enhancing their consumption.

First of all, it is evident that consumers are still not very well aware of the links between livestock production and climate change (de Boer et al., 2016; MacDiarmid et al., 2016). A study indicated that only 12% of the Dutch and 6% of the US sample recognized the effectiveness of eating less meat in mitigating climate change; and limiting one's meat consumption was considered to be less effective than buying local and seasonal food in both countries (de Boer et al., 2016). In a similar vein, de Boer et al. (2013) found that consumers who were skeptical about climate change were more unwilling than others to reduce their meat eating, and Vainio et al. (2013) discovered that a disbelief in the effects of food consumption on climate was associated with nonclimate-friendly food choices. In a qualitative study by McDiarmid et al. (2016), consumers cited transportation, industrial pollution, and energy production as more damaging for the environment than food production and meat eating.

Second, people's food choices are associated with habit, motivation, goals, and beliefs about one's own capabilities (Guillaumie et al., 2010), as well as attitudes, social norms, self-efficacy, and intention (Rothman et al., 2009). A wide range of personal motives have been associated with food choices. For example, studies applying The Eating Motivation Survey have identified 15 motivations for food choices: liking the food, visual appeal, pleasure, affect regulation, need/hunger, sociability, social norms, social image, weight control, health, price, convenience, habits, traditional eating, and concern for nature/ethical aspects (Renner et al., 2012). Valuing price, taste, and convenience may act as barriers to consuming healthy food, particularly fruit and vegetables (Lappalainen et al., 1997), and the importance of these factors may vary in different socioeconomic groups. Konttinen et al. (2012) found that the less healthy dietary habits among people in disadvantaged socioeconomic groups were in part explained by the higher priority they gave to price and familiarity compared to health motives. In another study (Mäkiniemi and Vainio, 2014), price was perceived as the most important barrier to climate-friendly food choices, including the replacement of red meat and dairy with plant proteins. However, according to the results of a Finnish study reported in Table 10.1, barriers related to high prices and limited supply were rated as the least relevant, indicating that economic reasons may not be very prominent in hindering consumers from increasing their use of pulses (see also Jallinoja et al., 2016; Vainio et al., 2016).

Table 10.1   Perceived Barriers to Increasing the Consumption of Beans and Soya-Based Products Among the Adult Population Between 18 and 63 years of Age Living in Finland (N = 1048)[a]

Barrier	Beans		Soya-Based Products	
	Mean[b]	SD	Mean[b]	SD
Not used to eating pulses	3.54	1.23	3.82	1.25
Does not know pulse recipes	3.39	1.27	3.59	1.33
Not interested in pulses	3.22	1.32	3.58	1.33
Pulses do not replace meat and fish	3.02	1.35	3.10	1.38
Pulses do not fit into meals that I prepare	2.79	1.19	2.93	1.29
Pulses cause digestive problems	2.53	1.29	2.03	1.08
Pulses have an unpleasant taste	2.50	1.32	2.89	1.37
Pulses are difficult to prepare	2.34	1.11	2.62	1.16
A poor supply of pulses in cafeterias/restaurants	2.29	1.15	2.32	1.15
Pulses are expensive	2.29	1.03	2.77	1.25
A poor supply of pulses in supermarkets	2.16	1.00	2.31	1.12

[a]Previously unpublished results from the "Beans on Finnish dinner tables" study, data collected in 2013.
[b]Range between 1 and 4, high values indicate a high perceived relevance of a barrier.

It appears that certain personal motives may function as barriers to increasing plant protein consumption. In a Finnish study, the respondents whose diets included beans and soy products endorsed a higher level of natural concerns, health, and weight control motives and a lower level of convenience and price motives than the respondents who did not consume beans and soy products (Vainio et al., 2016). Moreover, participants who at the time of the survey were increasing their consumption of plant proteins endorsed a higher level of natural concerns, as well as health, sociability, social image, and price motives than those with an established diet that already included beans and soy products. At the same time, convenience and price motives were higher among devoted beef-eaters who did not consume any plant proteins as compared to those with an established diet including beans and soy products. In other words, it appears that health and natural concerns may function as motivational forces during the adoption of plant proteins, whereas convenience and price motives function as barriers.

The adoption of a diet rich in plant proteins requires replacing old behaviors with new ones, which has been found to be more demanding than initiating new behaviors. This is because motives associated with old behaviors may function as barriers (Holland et al., 2006). The adoption of new food habits can be divided into multiple stages and these stages include different automatic and reflective components. Reflective processes are important in initiating new behaviors, and the formation of a new habit involves automatic processes that operate beyond individuals' full awareness (Rothman et al., 2009). Therefore habits are likely to persist even after conscious motivation decreases (Gardner et al., 2011). The transtheoretical model of behavioral change suggests that a desired change is associated with an increased awareness and concern about an issue and an increased perceived importance of the motives associated with the desired change, as well as a decreased importance of the motives associated with the old behavior (Freestone and McGoldrick, 2007; Prochaska and DiClemente, 1983; Rossi et al., 2001).

According to the transtheoretical model, when individuals consider replacing meat with plant-based proteins in their diets, their awareness of the benefits of replacing meat with beans and soya-based products increases. At the same time, they probably start questioning meat as the main component of the meal, as well as its good taste and nutritional value. They begin to make concrete behavioral changes: they start searching for plant-based alternatives to meat in supermarkets and cafeterias, and for recipes and ways to integrate the new food items to their existing diets. Initially, all these efforts are relatively conscious and reflective. The repetition of these new behaviors is important for the formation of new habits, and it gradually leads to automaticity characterized by efficiency, lack of awareness, unintentionality, and uncontrollability (Bargh, 1994). When individuals have successfully found ways to integrate the new food elements into their existing eating patterns, they slowly develop routines that start operating largely beyond conscious efforts. Looking for plant-based alternatives in restaurants and supermarkets becomes a routinized activity, and ideally, social surroundings start supporting the new habits as well.

It appears that consumers perceive barriers related to their own everyday life as more relevant than barriers related to supply. A Finnish survey (Jallinoja et al., 2016;

Vainio et al., 2016) examining consumer views on beans and soya-based products showed that the barriers perceived as the most relevant were related to habit (i.e., the participants were not used to eating pulses), perceived lack of skills, and a low level of personal interest (Table 10.1). Similarly, studies conducted in Australia revealed that lack of knowledge about preparing vegetarian meals and the difficulties experienced in changing one's eating habits were perceived as the most important barriers to replacing meat with vegetarian foods (Lea et al., 2005, 2006b) together with the good taste of meat (Lea et al., 2006a).

Table 10.1 seems to indicate that for consumers, institutional and structural factors, such as price or a poor supply of pulses in various shopping and eating venues, are less significant barriers to using more pulses than more personal factors related to unfamiliarity, lack of knowledge, and lack of interest in pulses. This does not mean, however, that food supply, culture, and economy were insignificant in enabling and establishing the use of plant proteins, quite the contrary. Eating does take place in material, social, and cultural contexts, in which food choices are made possible and encouraged, while others are excluded and discouraged. This perspective is central in those accounts of social life suggesting that what may seem like individual behaviors are in fact performances of social practices and that individuals are "carriers" of those practices (Shove et al., 2012; Spurling et al., 2013). Shove et al. (2012) suggest that social practices are made up of three types of elements: *materials* (objects, tools, infrastructures), *competence* (knowledge, skills), and *meanings* (cultural conventions, expectations, shared meanings). Eating is a particularly complex practice as it is a "compound practice," which draws on other practices, such as those based on nutrition, cookery, etiquette, and taste; involves both social, bodily, and culinary dimensions; and is characterized by embodied habits, routines, and conventions (Warde, 2016; see also Warde, 2005). The transition to more plant-based diets is thus dependent on a variety of developments in many practices that are involved in or adjacent to eating, and these "adjacent" practices may either advance or hamper the embedding of pulses into Western food cultures.

For instance, when thinking of barriers to increasing the use of plant proteins, practice theories draw attention to sociocultural characteristics, such as cultural meanings associated with meat and vegetarian foods. Pohjolainen et al. (2015) note that because these change slowly, in meat-eating cultures, it is not easy to actualize an increase in plant-based food consumption. In Western countries, meat maintains a central position in culture and social relationships (Bohm et al., 2015), meals, and food purchases (Vinnari et al., 2010; Fiddes, 2004), and it is regarded as a healthy and necessary part of the diet (Verbeke et al., 2010; de Bakker and Dagevos, 2012). In contrast, pulses may be arduous to prepare, their taste may be regarded as strange, and they are known to cause digestive problems (Jallinoja et al., 2016). Furthermore, meat consumption has for long been culturally associated with power and masculinity (Fiddes, 2004), making it more difficult to reduce meat consumption among men, who on average consume larger amounts of meat than women. There are signs, however, that the masculinity image of meat may be weakening (de Bakker and Dagevos, 2012).

The food chain influences people's food choices by determining what foods are available and how they are marketed, positioned in shops, and priced. Context and availability have a large impact on food-related behaviors (Wansink and Sobal, 2007). For example, in the United States, access to supermarkets has been found to affect individuals' diets (Morland et al., 2002; Rose and Richards, 2004). At the same time, changes in agroindustry are slow to take place and difficult for several reasons. Many Western countries have well-established meat and dairy industries, whereas the vegetable protein industry is less developed. Schneider (2002) lists a low level of innovation and marketing of pulse products, lack of attractive food products, and the old-fashioned image of pulses as barriers of plant protein consumption in Europe. These kinds of barriers will be even more central with novel products such as algae and insects (Boland et al., 2013) that are not currently part of European diets. A transformation from animal protein production to plant protein production is difficult and costly both to farmers and the food processing industry, not least because of the heavily subsidized nature of meat and dairy production.

5. Solutions: How Could Plant Protein Consumption Increase?

Barriers to changing food consumption operate at multiple levels, and therefore, successful solutions are likely to be complex. A combination of multiple means is likely to be most effective, and it should take into account both individual-level motivations and practices as well as the structural characteristics of the food chain. Public information campaigns that stress the health and environmental benefits of replacing meat protein with plant proteins may increase public awareness of health issues related to a too high intake of meat and the role of livestock production in anthropogenic climate change, but because of the complexity of eating patterns, such campaigns are not likely to lead to substantial changes in meat consumption (de Boer et al., 2016; Jallinoja et al., 2016).

Also practice-theoretical perspectives into sustainable food consumption suggest that policy makers' efforts to inform and persuade individuals to make sacrifices for more sustainable diets will probably fail unless a wider culturally based transition takes place (Shove, 2010). In Table 10.2, we summarize, based on a practice-theoretical lens, possible ways of advancing plant protein consumption by looking at various actors' roles and potential activities in transforming meanings and enabling competences and infrastructures related to advancing plant protein consumption.

First, for bean, tofu and novel plant-based protein eating to become routinized as a practice, the products need to gain positive meanings as pleasurable and fulfilling food, suitable for both everyday and festive occasions; instead of being seen as a forced choice of vegetarians or other groups following special diets (Schyver and Smith, 2005). If such a change of meanings took place, the traditional and established meanings of meat and fish as the core of festive and fulfilling meals would be deconstructed, and vegetable proteins would become legitimate options for all kinds of eating occasions. When looking for

Table 10.2   Various Actors' Roles in Promoting Plant Protein Consumption and Potential Resulting Changes in Meanings, Competences, and Materials/Infrastructure Related to Plant Proteins

	Activities and Actors	Resulting Change
Meanings and images	The harms, such as climate change effects, caused by meat production and consumption are increasingly discussed in society, and people become more knowledgeable about them Vegetable proteins are promoted in the media as a palatable alternative Home economics education at schools promote a positive image of plant protein meals Celebrity chefs, food journalists, and bloggers develop and promote recipes based on plant proteins both for everyday and festive meals Workplace and school canteens and restaurants advance the use of plant proteins as the "default" option	The cultural image of plant proteins improves: plant proteins are considered ethical, sustainable, and healthy
Competence	Home economics education increasingly takes plant proteins to be the center of the meal and includes recipes from plant proteins both for everyday and festive meals Celebrity chefs, culinary magazines, bloggers, and food intermediaries promote easy dishes based on plant proteins	Consumers and food professionals are better skilled and enthusiastic in using plant proteins
Materials and infrastructure	Novel plant protein products are developed and marketed, and the supply of plant protein products is rich Public and private catering replace animal proteins with plant proteins Ready-made meals from plant proteins are palatable, affordable, and widely available Restaurants increase the variety of meals based on plant proteins on their menus Plant proteins are promoted in political strategies and action programs Price of meat increases either via taxation or increased costs of production	Food environments are increasingly based on plant proteins and decreasingly on animal proteins

Adapted from Jallinoja, P., Niva, M., Latvala, T., 2016. Towards more sustainable eating? Practices, competence, meanings and materialities of bean eating in a meat-eating culture. Futures 83, 4–14.

means to increase the demand for plant-based proteins, the social aspects of eating, the social image of eating particular foods, and various culturally shared ideas of "good" food need particular attention. From this perspective, social media campaigns initiated by, e.g., food bloggers, giving publicity to celebrities who adhere to vegan or vegetarian diets, might serve as part of normalizing meals without meat, particularly among adolescents and young adults.

Second, on an everyday level, new cooking skills for making tasty vegetarian food need to be taught and learned. This competence in a practice-theoretical sense might also mean consciously developing a taste for beans and products based on beans, i.e., learning to like them by tasting and experimenting, and bearing in mind that accommodating new flavors may take some time (Jallinoja et al., 2016). The competence aspect is equally pertinent in private and public settings, as it is not only the eaters and home cooks but also chefs and other staff in the catering business who would learn new skills, tastes, and routines. Home economics education at schools as well as the media have an important role to play in promoting both knowledge and skills, i.e., to improve what has been termed "food literacy" (Vaitkeviciute et al., 2014; Vidgen and Gallegos, 2014) related to vegetarian cooking.

Third, various institutional actors in the food system are significant in enabling a transition toward increasing the use of plant proteins. Food policy strategies and action programs need to take plant proteins onto the agenda, and policy measures need to be developed. For instance, it has been suggested that meat should be included in emissions trading and carbon tax schemes and that the general sales tax should be higher for meat and meat products than for nonmeat options (Raphaely and Marinova, 2014). Also public catering institutions in schools and workplaces have an important role in promoting plant proteins in both vegetarian dishes and dishes that combine meat and pulses. Keeping bean, tofu, and other pulse-based dishes systematically on the menus at school and workplace canteens, lunch cafeterias, and bistros serves as an active familiarization and positive image development (Vinnari, 2008). The accumulation of these kinds of incremental changes could serve to advance plant protein use in public catering and to gradually establish plant proteins also among those who are currently reluctant to eat vegetarian dishes.

Also actors in the food industry may facilitate a transition toward increased consumption of plant-based proteins by developing vegetable-based products in which meat is either totally or partly replaced by vegetable ingredients, such as new pulse-based foods the texture of which resembles meat, or so called "functional meat." The food industry and primary production have to both enable and accommodate to increased consumption of plant-based proteins. In many Western countries, meat and dairy industries are strong economic actors, and they are supported by agricultural subsidies more than plant protein production (Lehtonen and Irz, 2013). Agricultural policies taking environmental considerations better into account would enable a further development of plant protein production and product development.

As stressed earlier, policy measures are essential in fostering the consumption of plant proteins. Among those consumers who do not eat beans or soy products at all, effecting a transformation from animal to plant proteins may prove difficult because policy measures appealing to health, natural concerns, and weight control are not likely to be very effective (Vainio et al., 2016). This group could benefit from new food products in which meat has been only partly replaced with plant proteins, and that are relatively economical and easy to prepare. However, the results by Vainio et al. (2016) also show that, in fact, most beef-eaters do not object to eating plant proteins. Among these consumers, improving the availability of plant-based proteins that are easy to integrate into existing eating patterns would enable an increase in plant-based protein consumption.

A key question in the discussion on sustainable food consumption is whether, to what extent, and how it is possible to accelerate the replacement of meat with plant-based proteins and to turn plant proteins into a normalized, ordinary, and habitual component of Western diets. Some researchers have been rather skeptical about a voluntary substitution of plant proteins for meat (Smil, 2002). For instance, in Finland, vegetarian days at schools have met with noncompliance (Lombardini and Lankoski, 2013) and have been widely criticized in the media and by local politicians who have been opposing "green force-feeding." Consequently, interventions tailored differently for different target groups have been called for (Vinnari, 2008). For instance, Vinnari and Tapio (2009) suggest that those consumers who have very negative attitudes toward a reduction in meat consumption could benefit from campaigns about animal rights issues and about the possibilities of vegetarianism, whereas those who do not think that such a change would be necessary would probably need economic incentives to change their meat use.

Because the large majority of Western populations currently include animal proteins in their diets, it may well be that rather than promoting vegetarianism or veganism, political efforts to increase the use of vegetable proteins would be better placed if directed toward the promotion of replacing a part of meat with plant-based proteins and adding vegetables in the diet as is already suggested in many national nutrition recommendations (e.g., Nordic Nutrition Recommendations, 2012; Dietary guidelines for Americans, 2015–2020). Breaking down the dichotomy between meat consumption and vegetarianism and making visible multiple forms of combining moderate meat consumption and vegetable consumption could help this transition. This change might take place in the form of flexitarianism, referring to eating styles that reduce meat eating to healthy levels (Raphaely and Marinova, 2014) and that flexibly combine meat and vegetable-based proteins. It has been argued that flexitarianism "offers an immediate, accessible and effective opportunity to mitigate climate change and its negative impacts" (Raphaely and Marinova, 2014, p. 94). Others refer to reducetarianism, i.e., the reduction of the consumption of meat or "Eat vegan before 6 p.m." (VB6) (Bittman, 2013), indicating an increased interest in plant-based diets that do not totally abandon meat. However, for a more comprehensive understanding of the social and cultural conditions for meat-reducing strategies to succeed on an everyday level, more social scientific research is needed.

The adoption of new eating patterns with more plant proteins could be facilitated by offering instructions on how to make small and manageable changes in daily life, which have been found to be the key to successful adoption of new food habits (Gardner et al., 2011). In the long run, this may also facilitate the cultural acceptability of meat reduction and encourage people to reflect on the sustainability of their eating patterns. However, as has been emphasized in this chapter, sustainable culinary cultures (Mäkelä and Niva, 2016) for mitigating the environmental load of food production and consumption require more than a reliance in consumers making the change in their daily lives. Political, economic, structural, and cultural changes are needed for the transition to less animal-based diets to take place and for them to be a habitual and routinized part of everyday life.

References

Akibode, S., Maredia, M., March 27, 2011. Global and Regional Trends in Production, Trade and Consumption of Food Legume Crops. Department of Agricultural, Food and Resource Economics, Michigan State University. Report Submitted to SPIA.

de Bakker, E., Dagevos, H., 2012. Reducing meat consumption in today's consumer society: questioning the citizen-consumer gap. J. Agric. Environ. Ethics 25, 877–894.

Bargh, J.A., 1994. The four horsemen of automaticity: awareness, intention, efficiency, and control in social cognition. In: Wyer, R.S., Srull, T.K. (Eds.), Handbook of Social Cognition: Vol. 1 Basic Processes. Lawrence Erlbaum Associates, Hove, pp. 1–40.

Bittman, M., 2013. VB6: Eat Vegan Before 6:00 to Lose Weight and Restore Your Health … For Good. Clarkson Potter, New York.

de Boer, J., Schösler, H., Boersema, J.J., 2013. Climate change and meat eating: an inconvenient couple? J. Environ. Psychol. 33, 1–8.

de Boer, J., de Witt, A., Aiking, H., 2016. Help the climate, change your diet: a cross-sectional study on how to involve consumers in a transition to a low-carbon society. Appetite 98, 19–27.

Bohm, I., Lindblom, C., Åbacka, G., Bengs, C., Hörnell, A., 2015. "He just has to like ham" – the centrality of meat in home and consumer studies. Appetite 95, 101–112.

Boland, M.J., Rae, A.N., Vereijken, J.M., Meuwissen, M.P.M., Fischer, A.R.H., van Boekel, M.A.J.S., Rutherfurd, S.M., Gruppen, H., Moughan, P.J., Hendriks, W.H., 2013. The future supply of animal-derived protein for human consumption. Trends Food Sci. Technol. 29, 62–73.

Cross, A.J., Leitzmann, M.F., Gail, M.H., Hollenbeck, A.R., Schatzkin, A., Sinha, R., 2007. A prospective study of red and processed meat intake in relation to cancer risk. PLoS Med. 4 (12), e325.

Cubero, J.I., 2011. The faba bean: historic perspective. Grain Legum. (56), 5–7. Availabel at: http://www.ias.csic.es/grainlegumesmagazine/Grain_Legumes_issue_56.pdf.

Dietary Guidelines for Americans 2015–2020, eighth ed. Available at: http://health.gov/dietaryguidelines/2015/guidelines/.

Drewnowski, A., 2010. The Nutrient Rich Food Index helps to identify healthy, affordable foods. Am. J. Clin. Nutr. 91 (Suppl.), 1095S–1101S.

Elzerman, J.E., Hoek, A.C., van Boekel, M.A.J.S., Luning, P.A., 2011. Consumer acceptance and appropriateness of meat substitutes in a meal context. Food Qual. Prefer. 22, 233–240.

FAOSTAT, 2013. Food Balance Sheets. Pulses. Available at: http://faostat.fao.org/.

Fiddes, N., 2004. Meat: A Natural Symbol. Routledge.

Finley, J.W., Burrell, J.B., Reeves, P.G., 2007. Pinto bean consumption changes SCFA profiles in fecal fermentations, bacterial populations of the lower bowel, and lipid profiles in blood of humans. J. Nutr. 137, 2391–2398.

Fox, N., Ward, K., 2008. Health, ethics and environment: a qualitative study of vegetarian motivations. Appetite 50, 422–429.

Freestone, O.M., McGoldrick, P.J., 2007. Motivations of the ethical consumer. J. Bus. Ethics 79, 445–467.

Gardner, B., de Bruijin, G.J., Lally, P.A., 2011. A systematic review and meta-analysis of application of the self-report habit index to nutrition and physical activity behaviours. Ann. Behav. Med. 42, 174–187.

Guillaumie, L., Godin, G., Vézina-Im, L.A., 2010. Psychosocial determinants of fruit and vegetable intake in adult population: a systematic review. Int. J. Behav. Nutr. Phys. Act. 7, 2–12.

Hoek, A.C., Luning, P.A., Stafleu, A., de Graaf, C., 2004. Food-related lifestyle and health attitudes of Dutch vegetarians, non-vegetarian consumers of meat substitutes, and meat consumers. Appetite 42, 265–272.

Hoek, A.C., van Boekel, M.A.J.S., Voordouw, J., Luning, P.A., 2011. Identification of new food alternatives: how do consumers categorize meat and meat substitutes? Food Qual. Prefer. 22, 371–383.

Hoffmann, S.R., Stallings, S.F., Bessinger, R.C., Brooks, G.T., 2013. Differences between health and ethical vegetarians. Strength of conviction, nutrition knowledge, dietary restriction, and duration of adherence. Appetite 65, 139–144.

Holland, R.W., Aarts, H., Langendam, D., 2006. Breaking and creating habits on the working floor: a field-experiment on the power of implementation intentions. J. Exp. Soc. Psychol. 42, 776–783.

Jallinoja, P., Niva, M., Latvala, T., 2016. Towards more sustainable eating? Practices, competence, meanings and materialities of bean eating in a meat-eating culture. Futures 83, 4–14.

Johnston, J., Baumann, S., 2015. Foodies: Democracy and Distinction in the Gourmet Foodscape, second ed. Routledge, New York.

Konttinen, H., Sarlio-Lähteenkorva, S., Silventoinen, K., Männistö, S., Haukkala, A., 2012. Socio-economic disparities in the consumption of vegetables, fruit and energy-dense foods: the role of motive priorities. Public Health Nutr. 16, 873–882.

Lappalainen, R., Saba, A., Holm, L., Mykkänen, H., Gibney, M.J., Moles, A., 1997. Difficulties in trying to eat healthier: descriptive analysis of perceived barriers for healthy eating. Eur. J. Clin. Nutr. 51, 36–40.

Latvala, T., Niva, M., Mäkelä, J., Pouta, E., Heikkilä, J., Kotro, J., Forsman-Hugg, S., 2012. Diversifying meat consumption patterns: consumers' self-reported past behaviour and intentions for change. Meat Sci. 92, 71–77.

Lea, E., Worsley, A., Crawford, D., 2005. Australian adult consumers' beliefs about vegetarian foods: a qualitative study. Health Educ. Behav. 32, 795–808.

Lea, E., Crawford, D., Worsley, A., 2006a. Consumers' readiness to eat a plant-based diet. Eur. J. Clin. Nutr. 60, 342–351.

Lea, E., Crawford, D., Worsley, A., 2006b. Public views of the benefits and barriers to the consumption of a plant-based diet. Eur. J. Clin. Nutr. 60, 828–837.

Lehtonen, H., Irz, X., 2013. Impacts of reducing red meat consumption on agricultural production in Finland. Agric. Food Sci. 22, 345–370.

Leitzmann, C., 2014. Vegetarian nutrition: past, present, future. Am. J. Clin. Nutr. 100 (Suppl.), 496S–502S.

Lombardini, C., Lankoski, L., 2013. Forced choice restriction in promoting sustainable food consumption: intended and unintended effects of the mandatory vegetarian day in Helsinki schools. J. Consum. Policy 36, 159–178.

Macdiarmid, J.I., Douglas, F., Campbell, J., 2016. Eating like there's no tomorrow: public awareness of the environmental impact of food and reluctance to eat less meat as part of a sustainable diet. Appetite 96, 487–493.

Mäkelä, J., Niva, M., 2016. Citizens and sustainable culinary cultures. In: Paloviita, A., Järvelä, M. (Eds.), Climate Change Adaptation and Food Supply Chain Management. Routledge, London and New York, pp. 172–182.

Mäkiniemi, J.-P., Vainio, A., 2014. Barriers to climate-friendly food choices among young adults in Finland. Appetite 74, 12–19.

Morland, K., Wing, S., Diez, A.V., Roux, C., 2002. Poole neighborhood characteristics associated with the location of food stores and food service places. Am. J. Prev. Med. 22, 23–29.

Natural Resources Institute Finland (Luke), 2013. Balance Sheet for Food Commodities 2012, Preliminary and 2011 Final Figures. Available at: http://www.maataloustilastot.fi/en/balance-sheet-food-commodities-2012-preliminary-and-2011-final-figures_en.

Niva, M., Mäkelä, J., Kahma, N., Kjærnes, U., 2014. Eating sustainably? Practices and background factors of ecological food consumption in four Nordic countries. J. Consum. Policy 37, 465–484.

Nordic Food Recommendations, 2012. Part 1. Summary, Principles and Use. Nordic Council of Ministers, Copenhagen.

Paturi, M., Tapanainen, H., Reinivuo, H., Pietinen, P. (Eds.), 2008. The National FINDIET 2007 Survey. Publications B23. The National Public Health Institute, Helsinki.

Pohjolainen, P., Vinnari, M., Jokinen, P., 2015. Consumers' perceived barriers to following a plant-based diet. Br. Food J. 117, 1150–1167.

Pollard, T.M., Steptoe, A., Wardle, J., 1998. Motives underlying healthy eating: using the food choice questionnaire to explain variation in dietary intake. J. Biosoc. Sci. 30, 165–179.

Potts, A., White, M., 2008. New Zealand vegetarians: at odds with their nation. Soc. Animals 16, 336–353.

Prochaska, J.O., DiClemente, C.C., 1983. Stages and processes of self-change of smoking: toward an integrative model of change. J. Consult. Clin. Psychol. 31, 390–395.

Raphaely, T., Marinova, D., 2014. Flexitarianism: decarbonisng through flexible vegetarianism. Renew. Energy 67, 90–96.

Renner, B., Sproesser, G., Strohbach, S., Schupp, H.T., 2012. Why we eat what we eat. The eating motivation survey (TEMS). Appetite 59, 117–128.

Rizkalla, S.W., Bellisle, F., Slama, G., 2002. Health benefits of low glycaemic index foods, such as pulses, in diabetic patients and healthy individuals. Br. J. Nutr. 88 (3), 255–262.

Rose, D., Richards, R., 2004. Food store access and household fruit and vegetable use among participants in the US food stamp program. Public Health Nutr. 7, 1081–1088.

Rossi, S.R., Greene, G.W., Rossi, J.S., Plummer, B.A., Benisovich, S.V., Keller, S., Velicer, W.F., Redding, C.F., Prochaska, J.O., Pallonen, U.E., Meier, K.S., 2001. Validation of decisional balance and situational temptations: measures for dietary fat reduction in a large school-based population of adolescents. Eat. Behav. 2, 1–18.

Rothberger, H., 2014. A comparison of attitudes toward meat and animal among strict and semi-vegetarians. Appetite 72, 98–105.

Rothman, A.J., Sheeran, P., Wood, W., 2009. Reflective and automatic processes in the initiation and maintenance of dietary change. Ann. Behav. Med. 38, 4–17.

Schneider, A., 2002. Overview of the market and consumption of pulses in Europe. Br. J. Nutr. 88, S243–S250.

Schyver, T., Smith, C., 2005. Reported attitudes and beliefs toward soy food consumption of soy consumers versus nonconsumers in natural foods and mainstream grocery stores. J. Nutr. Educ. Behav. 37, 292–299.

Shove, E., Pantzar, M., Watson, M., 2012. The Dynamics of Social Practice: Everyday Life and How It Changes. Sage, London.

Shove, E., 2010. Beyond the ABC: climate change policy and theories of social change. Environ. Plan. A 42, 1273–1285.

Shurtleff, W., Aoyagi, A., 2013. History of Tofu and Tofu Products (965 CE To 2013): Extensively Annotated Bibliography and Sourcebook. SoyInfo Center. Available at: http://Www.Soyinfocenter.Com/Pdf/163/Tofu.Pdf.

Smil, V., 2002. Worldwide transformation of diets, burdens of meat production and opportunities for novel food proteins. Enzym. Microb. Tech. 30, 305–311.

Smith, C., Burke, L.E., Wing, R.R., 2000. Vegetarian and weight-loss diets among young adults. Obes. Res. 8, 123–129.

Spurling, N., McMeekin, A., Shove, E., Southerton, D., Welch, D., September 2013. Interventions in Practice: Re-framing Policy Approaches to Consumer Behavior. Sustainable Practices Research Group Report.

Steffen, W., Richardson, K., Rockström, J., Cornell, S., Fetzer, I., Bennett, E., Biggs, R., Carpenter, S., de Vries, W., de Wit, C., Folke, C., Gerten, D., Heinke, J., Mace, G., Persson, L., Ramanathan, V., Reyers, B., Sörlin, S., 2015. Planetary boundaries: guiding human development on a changing planet. Science 347 (6223). http://dx.doi.org/10.1126/science.1259855.

Stehfest, E., Bouwman, L., van Vuuren, D.P., den Elzen, M.G.J., Eickhout, B., Kabat, P., 2009. Climate benefits of changing diet. Clim. Change 95, 83–102.

Vainio, A., Mäkiniemi, J.-P., Paloniemi, R., 2013. System justification and the perception of food risks. Group Process. Intergr. Relat. 17, 510–524.

Vainio, A., Niva, M., Jallinoja, P., Latvala, T., 2016. From beef to beans: eating motives and the replacement of animal proteins with plant proteins among Finnish consumers. Appetite 106, 92–100.

Vaitkeviciute, R., Ball, L.E., Harris, N., 2014. The relationship between food literacy and dietary intake in adolescents: a systematic review. Public Health Nutr. 18, 649–658.

Verbeke, W., Pérez-Cueto, F.J.A., de Barcellos, M.D., Krystallis, A., Grunert, K.G., 2010. European citizen and consumer attitudes and preferences regarding beef and pork. Meat Sci. 84, 284–292.

Vidgen, H.A., Gallegos, D., 2014. Defining food literacy and its components. Appetite 76, 50–59.

Vinnari, M., Tapio, P., 2009. Future images of meat consumption in 2030. Futures 41, 269–278.

Vinnari, M., Mustonen, P., Räsänen, P., 2010. Tracking down trends in non-meat consumption in Finnish households, 1966–2006. Br. Food J. 112, 836–852.

Vinnari, M., 2008. The future of meat consumption - expert views from Finland. Technol. Forecast. Soc. Change 75, 893–904.

Virtanen, Y., Kurppa, S., Saarinen, M., Katajajuuri, J.-M., Usva, K., Mäenpää, I., Mäkelä, J., Grönroos, J., Nissinen, A., 2011. Carbon footprint of food – approaches from national input–output statistics and a LCA of a food portion. J. Clean. Prod. 19, 1849–1856.

Wansink, B., Sobal, J., 2007. Mindless eating: the 200 daily food decisions we overlook. Environ. Behav. 39, 106–123.

Warde, A., 2005. Consumption and theories of practice. J. Consum. Cult. 5, 131–153.

Warde, A., 2016. The Practice of Eating. Polity Press, Cambridge, UK.

World Cancer Research Fund, 2013. Food, Nutrition and Physical Activity, and the Prevention of Cancer: A Global Perspective. Available at: http://www.dietandcancerreport.org/expert_report/.

Setting the Scene – Specific Dietary Characteristics of Vegetarian Diet and Their Relation to Health

11

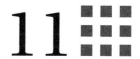

Dietary Patterns in Plant-Based, Vegetarian, and Omnivorous Diets

Stephen Walsh[1], Marcel Hebbelinck[1], Peter Deriemaeker[1,2], Peter Clarys[1,2]

[1]VRIJE UNIVERSITEIT BRUSSEL, BRUSSELS, BELGIUM; [2]ERASMUS UNIVERSITY COLLEGE, BRUSSELS, BELGIUM;

1. Introduction

Characterizing the quality of diets in such a way as to be able to predict long-term health outcomes is the core challenge for nutritional epidemiology. The vast majority of work on dietary quality models has been based on evidence from omnivorous diets. Typical examples include the Mediterranean Diet Score (MDS) (Trichopoulou et al., 2003), the Healthy Eating Index (Guenther et al., 2013), and the Global Burden of Disease diet model (Forouzanfar et al., 2015). The former two seek to score diet quality, while the latter seeks to predict explicitly the impact of dietary choices on healthy life expectancy.

The impact of vegetarian diets (which exclude animal flesh; for definition, see Chapter 1), vegan diets (which exclude all animal products), and other predominantly plant-based diets on health has been actively investigated for many years. Information on the effect of vegetarian dietary choices on death rates comes mainly from studies in the United States on Seventh-day Adventists, particularly Adventist Health Study 2 (AHS2) (Orlich et al., 2013), and from studies in the United Kingdom on vegetarians and "comparable"/"health-conscious" nonvegetarians, particularly the EPIC-Oxford study and the Oxford Vegetarian study (Appleby et al., 2016).

This chapter explores the interactions between these two research endeavors and seeks to answer the questions:

What are the defining and typical differences between plant-based, vegetarian, and omnivorous diets?

Can dietary quality models developed for measuring the quality of omnivorous diets be usefully applied to plant-based and vegetarian diets?

Do existing dietary quality models illuminate observed differences in health between plant-based, vegetarian, and omnivorous diets?

Are extensions needed to existing dietary quality models to more completely encompass plant-based and vegetarian diets?

2. Defining and Typical Differences Between Plant-Based, Vegetarian, and Omnivorous Diets

Vegan diets are defined by the complete absence of foods derived from animals, including meat, fish, eggs, milk, and honey. Vegetarian diets are defined by the absence of flesh foods: meat and fish. Vegan diets are therefore a special case of vegetarian diet along with lactovegetarian (includes milk and milk products), ovovegetarian (includes eggs and egg products), and ovolactovegetarian. The term semivegetarian is sometimes used to describe people who only occasionally eat flesh foods, while pesco-vegetarian is sometimes used for people who do not eat flesh foods other than fish and seafood. Both these terms are misnomers as by definition someone who eats flesh is not a vegetarian, and the terms occasional meat eater or fish eater/pescetarian would be preferable to avoid this inherent confusion. Chapter 1 sets out definitions of the terms generally used in this book. The threshold used to define regular meat eaters as opposed to occasional/low meat eaters is usually at least once a week, but a UK study (Appleby et al., 2016) used a threshold of at least five times a week, giving a reference group that had meat consumption closer to the general population.

The exclusions of certain foods that define the different diet groups are consistent with a wide range of possible substitutions and adaptations. These could include the following:

- scaling up of the use of *all* other foods;
- direct replacement of animal foods by plant milks and meat substitutes, leaving the rest of the diet unchanged;
- specific culturally supported changes, such as following recommendations from vegetarian and vegan associations and authors;
- adaptations based on personal tastes and preferences.

Such changes will vary according to the cultural setting. For example, among Seventh-day Adventists, vegetarianism is culturally linked to the promotion of health, and it was reported that as well as excluding animal products, Adventist vegans ate fewer fried potatoes and refined grains than any other diet group (Orlich et al., 2014).

2.1 Selection of a Representative Set of Vegetarians

A challenge in all dietary evaluations is finding a representative sample, and studies of vegetarians face special challenges. Almost all diet studies are subject to a healthy volunteer effect, though nationally representative surveys try to minimize this. The Adventist studies should be fairly representative of the Adventist community (of whom vegetarians make up a high proportion), but the Adventists differ in other respects from the general population, e.g., very low use of alcohol. Vegetarians are still rare enough in most countries that they must be sought out by some special route, e.g., via contacting members of vegetarian associations, who cannot be assumed to be representative of the overall vegetarian population.

Juan et al. (2015) looked at dietary intakes (assessed using a single-day record of diet intake) of self-identified vegetarians within the US NHANES study between 2007 and 2010. The self-identification was unreliable: about half the dietary records for self-identified vegetarians included flesh foods. Nevertheless, there were clear differences between the self-identified vegetarians and nonvegetarians. After expressing the results per 1000 kcal, the self-identified vegetarians ate more fruit, vegetables, legumes, soy products, grains, and whole grains and less solid fats (includes fat from meat and dairy) and added sugars. The self-identified vegetarians were thus consuming a more plant-based diet than the general population.

Kennedy et al. (2001), Farmer et al. (2011), and Farmer (2014) used earlier results from NHANES but classified vegetarians based on the absence of flesh foods from a one-day dietary record. Farmer et al. (2011) also found increased consumption by vegetarians of fruit and vegetables and higher fiber intakes: 23 g/day versus 16 g/day in individuals with normal calorie intake.

2.2 Reference Groups

While the NHANES studies had a nationally representative sample but struggled to identify true vegetarians among them, other studies may struggle to find an appropriate reference group for comparisons with a specially selected group of vegetarians. Studies may make comparisons between the selected vegetarians and either nationally representative samples or nonvegetarians matched in some way to the vegetarians.

Compared with the general population, the "comparable" nonvegetarians in many studies appear to be typically more health conscious, as shown by higher fruit and vegetable intake even in the regular meat eater category. Table 11.1 compares regular meat eaters in EPIC-Oxford (Appleby et al., 2016) with participants in the UK National Diet and Nutrition Survey (Bates et al., 2014). Note that in the UK studies, nonstarch polysaccharide (NSP) fiber was reported, while in other studies total fiber was reported.

The regular meat eaters in AHS-2 (consuming meat at least once a week) also consumed larger amounts of fruit and vegetables (Orlich et al., 2014) and fiber (Rizzo et al., 2013) than typical US diets (Daniel et al., 2011; Farmer, 2014). Furthermore, in contrast

Table 11.1 Food Consumption of EPIC-Oxford Regular Meat Eaters Versus National Diet and Nutrition Survey (g/day). Total fiber Has Been Estimated as 1.5 Times NSP Fiber (Aldwairji et al., 2012)

	EPIC-Oxford Men	NDNS Men	EPIC-Oxford Women	NDNS Women
Fruit	200	97	257	103
Vegetables	220	182	256	183
Meat	115	130	106	89
Red meat	84	86	70	56
NSP fiber	18	15	18	13
Total fiber	27	23	27	20

with the EPIC-Oxford regular meat eaters (consuming meat at least five times a week), the AHS-2 regular meat eaters consumed much less meat than a nationally representative sample in the United States (40.5 g/day vs. 128 g/day total meat and 17.5 g/day vs. 70 g/day red meat).

Reported fiber consumption for the regular meat eaters in AHS-2 and EPIC-Oxford is between 25 and 30 g/day (Rizzo et al., 2013; Appleby et al., 2016) and is consistently higher than national norms (15–20 g/day). It is also higher than the value of 23 g/day reported for nondieting vegetarians within the NHANES study (Farmer et al., 2011).

It is clear that the nonvegetarian comparison groups in the AHS-2 and EPIC-Oxford studies of vegetarians follow a diet richer in whole plant foods and sometimes also lower in meat than the general populations in their countries.

2.3 Composition of the Restricted Diets

With these caveats, we can characterize the typical differences as we move from regular meat eaters to low/occasional meat eaters, pescetarians, ovolactovegetarians, and vegans.

Vegan diets consistently show a much lower intake of saturated fats often accompanied by an increase in polyunsaturated fats (Davey et al., 2003; Rizzo et al., 2013). However, because some studies accept very infrequent consumption of animal products within "vegan" diets and because diet composition databases often assume animal products as a minor ingredient of prepared foods, nutritional analyses will often show vegans as consuming moderate amounts of animal-derived nutrients such as cholesterol. In fact, consumption of cholesterol in vegans should be zero.

Studies vary as to whether nonvegan vegetarians consume more or fewer dairy products than nonvegetarians. In AHS-2, lactovegetarians consumed about half the amount of animal milk products consumed by nonvegetarians (Orlich et al., 2014). Vegetarians in EPIC-Oxford also consumed about half as much milk as nonvegetarians but consumed slightly more cheese (Key et al., 2009). In Belgium (Clarys et al., 2013), vegetarians consumed more dairy foods than meat eaters. There does not seem to be a consistent pattern for animal milk consumption among vegetarians.

A broad substitution of plant foods for animal foods is consistently seen. For example, in AHS-2 (Orlich et al., 2014):

> *In the case of almost all the major plant food groups – legumes, soya foods and meat analogues, nuts and seeds, grains, potatoes, avocados, fruits and vegetables – vegans were found to consume the highest amounts of daily energy from these food groups, nonvegetarians the lowest amounts and the other vegetarian groups intermediate amounts.*

This is supported by other studies. For example, vegans generally consume about 40%–50% more fiber than nonvegetarians with other vegetarians showing intermediate values (Davey et al., 2003; Clarys et al., 2014; Rizzo et al., 2013). The absolute fiber intakes reported in different studies vary, but this variation is much reduced if NSP fiber values reported for the UK studies are multiplied by 1.5 to estimate the total fiber values (Aldwairji et al., 2012). With this adjustment, typical nonvegetarian fiber intake in these studies is around 25–30 g/day, while typical vegan intakes are about 40–45 g/day. Fiber values reported in AHS-2 may be exaggerated somewhat due to the rescaling of all nutrients to a calorie intake of 2000 kcal: for example, median unscaled fruit intake for the whole population was 260 g/day, while median scaled fruit intakes for each diet group ranged from 300 g/day for nonvegetarians to 480 g/day for vegans (Orlich et al., 2014), which will correspondingly increase estimates of fiber intakes.

There is less consistency in the observed changes between diet groups in intakes of plant foods considered to be unhealthy. In AHS-2 (Orlich et al., 2014), vegetarians consumed less of these.

Vegetarians also consumed lower amounts of added fats, sweets, snack foods and nonwater beverages: in each case, vegans consumed the lowest amounts, nonvegetarians the highest amounts and the other vegetarian groups intermediate amounts.

Adventist vegans also consumed the lowest amounts of fried potatoes (Orlich et al., 2014). The reduced intake of less healthy plant foods may be distinctive to the Adventist studies. In contrast, Clarys et al. (2013, 2014) found that vegetarians and vegans in Belgium consumed *more* refined grains than omnivores. Clearly the detail of substitution from animal foods to particular plant foods is modified by other factors such as the extent to which vegetarian choices are linked to the pursuit of health.

Satija et al. (2016) present a healthy plant-based diet index (hPDI) and show that diabetes incidence was reduced more strongly and consistently when intakes of healthy plant foods increased and intakes of unhealthy plant foods decreased than when intakes of all plant foods increased: the quality of the plant part of the diet is important.

Estimates of sodium intake on different diets also vary, with some studies suggesting a substantial decrease in sodium intake in vegan diets compared with nonvegetarian diets (Clarys et al., 2014), some suggesting an increase (Lau et al., 1998), and others suggesting little difference (Appleby et al., 2002; Rizzo et al., 2013; Sobiecki et al., 2016).

The variety in the differences observed between omnivorous and vegetarian diets raises the question as to how consistently vegetarian diets are associated with an improved diet quality. To address this, we need to look first at how diet quality can be measured.

3. Dietary Quality Models

USDA (2014) provides a useful overview of dietary quality models. This report found that dietary quality models including MDS, Dietary Approaches to Stop Hypertension, and Dietary Guidelines-related patterns (such as the HEI-2010) were convincingly successful in predicting risk of cardiovascular disease.

Dietary patterns associated with decreased risk of cardiovascular disease were characterized by regular consumption of fruits, vegetables, whole grains, low-fat dairy, and fish and were low in red and processed meat and sugar-sweetened foods and drinks. Regular consumption of nuts and legumes and moderate consumption of alcohol were also shown to be beneficial in most studies. Additionally, research that included specific nutrients in their description of dietary patterns indicated that patterns that were low in saturated fat, cholesterol, and sodium and rich in fiber and potassium may be beneficial for reducing cardiovascular disease risk.

3.1 Mediterranean Diet Score

The MDS set out by Trichopoulou et al. (2003) attempts to characterize Mediterranean diets, which have been associated with good health. The MDS targets high intake of vegetables, fruits and nuts, legumes, fish and seafood, and cereals; low intake of meat and dairy products; high ratio of monounsaturated to saturated fats; and moderate intake of alcohol. High and low are defined relative to the median intake in the population studied. Moderate alcohol intake is defined as 10–50 g/day of alcohol for men or 5–25 g/day for women. One point is given for falling in each desirable category, giving an overall score between 0 and 9. Against a background of typical Western diets, the choice of a vegan diet would get a score of 1 for low meat, a score of 0 for low fish, and a score of 1 for low dairy. A lactovegetarian diet could lose a point for high dairy, depending on the amounts consumed. If comparisons are limited to vegetarian diets, components such as meat and fish which have a consistently zero intake, could be assigned a score of 0.5.

In a recent meta-analysis, an increase of two points on the MDS was associated with an 8% reduction in overall death rate (Sofi et al., 2010), equivalent to living about 10 months longer. An analysis of death rates and MDS was carried out in participants over 60 in EPIC (Trichopoulou et al., 2005), and the analysis of the UK EPIC cohorts (Oxford and Norfolk) showed the same 8% reduction in death rates for a 2-unit increase in score.

3.2 The Healthy Eating Index

The HEI-2010 score (Guenther et al., 2013) is also widely used and has been confirmed to predict a reduction in all-cause mortality of about 15%–25% in the upper versus lower quintile of the HEI-2010 score (Liese et al., 2015). This score attempts to measure compliance with US Dietary Guidelines and explicitly tries to accommodate vegetarian and vegan diets. HEI-2010 assigns a score based on absolute levels of food/nutrient intake rather than based on population medians and includes a fixed intake beyond which the score will no longer improve. For fruit and vegetables, the thresholds are set in cups per day per 1000 kcal and for a 2000 kcal diet equate to about 240 g/day of fruit and 320 g/day of vegetables. It should be noted that the average intakes of regular meat eaters in EPIC-Oxford were close to these targets, while the average intakes of regular meat eaters in AHS-2 exceeded these targets. This again emphasizes that the reference meat-eating group in both these studies was eating larger amounts of healthy plant foods than the general populations in their countries. This may partly explain why the reference groups showed low death rates compared with the general population and may also limit differences in health outcomes and diet quality scores between the different diet groups within the studies.

The HEI-2010 score penalizes high sodium intake. It separates refined grains (less is better) and whole grains (more is better). The fatty acid score considers all unsaturated fats rather than just monounsaturated fats (with maximum points given for a ratio of 2.5 or more of unsaturated fat to saturated fat and minimum points for a ratio of 1.2 or less). The fat content of meat and dairy is added to solid fats and hence to empty calories. Unlike the MDS, HEI-2010 treats dairy products as a beneficial component, though their fat content will have an adverse impact on the fatty acid score and the empty calorie score. *Fortified* soya milk counts as equivalent to dairy. Beans and peas contribute both to total protein and to "seafood and plant proteins" unless the maximum score for total protein has already been reached, in which case they contribute to the "greens and beans" vegetable category. This means that the absence of fish does not incur an inevitable penalty for vegetarians as it does with the MDS. Alcohol is treated as neutral up to 13 g per 1000 kcal, above which it contributes to empty calories and is therefore penalized. Solid fats and added sugars also contribute to empty calories.

Processed meat substitutes can be high in saturated fat and salt, which would contribute toward empty calories and sodium under HEI-2000 as well as contributing to total protein. In the older HEI scores, which focus on meat as a source of protein, one cup of cooked legumes counts as the same as four-ounce equivalents of meat

3.3 Diet in Relation to Disability Adjusted Lost Years (DALYs): Adjustment of the Weight of the Components

An alternative approach to assessing diet quality is that of the Global Burden of Disease (GBD) study (Forouzanfar et al., 2015), which goes beyond the relatively uniform weighting of dietary characteristics used in the MDS and HEI scores by selecting dietary characteristics for which there is good evidence of an association with death or with DALYs due to specific causes. For each risk factor considered, a theoretical minimum risk exposure level (TMREL) is defined and relative risks for specific diseases due to deviations from the TMREL are used to estimate the impact of diet on DALYs and hence on the burden of disease. If the TMREL is considered to be uncertain, then it is given as a range, and the GBD model calculates the attributable DALYs assuming the TMREL varies uniformly over the given range.

The GBD model considers long chain omega-3 fatty acids (EPA and DHA) rather than fish (as in the MDS) or "seafood and plant proteins" (as in the HEI-2010 score). It treats alcohol as a drug rather than a component of diet and assigns it a high adverse impact, with zero intake as the TMREL.

The GBD model could, in principle, be applied to any measured diet in a given country to assign it a score in terms of DALYs lost. More broadly, it provides a guide to the appropriate weight to be attached to different dietary components.

Table 11.2   Age-Standardized DALYs Lost per 100,000 People per Year by Risk Factor

Risk Factor	Belgium	United Kingdom	United States	Global
Tobacco smoke	2154	1880	2363	2209
Alcohol use	1320	908	1140	1421
Diet low in fruits	427	484	588	1151
Diet high in processed meat	391	358	488	262
Diet high in sodium	300	309	489	1176
Diet low in vegetables	296	327	427	601
Diet low in whole grains	293	298	429	784
Diet low in nuts and seeds	227	297	373	416
Diet low in fiber	153	251	286	339
Diet low in polyunsaturated fatty acids	96	116	121	195
Diet low in seafood omega-3 fatty acids	79	95	242	343
Diet high in sugar-sweetened beverages	59	51	350	90
Diet high in red meat	58	66	77	62
Diet suboptimal in calcium	53	52	48	45
Diet high in trans-fatty acids	52	55	210	149
Diet low in milk	36	35	37	34
Diet sum (excluding tobacco and alcohol)	2520	2794	4165	5647

Table 11.2 shows DALYs (age-standardized rate per 100,000) attributed to each dietary cause in the GBD model for a selection of regions and countries. The table also includes DALYs attributed to smoking and alcohol to give a broader picture. In interpreting Table 11.2, it should be noted that an increase of about 1250 in the DALY rate equates to about 1 year less in Health Adjusted Life Expectancy (HALE), based on a regression analysis of DALYs versus HALE for those countries with a HALE above 68. Moving typical Western diets to the TMRELs in the GBD model could therefore potentially give 2–3 years' improvement in HALE. This projected impact is similar to the observed difference in death rates between top and bottom quintiles of the HEI-2010 and MDS dietary quality scores.

3.4 Comparison of Importance of the Components Over the Three Models

All three models (MDS, HEI-2010, and GBD) place a strong emphasis on increased consumption of fruit and vegetables. The GBD TMREL values for fruit and vegetables (200–400 g/day for fruit and 350–450 g/day for vegetables) are somewhat higher than the intakes required for maximum scores on HEI-2010 (240 g/day of fruit and 320 g/day of vegetables). Within Western countries, the GBD model assigns a particularly high impact to fruit intakes and slightly lower but significant impacts to vegetables, sodium, whole grains, and nuts/seeds. The only impact of animal foods of similar importance to these plant factors within Western diets is an adverse impact of processed meat consumption, but at a global level, lack of "seafood" omega-3s (EPA and DHA) also has a similar impact. The projected impact of red meat is relatively low as the only effects considered are an increase in colorectal cancer and diabetes. Fiber intake is not really an independent effect but depends on the other dietary factors listed, so it does not need to be considered as a separate component.

All three dietary quality measures include some component for fat quality that favors unsaturated fats, but the detail varies: MDS favors a high ratio of monounsaturated to saturated fats, HEI-2010 favors a high ratio of unsaturated fats to saturated fats, and GBD treats polyunsaturated fats as favorable, ignoring saturated fats. The HEI-2010 fat score would be expected to favor vegan diets most strongly, as they show a much lower saturated fat intake but similar or increased unsaturated fat. The GBD model singles out trans-fatty acids as a harmful component, though this appears to be a minor issue within Western Europe.

Fish is treated favorably in all three models, though HEI-2010 treats seafood and plant proteins as equivalent contributors to a "seafood and plant proteins" component, and the GBD study singles out the EPA and DHA fatty acids rather than protein as the relevant component with a TMREL of 200–300 mg/day. Zhao et al. (2016) present a meta-analysis of prospective cohort studies and fish intake that indicates a 6% reduction in all-cause mortality for the highest category of fish consumption.

The GBD model singles out red meat and processed meat as harmful components, but processed meat is estimated to have a much higher impact on DALYs than red meat. The MDS combines all meat as a harmful component, while the HEI-2010 score gives meat no special treatment beyond its contribution to protein and fat scores (fat from meat and dairy will have an adverse effect on the ratio of unsaturated to saturated fats and will also contribute to the solid fat category, which is a component of empty calories).

HEI-2010 and GBD favor whole grains, while MDS does not differentiate between whole and refined grains. This seems to be a clear weakness of the MDS, and some later variants of MDS use only whole grains as the favorable component. For example, Fung et al. (2005) present an alternate MDS (aMED):

> *We modified the original scale for this study by excluding potato products from the vegetable group, separating fruit and nuts into 2 groups, eliminating the dairy group, including whole-grain products only, including only red and processed meats for the meat group, and assigning alcohol intake between 5 and 15 g/day for 1 point.*

HEI-2010 and GBD treat high sodium intake as a strongly negative component, while the MDS is silent on this.

The MDS singles out legumes as a specific component, while HEI-2010 has three categories to which legumes can contribute (greens and beans, total protein, seafood and plant proteins), but the GBD model does not include legumes.

The GBD model treats nuts and seeds as a distinct and strongly beneficial component, while in HEI-2000 they are not separated out but contribute favorably to "seafood and plant proteins" and fatty acid scores. In the MDS, nuts are combined with fruit based on total weight, and therefore will have little impact. Fung et al. (2005) created a separate category for nuts and seeds as part of the aMED score.

The treatment of dairy varies considerably between these diet quality measures: MDS treats it as having an adverse effect, HEI-2010 treats it beneficial (especially if low-fat), while the GBD model attributes a beneficial but negligible impact. An analysis of the MDS by component in Greece also found negligible impact of the dairy component. The aMED score drops dairy as a component.

The divergence in the treatment of alcohol between the MDS, HEI-2010, and GBD models is particularly dramatic, ranging from strongly beneficial, in moderation, to strongly harmful. The harm reflects increased risks of injuries, cirrhosis, and cancer. The benefit comes mainly from apparent reductions in ischemic heart disease and stroke. The apparent reductions in risk for drinkers versus lifetime abstainers are found even in people consuming so little alcohol (<2 g/day) that a real effect seems physiologically implausible. The EPIC study (Bergmann et al., 2003) found further reduction (about 9%) in risk of death from all causes associated with higher but still moderate alcohol consumption. Whether this remaining reduction, after careful attempts to control for confounding, is causal or reflects residual confounding remains debatable.

The GBD model attributes a small reduction of risk of ischemic stroke and heart disease to alcohol, but overall this is far outweighed by increased injuries, cirrhosis, and cancer. The impact of injuries on DALYs is higher than their impact on deaths. HEI-2010 treats alcohol as neutral up to a certain intake and then slightly harmful (as a component of empty calories). The MDS takes an intermediate range of alcohol consumption as desirable with both minimal and high intakes penalized, and an analysis of the MDS by component in Greece (Trichopoulou et al., 2009) found moderate alcohol intake to be the score component with the most beneficial element within the MDS. The apparent effect of moderate alcohol consumption within the MDS score is probably exaggerated to some extent by reverse causation, with ill-health leading to abstention from alcohol. The aMED score retains a moderate alcohol category but shifts the desirable range of intakes to between 5 and 15 g/day, encompassing occasional drinkers and setting a tighter threshold for moderation.

3.5 Diet Quality and Relative Risks

There is very good evidence that a range of different diet quality indices predict all-cause mortality and cardiovascular mortality. A two-point increase in the MDS score was associated with an 8% reduction in all-cause mortality (Sofi et al., 2010).

Liese et al. (2015) compared four different diet quality measures, including HEI-2010 and aMED, in several different US cohorts using a prespecified standardized approach. Top versus bottom quintiles on HEI-2010 showed a relative risk (RR) for all-cause mortality of between 0.74 and 0.78 in men and between 0.76 and 0.89 for women. Results using the alternate Mediterranean score, aMED, were similar in men (0.76–0.77) but more consistent in predicting reduced mortality in women (0.74–0.78). The similarity in the results on the various scores is more striking than the relatively small differences.

4. Diet Quality Measures and Vegetarian Diets

Farmer et al. (2011) and Kennedy et al. (2001) compared HEI scores between vegetarians and nonvegetarians within the US NHANES participants, with conflicting results. In both cases, vegetarians were defined as those who reported eating no flesh foods during a single-day dietary record. This selection would be expected to include quite a few nonvegetarians and therefore to reflect less systematic adaptation of diets to replace meat and fish than in true vegetarians.

Kennedy et al. (2001) reported that vegetarian diets had a lower HEI score (60.8) than nonvegetarian diets (63.2). Very little detail was provided for the component scores, though it was apparent that vegetarians gained 0.7 points on the fruits score and lost 2.3 points on the variety score.

Farmer et al. (2011) used the HEI-2005 score and considered individuals with low reported calorie intake ("dieters") separately from nondieters. Farmer et al. (2011) provided full detail on the components of the score. Considering dieters and nondieters combined, essentially no differences were found: vegetarians had a score of 50.5 and nonvegetarians 50.1. Unlike the original HEI score, there was no component score for variety. As in Kennedy et al. (2001), the vegetarians gained 0.6 points on fruits. The largest difference in component score was on "meat and beans" where the vegetarians lost 4.8 points. Vegetarian consumption of beans was just a tenth of a cup more than that of nonvegetarians, which left them trailing far behind on the "meat and beans" component. Although Kennedy et al. (2001) did not report this individual component, a similar difference very probably applied.

Among nondieters, the vegetarians had a higher score than nonvegetarians (53 vs. 49.7), while among dieters the vegetarians had a lower score (47.3 vs. 51). The difference in the relative score of vegetarians and nonvegetarians as between dieters and nondieters centered on two individual categories—"solid fat, alcohol, and added sugar" (2.3 swing) and "meat and beans" (1.3 swing)—plus a swing of 2 on the combination of all the fruit and vegetable categories.

Overall the analyses based on NHANES indicate little difference in diet quality between daily diets with and without flesh, as measured by the older versions of the HEI. To consider the diets of people who have consciously chosen a vegetarian diet, we need to look elsewhere.

Clarys et al. (2013) investigated how the MDS and HEI-2010 diet quality measures worked in practice for matched vegetarians and omnivores. There were 69 vegetarians and 69 omnivores, and diets were assessed using a three-day food diary, including one weekend day.

The vegetarian diets scored more highly on both measures (see Table 11.3).

On the MDS score, the vegetarians all had a 0 score for fish but a compensating score of 1 for meat. As some omnivores also had zero intake of fish but none had a zero intake of meat, the net effect was an advantage of 0.4 to the vegetarians. The vegetarians had higher intakes of dairy and hence a lower score, but this was counterbalanced by higher scores from the plant components.

Table 11.5   All-Cause Death Rates by Diet Group Compared With Regular Meat Eaters[a]

	Vegan	Other Vegetarian	Pescetarian	Occasional/Low Meat Eaters
Pooled analysis (Key et al., 1999)	1.00	**0.84**	**0.82**	**0.84**
UK: EPIC-Oxford/ Oxford Vegetarian study (Appleby et al., 2016)	1.00	0.93	0.91	0.93
AHS-2 all (Orlich et al., 2013)	0.85	**0.91**	**0.81**	0.92
AHS-2 men	**0.72**	0.86	**0.73**	0.93
AHS-2 women	0.97	0.94	0.88	0.92

Results in bold were significant at $P < .05$.
[a]The UK results for vegetarians and vegans are based on participants who did not change diet group in the course of the studies (the relative risk of 0.93 for other vegetarians was not included in the published paper and was provided by the authors in a personal communication).

Results that included all participants, based on their last recorded diet group, showed less evidence of a benefit from vegetarian and vegan diets. This is to be expected, as participants changing diets would dilute any long-term effect of diet and could also reflect confounding by indication, changes in diet as a consequence of health changes.

Mean reported adherence to each diet group at baseline was high in AHS-2: 21 years for vegans, 39 years for other vegetarians, 24 years for pescetarians, 19 years for semivegetarians, and 48 years for meat eaters. In the Oxford studies, median adherence for vegans was 5 years and for other nonmeat-eating groups about 10 years. At baseline, the meat eaters in the AHS-2 cohort were about 6 years older than in EPIC-Oxford (56 vs. 50), and the vegans in AHS-2 were 20 years older than in EPIC-Oxford (58 vs. 38). Follow-up was much longer in the Oxford studies, narrowing the gap in age range.

Considering both sexes combined in AHS-2, ovolactovegetarians showed a statistically significant reduction in death rates (0.91), equivalent to living about 1 year longer, and pescetarians showed a significant reduction (0.81) equivalent to living 2 years longer. Occasional meat eaters (0.92) and vegans (0.85) showed numerically similar improvements, but these were not statistically significant. Appleby et al. (2016) showed similar improvements to AHS-2 for most diet groups. For vegans, there was a notable difference between the two studies (RR of 1.00 in the Oxford studies vs. 0.85 in AHS-2). The pooled analysis showed slightly larger (0.82–0.84) benefits for all diet groups compared with regular meat eaters, except for the vegans who again had a RR of 1.00.

The results match the conclusion from the MDS/HEI-2010 quality measures that vegetarian diets have an improved quality compared with omnivorous diets. The size of effect is modest but is broadly comparable with that expected based on dietary quality scores in other studies of vegetarians and vegans.

In AHS-2, both vegan men and pescetarian men showed a statistically significant reduction in death rates equivalent to living about 3 years longer. No other diet–sex combination showed statistically significant benefit in all-cause mortality.

Table 11.6   Death Rates From Cardiovascular Disease and Ischemic Heart Disease by Diet Group Compared With Regular Meat Eaters

Adventist Health Study 2	Cardiovascular Disease			Ischemic Heart Disease		
	All	Men	Women	All	Men	Women
Vegan	0.91	**0.58**	1.18	0.90	**0.45**	1.39
Other vegetarian	0.90	**0.77**	0.99	0.82	0.76	0.85
Pescetarian	0.80	**0.66**	0.90	**0.65**	0.77	**0.51**
Occasional meat eaters	0.85	0.75	0.93	0.92	0.73	1.09

Results in bold were significant at $P < .05$.

There was clear evidence from AHS-2 of a difference in the effect of diet type between men and women. This centered on cardiovascular disease and was particularly pronounced in vegans (Table 11.6).

This did not appear to be due to differences in diet between men and women. Orlich et al. (2013) note:

> *It is possible that within dietary groups the diets of men and women differ in important ways; however, a recent evaluation of the nutrient profile of the dietary patterns in this cohort did not reveal striking differences. Alternatively, the biological effect of dietary factors on mortality may be different in men and women.*

As previously noted, the reference group for the Oxford studies had higher levels of both meat and red meat consumption than the reference group for AHS-2, but this does not seem to have increased the differentials in mortality observed (Table 11.5).

It is notable that in all three studies, the pescetarians came out slightly (but nonsignificantly) ahead of the nearest vegetarian group, but the difference was small: a 2%–4% reduction in RR of death from all causes. This does not support a large overall effect of fish on death rates in these populations but is consistent with the reduction of 6% reported by Zhao et al. (2016).

The most striking specific advantage for pescetarians was for ischemic heart disease deaths in women, while the worst result for vegans was also for ischemic heart disease deaths in women. The poor result for vegan women in terms of ischemic heart disease echoes an earlier Adventist study in which vegan men showed 14% of the expected death rate from heart disease compared with the general population, but vegan women showed 94% of the expected death rate (Phillips et al., 1978).

There are few differences in dietary intakes between pescetarians and vegans in AHS-2 (Orlich et al., 2014). Indeed, in many respects the pescetarians were the closest of the other diet groups to the vegans and they were also very close in overall death rates. The vegans consumed slightly more fiber and fruit and slightly less saturated fat, but the differences were not dramatic.

The only clear difference was the defining one: consumption of fish. Median DHA intake in pescetarians (men and women combined) was about 100 mg/day. EPA intake is not reported, but EPA + DHA was probably comparable to the TMREL in the GBD model (200–300 mg/day of EPA + DHA). The MDS fish score would also favor the pescetarians. EPA and DHA can be consumed by vegetarians in the form of supplements derived from algae, but no such intake was recorded in AHS-2.

Although vegetarians showed similar overall RRs in the two recent studies, there are slight differences in specific causes of death. In the Oxford studies the main advantage was seen in cancer (Table 11.7).

In AHS-2 the advantage was more evenly spread (Table 11.8).

The AHS-2 vegans showed an advantage over regular meat eaters, while their counterparts in both the Oxford studies and the pooled analysis did not. A previous report based on earlier Adventist studies gave a very similar result to AHS-2 on all-cause mortality: vegans 0.84 and other vegetarians 0.87 compared with omnivores (Fraser, 2003).

While there is a risk of overinterpreting the limited data available, the consistency with earlier reports makes the observed difference between Adventist vegans and UK vegans credible and deserving of further consideration.

At baseline the vegans in EPIC-Oxford were much younger than in AHS-2 (mean of 38 vs. 58) and had followed their diet for less time (5 years vs. 21 years). The younger age may have reduced differentials in death rates, and the shorter duration of diet may reduce the impact of dietary differences and make future changes in diet more likely. However, the longer follow-up in the Oxford studies and the elimination of individuals known to have changed diet group should reduce the impact of these factors.

Table 11.7   Death Rates From Specific Causes by Diet Group Compared With Regular Meat Eaters in the Oxford Studies

EPIC and Oxford Vegetarian	All Causes	Cancer	Ischemic Heart Disease	Cerebrovascular Disease	Cardiovascular Disease	Respiratory Disease
Vegan	1.00	0.97	0.79	1.50	1.09	1.00
Other vegetarian	0.93	**0.83**	0.92	1.12	1.01	0.94
Pescetarian	0.91	**0.76**	0.89	1.23	1.10	0.79
Occasional meat eaters	0.93	0.93	1.00	0.91	1.02	**0.69**

Results in bold were significant at $P < .05$.

Table 11.8   Death Rates From Specific Causes by Diet Group Compared With Regular Meat Eaters in AHS-2

Adventist Health Study 2	All Causes	Cancer	Ischemic Heart Disease	Cardiovascular Disease	Other
Vegan	0.85	0.92	0.90	0.91	**0.74**
Other vegetarian	**0.91**	0.90	0.82	0.90	0.91
Pescetarian	**0.81**	0.94	**0.65**	0.80	**0.71**
Occasional meat eaters	0.92	0.94	0.92	0.95	0.99

Results in bold were significant at $P < .05$.

UK vegans consumed more alcohol than those in AHS-2 (4% of calories—about 1.5 units—vs. virtually none), but alcohol intakes were fairly uniform across dietary groups within each cohort so are unlikely to make much contribution to differences between diet groups within each cohort.

The baseline BMIs in AHS-2 ranged from 24 in vegans to 28 in meat eaters compared with 23 in vegans and 25 in regular meat eaters for EPIC-Oxford (Davey et al., 2003). Thirty-three percent of meat eaters in AHS-2 were obese compared with 9% of vegans (Rizzo et al., 2013). With an estimated RR of 1.45 for death due to grade 1 obesity (Global BMI Mortality Collaboration, 2016) and an additional 24% of the reference group being obese, obesity seems a plausible contributor to the vegan advantage in AHS-2. However, adjustment for BMI was reported to make little difference to overall death rates in either AHS-2 or the Oxford studies. Indeed, in AHS-2 adjustment for BMI strengthened the RR for vegans compared with meat eaters from 0.85 to 0.84, nudging it into statistical significance. Differences in BMI therefore seem unlikely to explain the differences in RR.

The analysis by Clarys et al. (2014) using the HEI-2010 score highlighted increased refined grain consumption and decreased total protein as potential weak points in diets excluding meat. Neither of these weaknesses is observed in AHS-2. Refined grain use *decreased* with increasing exclusion of animal products (Orlich et al., 2014), and total protein was 14%–15% of calories in all diet groups (Rizzo et al., 2013). Refined grain use has not been reported for different diet groups within EPIC-Oxford, but protein intakes appear to decline from 16 to 17% of calories in meat eaters down to 13% of calories in vegans (Davey et al., 2003; Sobiecki et al., 2016). A potentially relevant effect of lower protein intake in this cohort was confirmed by Allen et al. (2002), who reported reduced IGF-1 levels in vegans, particularly those consuming little soya milk, and by Schmidt et al. (2016) who reported lower plasma concentrations of some amino acids, particularly lysine, in vegans.

There is a very striking difference between Adventist and UK vegans in reported vitamin B_{12} intakes. Recommended vitamin B_{12} intakes are 1.5 µg in the UK and 2.4 µg in the United States. The median intake (including supplements) of AHS-2 vegans was about 6 µg/day. Much of this probably came from fortified foods: many fortified plant milks in the United States contain more than 1 µg of vitamin B_{12} per 100 mL, compared with about 0.4 µg in Europe. The mean vitamin B_{12} intake of EPIC-Oxford vegans from foods was less than 1 µg (Davey et al., 2003; Sobiecki et al., 2016), though this did not take full account of vitamin B_{12} fortification.

Blood measurements confirm a major difference between the Adventist and EPIC-Oxford vegans in vitamin B_{12} status. A previous study of B_{12} in Adventist vegans (Haddad et al., 1999) found normal average levels of vitamin B_{12} and homocysteine in blood. In contrast, a study based on the EPIC-Oxford cohort (Gilsing et al., 2010) found 52% of vegans to have blood B_{12} levels below 118 pmol/L, and homocysteine levels were elevated. Elevated homocysteine is strongly associated with increased death rates, though a lack of effect from homocysteine reduction trials calls into question how much of this association is causal. For a review, the readers may refer to Chapter 41. There is a particular association between elevated homocysteine and cerebrovascular disease. Although both estimates were not significantly different from 1, the RR for cerebrovascular disease was somewhat elevated (1.5; 0.84–2.68) in vegans in the Oxford studies but not in vegans in the pooled analysis (0.7; 0.25–1.98). The much better vitamin B_{12} status in the AHS-2 vegans relative to the UK vegans plausibly contributed to their more favorable results.

Calcium intakes in AHS-2 vegans with a median of 933 mg/day (Rizzo et al., 2013) were also higher than the reported baseline values in EPIC-Oxford vegans with a mean value of 600 mg/day (Davey et al., 2003). Vegans in EPIC-Oxford have been reported to show increased fracture rates, though this was not observed when the analysis was restricted to people with calcium intakes above 525 mg/day (Appleby et al., 2007). However, Sobiecki et al. (2016) reported a mean value of 850 mg/day based on a later follow-up of the EPIC-Oxford cohort that assumed standard levels of calcium fortification of various soya products.

Overall, vitamin B_{12} seems the most credible hypothesis to explain the difference in the RR for vegans in the Oxford and AHS-2 studies. Existing dietary indices are based on omnivores, among whom vitamin B_{12} deficiency is rare, and not surprisingly are insensitive to this consideration. As calcium-fortified plant milks usually also contain vitamin B_{12} and contribute to the dairy dimension in HEI-2010, this would *partly* reflect this important dimension of vegan diets, but the other models would not. Any model that truly encompasses vegan diets needs to capture this directly.

6. Recommendations for Dietary Quality Indices for Vegan and Other Vegetarian Diets

The first recommendation is to add a measure to capture the effective intake of vitamin B_{12}, as this may be a key contributor to the quality of vegetarian and vegan diets.

In capturing vitamin B_{12} intakes, supplements need to be included in the analysis, and a correction then needs to be applied for the nonlinear absorption characteristic of vitamin B_{12}. Without applying some correction, the impact of occasional use of high dose supplements will be greatly overestimated. An equation for vitamin B_{12} absorption was developed by Heinrich et al. (1965) to cover a wide range of intakes:

$$A = 1.5D/(1.5 + D) + 0.009 * (D - 1.5D/(1.5 + D))$$

where D is the intake in µg, and A is the absorbed amount in µg.

Applying this equation to FFQ data could slightly overestimate the absorbed amount from diet if multiple vitamin B_{12} sources are usually consumed at the same meal, as this will reduce the absorption from each individual source. Absorption of vitamin B_{12} from eggs is exceptionally poor and should be multiplied by a correction factor of about 0.2.

In terms of a diet quality score, an average absorbed amount of 1.5 µg would meet all official national and international guidelines, so it should get maximum points. The potential overestimation of absorption is unlikely to matter in practice for such a diet score, as whenever vitamin B_{12} intake is frequent enough to lead to overestimation of absorption due to multiple sources appearing in the same meal then a maximum score would be expected even if an analysis were carried out on a meal by meal basis.

Nuts and seeds should be included as a separate category, as in the GBD model and the aMED score, as they play a significant role in plant-based diets, and they have strong and consistent associations with health. Combining nuts with fruits by weight, as in the MDS, obscures any effect of nuts, as nuts are consumed in much smaller quantities.

If dairy/milk is included as a separate beneficial category in a diet quality model, then *calcium-fortified* plant milks should be treated as equivalents of dairy milk and *calcium-set* tofu should be treated as an equivalent of cheese since the main potential benefits relate to calcium content. If dairy/milk is included as a separate adverse category, then plant milks/tofu should not be treated as an equivalent as the harm anticipated relates to either saturated fat or sugar (lactose/galactose) content. Alternatively, dairy could simply be omitted from the scoring altogether, as in the aMED score.

If there is a general meat category in the quality score, then we need to consider how to treat meat substitutes, other than legumes and nuts that are generally treated as special cases. In relation to the MDS, which treats meat as a separate adverse component, the less healthy end of the meat substitutes should arguably be counted as meat equivalents. Clarys et al. (2014) treated processed meat substitutes as equivalent to meat for this reason.

Based on the GBD model, processed meat is considered to be the main harmful meat category through an effect on cancer risk. In this case, there is no obvious reason to expect meat substitutes to have an equivalent effect. Similarly, the red meat component of the GBD and other scores may act at least in part through the heme iron content, so meat substitutes would not be equivalent.

The treatment of fish is the most problematic area for two reasons. First, the mechanism and magnitude of its effect remains uncertain, though the EPA and DHA content of fish is the most plausible basis of any effect. Secondly, the equivalence of the plant omega-3 alpha-linolenic acid (ALA) to EPA/DHA is not clear, so it is difficult to create a score that encompasses all sources of omega-3. Dietary ALA predictably increases EPA levels in the blood, but conversion to DHA in the blood is very limited, at least in adults (Brenna et al., 2009). ALA also has its own direct effects. Based on the contribution of ALA intake versus EPA intake to EPA levels in blood (Finnegan et al., 2003; Walsh, 2003), about 7% of ALA intake should be counted as an EPA equivalent. In AHS-2, median vegan ALA intakes were 1.8 g/day (Rizzo et al., 2013), which would be equivalent to 126 mg/day of EPA.

7. Conclusions

Generally, existing diet quality indices seem to encompass vegan and other vegetarian diets, and they seem to favor increasingly plant-based diet choices. The trends in dietary quality scores are broadly consistent with observed death rates in plant-based and vegetarian diet groups.

Some small adjustments to particular scores could improve the application of diet quality scores to diets with restricted use of foods derived from animals.

A key gap in existing dietary quality indices is the lack of sensitivity to insufficient supply of vitamin B_{12}. Vitamin B_{12} intakes are often (but not always) low in vegan diets. They may also be low in other vegetarian diets, which are often accompanied by reduced intake of dairy products. Low vitamin B_{12} certainly has effects on health and may make a significant contribution to death rates among vegans.

Observations of diet groups that differ in their intakes of meat and fish do not support a *major* effect of fish/EPA+DHA, but the difference between vegan and pescetarian women in terms of ischemic heart disease in AHS-2 deserves further exploration, particularly if confirmed with longer follow-up or in other studies.

Further research on dietary patterns in plant-based and vegetarian diets could enhance our knowledge both of how best to measure dietary quality and of the implications of plant-based and vegetarian diet choices.

Conflicts of Interest

Stephen Walsh is Chair of The Vegan Society in the United Kingdom.

References

Aldwairji, M., Orfila, C., Burley, V.J., 2012. Degree of agreement between AOAC-based dietary fibre intake and Englyst-based dietary fibre intake in the UK Women's Cohort Study (UKWCS). Proc. Nutr. Soc. 71 (OCE2), E194.

Allen, N.E., Appleby, P.N., Davey, G.K., Kaaks, R., Rinaldi, S., Key, T.J., 2002. The associations of diet with serum insulin-like growth factor I and its main binding proteins in 292 women meat-eaters, vegetarians, and vegans. Cancer Epidemiol. Biomarkers Prev. 11 (11), 1441–1448.

Appleby, P.N., Davey, G.K., Key, T.J., 2002. Hypertension and blood pressure among meat eaters, fish eaters, vegetarians and vegans in EPIC–Oxford. Public Health Nutr. 5 (05), 645–654.

Appleby, P., Roddam, A., Allen, N., Key, T., 2007. Comparative fracture risk in vegetarians and nonvegetarians in EPIC-Oxford. Eur. J. Clin. Nutr. 61 (12), 1400–1406.

Appleby, P.N., Crowe, F.L., Bradbury, K.E., Travis, R.C., Key, T.J., 2016. Mortality in vegetarians and comparable nonvegetarians in the United Kingdom. Am. J. Clin. Nutr. 103 (1), 218–230.

Bates, B., Lennox, A., Prentice, A., Bates, C., Page, P., Nicholson, S., Swan, G. (Eds.), 2014. National Diet and Nutrition Survey Results from Years 1, 2, 3 and 4 (Combined) of the Rolling Programme (2008/2009–2011/2012): A Survey Carried Out on Behalf of Public Health England and the Food Standards Agency. (Appendices, Chapter 5 Tables 5.3 & 5.4).

Bergmann, M.M., Rehm, J., Klipstein-Grobusch, K., Boeing, H., Schütze, M., Drogan, D., Overvad, K., Tjønneland, A., Halkjær, J., Fagherazzi, G., Boutron-Ruault, M.C., 2013. The association of pattern of lifetime alcohol use and cause of death in the European prospective investigation into cancer and nutrition (EPIC) study. Int. J. Epidemiol. 42 (6), 1772–1790.

Brenna, J.T., Salem, N., Sinclair, A.J., Cunnane, S.C., 2009. α-Linolenic acid supplementation and conversion to n-3 long-chain polyunsaturated fatty acids in humans. Prostaglandins Leukot. Essent. Fat. Acids 80 (2), 85–91.

Clarys, P., Deriemaeker, P., Huybrechts, I., Hebbelinck, M., Mullie, P., 2013. Dietary pattern analysis: a comparison between matched vegetarian and omnivorous subjects. Nutr. J. 12 (1), 1.

Clarys, P., Deliens, T., Huybrechts, I., Deriemaeker, P., Vanaelst, B., De Keyzer, W., Hebbelinck, M., Mullie, P., 2014. Comparison of nutritional quality of the vegan, vegetarian, semi-vegetarian, pesco-vegetarian and omnivorous diet. Nutrients 6 (3), 1318–1332.

Daniel, C.R., Cross, A.J., Koebnick, C., Sinha, R., 2011. Trends in meat consumption in the USA. Public Health Nutr. 14 (04), 575–583.

Davey, G.K., Spencer, E.A., Appleby, P.N., Allen, N.E., Knox, K.H., Key, T.J., 2003. EPIC–Oxford: lifestyle characteristics and nutrient intakes in a cohort of 33 883 meat-eaters and 31 546 non meat-eaters in the UK. Public Health Nutr. 6 (03), 259–268.

Farmer, B., Larson, B.T., Fulgoni, V.L., Rainville, A.J., Liepa, G.U., 2011. A vegetarian dietary pattern as a nutrient-dense approach to weight management: an analysis of the national health and nutrition examination survey 1999–2004. J. Am. Diet. Assoc. 111 (6), 819–827.

Farmer, B., 2014. Nutritional adequacy of plant-based diets for weight management: observations from the NHANES. Am. J. Clin. Nutr. 100 (Suppl. 1), 365S–368S.

Finnegan, Y.E., Howarth, D., Minihane, A.M., Kew, S., Miller, G.J., Calder, P.C., Williams, C.M., 2003. Plant and marine derived (n-3) polyunsaturated fatty acids do not affect blood coagulation and fibrinolytic factors in moderately hyperlipidemic humans. J. Nutr. 133 (7), 2210–2213.

Forouzanfar, M.H., Alexander, L., Anderson, H.R., Bachman, V.F., Biryukov, S., Brauer, M., Burnett, R., Casey, D., Coates, M.M., Cohen, A., Delwiche, K., 2015. Global, regional, and national comparative risk assessment of 79 behavioural, environmental and occupational, and metabolic risks or clusters of risks in 188 countries, 1990–2013: a systematic analysis for the Global Burden of Disease Study 2013. Lancet 386 (10010), 2287–2323.

Fraser, G., 2003. Diet, Life Expectancy, and Chronic Disease: Studies of Seventh-day Adventists and Other Vegetarians. Oxford University Press.

Fung, T.T., McCullough, M.L., Newby, P.K., Manson, J.E., Meigs, J.B., Rifai, N., Willett, W.C., Hu, F.B., 2005. Diet-quality scores and plasma concentrations of markers of inflammation and endothelial dysfunction. Am. J. Clin. Nutr. 82 (1), 163–173.

Gilsing, A.M., Crowe, F.L., Lloyd-Wright, Z., Sanders, T.A., Appleby, P.N., Allen, N.E., Key, T.J., 2010. Serum concentrations of vitamin B12 and folate in British male omnivores, vegetarians and vegans: results from a cross-sectional analysis of the EPIC-Oxford cohort study. Eur. J. Clin. Nutr. 64 (9), 933–939.

Global BMI Mortality Collaboration, 2016. Body-mass index and all-cause mortality: individual-participant-data meta-analysis of 239 prospective studies in four continents. Lancet 388 (10046), 776–786.

Guenther, P.M., Casavale, K.O., Reedy, J., Kirkpatrick, S.I., Hiza, H.A., Kuczynski, K.J., Kahle, L.L., Krebs-Smith, S.M., 2013. Update of the healthy eating index: HEI-2010. J. Acad. Nutr. Diet. 113 (4), 569–580.

Haddad, E.H., Berk, L.S., Kettering, J.D., Hubbard, R.W., Peters, W.R., 1999. Dietary intake and biochemical, hematologic, and immune status of vegans compared with nonvegetarians. Am. J. Clin. Nutr. 70 (3), 586s–593s.

Heinrich, H.C., Gabbe, E.E., Whang, D.D., Wolfsteller, E., 1965. Eine für die Berechnung der intestinalen Vitamin B_{12}-Resorption beim Menschen sowohl im physiologischen, Intrinsic Factor-abhängigen als auch im unphysiologisch hohen, diffusionsbedingten Dosisbereich allgemein gültige Formel. Z. für Naturforsch. B 20 (11), 1067–1069.

Juan, W., Yamini, S., Britten, P., 2015. Food intake patterns of self-identified vegetarians among the US population, 2007–2010. Procedia Food Sci. 4, 86–93.

Kennedy, E.T., Bowman, S.A., Spence, J.T., Freedman, M., King, J., 2001. Popular diets: correlation to health, nutrition, and obesity. J. Acad. Nutr. Diet. 101 (4), 411–420.

Key, T.J., Fraser, G.E., Thorogood, M., Appleby, P.N., Beral, V., Reeves, G., Burr, M.L., Chang-Claude, J., Frentzel-Beyme, R., Kuzma, J.W., Mann, J., 1999. Mortality in vegetarians and nonvegetarians: detailed findings from a collaborative analysis of 5 prospective studies. Am. J. Clin. Nutr. 70 (3), 516S–524S.

of diseases to meat is challenging, owing to the fact that meat is typically consumed as part of a composite meal, often containing nonmeat components such as vegetables, starchy foods (rice, pasta, or potatoes), or legumes (Wyness et al., 2011). Therefore, an increasing number of studies investigated overall dietary behaviors using dietary patterns rather than considering only meat products.

Meat provides little if any carbohydrate, and it is mostly composed of protein and fat. Red meat contains a range of important nutrients including high-quality protein, fatty acids, iron, zinc, selenium, potassium, and a range of B-vitamins especially vitamin B_{12} (Wyness et al., 2011). Red meat (and in some cases, meat products), as well as other animal foods, is an important source of the nine indispensable amino acids for humans (Wyness et al., 2011). Meat contains fat in varying amounts. Besides a small amount of long-chain n-3 polyunsaturated fatty acids (PUFAs), red meat contains monounsaturated fatty acids (MUFAs) (30%–40% of total fatty acids) and saturated fatty acids, one-third of them being stearic acid, neutral on total cholesterol, and low-density lipoprotein plasmatic levels (Wyness et al., 2011; McNeill, 2014).

As meat- and animal-derived foods (such as dairy products) and fish are the only foods that naturally provide vitamin B_{12}, individuals who totally exclude such foods from their diet are at risk of inadequate intakes (Wyness et al., 2011). The readers can refer to Chapter 43 for a detailed review. Dietary iron is found in two forms: heme and nonheme iron. Red meat (beef, lamb, and pork) has a 10-fold higher heme content than white meat (e.g., chicken) (Hooda et al., 2014). Ferric iron, which is present in hemoglobin and myoglobin within the heme molecule, has strong oxidative properties but is better absorbed than nonheme iron, present in foods of plant origin. In Western countries, heme iron derived from myoglobin and hemoglobin makes up two-thirds of the average person's total iron stores, although it constitutes only one-third of the ingested iron (Hooda et al., 2014). The readers can refer to Chapter 39 for a detailed review on iron status in a plant-based diet.

2. Meat Consumption and Obesity

Rouhani et al. (2014) performed a meta-analysis of transversal studies on the relationship between red meat intake (21 studies) and processed meat intake (18 studies) and obesity. When comparing extreme quantiles of red or processed meat intake, those in the highest quantile had an approximately 37% increased risk of obesity (Rouhani et al., 2014), and they had higher body mass index (BMI) and higher waist circumference. Associations were similar for nonprocessed and processed meat.

Red meat and by-products are categorized as energy-dense foods, and energy density of the diet has been directly associated with obesity (Rouhani et al., 2014). Read meat is also an important component of the Western diet, which has been consistently associated with obesity, but it is difficult to assess what is due to meat consumption and what is related to other components of the Western diet, such as low dietary fiber intake and high-sugar and high-fat processed foods. Vegetarians have been found to have somewhat lower energy intakes that are associated with higher fiber and lower fat intakes (Wyness et al., 2011).

The energy content of meat widely varies according to the fat content. Although there is no international consensus, lean meat is usually defined as meat containing 5%–10% fat (Wyness et al., 2011). Thus, lean red meat has been considered a useful component of weight loss diets because of the satiating effect (Wyness et al., 2011). High-protein, low-fat diets compared with standard-protein, low-fat diets produced more favorable changes in weight loss and fat mass over the short-term, and the suggested reasons include increased satiating properties of protein and protein effects on thermogenesis, body composition, and decreased energy efficiency (Wyness et al., 2011).

The importance of the microbiota in the development of obesity receives growing interest and evidence. As discussed in a review (Ramakrishna, 2013), "alteration of the microbiota composition may stimulate development of obesity and other metabolic diseases via several mechanisms: increasing gut permeability with subsequent metabolic inflammation; increasing energy harvest from the diet; impairing short-chain fatty acids synthesis; and altering bile acids metabolism and FXR/TGR5 signaling." The relationship between the red meat-associated microbiota and obesity-associated microbiota is complex and requests further investigation. A diet high in animal protein and fat has been associated with a development of the *Bacteroides* enterotype, but the latter has been diversely associated with weight changes in different parts of the world (Ramakrishna, 2013).

Altogether, high consumption of red and/or processed meat is likely to be associated with higher risk of obesity, either directly or via other components of the Western diet.

3. Red and Processed Meat Consumptions and Cancer Risk

3.1 Epidemiological Evidence

In October 2015, the International Agency for Research on Cancer (IARC) evaluated the carcinogenicity of red meat and processed meat consumptions (Bouvard et al., 2015). The working group classified consumption of red meat as "probably carcinogenic to humans" (Group 2A) and consumption of processed meat as "carcinogenic to humans" (Group 1). IARC has based this classification on substantial epidemiological evidence for a positive association between consumption of processed and red meat and risk of several cancers, especially colorectal cancer.

Associations between consumption of red and processed meat (including processed red meat, but also processed poultry) and the risk of various cancers have been jointly summarized by the World Cancer Research Fund (WCRF) and the American Institute for Cancer Research (AICR) in the 2007 report and the 2010–14 Continuous Update Program (CUP).

Concerning the association with red and/or processed meat consumption, the largest body of epidemiological data concerned colorectal cancer. Results of the meta-analysis on the association between consumption of red and processed meat and colorectal cancer risk, reported in the 2011 WCRF/AICR CUP report (World Cancer Research Fund American Institute for Cancer Research, 2016), confirmed those presented in the 2007 report and considered the increased colorectal cancer risk as convincing for both red and processed meats. The meta-analysis (Chan et al., 2011), on which the report was based, included 11 cohort studies. The dose–response meta-analysis concluded an increase in risk of colorectal cancer with the consumption of red and processed meats: per 100 g total red meat/day, increases in risks of proximal colon, distal colon, and rectum were 11%, 22%, and 23%, respectively. For processed meat, the increased risk of colorectal cancer was 18% per 50 g/day, while for unprocessed red meat the increased risk of colorectal cancer was 17% per 100 g/day. A further meta-analysis of 25 cohort studies (Alexander et al., 2011) reported associations that were not as strong and some heterogeneity between studies.

Other cancer sites have been associated with red and/or processed meat intakes as summarized by the WCRF/AICR reports. The meta-analysis of available data on the relationship between consumption of red and/or processed meats and pancreatic cancer risk presented in the 2012 WCRF report (World Cancer Research Fund American Institute for Cancer Research, 2016) is in favor of an increased risk with a level of evidence qualified as "limited-suggestive." The dose–response meta-analysis per 100 g/day of red meat consumption (8 cohort studies) and 50 g/day of processed meat consumption (7 cohort studies) reported increased risks by 43% and 21%, respectively, in men. No statistically significant association was observed in women, but this may be due to a lack of statistical power since the disease is less common in women. In a meta-analysis (Larsson and Wolk, 2012), pancreatic cancer risk increased by 29% per 120 g/day increment of red meat consumption (11 cohort studies) and by 19% per 50 g/day increment of processed meat consumption (7 cohort studies).

For esophageal cancer, a positive association has been observed in Western countries (the United States and Europe) with red and processed meat. Three meta-analyses have investigated the association between esophageal cancer and red or processed meat intake. A meta-analysis of three cohort and six case–control studies on esophageal adenocarcinoma reported a 31% increase between extreme quantiles (Huang et al., 2013). A meta-analysis of 4 cohorts and 31 case–control studies reported a 40% increased risk of esophageal cancer between extreme quantiles of red meat and a 41% increase for processed meat. Squamous cell carcinoma was associated with high red meat intake, while adenocarcinoma was associated with processed meat intake (Salehi et al., 2013). In a meta-analysis separately investigating the included 4 cohort and 23 case–control studies, the highest versus lowest quantiles of intake were associated with a 26% and 25% increased risk of esophageal cancer in the cohort studies, while the corresponding figures were higher, 44% and 36%, respectively, for the case–control studies (Choi et al., 2013). In another meta-analysis of three cohort and seven case–control studies on esophageal adenocarcinoma, the dose–response analysis reported a 45% increased risk per 100 g/day of red meat intake and 37% per 50 g/day of processed meat intake (Huang et al., 2013). In a study focused on squamous cell carcinoma, summary estimates provided 42% and 41% increased risks with red and processed meats, respectively (Qu et al., 2013; Zhu et al., 2014). In a study including 7 cohort and 23 case–control studies, total meat, poultry, or fish intakes were not associated with esophageal cancer risk, and white meat intake was associated with a decreased risk, while a 55% increased risk comparing extreme categories was reported with red meat and a 33% increase for processed meat. When considering histological types, esophageal squamous cell carcinoma was positively associated with red meat, and inversely with white meat and poultry, while esophageal adenocarcinoma was associated with total meat and processed meat (Zhu et al., 2014).

The results from the meta-analyses on the link between consumption of processed meats and stomach cancer risk presented in the 2007 WCRF report are in favor of an increased risk with a level of evidence considered as "limited-suggestive" (World Cancer Research Fund American Institute for Cancer Research, 2007). The dose–response meta-analysis per 20 g/day of processed meat (nine case–control studies) showed a 13% increased risk (World Cancer Research Fund American Institute for Cancer Research, 2007). These results were confirmed in more recent meta-analyses with increases of 24% (7 cohort studies) (D'Elia et al., 2012), 45% (12 cohort studies, 30 case–control studies) (Zhu et al., 2013), and 15% (13 cohort studies) (Fang et al., 2015) of stomach cancer risk associated with higher consumption of processed meat. In the 2016 CUP report, the finding on processed meat has been upgraded to strong evidence, and it is now specific to stomach noncardia cancer. The report stated that "there is strong evidence that consuming processed meat increases the risk of stomach non-cardia cancer."

The level of evidence was judged "limited-suggestive" for an increased risk of lung cancer (World Cancer Research Fund American Institute for Cancer Research, 2007) associated with both red and processed meats; this was confirmed by a meta-analysis of 13 case–control studies and 5 cohort studies, with a 34% increase in lung cancer risk associated with the highest quantile of red meat consumption (Yang et al., 2012). A 20% increase was observed for the five cohort studies (including two not adjusted for BMI and fruit and vegetable intake). High red meat consumption was associated with a 30% increased risk in men, while the 23% increase in women was only borderline statistically significant. Pork consumption was not associated with lung cancer risk.

Levels of evidence for breast, oral cavity, and oropharynx cancers were evaluated as "not conclusive" in 2007 (World Cancer Research Fund American Institute for Cancer Research, 2007). Further meta-analyses (World Cancer Research Fund American Institute for Cancer Research, 2007; Alexander et al., 2010; Guo et al., 2015; Taylor et al., 2009) suggest an association between the consumption of red meat and increased breast cancer risk with a level of evidence judged as "suggestive," however with significant heterogeneity between studies that precludes final conclusions. Regarding oral cavity and oropharynx cancers, a meta-analysis updated in 2014 (1 cohort and 12 case–control studies) reported a 91% increased risk with high consumption of processed meat but no association with total or red meat intakes (Xu et al., 2014).

Recent publications have investigated the associations between red and processed meats and bladder, kidney, thyroid, and liver cancers. For bladder cancer (Wang and Jiang, 2012) the evidence regarding an association was judged "suggestive." Considering the heterogeneity of results between meta-analyses or the limited number of studies, the level of evidence is considered "not conclusive" for kidney, liver (World Cancer Research

Fund American Institute for Cancer Research, 2016; Luo et al., 2014), and thyroid (Liu and Lin, 2014) cancers, and red and processed meat intakes (World Cancer Research Fund American Institute for Cancer Research, 2016; Alexander and Cushing, 2009; Faramawi et al., 2007; Lee et al., 2008), and for bladder cancer (Wang and Jiang, 2012) and processed meat.

In addition, the evidence for endometrial cancer in 2013 (World Cancer Research Fund American Institute for Cancer Research, 2016) and ovarian and prostate cancer in 2014 (World Cancer Research Fund American Institute for Cancer Research, 2016), for which no new studies were identified, remains "not conclusive."

Altogether, there is strong evidence that high consumption of red meat or processed meat is associated with increased incidence of several frequent cancer sites, therefore justifying the WCRF/AICR recommendations at the individual level as "People who eat red meat should consume less than 500 g a week (18 oz), and very little if any of processed meat," and at the population level "consumption of red meat should be no more than 300 g (11 oz) a week, and very little if any of processed meat" (World Cancer Research Fund American Institute for Cancer Research, 2007). The panel of experts in charge of elaborating the European Code Against Cancer in 2015 endorsed these recommendations (Norat et al., 2015).

3.2 Meat and Cancer-Specific Mortality

The only meta-analysis on the association between meat consumption and risk of cancer death reports an increased cancer mortality associated with higher total and processed meat intakes. High consumptions of total meat (four cohort studies) and processed meat (three cohort studies) were associated with 14% and 13% higher risks of cancer death, respectively (O'Sullivan et al., 2013). In the dose–response meta-analysis, there was a 2% increase risk per 120 g/day of total meat and a borderline statistically significant 4% increased risk per 50 g/day of processed meat.

3.3 Red and Processed Meat Consumptions and Cancer Risk: Mechanistic Hypotheses

For colon cancer, mechanisms proposed to explain the association with red and processed meat consumptions largely involve the effect of heme iron, lipid peroxidation, and the formation of aldehydes. Unsaturated aldehydes are able to make covalent adducts with DNA bases (Chung et al., 1996) and to provoke DNA lesions at low dosages, and micronuclei and chromosomal aberrations at higher dosages (Eckl et al., 1993; Eckl, 2003). Beside DNA, unsaturated aldehydes can make covalent binding with proteins and modify their function. Furthermore, in vitro studies showed that the single Apc mutation, an initiating event in many human colorectal cancers, rendered the cells strongly resistant to aldehyde-induced cytotoxicity (Pierre et al., 2007). This would give the Apc-mutated cells a clear survival advantage over nonmutated cells when subjected to aldehydes after meat consumption. Those conditions may act as a selective factor for precancerous Apc-mutated cells and induce colon cancer promotion. Moreover, cancer cells require increased intracellular heme biosynthesis and uptake to meet the increased demand for oxygen-utilizing hemoproteins. Increased levels of hemoproteins in turn lead to intensified oxygen consumption and cellular energy generation, thereby fueling cancer cell progression (Hooda et al., 2014). For processed meats, nitrates and nitrites used during meat processing may represent an additional important part of the carcinogenic effect via N-nitroso compounds (NOCs) formation facilitated by the presence of heme iron (Bastide et al., 2011). NOCs, which are alkylating agents that can react with DNA, are produced by the reaction of nitrite and nitrogen oxides with secondary amines and N-alkylamides. Many NOCs, including nitrosamines and nitrosamides, are carcinogenic in experimental animals. And for all cancer sites, mechanisms proposed can be multiple. In addition to the heme-iron hypothesis, the effect on cancers may be related to neoformed mutagenic compounds such as heterocyclic amines (HCA) and polycyclic aromatic hydrocarbons (PAHs) (Bouvard et al., 2015). HCAs and PAHs are formed during the cooking of meat. HCAs are formed by pyrolysis of creati(ni)ne with specific amino acids. Since a high temperature is needed, only fried, broiled, or barbecued meat contains significant amounts of HCAs. In contrast with HCAs, PAHs are produced from the incomplete combustion of organic compounds. Many tested PAHs and HCAs are mutagens and animal carcinogens (World Cancer Research Fund American Institute for Cancer Research, 2016, 2007). However, similar compounds are found in chicken or fish cooked in similar ways, thus these compounds are by no means specific of red meat. In addition, it has been suggested that only subjects with a fast acetylator status could be at high risk of colorectal cancer when consuming overdone meat, but recent evidence is less strong (Liu et al., 2012). A recent publication reviews the various hypotheses related to red meat–associated disease risk. It reports a novel hypothesis that involves a human-specific mechanism associated with the presence in red meat of a nonhuman glycan, a particular variant of sialic acid called N-glycolylneuraminic acid (Neu5Gc) (Alisson-Silva et al., 2016).

4. Meat Consumption and Risk of Type 2 Diabetes

4.1 Epidemiological Evidence

Several meta-analyses have investigated the association between risk of type 2 diabetes (T2D) and meat intake; they suggest that a high consumption of processed meat, rather than that of unprocessed red meat, may increase the risk of developing T2D (Aune et al., 2009; Feskens et al., 2013; Micha et al., 2010, 2012; Pan et al., 2011).

In each of the included cohorts, higher meat consumption was associated with less favorable lifestyle and dietary behaviors, including, for example, less physical activity, higher smoking, higher total energy intake, and lower fruit, vegetable, dietary fiber, whole grains, and fish intakes, and higher alcohol and trans fat intakes. Most of the included studies took into account these lifestyle habits or dietary patterns (Micha et al., 2012).

The consumption of total red meat was associated with a 20% increase of T2D risk per 120 g/day in Aune et al.'s (2009) meta-analysis of 9 cohort studies and 13% per 100 g/day in Feskens et al.'s (2013) meta-analysis of 14 cohort studies, while Micha et al.'s (2010) meta-analysis of 5 studies reported a nonstatistically significant 16% increase per 100 g/day. For poultry, a meta-analysis of 10 cohort studies (Feskens et al., 2013) reported a non-statistically significant 4% excess risk per 100 g/day. The association between consumption of red meat and diabetes risk was stronger with processed meat than with nonprocessed meat, with 57% (Aune et al., 2009), 32% (Feskens et al., 2013), and 19% (Micha et al., 2010) increased risks per 50 g/day. In another meta-analysis of 10 prospective studies, diabetes risk increased by 19% per 100 g/day of unprocessed red meat and 51% per 50 g/day of processed red meat (Pan et al., 2011). Elevated risks of diabetes were specifically reported for hamburgers (9% increase per serving/week), bacon (14% increase per serving/week), and hot dogs and other processed meats (9% increase per serving/week for both) (Aune et al., 2009). Concordant estimates were reported for bacon (twofold increased risk per 2 slices/day), hot dogs (close to a twofold increase per hot dog unit/day), and "other processed meat" consumption (66% increase per 1 piece/day) (Micha et al., 2010).

However, between-studies heterogeneity was high in most meta-analyses for red meat (Aune et al., 2009), white meat (Feskens et al., 2013), processed meat (Aune et al., 2009; Feskens et al., 2013; Micha et al., 2010), processed red meat (Pan et al., 2011), or unprocessed red meat (Pan et al., 2011). In some meta-analyses, heterogeneity was reduced (Aune et al., 2009) or associations were stronger (Micha et al., 2010) after the exclusion of Asian studies.

4.2 Meat and Type 2 Diabetes Risk: Mechanistic Hypotheses

Several hypotheses have been considered regarding the positive association of meat consumption with incidence of T2D.

Saturated and trans-fatty acids present in meat could play a role in the onset of T2D. Several studies suggested a detrimental effect of saturated fat (main sources are animal foods) or trans-fatty acids (industrial products as well as some red meats) in the development of T2D due to adverse metabolic effects on insulin sensitivity (The InterAct Consortium, 2012). A diet rich in meat and meat products could lead to an increase in the body's iron stores, which can promote oxidative stress and cause damage to tissues, in particular the pancreatic beta cells. Excessive heme intake leads to deposits of iron in tissues, which damage the DNA and cell integrity and interfere with glucose uptake by various tissues, and thus may impair insulin sensitivity (Hooda et al., 2014). The higher fat and iron contents of red compared to white meat could explain the stronger association of diabetes risk with the former.

However, differences in fat and iron cannot account for different associations of unprocessed and processed meat with diabetes risk since processed red meats contain, on average, similar saturated fat and iron as unprocessed red meats, at least in the United States, where most of the studies were performed (Micha et al., 2010).

On average, processed meats contain about 400% more sodium and 50% more nitrates per gram, which could plausibly account, at least in part, for these differences (Micha et al., 2010; Männistö et al., 2010). Nitrites may have a toxic effect on pancreatic beta cells, mediated by the formation of nitrosamines in the stomach or in the meat product itself. Nitrosamines could also be produced in well-cooked meat from HCA or PAHs. Some nitrosamines were found to be associated with type 1 diabetes in humans, while streptozotocin, a nitrosamine-related compound, was found to be associated with T2D in animal models (Aune et al., 2009; Micha et al., 2010; The InterAct Consortium, 2012). Advanced glycation end-products, present in meat and meat products as a result of cooking or processing, have been associated with insulin resistance or T2D both in animal models and in humans (Aune et al., 2009; The InterAct Consortium, 2012). However, a review found conflicting evidence of an effect of a diet low in advanced glycation end-products on markers of insulin resistance in healthy individuals (Kellow and Savige, 2013). Other possible mechanisms could involve increased levels of inflammatory mediators and γ glutamyl-transferase and lower levels of adiponectin with high meat intake (Aune et al., 2009).

5. Meat Consumption and Cardiovascular Risk and Mortality

5.1 Meat Consumption and the Risk of Coronary Heart Disease (CHD)

Mente et al. (2009) concluded at insufficient evidence of an association between meat intake and CHD risk, with a nonstatistically significant 23% increase in risk associated with higher compared with lower meat intakes (12 cohort studies, c. 230,000 subjects).

In another meta-analysis including case–control and cohort studies (Micha et al., 2012), unprocessed red meat intake was not associated with CHD risk, while processed meat intake was associated with a 42% higher risk of CHD per 50 g/day. Restricting the analysis to cohort studies resulted in similar findings. With the exclusion of one large US study that evaluated only total CVD mortality and not CHD alone, each serving per day of processed meat consumption was associated with a nearly twofold higher risk of CHD. There was no evidence for between-studies heterogeneity (Micha et al., 2010).

5.2 Meat Consumption and the Risk of Stroke

Consumption of unprocessed or processed red meat was not associated with stroke in Micha et al.'s (2010) meta-analysis, including ~2300 stroke events in 3 cohorts. A larger study including 6 cohorts and ~10,600 cases of stroke (Kaluza et al., 2012) reported an 11% increase in the risk of total stroke per each daily serving (100–120 g) of unprocessed red meat and 13% for processed meat per each 50-g daily serving. When stratifying by geographic region, there were positive associations between risk of stroke and unprocessed red meat and processed meat consumptions in studies conducted in Europe and in the United States, but not in Japan. In the studies that investigated stroke subtypes, the consumption of unprocessed red meat and processed meat was associated with the risk of ischemic stroke (respectively, 13% and 15% increase per serving/day) but not with the risk of hemorrhagic stroke (respectively, 8% and 16% nonstatistically significant increases per serving/day). These results were confirmed in a meta-analysis of five cohort studies including c. 9500 stroke events (Chen et al., 2013). In the dose–response analysis, the risk of stroke increased by 13% per 100-g increment in daily red meat consumption and by 11% per 50-g increment in daily processed meat consumption. Consumption of red and/or processed meat was not associated with hemorrhagic stroke.

5.3 Meat Consumption and Cardiovascular Mortality

Processed meat intake, but not total meat intake, has been associated with CVD mortality in two meta-analyses (Abete et al., 2014; O'Sullivan et al., 2013).

In O'Sullivan et al.'s (2013) analysis of four cohort studies, the highest versus lowest category of processed meat consumption was associated with a 17% increased CVD mortality. For total meat consumption, although the increased CVD mortality was nonstatistically significant (9% increase, nine cohort studies), the association was stronger and statistically significant in a pooled analysis of non-Asian cohorts (29% increase, three cohorts). In the opposite, there was an 18% decrease in CVD mortality with higher total meat consumption in the Asian studies. In the dose–response analysis, the authors reported a 1% nonstatistically significant increased CVD mortality per 120 g/day of total meat (nine cohort studies) and a statistically significant 2% increase per 50 g/day of processed meat (two cohort studies).

In a further meta-analysis (Abete et al., 2014), the highest levels of processed and unprocessed red meat consumptions were associated with 18% and 16% increased risks of CVD mortality, respectively, while there was no association with total or white meat consumption. For unprocessed red meat, the heterogeneity substantially decreased and the association was strengthened (33% increase) when Asian studies were excluded. In the dose–response meta-analysis, a 50-g/day increase in processed meat intake and a 100-g/day increase in unprocessed red meat intake were, respectively, associated with 24% and 15% significant increases in CVD mortality, while no associations were observed for total and white meat consumption. Associations were similar in men and women. CHD mortality was not associated with consumption of any type of meat.

Several hypotheses have been proposed to explain differences in the associations between meat intake and diabetes risk or CVD risk/mortality in Asian and Western studies. First, meat consumption in Asian countries is considerably lower than in Western countries, which would result in differences in intake of some nutrients such as heme iron, saturated fatty acids, and cholesterol (Kaluza et al., 2012). Furthermore, in Western countries, red meat consumption is correlated with consumption of refined cereal products, full-fat dairy products, and soft drinks, while meat consumption is correlated with consumption of fish and deep-fried foods or tempura in Japan (Kaluza et al., 2012). Otherwise, the dietary and lifestyle transition is still under way in many parts of Asia, and meat consumption may not be at this stage as large a contributor to risk of CVD risk or death as the socioeconomic status, a sedentary lifestyle, smoking, or adiposity (Lee et al., 2013). A higher intake of meat may also be a marker for protective factors, such as normal-level energy intake or access to medical care (Lee et al., 2013). The food preparation technique could also play a role (Abete et al., 2014).

5.4 Meat and CVD Risk/Mortality: Mechanistic Hypotheses

Associations between meat intake and CVD risk and mortality are partly driven by the impact of meat intake, especially processed meat, on obesity or diabetes risk, as previously described. Meat intake has also been associated with risk of hypertension, with some discrepancies according to type of meat: the association was restricted to processed red meat in a French prospective study (Lajous et al., 2012), while it was observed for consumptions of processed meat, unprocessed red meat, and even poultry in three US prospective studies (Borgi et al., 2015). Conversely, changes in the fasting lipid profile were not significantly different with beef than with poultry and/or fish consumptions in randomized controlled trials (Maki et al., 2012). Likewise, a meta-analysis of 21 studies including more than 11,000 CV events found that dietary intake of saturated fat was not associated with any increased risk of CHD, stroke, or CVD (Siri-Tarino et al., 2010).

Beside the aforementioned mechanisms involved in the associations between meat intake and diabetes risk, some mechanisms could be more specifically involved in the associations between processed meat intake and hypertension and CVD risks.

Dietary sodium increases blood pressure, and it may also increase peripheral vascular resistance and impair arterial compliance. Based on the relationship between blood pressure and CVD risk, the sodium content has been hypothesized to account for a substantial portion of the observed CHD or stroke risk with processed meat consumption (Micha et al., 2012). Advanced glycation end-products produced at high cooking temperatures increase oxidative stress and inflammation, both potential factors in the development of hypertension and atherosclerosis (Borgi et al., 2015). PAHs from smoked meat have atherogenic effects (Kaluza et al., 2012). Phosphate-containing food additives can impair the calcium-phosphate metabolism. Among CHD patients, higher levels of serum phosphate have been associated with increased risk of new CHD events compared with participants with lower levels (Kaluza et al., 2012). L-carnitine, principally found in red meat, is converted by the gut microflora to trimethylamine, then absorbed and converted in the liver to trimethylamine-*N*-oxide. This product, which is also present in large quantities in saltwater fish, is proatherogenic in animals and humans by increasing two proatherogenic scavenger receptors, specifically CD36 and scavenger receptor A (Borgi et al., 2015).

6. Meat Consumption and All-Cause Mortality

In line with the increased risks of cancer and cardiovascular mortality associated with high meat intake, high meat consumption has been positively associated with all-cause mortality in three meta-analyses (Abete et al., 2014; O'Sullivan et al., 2013; Larsson and Orsini, 2014).

High consumptions of both total meat (seven cohort studies) and processed meat (three cohort studies) were associated with 17% and 21% increases in all-cause mortality, respectively (O'Sullivan et al., 2013). The dose–response meta-analysis concluded that 120 g/day of total meat, and 50 g/day of processed meat were associated with a 2%, and 4% (the latter with borderline statistical significance) increased all-cause mortality, respectively.

With a different assessment of the included types of meat, two other meta-analyses of prospective studies (Abete et al., 2014; Larsson and Orsini, 2014) reported 22% and 23% increases of all-cause mortality for the highest quantiles of processed red meat consumption in both men and women. Associations were similar with total red meat. Unprocessed red meat was not associated with mortality overall, or in women, but it was associated with all-cause mortality in men in the two meta-analyses. Results from the dose–response meta-analysis suggested that processed red meat consumption is associated with all-cause mortality in a nonlinear fashion with a 22% increased risk for two servings per day (60 g/day) compared with less than two servings per week (10 g/day) (Larsson and Orsini, 2014). When considering the study locations, associations between mortality and processed red meat consumption were restricted to US and European studies, and associations with unprocessed red meat to US studies.

Abete et al. (2014) also investigated the relationship between white meat intake and all-cause mortality; in women only, there was a 5% lower risk of all-cause mortality in the highest quantile of white meat consumption. However, this weak inverse association is to be considered with caution since subjects consuming more white meat were also lower red meat consumers (Abete et al., 2014).

7. Meat Consumption and Bone Health

There is little evidence for a direct effect of meat consumption on bone health. Evidence mostly relates dietary protein intake to bone metabolism, but meat is far from being the main source of protein involved. However, while insufficient dietary protein intake is deleterious for bone health, an excess of dietary protein has also been associated with osteoporosis. Because most studies did not directly investigate the association between meat consumption and bone health, we will only briefly summarize the available evidence relating dietary protein intake to bone health.

7.1 Protein Intake and Risk of Bone Mineral Density (BMD) or Bone Mineral Content (BMC)

A systematic review in 2009 quantitatively analyzed 18 cross-sectional surveys (Darling et al., 2009). Total protein intake was associated with higher BMD or BMC at the main clinically relevant sites; protein intake explained 1%–2% of BMD. A meta-analysis of six randomized placebo-controlled trials indicated a positive influence of protein supplementation on lumbar spine BMD (Darling et al., 2009).

7.2 Protein Intake, Including Meat, and Risk of Fracture

In 2009, a meta-analysis of four cohort studies did not find any association between total protein, animal protein, or vegetable protein intake and the risk of hip fracture (Darling et al., 2009). In a further meta-analysis in 2015, higher total protein intake was associated with a statistically significant 11% decrease of hip fracture risk (Wu et al., 2015), with no difference between animal and vegetable protein. A case–control study suggested a higher fracture risk in elderly Chinese with higher red meat intake, but not with poultry or eggs (Zeng et al., 2013).

7.3 Protein Intake and Bone Health: Mechanistic Hypotheses

The observed beneficial effects of long-term high protein intake, including that provided by meat, on bone mass (Darling et al., 2009) and fracture risk (Wu et al., 2015) may be partially the result of increased circulating concentration of IGFI and lower serum parathyroid hormone (Cao and Nielsen, 2010). Higher protein intake has been suggested to protect against sarcopenia, although several cross-sectional studies failed to show any association between protein intake and sarcopenia (Millward and Garnett, 2010).

High-meat diets have been suggested to increase renal acid load and urinary calcium excretion (Wyness et al., 2011; Nicoll and McLaren Howard, 2014). This could be modulated by calcium intake: high protein consumption could reduce fracture risk when calcium intake is high, while it may contribute to bone erosion when calcium intake is low (Cao and Nielsen, 2010; Nicoll and McLaren Howard, 2014). In a large cohort of French menopausal women, in the lowest quartile of calcium (<400 mg/1000 kcal), high protein intake, especially high animal protein intake, was associated with an increased fracture risk (Dargent-Molina et al., 2008). Buffering the dietary acid load by high intakes of alkalinizing and potassium-rich foods such as fruits and vegetables may ensure that a high protein or meat intake is beneficial rather than detrimental to bone health (Nicoll and McLaren Howard, 2014). A recent report summarized advice for optimal bone and cardiovascular health (Wyness et al., 2011): "calcium is best obtained from dietary sources rather than supplements (Abete et al., 2014); ensure that adequate animal protein intake is coupled with calcium intake of 1000 mg/day (Fardet and Boirie, 2014); maintain vitamin D levels in the normal range (Lee et al., 2013); increase intake of fruits and vegetables to alkalinize the system and promote bone health (McNeill, 2014); concomitantly increase potassium consumption while reducing sodium intake (Hooda et al., 2014); consider increasing the intake of foods rich in vitamins K_1 and K_2 (Rouhani et al., 2014); consider including bones in the diet; they are a rich source of calcium-hydroxyapatite and many other nutrients needed for building bone" (O'Keefe et al., 2016). The readers may also consult Chapter 17.

8. Conclusion and Future Trends

Recommendations to limit red meat intake were originally intended to reduce saturated fat intake (Battaglia Richi et al., 2015) and further based on the association of animal production with greenhouse gas emissions (Millward and Garnett, 2010) and on the association of the consumption of red and processed meat with colorectal cancer (World Cancer Research Fund American Institute for Cancer Research, 2007). Most dietary guidelines recommended limiting saturated fat but did not specify the replacement nutrient (O'Sullivan et al., 2013). As unintentional negative consequences, a decline in energy from nutrient-rich foods such as beef, milk, and eggs has been accompanied by an excessive increase in energy from fats (including trans fats) and refined carbohydrates found in many processed foods (Battaglia Richi et al., 2015).

However, the findings of this review suggest that strong reductions of processed meat consumption, including processed chicken or turkey, resulting in reduction of sodium and other preservatives of processed meats, is likely to produce the largest net benefits for both individual and population health (Micha et al., 2012). There is also quite a lot of evidence for an impact of unprocessed red meat consumption on risk of colorectal cancer, diabetes, and stroke, although not as strong as for processed meat. Based on these findings, the WCRF/AICR recommendation for red meat intake at the individual level is: "less than 500 g a week (18 oz), and very little if any of processed meat." However, men often have higher red meat intake in Western countries (Wyness et al., 2011). There is insufficient evidence for associations of unprocessed white meat with chronic diseases.

Meat, especially red and processed meat intake, is an important component of the Western diet, which includes several unhealthy behaviors such as high alcohol intake, high processed food intake (often high in sugar and fat and with low nutritional density), and low fruit and vegetable intake, and it is often associated with sedentary lifestyle and smoking (Micha et al., 2012). It is therefore difficult to disentangle the exact responsibility of a specific behavior such as high meat intake. On the other hand, it also suggests that inducing changes in dietary habits may also encourage modifying other unhealthy lifestyle components and/or adopting healthy ones. Public health authorities should therefore consider high red meat intake as part of an overall behavior that has to be tackled comprehensively for inducing optimal reductions in chronic diseases.

References

Abete, I., Romaguera, D., Vieira, A.R., de Munain, A.L., Norat, T., 2014. Association between total, processed, red and white meat consumption and all-cause, CVD and IHD mortality: a meta-analysis of cohort studies. Br. J. Nutr. 112 (05), 762–775.

Alexander, D.D., Cushing, C.A., 2009. Quantitative assessment of red meat or processed meat consumption and kidney cancer. Cancer Detect. Prev. 32 (5–6), 340–351.

Alexander, D.D., Morimoto, L.M., Mink, P.J., Cushing, C.A., 2010. A review and meta-analysis of red and processed meat consumption and breast cancer. Nutr. Res. Rev. 23 (02), 349–365.

Alexander, D.D., Weed, D.L., Cushing, C.A., Lowe, K.A., 2011. Meta-analysis of prospective studies of red meat consumption and colorectal cancer. Eur. J. Cancer Prev. 20 (4).

Alisson-Silva, F., Kawanishi, K., Varki, A., July 12, 2016. Human risk of diseases associated with red meat intake: analysis of current theories and proposed role for metabolic incorporation of a non-human sialic acid. Mol. Asp. Med. 51, 16–30.

Aune, D., Ursin, G., Veierød, M.B., 2009. Meat consumption and the risk of type 2 diabetes: a systematic review and meta-analysis of cohort studies. Diabetologia 52 (11), 2277–2287.

Bastide, N.M., Pierre, F.H.F., Corpet, D.E., February 1, 2011. Heme iron from meat and risk of colorectal cancer: a meta-analysis and a review of the mechanisms involved. Cancer Prev. Res. 4 (2), 177–184.

Battaglia Richi, E., Baumer, B., Conrad, B., Darioli, R., Schmid, A., Keller, U., December 1, 2015. Health risks associated with meat consumption: a review of epidemiological studies. Int. J. Vitam. Nutr. Res. 85 (1–2), 70–78.

Borgi, L., Curhan, G.C., Willett, W.C., Hu, F.B., Satija, A., Forman, J.P., 2015. Long-term intake of animal flesh and risk of developing hypertension in three prospective cohort studies. J. Hypertens. 33 (11).

Bouvard, V., Loomis, D., Guyton, K.Z., Grosse, Y., Ghissassi, F.E., Benbrahim-Tallaa, L., et al., December 2015. Carcinogenicity of consumption of red and processed meat. Lancet Oncol. 16 (16), 1599–1600.

Cao, J.J., Nielsen, F.H., 2010. Acid diet (high-meat protein) effects on calcium metabolism and bone health. Curr. Opin. Clin. Nutr. Metab. Care 13 (6), 698–702.

Chan, D.S.M., Lau, R., Aune, D., Vieira, R., Greenwood, D.C., Kampman, E., et al., June 6, 2011. Red and processed meat and colorectal cancer incidence: meta-analysis of prospective studies. PLoS One 6 (6), e20456.

Chen, G.C., Lv, D.B., Pang, Z., Liu, Q.F., January 2013. Red and processed meat consumption and risk of stroke: a meta-analysis of prospective cohort studies. Eur. J. Clin. Nutr. 67 (1), 91–95.

Choi, Y., Song, S., Song, Y., Lee, J.E., 2013. Consumption of red and processed meat and esophageal cancer risk: meta-analysis. World J. Gastroenterol. 19 (7), 1020–1029.

Chung, F.L., Chen, H.J.C., Nath, R.G., October 1, 1996. Lipid peroxidation as a potential endogenous source for the formation of exocyclic DNA adducts. Carcinogenesis 17 (10), 2105–2111.

D'Elia, L., Rossi, G., Ippolito, R., Cappuccio, F.P., Strazzullo, P., August 2012. Habitual salt intake and risk of gastric cancer: a meta-analysis of prospective studies. Clin. Nutr. 31 (4), 489–498.

Dargent-Molina, P., Sabia, S., Touvier, M., Kesse, E., Bréart, G.+, Clavel-Chapelon, F., et al., December 1, 2008. Proteins, dietary acid load, and calcium and risk of postmenopausal fractures in the E3N French women prospective study. J. Bone Miner. Res. 23 (12), 1915–1922.

Darling, A.L., Millward, D.J., Torgerson, D.J., Hewitt, C.E., Lanham-New, S.A., December 1, 2009. Dietary protein and bone health: a systematic review and meta-analysis. Am. J. Clin. Nutr. 90 (6), 1674–1692.

Eckl, P.M., August 2003. Genotoxicity of HNE. Mol. Aspects Med. 24 (4ГÇô5), 161–165.

Eckl, P.M., Ortner, A., Esterbauer, H., December 1993. Genotoxic properties of 4-hydroxyalkenals and analogous aldehydes. Mutat. Res./Fund. Mol. Mech. Mutagen. 290 (2), 183–192.

Fang, X., Wei, J., He, X., An, P., Wang, H., Jiang, L., et al., December 2015. Landscape of dietary factors associated with risk of gastric cancer: a systematic review and dose-response meta-analysis of prospective cohort studies. Eur. J. Cancer 51 (18), 2820–2832.

Faramawi, M.F., Johnson, E., Fry, M.W., Sall, M., Yi, Z., 2007. Consumption of different types of meat and the risk of renal cancer: meta-analysis of case–control studies. Cancer Causes Control 18 (2), 125–133.

Fardet, A., Boirie, Y., December 19, 2014. Associations between food and beverage groups and major diet-related chronic diseases: an exhaustive review of pooled/meta-analyses and systematic reviews. Nutr. Rev. 72 (12), 741–762.

Feskens, E.J.M., Sluik, D., Woudenbergh, G.J., 2013. Meat consumption, diabetes, and its complications. Curr. Diabetes Rep. 13 (2), 298–306.

Guo, J., Wei, W., Zhan, L., 2015. Red and processed meat intake and risk of breast cancer: a meta-analysis of prospective studies. Breast Cancer Res. Treat. 151 (1), 191–198.

Hooda, J., Shah, A., Zhang, L., 2014. Heme, an essential nutrient from dietary proteins, critically impacts diverse physiological and pathological processes. Nutrients 6 (3), 1080–1102.

Huang, W., Han, Y., Xu, J., Zhu, W., Li, Z., 2013. Red and processed meat intake and risk of esophageal adenocarcinoma: a meta-analysis of observational studies. Cancer Causes Control 24 (1), 193–201.

Kaluza, J., Wolk, A., Larsson, S.C., October 1, 2012. Red meat consumption and risk of stroke: a meta-analysis of prospective studies. Stroke 43 (10), 2556–2560.

Kellow, N.J., Savige, G.S., March 2013. Dietary advanced glycation end-product restriction for the attenuation of insulin resistance, oxidative stress and endothelial dysfunction: a systematic review. Eur. J. Clin. Nutr. 67 (3), 239–248.

Lajous, M., Tondeur, L., Fagherazzi, G., de Lauzon-Guillain, B., Boutron-Ruaualt, M.C., Clavel-Chapelon, F., January 1, 2012. Processed and unprocessed red meat consumption and incident type 2 diabetes among French women. Diabetes Care 35 (1), 128–130.

Larsson, S.C., Orsini, N., February 1, 2014. Red meat and processed meat consumption and all-cause mortality: a meta-analysis. Am. J. Epidemiol. 179 (3), 282–289.

Larsson, S.C., Wolk, A., January 31, 2012. Red and processed meat consumption and risk of pancreatic cancer: meta-analysis of prospective studies. Br. J. Cancer 106 (3), 603–607.

Lee, J.E., Spiegelman, D., Hunter, D.J., Albanes, D., Bernstein, L., van den Brandt, P.A., et al., December 3, 2008. Fat, protein, and meat consumption and renal cell cancer risk: a pooled analysis of 13 prospective studies. J. Natl. Cancer Inst. 100 (23), 1695–1706.

Lee, J.E., McLerran, D.F., Rolland, B., Chen, Y., Grant, E.J., Vedanthan, R., et al., 2013. Meat intake and cause-specific mortality: a pooled analysis of Asian prospective cohort studies. Am. J. Clin. Nutr. 98 (4), 1032–1041.

Liu, Z.T., Lin, A.H., 2014. Dietary factors and thyroid cancer risk: a meta-analysis of observational studies. Nutr. Cancer 66 (7), 1165–1178.

Liu, H., Fu, Z.X., Wang, C.Y., Qian, J., Xing, L., Liu, Y.W., 2012. A meta-analysis of the relationship between NAT2 polymorphism and colorectal cancer susceptibility. Medicina (Kaunas) 48 (3), 117–131.

Luo, J., Yang, Y., Liu, J., Lu, K., Tang, Z., Liu, P., et al., May 1, 2014. Systematic review with meta-analysis: meat consumption and the risk of hepatocellular carcinoma. Aliment. Pharmacol. Ther. 39 (9), 913–922.

Maki, K.C., Van Elswyk, M.E., Alexander, D.D., Rains, T.M., Sohn, E.L., McNeill, S., July 2012. A meta-analysis of randomized controlled trials that compare the lipid effects of beef versus poultry and/or fish consumption. J. Clin. Lipidol. 6 (4), 352–361.

Männistö, S., Kontto, J., Kataja-Tuomola, M., Albanes, D., Virtamo, J., 2010. High processed meat consumption is a risk factor of type 2 diabetes in the Alpha-Tocopherol, Beta-Carotene Cancer Prevention study. Br. J. Nutr. 103 (12), 1817–1822.

McNeill, S.H., November 2014. Inclusion of red meat in healthful dietary patterns. Meat Sci. 98 (3), 452–460.

Mente, A., de Koning, L., Shannon, H.S., Anand, S.S., 2009. A systematic review of the evidence supporting a causal link between dietary factors and coronary heart disease. Arch. Intern. Med. 169 (7), 659–669.

Micha, R., Wallace, S.K., Mozaffarian, D., June 1, 2010. Red and processed meat consumption and risk of incident coronary heart disease, stroke, and diabetes mellitus: a systematic review and meta-analysis. Circulation 121 (21), 2271–2283.

Micha, R., Michas, G., Mozaffarian, D., 2012. Unprocessed red and processed meats and risk of coronary artery disease and type 2 diabetes – an updated review of the evidence. Curr. Atheroscler. Rep. 14 (6), 515–524.

Millward, D., Garnett, T., 2010. Plenary Lecture 3 Food and the planet: nutritional dilemmas of greenhouse gas emission reductions through reduced intakes of meat and dairy foods. Proc. Nutr. Soc. 69 (01), 103–118.

Nicoll, R., McLaren Howard, J., 2014. The acid–ash hypothesis revisited: a reassessment of the impact of dietary acidity on bone. J. Bone Miner. Metab. 32 (5), 469–475.

Norat, T., Scoccianti, C., Boutron-Ruault, M.C., Anderson, A., Berrino, F., Cecchini, M., et al., December 2015. European Code Against Cancer 4th Edition: diet and cancer. Cancer Epidemiol. 39 (Suppl. 1), S56–S66.

O'Keefe, J.H., Bergman, N., Carrera-Bastos, P., Fontes-Villalba, M., DiNicolantonio, J.J., Cordain, L., March 1, 2016. Nutritional strategies for skeletal and cardiovascular health: hard bones, soft arteries, rather than vice versa. Open Heart 3 (1).

O'Sullivan, T.A., Hafekost, K., Mitrou, F., Lawrence, D., July 18, 2013. Food sources of saturated fat and the association with mortality: a meta-analysis. Am. J. Public Health 103 (9), e31–e42.

Pan, A., Sun, Q., Bernstein, A.M., Schulze, M.B., Manson, J.E., Willett, W.C., et al., October 1, 2011. Red meat consumption and risk of type 2 diabetes: 3 cohorts of US adults and an updated meta-analysis. Am. J. Clin. Nutr. 94 (4), 1088–1096.

Pierre, F., Tache, S., Guéraud, F., Rerole, A.L., Jourdan, M.L., Petit, C., 2007. Apc mutation induces resistance of colonic cells to lipoperoxide-triggered apoptosis induced by faecal water from haem-fed rats. Carcinogenesis 28 (2), 321–327.

Qu, X., Ben, Q., Jiang, Y., December 2013. Consumption of red and processed meat and risk for esophageal squamous cell carcinoma based on a meta-analysis. Ann. Epidemiol. 23 (12), 762–770.

Ramakrishna, B.S., December 1, 2013. Role of the gut microbiota in human nutrition and metabolism. J. Gastroenterol. Hepatol. 28, 9–17.

Rouhani, M.H., Salehi-Abargouei, A., Surkan, P.J., Azadbakht, L., September 1, 2014. Is there a relationship between red or processed meat intake and obesity? A systematic review and meta-analysis of observational studies. Obes. Rev. 15 (9), 740–748.

Salehi, M., Moradi-Lakeh, M., Salehi, M.H., Nojomi, M., Kolahdooz, F., May 1, 2013. Meat, fish, and esophageal cancer risk: a systematic review and dose-response meta-analysis. Nutr. Rev. 71 (5), 257–267.

Siri-Tarino, P.W., Sun, Q., Hu, F.B., Krauss, R.M., March 2010. Meta-analysis of prospective cohort studies evaluating the association of saturated fat with cardiovascular disease. Am. J. Clin. Nutr. 91 (3), 535–546.

Taylor, V.H., Misra, M., Mukherjee, S.D., 2009. Is red meat intake a risk factor for breast cancer among premenopausal women? Breast Cancer Res. Treat. 117 (1), 1–8.

The InterAct Consortium, 2012. Association between dietary meat consumption and incident type 2 diabetes: the EPIC-InterAct study. Diabetologia 56 (1), 47–59.

Wang, C., Jiang, H., 2012. Meat intake and risk of bladder cancer: a meta-analysis. Med. Oncol. 29 (2), 848–855.

World Cancer Research Fund, American Institute for Cancer Research, 2007. Second Expert Report, Food, Nutrition, Physical Activity, and the Prevention of Cancer: A Global Perspective. http://www.wcrf.org/int/research-we-fund/continuous-update-project-findings-reports.

World Cancer Research Fund, American Institute for Cancer Research, 2016. Continuous Update Project Findings & Reports. http://www.wcrf.org/int/research-we-fund/continuous-update-project-findings-reports.

Wu, A.M., Sun, X.L., Lv, Q.B., Zhou, Y., Xia, D.D., Xu, H.Z., et al., March 16, 2015. The relationship between dietary protein consumption and risk of fracture: a subgroup and dose-response meta-analysis of prospective cohort studies. Sci. Rep. 5, 9151.

Wyness, L., Weichselbaum, E., O'Connor, A., Williams, E.B., Benelam, B., Riley, H., et al., 2011. Red meat in the diet: an update. Nutr. Bull. 36 (1), 34–77.

Xu, J., Xx, Y., Yg, W., Li Xy, B.B., April 15, 2014. Meat consumption and risk of oral cavity and oropharynx cancer: a meta-analysis of observational studies. PLoS One 9 (4), c95048.

Yang, W.S., Wong, M.Y., Vogtmann, E., Tang, R.Q., Xie, L., Yang, Y.S., et al., December 1, 2012. Meat consumption and risk of lung cancer: evidence from observational studies. Ann. Oncol. 23 (12), 3163–3170.

Zeng, F.F., Fan, F., Xue, W.Q., Xie, H.L., Wu, B.H., Tu, S.L., et al., October 2013. The association of red meat, poultry, and egg consumption with risk of hip fractures in elderly Chinese: a case-control study. Bone 56 (2), 242–248.

Zhu, H., Yang, X., Zhang, C., Zhu, C., Tao, G., Zhao, L., et al., August 14, 2013. Red and processed meat intake is associated with higher gastric cancer risk: a meta-analysis of epidemiological observational studies. PLoS One 8 (8), e70955.

Zhu, H.C., Yang, X., Xu, L.P., Zhao, L.J., Tao, G.Z., Zhang, C., et al., 2014. Meat consumption is associated with esophageal cancer risk in a meat- and cancer-histological-type dependent manner. Dig. Dis. Sci. 59 (3), 664–673.

13

Fruits, Vegetables, and Health: Evidence From Meta-analyses of Prospective Epidemiological Studies

Marine van Berleere[1], Luc Dauchet[1,2]

[1]CHRU LILLE UNIVERSITY MEDICAL CENTER, LILLE, FRANCE; [2]LILLE UNIVERSITY, LILLE, FRANCE

1. Introduction

By the end of the 1980s, the evidence from laboratory, clinical, and epidemiological studies indicated that the consumption of fruits and vegetables prevented several major diseases (such as cancer and heart disease) and thus prompted the health authorities to promote this health behavior. However, the optimal level of consumption (above which there is no further benefit of increased consumption) is unknown. Until recently, the available data suggested that the association between fruit and vegetable consumption and decreased risk was proportional (i.e., with no identified threshold); this conclusion has led to different recommendations. For example, the Dietary Guidelines for Americans recommend that most people should eat at least nine servings of fruits and vegetables a day (US Department of Agriculture and US Department of Health and Human Services, 2010), whereas the American Heart Association recommends the consumption of at least eight fruits and vegetables a day (Carnethon et al., 2009), and many countries recommend five servings of fruits and vegetables per day (WHO, 2013). In the absence of evidence of a threshold effect for fruit and vegetable consumption, the message "five a day" has switched to "more is better" in the United States (Ungar et al., 2013).

The putative health benefits of fruits and vegetables are underpinned by a number of physiologic hypotheses. Fruits and vegetables have a low energy density and a low glycemic index. Conversely, they are rich in vitamins, minerals, and micronutrients. Therefore, fruits and vegetables contribute to micronutrient intake, provide a satiating volume of food, and have a low impact on energy intake. Moreover, many components of fruits and vegetables may act (through a variety of mechanisms) to prevent chronic disease. For example, dietary fiber may delay the postprandial absorption of carbohydrates after a meal, decrease the insulinemic response, and increase satiety (Bazzano et al., 2003a,b). Dietary fiber may also protect against colon cancer by promoting the fermentative formation of short-chain fatty acids by colonic bacteria, increasing fecal bulk, and reducing secondary bile acid production, intestinal transit time, and insulin resistance (Murphy et al., 2012). Potassium in fruits and vegetables may lower blood pressure (Whelton and He, 2014). Folate may reduce the cardiovascular risk through the lowering of plasma homocysteine and the improvement of endothelial dysfunction (Bazzano et al., 2003a,b), and it may prevent cancer by acting on DNA synthesis (WCRF/AICR, 2007).

Furthermore, fruits and vegetables contain numerous micronutrients with antioxidant properties, including beta-carotene, vitamin A, vitamin C, vitamin E, and selenium. Oxidative damage to cells and tissues is thought to be involved in the aging process and in the development of chronic disease. The imbalance between oxidants and antioxidants in our body is defined as oxidative stress (Bjelakovic et al., 2004). The antioxidant effect is one of the major physiologic hypotheses supporting the beneficial health effects of fruits and vegetables. Last, fruits and vegetables contain a wide range of biologically active, structurally varied phytochemicals (e.g., polyphenols, phytosterols, lectins) whose functional characteristics may contribute to the aforementioned health benefits (WCRF/AICR, 2007).

The effects of these nutrients on biologic processes have been tested in animal models and in vitro cell culture systems (Van Duyn and Pivonka, 2000). Randomized controlled trials are required for robust demonstrations of health effects in humans. Furthermore, evaluating the effects of these nutrients on disease incidence in randomized controlled clinical trials requires large sample sizes and long follow-up times. This demonstration is only possible when pharmacological supplementation is available. Unexpectedly, the results of the first large trials suggested that beta-carotene supplementation was associated with an increase in the incidence of cancer (Omenn et al., 1996). Further to these two important studies, antioxidant supplementation has been extensively evaluated in randomized controlled clinical trials (Bjelakovic et al., 2014). Meta-analyses of these trials' results have failed to demonstrate an effect of antioxidant supplementation on cancer (Myung et al., 2010) [and specifically gastrointestinal cancer (Bjelakovic et al., 2004) and lung cancer (Cortés-Jofré et al., 2012)], cardiovascular disease (Myung et al., 2013; Ye et al., 2013), cataracts (Mathew et al., 2012), and macular degeneration (Evans and Lawrenson, 2012). Moreover, meta-analyses have evidenced an increase in the risk of mortality associated with supplementation with beta-carotene, vitamin E, and the highest doses of vitamin A (Bjelakovic et al., 2012). Even though meta-analyses have identified significant associations in specific subgroups (Jiang et al., 2014; Loffredo et al., 2015) or for intermediate markers (such as arterial stiffness) (Ashor et al., 2014), the results of randomized clinical trials have mostly failed to demonstrate an effect of antioxidant supplementation; positive results remain scarce. The safety of supplementation has also been questioned. On the basis of these findings, antioxidant supplementation cannot be recommended for additional disease prevention (Bjelakovic et al., 2014). However, the lack of positive results for antioxidant supplementation does not rule out a positive effect of the antioxidants provided by fruits and vegetables. Clinical trials often use doses that are higher than those provided by fruits and vegetables; simulating the cocktail of antioxidants delivered by fruits and vegetables is difficult, and the wrong supplements may have been chosen (Liu, 2013; Steinhubl, 2008). However, the effect of antioxidants on health has not yet been demonstrated.

Last, clinical trials provide little evidence of an effect of a single fruit or vegetable component on the chronic disease risk. The interactions between the variety of nutrients found in fruits and vegetables need to be explored and are rarely evaluated when modeling physiopathologic process in the laboratory. Given that pathophysiologic factors arise and act at different time points (often years before the clinical manifestations), determining the respective contributions of various pathways to the final event is complex. Thus, identifying the mechanisms through which fruits and vegetables exert a putative protective impact on multifactorial disease processes is also complex. Moreover, differences in fruit and vegetable varieties, growing techniques, industrial processing techniques, and storage and cooking conditions can strongly affect the nutrients' composition and properties (Dauchet et al., 2009). In view of these variables, determining the biological plausibility of the observed association between fruit and vegetable intake and health is particularly challenging and lies beyond the scope of this review.

Clinical trial evidence is required to support the effect of fruits and vegetables on health. The gold standard in evidence-based medicine is the randomized clinical trial. Only randomized, disease-prevention trials can be used to draw firm conclusions about causal relationships. Fruits and vegetables per se can be evaluated in short-term randomized trials of controlled diets. With longer-term follow-up, only the effect of nutritional counseling (aimed at increasing fruit and vegetable consumption) can be evaluated. However, randomized nutritional prevention trials are difficult to perform and not always feasible. The success of these studies relies on the participants' compliance throughout the duration of the study, which can be several years. Even with appropriate interventions, changes in fruit and vegetable intake are generally modest, barely one additional portion per day on average, according to published trials (Brunner et al., 2007). Not surprisingly (given these difficulties), few randomized prevention trials have evaluated the effect of high fruit and vegetable intake in primary prevention. For example, in the Women's Health Initiative randomized controlled dietary modification trial (Liu et al., 2000), dietary advice was provided to 40% of 48,835 postmenopausal women aged 50–70 years, with the goal of reducing their fat intake and increasing their consumption of fruit, vegetables, and grains. After 6 years, the fruit and vegetable intake in the group that received nutritional advice had increased only slightly (by 1.2 servings per day), compared with the control group (Howard et al., 2006). The two groups did not differ significantly in terms of the frequency of major coronary heart disease relative risk (RR) [95% confidence interval (CI)] = 0.94 (0.86; 1.02), stroke [1.02 (0.90; 1.17)] (Howard et al., 2006), breast cancer [0.91 (0.83–1.01)] (Prentice et al., 2006), colorectal cancer [1.08(0.90; 1.29)], or total cancer [0.95 (0.89; 1.01)] (Prentice et al., 2007). Despite the large number of study participants, the statistical power of this type of study is limited by how difficult it is to change long-term fruit and vegetable intake. Hence, long-term prevention trials may not be able to show an effect of fruit and vegetable intake. Greater increases in fruit and vegetable consumption could be achieved in short-term randomized trials, although the outcome might only be a biomarker of risk factors. These trials have mainly studied cardiovascular risk factors or weight, and they will be described when discussing the biological plausibility of these outcomes.

Given the complexity of biological hypotheses and the limited feasibility of clinical trials, the main evidence for an effect of fruits and vegetables on health comes from epidemiological, observational studies. The latter can have ecological, case–control, or prospective cohort designs. Ecological studies are designed to explore relationships between environmental factors and diseases in human populations. They do not provide precise information about individuals within a population and are subject to many non-controlled sources of bias. In contrast, case–control studies compare diagnosed patients with disease-free individuals. Case–control nutrition studies rely on the retrospective assessment of an individual's diet and are therefore particularly subject to selection and recall bias, especially in nutrition studies (Willett, 2005). In prospective cohort studies, diets of people who are assumed to be healthy are assessed, and the group is monitored over time. During the follow-up period, some individuals will develop diseases. Given that measurements are made before any disease is diagnosed, cohort studies are not subject to recall bias. Hence, most of the epidemiological evidence has been generated in cohort studies (Dauchet et al., 2009). The results of many cohort studies have been published over the last decade and have been summarized by recent meta-analyses. In parallel, the methodology of meta-analyses has improved, notably with better analysis of the dose–response relationship.

In the present work, we therefore focused on recent meta-analyses of cohort studies dealing with the putative associations between fruits and vegetables and health outcomes. For each meta-analysis, we evaluated the strength of the association and the dose–response relationship. Given the importance (in terms of potential causality) of obtaining reproducible results across heterogeneous populations, we focused on geographic variations (see Fig. 13.1).

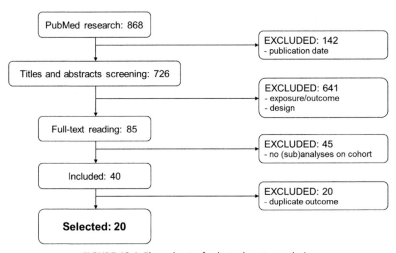

FIGURE 13.1 Flow chart of selected meta-analysis.

2. Search Strategy

We searched the PubMed database between January 2006 and December 2015, using the following keywords [including both medical subject heading (MeSH) terms and free text keywords]: ["Fruit"(MeSH) OR "Vegetables"(MeSH) OR vegetable OR fruit] AND ["Meta-Analysis"(Publication Type) OR "meta-analysis" OR "systematic review"]. The reference lists of retrieved articles were also hand-searched to identify further relevant reports.

Meta-analyses of prospective cohort studies investigating the relationship between fruit and/or vegetables and any outcome related to health status (e.g., risk factors, disease, health events, etc.) were eligible for inclusion. Fruit and/or vegetable intake constituted the exposure. We excluded reports of exposure to subtypes, specific types, or by-products of fruits and vegetables. We also excluded studies focusing on macro- or microconstituents (e.g., fibers or antioxidants) and publications not considering fruits and vegetables as an independent exposure (e.g., dietary patterns). Last, we excluded (1) systematic reviews lacking a meta-analysis, (2) meta-analyses of clinical trials only, and (3) meta-analyses of observational studies that did not report separate results for cohort studies and case–control studies. To be included in this review, the eligible meta-analyses had to report RRs summarized for at least two cohorts of fruit and/or vegetables.

The following data were collected for each eligible meta-analysis: authors; year of publication; design; number, names and location of the included cohorts; inclusion dates; total number of cases and subjects (if extractable); reported use of a quality assessment tool for the cohorts; outcome; exposure (fruits, vegetables, or fruits and vegetables); and confounding factors.

The following data were also collected, when available:

- the RR (95% CI) for the highest versus lowest fruit and vegetable intakes
- the RR for each incremental unit of fruits and vegetables, together with the details of the quantitation method used, the standard portion and the intake units
- any dose–response relationships, associated plots and nonlinearity tests
- the results by continent or geographic area
- heterogeneity assessments, specific investigations of publication bias, and the results of metaregressions and sensitivity analyses

The review's results were classified by outcome. Several meta-analyses may investigate the same outcome since they are based on the systematic review of the same studies and thus produce redundant results. Hence, when several meta-analyses were available for a single outcome, we focused on the analysis that met the most of the following criteria: (1) the most recent year of publication, (2) the greatest number of cohorts/subjects included, (3) the greatest number of exposure categories (from "fruit intake," "vegetable intake," and "fruit and vegetable intake"), (4) the inclusion of dose–response analyses, and (5) assessment of the influence of geographic location. In studies of cancer, we always selected meta-analyses that were part of the WCRF/AICR International Continuous Update Project.

Since different units could be used in reports of the RR for one supplementary unit of fruits and vegetables, we standardized these results for a 100 g/day increment (using Microsoft Excel software) according to the standard serving size quoted by the authors or by assuming that the standard portion was 100 g.

3. Results

Our PubMed search retrieved 868 articles: 142 were excluded because of their publication date, and 641 were excluded after the title and abstract had been screened. Eighty-five were eligible and thus were read fully; 40 of the latter were then included. Last, to keep just one meta-analysis per outcome, 20 studies were selected for final analysis.

3.1 Mortality

Fruit and vegetable consumption was significantly associated with lower overall mortality in a meta-analysis (Wang et al., 2014b), with a significant decrease of 6% for 100 g/day of fruits and vegetables, 7% for fruits, and 6% for vegetables (Table 13.1). The associations did not differ substantially as a function of study location, gender, the number of participants, the duration of follow-up, or the study quality. However, significant interstudy heterogeneity was observed (mostly due to the EPIC cohort, which contributed more than half of subjects in the meta-analysis). In the latter study, a weak association and a low decrease in risk were observed (ranging from 1% for fruits and vegetables to 3% for vegetables). Thanks to the very high power of this study, the association remains significant; this discrepancy might be due to a healthier diet in the EPIC population (Leenders et al., 2013) or by publication bias. Nevertheless, the strength of the association remains uncertain. For fruits and vegetables, similar associations have been observed in Europe and in the United States. Data from Asia are scarcer. The dose–response analysis suggested that there was no supplementary decrease in risk beyond four or five portions a day. In this meta-analysis, a significant association was observed for fruits and vegetables and cardiovascular mortality. Conversely, no association with cancer mortality was seen. The association between fruits and vegetables and mortality could be biased by the treatment of incident disease. Furthermore, consumption of fruits and vegetables may be associated with better access to care through higher socioeconomic status. However, many studies adjusted for socioeconomic status, and the results of the meta-analysis did not differ markedly when only status-adjusted studies were included.

3.2 Cardiovascular Disease

3.2.1 Coronary Heart Disease

Consumption of fruits and/or vegetables was significantly associated with a decrease in the risk of coronary heart disease (Gan et al., 2015). The RR (95% CI) per 100 g/day increment in fruit, vegetable, and fruit and vegetable intake were respectively 0.94 (0.91–0.98), 0.95 (0.91–0.99), and 0.97 (0.97–0.98) (Table 13.1). These associations were found to be

Table 13.1 Associations Between Fruit and/or Vegetable Intake and Mortality, Cardiovascular Disease, Cardiovascular Risk Factors and Other Diseases: Data From the Selected Meta-analyses

OUTCOME	Authors	Year	Cohorts	RR for "Highest Versus Lowest"	Egger Test	Cohorts Increment	RR per 100 g/day	Linearity	Threshold	Geographic Location(s)	Geographic Heterogeneity
Mortality			FV: 16	RR: 0.84 [0.79–0.90]–P heter: 0.35–I²: 9%	P=.18	FV: 7	RR: 0.94 [0.90–0.98]–P heter<0.01–I²: 82%	Nonlinear	<400 g/day	Europe/USA	No heterogeneity
			F:26	RR: 0.86 [0.82–0.91]–P heter: 0.76–I²: 0%	P=.15	F: 7	RR: 0.93 [0.86–0.98]–P heter<0.01–I²: 77%	Nonlinear	<150 g/day	Europe/USA/Asia	No heterogeneity
			V: 22	RR: 0.87 [0.81–0.93]–P heter: 0.28–I²: 13%	P=.10	V: 7	RR: 0.94 [0.89–0.99]–P heter<0.01–I²: 86%	Nonlinear	<200–250 g/day	Europe/USA/Asia	No heterogeneity
Cancer mortality	Wang X, Ouyang Y, et al.	2014b	FV: 24	RR: 0.79 [0.75–0.84]–P heter: 0.23–I²: 17%	P<.01	FV: 24	RR: 0.96 [0.88–1.04]–P heter: 0.08–I²: 68%	N/A			
			F: 19	RR: 0.77 [0.71–0.84]–P heter<0.01–I²: 52%	P=.02	F: 7	RR: 0.99 [0.96–1.00]–P heter: 0.33–I²: 14%	N/A			
			V: 16	RR: 0.86 [0.79–0.93]–P heter: 0.05–I²: 40%	P=.36	V: 8	RR: 0.99 [0.96–1.01]–P heter: 0.13–I²: 37%	N/A			
Cardiovascular mortality					P=.08	FV: 4	RR: 0.95 [0.90–0.99]–P heter: 0.16–I²: 42%	N/A			
					P=.28	F: 6	RR: 0.94 [0.89–1.00]–P heter<0.01–I²: 71%	N/A			
					P=.74	V: 6	RR: 0.95 [0.91–0.99]–P heter: 0.02–I²: 63%	N/A			
Coronary heart disease	Gan Y, Tong X, et al.	2015			P=.53	FV: 14	RR: 0.97 [0.97–0.98]–P heter: 0.64–I²: 0%	Linear		Western/Eastern	P>.05
					P=.95	F: 22	RR: 0.94 [0.91–0.98]–P heter: 0.08–I²: 32%	Nonlinear	<200 g/day	Western/Eastern	P>.05
					P=.89	V: 18	RR: 0.95 [0.92–0.98]–P heter: 0.07–I²: 36%	Nonlinear	<250 g/day	Western/Eastern	P>.05
Stroke	Hu D, Huang J, et al.	2014	FV: 24		P=.05	-				Europe/USA/Asia	P>.05
			F: 19	RR: 0.82 [0.75–0.91]	P=.02	F: 8		Linear			
			V: 16	RR: 0.94 [0.90–0.99]	P=.78	V: 6		Linear			

Continued

Table 13.1 Associations Between Fruit and/or Vegetable Intake and Mortality, Cardiovascular Disease, Cardiovascular Risk Factors and Other Diseases: Data From the Selected Meta-analyses—cont'd

OUTCOME	Authors	Year	Cohorts	RR for "Highest Versus Lowest"	Egger Test	Cohorts	RR per 100 g/day Increment	Linearity	Threshold	Geographic Location(s)	Geographic heterogeneity
Diabetes [type 2]	Wu Y, Zhang D, et al.	2015b	FV: 7		P=.33	FV: 7	RR: 0.99 [0.98–1.00]–P heter: 0.03–I²: 56%	Linear		Europe/USA/Asia	No heterogeneity
			F: 9		P=.68	F: 9	N/A–P heter: 0.28–I²: 19%	U Curve	200 g/day	Europe/USA/Asia	No heterogeneity
			V: 7		P=.15	V: 7	N/A–P heter< 0.01–I²: 78%	U Curve	200–300 g/day	Europe/USA/Asia	Not comparable
Obesity	Schwingshackl L, Hoffmann G, et al.	2015	FV: 5	RR: 0.91 [0.84–0.99]–P heter: 0.08–I²: 53%	N/A						
			F: 5	RR: 0.83 [0.71–0.99]–P heter: 0.24–I²: 28%	N/A						
			V: 7	RR: 0.83 [0.70–0.99]–P heter< 0.01–I²: 75%	N/A						
Asthma	Seyedrezazadeh E, Moghaddam MP, et al.	2014	F: 3	RR: 0.71 [0.61–0.82]–P heter: 0.27–I²: 23%	N/A						
Dementia	Cao L, Tan L, et al.	2015	FV: 2	RR: 0.46 [0.16–1.32]–P heter: 0.03–I²: 78%	N/A						
Depression	Liu X, Yan Y, et al.	2015	F:4	RR: 0.83 [0.77–0.91]–P heter: 0.16–I²: 41%	P=.02[a]					Europe/America/Asia/Oceania	P >.05[a]
			V: 4	RR: 0.88 [0.79–0.96]–P heter: 0.92–I²: 0%	P=.05[a]					Europe/America/Asia/Oceania	P >.05[a]

F, fruits; V, vegetables; FV, fruits and vegetables combined; RR, relative risk.
[a]Pooled results for case–control studies and cohort studies.

nonlinear for fruit consumption and for vegetable consumption but not for total fruit and vegetable consumption. Threshold effects were seen; the risk reduction was mainly observed for intakes up to around 200 g/day of fruits and 250 g/day of vegetables, with a smaller decrease thereafter. Levels of heterogeneity were moderate in both cases. Metaregression identified the year of publication as a significant source of heterogeneity for studies of vegetable intake; the inverse association with coronary heart disease risk was stronger in studies published after 2006. There were no significant differences between Western countries and Asian countries, and there was no evidence for publication bias. These results confirmed the previously reported significant, inverse associations between fruit and/or vegetable consumption and the risk of coronary heart disease (Dauchet et al., 2006; He et al., 2007).

3.2.2 Stroke

Linear inverse associations have been observed for the stroke risk on one hand and fruit intake and vegetable intake on the other (Hu et al., 2014), with risk reductions of 18% and 6% per 100 g/day, respectively (Table 13.1). The level of heterogeneity was not evaluated for these dose–response analyses. However, a "highest versus lowest" analysis revealed a significant association between a decreased stroke risk and intakes of fruits, vegetables, and fruits and vegetables. There were moderate to high levels of heterogeneity (mainly attributable to publication bias). In an earlier meta-analysis, fruit and/or vegetable consumption had been associated with a significant risk reduction (He et al., 2006).

In contrast to the modest association observed in meta-analyses of studies performed in Western countries, a strong association with fresh fruit was observed in a very large Chinese cohort study [RR (95% CI) = 0.60 (0.54–0.67) for cardiovascular death, in daily consumers versus nonconsumers] (Du et al., 2016). The strength of this association might be due to the very low mean consumption in this population. Most of the benefit could be achieved by moderate consumption, and nonconsumers may have been too rare to observe this effect. Another possible explanation relates to the very great difference in the social and behavioral characteristics when comparing consumers with nonconsumers, suggesting the presence of residual confounding factors.

Interventional studies have evidenced that increased consumption of fruits and vegetables is associated with significantly lower hypertension (a well-known cardiovascular risk factor). In the Dietary Approaches to Stop Hypertension Study in 1997 (Appel et al., 1997), both systolic and diastolic blood pressures were lower in the intervention group (assigned to a fruit- and vegetable-rich diet) than in the control group. In 2002, a randomized controlled trial also found evidence of a protective effect of fruits and vegetables on blood pressure in the general population (John et al., 2002). In 2013, a Cochrane review of interventional, randomized, controlled trials of primary prevention of cardiovascular disease (based on recommending greater consumption of fruits and vegetables or on actual provision of fruits and vegetables to facilitate greater intake) concluded that dietary advice may have beneficial effects on blood pressure and low-density lipoprotein cholesterol levels (Hartley et al., 2013). However, these data came from only two trials and thus did not provide strong evidence of a protective effect.

Last, a moderately significant decrease in the risk of coronary heart disease and stroke is associated with fruit and vegetable consumption. A causal relationship is supported by the observed effect of fruits and vegetables on blood pressure in intervention trials, and it has been discussed in detail elsewhere (Dauchet et al., 2009).

3.3 Obesity

Fruit and/or vegetable consumption was significantly associated with a decrease in the risk of weight gain, obesity, or overweight when comparing highest versus lowest intake categories (Schwingshackl et al., 2015) (Table 13.1). Significant associations were also found between increased fruit intakes and decreased weight and waist circumference. However, the outcome parameters and exposures (e.g., consumption at baseline or changes in consumption) differed from one study to another and prevented the reliable calculation of an effect size. Furthermore, a causal relationship is questionable.

The impact of fruits and vegetables on weight is controversial. On one hand, increased consumption of fruits and vegetables in the absence of a compensatory reduction in the intake of other foods will lead to weight gain. On the other, fruits and vegetables have low energy density and satiating properties; this might lead to lower consumption of other foods and thus a decrease in total energy intake (Kaiser et al., 2014). In contrast to the results of observational studies, clinical trials have failed to demonstrate an effect of fruit and vegetable intake on weight loss. Kaiser et al.'s meta-analysis evaluated randomized clinical trials of the effect of fruits and vegetables on either weight or fat loss or the prevention of weight or fat gain. None of the seven included studies yielded significant results for fruits and vegetables, and the meta-analysis was also negative. Another meta-analysis from 2014 studied randomized clinical trials that sought to increase fruit and vegetable consumption in the absence of advice or specific encouragement to remove other foods from diet (and regardless of whether or not the intervention's primary objective was weight loss) (Mytton et al., 2014). In this latter meta-analysis, our interpretation is that fruits and vegetables had no effect on weight gain or loss. In the original paper by Mytton et al., fruits and vegetables were associated with a small but significant decrease in weight. However, the effect size variance of some of the included studies in that paper appears to be incorrectly derived, and the decrease was no longer significant after application of a correction suggested by Kaiser et al. Despite the small number of clinical trials, the data suggest that supplemental energy intake from fruits and vegetables is balanced by an equivalent reduction in the intake of other food, leading to neither weight gain nor loss. Hence, fruits and vegetables per se seem to have a small or negligible effect on weight.

Public health recommendations aimed at increasing fruit and vegetable intake do not seem to have prompted weight gain, whereas greater fruit and vegetable intake is not expected to lead to a reduction in obesity. The associations between fruits and vegetables and weight found in observational studies are probably not causal. Fruit and vegetable consumption is probably a marker of a healthy diet and healthy behavior. Although fruit and vegetable consumption is not sufficient for weight loss, fruits and vegetables might be an important component of a dietary strategy that helps individuals to control hunger by eating satisfying amounts of food and therefore to improve their adherence to a weight loss program (Ello-Martin et al., 2007). In a randomized, controlled trial (Ello-Martin et al., 2007), two groups were encouraged to lower their fat intake. In one of the groups, the participants also received advice on increasing water-rich foods in general and fruits and vegetables in particular; greater weight loss and lower hunger levels were reported in this latter group.

Therefore, fruits and vegetables probably contribute to weight loss more by improving acceptability and adherence to weight loss programs than through a direct impact on body weight.

3.4 Diabetes

Fruit intake and vegetable intake were shown to be associated (in a nonlinear manner) with a decreased risk of type 2 diabetes (Wu et al., 2015b) (Table 13.1). A decreased diabetes risk was associated with increasing fruit intakes up to around 200 g/day of fruit [with an RR (95% CI) of 0.88 (0.85–0.92) for two 106 g servings] and increasing vegetable intakes up to 250–300 g/day [with an RR (95% CI) of 0.94 (0.90–0.98) and 0.94 (0.89–0.98) for two and three 106 g servings, respectively]. Above these cut-offs, the risk increased with the level of intake and thus suggested the presence of a U-shaped curve. Similar curvilinear relationships and thresholds were described in two other meta-analyses for fruit consumption and risk of type 2 diabetes (Li et al., 2014b; Li et al., 2015). There was no significant association with the total fruit and vegetable intake.

The inverse association between the risk of type 2 diabetes and fruits and vegetables is thought to be mediated by weight loss, antioxidants, and dietary fiber. The lack of a further decrease in risk after a certain cut-off might be due to changes in the availability of nutrients and the digestibility of fruits and vegetables. Furthermore, one can hypothesize that fruits increase the total intake of fructose (which is also provided by sugar-sweetened beverages and sweets). Fructose might decrease insulin sensitivity and increase risk factors for metabolic syndrome (Moreno and Hong, 2013; Stanhope, 2012; Stanhope et al., 2013). However, the contribution of fruits and vegetables to fructose intake is small, –17.1% in the NHANES study, for example (Marriott et al., 2009). Therefore, the impact of fruits and vegetables on a supplemental increase in fructose intake may be weak. Another hypothesis relates to the adverse impact of fruit juice. Some studies include fruit juice in their definition of fruit. However, fruit juice and whole fruit may differ in their impact on diabetes. Due to the juicing process, fruit juices have a relatively high glycemic load and lower levels of some potentially beneficial nutrients (Muraki et al., 2013). Indeed, in three pooled cohorts in the United States, whole fruit intake was significantly associated with a lower diabetes risk, whereas the consumption of fruit juice was associated with a higher risk. Furthermore, the U-shaped association was absent in studies that explicitly excluded fruit juice from their definition (Bazzano et al., 2008; Cooper et al., 2012; Muraki et al., 2013; Mursu et al., 2014) and present in studies that did include fruit juice (Kurotani et al., 2013) or did not specify whether juices were included (Villegas et al., 2008). Therefore, many high fruit juice consumers may be included in the group of high fruit or fruit and vegetable consumers. An adverse effect of fruit juice may therefore explain the observed U-shaped relationship. To rule out this hypothesis, results concerning fruit juice and whole fruits should always be reported separately.

There was a high level of heterogeneity in the analysis of vegetable intake, with significant geographic heterogeneity. The intake ranges differed highly when comparing Europe, the Unites States, and Asia. For fruit intake, a U-shaped curve was observed in the United States and Asia but not in Europe (where no data on high levels of consumption were available). Inclusion (or not) of fruit juice may explain this discrepancy between continents. Geographic location was not found to be a significant source of heterogeneity.

Earlier meta-analyses (of fewer studies) did not report any significant associations between fruit and/or vegetable consumption and the risk of type 2 diabetes, regardless of the serving size (Carter et al., 2010; Cooper et al., 2012; Hamer and Chida, 2007). A decreased risk of diabetes is observed for the moderate consumption of fruits and vegetables but not for higher intakes. To clarify this issue, the association with juice should be separated more clearly from that with fruit.

3.5 Other Diseases

3.5.1 Asthma

Asthma is considered to be a multifactorial disease with genetic and environmental factors, whose physiopathology involves hypersensitivity and inflammatory reactions. Nutrition has been cited as one of the environmental factors responsible for an increase in the prevalence of asthma over recent decades (McKeever and Britton, 2004). In this context, a meta-analysis of adult cohort studies (Seyedrezazadeh et al., 2014) (Table 13.1) found a significant (29%) reduction in the risk of asthma when comparing highest versus lowest levels of fruit intake. This association might be due to fruit components with antiinflammatory properties, such as flavonoids (Middleton and Kandaswami, 1992). This association could also be explained by a confounding effect of obesity. Of the three cohorts included in this analysis, two had adjusted for BMI but only one (Uddenfeldt et al., 2010) took account of the nonlinear, U-shaped relationship between BMI and asthma. For a detailed review of the relationship between the intake of vegetables (and especially raw vegetables) and asthma, the reader may refer to Chapter 27.

3.5.2 Dementia

Fruit and vegetable consumption might conceivably be related to risk of dementia via an effect on oxidative stress and thus on age-related cognitive decline; however, a clear, protective role for dietary antioxidants has yet to be established (Crichton et al., 2013).

A 2015 meta-analysis did not find an association between fruits and vegetables and the risk of dementia (Cao et al., 2015) (Table 13.1). However, there was a high level of heterogeneity and only two cohorts were included. In 2012, a systematic review identified nine cohort studies of fruit and vegetable consumption and Alzheimer's disease; unfortunately, heterogeneity in the outcome assessments prevented meta-analysis of these data (Loef and Walach, 2012). According to the systematic review, five out of six studies of vegetable intake reported a significant inverse association with the risk of dementia or cognitive decline. Hence, these findings appear to be weak and inconsistent.

Although dementia is a very common disease and places a very high burden on healthcare systems, the quantity of data is limited by the heterogeneity of outcome measurements in cohort studies.

3.5.3 Depression
Chronic inflammation and oxidative stress are thought to be involved in the pathogenesis of depression (Khanzode et al., 2003; Maes et al., 2000; Schiepers et al., 2005). Hence, the antioxidant and antiinflammatory properties of fruits and vegetables might protect against depression.

A meta-analysis of highest versus lowest intake groups revealed significant inverse associations between fruit intake, vegetable intake, and the risk of depression [RR (95% CI): 0.83 (0.77–0.91) and 0.88 (0.79–0.96), respectively] (Liu et al., 2016) (Table 13.1). There was a moderate level of heterogeneity in the data on fruit intake. As was the case for other potential sources of heterogeneity, geographic heterogeneity within a subgroup of cohorts was not analyzed. However, metaregressions in case–control and cohort studies failed to detect significant differences between Europe, America, Asia, and Oceania for both fruits and vegetables.

3.6 Cancer

3.6.1 Bladder Cancer
In a linear dose–response analysis, the bladder cancer risk decreased significantly (by 4% per 100 g/day increment in fruit and vegetable intake) (Vieira et al., 2015b) (Table 13.2). No significant reductions were reported for increased intakes of fruits alone or vegetables alone. The results of "highest versus lowest intake" analyses were not significant. In a nonlinear dose–response analysis, the decrease in risk for fruits and vegetables was observed for intakes of more than 400 g/day and was probably driven by two studies with higher reported intakes (the Multiethnic Cohort Study and the Netherlands Cohort Study). Furthermore, the nonlinearity test was not significant ($P = .06$).

Even though the associations indicated by this meta-analysis were attenuated after adjustment for smoking status, there was no evidence that the pooled results differed by smoking status in stratified analyses. Neither was there evidence of geographic heterogeneity.

This meta-analysis was part of the WCRF/AICR Continuous Update Project (CUP). The two main risk factors for bladder cancer are smoking and professional exposure to carcinogens. All but one of the studies included in the meta-analysis adjusted for smoking.

Table 13.2 Associations Between Fruit and/or Vegetable Intake and Various Types of Cancer: Data From the Selected Meta-analyses

Outcome	Authors	Year	Cohorts	RR for "Highest Versus Lowest"	Egger Test	Cohorts Increment	RR per 100g/day	Linearity	Threshold	Geographic Location[s]	Geographic Heterogeneity
Bladder cancer	Vieira AR, Vingeliene S, et al.	2015b	FV: 9	RR: 0.89 [0.75–1.05]–P heter: 0.16–I^2: 34%	$P=.09$	FV: 8	RR: 0.96 [0.94–0.99]–P heter: 0.76–I^2: 0%	Linear		Europe/USA	no heterogeneity
			F: 12	RR: 0.91 [0.82–1.00]–P heter: 0.34–I^2: 11%	$P=.48$	F: 12	RR: 0.98 [0.95–1.00]–P heter: 0.51–I^2: 0%	Linear		Europe/USA	no heterogeneity
			V: 10	RR: 0.92 [0.84–1.01]–P heter: 0.39–I^2: 5%	$P=.02$	V: 10	RR: 0.96 [0.93–1.00]–P heter: 0.35–I^2: 10%	Nonlinear	>350g/day	Europe/USA/Asia	no heterogeneity
Breast cancer	Aune D, Chan DSM, et al.	2012	FV: 7	RR: 0.89 [0.80–0.99]–P heter: 0.67–I^2: 0%	$P=.44$	FV: 6	RR: 0.98 [0.96–1.00]–P heter: 0.41–I^2: 2%	Linear		Europe/America	$P>.05$
			F: 10	RR: 0.92 [0.86–0.98]–P heter: 0.36–I^2: 9%	$P=.41$	F: 10	RR: 0.97 [0.94–1.00]–P heter: 0.10–I^2: 39%	Linear		Europe/America/Asia	$P>.05$
			V: 10	RR: 0.99 [0.92–1.06]–P heter: 0.26–I^2: 20%	$P=.23$	V: 9	RR: 1.00 [0.97–1.03]–P heter: 0.29–I^2: 17%	Linear		Europe/America/Asia	$P>.05$
Lung cancer	Vieira AR, Abar L, et al.	2015a	FV: 18	RR: 0.86 [0.78–0.94]–P heter: 0.08–I^2: 37%	$P<.01$	FV: 14	RR: 0.96 [0.94–0.98]–P heter< 0.01–I^2: 67%	Nonlinear	<400g/day	Europe/North America/Asia	heterogeneity
			F: 29	RR: 0.82 [0.76–0.89]–P heter: 0.07–I^2: 32%	$P<.01$	F: 23	RR: 0.92 [0.88–0.95]–P heter< 0.01–I^2: 57%	Nonlinear	<300g/day	Europe/North America/Asia	heterogeneity
			V: 25	RR: 0.92 [0.87–0.97]–P heter: 0.54–I^2: 0%	$P<.01$	V: 20	RR: 0.94 [0.89–0.98]–P heter< 0.01–I^2: 48%	Nonlinear	<300g/day	Europe/North America/Asia	heterogeneity
Colorectal cancer			FV: 10	RR: 0.92 [0.86–0.99]–P heter: 0.24–I^2: 22%	$P=.52$	FV: 11	RR: 0.99 [0.98–1.00]–P heter: 0.10–I^2: 38%	N/A		Europe/America/Asia	$P<.05$
			F: 14	RR: 0.90 [0.83–0.98]–P heter: 0.05–I^2: 42%	$P=.79$	F:13	RR: 0.98 [0.94–1.01]–P heter< 0.01–I^2: 64%	Nonlinear	<100g/day	Europe/America/Asia	$P>.05$
			V: 15	RR: 0.91 [0.86–0.96]–P heter: 0.54–I^2: 0%	$P=.14$	V: 12	RR: 0.98 [0.97–0.99]–P heter: 0.69–I^2: 0%	Nonlinear	<100–200g/day	Europe/America/Asia	$P>.05$
Colon cancer	Aune D, Lau R, et al.	2011	FV: 11	RR: 0.91 [0.84–0.99]–P heter: 0.32–I^2: 13%		FV: 11	RR: 0.99 [0.97–1.00]–P heter: 0.21–I^2: 25%	N/A			
			F: 11	RR: 0.89 [0.81–0.97]–P heter: 0.16–I^2: 30%		F: 11	RR: 0.98 [0.96–1.01]–P heter: 0.10–I^2: 38%	N/A			
			V: 11	RR: 0.87 [0.81–0.94]–P heter: 0.70–I^2: 0%		V: 11	RR: 0.96 [0.94–0.98]–P heter: 0.65–I^2: 0%	N/A			
Rectal cancer			FV: 9	RR: 0.97 [0.86–1.09]–P heter: 0.65–I^2: 0%		FV: 10	RR: 0.99 [0.97–1.01]–P heter: 0.48–I^2: 0%	N/A			
			F: 7	RR: 0.91 [0.76–1.09]–P heter: 0.09–I^2: 45%		F: 8	RR: 0.99 [0.95–1.03]–P heter: 0.04–I^2: 54%	N/A			
			V: 8	RR: 0.94 [0.85–1.04]–P heter: 0.59–I^2: 0%		V: 8	RR: 1.00 [0.96–1.03]–P heter: 0.88–I^2: 0%	N/A			

Cancer	Author(s)	Year	Exposure	RR [95% CI] – P heter – I²	P	Exposure	RR [95% CI] – P heter – I²	Dose–response	Threshold	Subgroup	Subgroup P
Colorectal adenoma	Ben Q, Zhong J, et al.	2015	FV: 3	RR: 0.82 [0.74–0.90]–P heter: 0.99–I²: 0%	P=.04a	FV: 3	RR: 0.99 [0.98–0.99]–P heter: 0.53–I²: 0%	Linear a		Western/Japan	P <.10a
			F: 4	RR: 0.79 [0.68–0.92]–P heter: 0.15–I²: 38%	P <.01a	F: 4	RR: 0.95 [0.93–0.96]–P heter: 0.68–I²: 0%	Linear a		Western/Japan	P <.10a
			V: 6	RR: 0.95 [0.81–1.10]–P heter: 0.08–I²: 49%	P=.28a	V: 4	RR: 0.99 [0.96–1.02]–P heter: 0.02–I²: 68%	Nonlinear a	>350 g/day a		
Prostate cancer	Meng H, Hu W, et al.	2014	F: 14	RR: 1.02 [0.98–1.07]–P heter: 0.93–I²: 0%	P=.09					Europe/North America/Japan/Oceania	no heterogeneity
			V: 12	RR: 0.97 [0.93–1.01]–P heter: 0.51–I²: 0%	P=.55					Europe/North America/Japan/Oceania	no heterogeneity
Gastric cancer	Wang Q, Chen Y, et al.	2014a	F: 22	RR: 0.90 [0.83–0.98]–P heter: 0.45–I²: 1%	P=.19	F: 16	RR: 0.95 [0.91–0.99]–P heter: 0.06–I²: 38%	Nonlinear	<100 g/day	Europe/USA/Asia	P >.05
			V: 19	RR: 0.96 [0.88–1.06]–P heter: 0.20–I²: 21%	P=.15	V: 16	RR: 0.96 [0.91–1.01]–P heter< 0.01–I²: 50%	Linear		Europe/USA/Asia	P >.05
Esophageal adenocarcinoma	Li B, Jiang G, et al.	2014a	F: 3	RR: 0.99 [0.72–1.36]–P heter: 0.97–I²: 0%	P=.06a					Europe/USA	P >.05a
			V: 3	RR: 0.76 [0.54–1.05]–P heter: 0.51–I²: 0%	P=.63a					Europe/USA	P >.05a
Esophageal squamous cell carcinoma	Liu J, Wang J, et al.	2013	F: 5	RR: 0.68 [0.55–0.86]–P heter: 0.25–I²: 25%	P=.13a	F: 4	RR: 0.87 [0.82–0.91]–P heter: 0.82–I²: 0%	N/A		Europe/USA/South America/Asia	P >.05a
			V: 5	RR: 0.80 [0.60–1.06]–P heter: 0.18–I²: 36%	P=.83a	V: 4	RR: 0.92 [0.84–1.01]–P heter: 0.05–I²: 61%	N/A		Europe/USA/South America/Asia	P >.05a
Hepatocellular carcinoma	Yang Y, Zhang D, et al.	2014	F: 6	RR: 1.04 [0.91–1.20]–P heter: 0.10–I²: 0%	P=.70a					Asian/Non-Asian	P <.05a
			V: 9	RR: 0.66 [0.51–0.86]–P heter< 0.01–I²: 75%	P=.06a					Asian/Non-Asian	P >.05a
Non-Hodgkin's lymphoma	Chen G-C, Lv D-B, et al.	2013	FV: 3	RR: 0.79 [0.65–0.96]–P heter: 0.32–I²: 11%	P=.28a	FV: 3	RR: 0.94 [0.85–1.03]–P heter: 0.14–I²: 49%	N/A		Europe/North America	P >.05a
			F: 5	RR: 1.01 [0.88–1.16]–P heter: 0.18–I²: 36%	P=.02a	F: 5	RR: 1.01 [0.96–1.06]–P heter: 0.12–I²: 46%	N/A		Europe/North America	P >.05a
			V: 5	RR: 0.90 [0.81–1.00]–P heter: 0.57–I²: 0%	P=.24a	V: 5	RR: 0.95 [0.90–1.00]–P heter: 0.14–I²: 43%	N/A		Europe/North America	P >.05a
Pancreatic cancer	Wu Q-J, Wu L, et al.	2015a	FV: 3	RR: 0.90 [0.77–1.05]	P=.40a					Europe/North America/Asia	-
			F: 8	RR: 0.93 [0.83–1.03]–P heter: 0.13–I²: 35%	P=.66a					Europe/North America/Asia	P >.05a
			V: 7	RR: 0.89 [0.80–1.00]–P heter: 0.60–I²: 0%	P=.66a					Europe/North America/Asia	P >.05a

F, fruits; V, vegetables; FV, fruits and vegetables combined; RR, relative risk.

aPooled results for case–control studies and cohort studies.

Conversely, only one study (Nagano et al., 2000) adjusted for exposure to radiation, and only the Multiethnic Cohort Study (Park et al., 2013) adjusted for "employment in high-risk industry." Interestingly, the Multiethnic Cohort Study is the only study to have reported a significantly lower risk associated with fruit and vegetable consumption. However, this association was observed only in women with a very low prevalence of exposure (1%). Furthermore, the hypothesis whereby professional exposure to carcinogens (as a confounding factor) might explain the overall lack of statistical significance supposes that this exposure reduces fruit and vegetable consumption and counters the latter's effect, which seems unlikely.

Other meta-analyses of observational studies were published around the same time (Liu et al., 2015; Xu et al., 2015; Yao et al., 2014). Yao et al. (2014) reported significant decreases in the bladder cancer risk for increasing intakes of fruits, vegetables, and fruits and vegetables but included both case–control and cohort studies. When analyzing only cohort studies, no significant associations were found for a 100 g/day increment in fruit, vegetable (Liu et al., 2015), or fruit and vegetable intake (Xu et al., 2015).

Overall, there is limited evidence of a protective association between fruit and vegetable intake and bladder cancer.

3.6.2 Breast Cancer

The CUP meta-analysis on breast cancer detected borderline-significant, linear dose–response associations for fruits and vegetables [RR (95% CI) per 100 g/day increment: 0.98 (0.96–1.00)] and for fruit alone [0.97 (0.94–1.00)] (Aune et al., 2012) (Table 13.2). In "highest versus lowest" analyses, fruit and vegetable consumption and fruit consumption (but not vegetable consumption) were significantly associated with a lower risk of breast cancer. There was little to no heterogeneity and no evidence of publication bias in any of these analyses. Furthermore, there were no significant differences between the results stratified by geographic location.

More recently, a pooled meta-analysis (Jung et al., 2013) found that fruit and vegetable consumption was associated with a significant lower risk of estrogen-negative breast cancer (ER–) [RR (95% CI) = 0.90 (0.81–1.01) for the fifth quintile versus the first quintile; P-trend = 0.03], as was vegetable consumption [RR (95% CI) = 0.82 (0.74–0.90); P-trend < 0.001]. In contrast, neither was associated with estrogen-positive breast cancer (ER+). Although fiber intake can lower sex hormone levels (Maskarinec et al., 2006), fruits and vegetables are less associated with the hormone-dependent ER+ cancers. The difference in the associations with ER+ and ER– cancers may be due to the difficulty in detecting a modest effect of fruit and vegetable intake (relative to hormonal factors) or to the differing mechanistic effects of phytochemicals in vegetables (Jung et al., 2013).

This suggests that there is weak association (may be only for subtypes of cancer) between fruit and vegetable consumption and breast cancer.

3.6.3 Lung Cancer

Increased intakes of fruits, vegetables, and fruits and vegetables were significantly associated with a lower risk of lung cancer in a WCRF/AICR-CUP meta-analysis (Vieira et al., 2015):

decreases of 4%, 8%, and 6% in the lung cancer risk were respectively reported of 100 g/day fruits and vegetables, fruits, and vegetables, respectively (Table 13.2). The dose–response relationships were found to be nonlinear, with no supplemental benefits for intakes of more than 400 g/day for fruits and vegetables, 300 g/day for fruits, and 300 g/day for vegetables. All the results were marked by high levels of heterogeneity. There was also significant evidence of publication bias, together with possible geographic heterogeneity (with stronger relationships in Europe). When stratified by smoking status, the power of the study decreased because studies not presenting stratified results were excluded. However, associations with fruits or vegetables remained significant in smokers but were not significant in former and never smokers (excepted for fruit in current smokers, in a "highest versus lowest" consumption). This association (observed only in smokers) could be explained by the fact that the effect of fruits and vegetables may partially counteract that of tobacco. For example, oxidative DNA damage is one of the tobacco-related pathways that leads to a carcinogenic effect (Hecht, 1999); this effect may be reduced by the antioxidant compounds that are found in fruits and vegetables. Another possible explanation is that smoking exposure is not measured precisely enough in smokers. Hence, smoking status may have been a residual confounding factor. Interactions between fruits and vegetables are discussed more extensively later in this review.

Two other meta-analyses were published in 2015 but included fewer cohorts (Wang et al., 2015a, 2015b). The "highest versus lowest" analyses were all consistent. One of these meta-analyses did not find a significant decrease in risk for a 100 g increment of fruits and vegetables or of vegetables (Wang et al., 2015b). This discrepancy may be due to differences in statistical power. Only one meta-analysis featured a dose–response analysis (Wang et al., 2015b) but did not find a significant association for vegetables or for fruits and vegetables. However, it did not report heterogeneity data either.

Hence, the fruit and vegetable consumption seems to be associated with a lower lung cancer risk. However, the effect of residual confounding factors (smoking status) cannot be completely ruled out.

3.6.4 Colorectal Cancer

As part of the WCRF/AICR-CUP, a meta-analysis assessing the association between fruit and/or vegetable intake and colorectal cancer risk was conducted in 2011 (Aune et al., 2011) (Table 13.2). In the linear dose–response analysis, only vegetable consumption was significantly associated with a lower risk (with a 2% decrease per 100 g/day increment in vegetable intake). For fruits alone and for fruits and vegetables, the linear associations were borderline-significant [with RRs (95% CI) per 100 g/day increment of 0.98 (0.94–1.01) and 0.99 (0.98–1.00), respectively], whereas fruit, vegetable, and fruit and vegetable intakes were all significantly associated with a decrease in the colorectal cancer risk in "highest versus lowest" analyses. Nonlinearity tests evidenced nonlinear relationships for fruit consumption and vegetable consumption. For fruits, most of the risk reduction occurred for intakes up to 100 g/day; above this threshold, the decrease was more modest. For vegetables, a similar threshold around 100–200 g/day was observed.

In terms of the tumor's location in the body, the aforementioned associations were found for colon cancer; there was a significant relationship between an increasing vegetable intake and lower risk, a borderline-significant relationship for fruit and for fruit and vegetable intakes, and significant associations for fruits and/or vegetables in "highest versus lowest" analyses. In contrast, there was no evidence of any association for rectal cancer. In addition to having an effect on folate and antioxidants, the fiber present in fruits and vegetables may prevent colorectal cancer by increasing stool bulk, decreasing transit time in the colon, and diluting potential carcinogens (Aune et al., 2011; WCRF/AICR, 2007). Fiber may decrease the transit time in the colon without altering the storage time in the rectum, and it may account for the absence of a decreased risk of rectal cancer (Aune et al., 2011).

All the results for fruit consumption were moderately heterogeneous, but no predictors were identified by metaregression.

There was evidence of geographic heterogeneity for fruits and vegetables, with a strong association in Europe and no effect in Asia (metaregression: $P < .05$). This difference might be due to several factors. First, only two Asian cohorts were considered. Second, there were undoubtedly differences in cultural factors, production, storage, cooking methods, and possibly in genetic make-up. Furthermore, the types of fruits and vegetables differed from one study site to another. Last, given the nonlinear associations with thresholds for fruits and for vegetables, differences in the ranges of intake or between reference categories may have caused some effects to be missed.

Two other meta-analyses were found but did not report dose–response analyses and did not find any significant associations in "highest versus lowest" analyses (Huxley et al., 2009; Kashino et al., 2015).

Last, epidemiological evidence suggests a weak but significant decrease in the colorectal cancer risk associated with moderate fruit and vegetable consumption.

3.6.5 Colorectal Adenoma

The colorectal adenoma risk fell significantly by 1% per 100 g/day increment of fruit and vegetable intake and by 5% per 100 g/day increment in fruit intake (Ben et al., 2015) (Table 13.2). There was no significant association with vegetable intake. The meta-analysis included both case–control and cohort studies. Therefore, nonlinearity tests and metaregressions were not performed on a subgroup of cohorts separately from case–control studies, and so the results had to be interpreted accordingly. However, they suggested the presence of linear associations for fruit and for fruits and vegetables, geographic heterogeneity, and smoking and total energy intake as residual confounding factors. Publication bias was also detected. Hence, there is some evidence that fruit consumption (but not vegetable consumption) is associated with a lower risk of colorectal adenoma.

3.6.6 Prostate Cancer

When comparing highest versus lowest intakes, fruit and vegetable consumption were not associated with prostate cancer risk in a meta-analysis. There was no heterogeneity, no publication bias, and no geographic heterogeneity (Meng et al., 2014) (Table 13.2).

3.6.7 Gastric Cancer

In a linear dose–response analysis, a 100 g/day increment in fruit intake was significantly associated with a 5% decrease in the gastric cancer risk (Wang et al., 2014a) (Table 13.2). No association was found for vegetable consumption. The "highest versus lowest" analysis yielded similar results because only fruit consumption was significantly associated with a decrease in the gastric cancer risk. The dose–response relationship for fruit was nonlinear, with most of the risk reduction occurring for intakes up to 100 g/day and a modest decrease thereafter. The moderate level of heterogeneity was mainly imputable to the outcome (incidence vs. mortality) and study quality.

Another meta-analysis (Fang et al., 2015) failed to perform dose–response analyses for vegetable consumption and included two articles based on the same data from the EPIC cohort. However, this analysis gave consistent results for fruit consumption: a significant association in a "highest versus lowest" analysis, a 5% decrease in the risk per 100 g/day, and a nonlinear dose–response relationship with a threshold at 200 g/day.

Helicobacter pylori is the strongest risk factor for gastric cancer. Fruits and vegetables may protect against the effect of *H. pylori*. Constituents such as selenium, beta-carotene, and vitamins A, C, and E may protect the epithelium from *H. pylori*–induced inflammation. Furthermore, high-dose vitamin C has been shown to inhibit *H. pylori* growth and colonization and to block intragastric nitrosation (Wang et al., 2014a). One can conclude that fruit consumption is inversely associated with the gastric cancer risk. Most of the risk reduction occurs for small increments in daily intake.

3.6.8 Esophageal Cancer

The results for esophageal cancer differ according to the histological subtype (adenocarcinoma or squamous cell carcinoma). There were no dose–response analyses for esophageal adenocarcinoma, and the "highest versus lowest" analyses did not report any significant associations for fruits or for vegetables (Li et al., 2014a) (Table 13.2). The squamous cell carcinoma risk was not associated with vegetable intake (Liu et al., 2013). In contrast, a significant (13%) risk decrease per 100 g/day was reported for fruit intake. However, nonlinearity tests performed on the pooled results of case–control and cohort studies evidenced a nonlinear association, with little effect of fruit intakes above 20 g/day. For both types of esophageal cancer, metaregressions for geographic location were also only performed on the pooled results of case–control and cohort studies; no significant differences between continents were found. Hence, for esophageal cancer, the only significant association involved fruit and squamous cell carcinoma. However, the design of the corresponding meta-analysis was not robust enough to rule out residual confounding by known risk factors (such as smoking and alcohol consumption). In addition to a general effect of fruits and vegetables on cancer, vitamin C may protect against the development of esophageal squamous cell carcinoma by blocking intragastric nitrosation (Liu et al., 2013). The differences in association for squamous cell carcinoma versus adenocarcinoma are not surprising because these tumors have different biological mechanisms and risk factors (mainly alcohol and tobacco for squamous cell carcinoma and acid reflux for adenocarcinoma).

3.6.9 Hepatocellular Carcinoma

In a meta-analysis of both case–control and cohort studies, the "highest versus lowest" subgroup analysis of cohorts only showed that the intakes of vegetables (not fruits) was associated with a reduced risk of hepatocellular carcinoma (Yang et al., 2014) (Table 13.2). However, the level of heterogeneity was high, publication bias was highly probable, and there was no dose–response analysis of cohort results alone. Furthermore, geographic heterogeneity cannot be ruled out. In view of the many possible confounding factors, there were too few data to draw firm conclusions.

3.6.10 Non-Hodgkin Lymphoma

Intakes of fruits, vegetables, and fruits and vegetables were not significantly associated with non-Hodgkin lymphoma risk when considering 100 g/day increments (Chen et al., 2013) (Table 13.2). When considering "highest versus lowest" analyses, only fruit and vegetable consumption was significantly associated with a decrease in non-Hodgkin lymphoma risk. The meta-analysis included case–control and cohort studies, and the latter results were extracted from subanalyses of cohort studies. Only three cohorts examined fruit and vegetable consumption. Furthermore, there was moderate heterogeneity in the results of the dose–response analyses, and some publication bias was detected. Therefore, there was very little evidence of a role for fruits or vegetables in the prevention of non-Hodgkin lymphoma.

3.6.11 Pancreatic Cancer

No significant associations between fruit, vegetable, and fruit and vegetable intakes and the pancreatic cancer risk were found in "highest versus lowest" analyses of cohorts in a meta-analysis of observational studies (Wu et al., 2015a) (Table 13.2). Similar results had already been reported for fruits and for vegetables in 2012 (Paluszkiewicz et al., 2012). In a meta-analysis of studies of pancreatic diseases, a protective effect of fruit consumption on pancreatic cancer was suggested (Alsamarrai et al., 2014); however, only three cohorts were included (compared with eight for fruit only in Q.J. Wu et al.), and so the latter systematic review was probably not exhaustive.

4. Discussion

Fruit and vegetable consumption is inversely associated with all-cause mortality and cardiovascular mortality. Consistently, fruits and vegetables are associated with a decrease in the risk of cardiovascular diseases. In contrast, an association with the cancer risk is less clear: although there is no decrease in overall cancer mortality, a decrease in risk is observed for specific cancer sites: lung cancer for fruits and/or vegetables; colorectal cancer for vegetables; and gastric cancer, esophageal cancer, and colorectal adenoma for fruits. With the exception of colorectal cancer, there is no significant evidence of geographic heterogeneity for the risk of cancer or cardiovascular disease. Hence, geographic differences in consumption habits, storage, and cooking methods do not seem to have a major impact on these associations.

Although several significant, consistent associations have been identified, the effect sizes are all moderate. With the exception of stroke, all of these dose–response relationships are nonlinear and exhibit a threshold effect. Accordingly, there are cut-offs in fruit and vegetable intake above which little or no additional decrease in risk is observed. Even though the "five a day" guideline was developed before the latest studies highlighted the cut-off effects, five portions a day appear to be an appropriate target, and the real benefit of higher intakes can be questioned. However, accurate estimations of the shape of the dose–response relationship are impaired by the small number of people consuming truly high amounts of fruits and/or vegetables. Indeed, few cohorts have reported on high intakes and thus may have biased the results toward a nonlinear effect. Hence, more data is required before firm conclusions and additional public health guidelines can be formulated.

In addition to cancer and cardiovascular disease, comparisons of highest versus lowest levels of intake have highlighted significant, inverse associations between fruit intake and asthma and between fruit intake, vegetable intake, and depression. Furthermore, a small body of data suggests a weak inverse association with obesity.

4.1 Confounding Factors

In view of the difficulty in organizing randomized trials in this field, most of the evidence in favor of health benefits for fruits and vegetables comes from observational cohort studies. The results of these studies may be biased by confounding factors, such as behaviors associated with fruit and vegetable consumption and with particular diseases. This might create associations that are not causal relationships with fruits and vegetables. In fact, high fruit and vegetable consumers have specific social, economic, access to care, and behavioral characteristics. For example, higher fruit and vegetable consumption has been associated with less smoking, more vitamin consumption, lower alcohol consumption, lower physical activity, and a higher educational level (Bazzano et al., 2002; Crowe et al., 2011; Joshipura et al., 1999). Although most of the known confounding factors are included in multivariate analyses, they cannot all be identified or perfectly measured, leading to residual confounding.

Moreover, the separate assessment of fruits and vegetables is impaired by the fact that nutrients and food are consumed in combinations (Hu, 2002). Indeed, fruit and vegetable consumption is highly correlated with other food intakes. For example, fruit and vegetable intake was strongly correlated with prudent diet patterns in the Health Professionals Follow-up Study (Hu, 2002). Furthermore, fruits and vegetables are prime components of recommended dietary patterns, such as the Mediterranean diet (Trichopoulou et al., 2005). Given the complexity of modeling diets, cohort studies rarely adjust for other components. Last, dietary pattern may also explain the potential effect of fruits and vegetables on health as well as being a strong confounding factor. Indeed, fruits and vegetables may displace less healthy food and will therefore change the overall balance of diet (Fulton et al., 2014). In a meta-analysis of randomized intervention trials that required adult subjects to increase only their fruit and vegetable intake (i.e., in the absence of other dietary or lifestyle changes), a decrease in fat intake was observed in the intervention groups (Fulton et al., 2014). Therefore, it is hard to distinguish the effect of fruits and vegetables per se from associated changes in dietary patterns.

4.2 Interaction With Smoking

Smoking has an impact on the main diseases for which an association with fruit and vegetable consumption has been found (e.g., lung cancer and cardiovascular disease). Furthermore, stronger associations are observed among smokers. The associations between fruits and vegetables in the EPIC cohort study were observed only in current smokers (Linseisen et al., 2007), and not in former and never smokers. In the meta-analysis by Vieira et al., the associations were more consistent among smokers than among never or former smokers. In addition, several studies have reported larger reductions in the coronary heart disease risk with fruit and vegetable consumption in smokers than in nonsmokers (Dauchet et al., 2010; Hung et al., 2004; Liu et al., 2001). This interaction with tobacco might be explained by a partial prevention of tobacco's harmful effect by fruits and vegetables (Dauchet et al., 2010). For example, smoking products lower blood levels of antioxidant micronutrients (Bruno and Traber, 2006; Dietrich et al., 2003; Yanbaeva et al., 2007). The antioxidant content of some fruits and vegetables may reduce the oxidative damage caused by tobacco. Furthermore, fruit and vegetable consumption is associated with lower plasma C-reactive protein concentrations (Chun et al., 2008; Esmaillzadeh et al., 2006), which might attenuate the proinflammatory effects of smoking (Yanbaeva et al., 2007). However, the hypothesized effect of antioxidants has not been demonstrated (Bjelakovic et al., 2014), and beta-carotene has been associated with a higher risk of tobacco-related cancer among smokers only (Touvier et al., 2005).

Another hypothesis is that stronger association among smokers and for tobacco-induced pathologies may be due to residual confounding by smoking. Indeed, in general, high fruit and vegetable consumers are less likely to be smokers (Bazzano et al., 2002; Crowe et al., 2011; Joshipura et al., 1999; Poisson et al., 2012). Smoking status is therefore a major confounding factor. Thus, in the EPIC cohort study, the observed associations with lung cancer were dramatically modified after adjustment for smoking (Linseisen et al., 2007). Even if results of most of the studies adjusted for smoking, measurement of exposure to tobacco may not have been measured precisely enough. Furthermore, in the majority of cohorts, smoking status is analyzed only at baseline, and the consumption of fruits and vegetables may be associated with a greater likelihood of quitting smoking during the follow-up period (Poisson et al., 2012). Smoking cessation is a potential confounding factor that is rarely taken into account in cohort studies. Hence, one cannot rule out that residual confounding by smoker status explaining (at least in part) associations between fruits and vegetables and smoking-related diseases.

4.3 Subtypes of Fruits and Vegetables

We chose to focus on fruits and vegetables in general, and therefore we excluded studies of categories or subtypes of fruits and vegetables. For instance, we did not review meta-analyses of the putative association between cruciferous vegetables and the risk of renal cell carcinoma (Zhao and Zhao, 2013) or the risk of ovarian cancer (Hu et al., 2015). Our approach is consistent with most public health guidelines, which rarely include specific advice on subtypes of fruits and vegetables. However, fruits and vegetables constitute a wide, diverse group of foods, and their components (e.g., antioxidants) differ substantially from one type to another. Therefore, biological hypotheses and expected associations may also differ from type of fruit or vegetable to another. For example, Fang et al.'s (2015) "highest versus lowest" analyses of the gastric cancer risk found that there were significant associations for white vegetables (but not for total vegetables) and citrus fruits (but not for apples and pears). White vegetables and citrus fruits are rich sources of vitamin C, which was also significantly associated with a decrease in the gastric cancer risk in Fang et al.'s meta-analysis. *H. pylori* is a proven carcinogen in the development of gastric cancer (IARC, 1994), and high doses of vitamin C have been shown to inhibit *H. pylori* growth and colonization (Sezikli et al., 2012; Zhang et al., 1997). Furthermore, dietary vitamin C acts as a scavenger of carcinogenic *N*-nitroso compounds in the gastric lumen (Tannenbaum et al., 1991; Yamaguchi and Kakizoe, 2001). Therefore, different concentrations of vitamin C may account for different associations between types of fruits and vegetables and the gastric cancer risk.

4.4 Limitations

This review has several limitations. Even though most of the studies used validated food frequency questionnaires, there is still a large error in measuring food intake (whatever the method). Furthermore, as the dietary habits of cohort participants are usually only assessed at inclusion, misclassification of subsequent exposure cannot be ruled out. Hence, these errors may have weakened (or hidden) the associations between fruits and vegetables and disease. Moreover, classification of fruits and vegetables differs from one cohort study to another and may alter the results of subsequent meta-analyses.

Few cohorts are based on representative samples of the population, such as the cohort based on the follow-up of the US National Health and Nutrition survey (Bazzano et al., 2003a,b). Given that the inclusion and monitoring of the very large number of patients required in a cohort study are very difficult, most studies did not randomize their participants or included specific populations. For example, the Nagasaki Lifespan study includes atomic bomb survivors (Sauvaget et al., 2003), and the Nurse Health Study and the Health Professionals' Follow-up Study include health workers. The EPIC study merges cohorts from 10 European countries, which include both samples of the general population or specific samples (such as teachers and blood donors) (Leenders et al., 2013). Therefore, few cohorts include representative samples. Mean consumption or the incidence of disease cannot be evaluated in these studies. However, selection bias is reduced by comparing different intensities of exposure (e.g., to fruits and vegetables) within a single group (internal comparisons) (Rothman and Greenland, 1998). Nevertheless, an association observed in a single, specific cohort is not sufficient for robust conclusions and must be confirmed by the results from different types of cohorts.

In addition, by restricting this review to meta-analyses of cohorts, we restricted it to the health events widely examined in this type of study. Moreover, prospective cohorts mostly include middle-aged men and women. Hence, this design makes it difficult to study diseases that start earlier in life (such as chronic inflammatory bowel disease, for which no meta-analyses of prospective cohort studies were found). However, the diseases included in this review (such as cancer, cardiovascular disease, and diabetes) account for a large proportion of morbidity and mortality worldwide, so the results of the corresponding meta-analysis probably enable relevant public health conclusions to be drawn.

4.5 Causality

Associations highlighted by observational epidemiological studies can result from a true, health-promoting effect of fruits and vegetables or from a simple statistical relationship due to bias. Accordingly, the results of epidemiological studies should be examined in terms of causality before being used for nutrition guidelines. However, this examination is challenging and requires a specific review for each outcome. Potischman and Weed (1999) have adapted Hill's criteria for causation (Hill, 1965) to the field of nutritional epidemiology. We shall consider the main criteria and present the corresponding conclusions for fruits and vegetables. (1) *The association should be consistent.* On one hand, most associations seen in the meta-analyses are hampered by significant heterogeneity; this might be due to methodological differences in how diet is measured (Potischman and Weed, 1999). On the other hand, these associations are mostly similar for geographic areas, which suggests that they are consistent across populations with differing diets and behaviors. (2) *The association should be strong.* In nutritional epidemiology, strong associations are rarely found (notably because of measurement error). Furthermore, weak associations may have large public health effects because fruit and vegetable consumption concerns the whole population and targets prevalent diseases. The association between fruits and vegetables and mortality was measured earlier, for instance. The decrease in the mortality risk of 6% for a 100 g/day increment corresponds to a 22% decrease in risk for a 400 g/day increment; these weights more or less correspond to the observed range of daily intakes. Hence, this is equivalent to the 20% decrease considered to be a "positive finding" by Potischman and Weed (1999). However, almost none of these associations could be considered to be "strong" (>40%) decrease in risk. (3) *The dose–response relationship should be significantly linear or at least regularly decreasing.* Despite threshold effects, most associations (except for diabetes and bladder cancer) are linear across the most frequent portion size/consumption levels, so they are suggestive of a causal link. (4) *The exposure assessment must precede the onset of the disease.* This criterion is necessarily met by the studies' prospective design. (5) *When evaluating causality, the corner stone is biological plausibility, i.e., evidence collected from animal models, in vitro cell culture systems, and metabolic and clinical studies in humans.* The difficulty in examining physiologic hypothesis has been mentioned earlier. Data from clinical studies in humans are scarce and restricted to a few clinical markers (such as hypertension). Last, determining the causal nature of these associations is subject to debate and requires further research.

5. Conclusion

In meta-analyses of observational studies, fruit and vegetable consumption is associated with significantly lower risks of mortality and frequent diseases, such as cardiovascular disease, obesity, and some types of cancers. Although the observed associations are modest in size, they may explain part of the lower risk of disease reported for plant-based and vegetarian diets (see other sections of this book). Furthermore, these associations may be significantly important for public health because the decrease in risk might well concern (1) the whole population and (2) diseases that place a high burden on healthcare systems. Furthermore, the decrease in risk may have been underestimated for methodological reasons. Given how difficult it is to study the effects of fruits and vegetables in clinical trials, it is hard to demonstrate causal relationships between fruits and vegetables and health outcomes or to distinguish between an effect of fruits and vegetables per se and an effect of the associated dietary patterns. Advice on eating more fruits and vegetables should probably constitute one way of improving dietary patterns (by replacing unhealthy food by fruits and vegetables), rather than an isolated recommendation.

References

Alsamarrai, A., Das, S.L.M., Windsor, J.A., Petrov, M.S., 2014. Factors that affect risk for pancreatic disease in the general population: a systematic review and meta-analysis of prospective cohort studies. Clin. Gastroenterol. Hepatol. 12, 1635–1644.e5; quiz e103. http://dx.doi.org/10.1016/j.cgh.2014.01.038.

Appel, L.J., Moore, T.J., Obarzanek, E., Vollmer, W.M., Svetkey, L.P., Sacks, F.M., Bray, G.A., Vogt, T.M., Cutler, J.A., Windhauser, M.M., Lin, P.H., Karanja, N., 1997. A clinical trial of the effects of dietary patterns on blood pressure. DASH Collaborative Research Group. N. Engl. J. Med. 336, 1117–1124. http://dx.doi.org/10.1056/NEJM199704173361601.

Ashor, A.W., Siervo, M., Lara, J., Oggioni, C., Mathers, J.C., 2014. Antioxidant vitamin supplementation reduces arterial stiffness in adults: a systematic review and meta-analysis of randomized controlled trials. J. Nutr. 144, 1594–1602. http://dx.doi.org/10.3945/jn.114.195826.

Aune, D., Chan, D.S.M., Greenwood, D.C., Vieira, A.R., Rosenblatt, D.A.N., Vieira, R., Norat, T., 2012. Dietary fiber and breast cancer risk: a systematic review and meta-analysis of prospective studies. Ann. Oncol. 23, 1394–1402. http://dx.doi.org/10.1093/annonc/mdr589.

Aune, D., Lau, R., Chan, D.S.M., Vieira, R., Greenwood, D.C., Kampman, E., Norat, T., 2011. Nonlinear reduction in risk for colorectal cancer by fruit and vegetable intake based on meta-analysis of prospective studies. Gastroenterology 141, 106–118. http://dx.doi.org/10.1053/j.gastro.2011.04.013.

Bazzano, L.A., He, J., Ogden, L.G., Loria, C.M., Vupputuri, S., Myers, L., Whelton, P.K., 2002. Fruit and vegetable intake and risk of cardiovascular disease in US adults: the first national health and nutrition examination survey epidemiologic follow-up study. Am. J. Clin. Nutr. 76, 93–99.

Bazzano, L.A., Li, T.Y., Joshipura, K.J., Hu, F.B., 2008. Intake of fruit, vegetables, and fruit juices and risk of diabetes in women. Diabetes Care 31, 1311–1317. http://dx.doi.org/10.2337/dc08-0080.

Bazzano, L.A., Serdula, M.K., Liu, S., 2003a. Dietary intake of fruits and vegetables and risk of cardiovascular disease. Curr. Atheroscler. Rep. 5, 492–499.

Bazzano, L.A., He, J., Ogden, L.G., Loria, C.M., Whelton, P.K., 2003b. Dietary fiber intake and reduced risk of coronary heart disease in us men and women: the national health and nutrition examination survey i epidemiologic follow-up study. Arch. Intern. Med. 163, 1897–1904. http://dx.doi.org/10.1001/archinte.163.16.1897.

Ben, Q., Zhong, J., Liu, J., Wang, L., Sun, Y., Yv, L., Yuan, Y., 2015. Association between consumption of fruits and vegetables and risk of colorectal adenoma: a PRISMA-compliant meta-analysis of observational studies. Med. Baltim. 94, e1599. http://dx.doi.org/10.1097/MD.0000000000001599.

Bjelakovic, G., Nikolova, D., Gluud, C., 2014. Antioxidant supplements and mortality. Curr. Opin. Clin. Nutr. Metab. Care 17, 40–44. http://dx.doi.org/10.1097/MCO.0000000000000009.

Bjelakovic, G., Nikolova, D., Gluud, L.L., Simonetti, R.G., Gluud, C., 2012. Antioxidant supplements for prevention of mortality in healthy participants and patients with various diseases. Cochrane Database Syst. Rev. 3, CD007176. http://dx.doi.org/10.1002/14651858.CD007176.pub2.

Bjelakovic, G., Nikolova, D., Simonetti, R.G., Gluud, C., 2004. Antioxidant supplements for prevention of gastrointestinal cancers: a systematic review and meta-analysis. Lancet 364, 1219–1228. http://dx.doi.org/10.1016/S0140-6736(04)17138-9.

Brunner, E.J., Rees, K., Ward, K., Burke, M., Thorogood, M., 2007. Dietary advice for reducing cardiovascular risk. Cochrane Database Syst. Rev. CD002128. http://dx.doi.org/10.1002/14651858.CD002128.pub3.

Bruno, R.S., Traber, M.G., 2006. Vitamin E biokinetics, oxidative stress and cigarette smoking. Pathophysiology 13, 143–149. http://dx.doi.org/10.1016/j.pathophys.2006.05.003.

Cao, L., Tan, L., Wang, H.-F., Jiang, T., Zhu, X.-C., Lu, H., Tan, M.-S., Yu, J.-T., 2015. Dietary patterns and risk of dementia: a systematic review and meta-analysis of cohort studies. Mol. Neurobiol. http://dx.doi.org/10.1007/s12035-015-9516-4.

Carnethon, M., Whitsel, L.P., Franklin, B.A., Kris-Etherton, P., Milani, R., Pratt, C.A., Wagner, G.R., American Heart Association Advocacy Coordinating Committee, Council on Epidemiology and Prevention, Council on the Kidney in Cardiovascular Disease, Council on Nutrition, Physical Activity and Metabolism, 2009. Worksite wellness programs for cardiovascular disease prevention: a policy statement from the American Heart Association. Circulation 120, 1725–1741. http://dx.doi.org/10.1161/CIRCULATIONAHA.109.192653.

Carter, P., Gray, L.J., Troughton, J., Khunti, K., Davies, M.J., 2010. Fruit and vegetable intake and incidence of type 2 diabetes mellitus: systematic review and meta-analysis. BMJ 341, c4229.

Chen, G.-C., Lv, D.-B., Pang, Z., Liu, Q.-F., 2013. Fruits and vegetables consumption and risk of non-Hodgkin's lymphoma: a meta-analysis of observational studies. Int. J. Cancer 133, 190–200. http://dx.doi.org/10.1002/ijc.27992.

Chun, O.K., Chung, S.-J., Claycombe, K.J., Song, W.O., 2008. Serum C-reactive protein concentrations are inversely associated with dietary flavonoid intake in U.S. adults. J. Nutr. 138, 753–760.

Cooper, A.J., Forouhi, N.G., Ye, Z., Buijsse, B., Arriola, L., Balkau, B., Barricarte, A., Beulens, J.W.J., Boeing, H., Büchner, F.L., Dahm, C.C., de Lauzon-Guillain, B., Fagherazzi, G., Franks, P.W., Gonzalez, C., Grioni, S., Kaaks, R., Key, T.J., Masala, G., Navarro, C., Nilsson, P., Overvad, K., Panico, S., Ramón Quirós, J., Rolandsson, O., Roswall, N., Sacerdote, C., Sánchez, M.-J., Slimani, N., Sluijs, I., Spijkerman, A.M.W., Teucher, B., Tjonneland, A., Tumino, R., Sharp, S.J., Langenberg, C., Feskens, E.J.M., Riboli, E., Wareham, N.J., InterAct Consortium, 2012. Fruit and vegetable intake and type 2 diabetes: EPIC-InterAct prospective study and meta-analysis. Eur. J. Clin. Nutr. 66, 1082–1092. http://dx.doi.org/10.1038/ejcn.2012.85.

Cortés-Jofré, M., Rueda, J.-R., Corsini-Muñoz, G., Fonseca-Cortés, C., Caraballoso, M., Bonfill Cosp, X., 2012. Drugs for preventing lung cancer in healthy people. Cochrane Database Syst. Rev. 10, CD002141. http://dx.doi.org/10.1002/14651858.CD002141.pub2.

Crichton, G.E., Bryan, J., Murphy, K.J., 2013. Dietary antioxidants, cognitive function and dementia–a systematic review. Plant Foods Hum. Nutr. 68, 279–292. http://dx.doi.org/10.1007/s11130-013-0370-0.

Crowe, F.L., Roddam, A.W., Key, T.J., Appleby, P.N., Overvad, K., Jakobsen, M.U., Tjønneland, A., Hansen, L., Boeing, H., Weikert, C., Linseisen, J., Kaaks, R., Trichopoulou, A., Misirli, G., Lagiou, P., Sacerdote, C., Pala, V., Palli, D., Tumino, R., Panico, S., Bueno-de-Mesquita, H.B., Boer, J., van Gils, C.H., Beulens, J.W.J., Barricarte, A., Rodríguez, L., Larrañaga, N., Sánchez, M.-J., Tormo, M.-J., Buckland, G., Lund, E., Hedblad, B., Melander, O., Jansson, J.-H., Wennberg, P., Wareham, N.J., Slimani, N., Romieu, I., Jenab, M., Danesh, J., Gallo, V., Norat, T., Riboli, E., European Prospective Investigation into Cancer and Nutrition (EPIC)-Heart Study Collaborators, 2011. Fruit and vegetable intake and mortality from ischaemic heart disease: results from the European Prospective Investigation into Cancer and Nutrition (EPIC)-Heart study. Eur. Heart J. 32, 1235–1243. http://dx.doi.org/10.1093/eurheartj/ehq465.

Dauchet, L., Amouyel, P., Dallongeville, J., 2009. Fruits, vegetables and coronary heart disease. Nat. Rev. Cardiol. 6, 599–608. http://dx.doi.org/10.1038/nrcardio.2009.131.

Dauchet, L., Amouyel, P., Hercberg, S., Dallongeville, J., 2006. Fruit and vegetable consumption and risk of coronary heart disease: a meta-analysis of cohort studies. J. Nutr. 136, 2588–2593.

Dauchet, L., Montaye, M., Ruidavets, J.-B., Arveiler, D., Kee, F., Bingham, A., Ferrières, J., Haas, B., Evans, A., Ducimetière, P., Amouyel, P., Dallongeville, J., 2010. Association between the frequency of fruit and vegetable consumption and cardiovascular disease in male smokers and non-smokers. Eur. J. Clin. Nutr. 64, 578–586. http://dx.doi.org/10.1038/ejcn.2010.46.

Dietrich, M., Block, G., Norkus, E.P., Hudes, M., Traber, M.G., Cross, C.E., Packer, L., 2003. Smoking and exposure to environmental tobacco smoke decrease some plasma antioxidants and increase gamma-tocopherol in vivo after adjustment for dietary antioxidant intakes. Am. J. Clin. Nutr. 77, 160–166.

Du, H., Li, L., Bennett, D., Guo, Y., Key, T.J., Bian, Z., Sherliker, P., Gao, H., Chen, Y., Yang, L., Chen, J., Wang, S., Du, R., Su, H., Collins, R., Peto, R., Chen, Z., China Kadoorie Biobank study, April 2016. Fresh fruit consumption and major cardiovascular disease in China. N. Engl. J. Med. 374 (14), 1332–1343. http://dx.doi.org/10.1056/NEJMoa1501451.

Ello-Martin, J.A., Roe, L.S., Ledikwe, J.H., Beach, A.M., Rolls, B.J., 2007. Dietary energy density in the treatment of obesity: a year-long trial comparing 2 weight-loss diets. Am. J. Clin. Nutr. 85, 1465–1477.

Esmaillzadeh, A., Kimiagar, M., Mehrabi, Y., Azadbakht, L., Hu, F.B., Willett, W.C., 2006. Fruit and vegetable intakes, C-reactive protein, and the metabolic syndrome. Am. J. Clin. Nutr. 84, 1489–1497.

Evans, J.R., Lawrenson, J.G., 2012. Antioxidant vitamin and mineral supplements for preventing age-related macular degeneration. Cochrane Database of Syst. Rev. John Wiley and Sons, Ltd.

Fang, X., Wei, J., He, X., An, P., Wang, H., Jiang, L., Shao, D., Liang, H., Li, Y., Wang, F., Min, J., 2015. Landscape of dietary factors associated with risk of gastric cancer: a systematic review and dose-response meta-analysis of prospective cohort studies. Eur. J. Cancer 51, 2820–2832. http://dx.doi.org/10.1016/j.ejca.2015.09.010.

Fulton, S.L., McKinley, M.C., Young, I.S., Cardwell, C.R., Woodside, J.V., 2014. The effect of increasing fruit and vegetable consumption on overall diet: a systematic review and meta-analysis. Crit. Rev. Food Sci. Nutr. http://dx.doi.org/10.1080/10408398.2012.727917.

Gan, Y., Tong, X., Li, L., Cao, S., Yin, X., Gao, C., Herath, C., Li, W., Jin, Z., Chen, Y., Lu, Z., 2015. Consumption of fruit and vegetable and risk of coronary heart disease: a meta-analysis of prospective cohort studies. Int. J. Cardiol. 183, 129–137. http://dx.doi.org/10.1016/j.ijcard.2015.01.077.

Hamer, M., Chida, Y., 2007. Intake of fruit, vegetables, and antioxidants and risk of type 2 diabetes: systematic review and meta-analysis. J. Hypertens. 25, 2361–2369. http://dx.doi.org/10.1097/HJH.0b013e3282efc214.

Hartley, L., Igbinedion, E., Holmes, J., Flowers, N., Thorogood, M., Clarke, A., Stranges, S., Hooper, L., Rees, K., 2013. Increased consumption of fruit and vegetables for the primary prevention of cardio-vascular diseases. Cochrane Database Syst. Rev. 6, CD009874. http://dx.doi.org/10.1002/14651858. CD009874.pub2.

He, F.J., Nowson, C.A., Lucas, M., MacGregor, G.A., 2007. Increased consumption of fruit and vegetables is related to a reduced risk of coronary heart disease: meta-analysis of cohort studies. J. Hum. Hypertens. 21, 717–728. http://dx.doi.org/10.1038/sj.jhh.1002212.

He, F.J., Nowson, C.A., MacGregor, G.A., 2006. Fruit and vegetable consumption and stroke: meta-analysis of cohort studies. Lancet lond. Engl. 367, 320–326. http://dx.doi.org/10.1016/S0140-6736(06)68069-0.

Hecht, S.S., 1999. Tobacco smoke carcinogens and lung cancer. J. Natl. Cancer Inst. 91, 1194–1210. http://dx.doi.org/10.1093/jnci/91.14.1194.

Hill, A.B., 1965. The environment and disease: association or causation? Proc. R. Soc. Med. 58, 295–300.

Howard, B.V., Van Horn, L., Hsia, J., Manson, J.E., Stefanick, M.L., Wassertheil-Smoller, S., Kuller, L.H., LaCroix, A.Z., Langer, R.D., Lasser, N.L., Lewis, C.E., Limacher, M.C., Margolis, K.L., Mysiw, W.J., Ockene, J.K., Parker, L.M., Perri, M.G., Phillips, L., Prentice, R.L., Robbins, J., Rossouw, J.E., Sarto, G.E., Schatz, I.J., Snetselaar, L.G., Stevens, V.J., Tinker, L.F., Trevisan, M., Vitolins, M.Z., Anderson, G.L., Assaf, A.R., Bassford, T., Beresford, S.A.A., Black, H.R., Brunner, R.L., Brzyski, R.G., Caan, B., Chlebowski, R.T., Gass, M., Granek, I., Greenland, P., Hays, J., Heber, D., Heiss, G., Hendrix, S.L., Hubbell, F.A., Johnson, K.C., Kotchen, J.M., 2006. Low-fat dietary pattern and risk of cardiovascular disease: the women's health initiative randomized controlled dietary modification trial. JAMA 295, 655–666. http://dx.doi. org/10.1001/jama.295.6.655.

Hu, D., Huang, J., Wang, Y., Zhang, D., Qu, Y., 2014. Fruits and vegetables consumption and risk of stroke: a meta-analysis of prospective cohort studies. Stroke J. Cereb. Circ. 45, 1613–1619. http://dx.doi. org/10.1161/STROKEAHA.114.004836.

Hu, F.B., 2002. Dietary pattern analysis: a new direction in nutritional epidemiology. Curr. Opin. Lipidol. 13, 3–9.

Hu, J., Hu, Y., Hu, Y., Zheng, S., 2015. Intake of cruciferous vegetables is associated with reduced risk of ovarian cancer: a meta-analysis. Asia Pac. J. Clin. Nutr. 24, 101–109.

Hung, H.-C., Joshipura, K.J., Jiang, R., Hu, F.B., Hunter, D., Smith-Warner, S.A., Colditz, G.A., Rosner, B., Spiegelman, D., Willett, W.C., 2004. Fruit and vegetable intake and risk of major chronic disease. J. Natl. Cancer Inst. 96, 1577–1584. http://dx.doi.org/10.1093/jnci/djh296.

Huxley, R.R., Ansary-Moghaddam, A., Clifton, P., Czernichow, S., Parr, C.L., Woodward, M., 2009. The impact of dietary and lifestyle risk factors on risk of colorectal cancer: a quantitative overview of the epidemiological evidence. Int. J. Cancer J. Int. Cancer 125, 171–180. http://dx.doi.org/10.1002/ijc.24343.

IARC, 1994. IARC Working Group on the Evaluation of Carcinogenic Risks to Humans. Schistosomes, Liver Flukes and *Helicobacter pylori*: Views and Expert Opinions of an IARC Working Group on the Evaluation of Carcinogenic Risks to Humans. IARC, Lyon.

Jiang, S., Pan, Z., Li, H., Li, F., Song, Y., Qiu, Y., 2014. Meta-analysis: low-dose intake of vitamin E combined with other vitamins or minerals may decrease all-cause mortality. J. Nutr. Sci. Vitaminol. (Tokyo) 60, 194–205.

John, J.H., Ziebland, S., Yudkin, P., Roe, L.S., Neil, H.A., Oxford Fruit and Vegetable Study Group, 2002. Effects of fruit and vegetable consumption on plasma antioxidant concentrations and blood pressure: a randomised controlled trial. Lancet lond. Engl. 359, 1969–1974.

Joshipura, K.J., Ascherio, A., Manson, J.E., Stampfer, M.J., Rimm, E.B., Speizer, F.E., Hennekens, C.H., Spiegelman, D., Willett, W.C., 1999. Fruit and vegetable intake in relation to risk of ischemic stroke. JAMA 282, 1233–1239.

Jung, S., Spiegelman, D., Baglietto, L., Bernstein, L., Boggs, D.A., van den Brandt, P.A., Buring, J.E., Cerhan, J.R., Gaudet, M.M., Giles, G.G., Goodman, G., Hakansson, N., Hankinson, S.E., Helzlsouer, K., Horn-Ross, P.L., Inoue, M., Krogh, V., Lof, M., McCullough, M.L., Miller, A.B., Neuhouser, M.L., Palmer, J.R., Park, Y., Robien, K., Rohan, T.E., Scarmo, S., Schairer, C., Schouten, L.J., Shikany, J.M., Sieri, S., Tsugane, S., Visvanathan, K., Weiderpass, E., Willett, W.C., Wolk, A., Zeleniuch-Jacquotte, A., Zhang, S.M., Zhang, X., Ziegler, R.G., Smith-Warner, S.A., 2013. Fruit and vegetable intake and risk of breast cancer by hormone receptor status. J. Natl. Cancer Inst. 105, 219–236. http://dx.doi.org/10.1093/jnci/djs635.

Kaiser, K.A., Brown, A.W., Bohan Brown, M.M., Shikany, J.M., Mattes, R.D., Allison, D.B., 2014. Increased fruit and vegetable intake has no discernible effect on weight loss: a systematic review and meta-analysis. Am. J. Clin. Nutr. 100, 567–576. http://dx.doi.org/10.3945/ajcn.114.090548.

Kashino, I., Mizoue, T., Tanaka, K., Tsuji, I., Tamakoshi, A., Matsuo, K., Wakai, K., Nagata, C., Inoue, M., Tsugane, S., Sasazuki, S., Research Group for the Development and Evaluation of Cancer Prevention Strategies in Japan, 2015. Vegetable consumption and colorectal cancer risk: an evaluation based on a systematic review and meta-analysis among the Japanese population. Jpn. J. Clin. Oncol. 45, 973–979. http://dx.doi.org/10.1093/jjco/hyv111.

Khanzode, S.D., Dakhale, G.N., Khanzode, S.S., Saoji, A., Palasodkar, R., 2003. Oxidative damage and major depression: the potential antioxidant action of selective serotonin re-uptake inhibitors. Redox Rep. 8, 365–370. http://dx.doi.org/10.1179/135100003225003393.

Kurotani, K., Nanri, A., Goto, A., Mizoue, T., Noda, M., Oba, S., Kato, M., Matsushita, Y., Inoue, M., Tsugane, S., Japan Public Health Center-based Prospective Study Group, 2013. Red meat consumption is associated with the risk of type 2 diabetes in men but not in women: a Japan Public Health Center-based Prospective Study. Br. J. Nutr. 110, 1910–1918. http://dx.doi.org/10.1017/S0007114513001128.

Leenders, M., Sluijs, I., Ros, M.M., Boshuizen, H.C., Siersema, P.D., Ferrari, P., Weikert, C., Tjønneland, A., Olsen, A., Boutron-Ruault, M.-C., Clavel-Chapelon, F., Nailler, L., Teucher, B., Li, K., Boeing, H., Bergmann, M.M., Trichopoulou, A., Lagiou, P., Trichopoulos, D., Palli, D., Pala, V., Panico, S., Tumino, R., Sacerdote, C., Peeters, P.H.M., van Gils, C.H., Lund, E., Engeset, D., Redondo, M.L., Agudo, A., Sánchez, M.J., Navarro, C., Ardanaz, E., Sonestedt, E., Ericson, U., Nilsson, L.M., Khaw, K.-T., Wareham, N.J., Key, T.J., Crowe, F.L., Romieu, I., Gunter, M.J., Gallo, V., Overvad, K., Riboli, E., Bueno-de-Mesquita, H.B., 2013. Fruit and vegetable consumption and mortality: European prospective investigation into cancer and nutrition. Am. J. Epidemiol. 178, 590–602. http://dx.doi.org/10.1093/aje/kwt006.

Li, B., Jiang, G., Zhang, G., Xue, Q., Zhang, H., Wang, C., Zhao, T., 2014a. Intake of vegetables and fruit and risk of esophageal adenocarcinoma: a meta-analysis of observational studies. Eur. J. Nutr. 53, 1511–1521. http://dx.doi.org/10.1007/s00394-014-0656-5.

Li, M., Fan, Y., Zhang, X., Hou, W., Tang, Z., 2014b. Fruit and vegetable intake and risk of type 2 diabetes mellitus: meta-analysis of prospective cohort studies. BMJ Open 4, e005497. http://dx.doi.org/10.1136/bmjopen-2014-005497.

Li, S., Miao, S., Huang, Y., Liu, Z., Tian, H., Yin, X., Tang, W., Steffen, L.M., Xi, B., 2015. Fruit intake decreases risk of incident type 2 diabetes: an updated meta-analysis. Endocrine 48, 454–460. http://dx.doi.org/10.1007/s12020-014-0351-6.

Linseisen, J., Rohrmann, S., Miller, A.B., Bueno-de-Mesquita, H.B., Büchner, F.L., Vineis, P., Agudo, A., Gram, I.T., Janson, L., Krogh, V., Overvad, K., Rasmuson, T., Schulz, M., Pischon, T., Kaaks, R., Nieters, A., Allen, N.E., Key, T.J., Bingham, S., Khaw, K.-T., Amiano, P., Barricarte, A., Martinez, C., Navarro, C., Quirós, R., Clavel-Chapelon, F., Boutron-Ruault, M.-C., Touvier, M., Peeters, P.H.M., Berglund, G., Hallmans, G., Lund, E., Palli, D., Panico, S., Tumino, R., Tjønneland, A., Olsen, A., Trichopoulou, A., Trichopoulos, D., Autier, P., Boffetta, P., Slimani, N., Riboli, E., 2007. Fruit and vegetable consumption and lung cancer risk: updated information from the European Prospective Investigation into Cancer and Nutrition (EPIC). Int. J. Cancer 121, 1103–1114. http://dx.doi.org/10.1002/ijc.22807.

Liu, H., Wang, X.-C., Hu, G.-H., Guo, Z.-F., Lai, P., Xu, L., Huang, T.-B., Xu, Y.-F., 2015. Fruit and vegetable consumption and risk of bladder cancer: an updated meta-analysis of observational studies. Eur. J. Cancer Prev. 24, 508–516. http://dx.doi.org/10.1097/CEJ.0000000000000119.

Liu, J., Wang, J., Leng, Y., Lv, C., 2013. Intake of fruit and vegetables and risk of esophageal squamous cell carcinoma: a meta-analysis of observational studies. Int. J. Cancer J. Int. Cancer 133, 473–485. http://dx.doi.org/10.1002/ijc.28024.

Liu, R.H., 2013. Health-promoting components of fruits and vegetables in the Diet. Adv. Nutr. 4, 384S–392S. http://dx.doi.org/10.3945/an.112.003517.

Liu, S., Lee, I.M., Ajani, U., Cole, S.R., Buring, J.E., Manson, J.E., Physicians' Health Study, 2001. Intake of vegetables rich in carotenoids and risk of coronary heart disease in men: the Physicians' Health Study. Int. J. Epidemiol. 30, 130–135.

Liu, S., Manson, J.E., Lee, I.M., Cole, S.R., Hennekens, C.H., Willett, W.C., Buring, J.E., 2000. Fruit and vegetable intake and risk of cardiovascular disease: the women's health study. Am. J. Clin. Nutr. 72, 922–928.

Liu, X., Yan, Y., Li, F., Zhang, D., 2016. Fruit and vegetable consumption and the risk of depression: a meta-analysis. Nutrition 32, 296–302. http://dx.doi.org/10.1016/j.nut.2015.09.009.

Loef, M., Walach, H., 2012. Fruit, vegetables and prevention of cognitive decline or dementia: a systematic review of cohort studies. J. Nutr. Health Aging 16, 626–630.

Loffredo, L., Perri, L., Di Castelnuovo, A., Iacoviello, L., De Gaetano, G., Violi, F., 2015. Supplementation with vitamin E alone is associated with reduced myocardial infarction: a meta-analysis. Nutr. Metab. Cardiovasc. Dis. 25, 354–363. http://dx.doi.org/10.1016/j.numecd.2015.01.008.

Maes, M., De Vos, N., Pioli, R., Demedts, P., Wauters, A., Neels, H., Christophe, A., 2000. Lower serum vitamin E concentrations in major depression: another marker of lowered antioxidant defenses in that illness. J. Affect. Disord. 58, 241–246. http://dx.doi.org/10.1016/S0165-0327(99)00121-4.

Marriott, B.P., Cole, N., Lee, E., 2009. National estimates of dietary fructose intake increased from 1977 to 2004 in the United States. J. Nutr. 139, 1228S–1235S. http://dx.doi.org/10.3945/jn.108.098277.

Maskarinec, G., Morimoto, Y., Takata, Y., Murphy, S.P., Stanczyk, F.Z., 2006. Alcohol and dietary fibre intakes affect circulating sex hormones among premenopausal women. Public Health Nutr. 9, 875–881. http://dx.doi.org/10.1017/PHN2005923.

Mathew, M.C., Ervin, A.-M., Tao, J., Davis, R.M., 2012. Antioxidant vitamin supplementation for preventing and slowing the progression of age-related cataract. Cochrane Database Syst. Rev. 6, CD004567. http://dx.doi.org/10.1002/14651858.CD004567.pub2.

McKeever, T.M., Britton, J., 2004. Diet and asthma. Am. J. Respir. Crit. Care Med. 170, 725–729. http://dx.doi.org/10.1164/rccm.200405-611PP.

Meng, H., Hu, W., Chen, Z., Shen, Y., 2014. Fruit and vegetable intake and prostate cancer risk: a meta-analysis. Asia Pac. J. Clin. Oncol. 10, 133–140. http://dx.doi.org/10.1111/ajco.12067.

Middleton, E., Kandaswami, C., 1992. Effects of flavonoids on immune and inflammatory cell functions. Biochem. Pharmacol. 43, 1167–1179.

Moreno, J.A., Hong, E., 2013. A single oral dose of fructose induces some features of metabolic syndrome in rats: role of oxidative stress. Nutr. Metab. Cardiovasc. Dis. 23, 536–542. http://dx.doi.org/10.1016/j.numecd.2011.10.008.

Muraki, I., Imamura, F., Manson, J.E., Hu, F.B., Willett, W.C., van Dam, R.M., Sun, Q., 2013. Fruit consumption and risk of type 2 diabetes: results from three prospective longitudinal cohort studies. BMJ 347, f5001.

Murphy, N., Norat, T., Ferrari, P., Jenab, M., Bueno-de-Mesquita, B., Skeie, G., Dahm, C.C., Overvad, K., Olsen, A., Tjønneland, A., Clavel-Chapelon, F., Boutron-Ruault, M.C., Racine, A., Kaaks, R., Teucher, B., Boeing, H., Bergmann, M.M., Trichopoulou, A., Trichopoulos, D., Lagiou, P., Palli, D., Pala, V., Panico, S., Tumino, R., Vineis, P., Siersema, P., van Duijnhoven, F., Peeters, P.H.M., Hjartaker, A., Engeset, D., González, C.A., Sánchez, M.-J., Dorronsoro, M., Navarro, C., Ardanaz, E., Quirós, J.R., Sonestedt, E.,

Ericson, U., Nilsson, L., Palmqvist, R., Khaw, K.-T., Wareham, N., Key, T.J., Crowe, F.L., Fedirko, V., Wark, P.A., Chuang, S.-C., Riboli, E., 2012. Dietary fibre intake and risks of cancers of the colon and rectum in the European prospective investigation into cancer and nutrition (EPIC). PLoS One 7, e39361. http://dx.doi.org/10.1371/journal.pone.0039361.

Mursu, J., Virtanen, J.K., Tuomainen, T.-P., Nurmi, T., Voutilainen, S., 2014. Intake of fruit, berries, and vegetables and risk of type 2 diabetes in Finnish men: the Kuopio ischaemic heart disease risk factor study. Am. J. Clin. Nutr. 99, 328–333. http://dx.doi.org/10.3945/ajcn.113.069641.

Mytton, O.T., Nnoaham, K., Eyles, H., Scarborough, P., Ni Mhurchu, C., 2014. Systematic review and meta-analysis of the effect of increased vegetable and fruit consumption on body weight and energy intake. BMC Public Health 14, 886. http://dx.doi.org/10.1186/1471-2458-14-886.

Myung, S.-K., Ju, W., Cho, B., Oh, S.-W., Park, S.M., Koo, B.-K., Park, B.-J., Korean meta-analysis study group, 2013. Efficacy of vitamin and antioxidant supplements in prevention of cardiovascular disease: systematic review and meta-analysis of randomised controlled trials. BMJ 346, f10.

Myung, S.-K., Kim, Y., Ju, W., Choi, H.J., Bae, W.K., 2010. Effects of antioxidant supplements on cancer prevention: meta-analysis of randomized controlled trials. Ann. Oncol. 21, 166–179. http://dx.doi.org/10.1093/annonc/mdp286.

Nagano, J., Kono, S., Preston, D.L., Moriwaki, H., Sharp, G.B., Koyama, K., Mabuchi, K., 2000. Bladder-cancer incidence in relation to vegetable and fruit consumption: a prospective study of atomic-bomb survivors. Int. J. Cancer 86, 132–138.

Omenn, G.S., Goodman, G.E., Thornquist, M.D., Balmes, J., Cullen, M.R., Glass, A., Keogh, J.P., Meyskens, F.L., Valanis, B., Williams, J.H., Barnhart, S., Cherniack, M.G., Brodkin, C.A., Hammar, S., 1996. Risk factors for lung cancer and for intervention effects in CARET, the beta-carotene and retinol efficacy trial. J. Natl. Cancer Inst. 88, 1550–1559. http://dx.doi.org/10.1093/jnci/88.21.1550.

Paluszkiewicz, P., Smolińska, K., Dębińska, I., Turski, W.A., 2012. Main dietary compounds and pancreatic cancer risk. The quantitative analysis of case-control and cohort studies. Cancer Epidemiol. 36, 60–67. http://dx.doi.org/10.1016/j.canep.2011.05.004.

Park, S.-Y., Ollberding, N.J., Woolcott, C.G., Wilkens, L.R., Henderson, B.E., Kolonel, L.N., 2013. Fruit and vegetable intakes are associated with lower risk of bladder cancer among women in the multiethnic cohort study. J. Nutr. 143, 1283–1292. http://dx.doi.org/10.3945/jn.113.174920.

Poisson, T., Dallongeville, J., Evans, A., Ducimetierre, P., Amouyel, P., Yarnell, J., Bingham, A., Kee, F., Dauchet, L., 2012. Fruit and vegetable intake and smoking cessation. Eur. J. Clin. Nutr. 66, 1247–1253. http://dx.doi.org/10.1038/ejcn.2012.70.

Potischman, N., Weed, D.L., 1999. Causal criteria in nutritional epidemiology. Am. J. Clin. Nutr. 69, 1309S–1314S.

Prentice, R.L., Caan, B., Chlebowski, R.T., Patterson, R., Kuller, L.H., Ockene, J.K., Margolis, K.L., Limacher, M.C., Manson, J.E., Parker, L.M., Paskett, E., Phillips, L., Robbins, J., Rossouw, J.E., Sarto, G.E., Shikany, J.M., Stefanick, M.L., Thomson, C.A., Van Horn, L., Vitolins, M.Z., Wactawski-Wende, J., Wallace, R.B., Wassertheil-Smoller, S., Whitlock, E., Yano, K., Adams-Campbell, L., Anderson, G.L., Assaf, A.R., Beresford, S.A.A., Black, H.R., Brunner, R.L., Brzyski, R.G., Ford, L., Gass, M., Hays, J., Heber, D., Heiss, G., Hendrix, S.L., Hsia, J., Hubbell, F.A., Jackson, R.D., Johnson, K.C., Kotchen, J.M., LaCroix, A.Z., Lane, D.S., Langer, R.D., Lasser, N.L., Henderson, M.M., 2006. Low-fat dietary pattern and risk of invasive breast cancer: the women's health initiative randomized controlled dietary modification trial. JAMA 295, 629–642. http://dx.doi.org/10.1001/jama.295.6.629.

Prentice, R.L., Thomson, C.A., Caan, B., Hubbell, F.A., Anderson, G.L., Beresford, S.A.A., Pettinger, M., Lane, D.S., Lessin, L., Yasmeen, S., Singh, B., Khandekar, J., Shikany, J.M., Satterfield, S., Chlebowski, R.T., 2007. Low-fat dietary pattern and cancer incidence in the women's health initiative dietary modification randomized controlled trial. J. Natl. Cancer Inst. 99, 1534–1543. http://dx.doi.org/10.1093/jnci/djm159.

Rothman, K.J., Greenland, S., 1998. Accuracy consideration in study design. In: Modern Epidemiology. Lippincott-Raven Publishers, Philadelphia, pp. 135–145.

Sauvaget, C., Nagano, J., Hayashi, M., Spencer, E., Shimizu, Y., Allen, N., 2003. Vegetables and fruit intake and cancer mortality in the Hiroshima/Nagasaki life span study. Br. J. Cancer 88, 689–694. http://dx.doi.org/10.1038/sj.bjc.6600775.

Schiepers, O.J.G., Wichers, M.C., Maes, M., 2005. Cytokines and major depression. Prog. Neuropsychopharmacol. Biol. Psychiatry 29, 201–217. http://dx.doi.org/10.1016/j.pnpbp.2004.11.003.

Schwingshackl, L., Hoffmann, G., Kalle-Uhlmann, T., Arregui, M., Buijsse, B., Boeing, H., 2015. Fruit and vegetable consumption and changes in anthropometric variables in adult populations: a systematic review and meta-analysis of prospective cohort studies. PLoS One 10, e0140846. http://dx.doi.org/10.1371/journal.pone.0140846.

Seyedrezazadeh, E., Moghaddam, M.P., Ansarin, K., Vafa, M.R., Sharma, S., Kolahdooz, F., 2014. Fruit and vegetable intake and risk of wheezing and asthma: a systematic review and meta-analysis. Nutr. Rev. 72, 411–428. http://dx.doi.org/10.1111/nure.12121.

Sezikli, M., Çetinkaya, Z.A., Güzelbulut, F., Çimen, B., Özcan, Ö., Özkara, S., Yeşil, A., Gümrükçü, G., İpçioğlu, O.M., Sezikli, H., Övünç, A.O.K., 2012. Effects of alpha tocopherol and ascorbic acid on *Helicobacter pylori* colonization and the severity of gastric inflammation. Helicobacter 17, 127–132. http://dx.doi.org/10.1111/j.1523-5378.2011.00925.x.

Stanhope, K.L., 2012. Role of fructose-containing sugars in the epidemics of obesity and metabolic syndrome. Annu. Rev. Med. 63, 329–343. http://dx.doi.org/10.1146/annurev-med-042010-113026.

Stanhope, K.L., Schwarz, J.-M., Havel, P.J., 2013. Adverse metabolic effects of dietary fructose: results from the recent epidemiological, clinical, and mechanistic studies. Curr. Opin. Lipidol. 24, 198–206. http://dx.doi.org/10.1097/MOL.0b013e3283613bca.

Steinhubl, S.R., 2008. Why have antioxidants failed in clinical trials? Am. J. Cardiol. 101, 14D–19D. http://dx.doi.org/10.1016/j.amjcard.2008.02.003.

Tannenbaum, S.R., Wishnok, J.S., Leaf, C.D., 1991. Inhibition of nitrosamine formation by ascorbic acid. Am. J. Clin. Nutr. 53 (Suppl. 1), 247S–250S.

Touvier, M., Kesse, E., Clavel-Chapelon, F., Boutron-Ruault, M.-C., 2005. Dual Association of beta-carotene with risk of tobacco-related cancers in a cohort of French women. J. Natl. Cancer Inst. 97, 1338–1344. http://dx.doi.org/10.1093/jnci/dji276.

Trichopoulou, A., Orfanos, P., Norat, T., Bueno-de-Mesquita, B., Ocké, M.C., Peeters, P.H.M., van der Schouw, Y.T., Boeing, H., Hoffmann, K., Boffetta, P., Nagel, G., Masala, G., Krogh, V., Panico, S., Tumino, R., Vineis, P., Bamia, C., Naska, A., Benetou, V., Ferrari, P., Slimani, N., Pera, G., Martinez-Garcia, C., Navarro, C., Rodriguez-Barranco, M., Dorronsoro, M., Spencer, E.A., Key, T.J., Bingham, S., Khaw, K.-T., Kesse, E., Clavel-Chapelon, F., Boutron-Ruault, M.-C., Berglund, G., Wirfalt, E., Hallmans, G., Johansson, I., Tjonneland, A., Olsen, A., Overvad, K., Hundborg, H.H., Riboli, E., Trichopoulos, D., 2005. Modified Mediterranean diet and survival: EPIC-elderly prospective cohort study. BMJ 330, 991. http://dx.doi.org/10.1136/bmj.38415.644155.8F.

Uddenfeldt, M., Janson, C., Lampa, E., Leander, M., Norbäck, D., Larsson, L., Rask-Andersen, A., 2010. High BMI is related to higher incidence of asthma, while a fish and fruit diet is related to a lower. Respir. Med. 104, 972–980. http://dx.doi.org/10.1016/j.rmed.2009.12.013.

Ungar, N., Sieverding, M., Stadnitski, T., 2013. Increasing fruit and vegetable intake. "Five a day" versus "just one more.". Appetite 65, 200–204. http://dx.doi.org/10.1016/j.appet.2013.02.007.

U.S. Department of Agriculture, U.S. Department of Health and Human Services, December 2010. Dietary Guidelines for Americans, 2010, seventh ed. U.S. Government Printing Office, Washington, DC.

Van Duyn, M.A., Pivonka, E., 2000. Overview of the health benefits of fruit and vegetable consumption for the dietetics professional: selected literature. J. Am. Diet. Assoc. 100, 1511–1521. http://dx.doi.org/10.1016/S0002-8223(00)00420-X.

Vieira, A.R., Abar, L., Vingeliene, S., Chan, D.S.M., Aune, D., Navarro-Rosenblatt, D., Stevens, C., Greenwood, D., Norat, T., 2015a. Fruits, vegetables and lung cancer risk: a systematic review and meta-analysis. Ann. Oncol. http://dx.doi.org/10.1093/annonc/mdv381.

Vieira, A.R., Vingeliene, S., Chan, D.S.M., Aune, D., Abar, L., Navarro Rosenblatt, D., Greenwood, D.C., Norat, T., 2015b. Fruits, vegetables, and bladder cancer risk: a systematic review and meta-analysis. Cancer Med. 4, 136–146. http://dx.doi.org/10.1002/cam4.327.

Villegas, R., Shu, X.O., Gao, Y.-T., Yang, G., Elasy, T., Li, H., Zheng, W., 2008. Vegetable but not fruit consumption reduces the risk of type 2 diabetes in Chinese women. J. Nutr. 138, 574–580.

Wang, M., Qin, S., Zhang, T., Song, X., Zhang, S., 2015a. The effect of fruit and vegetable intake on the development of lung cancer: a meta-analysis of 32 publications and 20 414 cases. Eur. J. Clin. Nutr. 69, 1184–1192. http://dx.doi.org/10.1038/ejcn.2015.64.

Wang, Q., Chen, Y., Wang, X., Gong, G., Li, G., Li, C., 2014a. Consumption of fruit, but not vegetables, may reduce risk of gastric cancer: results from a meta-analysis of cohort studies. Eur. J. Cancer 50, 1498–1509. http://dx.doi.org/10.1016/j.ejca.2014.02.009.

Wang, X., Ouyang, Y., Liu, J., Zhu, M., Zhao, G., Bao, W., Hu, F.B., 2014b. Fruit and vegetable consumption and mortality from all causes, cardiovascular disease, and cancer: systematic review and dose-response meta-analysis of prospective cohort studies. BMJ 349, g4490.

Wang, Y., Li, F., Wang, Z., Qiu, T., Shen, Y., Wang, M., 2015b. Fruit and vegetable consumption and risk of lung cancer: a dose-response meta-analysis of prospective cohort studies. Lung Cancer 88, 124–130. http://dx.doi.org/10.1016/j.lungcan.2015.02.015.

WCRF/AICR, 2007. World Cancer Research Fund/American Institute for Cancer Research. Food, Nutrition, Physical Activity, and the Prevention of Cancer: A Global Perspective. AICR, Washington, DC.

Whelton, P.K., He, J., 2014. Health effects of sodium and potassium in humans. Curr. Opin. Lipidol. 25, 75–79. http://dx.doi.org/10.1097/MOL.0000000000000033.

WHO, 2013. Global Action Plan for the Prevention and Control of Noncommunicable Diseases 2013-2020. World Health Organization.

Willett, W.C., 2005. Diet and cancer: an evolving picture. JAMA 293, 233–234. http://dx.doi.org/10.1001/jama.293.2.233.

Wu, Q.-J., Wu, L., Zheng, L.-Q., Xu, X., Ji, C., Gong, T.-T., 2015a. Consumption of fruit and vegetables reduces risk of pancreatic cancer: evidence from epidemiological studies. Eur. J. Cancer Prev. http://dx.doi.org/10.1097/CEJ.0000000000000171.

Wu, Y., Zhang, D., Jiang, X., Jiang, W., 2015b. Fruit and vegetable consumption and risk of type 2 diabetes mellitus: a dose-response meta-analysis of prospective cohort studies. Nutr. Metab. Cardiovasc. Dis. 25, 140–147. http://dx.doi.org/10.1016/j.numecd.2014.10.004.

Xu, C., Zeng, X.-T., Liu, T.-Z., Zhang, C., Yang, Z.-H., Li, S., Chen, X.-Y., 2015. Fruits and vegetables intake and risk of bladder cancer: a PRISMA-compliant systematic review and dose-response meta-analysis of prospective cohort studies. Med. Baltim. 94, e759. http://dx.doi.org/10.1097/MD.0000000000000759.

Yamaguchi, N., Kakizoe, T., 2001. Synergistic interaction between Helicobacter pylori gastritis and diet in gastric cancer. Lancet Oncol. 2, 88–94. http://dx.doi.org/10.1016/S1470-2045(00)00225-4.

Yanbaeva, D.G., Dentener, M.A., Creutzberg, E.C., Wesseling, G., Wouters, E.F.M., 2007. Systemic effects of smoking. Chest 131, 1557–1566. http://dx.doi.org/10.1378/chest.06-2179.

Yang, Y., Zhang, D., Feng, N., Chen, G., Liu, J., Chen, G., Zhu, Y., 2014. Increased intake of vegetables, but not fruit, reduces risk for hepatocellular carcinoma: a meta-analysis. Gastroenterology 147, 1031–1042. http://dx.doi.org/10.1053/j.gastro.2014.08.005.

Yao, B., Yan, Y., Ye, X., Fang, H., Xu, H., Liu, Y., Li, S., Zhao, Y., 2014. Intake of fruit and vegetables and risk of bladder cancer: a dose-response meta-analysis of observational studies. Cancer Causes Control 25, 1645–1658. http://dx.doi.org/10.1007/s10552-014-0469-0.

Ye, Y., Li, J., Yuan, Z., 2013. Effect of antioxidant vitamin supplementation on cardiovascular outcomes: a meta-analysis of randomized controlled trials. PLoS One 8, e56803. http://dx.doi.org/10.1371/journal.pone.0056803.

Zhang, H.-M., Wakisaka, N., Maeda, O., Yamamoto, T., 1997. Vitamin C inhibits the growth of a bacterial risk factor for gastric carcinoma: *Helicobacter pylori*. Cancer 80, 1897–1903. http://dx.doi.org/10.1002/(SICI)1097-0142(19971115)80:10<1897::AID-CNCR4>3.0.CO;2-L.

Zhao, J., Zhao, L., 2013. Cruciferous vegetables intake is associated with lower risk of renal cell carcinoma: evidence from a meta-analysis of observational studies. PLoS One 8, e75732. http://dx.doi.org/10.1371/journal.pone.0075732.

14

Whole Grains and Disease Risk

Frank Thies

UNIVERSITY OF ABERDEEN, ABERDEEN, UNITED KINGDOM

1. Introduction

Humans included whole grains (WGs) in their diet with the advent of agriculture around 10,000 years ago to become one of our major dietary components for the last 4000 years (Spiller, 2002). However, the development of the refining process in the late 18th century to produce refined flour with longer shelf life compared with nonrefined flour led to a dramatic increase in refined products consumption within the last century.

The health benefits of eating WG products had been suggested a long time ago by Hippocrates in the 4th century BC and more recently in the 18th and 19th centuries (Räsänen, 2007; Thomas, 1894). In early 1970s, the fiber hypothesis (Burkitt, 1983; Trowell, 1975) led the path to many quantitative population-based studies, which underlined the positive association between higher intake of WG foods and reduced risk for major chronic diseases such as cardiovascular disease (CVD), type 2 diabetes, and some cancers. Large prospective studies investigating the relationship between WG intake and the risk of mortality (all cause and cause-specific) consistently suggested a protective role of high intake of WG products against early death (Huang et al., 2015; Wu et al., 2015; Johnsen et al., 2015). Only evidence from epidemiological studies associated high whole grain intake with reduced cancer risk, and there is no evidence from intervention studies to support these findings. Therefore this chapter will focus mainly on CVD and associated risk factors.

2. Whole Grain Definition and Types

Cereals are grasses from the Poaceae family, producing edible grains. The term also includes grains from nongrass plants (pseudo cereals, wild rice), which are referred to as pseudo cereals because they are grown and used like cereal grains and have a similar composition to "true" grains.

2.1 Definition

WGs or WG products should contain all the essential parts and naturally occurring nutrients of the entire grain seed in their original proportions. If the grain has been processed (e.g., cracked, crushed, rolled, extruded, and/or cooked), the food product should contain the same relative proportion of components (endosperm, germ, and bran) that are found in the original grain seed. This first formal definition for "whole grain" was proposed in 1999 by the American Association for Cereal Chemists. This definition has been since modified to take into account the degree of sprout length, which if too long would affect nutrient value (Slavin et al., 2013). The European HEALTHGRAIN consortium also recently issued a similar definition of WG, which, however, allows for a minimal loss of bran, germ, and endosperm during grain processing (van der Kamp et al., 2014). Several definitions for WG foods have also been issued and all overall agree that a WG food should contain at least over half its weight from WG sources. Additional characterization for WG food has been proposed, which indicates that "A WG food must contain 8 grams or more of WG per 30 grams of product to be labeled as 'whole-grain' food" (Ferruzzi et al., 2014).

2.2 Structure and Composition of a Grain

A grain or kernel is constituted of three main parts: the endosperm, the bran, and the germ (Fig. 14.1). The endosperm usually represents over 80% of the kernel, and it contains mostly starch that provides the energy required for germination. The germ and bran fractions, which represent around 4% and 15% of the dry weight of most grains, respectively, contain in relatively high concentrations most of the biologically active compounds found in a grain. These include B vitamins (thiamine, niacin, riboflavin, and pantothenic acid) and minerals (phosphorus, magnesium, calcium, iron, and sodium), amino acids, essential fatty acids (n-6 linoleic and n-3 γ-linolenic acids), and vitamin E (α-tocopherols). The bran also contains a range of insoluble and soluble fibers and numerous phytochemicals (phytates, phenolics, phytosterols). Phytochemical composition differs between WGs, and some phenolic compounds are specific to particular grains, such as avenanthramides, which are found in oats and barley.

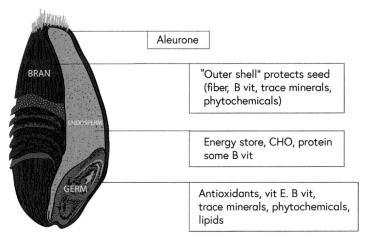

FIGURE 14.1 Structure of a cereal grain.

2.3 Whole Grain in Human Diet

The main WGs used for human consumption are listed in Table 14.1.

WG intake in the United Kingdom has been evaluated using data obtained from the National Diet and Nutrition Survey rolling program (2008–11) (Mann et al., 2015). UK adults and children/teenager populations consume 20 g/day and 13 g/day of WG products, respectively. Wheat and to a lesser extent oats are the major WG consumed in the United Kingdom and represent 77% and 15%, respectively, of the overall WG consumption. Wheat is mainly consumed as ready-to-eat cereals and whole meal breads, while porridge, oat-based ready-to-eat cereals, or other cereals represent the main source of oat intake in the UK population. Some countries like the United States (USDA and US Department of Health and Human Services, 2010) and Denmark (DTU National Food Institute, 2008) issued specific dietary recommendations for WG intake (three to five servings of WG per day or 75 g/day per 10 MJ energy intake, respectively). In the United Kingdom, there is currently no specific recommendation for WG intake other than the general advice to choose the WG variety of starchy foods (NHS Choices, 2015).

2.4 Effect of Refining on Chemical Composition

The removal of the bran and germ fractions during the milling process has drastic effects on the chemical composition of the resulting refined flour (Fig. 14.2). Most of the B vitamins, vitamin K, dietary fiber, zinc, vitamin E, magnesium, manganese, and potassium are lost, while content in pantothenic acid, copper, iron, and folate is significantly reduced. However, this is compensated to some extent by the voluntary fortification of white flour with thiamin, niacin, and iron in the United Kingdom. Food fortification with folate to help reducing the incidence of neural tube defects is mandatory and regulated in some countries like the United States, but it is currently voluntary in the United Kingdom.

Table 14.1 Main Whole Grains Available for Human Consumption[a]

Amaranth[b]	Millet	Whole corn
Barley	Oatmeal and whole oats	Whole grain pasta
Brown rice	Popcorn	Whole grain barley
Buckwheat[b]	Quinoa[b]	Whole rye
Bulgur	Sorghum	Whole wheat
Emmer/farro	Spelt	Whole wheat couscous
Grano WG	Teff	Wild rice
Kamut	Triticale	

[a]This list is not exhaustive.
[b]Pseudo cereals.

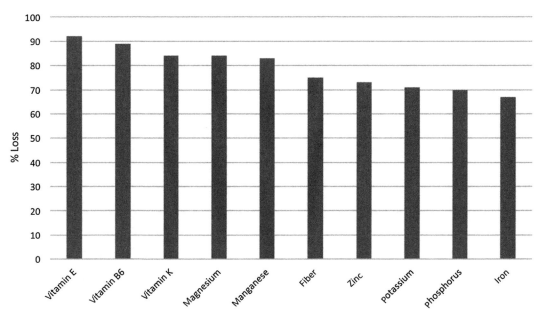

FIGURE 14.2 Effect of milling on wheat flour nutrient composition. Results are expressed as percent loss compared with whole meal flour. *Data from USDA National Nutrient Database for Standard Reference, Release 28.* http://www.ars.usda.gov/Services/docs.htm?docid=8964.

3. Whole Grain and Cardiovascular Disease

3.1 Cardiovascular Disease

CVD is the main cause of death worldwide. In 2012, around 17.5 million people died from CVD, which represented 31% of all global deaths. An estimated 7.4 million were due to coronary heart disease, and 6.7 million were due to stroke (WHO, 2015). CVD is a general term encompassing pathologies affecting the heart and circulation. These include coronary (or ischemic) heart disease, cerebrovascular disease, peripheral arterial disease, rheumatic heart disease, congenital heart disease, deep vein thrombosis, and pulmonary embolism. One of the main underlying causes for CVD is atherosclerosis, a chronic inflammatory condition leading to the thickening of arterial lining in places by atheromatous plaques. The process starts with the formation of fatty streaks (accumulation of modified lipids within the arterial wall), which can progress into mature plaque with proliferation of connective tissue, adhesion of platelets, proliferation, and migration of smooth muscle cells and infiltration of immune cells. The plaque can become sufficiently big to induce a significant reduction of the blood flow, which can lead to ischemia with or without associated symptoms, such as angina, when coronary arteries are affected. The inflammatory process can also make the plaque unstable, increasing the risk of rupture. In this case, the modified lipids present in atheromatous plaques are highly thrombotic, and they can induce the immediate formation of a thrombus that can occlude the artery and provoke a myocardial infarction or stroke if the coronary or cerebral arteries are affected respectively. The main risk factors for CVD are shown in Fig. 14.3.

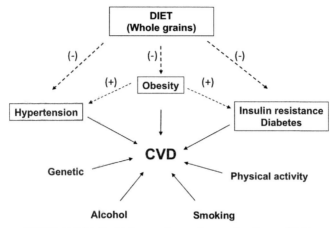

FIGURE 14.3 Main risk factors for cardiovascular disease (CVD).

3.2 Epidemiological Evidence

Large prospective studies carried out over the last 25 years mainly in the United States and Europe found a strong association between high consumption of whole grain foods and reduced risk of chronic diseases including coronary heart disease, hypertension, type 2 diabetes, and some cancers.

3.2.1 Coronary Heart Disease/Stroke

Findings from the Iowa Women's Health Study, a prospective cohort study of over 30,000 postmenopausal women, suggested that the risk of ischemic heart disease would be reduced by 30%–36%, or by 26% after controlling for fiber intake, in women eating one serving or more of WG foods daily compared with those rarely eating any WG products (Jacobs et al., 1998). Another large prospective study, the Harvard Nurses' Health Study found a similar association between increased WG intake and reduced risk of coronary heart disease (Liu et al., 1999). The results suggested that three servings of WG food per day would result in 25% decreased risk of coronary heart disease (21% after adjusting for fiber intake). The Atherosclerosis Risk in Communities (ARIC) study, which included 15,762 middle-aged adults followed up over 11 years, also showed an inverse relationship between WG intake and risk of incident coronary artery disease and mortality. The data also suggested that three servings per day could confer cardiovascular protection (28% decreased risk of coronary artery disease) (Steffen et al., 2003). This was further supported by the results of the Health Professional Follow-up study involving over 42,000 mostly middle-aged men, which suggested that three servings per day could decrease coronary heart disease risk by 18% (Jensen et al., 2004). Several meta-analyses including the results of numerous observational studies conducted to date have been carried out, and the results consistently showed an inverse association between dietary WG intake and incident CVD. Based on the meta-analysis of seven prospective cohort studies with quantitative measure of dietary WG and clinical cardiovascular outcomes, an average of daily intake of 2.5 servings would reduce risk of CVD events by 21% compared with 0.2 servings per day (Mellen et al., 2008). The meta-analysis carried out by Ye et al. (2012), which integrated results from 45 observational studies and 21 randomized trials, estimated that people consuming three to five servings per day of WG had a 25% lower risk of CVD compared with people eating WG only occasionally.

The studies reporting the association between dietary WG intake and risk of stroke have produced inconsistent results. The Physicians' Health Study (Liu et al., 2003a,b) and the Finnish Mobile Clinic Health Examination Survey (Mizrahi et al., 2009) found no association between WG intake and risk of stroke, while the results of other large prospective studies suggested otherwise (Steffen et al., 2003; Jacobs et al., 2007). The results from a meta-analysis that pooled the results of six prospective studies involving 1635 stroke cases and 247,487 participants suggest that higher intake of WG might have a protective effect on stroke (Fang et al., 2015). However, all the studies but one originated from the United States, and therefore, the results and conclusions may only be applied to American populations and cannot be extrapolated to populations from other countries. Interestingly, the authors found a significant association in the follow-up duration over 10 years, but not below, suggesting that further follow-up studies should be carried out over 10 years to assess the association between WG intake and the risk of stroke. Although current evidence is limited, increased intake may be associated with a modest but significant reduced risk of hypertension, one of the most important independent risk factor for CVD, and for particularly stroke. Lairon et al. (2005) found in a cross-sectional study involving 2532 men and 3429 women that high quintile of cereal fiber intake was associated with lower risk of hypertension compared with lower quintile of intake [odds ratio (OR) 0.86, 95% CIs 0.67, 1.10; $P = .02$]. Similar results were described by Wang et al. (2007), who found that women who consumed 0.5 to <1, 1 to <2, 2 to <4, and 4 or more whole grain servings per day had multivariate relative risks (95% CIs) of 0.93 (0.87, 1.00), 0.93 (0.87, 0.99), 0.92 (0.85, 0.99), and 0.77 (0.66, 0.89), respectively, compared with those who consumed less than 0.5 whole grain servings per day. Similar results were described in a prospective cohort of male health professionals (Flint et al., 2009), where WG intake was inversely associated with risk of hypertension among quintiles, showing a relative risk of 0.81 (95% CI: 0.75, 0.87) in the highest compared with the lowest quintile.

3.2.2 Diabetes/Insulin Resistance

Increased intake of food with high glycemic index is associated with a higher incidence of type 2 diabetes mellitus (RR 1.03, 95% CI 1.01, 1.06 for each two GI unit increase per day; SACN, 2015). The reverse was found in many observations looking at the association between WG intake and the risk of type 2 diabetes (Meyer et al., 2000; van Dam et al., 2002; Sun et al., 2010; Wirstrom et al., 2013). A meta-analysis of 16 prospective studies suggested that three servings per day could reduce the risk of type 2 diabetes by 32% (Aune et al., 2013). Results from the Women's Health Initiative Observational Study also showed an inverse dose–response relationship between WG consumption and incident type 2 diabetes in ever nonsmoker postmenopausal women (Parker et al., 2013). Further evidence has recently been gathered from the EPIC-InterAct study that suggested an inverse relationship between cereal fiber intake and the risk of type 2 diabetes (Kuijsten et al., 2015).

3.3 Intervention Trials

Many intervention trials looking at the effects of increased WG consumption on markers of cardiovascular and metabolic health have been conducted over the last 15 years. However, the findings from these studies are far less consistent compared with those from epidemiological studies. One of the reasons for such variability in study outcomes may relate to the diversity of study design considered (type of WG, control diet, length of intervention, doses, etc.) (Ferruzzi et al., 2014). Processing of WG can lead to the production of WG products with a lower glycemic index compared with similar refined foods (Atkinson et al., 2008; Brand-Miller et al., 2008). This would affect insulin response and blood glucose, and it could confound the results from intervention trials looking at these parameters. Furthermore, the methods for reporting the results and calculating WG intake also greatly vary between studies, making comparison between studies very difficult (Ross et al., 2015). The heterogeneity of treatments used as control in intervention studies with WGs has been highlighted (Thies et al., 2014). The authors suggested that an ideal control group should at least consider unchanged total energy intake during the intervention, substituting WG food items with a similar amount of refined cereal products. Furthermore, the level of WG intake in the control group should match the lowest quartile of consumption observed in the population studied. The main markers for cardiovascular health considered in intervention studies are shown in Fig. 14.4.

Most studies carried out in humans focused on serum lipids, insulin sensitivity, inflammation, and weight loss.

3.3.1 Whole Grain and Lipid Profile

A meta-analysis of 21 randomized control trials indicated that whole grain intervention significantly lowered LDL cholesterol concentrations compared with controls

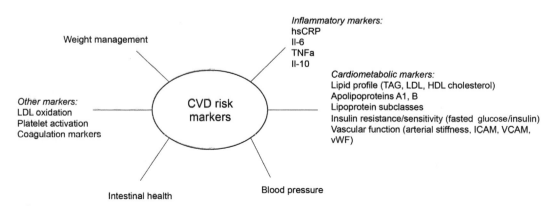

FIGURE 14.4 Main markers for cardiovascular disease (CVD) risk considered in whole grain intervention trials.

[differences in fasting LDL cholesterol: –0.82 mmol/L (–1.31, –0.33)] (Ye et al., 2012). Another meta-analysis recently carried by Hollaender et al. (2015) found similar results. The authors reviewed the effects of interventions including WG groups compared with non-WG groups on blood lipid, and they suggested that the consumption of 28–213 g WG daily for 2–16 weeks could significantly reduce plasma concentrations of total and LDL cholesterol. However, plasma triglyceride and HDL cholesterol concentrations were not affected. This review also highlighted the fact that interventions with oats were mostly effective. Indeed, the type of WG used in intervention studies seems to determine the lipid response, WG containing a high amount of viscous soluble fibers such as barley and oats being among the most effective (Behall et al., 2004; Karmally et al., 2005; Smith et al., 2008; Queenan et al., 2007). The many interventions studies using β-glucan-enriched foods or supplements have had variable outcomes, but 3 g β-glucan per day, which is equivalent to around 60 g oatmeal, appears to be the minimum amount required to achieve a clinically significant reduction in serum cholesterol (Whitehead et al., 2014). The size of the effect would also depend on the cholesterol status of the individuals intervened on. Interventions with oats seem more effective in hypercholesterolemic subjects compared with volunteers with "normal" LDL cholesterol concentrations (Thies et al., 2014).

Only a few numbers of studies have reported on the effects of WG intervention on lipoprotein subclass size and concentration (Davy et al., 2002), and the results were generally negative. This has been recently confirmed by Tighe et al. (2013), who conducted the most comprehensive randomized controlled intervention with WGs conducted to date looking at serum lipoprotein subclass size and distribution. However, the study had been carried out in overweight but otherwise healthy individuals. The effects of such intervention, particularly if it involves oats and barley products, on lipoprotein subclasses profile remains to be adequately investigated in hypercholesterolemic subjects. Interestingly, findings from a cross-sectional study using data from 4284 adults enrolled in the 2003–06 cycle of the NHANES study suggested that combining WG with statin treatment may improve the efficacy of statin treatment for cholesterol lowering (Wang et al., 2014).

3.3.2 Whole Grain, Blood Glucose, and Insulin Sensitivity

The substantial evidence linking WG consumption with lower risk of diabetes and improvement in blood glucose and insulin concentrations demonstrated in prospective studies is only partially supported by the results obtained from intervention trials. The results from two well-designed, large-scale, comprehensive studies carried out in the United Kingdom in overweight but otherwise healthy volunteers were negative. Brownlee et al. (2010) carried out a 16-week dietary intervention trial with three groups (control, 60 g WG per day, 60 g WG per day for 8 weeks incremented to 120 g WG per day for the last 8 weeks of the intervention). The study involved 316 overweight participants, aged 18–65 years, usually eating less than 30 g WG per day. Participants were asked to substitute WG foods provided for similar refined grain foods in their diet. Despite an excellent compliance, the results showed no improvement for any conventional markers for cardiovascular risk, including fasting plasma lipids, inflammatory and coagulation markers, endothelial function, and fasting blood glucose and insulin. The second trial involved 233 overweight subjects, also otherwise healthy, who after a 4-week run-in period on a refined diet, were randomly allocated to a control (refined diet), wheat, or wheat+oats group for 12 weeks (three portions of refined or WG per day). No beneficial changes for all the systemic markers of CVD risk measured including serum glucose and insulin concentrations and homeostasis model assessment-estimated insulin resistance (HOMA-IR) index were observed (Tighe et al., 2010).

However, intervention trials with WG foods suggested that WG favorably influences metabolic risk factors and insulin sensitivity in patients with type 2 diabetes (Rave et al., 2007). Giacco et al. (2014) showed that a 12-week dietary intervention with WG in subjects with metabolic syndrome improved postprandial insulinemic response to a test meal, with a reduction of 29% compared with the control group assigned to a refined cereal diet. However, the intervention had no effect on blood glucose levels. Other studies, involving the consumption of whole rye products (Magnusdottir et al., 2014) or a composite diet including WG (Poulsen et al., 2014), found similar results. Another 12-week intervention study comparing white rice with WGs, barley, and legumes carried out in newly diagnosed type 2 diabetics and subjects with impaired glucose control showed improvement in both fasting blood insulin and glucose concentrations as well as HOMA-IR index in the WG, barley, and legume group (Kang et al., 2014). Overall, these findings suggest that increased WG consumption, particularly if part of a healthier dietary pattern, could reduce the risk of type 2 diabetes by improving insulin sensitivity (Seal and Brownlee, 2015). The results of a dose–response metaregression analysis between WG intake and type 2 diabetes occurrence has estimated a reduction of 0.3% in the type 2 diabetes rate for each additional 10 g of WG ingredient consumed daily (Chanson-Rolle et al., 2015). Considering these data, consuming three servings of WG foods per day (defined here as 45 g of WG ingredients) would reduce the risk of type 2 diabetes by 20% compared with consuming a half serving.

3.3.3 Whole Grain, Inflammatory Markers, and Blood Pressure

The only established systemic inflammatory marker for CVD risk is C reactive protein (CRP). Other inflammatory risk markers as well as markers of coagulation and endothelial dysfunction have also been considered in intervention studies with WGs, such as interleukin 6 (IL-6), tumor necrosis factor alpha (TNF-α), interleukin 10 (IL-10), serum amyloid A (SAA), intercellular adhesion molecule 1 (ICAM-1), vascular cellular adhesion molecule 1 (VCAM-1), fibrinogen, and von Willebrand factor. The effects of WG consumption on markers of subclinical inflammation have been reviewed (Lefevre and Jonnalagadda, 2012). Data derived from 13 epidemiological studies show a moderate association between high WG intake and lower CRP concentrations. The authors estimated that each serving of WG would reduce CRP concentrations by approximately 7%. However, the evidence is generally not substantiated by the results obtained from intervention trials carried out in healthy, normal, overweight, or obese subjects (Andersson et al., 2007; Brownlee et al., 2010; Giacco et al., 2010; Nelson et al., 2016; Tighe et al., 2010). Results from a small crossover trial in healthy, low whole grain consumers showed that increased consumption of mixed

WGs (mean intake of 168 g/day) for 6 weeks had no effect on systemic markers of inflammation (IL-10, TNF-α, CRP) or on absolute counts of blood immune cells or on ex vivo phagocytic activities of these cells compared to low whole grain consumption (<16 g/day) (Ampatzoglou et al., 2015). Only a few studies reported positive effects of WG intervention in inflammatory markers. Increased WG intake (five servings per day compared with less than one serving per day) integrated within a hypocaloric diet for 12 weeks decreased serum CRP concentrations by 38% in obese subjects with metabolic syndrome, while IL-6 and TNF-α concentrations remained unchanged (Katcher et al., 2008). Vitaglione et al. (2015) recently showed in overweight and obese subjects that the replacement of refined products in the habitual diet by WG wheat products for 8 weeks significantly reduced blood TNF-α concentration, while IL-6 concentration remained unchanged. A transient increase in antiinflammatory IL-10 was also observed. Interestingly, the reduction in TNF-α concentration was associated with changes in gut microbiota composition, with increased *Bacteroides* and *Lactobacillus* bacterial species. Beneficial effect of WG intervention on inflammatory markers has also been described in overweight and obese children (Hajihashemi et al., 2014). Serum CRP, ICAM1, SAA, and leptin concentrations were significantly reduced by 21.8%, 28.4%, 17.4%, and 9.7%, respectively, after 6 weeks intervention with daily intakes of 98 g of WG products compared with the control (11 g/day). Serum VCAM-1 concentrations also tended to decrease (−36.2%, $P = .07$).

With regard to blood pressure, two meta-analyses concluded that an increase in fiber intake of 10–15 g fiber per day for 8 weeks was associated with a fall in systolic blood pressure of between 1 and 3 mm Hg (Whelton et al., 2005; Streppel et al., 2005). WG diets containing brown rice/whole wheat, and/or barley (20% of energy intake) significantly reduced systolic, diastolic, and mean arterial pressures in mildly hypercholesterolemic men and women (Behall et al., 2006). Tighe et al. (2010) reported that a 12-week intervention with three daily portions of WG (wheat or oats and wheat products) significantly decreased systolic blood pressure in overweight middle-aged subjects by around 5 mm Hg. The observed decrease in systolic blood pressure was not related to changes in heart rates or weight loss. However, many other interventions with WG failed to report any significant effect on blood pressure (Brownlee et al., 2010). The disparity of results might be due to the different methodologies used to measure blood pressure (Tighe et al., 2010), and there is a requirement for conducting relevant standardized, well-controlled intervention studies.

3.3.4 Whole Grain and Body Weight Regulation

Consumption of WG foods may benefit obesity prevention by potentially regulating satiety and food intake. Indeed, increased WG intake (at least three servings per day) has been associated with lower body mass index (Sahyoun et al., 2006; Liu et al., 2003a,b; Cho et al., 2013), decreased body weight gain (Bazzano et al., 2005; Newby et al., 2007), reduced abdominal adiposity (McKeown et al., 2009), and lower visceral adipose tissue (McKeown et al., 2010). However, findings from a large number of randomized controlled studies published in recent years have been less consistent. The results of a meta-analysis of 26 randomized controlled trials indicated that WG consumption (18.2 g/day to 150 g/day for 2–16 weeks) does not reduce body weight (Pol et al., 2013). However, the authors suggested that a small beneficial effect on body fat may be present. Small reductions of body fat have been observed after WG interventions within energy-restricted dietary patterns (Katcher et al., 2008; Kristensen et al., 2012). The clinical benefit of such reduction remains to be established. However, the results of a 12-week randomized controlled trial involving 50 overweight/obese individuals with metabolic syndrome showed that replacing refined grain products with WGs (6–12 servings per day) does not improve the efficacy of a weight loss diet on body weight, percentage of body fat, and abdominal adipose tissue beyond the reductions also observed with consumption of refined grains (Harris Jackson et al., 2014). Further investigation is required to clarify whether WG consumption could play a significant role in appetite and body weight regulation, but the size of the effects and related clinical benefits are likely to be small, if any.

3.4 Mechanisms of Action

The mechanisms by which WG could modulate cardiovascular risk markers and confer protection against heart disease are still putative and mainly related to various components present in the bran. It is also likely that the potential cardiovascular health benefits of eating WGs lies within many components present in the grain acting synergistically. Readers may refer to Chapter 16, which presents synergy and food complexity. In recent years, interest has focused on the potential role of compounds with antioxidant-related properties and dietary fibers in modulating insulin resistance, cholesterol metabolism, low density lipoprotein oxidizability, and regulation of vascular endothelial function. The importance of the critical role played by the gut microbiota in the process is also emerging, and there is increasing evidence that the release of short chain fatty acids (SCFA) and fiber-related phenolic metabolites in the gut is a contributing factor.

3.4.1 Compounds With Antioxidant-Related Properties

The main nutritionally relevant antioxidant present in WGs is α-tocopherol. However, WG products also contain a relatively large amount of various chemicals such as carotenoids, γ-tocopherols, tocotrienols, and phenolic compounds that have important antioxidant capacity (Adom et al., 2005). The refining process leads to a substantial loss of phytochemicals (over 70%–90% loss of phenolic acids and carotenoids). Generally, most of these compounds tend to be poorly absorbed in the small intestine, and they are metabolized and excreted very quickly. However, most of these chemicals are bound covalently to fibers, and they are consequently released in the large intestine during fermentation by the gut microbiota. Wheat bran–based cereals deliver substantially higher amounts of bound hydroxycinnamic acids such as ferulic, sinapic, and *p*-coumaric acids and their dimers compared to soft fruits and commonly consumed vegetables and fruits when equivalent amounts are consumed (Neacsu et al., 2013). Some phenolics are particularly associated to one or few plant species, such as the oat avenanthramides (Collins, 1989). Much research to date on phenolics has focused on the antioxidant potential of easily solubilized compounds. Recent evidence suggests that cereal grains could have a much more significant impact on total dietary intake of phenolics than previously considered and that their biological effects could be more extensive than just their ability to inhibit oxidation (Anson et al., 2010; Russell et al., 2008). Most of the in vitro or animal studies carried out with plant phenolics focused mainly on those in fruits, vegetables, wines, and teas (Dykes and Rooney, 2007). However, many of these compounds are also found in cereals. Many phenolics inhibit LDL oxidation (Aviram et al., 2000) and platelet aggregation (Kim and Ynu-Choi, 2008; Pignatelli et al., 2000; Harikumar and Aggarwal, 2008; Wright et al., 2010) and can improve endothelial function (García-Lafuente et al., 2009; Macready et al., 2014). Other flavonoids such as quercetin and tea catechins have been suggested to help stabilize atherosclerotic plaques via the inhibition of metalloproteinase expression and inhibition of smooth muscle proliferation (Maeda et al., 2003). Curcumin, resveratrol, genistein, and epigallocatechin-3-gallate could have antiinflammatory properties by downregulating inducible nitric oxide synthase and cyclooxygenase 2 expressions and by inhibiting inflammatory cytokines production via the inhibition of the transcription factors NF-κB and STAT-3 (Kim et al., 2011). Molecular mechanisms by which flavonoids could exert their cardiovascular benefits include the modulation of cell signaling pathways by blocking kinase activities that drive these processes. For example, flavonoids attenuate activities of kinases including phosphoinositide-3-kinase (PI3K), Fyn, Lyn, Src, Syk, PKC, PIM1/2, ERK, JNK, and PKA (Wright et al., 2015). Many phytochemicals are available in the colon from the action of the gut microbiota where they are metabolized. However, the molecular transformations of bioactive phytochemicals in the gut and the identification of the bacteria responsible remain to be fully elucidated.

3.4.2 Cereal Fibers

The main fibers found in cereals are cellulose (main component of cell wall), hemicelluloses (cell wall polysaccharides soluble in dilute alkali), lignins (nonpolysaccharides cell wall components), fructans, and resistant starch (Bernstein et al., 2013). Hemicelluloses present in cereals mainly include arabinoxylans and β-glucans and to a lesser extent pectins and arabinogalactans. As indicated previously in Section 3.3.1, serum cholesterol is the only marker for CVD risk for which the benefit of increasing β-glucan-rich foods intake is well substantiated by the results of intervention trials. The mechanisms are not fully understood, but the reduction of cholesterol is possibly a sum of several effects. The main mechanism is the reduction of bile acids reabsorption in the ileum. This leads to the removal of steroids from the body by fecal excretion, thus diverting hepatic cholesterol toward bile acid production. Consequently, the body pool of cholesterol, as well as cholesterol secretion in lipoproteins, is reduced (Malkki, 2001). Other mechanisms suggested include delaying gastric emptying rate and small bowel transit time (Malkki, 2001) as well as the modulation of satiety by the regulation of gut hormones secretion such as cholecystokinin (Beck et al., 2009), glucagon-like peptide 1, peptide YY, and ghrelin (Juvonen et al., 2009).

In addition to the release of bound phytochemicals in the large intestine, the fermentation of fiber decreases pH and increases bacterial biomass, leading to an increase in fecal output and the production of SCFA, primarily acetate, propionate, and butyrate (Bernstein et al., 2013). Soluble fibers, as well as resistant starch and inulin-like fructans, are fermented in the colon to SCFAs (Jenkins et al., 2000). SCFAs, particularly butyrate, are the main energy source for the gut epithelial cells, and they can modulate gut morphology and function (http://www.nature.com/nm/journal/v20/n2/full/nm.3444.html; Binder and Mehta, 1989). Fermentation of the carbohydrates reaching the cecum yield 400–600 mmol SCFAs/day, which represents around 10% of the human energy requirements (Bergman, 1990). The potential mechanisms by which the gut microbiota can impact cardiovascular health are summarized in Fig. 14.5.

It has been suggested that SCFAs produced in the large intestine might play a critical role in the prevention and treatment of chronic disease. Butyrate seems particularly associated with colon cancer prevention (Scharlau et al., 2009; Donohoe et al., 2011; Blouin et al., 2011) via mechanisms involving the activation of G protein–coupled receptors specific for SCFA (Tang et al., 2011). Butyrate may improve insulin sensitivity in mice (Gao et al., 2009). The results of a study carried out in a mouse model showed that propionate had potent hypotensive properties (Pluznick et al., 2013). Furthermore, the authors found that these effects were mediated by olfactory receptors (GPR41) present in the animal's tissues which respond to propionate. It is therefore possible that the beneficial effects of increasing WG consumption on systolic BP described in Section 3.3.3 originated from the production of SCFA, particularly propionate, after fermentation of WG-derived indigestible carbohydrates in the colon by the gut microflora. Further evidence suggested that SCFA could act directly centrally, via gut–brain neural signaling activated by SCFA receptors (De Vadder et al., 2014; Bindels et al., 2013). Activation of GPR43 by SCFA on enteroendocrine cells induces the production of peptide YY and glucagon-like peptide 1, which

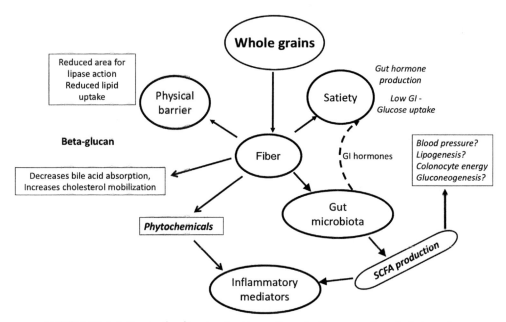

FIGURE 14.5 Putative mechanisms involved in cardioprotective properties of whole grains.

modulates intestinal transit and appetite and stimulates insulin secretion (Bindels et al., 2013). However, the involvement of receptors specific for SCFA such as GRP41 and GRP43 in the beneficial effects of dietary fibers remains to be demonstrated in human studies. The fiber composition differs between WGs and can impact on the growth of different bacterial groups. Human intervention studies suggested a possible bifidogenic effect of WG products (Graf et al., 2015). However, since the studies carried out were mostly of short-term duration, not well controlled, and lacking statistical power, further evaluation is required using long-term, placebo-controlled studies comparing various WG foods.

4. Whole Grain and Cancer

Many prospective studies carried out over the last 15 years showed an inverse relationship between high WG intake and cancer rate, with a particular focus on colon cancer. A meta-analysis of 16 prospective studies showed that the relative risk (95% CIs) of developing colorectal cancer for 10 g daily of total dietary fiber was 0.90 (0.86, 0.94) which is similar to that calculated for cereal fiber (Aune et al., 2011). The authors also indicated that the relative risk would decrease by 17% (RR 0.83; CIs: 0.78, 0.89) when consuming three servings of WGs per day. Considering the variability inherent to dietary assessment methods usually used in prospective study, Knudsen et al. (2014) evaluated the association between incidence of colorectal cancer and systemic markers of wheat and rye intake. Interestingly, the authors found that plasma alkylresorcinol concentrations alone were inversely associated with the incidence of distal colon cancer when the highest quartile was compared with the lowest (incidence rate ratio = 0.34, 95% CIs: 0.13, 0.92). However, the authors found no association between WG intake and any colorectal cancer when using WG intake data from a food frequency questionnaire, suggesting that using both dietary assessment data and biomarkers would improve the precision in estimating disease risk. Using plasma alkylresorcinol concentrations as a surrogate marker of WG wheat and rye intake collected from participants of the multicenter European Prospective Investigation into Cancer and Nutrition for a nested case–control study, Kyro et al. (2014) showed that the highest quartile of WG intake was associated with a 52% lower incidence of distal colon cancer compared with lowest quartile of intake. A 10-g increase in whole wheat intake has been associated with a 50% lower risk of esophageal cancer (Skeie et al., 2015).

With regard to breast cancer, a meta-analysis of 16 prospective studies showed that each 10 g/day increment of fiber intake would result into a 5% lower risk of breast cancer (Aune et al., 2012). The top quintile of fiber intake, particularly from cereals, has been associated with decreased risk of breast cancer in premenopausal women (hazard ratio 0.48, CIs: 0.24, 0.96) compared with the lowest quintile of intake (Cade et al., 2007). The results of a recent case–control study involving 250 breast cancer female patients and 250 aged-matched control suggested that eating WGs more than seven times/week was associated with a twofold (odds ratio = 0.49; CIs: 0.29, 0.82) lower likelihood of having breast cancer (Mourouti et al., 2016). Increasing WG daily intake during adolescence and early adulthood might be particularly important for breast cancer risk. Indeed, results from the Nurses' Health Study II suggested that every daily intake of 10 g of fiber during adolescence and young adulthood would lower the risk of breast cancer by 14% and 13%, respectively. Furthermore, the results also suggested that subjects eating around 25 g/day during these life periods were 25% (RR 0.75, 95% CIs 0.62–0.91) less likely to get breast cancer than those consuming 12 g fiber per day (Farvid et al., 2016).

However, there is no evidence from intervention studies whether high WG intake could decrease cancer risk, mainly due to the lack of well-defined relevant biomarkers (Seal and Brownlee, 2015).

5. Conclusion

The identification of relevant and specific biomarkers to evaluate cancer risk is essential to further evaluate the impact of WG consumption on cancer risk. There is some evidence that increasing WG consumption to at least three portions (equivalent to three medium slices of whole meal bread, for example) per day can provide some cardiovascular benefit. WG contains many components that have been associated with disease risk reduction. However, latest findings suggest that WG fibers, particularly via the action of the gut bacteria releasing potential bioactive phytochemicals bound to fiber and producing SCFA, are mainly responsible for the health effects. Further studies looking at interactions between host, gut bacteria, and fiber components are warranted.

References

Adom, K.K., Sorrells, M.E., Liu, R.H., 2005. Phytochemicals and antioxidant activity of milled fractions of different wheat varieties. J. Agric. Food Chem. 53, 2297–2306.

American Association of Cereal Chemists, 1999. Wholegrain definition. Cereal Foods World 45, 79.

Ampatzoglou, A., Atwal, K., Maidens, C., et al., 2015. Increased whole grain consumption does not affect blood biochemistry, body composition or gut microbiology in healthy low habitual whole grain consumers. J. Nutr. 145 (2), 215–221.

Andersson, A., Tengblad, S., Karlstrom, B., et al., 2007. Whole-grain foods do not affect insulin sensitivity or markers of lipid peroxidation and inflammation in healthy, moderately overweight subjects. J. Nutr. 137 (6), 1401–1407.

Anson, N.M., Havenaar, R., Bast, A., et al., 2010. Antioxidant and anti-inflammatory capacity of bioaccessible compounds from wheat fractions after gastrointestinal digestion. J. Cereal Sci. 51, 110–114.

Atkinson, F.S., Foster-Powell, K., Brand-Miller, J.C., 2008. International tables of glycemic index and glycemic load values: 2008. Diab. Care 31, 2281–2283.

Aune, D., Chan, D.S.M., Lau, R., et al., 2011. Dietary fibre, whole grains, and risk of colorectal cancer: systematic review and dose-response meta-analysis of prospective studies. BMJ 343, d6617.

Aune, D., Chan, D.S., Greenwood, D.C., et al., 2012. Dietary fiber and breast cancer risk: a systematic review and meta-analysis of prospective studies. Ann. Oncol. 23 (6), 1394–1402.

Aune, D., Norat, T., Romundstad, P., et al., 2013. Whole grain and refined grain consumption and the risk of type 2 diabetes: a systematic review and dose-response meta-analysis of cohort studies. Eur. J. Epidemiol. 28, 845–858.

Aviram, M., Dornfeld, L., Rosenblat, M., et al., 2000. Pomegranate juice consumption reduces oxidative stress, atherogenic modifications to LDL, and platelet aggregation: studies in humans and in atherosclerotic apolipoprotein E-deficient mice. Am. J. Clin. Nutr. 71 (5), 1062–1076.

Bazzano, L.A., Song, Y., Bubes, V., et al., 2005. Dietary intake of whole and refined grain breakfast cereals and weight gain in men. Obes. Res. 13, 1952–1960.

Beck, E., Tosh, S.M., Batterham, M.J., et al., 2009. Oat beta-glucan increases postprandial cholecystokinin levels, decreases insulin response and extends subjective satiety in overweight subjects. Mol. Nutr. Food Res. 53, 1343–1351.

Behall, K.M., Schoffield, D.J., Hallfrish, J., 2004. Diet containing barley significantly reduce lipids in mildly hypercholesterolemic men and women. Am. J. Clin. Nutr. 80, 1185–1193.

Behall, K.M., Schoffield, D.J., Hallfrish, J., 2006. Whole-grain diets reduce blood pressure in mildly hypercholesterolemic men and women. J. Am. Diet. Assoc. 106 (9), 1445–1449.

Bergman, E.N., 1990. Energy contributions of volatile fatty acids from the gastrointestinal tract in various species. Physiol. Rev. 70, 567–590.

Bernstein, A.M., Titgemeier, B., Kirkpatrick, K., Golubic, M., RoizenMajor, M.F., 2013. Cereal grain fibers and psyllium in relation to cardiovascular health. Nutrients 5, 1471–1487.

Bindels, L., Dewulf, E.M., Delzenne, N.M., 2013. GPR43/FFA2: physiopathological relevance and therapeutic prospects. Trends Pharm. Sci. 34 (4).

Binder, H.J., Mehta, P., 1989. Short-chain fatty acids stimulate active sodium and chloride absorption in vitro in the rat distal colon. Gastroenterology 96, 989–996.

Blouin, J.M., Penot, G., Collinet, M., et al., 2011. Butyrate elicits a metabolic switch in human colon cancer cells by targeting the pyruvate dehydrogenase complex. Int. J. Cancer 128, 2591–2601.

Brand-Miller, J., McMillan-Price, J., Steinbeck, K., et al., 2008. Carbohydrates-the good, the bad and the whole grain. Asia Pac. J. Clin. Nutr. 17, 16–19.

Brownlee, I.A., Moore, C., Chatfield, M., et al., 2010. Markers of cardiovascular risk are not changed by increased whole-grain intake: the WHOLEheart study, a randomised, controlled dietary intervention. Brit. J. Nutr. 104, 125–134.

Burkitt, D.P., 1983. The development of the fibre hypothesis. In: Birch, G.G., Parker, K.J. (Eds.), Dietary Fibre. Applied Science Publishers, London, pp. 21–27.

Cade, J.E., Burley, V.J., Greenwood, D.C., 2007. Dietary fibre and risk of breast cancer in the UK Women's Cohort Study. Int. J. Epidemiol. 36 (2), 431–438.

Chanson-Rolle, A., Meynier, A., Aubin, F., et al., 2015. Systematic review and meta-analysis of human studies to support a quantitative recommendation for whole grain intake in relation to type 2 diabetes. PLoS One 10 (6), e0131377.

Cho, S.S., Qi, L., Fahey, G.C., et al., 2013. Consumption of cereal fiber, mixtures of whole grains and bran, and whole grains and risk reduction in type 2 diabetes, obesity, and cardiovascular disease. Am. J. Clin. Nutr. 98 (2), 594–619.

Collins, F.W., 1989. Oat phenolics: avenanthramides, novel substituted N-cinnamoylanthranilate alkaloids from oat groats and hulls. J. Agric. Food Chem. 37, 60.

Davy, B.M., Davy, P.D., Ho, R.C., et al., 2002. High-fiber oat cereal compared with wheat cereal consumption favourably alters LDL cholesterol subclass and particle numbers in middle-aged and older men. Am. J. Clin. Nutr. 76, 350–358.

De Vadder, F., Kovatcheva-Datchary, P., Goncalves, D., et al., 2014. SCFAs could also act directly centrally microbiota-generated metabolites promote metabolic benefits via gut-brain neural circuits. Cell 156, 84–96.

Donohoe, D.R., Garge, N., Zhang, X., et al., 2011. The microbiome and butyrate regulate energy metabolism and autophagy in the mammalian colon. Cell Metab. 13, 517–526.

DTU (National Food Institute), 2008. Report of the National Food Institute. English summary available at: http://whole.grainscouncil.org/files/WholeGrainsinDenmark.pdf.

Dykes, L., Rooney, L.W., 2007. Phenolic compounds in cereal grains and their health benefits. Cereal Foods World 52 (3), 105–111.

Fang, L., Li, W., Zhang, W., et al., 2015. Association between whole grain intake and stroke risk: evidence from a meta-analysis. Int. J. Clin. Exp. Med. 8 (9), 16978–16983.

Farvid, M.S., Eliassen, A.H., Cho, E., et al., 2016. Dietary fiber intake in young adults and breast cancer risk. Pediatrics 137 (3), 1–11.

Ferruzzi, M.G., Jonnalagadda, S.S., Liu, S., et al., 2014. Developing a standard definition of whole-grain foods for dietary recommendations: summary report of a multi-disciplinary expert roundtable discussion. Adv. Nutr. 5, 164–176.

Flint, A.J., Hu, F.B., Glynn, R.J., et al., 2009. Whole grains and incident hypertension in men. Am. J. Clin. Nutr. 90 (3), 493–498.

Gao, Z., Yin, J., Zhang, J., Ward, R.E., et al., 2009. Butyrate improves insulin sensitivity and increases energy expenditure in mice. Diabetes 58, 1509–1517.

García-Lafuente, A., Guillamón, E., Villares, A., et al., 2009. Flavonoids as anti-inflammatory agents: implications in cancer and cardiovascular disease. Inflamm. Res. 58, 537–552.

Giacco, R., Clemente, G., Cipriano, D., et al., 2010. Effects of the regular consumption of wholemeal wheat foods on cardiovascular risk factors in healthy people. Nutr. Metab. Cardiovasc. Dis. 20 (3), 186–194.

Giacco, R., Costabile, G., Della Pepa, G., et al., 2014. A wholegrain cereal-based diet lowers postprandial plasma insulin and triglyceride levels in individuals with metabolic syndrome. Nutr. Metab. Cardiovasc. Dis. 24, 837–844.

Graf, D., Di Cagno, R., Fak, F., et al., 2015. Contribution of diet to the composition of the human gut microbiota. Microb. Ecol. Health Dis. 26, 26164.

Hajihashemi, P., Azadbakht, L., Hashemipor, M., et al., 2014. Whole-grain intake favorably affects markers of systemic inflammation in obese children: a randomized controlled crossover clinical trial. Mol. Nutr. Food Res. 58 (6), 1301–1308.

Harikumar, K.B., Aggarwal, B.B., 2008. Resveratrol: a multitargeted agent for age-associated chronic diseases. Cell Cycle 7, 1020–1035.

Harris Jackson, K., West, S.G., Vanden Heuvel, J.P., et al., 2014. Effects of whole and refined grains in a weight-loss diet on markers of metabolic syndrome in individuals with increased waist circumference: a randomized controlled-feeding trial. Am. J. Clin. Nutr. 100 (2), 577–586.

Hollaender, P.L., Ross, A.B., Kristensen, M., 2015. Whole-grain and blood lipid changes in apparently healthy adults: a systematic review and meta-analysis of randomized controlled studies. Am. J. Clin. Nutr. 102 (3), 556–572.

Huang, T., Xu, M., Lee, A., et al., 2015. Consumption of whole grains and cereal fiber and total and cause-specific mortality: prospective analysis of 367,442 individuals. BMC Med. 13, 59.

Jacobs, D.R., Meyer, K.A., Hushi, L.H., et al., 1998. Whole grain intake may reduce the risk of ischaemic heart disease death in postmenopausal women: the Iowa Women's Health Study. Am. J. Clin. Nutr. 68, 248–257.

Jacobs Jr., D.R., Andersen, L.F., Blomhoff, R., 2007. Whole-grain consumption is associated with a reduced risk of non-cardiovascular, non-cancer death attributed to inflammatory diseases in the Iowa Women's Health Study. Am. J. Clin. Nutr. 85, 1606–1614.

Jenkins, D.J., Kendall, C.W., Axelsen, M., et al., 2000. Viscous and nonviscous fibres, nonabsorbable and low glycaemic index carbohydrates, blood lipids and coronary heart disease. Curr. Opin. Lipidol. 11, 49–56.

Jensen, M.K., Koh-Banerjee, P., Hu, F.B., et al., 2004. Intakes of whole grains. Bran and germ and the risk of coronary heart disease in men. Am. J. Clin. Nutr. 80 (6), 1492–1499.

Johnsen, N.F., Frederiksen, K., Christensen, J., et al., 2015. Whole-grain products and whole-grain types are associated with lower all-cause and cause-specific mortality in the Scandinavian HELGA cohort. Br. J. Nutr. 114 (4), 608–623.

Juvonen, K.R., Purhonen, A.K., Salmenkallio-Marttila, M., et al., 2009. Viscosity of oat bran-enriched beverages influences gastrointestinal hormonal responses in healthy humans. J. Nutr. 139, 461–466.

Kang, R., Kim, M., Chae, J.S., et al., 2014. Consumption of whole grains and legumes modulates the genetic effect of the APOA5 -1131C variant on changes in triglyceride and apolipoprotein A-V concentrations in patients with impaired fasting glucose or newly diagnosed type 2 diabetes. Trials 15, 100.

Karmally, W., Montez, M.G., Palmas, W., et al., 2005. Cholesterol-lowering benefits of oat-containing cereal in Hispanic Americans. J. Am. Diet. Assoc. 105, 967–970.

Katcher, H.I., Legro, R.S., Kunselman, A.R., et al., 2008. The effects of a whole grain-enriched hypocaloric diet on cardiovascular disease risk factors in men and women with metabolic syndrome. Am. J. Clin. Nutr. 87 (1), 79–90.

Kim, J.M., Ynu-Choi, H.S., 2008. Anti-platelet effects of flavonoids and flavonoid-glycosides from *Sophora japonica*. Arch. Pharm. Res. 31 (7), 886.

Kim, M.K., Kidong Kim, K., Jae Yong Han, J.Y., et al., 2011. Modulation of inflammatory signaling pathways by phytochemicals in ovarian cancer. Genes Nutr. 6 (2), 109–115.

Knudsen, M.D., Kyrø, C., Olsen, A., et al., 2014. Self-reported whole-grain intake and plasma alkylresorcinol concentrations in combination in relation to the incidence of colorectal cancer. Am. J. Epidemiol. 179, 1188–1196.

Kristensen, M., Toubro, S., Jensen, M.G., et al., 2012. Whole grain compared with refined wheat decreases the percentage of body fat following a 12-week, energy-restricted dietary intervention in postmenopausal women. J. Nutr. 142 (4), 710–716.

Kuijsten, A., InterAct Consortium, et al., 2015. Dietary fibre and incidence of type 2 diabetes in eight European countries: the EPIC-InterAct Study and a meta-analysis of prospective studies. Diabetologia 58, 1394–1408.

Kyro, C., Olsen, A., Landberg, R., et al., 2014. Plasma alkylresorcinols, biomarkers of whole-grain wheat and rye intake and incidence of colorectal cancer. J. Natl. Cancer Inst. 106 (1), djt352.

Lairon, D., Arnault, N., Bertrais, S., et al., 2005. Dietary fiber intake and risk factors for cardiovascular disease in French adults. Am. J. Clin. Nutr. 82, 1185–1194.

Lefevre, M., Jonnalagadda, S., 2012. Effect of whole grains on markers of subclinical inflammation. Nutr. Rev. 70 (7), 387–396.

Liu, S., Stampfer, M.J., Hu, F.B., et al., 1999. Whole-grain consumption and risk of CHD: results from the Nurses' health study. Am. J. Clin. Nutr. 70, 412–419.

Liu, S., Sesso, H.D., Manson, J.E., et al., 2003a. Is intake of breakfast cereals related to total and cause-specific mortality in men? Am. J. Clin. Nutr. 77, 594–599.

Liu, S., Willett, W.C., Manson, J.E., et al., 2003b. Relation between changes in intakes of dietary fiber and grain products and changes in weight and development of obesity among middle-aged women. Am. J. Clin. Nutr. 78, 920–927.

Macready, A.L., George, T.W., Chong, M.F., et al., 2014. Flavonoid-rich fruit and vegetables improve microvascular reactivity and inflammatory status in men at risk of cardiovascular disease — FLAVURS: a randomized controlled trial. Am. J. Clin. Nutr. 99 (3), 479–489.

Maeda, K., Kuzuya, M., Cheng, X.W., et al., 2003. Green tea catechins inhibit the cultured smooth muscle cell invasion through the basement barrier. Atherosclerosis 166, 23–30.

Magnusdottir, O.K., Landberg, R., Gunnarsdottir, I., et al., 2014. Whole grain rye intake, reflected by a biomarker, is associated with favorable blood lipid outcomes in subjects with the metabolic syndrome – a randomized study. PLoS One 9, e110827.

Malkki, Y., 2001. Oat Fiber. Handbook of Dietary Fiber. In: Cho, S.S., Dreher, M.L. (Eds.). Macrel Dekker, New York, pp. 497–512.

Mann, K.D., Pearce, M.S., McKevith, B., et al., 2015. Low whole grain intake in the UK: results from the National Diet and Nutrition Survey rolling programme 2008-11. Brit. J. Nutr. 113, 1643–1651.

McKeown, N.M., Yoshida, M., Shea, M.K., et al., 2009. Whole-grain intake and cereal fiber are associated with lower abdominal adiposity in older adults. J. Nutr. 139, 1950–1955.

McKeown, N.M., Troy, L.M., Jacques, P.F., et al., 2010. Whole- and refined-grain intakes are differentially associated with abdominal visceral and subcutaneous adiposity in healthy adults: the Framingham Heart Study. Am. J. Clin. Nutr. 92, 1165–1171.

Mellen, P.B., Walsh, T.F., Herrington, D.M., 2008. Whole grain intake and cardiovascular disease: a meta-analysis. Nutr. Metab. Cardiovasc. Dis. 18, 283–290.

Meyer, K.A., Kushi, L.H., Jacobs Jr., D.R., Slavin, J., Sellers, T.A., Folsom, A.R., 2000. Carbohydrates, dietary fiber, and incident type 2 diabetes in older women. Am. J. Clin. Nutr. 71, 921–930.

Mizrahi, A., Knekt, P., Montonen, J., et al., 2009. Plant foods and the risk of cerebrovascular diseases: a potential protection of fruit consumption. Br. J. Nutr. 102, 1075–1083.

Mourouti, N., Kontogianni, M.D., Papavagelis, C., et al., 2016. Whole grain consumption and breast cancer: a case-control study in women. J. Am. Coll. Nutr. 35 (2), 143–149.

Neacsu, M., McMonagle, J., Fletcher, R.J., et al., 2013. Bound phytophenols from ready-to-eat cereals: comparison with other plant-based foods. Food Chem. 141, 2880–2886.

Nelson, K., Mathai, M.L., Ashton, J.F., et al., 2016. Effects of malted and non-malted whole-grain wheat on metabolic and inflammatory biomarkers in overweight/obese adults: a randomised crossover pilot study. Food Chem. 194, 495–502.

Newby, P.K., Maras, J., Bakun, P., et al., 2007. Intake of whole grains, refined grains, and cereal fiber measured with 7-d diet records and associations with risk factors for chronic disease. Am. J. Clin. Nutr. 86, 1745–1753.

NHS Choices, 2015. Starchy Foods. http://www.nhs.uk/Livewell/Goodfood/Pages/starchy-foods.aspx.

Parker, E.D., Liu, S., Van Horn, L., Tinker, L.F., et al., 2013. The association of whole grain consumption with incident type 2 diabetes: the Women's Health Initiative Observational Study. Ann. Epidemiol. 23 (6), 321–327.

Pignatelli, P., Pulcinelli, F.M., Celestini, A., et al., 2000. The flavonoids quercetin and catechin synergistically inhibit platelet function by antagonizing the intracellular production of hydrogen peroxide. Am. J. Clin. Nutr. 72 (5), 1150–1155.

Pluznick, J.L., Protzko, R.J., Gevorgyan, H., et al., 2013. Olfactory receptor responding to gut microbiota-derived signals plays a role in renin secretion and blood pressure regulation. PNAS 110, 4410–4415.

Pol, K., Christensen, R., Bartels, E.M., et al., 2013. Whole grain and body weight changes in apparently healthy adults: a systematic review and meta-analysis of randomized controlled studies. Am. J. Clin. Nutr. 98 (4), 872–884.

Poulsen, S.K., Due, A., Jordy, A.B., et al., 2014. Health effect of the New Nordic Diet in adults with increased waist circumference: a 6-mo randomized controlled trial. Am. J. Clin. Nutr. 99, 35–45.

Queenan, K.M., Stewart, M.L., Smith, K.N., et al., 2007. Concentrated oat b-glucan, a fermentable fiber, lowers serum cholesterol in hypercholesterolemic adults in a randomised controlled trial. Nutr. J. 6, 6.

Räsänen, L., 2007. Of all foods bread is the most noble: Carl von Linné (Carl Linneaus) on bread. Scand. J. Food Nutr. 51, 91–99.

Rave, K., Roggen, K., Dellweg, S., et al., 2007. Improvement of insulin resistance after diet with a wholegrain based dietary product: results of a randomized, controlled cross-over study in obese subjects with elevated fasting blood glucose. Br. J. Nutr. 98, 929–936.

Ross, A.B., Kristensen, M., Seal, C.J., et al., 2015. Recommendations for reporting whole-grain intake in observational and intervention studies. Am. J. Clin. Nutr. 101, 903–907.

Russell, W.R., Scobbie, L., Chesson, A., et al., 2008. Anti-inflammatory implications of the microbial transformation of dietary phenolic compounds. Nutr. Cancer 60 (5), 636–642.

Sahyoun, N.R., Jacques, P.F., Zhang, X.L., et al., 2006. Wholegrain intake is inversely associated with the metabolic syndrome and mortality in older adults. Am. J. Clin. Nutr. 83, 124–131.

Scharlau, D., Borowicki, A., Habermann, N., et al., 2009. Mechanisms of primary cancer prevention by butyrate and other products formed during gut flora-mediated fermentation of dietary fibre. Mutat. Res. 682, 39–53.

Scientific Advisory Committee on Nutrition, 2015. SACN Carbohydrates and Health Report. https://www.gov.uk/government/publications/sacn-carbohydrates-and-health-report.

Seal, C.J., Brownlee, I.A., 2015. Whole-grain foods and chronic disease: evidence from epidemiological and intervention studies. Proc. Nutr. Soc. 74, 313–319.

Skeie, G., Braaten, T., Olsen, A., et al., 2015. Intake of whole grains and incidence of oesophageal cancer in the HELGA Cohort. Eur. J. Epidemiol.. ISSN: 0393-2990. http://dx.doi.org/10.1007/s10654-015-0057-y. Published ahead of print.

Slavin, J., Tucker, M., Harriman, C., et al., 2013. Whole grains: definition, dietary recommendations and health benefits. Cereal Foods World 5, 191–198.

Smith, K.N., Queenan, K.M., Thomas, W., et al., 2008. Physiological effects of concentrated barley beta-glucan in mildly hypercholesterolemic adults. J. Am. Coll. Nutr. 27, 434–440.

Spiller, G.A., 2002. Whole grains, whole wheat and white flours in history. In: Marquart, Slavib, Flutcher (Eds.), Wholegrain Foods in Health and Disease. Eagan Press, St Paul, Minnesota, pp. 1–7.

Steffen, L.M., Jacobs Jr., D.R., Stevens, J., et al., 2003. Associations of whole-grain, refined-grain, and fruit and vegetable consumption with risks of all-cause mortality and incident coronary artery disease and ischemic stroke: the Atherosclerosis Risk in Communities (ARIC) Study. Am. J. Clin. Nutr. 78 (3), 383–390.

Streppel, M.T., Arends, L.R., van't Veer, P., et al., 2005. Dietary fiber and blood pressure: a meta-analysis of randomized placebo-controlled trials. Arch. Intern. Med. 165, 150–156.

Sun, Q., Spiegelman, D., van Dam, R.M., Holmes, M.D., Malik, V.S., Willett, W.C., Hu, F.B., 2010. White rice, brown rice, and risk of type 2 diabetes in US men and women. Arch. Intern. Med. 170 (11), 961–969.

Tang, Y., Chen, Y., Jiang, H., et al., 2011. G-protein-coupled receptor for short-chain fatty acids suppresses colon cancer. Int. J. Cancer 128, 847–856.

Thies, F., Masson, L.F., Boffetta, P., et al., 2014. Oats and CVD risk markers: a systematic literature review. Br. J. Nutr. 112 (Suppl. 2), S19–S30.

Thomas, R.A., 1894. Medical Essays. F. Pitman, London, UK.

Tighe, P., Vaughan, N., Duthie, G., et al., 2010. Effect of increased consumption of whole-grain foods on blood pressure and other cardiovascular risk markers in healthy middle-aged persons: a randomized controlled trial. Am. J. Clin. Nutr. 92, 733–740.

Tighe, P., Duthie, G., Brittenden, J., et al., 2013. Effects of wheat and oat-based whole grain foods on serum lipoprotein size and distribution in overweight middle aged people: a randomised controlled trial. PLoS One 8 (8), e70436.

Trowell, H.C., 1975. Dietary-fiber hypothesis of the etiology of diabetes mellitus. Diabetes 24 (8), 762–765.

USDA and US Department of Health and Human Services (2010). Dietary Guidelines for Americans 2010. US Government Printing Office, Washington, DC. http://www.cnpp.usda.gov/DietaryGuidelines.htm.

USDA National Nutrient Database for Standard Reference, Release 28. http://www.ars.usda.gov/Services/docs.htm?docid=8964.

van Dam, R.M., Rimm, E.B., Willett, W.C., Stampfer, M.J., Hu, F.B., 2002. Dietary patterns and risk for type 2 diabetes mellitus in U.S. men. Ann. Intern. Med. 136, 201–209.

van der Kamp, J.W., Poutanen, K., Seal, C.J., et al., 2014. The HEALTHGRAIN definition of 'whole grain'. Food Nutr. Res. 58, 22100.

Vitaglione, P., Mennella, I., Ferracane, R., et al., 2015. Whole-grain wheat consumption reduces inflammation in a randomized controlled trial on overweight and obese subjects with unhealthy dietary and lifestyle behaviors: role of polyphenols bound to cereal dietary fiber. Am. J. Clin. Nutr. 101 (2), 251–261.

Wang, L., Gaziano, J.M., Liu, S., et al., 2007. Whole- and refined-grain intakes and the risk of hypertension in women. Am. J. Clin. Nutr. 86 (2), 472–479.

Wang, H., Lichtenstein, A.H., Lamon-Fava, S., et al., 2014. Association between statin use and serum cholesterol concentrations is modified by whole-grain consumption : NHANES 2003-2006. Am. J. Clin. Nutr. 100, 1149–1157.

Whelton, S.P., Hyre, A.D., Pedersen, B., et al., 2005. Effect of dietary fiber intake on blood pressure; a meta-analysis of randomised, controlled clinical trials. J. Hypertens. 23, 475–481.

Whitehead, A., Beck, E.J., Tosh, S., et al., 2014. Cholesterol-lowering effects of oat b-glucan: a meta-analysis of randomized controlled trials. Am. J. Clin. Nutr. 100, 1413–1421.

Wirstrom, T., Hilding, A., Gu, H.F., Ostenson, C.G., Bjorklund, A., 2013. Consumption of whole grain reduces risk of deteriorating glucose tolerance, including progression to prediabetes. Am. J. Clin. Nutr. 97 (1), 179–187.

World Health Organisation, Cardiovascular Diseases (CVDs), http://www.who.int/mediacentre/factsheets/fs317/en/.

Wright, B., Moraes, L.A., Kemp, C.F., et al., 2010. A structural basis for the inhibition of collagen-stimulated platelet function by quercetin and structurally related flavonoids. Brit. J. Pharm. 159, 1312–1325.

Wright, B., Watson, K.A., McGuffin, et al., 2015. GRID and docking analyses reveal a molecular basis for flavonoid inhibition of src-family kinase activity. J. Nutr. Biochem. 26 (11), 1156–1165.

Wu, H., Flint, A.J., Qi, Q., et al., 2015. Association between dietary whole grain intake and risk of mortality: two large prospective studies in US men and women. JAMA Intern. Med. 175 (3), 373–384.

Ye, E.Q., Chacko, S.A., Chou, E.L., et al., 2012. Greater wholegrain intake is associated with lower risk of Type 2 diabetes, cardiovascular disease, and weight gain. J. Nutr. 142, 1304–1313.

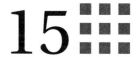

15

Nut Intake and Health

Michelle Wien

CALIFORNIA STATE POLYTECHNIC UNIVERSITY, POMONA, POMONA, CA, UNITED STATES

1. Introduction

The definition of the term "nut" varies considerably across botanical and culinary disciplines as well as in the minds of consumers. A botanist would define a nut as a dry fruit with one seed that remains free within a very hard mature ovary wall, whereas a culinologist would apply the term to any oily kernel found within a shell (e.g., nuts, seeds). Commonly consumed tree nuts include almonds, Brazil nuts, cashews, chestnuts, hazelnuts, macadamias, pecans, pine nuts, pistachios, and walnuts, which all have a rather similar nutrient profiles with the exception of chestnuts. The consumer typically includes peanuts in the "nuts" food group, but peanuts are botanically classified as a groundnut and part of the legume family. In light of their similar nutrient profile to tree nuts, the term "nuts" in this chapter will hereafter be referred to as peanuts plus the commonly consumed tree nuts (excluding chestnuts).

Nuts have been consumed by animals and humans as an energy dense food since Paleolithic times (Eaton and Konner, 1985). In general, nuts are rich sources of plant protein (10%–25%), polyunsaturated (PUFA) and monounsaturated (MUFA) fatty acids (Ros and Mataix, 2006), dietary fiber, vitamins (e.g., niacin, folate, E, B_6), minerals (e.g., magnesium, copper, selenium, and potassium) (Segura et al., 2006), phenolic antioxidants, and phytosterols (Bolling et al., 2010) (Tables 15.1 and 15.2). Trends in nut intake have varied over the past several decades in industrialized nations with the exception of vegetarians and Seventh-day Adventists, both of whom are health conscious populations that have consistently included nuts in their dietary patterns. More recently, global nut consumption has been trending upward, which may be due to the media reports connecting nut intake to health benefits based on the favorable scientific findings from studies being conducted worldwide. According to the 2007–12 Global Statistical Review published by the International Nut and Dried Fruit Council, a 7% and 5.5% increase in peanut and tree nut consumption was found in 2011 as compared to the previous year, respectively, which confirmed the previous year's rising trend on global consumption (International Nut and Dried Fruit Council, 2015). Hence, The focus of this chapter will include the scientific evidence surrounding the role of nuts as a whole food for preventing, reducing, and/or managing disease risk (e.g., cardiovascular, diabetes, obesity, metabolic syndrome, and cognitive decline) and thus promoting optimal health.

Vegetarian and Plant-Based Diets in Health and Disease Prevention. http://dx.doi.org/10.1016/B978-0-12-803968-7.00015-0

Table 15.1 Nutrients in 100 g of Tree Nuts[a]

Nutrient	Units	Almonds	Brazils	Cashews	Hazelnuts	Macadamias	Pecans	Pine Nuts	Pistachios	Walnuts
Calories	kcal	580	660	570	630	720	690	670	570	650
Protein	g	21	14	15	15	8	9	14	21	15
Total fat	g	50	67	46	61	76	72	68	45	65
Saturated fat	g	4	16	9	4	12	6	5	5	6
Monounsaturated fat	g	32	24	27	46	59	41	19	24	9
Polyunsaturated fat	g	12	24	8	8	1.5	22	34	13	47
Linoleic acid (18:2)	g	12	24	8	8	1.30	21	33	13	38
Linolenic acid (18:3)	g	0	0.04	0.16	0.09	0.20	1	0.16	0.24	9
Cholesterol	mg	0	0	0	0	0	0	0	0	0
Carbohydrate	g	22	12	33	17	13	14	13	29	14
Fiber	g	12	8	3	10	8	10	4	10	7
Calcium	mg	269	160	45	114	70	70	16	107	98
Iron	mg	3.71	2.43	6.00	4.70	2.65	2.53	5.53	4.03	2.91
Magnesium	mg	270	376	260	163	118	121	251	109	158
Phosphorus	mg	481	725	490	290	198	277	575	469	346
Potassium	mg	733	659	565	680	363	410	597	1007	441
Sodium	mg	1	3	16	0	4	0	2	6	2
Zinc	mg	3.12	4.06	5.60	2.45	1.29	4.53	6.45	2.34	3.09
Copper	mg	1.03	1.74	2.22	1.73	0.57	1.20	1.32	1.29	1.59
Manganese	mg	2.18	1.22	0.83	6.18	3.04	4.50	8.80	1.24	3.41
Selenium	mcg	4.10	1917	11.70	2.40	11.70	3.80	0.70	10	4.90
Vitamin C	mg	0	0.70	0	6.30	0.70	1.10	0.80	3	1.30
Thiamin	mg	0.21	0.62	0.20	0.64	0.71	0.66	0.36	0.70	0.34
Riboflavin	mg	1.14	0.04	0.20	0.11	0.09	0.13	0.23	0.23	0.15
Niacin	mg	3.62	0.30	1.40	1.80	2.27	1.17	4.39	1.37	1.13
Pantothenic acid	mg	0.47	0.18	1.22	0.92	0.60	0.86	0.31	0.51	0.57
Vitamin B6	mg	0.14	0.10	0.26	0.56	0.36	0.21	0.09	1.12	0.54
Folate	mcg	44	22	69	113	10	22	34	51	98
Choline, total	mg	52	29	61	46	45	41	56	71	39
Betaine	mg	0.5	0.4	n/a	0.4	0.3	0.7	0.4	0.8	0.3

Vitamin B12	mcg	0	0	0	0	0	0	0	0	0
Vitamin A	IU	2	0	0	20	0	56	29	266	20
Vitamin K	mcg	0	0	34.70	14.20	0	3.50	53.90	13.20	2.70
Vitamin E										
Tocopherol, alpha	mg	25.63	5.65	0.92	15.03	0.57	1.40	9.33	2.17	0.70
Tocopherol, beta	mg	0.23	0	n/a	0.33	0	0.39	0	0.13	0.15
Tocopherol, gamma	mg	0.64	9.56	n/a	0	0	24.44	11.15	23.42	20.83
Tocopherol, delta	mg	0.07	0.63	n/a	0	0	0.47	0	0.55	1.89
Carotenoids										
Carotene, beta	mcg	1	0	0	11	0	29	17	159	12
Carotene, alpha	mcg	0	0	0	3	0	0	0	0	0
Cryptoxanthin, beta	mcg	0	0	0	0	0	9	0	0	0
Lutein + zeaxanthin	mcg	1	0	23	92	0	17	9	1160	9

aAll of the nuts are unsalted; almonds, Brazil nuts, hazelnuts, pecans, pine nuts and walnuts are unroasted; cashews, macadamias and pistachios are dry roasted.

g, gram; *IU*, International Units; *mcg*, microgram; *mg*, milligram.

USDA National Nutrient Database for Standard Reference, Release 28, Full Report, 2015. Prepared by the International Tree Nut Council Nutrition Research & Education Foundation, 10/15.

Table 15.2 Flavonoids and Phytosterols in 100 g of Tree Nuts

Phytochemical	Units	Almonds	Brazils	Cashews	Hazelnuts	Macadamias	Pecans	Pine Nuts	Pistachios	Walnuts
Flavonoids										
Anthocyanidins										
Cyanidin	mg	2.45	0	0	6.70	0	10.73	0	7.33	2.70
Delphinidin	mg	0	0	0	0	0	7.27	0	0	0
Flavan-3-ols										
Epicatechin	mg	0.60	0	0.93	0.21	0	0.81	0	0.83	0
Epicatechin 3-gallate	mg	0	0	0.15	0	0	0	0	0	0
Epigallocatechin	mg	2.59	0	0	2.78	0	5.62	0.49	2.05	0
Epigallocatechin 3-gallate	mg	0	0	0	1.06	0	2.29	0	0.40	0
Catechin	mg	1.27	0	0.90	1.18	0	7.23	0	3.57	0
Flavanones										
Eriodictyol	mg	0.25	n/a	n/a	n/a	n/a	n/a	n/a	n/a	n/a
Naringenin	mg	0.42	0	0	0	0	0	0	0	0
Flavonols										
Isorhamnetin	mg	2.63	n/a	n/a	n/a	n/a	n/a	n/a	n/a	n/a
Kaempferol	mg	0.39	n/a	n/a	n/a	n/a	n/a	n/a	n/a	n/a
Quercetin	mg	0.36	0	0	0	0	0	0	1.46	0
Total Proanthocyanidins	mg	184	0	9	501	0	494	0	237	67
Monomers	mg	7.77	0	6.66	9.83	0	17.22	0	10.94	6.93
Dimers	mg	9.52	0	2.02	12.51	0	42.13	0	13.26	5.65
Trimers	mg	8.82	0	0	13.56	0	26.03	0	10.51	7.19
4–6mers	mg	39.97	0	0	67.72	0	101.43	0	42.24	22.05
7–10mers	mg	37.68	0	0	74.60	0	84.23	0	37.93	5.41
Polymers	mg	80.26	0	0	322.44	0	223.01	0	122.46	20.02
Total Phytosterols	mg	n/a	n/a	158	n/a	n/a	n/a	n/a	n/a	n/a
Stigmasterol	mg	4	6	n/a	1	0	3	0	2	0
Campesterol	mg	5	2	n/a	7	10	6	20	10	5
Beta-sitosterol	mg	130	64	n/a	102	145	117	132	210	87

mg, milligram; *n/a*, not available.

Flavonoid data from USDA Database for the Flavonoid Content of Selected Foods, Release 3.1, 2014; Phytosterol data from USDA Database for Standard Reference, Release 28, Full Report, 2015; Proanthocyanidin data from USDA Database for the Proanthocyanidin Content of Selected Foods, 2004. Prepared by the International Tree Nut Council Nutrition Research & Education Foundation, 10/15.

2. Coronary Heart Disease

2.1 Epidemiological Studies

Epidemiologic evidence of a potential protective role for nuts in coronary heart disease (CHD) emerged in 1992 with the findings from the Adventist Health Study-1 (Fraser et al., 1992), which found that frequent consumption of nuts (>4 times per week) was associated with a reduction in fatal CHD events [relative risk, 0.52; 95% confidence interval (CI) 0.36–0.76] and nonfatal myocardial infarctions (relative risk, 0.49; 95% CI 0.28–0.85) when compared with nut consumption of less than once per week. Both vegetarians and non-vegetarians were found to experience protective effects from frequent nut consumption in a subsequent analysis (Sabaté, 1999); however, the beneficial effects were attenuated among omnivores. During the following decade, three additional large US-based prospective cohort studies (Albert et al., 2002; Ellsworth et al., 2001; Hu et al., 1998) reported similar findings, which provided support for the cardioprotective role of frequent nut consumption in the background Western-type diet. More specifically, there was a 37% reduction in mean CHD risk among subjects who consumed four or more servings of nuts weekly compared to subjects who rarely or never consumed nuts (Kelly and Sabate, 2006).

2.2 Nut Intervention Trials

One year after the first epidemiological findings were shown, Sabaté et al. (1993) reported that a walnut-enriched diet (20% of energy) produced a 12.4% reduction in total cholesterol (TC) and 16.3% reduction in low density lipoprotein cholesterol (LDL-C) compared to a National Cholesterol Education Program (NCEP) Step 1 diet among 18 healthy males. This seminal clinical trial paved the way for a multitude of controlled clinical nut intervention trials that were designed to investigate the effects of nut intake on a variety of health outcomes. In light of the consistency of findings across more than 30 studies that supported the role of nuts in cardiovascular health between 1992 and 2002, the US Food and Drug Administration approved the first qualified health claim in 2003 for specific nuts (almonds, hazelnuts, pecans, pistachios, walnuts, and peanuts) stating, "Scientific evidence suggests but does not prove that eating 1.5 ounces per day of most nuts, as part of a diet low in saturated fat and cholesterol, may reduce the risk of heart disease." (Food and Drug Administration, 2003).

2.2.1 Nut Intake and Blood Lipids

Almonds and walnuts have been the most extensively evaluated nuts in human dietary intervention studies since the findings from the first nut trial were reported in 1993 (Sabaté et al., 1993). A meta-analysis was more recently conducted on 13 walnut intervention trials representing 365 subjects to evaluate the changes in lipid levels from the consumption of walnut-enriched diets versus nut-free control diets (Banel and Hu, 2009). Compared to the nut-free control diets, the walnut-enriched diets produced a greater reduction in both the TC and LDL-C levels of 10.3 and 9.2 mg/dL, respectively ($Ps < .001$). However, high density lipoprotein cholesterol (HDL-C) and triglyceride (TG) levels were not significantly different between the walnut-enriched and the nut-free control diet.

Since there have been differences among nut studies in the quantity and type of nut consumed, study design, type of analysis, subject inclusion and exclusion criteria, and study duration, Sabaté et al. (2010) explored the possibility of finding a dose–response relationship between blood lipid levels and nut intake by conducting a pooled analysis of 25 nut intervention trials performed between 1992 and 2004 that were identified using a comprehensive MEDLINE search. The change in the standards of care related to prescribing statins that occurred with the release of the Third Report of the NCEP Adult Treatment Panel (ATP III) guidelines was the rationale for the 2004 cutoff because of potential confounding among individuals taking statin medications. The primary data that was collected were from 7 countries and included 583 men and women with normal lipid levels or hypercholesterolemia who were not taking any lipid lowering medications. A mean daily nut intake of 67 g yielded greater reductions in TC, LDL-C, ratio of LDL-C to HDL-C, and TC:HDL-C of 10.9 mg/dL, 10.2 mg/dL, 0.22, and 0.24 ($Ps < .001$), respectively. Also, TG levels showed a 20.6 mg/dL reduction among subjects with baseline TG levels ≥150 mg/dL. It is worth noting that the estimated reductions in TC and LDL-C that were found in the pooled analysis are consistent with the findings of the aforementioned meta-analysis of walnut intervention trials, which confirms the validity of the pooled analysis findings. Neither the type of nut consumed nor gender or age of the subjects influenced the blood lipid findings; however, nut intake was found to be dose related and significantly modified by baseline LDL-C levels, body mass index (BMI), and the background diet of the subjects. Subjects with higher baseline LDL-C levels (>160 mg/dL) showed a greater decrease in TC and LDL-C levels versus those with lower baseline LDL-C (<130 mg/dL) levels. Further, a nut intake × BMI interaction was found for subjects with a lower BMI (<25 kg/m^2) compared to subjects with a BMI of 25–30 kg/m^2 or a BMI greater than 30 kg/m^2 ($P = .02$ for both). More specifically, a high BMI reduces the effect of nut intake on blood lipids. Last, nut intake lowered TC and LDL-C levels (−7.4% and −9.6%, respectively) if the subjects were consuming a Western-type background diet as compared to a Mediterranean-type (−4.3% and −6.7%, respectively) or low-fat (−4.1% and −6.0%, respectively) background diet.

2.3 Other Coronary Heart Disease Risk Factors

Nut intake and mortality risk was evaluated among 7216 subjects aged 55–80 years at high cardiovascular risk residing in Spain that were enrolled in the Prevención con Dieta Mediterráneá trial (PREDIMED) (Guasch-Ferre et al., 2013). Subjects completed a food frequency questionnaire at baseline and reported the frequency of their nut intake. After a median of 4.8 years of follow-up, subjects who consumed nuts with a frequency of more than three servings per week had a 39% lower all-cause mortality risk and a 55% lower cardiovascular disease (CVD) mortality risk compared to nonconsumers. Hence, it is important to briefly discuss the findings of nut studies that have evaluated other CHD risk factors, i.e., LDL-C oxidation and inflammatory markers, which are known to be associated with CVD risk.

Oxidative stress is a hallmark feature of CVD beyond blood lipids and has been evaluated in nut intervention trials using one or more markers among subjects consuming walnuts, pecans, pistachios, or Brazil nuts. Three walnut trials measured LDL-C conjugated diene formation and found no effect on in vitro lag time (Davis et al., 2007; Iwamoto et al., 2002; Zambon et al., 2000), and three additional walnut trials did not observe any change in levels of oxidized LDL-C, malondialdehyde, lipid peroxidation, and/or uric acid (Canales et al., 2007; Mukuddem-Petersen et al., 2007; Ros et al., 2004). However, two of these studies found significant reductions in oxidized glutathione during the walnut-enriched diet intervention versus the control nut-free diet (Canales et al., 2007; Davis et al., 2007). Reductions in postprandial levels of oxidized LDL-C have been observed after consumption of pecans (Hudthagosol et al., 2011), pistachios (Kay et al., 2010), and Brazil nuts (Maranhao et al., 2011). Postprandial studies are unable to evaluate changes in total LDL-C; however, these findings demonstrate that the bioactive constituents in nuts are bioavailable and contribute to postprandial antioxidant defense mechanisms that reduce oxidative damage involved in CHD and other inflammatory and degenerative diseases.

3. Diabetes Mellitus

The World Health Organization's 2014 status report on noncommunicable diseases has estimated the global prevalence of diabetes mellitus (DM) to be 9% among adults aged 18+ years (World Health Organization, 2012). Further, a 50% increase in the global prevalence of DM is predicted to occur between 2010 and 2030 (Shaw et al., 2010) with a particularly rapid growth in the Middle East as well as in the Indian subcontinent, China, Central and South America, and Africa (Adeghate et al., 2006). This increased DM prevalence has the potential to have a devastating impact on the public health and economies in the Western world and aforementioned regions.

3.1 Epidemiological Studies

Several large prospective cohort studies have investigated the risk for developing type 2 DM (T2DM) in the context of the frequency of nut consumption and have shown inconsistent findings. Two of the three studies that included only women, the Nurses Health Study (Jiang et al., 2002) and the Shanghai Women Health Study (Villegas et al., 2008), have shown a 27% and 20% T2DM risk reduction among women who consumed nuts frequently compared to women who rarely consume nuts during 16 and 11 years of follow-up, respectively. However, the Iowa Women's Health Study (Parker et al., 2003) failed to find an association among postmenopausal women during 11 years of follow-up, and null findings were also reported for a cohort of US male physicians enrolled in the Physicians' Health Study during 19 years of follow-up (Kochar et al., 2010). Although further studies must be conducted prior to the confirmation of any protective role of nuts on T2DM risk, the inclusion of a highly nutritious whole food may have direct health benefits in the prevention and management of T2DM. For example, the PREDIMED study found a 52% reduction in risk of developing T2DM among participants that were randomized to consume a Mediterranean diet enriched with 30 g/day of mixed nuts (15 g walnuts, 7.5 g almonds, and 7.5 g hazelnuts) (Salas-Salvado et al., 2011) compared to participants advised to consume a nut-free low-fat Mediterranean diet. These findings provide us with reasons to believe that specific nuts may reduce the risk of developing T2DM in persons consuming a healthy background dietary pattern.

3.2 Nut Intervention Trials

Nuts are a low glycemic food with a low available carbohydrate content, which makes them desirable as a snack or when consumed with carbohydrate-rich foods. Two studies using almonds have demonstrated that they are capable of lowering the postprandial glucose and insulin responses either consumed alone or in combination with carbohydrate-rich foods among persons with T2DM (Jenkins et al., 2006; Josse et al., 2007). Studies that have been conducted to date to evaluate the effect the role of nuts on long-term glycemic control (e.g., HgbA1c) have reported mixed findings, which may be due to the varying duration of T2DM and existing comorbidities among the study participants. In addition to dietary approaches that confer benefits for blood glucose control, it is also important to determine if nut intake can produce cardioprotective effects among this population of individuals that is at high risk of developing CHD. The liberalization of fat intake, more specifically MUFA, has been shown to be effective in optimizing dyslipidemia among persons with T2DM as compared to a diet containing a higher level of carbohydrate without affecting plasma insulin levels (Garg et al., 1992). Therefore, a study was conducted to evaluate the effect of consuming 2 ounces of mixed nuts (raw almonds, pistachios, walnuts, pecans, hazelnuts, peanuts, cashews, and macadamias) for 3 months as a source of daily fat intake on blood lipids and HbA1c in adults with T2DM (Jenkins et al., 2011). Compared to participants assigned to consume an isocaloric reference muffin or a half-dose of both muffin and mixed nuts, the participants consuming a full dose of mixed nuts had a reduced HbA1c (−0.21% absolute HbA1c, 95% CI −0.30 to −0.11, $P < .001$) and significant improvement in measures of dyslipidemia. The investigators concluded that the replacement of a food high in dietary starch with mixed nuts as a source of MUFA and PUFA favorably reduced both HbA1c and improved dyslipidemia among adults with T2DM. This study's findings contribute to the body of evidence that exists supporting the beneficial effects of nuts on blood lipids (Tapsell et al., 2004; Wien et al., 2014) and endothelial function (Ma et al., 2010) in persons with T2DM.

Conversely, other studies have found no benefits of nut consumption on blood lipid management in participants with T2DM (Lovejoy et al., 2002; Tapsell et al., 2009). Some possible reasons for the null findings found in some of the nut intervention trials is that the study participant's baseline LDL-C levels may be very low or the baseline HDL-C levels may be very high, which would make it difficult to attain statistically significant beneficial changes in the lipid levels. Further, use of a "heart healthy" control diet would also make it difficult to achieve statistically significant results using a nut intervention compared to a healthy control diet.

The role of tree nuts under isocaloric conditions on glycemic control was the focus of a systematic review and meta-analysis of 12 randomized controlled trials (RCTs) with 450 persons with T2DM (Viguiliouk et al., 2014). A pooled analysis for the endpoints HbA1c, fasting glucose, fasting insulin, and homeostasis model assessment of insulin resistance (HOMA-IR) in individuals with diabetes revealed that tree nuts at a median dose (MD) of 56 g/day significantly lowered HbA1c (MD = −0.07%, 95% CI −0.10% to −0.03%; P = .0003) and fasting glucose (MD = −0.15 mmol/L, 95% CI −0.27 to −0.02 mmol/L; P = .03) compared with tree nut–free control diets. Further, no significant treatment effects were demonstrated for fasting insulin and HOMA-IR; however, there was a favorable direction of effect for the tree nut inclusive diets.

3.3 Polycystic Ovary Syndrome

Since polycystic ovary syndrome (PCOS) is associated with insulin resistance, it is worth discussing the most notable findings of a randomized parallel design study that examined the effects of exchanging 31 g of habitual fats per 1800 kcal with 36 g/day walnuts versus 46 g/day almonds for 6 weeks on metabolic and endocrine parameters among 31 participants with PCOS (Kalgaonkar et al., 2011). Participants in the walnut group experienced a 6% reduction in LDL-C (P = .05) and an 11% reduction in apoB (P < .03) compared to the almond group. Additionally, walnut intake increased the insulin response by 26% as measured by an oral glucose tolerance test (P < .02). Further, increased levels of adiponectin were observed in both groups, walnuts increased sex hormone-binding globulin levels, and almonds reduced the free androgen index. Lastly, walnuts decreased the HbA1c from $5.7 \pm 0.1\%$ to $5.5 \pm 0.1\%$ (P < .001).

In light of the availability of continuous glucose monitoring devices and the discovery that the oxidative stress of hyperglycemia promotes glucose-mediated vascular damage and an increased risk for long-term complications, future studies should be designed to evaluate the daily glucose variations in participants with T2DM consuming nut-enriched snacks and meals.

4. Weight Management

Based on existing prevalence and trend data for 2015, at least one-third of the world's adult population are classified as overweight or obese (Seidell and Halberstadt, 2015). Further, the prevalence of obesity is on a trajectory in low- and middle-income countries compared to high-income countries. Global overweight and obesity ("globesity") is a public health crisis that negatively influences the population's health and quality of life and adds a considerably financial burden to national healthcare budgets.

A common perception by the general public is that foods containing fat promote obesity. Although the fat content of nuts ranges from 49% to 76%, the majority of the fat comes from MUFA and PUFA. Additionally, nuts are a source of protein and fiber, which are characteristics known to increase satiety and prolong feelings of fullness after consumption (Burton-Freeman, 2000; Holt et al., 1995). Thus, the role of nuts in weight management continues to be investigated as a nutrient dense food that may be a useful adjunct for individuals struggling with weight management.

4.1 Epidemiological Studies

The association between frequent nut consumption and BMI has been previously investigated in four large epidemiological studies. The investigative team of the Adventist Health Study-1 was the first to report their findings of a statistically significant lower BMI with higher frequency of nut consumption among 31,208 Adventists residing in California (Fraser et al., 1992). Inverse trends between BMI and frequency of nut intake were also observed among women participants of the Nurses Health Study-1 (N=83,818) (Hu et al., 1998) and the Iowa Women's Health Study (N=34,111) (Ellsworth et al., 2001). Alternatively, there was no association found between frequent nut consumption and BMI among the 21,454 male participants in the Physician's Health Study (Albert et al., 2002). Overall, the evidence from US-based epidemiological studies does not support the general public's concern that nuts may cause weight gain.

Similar findings showing an inverse association between BMI and frequent nut consumption from two large prospective cohort and cross-sectional trials have been reported. In the Seguimiento University de Navarra (SUN) trial, a Spanish prospective cohort study designed in collaboration with the Harvard School of Public Health, participants (N=8865) that consumed nuts ≥2 times per week had a 31% reduced risk of gaining ≥2.5 kg during 28 months of follow-up, and frequent nut consumption yielded an average 0.42 kg less weight gain versus participants who rarely consumed nuts after multivariate adjustment (Bes-Rastrollo et al., 2007). Women participants in the Nurses Health Study (N=51,188) that reported consuming nuts ≥2 times per week had 0.4 kg less mean weight gain compared to women that rarely consumed nuts (Bes-Rastrollo et al., 2009). Further, consumption of nuts ≥2 times per week was associated with a 23% lower risk of obesity (hazard ratio 0.77, 95% CI 0.57–1.02). Lastly, cross-sectional findings from 847 participants enrolled in the PREDIMED study showed that BMI and waist circumference (WC) were inversely associated with frequent nut consumption (Casas-Agustench et al., 2011). More specifically, regression coefficients of nut intake versus BMI and WC variables predicted a decrease of 0.78 kg/m^2 and 2.1 cm, respectively, for each 30 g/day serving of nuts.

The following four plausible reasons have been postulated to explain why nut consumption is inversely associated with BMI in free-living individuals (Sabaté, 2003): reverse causation; higher physical activity or resting metabolic rate; increased satiety and corresponding diminished intake of other foods (e.g., dietary compensation); and reduced bioaccessibility of energy from nuts. First, reverse causation is possible since individuals with a normal BMI may have reduced inhibitions about consuming energy-dense nuts, whereas overweight or obese individuals may avoid nuts due to their high fat and energy content. Second, evidence from the Nurses Health Study (Hu et al., 1998) and the Physicians' Health Study (Albert et al., 2002) has shown nut consumption to be associated with engagement in higher levels of physical activity. Alternatively, a 6-month study that supplemented the habitual diet of free-living participants with almonds did not find any change in self-reported vigorous exercise (Fraser et al., 2002). Regarding resting metabolic activity, an 11% increase in resting energy expenditure was observed in 15 subjects after 19 weeks of peanut supplementation (Alper and Mattes, 2002); however, no changes in resting energy expenditure have been reported in two separate almond supplementation trials (Fraser et al., 2002; Hollis and Mattes, 2007). Third, the lack of predicted weight gain may be partially attributed to the dietary compensation that has been observed in nut trials of varying duration. In a 6-month almond supplementation trial among free-living participants, 54%–78% of the additional energy from almonds was displaced by reduced consumption of other foods (Fraser et al., 2002), which was consistent with the findings from a peanut supplementation trial of 8 weeks duration (Alper and Mattes, 2002). These compensatory findings may be a result of the satiating attributes in nuts (e.g., low glycemic index, good protein and fiber content). Fourth, the first indication of fecal fat loss from whole peanut intake was observed in 1980 (Levine and Silvis, 1980). Participants that consumed whole peanuts excreted 17% of the dietary fat in their stool compared to only 4%–7% fat excretion while consuming peanut butter. During a pecan feeding trial, participants excreted 8% of dietary fat in their stools compared to only 3% during the nut-free control diet (Rajaram et al., 2001). Further, three studies conducted at the Beltsville Human Nutrition Research Center that were supported by the US Department of Agriculture have shown that 5%, 23%, and 21% of the energy from pistachios, almonds, and walnuts is unabsorbed, respectively (Baer et al., 2012, 2015; Novotny et al., 2012).

4.2 Nut Intervention Trials

Four trials have been conducted to date that explored the effect on body weight of supplementing habitual diets with nuts in free-living subjects without providing dietary guidance or energy restriction (Alper and Mattes, 2002; Fraser et al., 2002; Hollis and Mattes, 2007; Sabaté et al., 2005). The amount of peanuts, almonds, or walnuts that were provided for daily consumption ranged between approximately 230 and 500 kcal, and study duration ranged from 8 weeks to 6 months. No significant increases or changes in body weight were observed after consumption of the nut diets compared to the corresponding control diet periods.

Four RCTs have also been conducted to date that investigated the effect of nut intake within structured weight loss programs (Foster et al., 2012; Li et al., 2010; Pelkman et al., 2004; Wien et al., 2003), but only one of these four trials also evaluated the effect of nut intake during a structured weight maintenance program (Foster et al., 2012). In 2003, the findings from a study that was designed to evaluate the effectiveness of using raw or dry roasted almonds with a liquid formula–based low calorie diet versus a liquid formula–based low calorie diet with self-selected complex carbohydrate foods among 65 overweight and overweight were reported (Wien et al., 2003). The participants in the almond group lost an average of 18% body weight compared to an 11% loss of body weight in the complex carbohydrate group over the 24-week study duration. A more recent almond trial was conducted with 123 overweight and obese participants randomized to an almond-enriched hypocaloric diet or a nut-free hypocaloric diet for 6 months with an additional 12 months of weight maintenance follow-up (Foster et al., 2012). Greater weight loss was observed in the nut-free group after 6 months; however, clinically significant and equivalent weight loss was observed at 18 months. Further, the almond-enriched group experienced significantly great improvements in blood lipids (TC, TC:HDL-C, and TG). Similarly, trials using pistachios or peanuts failed to show differences in weight change as compared to their respective nut-free control diets; however, the nut-enriched diets resulted in an improvement in blood lipids (Li et al., 2010; Pelkman et al., 2004). Hence, the inclusion of nuts in portion-controlled amounts does not lead to weight gain as long as total daily energy level is controlled, and nut intake may confer an improvement in markers of cardiovascular disease risk among select populations.

5. Metabolic Syndrome

Metabolic syndrome (MetS) is defined by a constellation of several associated physiological, biochemical, clinical, and metabolic factors that directly increases the risk of atherosclerotic CVD, T2DM, and all-cause mortality (Wilson et al., 2005). The prevalence of MetS ranges from <10% to 84%, depending on the region, urban or rural environment, demographic composition (e.g., gender, age, race, and ethnicity) of the population studied, and the diagnostic criteria that is used to define MetS (Desroches and Lamarche, 2007). Currently, the International Diabetes Federation (IDF) estimates that 25% of the world's adult population has MetS (International Diabetes Federation, 2006).

5.1 Epidemiological Studies

Consistent with the body of epidemiological evidence supportive of the protective role of nuts in the development of CHD, T2DM, and obesity, there is emerging evidence to suggest a role of nuts in the prevention of MetS and other cardiometabolic conditions. A cross-sectional study of 13,292 participants in the 1999–2004 National Health and Examination Survey (NHANES) found that nut consumption (greater than or equal to one-fourth ounce per day) was associated with a reduced BMI, WC, systolic blood pressure, hypertension, and low HDL-C (all $P<.05$) as compared to no nut consumption (O'Neil et al., 2011). Further, participants consuming tree nuts had a reduced prevalence of four MetS risk factors (abdominal obesity, hypertension, low HDL-C, and high fasting glucose) and a lower prevalence of MetS ($21.2 \pm 2.1\%$ vs. $26.6 \pm 0.7\%$, $P<.05$).

The investigative team of the Adventist Health Study-2 (AHS-2) explored the association of a wide range of tree nut and peanut intake and incidence of MetS among 803 participants enrolled in the AHS-2 Calibration Substudy (Jaceldo-Siegl et al., 2014). Thirty-two percent of the participants had a diagnosis of MetS using the criteria established by the American Heart Association and the National Heart, Lung, and Blood Institute diagnostic criteria. Compared to low consumers of tree nuts and peanuts, odds ratios (95% CI) for MetS were 0.77 (0.47, 1.28), 0.65 (0.42, 1.00), and 0.68 (0.43, 1.07) for low tree nut/high peanut, high tree nut/high peanut, and high tree nut/low peanut intake, respectively. Further, tree nut intake at a frequency of once per week was inversely associated with MetS (3% less for tree nuts and 2% less for total nuts). Thus, tree nuts were found to have a strong inverse association with MetS independent of demographic, lifestyle, and dietary factors.

The PREDIMED team also conducted a cross-sectional study of 7210 participants (mean age of 67 years) to evaluate the association between frequency of nut consumption (<1, 1–3, and >3 servings per week) and prevalence of cardiometabolic risk factors (Ibarrola-Jurado et al., 2013). The operational definition of MetS was based upon a blend of the ATP III and IDF criteria. Participants consuming more than three servings of nuts on a weekly basis had lower adjusted odds ratios compared to those consuming less than one serving per week for obesity (OR 0.61; 95% CI 0.54, 0.68; P-trend <.0001), MetS (OR 0.74; 95% CI 0.65, 0.85; P-trend <.0001) and diabetes (OR 0.87; 95% CI 0.78–0.99; P-trend = .043). Additionally, frequent nut intake was associated with a reduced risk of the abdominal obesity MetS criterion (OR 0.68; 95% CI 0.60, 0.79; P-trend <.001) in the context of no significant associations observed for hypertension, dyslipidemia, or elevated fasting glucose. Lastly, the long-term relationship between tree nut consumption and risk of developing MetS was evaluated among the 9887 Spanish university graduates participating in the SUN Project prospective cohort study (Fernandez-Montero et al., 2013). Using the same operational definition of MetS as the PREDIMED team, participants who consumed ≥2 servings of nuts weekly after 6 years of follow-up had a 32% reduced risk of developing MetS as compared to those who never or rarely consumed nuts (adjusted OR = 0.68; 95% CI 0.50, 0.92).

5.2 Nut Intervention Trials

Studies exploring the effect of a combination of a specific nut(s) on the status of MetS are slowing emerging. The PREDIMED team compared the 1-year effects of three diets as follows: a Mediterranean diet supplemented with 30 g/day of mixed nuts; a Mediterranean diet supplemented with 1 L/week of virgin olive oil (VOO); and a low-fat diet (Salas-Salvado et al., 2008). Approximately 61% of participants (*N* = 1224) met the criteria for MetS. After 1 year of follow-up, MetS prevalence was reduced by 6.7%, 13.7%, and 2.0% in the Mediterranean diet with VOO, Mediterranean diet with mixed nuts, and the control low-fat diet, respectively. The authors concluded that a

Mediterranean diet enriched with mixed nuts can be an effective dietary approach in the management of MetS.

A systematic review and meta-analysis of RCTs reporting at least one criterion of the MetS was conducted to evaluate the effect of tree nuts on MetS criteria (Blanco Mejia et al., 2014). Forty-nine RCTs of ≥3 weeks duration met the eligibility criteria and included 2226 participants who were healthy or had dyslipidemia, MetS, or T2DM. The tree nut interventions reduced TG and fasting glucose as compared to the control diet interventions. Further, no adverse effects were observed for WC, HDL-C, or blood pressure.

6. Cognition

The consumption of a Mediterranean diet has been shown to be associated with a lower rate of dementia (Feart et al., 2009) and other neurodegenerative diseases such as Alzheimer's disease (AD) (Scarmeas et al., 2006). During the aging process the central nervous system is highly susceptible to inflammation and oxidative stress, which may lead to the injury or death of neurons and increase the risk of developing neurodegenerative diseases (Floyd and Hensley, 2002; Joseph et al., 2009). Therefore, antioxidant-rich foods may have the potential to preserve cognitive function.

Studies that have been published to date that were designed to evaluate the effect of nuts on cognition have predominantly used walnuts, which are a rich source of neuroprotective compounds (e.g., polyphenols, alpha-linolenic acid, melatonin, folate, vitamin E). The main component of the amyloid plaques in the brains of patients with AD is amyloid beta-protein (Chauhan et al., 2004), which has been shown in cell line studies to undergo reduced oxidative stress and apoptosis with exposure to walnut extract (Muthaiyah et al., 2011). Cellular (Willis et al., 2010) and animal studies (Willis et al., 2009) have shown beneficial effects of walnut oil extract or ground English walnuts on brain cells and cognitive behavior in aged rats, respectively.

6.1 Epidemiological Studies

Human studies are emerging suggesting that the naturally occurring phenolic compounds found in nuts may have the potential to inhibit or slow down neurodegeneration and improve cognitive function. The long-term effect of nut intake on cognitive function was evaluated among 15,467 women age 70 years or older that were participating in the Nurses Health Study-1 (O'Brien et al., 2014). Four telephone-based cognitive interviews were conducted using several cognitive tests over 6 years in parallel with the administration of a validated food frequency questionnaire to assess nut consumption. Better mean cognitive status was observed among participants reporting a higher long-term total nut intake, and participants consuming ≥5 servings of nuts per week had higher global composite scores that combined all of the cognitive tests. More specifically, a mean difference of 0.08 was observed, which is equivalent to the mean difference found between women 2 years apart in age.

A cross-sectional study using 24-h diet recalls from a representative weighted sample of adults aged 20–90 years participating in the 1988–1994 and 1999–2002 NHANES rounds was conducted to evaluate the association between walnut consumption and cognitive function (O'Brien et al., 2014). Higher daily walnut intake was associated with better cognitive functioning in participants 20–59 years and those 60 years and older, suggesting that consuming walnuts on a daily basis may be beneficial to brain health across the life cycle.

To evaluate whether the consumption of antioxidant-rich foods is associated with cognitive function in an elderly population at high cardiovascular risk, the PREDIMED team administered neuropsychological tests to 447 of their participants (52% women; aged 55–80 years) (Valls-Pedret et al., 2012). Better memory function and global cognition were observed in the participants with higher intakes of olive oil, coffee, wine, and walnuts. Further, increased intake of walnuts, but not of other nuts, was associated with better working memory scores.

6.2 Nut Intervention Trials

To explore the effects of daily walnut supplementation on cognitive performance among young adults, a crossover design approach was utilized with a 6-week washout period between 8 weeks of walnut supplementation (60 g/day) versus an 8-week walnut-free period (Pribis et al., 2012). Although no effect on mood, nonverbal reasoning, or memory was found, significant increases in inferential verbal reasoning occurred after the walnut supplementation period. Hence, small improvements associated with walnut intake in cognitively intact young adults could translate into important outcomes among aging populations. However, further studies are needed because this is the only study that has been conducted to date, and it has yielded mixed findings.

7. Conclusion and Future Trends

Although nuts have been a part of the human diet for thousands of years, we are only beginning to understand how the components in nuts influence health. Nuts clearly have many health benefits; however, more research is needed to further our knowledge of the health effects of nuts and the underlying mechanisms involved.

Nuts are typically placed in the "protein category" when dietary guidelines are released for professionals to assist individuals in making food choices to achieve a healthy and nutritionally adequate diet. Further, 1 ounce of tree nuts can contribute toward the percent daily value (%DV) of macronutrient and micronutrient goals (Table 15.3). Interestingly, approximately 60% of the nuts consumed in the United States are consumed as snacks (King et al., 2008), which has fueled the idea to position nuts and seeds into a separate category when dietary guidelines are being developed in the future. Building the scientific evidence base through continued nut research will provide additional information for future dietary guidelines committees to consider for positioning and promoting nuts to improve the health of the world's population.

Table 15.3 Nutrients and %DV in 1 oz of Tree Nuts[a]

Nutrient	Units	Almonds	Brazils	Cashews	Hazelnuts	Macadamias	Pecans	Pine Nuts[b]	Pistachios	Walnuts
	# of kernels/oz	23	6	18	21	10–12	19 halves	167	49	14 halves
Calories	kcal	160	190	160	180	200	200	190	160	190
Protein	g	6	4	4	4	2	3	4	6	4
Total fat	g	14	19	13	17	22	20	20	13	18
Saturated fat	g	1	4.5	3	1.5	3.5	2	1.5	1.5	1.5
Monounsaturated fat	g	9	7	8	13	17	12	5.5	7	2.5
Polyunsaturated fat	g	3.5	7	2	2	0.5	6	10	4	13
Linoleic acid (18:2)	g	3.5	7	2	2	0.5	6	9	3.5	11
Linolenic acid (18:3)	g	0	0	0	0	0	0.5	0	0	2.5
Cholesterol	mg	0	0	0	0	0	0	0	0	0
Carbohydrate	g	6	3	9	5	4	4	4	8	4
Fiber	g	4	2	1	3	2	3	1	3	2
Calcium	mg (%DV)	76 (8)	45 (4)	13 (0)	32 (4)	20 (2)	20 (2)	5 (0)	30 (4)	28 (2)
Iron	mg (%DV)	1.05 (6)	0.69 (4)	1.7 (10)	1.33 (8)	0.75 (4)	0.72 (4)	1.57 (8)	1.14 (6)	0.82 (4)
Magnesium	mg (%DV)	77 (20)	107 (25)	74 (20)	46 (10)	33 (8)	34 (8)	71 (18)	31 (8)	45 (10)
Phosphorus	mg (%DV)	136 (15)	206 (20)	139 (15)	82 (8)	56 (6)	79 (8)	163 (16)	133 (15)	98 (10)
Potassium	mg (%DV)	208 (6)	187 (4)	160 (4)	193 (6)	103 (2)	116 (4)	169 (4)	285 (8)	125 (4)
Sodium	mg (%DV)	0 (0)	1 (0)	5 (0)	0 (0)	1 (0)	0 (0)	1 (0)	2 (0)	1 (0)
Zinc	mg (%DV)	0.88 (6)	1.15 (8)	1.59 (10)	0.69 (4)	0.37 (2)	1.28 (8)	1.83 (12)	0.66 (4)	0.88 (6)
Copper	mg (%DV)	0.29 (15)	0.49 (25)	0.63 (30)	0.49 (25)	0.16 (8)	0.34 (15)	0.38 (20)	0.37 (20)	0.45 (25)
Manganese	mg (%DV)	0.62 (30)	0.35 (15)	0.23 (10)	1.75 (90)	0.86 (45)	1.28 (60)	2.5 (120)	0.35 (20)	0.97 (50)
Selenium	mcg (%DV)	1.2 (2)	543.5 (780)	3.3 (4)	0.7 (0)	3.3 (4)	1.1 (2)	0.2 (0)	2.8 (4)	1.4 (2)
Vitamin C	mg (%DV)	0 (0)	0.2 (0)	0 (0)	1.8 (2)	0.2 (0)	0.3 (0)	0.2 (0)	0.9 (2)	0.4 (0)
Thiamin	mg (%DV)	0.06 (4)	0.18 (12)	0.06 (4)	0.18 (10)	0.2 (15)	0.19 (10)	0.1 (6)	0.2 (15)	0.1 (6)
Riboflavin	mg (%DV)	0.32 (20)	0.01 (0)	0.06 (4)	0.03 (2)	0.03 (2)	0.04 (2)	0.06 (4)	0.07 (4)	0.04 (2)
Niacin	mg (%DV)	1.03 (6)	0.08 (0)	0.4 (2)	0.51 (2)	0.65 (4)	0.33 (2)	1.24 (6)	0.39 (2)	0.32 (2)
Pantothenic acid	mg (%DV)	0.13 (2)	0.05 (0)	0.35 (4)	0.26 (2)	0.17 (2)	0.25 (2)	0.09 (0)	0.15 (2)	0.16 (2)
Vitamin B6	mg (%DV)	0.04 (2)	0.03 (0)	0.07 (4)	0.16 (8)	0.1 (6)	0.06 (2)	0.03 (0)	0.32 (15)	0.15 (8)
Folate	mcg (%DV)	12 (4)	6 (2)	20 (4)	32 (8)	3 (0)	6 (2)	10 (2)	14 (4)	28 (6)
Choline, total	mg (%DV)	14.8 (2)	8.2 (0)	17.3 (4)	12.9 (2)	12.6 (2)	11.5 (2)	15.8 (2)	20.2 (4)	11.1 (2)
Betaine	mg	0.1	0.1	n/a	0.1	0.1	0.2	0.1	0.2	0.1
Vitamin B12	mcg (%DV)	0 (0)	0 (0)	0 (0)	0 (0)	0 (0)	0 (0)	0 (0)	0 (0)	0 (0)
Vitamin A	IU (%DV)	1 (0)	0 (0)	0 (0)	6 (0)	0 (0)	16 (0)	8 (0)	75 (2)	6 (0)

Vitamin K	mcg	0	0	9.8	4	0	1	15.3	3.7	0.8
Vitamin D	IU (%DV)	0 (0)	0 (0)	0 (0)	0 (0)	0 (0)	0 (0)	0 (0)	0 (0)	0 (0)
Vitamin E	(%DV)	(35)	(8)	(0)	(20)	(0)	(2)	(10)	(2)	(0)
Tocopherol, alpha	mg	7.27	1.60	0.26	4.26	0.16	0.40	2.65	0.62	0.20
Tocopherol, beta	mg	0.07	0	n/a	0.09	0	0.11	0	0.04	0.04
Tocopherol, gamma	mg	0.18	2.71	n/a	0	0	6.93	3.16	6.64	5.91
Tocopherol, delta	mg	0.02	0.18	n/a	0	0	0.13	0	0.16	0.54
Carotenoids										
Carotene, beta	mcg	0	0	0	3	0	8	5	45	3
Carotene, alpha	mcg	0	0	0	1	0	0	0	0	0
Cryptoxanthin, beta	mcg	0	0	0	0	0	3	0	0	0
Lutein+zeaxanthin	mcg	0	0	7	26	0	5	3	329	3

[a]All of the nuts are unsalted; almonds, Brazil nuts, hazelnuts, pecans, pine nuts and walnuts are unroasted; cashews, macadamias and pistachios are dry roasted.
[b]Pignolia variety.

%DV, % daily value; *g*, gram; *IU*, International Unit; *mcg*, microgram; *mg*, milligram.
USDA National Nutrient Database for Standard Reference, Release 28, Full Report, 2015. Prepared by the International Tree Nut Council Nutrition Research & Education Foundation, 10/15.

References

Adeghate, E., Schattner, P., Dunn, E., 2006. An update on the etiology and epidemiology of diabetes mellitus. Ann. N. Y. Acad. Sci. 1084, 1–29.

Albert, C.M., Gaziano, J.M., Willett, W.C., Manson, J.E., 2002. Nut consumption and decreased risk of sudden cardiac death in the Physicians' Health Study. Arch. Intern. Med. 162, 1382–1387.

Alper, C.M., Mattes, R.D., 2002. Effects of chronic peanut consumption on energy balance and hedonics. Int. J. Obes. Relat. Metab. Disord. 26, 1129–1137.

Baer, D.J., Gebauer, S.K., Novotny, J.A., 2012. Measured energy value of pistachios in the human diet. Br. J. Nutr. 107, 120–125.

Baer, D.J., Gebauer, S.K., Novotny, J.A., 2015. Walnuts consumed by healthy adults provide less available energy than predicted by the Atwater factors. J. Nutr. 146.

Banel, D.K., Hu, F.B., 2009. Effects of walnut consumption on blood lipids and other cardiovascular risk factors: a meta-analysis and systematic review. Am. J. Clin. Nutr. 90, 56–63.

Bes-Rastrollo, M., Sabaté, J., Gomez-Gracia, E., Alonso, A., Martinez, J.A., Martinez-Gonzalez, M.A., 2007. Nut consumption and weight gain in a Mediterranean cohort: the SUN study. Obesity (Silver Spring) 15, 107–116.

Bes-Rastrollo, M., Wedick, N.M., Martinez-Gonzalez, M.A., Li, T.Y., Sampson, L., Hu, F.B., 2009. Prospective study of nut consumption, long-term weight change, and obesity risk in women. Am. J. Clin. Nutr. 89, 1913–1919.

Blanco Mejia, S., Kendall, C.W., Viguiliouk, E., Augustin, L.S., Ha, V., Cozma, A.I., Mirrahimi, A., Maroleanu, A., Chiavaroli, L., Leiter, L.A., De Souza, R.J., Jenkins, D.J., Sievenpiper, J.L., 2014. Effect of tree nuts on metabolic syndrome criteria: a systematic review and meta-analysis of randomised controlled trials. BMJ Open 4, e004660.

Bolling, B.W., Mckay, D.L., Blumberg, J.B., 2010. The phytochemical composition and antioxidant actions of tree nuts. Asia Pac. J. Clin. Nutr. 19, 117–123.

Burton-Freeman, B., 2000. Dietary fiber and energy regulation. J. Nutr. 130, 272S–275S.

Canales, A., Benedi, J., Nus, M., Librelotto, J., Sanchez-Montero, J.M., Sanchez-Muniz, F.J., 2007. Effect of walnut-enriched restructured meat in the antioxidant status of overweight/obese senior subjects with at least one extra CHD-risk factor. J. Am. Coll. Nutr. 26, 225–232.

Casas-Agustench, P., Bullo, M., Ros, E., Basora, J., Salas-Salvado, J., Nureta, P.I., 2011. Cross-sectional association of nut intake with adiposity in a Mediterranean population. Nutr. Metab. Cardiovasc. Dis. 21, 518–525.

Chauhan, N., Wang, K.C., Wegiel, J., Malik, M.N., 2004. Walnut extract inhibits the fibrillization of amyloid beta-protein, and also defibrillizes its preformed fibrils. Curr. Alzheimer Res. 1, 183–188.

Davis, L., Stonehouse, W., Loots Du, T., Mukuddem-Petersen, J., Van Der Westhuizen, F.H., Hanekom, S.M., Jerling, J.C., 2007. The effects of high walnut and cashew nut diets on the antioxidant status of subjects with metabolic syndrome. Eur. J. Nutr. 46, 155–164.

Desroches, S., Lamarche, B., 2007. The evolving definitions and increasing prevalence of the metabolic syndrome. Appl. Physiol. Nutr. Metab. 32, 23–32.

Eaton, S.B., Konner, M., 1985. Paleolithic nutrition. A consideration of its nature and current implications. N. Engl. J. Med. 312, 283–289.

Ellsworth, J.L., Kushi, L.H., Folsom, A.R., 2001. Frequent nut intake and risk of death from coronary heart disease and all causes in postmenopausal women: the Iowa Women's Health Study. Nutr. Metab. Cardiovasc. Dis. 11, 372–377.

Feart, C., Samieri, C., Rondeau, V., Amieva, H., Portet, F., Dartigues, J.F., Scarmeas, N., Barberger-Gateau, P., 2009. Adherence to a Mediterranean diet, cognitive decline, and risk of dementia. JAMA 302, 638–648.

Fernandez-Montero, A., Bes-Rastrollo, M., Beunza, J.J., Barrio-Lopez, M.T., De La Fuente-Arrillaga, C., Moreno-Galarraga, L., Martinez-Gonzalez, M.A., 2013. Nut consumption and incidence of metabolic syndrome after 6-year follow-up: the SUN (Seguimiento Universidad de Navarra, University of Navarra Follow-up) cohort. Public Health Nutr. 16, 2064–2072.

Floyd, R.A., Hensley, K., 2002. Oxidative stress in brain aging. Implications for therapeutics of neurodegenerative diseases. Neurobiol. Aging 23, 795–807.

Food and Drug Administration, 2003. Qualified Health Claims: Letter of Enforcement Discretion – Nuts and Coronary Heart Disease. Available from: http://www.fda.gov/Food/IngredientsPackagingLabeling/LabelingNutrition/ucm072926.htm.

Foster, G.D., Shantz, K.L., Vander Veur, S.S., Oliver, T.L., Lent, M.R., Virus, A., Szapary, P.O., Rader, D.J., Zemel, B.S., Gilden-Tsai, A., 2012. A randomized trial of the effects of an almond-enriched, hypocaloric diet in the treatment of obesity. Am. J. Clin. Nutr. 96, 249–254.

Fraser, G.E., Sabaté, J., Beeson, W.L., Strahan, T.M., 1992. A possible protective effect of nut consumption on risk of coronary heart disease. The Adventist Health Study. Arch. Intern. Med. 152, 1416–1424.

Fraser, G.E., Bennett, H.W., Jaceldo, K.B., Sabaté, J., 2002. Effect on body weight of a free 76 Kilojoule (320 calorie) daily supplement of almonds for six months. J. Am. Coll. Nutr. 21, 275–283.

Garg, A., Grundy, S.M., Unger, R.H., 1992. Comparison of effects of high and low carbohydrate diets on plasma lipoproteins and insulin sensitivity in patients with mild NIDDM. Diabetes 41, 1278–1285.

Guasch-Ferre, M., Bullo, M., Martinez-Gonzalez, M.A., Ros, E., Corella, D., Estruch, R., Fito, M., Aros, F., Warnberg, J., Fiol, M., Lapetra, J., Vinyoles, E., Lamuela-Raventos, R.M., Serra-Majem, L., Pinto, X., Ruiz-Gutierrez, V., Basora, J., Salas-Salvado, J., Group, P.S., 2013. Frequency of nut consumption and mortality risk in the PREDIMED nutrition intervention trial. BMC Med. 11, 164.

Hollis, J., Mattes, R., 2007. Effect of chronic consumption of almonds on body weight in healthy humans. Br. J. Nutr. 98, 651–656.

Holt, S.H., Miller, J.C., Petocz, P., Farmakalidis, E., 1995. A satiety index of common foods. Eur. J. Clin. Nutr. 49, 675–690.

Hu, F.B., Stampfer, M.J., Manson, J.E., Rimm, E.B., Colditz, G.A., Rosner, B.A., Speizer, F.E., Hennekens, C.H., Willett, W.C., 1998. Frequent nut consumption and risk of coronary heart disease in women: prospective cohort study. BMJ 317, 1341–1345.

Hudthagosol, C., Haddad, E.H., Mccarthy, K., Wang, P., Oda, K., Sabaté, J., 2011. Pecans acutely increase plasma postprandial antioxidant capacity and catechins and decrease LDL oxidation in humans. J. Nutr. 141, 56–62.

Ibarrola-Jurado, N., Bullo, M., Guasch-Ferre, M., Ros, E., Martinez-Gonzalez, M.A., Corella, D., Fiol, M., Warnberg, J., Estruch, R., Roman, P., Aros, F., Vinyoles, E., Serra-Majem, L., Pinto, X., Covas, M.I., Basora, J., Salas-Salvado, J., Investigators, P.S., 2013. Cross-sectional assessment of nut consumption and obesity, metabolic syndrome and other cardiometabolic risk factors: the PREDIMED study. PLoS One 8, e57367.

International Diabetes Federation, 2006. The IDF Consensus Worldwide Definition of the Metabolic Syndrome. Available from: http://www.idf.org/metabolic-syndrome.

International Nut and Dried Fruit Council, 2015. 2007–2012 Global Statistics Review. Available from: https://www.nutfruit.org/en/inc-global-statistical-review-reflects-the-continued-increase-of-the-global-consumption-of-nuts-and-dried-fruits_70983.

Iwamoto, M., Imaizumi, K., Sato, M., Hirooka, Y., Sakai, K., Takeshita, A., Kono, M., 2002. Serum lipid profiles in Japanese women and men during consumption of walnuts. Eur. J. Clin. Nutr. 56, 629–637.

Jaceldo-Siegl, K., Haddad, E., Oda, K., Fraser, G.E., Sabaté, J., 2014. Tree nuts are inversely associated with metabolic syndrome and obesity: the Adventist health study-2. PLoS One 9, e85133.

Jenkins, D.J., Kendall, C.W., Josse, A.R., Salvatore, S., Brighenti, F., Augustin, L.S., Ellis, P.R., Vidgen, E., Rao, A.V., 2006. Almonds decrease postprandial glycemia, insulinemia, and oxidative damage in healthy individuals. J. Nutr. 136, 2987–2992.

Jenkins, D.J., Kendall, C.W., Banach, M.S., Srichaikul, K., Vidgen, E., Mitchell, S., Parker, T., Nishi, S., Bashyam, B., De Souza, R., Ireland, C., Josse, R.G., 2011. Nuts as a replacement for carbohydrates in the diabetic diet. Diabetes Care 34, 1706–1711.

Jiang, R., Manson, J.E., Stampfer, M.J., Liu, S., Willett, W.C., Hu, F.B., 2002. Nut and peanut butter consumption and risk of type 2 diabetes in women. JAMA 288, 2554–2560.

Joseph, J., Cole, G., Head, E., Ingram, D., 2009. Nutrition, brain aging, and neurodegeneration. J. Neurosci. 29, 12795–12801.

Josse, A.R., Kendall, C.W., Augustin, L.S., Ellis, P.R., Jenkins, D.J., 2007. Almonds and postprandial glycemia – a dose-response study. Metabolism 56, 400–404.

Kalgaonkar, S., Almario, R.U., Gurusinghe, D., Garamendi, E.M., Buchan, W., Kim, K., Karakas, S.E., 2011. Differential effects of walnuts vs almonds on improving metabolic and endocrine parameters in PCOS. Eur. J. Clin. Nutr. 65, 386–393.

Kay, C.D., Gebauer, S.K., West, S.G., Kris-Etherton, P.M., 2010. Pistachios increase serum antioxidants and lower serum oxidized-LDL in hypercholesterolemic adults. J. Nutr. 140, 1093–1098.

Kelly Jr., J.H., Sabate, J., 2006. Nuts and coronary heart disease: an epidemiological perspective. Br. J. Nutr. 96 (Suppl. 2), S61–S67.

King, J.C., Blumberg, J., Ingwersen, L., Jenab, M., Tucker, K.L., 2008. Tree nuts and peanuts as components of a healthy diet. J. Nutr. 138, 1736S–1740S.

Kochar, J., Gaziano, J.M., Djousse, L., 2010. Nut consumption and risk of type II diabetes in the Physicians' Health Study. Eur. J. Clin. Nutr. 64, 75–79.

Levine, A.S., Silvis, S.E., 1980. Absorption of whole peanuts, peanut oil, and peanut butter. N. Engl. J. Med. 303, 917–918.

Li, Z., Song, R., Nguyen, C., Zerlin, A., Karp, H., Naowamondhol, K., Thames, G., Gao, K., Li, L., Tseng, C.H., Henning, S.M., Heber, D., 2010. Pistachio nuts reduce triglycerides and body weight by comparison to refined carbohydrate snack in obese subjects on a 12-week weight loss program. J. Am. Coll. Nutr. 29, 198–203.

Lovejoy, J.C., Most, M.M., Lefevre, M., Greenway, F.L., Rood, J.C., 2002. Effect of diets enriched in almonds on insulin action and serum lipids in adults with normal glucose tolerance or type 2 diabetes. Am. J. Clin. Nutr. 76, 1000–1006.

Ma, Y., Njike, V.Y., Millet, J., Dutta, S., Doughty, K., Treu, J.A., Katz, D.L., 2010. Effects of walnut consumption on endothelial function in type 2 diabetic subjects: a randomized controlled crossover trial. Diabetes Care 33, 227–232.

Maranhao, P.A., Kraemer-Aguiar, L.G., De Oliveira, C.L., Kuschnir, M.C., Vieira, Y.R., Souza, M.G., Koury, J.C., Bouskela, E., 2011. Brazil nuts intake improves lipid profile, oxidative stress and microvascular function in obese adolescents: a randomized controlled trial. Nutr. Metab. (Lond.) 8, 32.

Mukuddem-Petersen, J., Stonehouse Oosthuizen, W., Jerling, J.C., Hanekom, S.M., White, Z., 2007. Effects of a high walnut and high cashew nut diet on selected markers of the metabolic syndrome: a controlled feeding trial. Br. J. Nutr. 97, 1144–1153.

Muthaiyah, B., Essa, M.M., Chauhan, V., Chauhan, A., 2011. Protective effects of walnut extract against amyloid beta peptide-induced cell death and oxidative stress in PC12 cells. Neurochem. Res. 36, 2096–2103.

Novotny, J.A., Gebauer, S.K., Baer, D.J., 2012. Discrepancy between the Atwater factor predicted and empirically measured energy values of almonds in human diets. Am. J. Clin. Nutr. 96, 296–301.

O'Brien, J., Okereke, O., Devore, E., Rosner, B., Breteler, M., Grodstein, F., 2014. Long-term intake of nuts in relation to cognitive function in older women. J. Nutr. Health Aging 18, 496–502.

O'Neil, C.E., Keast, D.R., Nicklas, T.A., Fulgoni 3rd, V.L., 2011. Nut consumption is associated with decreased health risk factors for cardiovascular disease and metabolic syndrome in US adults: NHANES 1999–2004. J. Am. Coll. Nutr. 30, 502–510.

Parker, E.D., Harnack, L.J., Folsom, A.R., 2003. Nut consumption and risk of type 2 diabetes. JAMA 290, 38–39 author reply 39–40.

Pelkman, C.L., Fishell, V.K., Maddox, D.H., Pearson, T.A., Mauger, D.T., Kris-Etherton, P.M., 2004. Effects of moderate-fat (from monounsaturated fat) and low-fat weight-loss diets on the serum lipid profile in overweight and obese men and women. Am. J. Clin. Nutr. 79, 204–212.

Pribis, P., Bailey, R.N., Russell, A.A., Kilsby, M.A., Hernandez, M., Craig, W.J., Grajales, T., Shavlik, D.J., Sabaté, J., 2012. Effects of walnut consumption on cognitive performance in young adults. Br. J. Nutr. 107, 1393–1401.

Rajaram, S., Burke, K., Connell, B., Myint, T., Sabate, J., 2001. A monounsaturated fatty acid-rich pecan-enriched diet favorably alters the serum lipid profile of healthy men and women. J. Nutr. 131, 2275–2279.

Ros, E., Mataix, J., 2006. Fatty acid composition of nuts–implications for cardiovascular health. Br. J. Nutr. 96 (Suppl. 2), S29–S35.

Ros, E., Nunez, I., Perez-Heras, A., Serra, M., Gilabert, R., Casals, E., Deulofeu, R., 2004. A walnut diet improves endothelial function in hypercholesterolemic subjects: a randomized crossover trial. Circulation 109, 1609–1614.

Sabaté, J., Fraser, G.E., Burke, K., Knutsen, S.F., Bennett, H., Lindsted, K.D., 1993. Effects of walnuts on serum lipid levels and blood pressure in normal men. N. Engl. J. Med. 328, 603–607.

Sabaté, J., Cordero-Macintyre, Z., Siapco, G., Torabian, S., Haddad, E., 2005. Does regular walnut consumption lead to weight gain? Br. J. Nutr. 94, 859–864.

Sabaté, J., Oda, K., Ros, E., 2010. Nut consumption and blood lipid levels: a pooled analysis of 25 intervention trials. Arch. Intern. Med. 170, 821–827.

Sabaté, J., 1999. Nut consumption, vegetarian diets, ischemic heart disease risk, and all-cause mortality: evidence from epidemiologic studies. Am. J. Clin. Nutr. 70, 500S–503S.

Sabaté, J., 2003. Nut consumption and body weight. Am. J. Clin. Nutr. 78, 647S–650S.

Salas-Salvado, J., Fernandez-Ballart, J., Ros, E., Martinez-Gonzalez, M.A., Fito, M., Estruch, R., Corella, D., Fiol, M., Gomez-Gracia, E., Aros, F., Flores, G., Lapetra, J., Lamuela-Raventos, R., Ruiz-Gutierrez, V., Bullo, M., Basora, J., Covas, M.I., Investigators, P.S., 2008. Effect of a Mediterranean diet supplemented with nuts on metabolic syndrome status: one-year results of the PREDIMED randomized trial. Arch. Intern. Med. 168, 2449–2458.

Salas-Salvado, J., Bullo, M., Babio, N., Martinez-Gonzalez, M.A., Ibarrola-Jurado, N., Basora, J., Estruch, R., Covas, M.I., Corella, D., Aros, F., Ruiz-Gutierrez, V., Ros, E., Investigators, P.S., 2011. Reduction in the incidence of type 2 diabetes with the Mediterranean diet: results of the PREDIMED-Reus nutrition intervention randomized trial. Diabetes Care 34, 14–19.

Scarmeas, N., Stern, Y., Tang, M.X., Mayeux, R., Luchsinger, J.A., 2006. Mediterranean diet and risk for Alzheimer's disease. Ann. Neurol. 59, 912–921.

Segura, R., Javierre, C., Lizarraga, M.A., Ros, E., 2006. Other relevant components of nuts: phytosterols, folate and minerals. Br. J. Nutr. 96 (Suppl. 2), S36–S44.

Seidell, J.C., Halberstadt, J., 2015. The global burden of obesity and the challenges of prevention. Ann. Nutr. Metab. 66 (Suppl. 2), 7–12.

Shaw, J.E., Sicree, R.A., Zimmet, P.Z., 2010. Global estimates of the prevalence of diabetes for 2010 and 2030. Diabetes Res. Clin. Pract. 87, 4–14.

Tapsell, L.C., Gillen, L.J., Patch, C.S., Batterham, M., Owen, A., Bare, M., Kennedy, M., 2004. Including walnuts in a low-fat/modified-fat diet improves HDL cholesterol-to-total cholesterol ratios in patients with type 2 diabetes. Diabetes Care 27, 2777–2783.

Tapsell, L.C., Batterham, M.J., Teuss, G., Tan, S.Y., Dalton, S., Quick, C.J., Gillen, L.J., Charlton, K.E., 2009. Long-term effects of increased dietary polyunsaturated fat from walnuts on metabolic parameters in type II diabetes. Eur. J. Clin. Nutr. 63, 1008–1015.

Valls-Pedret, C., Lamuela-Raventos, R.M., Medina-Remon, A., Quintana, M., Corella, D., Pinto, X., Martinez-Gonzalez, M.A., Estruch, R., Ros, E., 2012. Polyphenol-rich foods in the Mediterranean diet are associated with better cognitive function in elderly subjects at high cardiovascular risk. J. Alzheimers Dis. 29, 773–782.

Viguiliouk, E., Kendall, C.W., Blanco Mejia, S., Cozma, A.I., Ha, V., Mirrahimi, A., Jayalath, V.H., Augustin, L.S., Chiavaroli, L., Leiter, L.A., De Souza, R.J., Jenkins, D.J., Sievenpiper, J.L., 2014. Effect of tree nuts on glycemic control in diabetes: a systematic review and meta-analysis of randomized controlled dietary trials. PLoS One 9, e103376.

Villegas, R., Gao, Y.T., Yang, G., Li, H.L., Elasy, T.A., Zheng, W., Shu, X.O., 2008. Legume and soy food intake and the incidence of type 2 diabetes in the Shanghai Women's Health Study. Am. J. Clin. Nutr. 87, 162–167.

Wien, M.A., Sabaté, J., Ikle, D.N., Cole, S.E., Kandeel, F.R., 2003. Almonds vs complex carbohydrates in a weight reduction program. Int. J. Obes. Relat. Metab. Disord. 27, 1365–1372.

Wien, M., Oda, K., Sabaté, J., 2014. A randomized controlled trial to evaluate the effect of incorporating peanuts into an American Diabetes Association meal plan on the nutrient profile of the total diet and cardiometabolic parameters of adults with type 2 diabetes. Nutr. J. 13, 10.

Willis, L.M., Shukitt-Hale, B., Cheng, V., Joseph, J.A., 2009. Dose-dependent effects of walnuts on motor and cognitive function in aged rats. Br. J. Nutr. 101, 1140–1144.

Willis, L.M., Bielinski, D.F., Fisher, D.R., Matthan, N.R., Joseph, J.A., 2010. Walnut extract inhibits LPS-induced activation of BV-2 microglia via internalization of TLR4: possible involvement of phospholipase D2. Inflammation 33, 325–333.

Wilson, P.W., D'agostino, R.B., Parise, H., Sullivan, L., Meigs, J.B., 2005. Metabolic syndrome as a precursor of cardiovascular disease and type 2 diabetes mellitus. Circulation 112, 3066–3072.

World Health Organization, 2012. Global Status Report on Noncommunicable Diseases 2014. Geneva.

Zambon, D., Sabaté, J., Munoz, S., Campero, B., Casals, E., Merlos, M., Laguna, J.C., Ros, E., 2000. Substituting walnuts for monounsaturated fat improves the serum lipid profile of hypercholesterolemic men and women. A randomized crossover trial. Ann. Intern. Med. 132, 538–546.

16

New Concepts and Paradigms for the Protective Effects of Plant-Based Food Components in Relation to Food Complexity

Anthony Fardet

INRA, UMR 1019, UNH, CRNH AUVERGNE, CLERMONT-FERRAND, FRANCE; CLERMONT UNIVERSITÉ, UNIVERSITÉ D'AUVERGNE, CLERMONT-FERRAND, FRANCE

1. Introduction

Plant-based foods are generally classified into fruits, vegetables, legumes, grains, nuts, and seeds; their derived processed counterparts such as breads, pasta, breakfast cereals, cooked and fermented vegetables and legumes, and fruit purées, juices, and jams; and their derived ingredients such as oleaginous seed–derived oils, sugars, and some herbs and spices. What differentiates them from animal-based foods is that their fiber fraction is made of indigestible compounds, mainly cellulose, hemicellulose, pectins, and/or resistant starch. Among grain products, legumes, cereals/pseudocereals, and nuts/seeds are characterized by their high carbohydrate, protein, and lipid contents, respectively. In addition to fiber, plant-based foods all possess macro- (proteins, lipids, and carbohydrates), micro- (minerals, trace elements, and vitamins), and phytonutrients (e.g., polyphenols and carotenoids). Each of them helps the plant to survive within its environment and reproduce itself.

By definition, a bioactive compound has biological effect within a human organism, tissues, or cells, being likely to have preventive effects toward pathophysiological processes. In plant-based foods, all compounds or nutrients are therefore potentially bioactive within human organisms, but their protective effect will depend on several factors such as the health status or physiological state, the degree of food processing, the presence of other compounds within the food matrix, and the quantity consumed. Even antinutritional factors, such as phytates, may have potential protective effects (Kumar et al., 2010), emphasizing the dual nature of plant bioactive compounds. Additionally, a bioactive compound is rarely protective alone but in synergy with other compounds, as emphasized with compounds with antioxidant (Fardet, 2015a,b; Wang et al., 2011) and lipotropic (Fardet and Chardigny, 2013) related properties.

Vegetarian and Plant-Based Diets in Health and Disease Prevention. http://dx.doi.org/10.1016/B978-0-12-803968-7.00016-2

Plant-based foods may be eaten raw, but most of the time, they undergo processing to render them secure, edible, and/or more palatable, especially grain-based foods. Processing may be minimal, such as soaking of leguminous seeds, to very drastic, such as extrusion-cooking of white cereal flour. Processing may also include the blending of plant-based foods with ingredients such as fats and cooking agents. In all cases, the potential package of bioactive compounds is obviously modified in different ways, either positively or negatively, notably when refining removes most of the minerals and vitamins in cereal products (Fardet, 2014d).

This chapter is not intended to review in detail each protective class of plant-based compounds. Many of these reviews can be easily found in the literature. Instead, this chapter is intended to develop and discuss some important concepts and paradigms of the protective effects of plant-based food components in relation to food complexity. This chapter is divided into three sections. In the first part, emphasis will be placed on the role of plant-based food structure in determining the protective effects of bioactive compounds. In the second part, the concept of synergy of biological effects will be developed, notably through examples of antioxidant and lipotropic packages. In the third part, the effect of processing on the bioactivity of protective compounds will be discussed, with a particular emphasis on thermal, refining, and fermentation treatments.

2. Plant-Based Food Groups and Their Bioactive Compounds: An Emphasis on Food Structure

It is not sufficient that a compound be present in plant-based foods to be protective; it has to be bioavailable within the human organism. Indeed, plant-based foods are more than the sum of nutrients; they are also complex structures involving more or less strong interactions between compounds that determine their bioaccessibility within the digestive tract and then their bioavailability (Fardet, 2014b, 2015c). Notably, the fiber fraction plays an important role in shaping plant-based food structure, conferring a very wide diversity of forms and physical properties that further condition nutrients' digestive fates and thus their health effects.

For example, considering wheat grain and excluding macronutrients, the fraction of bioactive compounds is more than 15% by weight including fiber, and of that, wheat bran is more than 50% by weight (Table 16.1; Fardet, 2010). However, due to the food structure, not all are fully bioavailable within the digestive tract.

In this section, the influence of the food structure of plant-based foods will be considered in its relation to the protective and health effects of their numerous bioactive nutrients, such as macro-, micro-, and phytonutrients.

2.1 Carbohydrates, Proteins, and Lipids

First, food structure plays an important role in the metabolic fate and health effects of macronutrients, i.e., carbohydrates, proteins, and lipids (Fardet et al., 2013).

Table 16.1 Average Percentages of the Major Bioactive Compounds in Whole Grain Wheat and Wheat Bran and Germ Fractions[a]

Bioactive Compound	Whole Grain Wheat (%)[b]	Wheat Bran (%)[b]	Wheat Germ (%)[b]
α-linolenic acid (18: 3n-3)	—[c]	0.16	0.53
Sulfur compounds	0.5	0.7	1.2
Total free glutathione[d]	0.007	0.038	0.270
Dietary fiber[e]	13.2	44.6	17.7
Lignins	1.9	5.6	1.5
Oligosaccharides[f]	1.9	3.7	10.1
Phytic acid	0.9	4.2	1.8
Minerals and trace elements	1.12	3.39	2.51
Vitamins	0.0138	0.0398	0.0394
B vitamins	0.0091	0.0303	0.0123
Vitamin E (tocopherols and tocotrienols)	0.0047	0.0095	0.0271
Carotenoids	0.00034	0.00072	—[c]
Polyphenols	0.15	1.10	>0.37
Phenolic acids	0.11	1.07	>0.07
Flavonoids	0.037	0.028	0.300
Lignans	0.0004	0.0050	0.0005
Alkylresorcinol	0.07	0.27	—[c]
Betaine	0.16	0.87	0.85
Total choline	0.12	0.17	0.24
Total free inositols (*myo*- and total *chiro*-inositols)	0.022	0.025	>0.011
Phytosterols	0.08	0.16	0.43
Policosanol + melatonin + *para*-aminobenzoic acid	0.00341	0.00290	>0.00186
Total	>15.4	51.5	>23.9
Subtotal (without dietary fiber)	>2.2	6.9	>6.2

[a]Mean percentages of bioactive compounds found in wheat bran, whole grain wheat and wheat germ are calculated as follows: % = (min.-value + max.-value)/2.

[b]Expressed as g/100 g of food.

[c]no data found.

[d]Total free glutathione is given as GSH (reduced form of glutathione) equivalents = GSH + (GSSG*2) (GSSG is the oxidized form of glutathione, i.e., glutathione disulfide).

[e]Dietary fiber content is measured according to the original or modified AOAC method (for details, see AACC, 2001, Association of Official Agricultural Chemists).

[f]Oligosaccharides include fructans, raffinose and stachyose.

From Fardet, A., 2010. New hypotheses for the health-protective mechanisms of whole-grain cereals: what is beyond fibre? Nutr. Res. Rev. 23, 65–134 with permission of Cambridge University Press.

2.1.1 The Carbohydrate Fraction

Carbohydrates in plant-based foods are mainly starch, fructose, glucose, sucrose, and other oligosaccharides such as raffinose and stachyose. Whereas simple sugars are generally more typical of fruits and, to a lesser extent, vegetables, starch is generally found in grain-based foods and tubers and needs to be gelatinized before eating.

The literature has shown that slowly digestible starch is more beneficial to health than rapidly digested starch, notably for controlling glucose homeostasis as in the case of diabetes (Miao et al., 2013). This feature can be achieved through several means. First, it can be achieved at the molecular level by limiting the degree of starch gelatinization (Holm et al., 1988). Second, it can be achieved at the microscopic level by entrapping starch within a fiber or protein network such as in leguminous seeds (Noah et al., 1998) and pasta (Fardet et al., 1998). Third, it can be achieved at the macroscopic level by increasing the particle size of the food eaten (Fardet, 2015c).

Concerning simple sugars, they appear more slowly released from intact complex foods than from more unstructured foods such as purées or refined juices, as notably shown with apples (Haber et al., 1977) and suggested by the comparisons of some glycemic index values of intact fruits versus juices (Foster-Powell et al., 2002). This difference has to be attributed to the role played by the fiber network trapping vegetable cells containing simple sugars, as the cell wall is more disrupted in fruit purées or juices than in the natural, complex food.

2.1.2 The Lipid Fraction

As for carbohydrates, the lipid fraction of plant-based foods may be more or less rapidly digested according to the food structure features. For example, chewing increases the release of lipids in almonds (Ellis et al., 2004), and the proportion of lipid lost in the stool is higher after 10 chews (44%) than after 40 chews (31%) in humans (Cassady et al., 2009). Similarly, higher fat losses were found after eating whole peanut seeds compared with peanut oil, butter, or flour, probably demonstrating reduced lipid availability (Traoret et al., 2008). These results suggest that most oilseeds could exhibit quite similar lipid digestive fate depending on food structure integrity (Fardet, 2015c). More generally, little is known about the effect of plant-based food structure on lipid bioavailability in humans.

2.1.3 The Protein Fraction

Protein fraction bioavailability in humans has been less studied than carbohydrate fraction bioavailability in relation to plant-based food structure. It is recognized that the cell wall may restrict protein accessibility by proteolytic enzymes, thus reducing amino acid bioavailability, as in leguminous seeds (Fardet et al., 2013). Antinutritional factors can also cause a reduction in protein bioavailability, as shown with vegetable peas (Habiba, 2002). In vitro, the increased protein digestibility of sorghum by including oral processing also indicates that physical breakdown of the plant cell walls and starch is important in enhancing protein digestibility and absorption in the small intestine (Lu et al., 2014). However, data in humans show that the availability and utilization of dietary protein vary little according to the presence of antinutritional factors or the nature and structure of the protein type (Mariotti et al., 2001).

2.2 Vitamins, Minerals, and Trace Elements

2.2.1 Vitamins

Plant-based foods are generally considered rich sources of vitamins, except for vitamin D (Japelt and Jakobsen, 2013) and vitamin B_{12} (Watanabe, 2007). Briefly, the main sources of B vitamins are whole grain–based foods; cereal germs; legumes; brown rice; some fresh vegetables, notably green leafy vegetables (rich in folates) such as spinach, watercress, green cabbage, mash, and other salads; and some dried fruits. Provitamin A (i.e., carotenes, precursor of vitamin A or retinol) is found primarily in colored plants, specifically orange, yellow, and green plants. Vitamin C (ascorbic acid) is found in high amounts in fruits and vegetables, specifically, citrus fruits, red berries (e.g., cassis, strawberries, and currants), papayas, guavas, and the green parts of leafy vegetables. Concerning vegetables, particularly good sources of vitamin C are peppers, watercress, spinach, cabbage, tomatoes, potatoes marketed before full maturity (i.e., "pommes de terre nouvelles"), onions, broccoli, parsley, chives, and sorrel. Vitamin E (notably tocopherols) is found mainly in oils (e.g., sunflower, corn, and grapeseed), margarines, oleaginous seeds (e.g., almonds and hazelnuts), green vegetables, and some other vegetables such as fennel, asparagus, and salsify. The main plant sources of vitamin K are cauliflower, brussels sprouts, red cabbage, sauerkraut, broccoli, spinach, asparagus, soya, and tomatoes. Plant-based foods do not significantly contain vitamin D. However, microalgae contain both vitamin D_3 and provitamin D_3, which suggests that vitamin D_3 exists in the plant kingdom, and vitamin D_2 and D_3 have also been identified in several plant species as a surprise to many (Japelt and Jakobsen, 2013).

Once the sources of vitamins are known, the real issue is their percent bioavailability within human organisms. This is a complex issue because bioavailability depends on many factors in relation to the individual, the form of the molecule, the food matrix, the presence and biological form of the fiber fraction and the degree of plant transformation. First, it is worth recalling that B vitamins may be present in both free and bound forms in plant-based foods, each form being likely to have a different digestive fate (Institute of Medicine, 1998). For example, vitamin B_6 (niacin) in mature cereal grains is largely bound and thus is only approximately 30% available (Institute of Medicine, 1998). No recent systematic reviews about vitamin B bioavailability from plant-based food sources could be found. However, a study in pigs with vitamin B_6 can provide an idea of vitamin B bioavailability because all B vitamins are water-soluble and are likely to behave similarly (Roth-Maier et al., 2002). The main results of that study showed that prececal digestibility of vitamin B_6 ranged from 51% to 91% from different food sources in the following order: cabbage > banana > fish > milk powder > brewer's yeast > soybeans > soybean meal > egg/corn > barley > wheat bran > rye. Only boiled brown rice had very low vitamin B_6 bioavailability at 16%. The authors concluded that the digestibility of vitamin B_6 from plant products (excluding rice) was on average 10% lower when compared with animal products (71% vs. 79%).

The absorption of β-carotene from plant sources has been reported to range from 5% to 65% in humans (Haskell, 2012). Otherwise, vitamin A equivalency ratios for β-carotene to vitamin A from plant sources range from 3.8:1 to 28:1 by weight (Haskell, 2012). It was also shown that the apparent uptake of β-carotene from raw vegetables in salads was significantly greater when salads were consumed with dressings containing

28 g fat compared with dressings with 6 g fat in US adults (Brown et al., 2004). In her review, Haskell also reported that "conversion to vitamin A decreases as the dose of β-carotene increases, but that absorption does not appear to be affected (Novotny et al., 2010)" (Haskell, 2012).

Vitamin C bioavailability percentages from plant-based foods have not been reviewed yet. In the most recent review discussing vitamin C bioavailability from kiwifruit (one of the richest sources), Vissers et al. (2013) concluded that vitamin C "plasma levels generally reflect the amount consumed, regardless of its origin." In an older study carried out in 68 male nonsmokers, the relative bioavailability of ascorbic acid from several sources (i.e., tablets with or without iron, orange segments or juice, and raw or cooked broccoli) was compared (Mangels et al., 1993). The authors reported that ascorbic acid seems to be equally bioavailable from all sources and that the "lower relative bioavailability of ascorbic acid from raw broccoli is unlikely to be of practical importance in mixed diets" (Mangels et al., 1993).

In a recent review, it was concluded that the efficiency of vitamin E absorption is widely variable, though not accurately known (i.e., between 10% and 79%), and it is affected by several dietary factors (e.g., food matrix) (Borel et al., 2013), particularly the amount of fat in the meal, as has been seen for provitamin A (Bruno et al., 2006).

No review of percent bioavailability of vitamin K (or phylloquinone) from plant sources could be found. However, the study by Garber et al. (1999) gives some interesting indications. Over a 9-h period in 22- to 30-year-old human subjects, their results showed that the absorption of phylloquinone was higher after the consumption of a 500 μg phylloquinone tablet (27.55 ± 10.08 nmol/(L h), $n=8$) than after the ingestion of 495 μg phylloquinone as 150 g of raw spinach (4.79 ± 1.11 nmol/(L h), $n=3$) (Garber et al., 1999). Finally, there was no significant difference in the absorption of phylloquinone from fresh spinach, fresh broccoli, or fresh romaine lettuce and no difference in phylloquinone absorption from fresh or cooked broccoli or from fresh romaine lettuce consumed with a meal containing 30% or 45% energy as fat.

2.2.2 Minerals and Trace Elements

As for vitamins, plant-based foods are generally considered good and diversified sources of minerals and trace elements. The main concern is the presence of phytates that are well-known to chelate or trap minerals and/or trace elements, thus limiting their bioavailability within the human organism (Lopez et al., 2002). Thus, in some African populations consuming monotonous diets based on unrefined cereals and/or legumes, which are otherwise rich in phytates, mineral deficiencies have been observed (Harinarayan et al., 2007; Reinhold, 1971; Sandstead and Freeland-Graves, 2014) as a consequence of reduced dietary diversity that has led to biofortification of staple crops (Keatinge et al., 2011). As reported by Gibson et al. (2010) "dephytinization techniques were able to potentially enhance mineral absorption, but probably not to an extent sufficient to overcome deficits in iron, zinc and calcium contents of plant-based complementary foods used in low-income countries."

Contrary to vitamins, there are more reviews about minerals and trace elements and their bioavailability from plant-based foods, such as zinc (Hambidge et al., 2010), iron (Hurrell and Egli, 2010), selenium (Fairweather-Tait et al., 2010), and calcium (Camara-Martos and Amaro-Lopez, 2002; Gueguen and Pointillart, 2000). Bioavailability percentages may vary considerably depending on plant sources, presence of phytates, the nature of coingested foods, the physiological status of subjects, and other factors.

2.3 Fiber- and Phenolic-Type Compounds, Carotenoids, and Other Bioactive Phytochemicals

2.3.1 Fiber-Type Components

Today, there are several definitions for fiber (Jones, 2014). As stated by Jones, "Currently, existing definitions may fail to capture all the nondigestible material in food" (Jones, 2013). However, taking a very broad perspective, one can consider that fiber-type compounds include all plant-based compounds that escape digestion to reach the colon, mainly soluble and insoluble fibers and resistant starch, but also other phytonutrients, such as lignin and polyphenols, and some lipids and proteins that remain undigested. For example, as presented earlier, important lipid fractions have been observed in the stool of subjects consuming almonds with different degrees of chewing (Cassady et al., 2009).

Although not digested within the upper digestive tract, fibers are a highly diversified package of bioactive and protective compounds. The main concern of this chapter is not to review the concept of fiber or to describe the fiber content of plant-based foods. What appears more interesting is two current issues surrounding fiber that deserve to be further studied.

2.3.1.1 SOLUBLE VERSUS INSOLUBLE FIBER

The first issue is the dual nature of fiber: either soluble or insoluble. Such a feature is crucial because it will determine the fermentative fate within the colon and further health effects (Fardet, 2015c). Again, this is the fiber structure that counts more than the simple chemical composition. Fiber physicochemical properties include porosity, solubility, water-holding capacity, degree of polymerization, particle size, and interaction with other food components. These factors led me to develop the concept of "slow"" versus "rapid" fiber because, globally, soluble fibers (e.g., pectins and arabinoxylans) are more or less fully and rapidly fermented (Rumpagaporn et al., 2015), whereas insoluble fibers (e.g., cellulose and some hemicelluloses) are only partially and very progressively fermented with different fermentation patterns and profiles of short-chain fatty acids (Monro, 2014). The main short-chain fatty acids, i.e., propionate, butyrate, and acetate, exert very different physiological effects within the human organism (Cherbut, 2003; Topping and Clifton, 2001). Otherwise, whereas soluble fiber plays a role in increased digesta viscosity by reducing either hyperglycemia (McIntosh, 2001) or hypercholesterolemia (Brown et al., 1999), insoluble fiber plays a role in increased fecal output and transit time and participates in diluting and adsorbing carcinogens, limiting their contact with colonic mucosa and thus playing a role in the prevention of colorectal cancer (Fardet, 2015c; Ferguson et al., 1995; Moore et al., 1998).

2.3.1.2 THE FIBER COPASSENGERS

The second important concept is that of fiber copassengers, first developed by Vitaglione et al. (2008) and furthered by others (Adlercreutz et al., 2007; Jones, 2010; Laerke and Knudsen, 2011). According to Vitaglione et al. (2008) fiber copassengers are all phenolic compounds with antioxidant-related properties bound to the fiber fraction and progressively released all along the digestive tract. In the case of cereal dietary fibers, "The dietary fiber-phenolic compounds (both soluble and insoluble dietary fiber) may exert in vivo antioxidant protection acting at the intestinal environment level. Free phenolic compounds, mainly released from soluble dietary fiber by the action of intestinal and microbial esterases, can be absorbed to various extents through the intestine and, passing in the bloodstream, can exert their health benefits in the whole body. The action performed on the cereal dietary fiber by the lower gut microflora causes a continuous absorption of phenolic compounds that may explain the epidemiological evidence relating a high intake of whole grain to a low incidence of cardiovascular diseases and diabetes" (Vitaglione et al., 2008).

Therefore, beyond their mere chemical composition, fiber structure and interactions with other compounds participate in enhanced health effects in human organisms. These findings raise the issue of whether it is better to use either isolated fiber from foods or natural intact fiber within the original food matrix.

2.3.2 Polyphenol-Type Components

Polyphenol-type components consist of hundreds of compounds. They are generally produced by the plant against external factors and stresses (e.g., climate and insects) and naturally confer their antioxidant related properties to the plant. Beyond the main four classes of polyphenols, phenolic acids, flavonoids, stilbenes, and lignans, other compounds are polyphenolics, such as phytosterols, curcumin, lignins, saponins, alkylresorcinols, and others (Fardet and Chardigny, 2013). According to the food matrix in which they are included, the relative urinary excretion of main classes of polyphenols ranged from 0.3% to 43% of the ingested dose, depending on the polyphenol. "Gallic acid and isoflavones are the most well-absorbed polyphenols, followed by catechins, flavanones, and quercetin glucosides, but with different kinetics" (Manach et al., 2005).

As for other plant-based food compounds, polyphenolic compounds may be in both free and bound form. For example, in whole grain cereal–based foods, ferulic acid exists in both free (<5%) and bound (>95%) form, with each fraction playing a different role: first, being rapidly released in the upper digestive tract and probably playing a role in cell signaling in relation to ferulic acid's antioxidant-related properties, and second, exerting a direct antioxidant related effect all along the digestive tract at different levels, notably within the colon to trap free radicals produced in high amounts by microbiota (Fardet, 2010).

The phytosterols/stanols deserve special attention because they have been used as supplements (generally at a very high daily dose of up to 3–6 g/day) in several foods for lowering cholesterol (Fardet et al., 2015a). However, based on 20 intervention studies, we showed that such high doses led to a significant mean reduced absorption of β-carotene of approximately 24% (Fardet et al., 2015a). The problem is that higher cardiovascular risk was observed for differences in plasma β-carotene concentrations of the same magnitude as the estimated average decrease by phytosterols/stanols consumption (Fardet et al., 2015a). As a result, people consuming high doses of phytosterols/stanols are advised to concomitantly consume more fruits and vegetables to compensate for the potentially reduced absorption of β-carotene. This is to say that isolating one compound for a presupposed beneficial health effect and incorporating it in high doses in foods is risky because synergy of action with other compounds is lost (Fardet, 2015a,b) and also because food protective compounds are not drugs and nutrition is not pharmacology (Fardet and Rock, 2014a).

2.3.3 Other Bioactive Phytochemicals

Other bioactive phytochemicals are carotenoids (carotenes and xanthophylls) and other minor compounds such as carnitine, organosulfur compounds, hydroxycitric acid, phytic acid, sugar-alcohol, melatonin, *para*-aminobenzoic acid, and others. They can all potentially have health effects, as we showed with the lipotropic potential of plant-based foods (Fardet and Chardigny, 2013), but their optimum health effect is probably found in synergy with other compounds. This leads us to the concept of synergy and compound packages.

3. Compound Packages and Synergistic Effects: A Holistic Picture of Plant-Based Foods

3.1 The Concept of Compound Packages

All plant-based foods are a complex matrix containing several hundred potentially protective compounds. Wheat grain illustrates this fact well (Fig. 16.1). Additionally, as illustrated in Figs. 16.2 and 16.3, whereas one compound may exert several physiological effects, several compounds may contribute to sustain one physiological function (Fardet, 2010). For example, ferulic acid may potentially have antioxidant, antiinflammatory, antidiabetic, anticancer, antiaging, antiapoptotic, hepatoprotective, neuroprotective, antiatherogenic, and/or hypotensive-related properties (Srinivasan et al., 2007). Conversely, more than 30 compounds in wheat grain have direct or indirect antioxidant-related properties, acting complementarily in synergy to sustain one physiological function (Fig. 16.3; Fardet, 2010). This is true for grain products but also for legumes, nuts and seeds, fruits, and vegetables. In the end, the literature clearly shows that many compounds at moderate doses is better than a few compounds at high doses to have the maximum protective effect (Fardet, 2015a,b; Thompson et al., 2006).

If antioxidant potential has been well studied, there are also other packages of compounds acting in synergy within an organism to express their full potential, as we showed with the lipotropic package (Fardet and Chardigny, 2013). It is not one compound that is protective but the whole package. Thus, in plant-based foods, several packages of

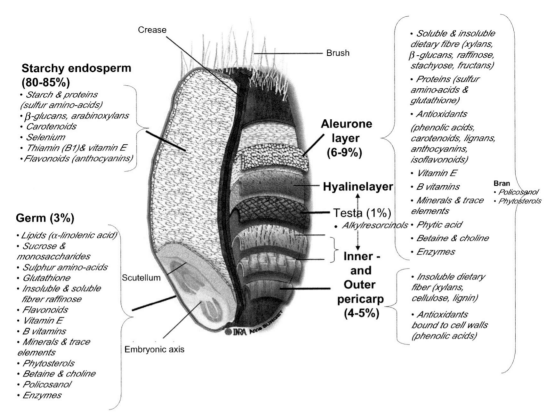

Crease

Brush

Starchy endosperm (80-85%)
- *Starch & proteins (sulfur amino-acids)*
- *β-glucans, arabinoxylans*
- *Carotenoids*
- *Selenium*
- *Thiamin (B1)& vitamin E*
- *Flavonoids (anthocyanins)*

Aleurone layer (6-9%)

Hyalinelayer

Testa (1%)
- *Alkylresorcinols*

Inner - and Outer pericarp (4-5%)

Germ (3%)
- *Lipids (α-linolenic acid)*
- *Sucrose & monosaccharides*
- *Sulphur amino-acids*
- *Glutathione*
- *Insoluble & soluble fibrer raffinose*
- *Flavonoids*
- *Vitamin E*
- *B vitamins*
- *Minerals & trace elements*
- *Phytosterols*
- *Betaine & choline*
- *Policosanol*
- *Enzymes*

Scutellum

Embryonic axis

- *Soluble & insoluble dietary fibre (xylans, β-glucans, raffinose, stachyose, fructans)*
- *Proteins (sulfur amino-acids & glutathione)*
- *Antioxidants (phenolic acids, carotenoids, lignans, anthocyanins, isoflavonoids)*
- *Vitamin E*
- *B vitamins*
- *Minerals & trace elements*
- *Phytic acid*
- *Betaine & choline*
- *Enzymes*

Bran
- *Policosanol*
- *Phytosterols*

- *Insoluble dietary fiber (xylans, cellulose, lignin)*
- *Antioxidants bound to cell walls (phenolic acids)*

© INRA Anne BURGET

FIGURE 16.1 The three wheat fractions (bran, germ, and endosperm) with their main bioactive compounds. Whole grain wheat has a heterogeneous structure with bioactive compounds unevenly distributed within its different parts. *From Fardet, A., 2010. New hypotheses for the health-protective mechanisms of whole-grain cereals: what is beyond fibre? Nutr. Res. Rev. 23, 65–134; Adapted from Surget, A., Barron, C., 2005. Histologie du grain de blé. Ind. Des. Céréales, 145, 3–7 for original image with permission of Cambridge University Press.*

protective compounds, e.g., hypolipemic or cholesterol-lowering packages or anticarcinogenic or antiinflammatory packages, can be found. These packages are the basis for the adage "Eat diversified."

3.2 Synergy, Complementarity, and Multifunctionality

Synergy means that $2 > 1 + 1$, not $2 = 1 + 1$: the whole is more than the sum of the parts (Fardet and Rock, 2014b; Jacobs and Tapsell, 2013). Each compound acts complementarily with other compounds. Thus, as regards antioxidant potential, vitamin C regenerates vitamin E tocopheryl radicals, and glutathione regenerates vitamin C ascorbyl radicals. Just missing a compound can disrupt the mechanics. This is also true for all compounds with antioxidant-related properties.

This leads us to the concept of multifunctionality, as illustrated in Fig. 16.3 for wheat grain and the fiber fraction. In recent decades, the development of functional foods has

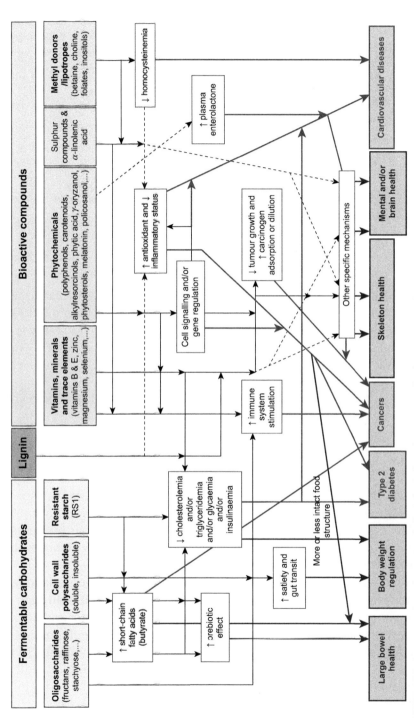

FIGURE 16.2 Current and newly proposed physiological mechanisms involved in protection by whole grain cereals as obtained via a reductionist approach. The *dotted thin arrows* indicate the link between whole grain bioactive compounds and protective physiological mechanisms, and the *plain arrows* indicate the relationship between physiological mechanisms and health outcomes. *From Fardet, A., 2010. New hypotheses for the health-protective mechanisms of whole-grain cereals: what is beyond fibre? Nutr. Res. Rev. 23, 65–134 with permission of Cambridge University Press.*

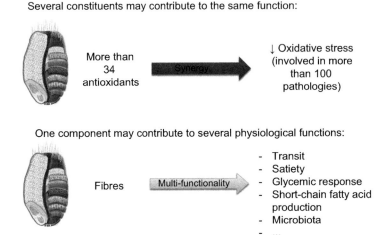

Several constituents may contribute to the same function:

More than 34 antioxidants → Synergy → ↓ Oxidative stress (involved in more than 100 pathologies)

One component may contribute to several physiological functions:

Fibres → Multi-functionality →
- Transit
- Satiety
- Glycemic response
- Short-chain fatty acid production
- Microbiota
- ...

FIGURE 16.3 Synergy and multifunctionality in wheat grain: the examples of antioxidants and fiber fractions.

been based on the enrichment of foods with one compound at a high dose based on the presumption of one compound versus one physiological effect. Monofunctionality is a reductionist view based on a linear cause–effect relationship, whereas reality is complex and based on nonlinear multicausal relationships (Fardet and Rock, 2014b). This should lead us to have a more holistic picture of foods.

3.3 From a Reductionist to a Holistic Picture of Plant-Based Bioactive Compounds

What does a holistic picture of plant-based foods mean? First, plant-based foods are primarily a complex matrix, and the health potential of the whole matrix is more than the health potential of isolated compounds. Second, food structure parameters (qualitative aspects), not just the composition in protective compounds (quantitative aspects), play a crucial role in the health potential of plant-based foods (Fardet and Rock, 2015). The health potential of the whole food is not the same as that of a mix of its nutrients without natural interactions, as shown with whole cooked carrots versus a mix of their nutrients on satiety responses (Moorhead et al., 2006).

The consequences of adopting a holistic picture of plant-based foods is to favor food biodiversity but also to better respect the complexity of food structure through soft processing, not drastic processes that denature the health potential (Fardet and Rock, 2014b). Indeed, refining and fractionating foods into isolated ingredients or compounds is part of a reductionist view of foods, forgetting that the whole is better than the sum of the parts (Scrinis, 2013, 2015). We have reached the paradox today of isolating ingredients from complex foods, then recombining them with the addition of vitamins and minerals that have been lost during refining. This is time- and cost-consuming, and complex foods have been shown to be better for health than the fractionated/recombined ones, usually called ultraprocessed foods (Monteiro et al., 2015; Moubarac et al., 2013)

4. Processing, Bioactive Compounds, and Plant Health Potential

Beyond genetic diversity and agricultural conditions, what probably plays the most important role in the plant-based food package of protective components is processing. To date, foods have been classified according to their botanical affiliation or animal species, e.g., fruits, vegetables, grains, dairy, white and red meats, and eggs. However, within one food group, there may exist simultaneously very different foods with opposite health potential. For example, within fruits, eating an intact complex apple compared to an apple purée or refined apple juice differently impact satiety and insulinemic response (Haber et al., 1977). In the same way, due to different food structure and nutrient density, eating minimally processed muesli compared to extrusion-cooked breakfast cereals enriched with sugar and/or fat will not impact health similarly. This categorization greatly underestimates the role of processing, and the increased risk of chronic diseases is above all associated with a great adherence to refined and ultraprocessed foods, not to a particular food group (Fardet et al., 2015b).

What is particularly interesting is that vegetarian, prudent, or other healthy diets are both health-protective and generally characterized by an adherence to minimally processed and complex foods. Therefore, a new typology based on the degree of food processing might be a very relevant typology for consumption (Fardet et al., 2015b). This typology was created by the research team of Monteiro et al. in their new Brazilian dietary guidelines released in December 2014. The categories were based, for the first time, on the degree of processing and a holistic vision of preventive nutrition and diets (Ministry of Health of Brazil, 2014; Monteiro et al., 2015). The categories were based on what they called the NOVA food classification (Moubarac et al., 2014).

Processing is quite indispensable to render foods secure, palatable, and/or edible for the human population. However, processing may alter bioactive compounds in either positive or negative ways (Fardet, 2014a,c). Globally, technological processes may be divided into three main categories: thermal, refining, and fermentative treatments. All modify both food structure and nutritional quality or composition to different extents.

4.1 Thermal Treatments and Bioactive Compounds

Thermal treatments are carried out either in dry or wet conditions. The influence of thermal treatment on plant-based food compounds has been studied considerably. A review of thermal treatment is not within the scope of this chapter.

In previous works, we studied the influence of thermal treatments on the lipotropic potential of plant-based foods (Fardet et al., 2011). The results provided an interesting idea of how such processes modify plant-based food components. Thus, considering raw versus boiled/canned products, thermal treatment with water decreases betaine, *myo*-inositol, and micronutrient contents (median changes $\leq -14\%$) and increases choline content without having a marked effect on methionine content. The sum of B vitamins was decreased (median change = −23%) (Fardet et al., 2011). Then, considering raw versus toasted/baked /dried products, thermal treatment without water tended to decrease betaine, methionine, *myo*-inositol, pantothenic acid, and folate content (median changes ≤ −12%) without having a marked effect on choline, magnesium, or niacin content. Finally, considering thermal treatment as a whole, with or without water, it tended to decrease betaine, *myo*-inositol, and micronutrient content (median changes ≤ −10%) without having a marked effect on choline or methionine content. We also showed that boiling, canning, and drying importantly reduced total polyphenol densities, especially in the case of transformation of fruits into juices. On a dry weight basis, thermal treatment reduced total polyphenol content by approximately 46%.

Therefore, thermal treatment tended to decrease nutrient densities. In addition, it rendered protein and starch more digestible. In addition to drastic hydrothermal treatments such as extrusion-cooking under high pressure and raw products, there are probably intermediary treatments to develop, i.e., minimal processing, that would render complex plant-based foods both more edible and healthier. An example is a cooked whole-meal pasta using minimal thermal processing that yields a healthy food product where starch is minimally gelatinized, carbohydrates slowly digested, and nutrient density well preserved.

4.2 Refining and Bioactive Compounds

Refining processes are all technological treatments that lead to ingredient losses, mainly in the fiber fraction. For example, they may include cereal milling, tomato and potato processing into ketchup and French fries, respectively, soybean flour defatting, or transformation of fruits into juices or soda or of peanut into peanut butter.

In our study on the influence of processing on the lipotropic potential of plant-based foods, we showed that refining tended to decrease choline, methionine, *myo*-inositol, and micronutrients (median changes ≤ −10%) and to increase betaine (median change = +24%) (Fardet et al., 2011). Conversely, transformation of tomatoes into canned sauce and canned condensed soup increased total polyphenol density, whereas the polyphenol density of catsup was severely reduced. On a dry weight basis, refining reduced the total polyphenol content by around 50%.

Refining is probably the worst of all technological treatments because it both destroys food structure and severely reduces nutrient density. Its use is justified to valorize food ingredients or to remove some pesticides, such as in whole grain cereals. However, scientifically speaking and based on epidemiological studies, the adherence to refined plant-based foods is rather deleterious to health (Louzada et al., 2015a,b,c; Monteiro et al., 2011; Moreira et al., 2015).

4.3 Fermentation, Germination and Soaking, and Bioactive Compounds

In our study on the lipotropic potential of plant-based foods, fermentation included baking, acidic fermentation, and alcoholic beverage production (Fardet et al., 2011).

Fermentation tended to decrease methionine, magnesium, and pantothenic acid content (median changes ≤ –12%) and to increase betaine, choline, and *myo*-inositol content (median changes ≥ +24%) without having a marked effect on niacin, folate, or the sum of B vitamins. On a dry weight basis, fermentation increased total polyphenol content by approximately 83% via the release of bound fractions into free fractions.

In a previous review, I discussed the impact of soaking, prefermentation, and germination on grain-based food health potential (Fardet, 2015c). I invite the reader to refer to it. Briefly, the scientific literature clearly shows that such minimal processing appears as one of the more beneficial for the health potential of plant-based foods. Indeed, plant-based food prefermentation has been shown to increase nutrient density, notably through releasing bound fractions of micronutrients and polyphenol compounds, and it may substantially degrade phytic acid, thus favoring further mineral bioavailability in humans. Prefermentation may also help preserve foods over longer times (Chavan and Kadam, 1989; Dordevic et al., 2010; Katina and Poutanen, 2013; Lioger et al., 2006; Nout, 2009; Poutanen et al., 2009; Singh et al., 2015), making it an inexpensive and efficient means of minimally transforming foods.

5. Conclusions

The topic of protective components in dietary plant-based foods is an immense issue to address. Indeed, there are numerous plant-based foods, numerous protective components within them, and highly diversified technological processes applied to them.

Globally, vegetarian diets are a rich source of protective components of all types provided that the processing applied to the foods is not too drastic. Beyond processing, which is generally minimal for foods in vegetarian diets, the main concern is probably that of bioavailability. Plant-based foods are characterized by a solid food structure due to the fiber network surrounding cells and the presence of antinutritional factors. This reality should encourage people eating a plant-rich diet to plan to diversify the foods in their diet to favor the maximum diversity of protective components but also to pay attention to fermented foods because this particular process tends to improve healthy food potential, either by generating new bioactive compounds or by releasing initially bound nutrient fractions into free and more available forms.

Finally, it is time to reconsider our vision of food toward a more holistic picture, taking into account synergistic effects of nutrients, complexity of food structure, and biodiversity of protective compounds. In addition, we know today that many compounds at a moderate dose is better than a few at higher doses. Otherwise, linear cause–effect concepts are not appropriate for foods, as plant-based foods are complex, and their relationship to health is likely nonlinear and multicausal. Taking into account these modern paradigms is required to develop more healthful plant-based foods.

References

AACC, 2001. The definition of dietary fiber. Cereal Foods World 46, 112–129.

Adlercreutz, H., Penalvo, J., Heinonen, S.M., Linko-Parvinen, A., 2007. Lignans and Other Co-passengers.

Borel, P., Preveraud, D., Desmarchelier, C., 2013. Bioavailability of vitamin E in humans: an update. Nutr. Rev. 319–331.

Brown, L., Rosner, B., Willett, W.W., Sacks, F.M., 1999. Cholesterol-lowering effects of dietary fiber: a meta-analysis. Am. J. Clin. Nutr. 69, 30–42.

Brown, M.J., Ferruzzi, M.G., Nguyen, M.L., Cooper, D.A., Eldridge, A.L., Schwartz, S.J., White, W.S., 2004. Carotenoid bioavailability is higher from salads ingested with full-fat than with fat-reduced salad dressings as measured with electrochemical detection. Am. J. Clin. Nutr. 80, 396–403.

Bruno, R.S., Leonard, S.W., Park, S.-I., Zhao, Y., Traber, M.G., 2006. Human vitamin E requirements assessed with the use of apples fortified with deuterium-labeled α-tocopheryl acetate. Am. J. Clin. Nutr. 83, 299–304.

Camara-Martos, F., Amaro-Lopez, M.A., 2002. Influence of dietary factors on calcium bioavailability – a brief review. Biol. Trace Elem. Res. 89, 43–52.

Cassady, B.A., Hollis, J.H., Fulford, A.D., Considine, R.V., Mattes, R.D., 2009. Mastication of almonds: effects of lipid bioaccessibility, appetite, and hormone response. Am. J. Clin. Nutr. 89, 794–800.

Chavan, J.K., Kadam, S.S., 1989. Nutritional improvement of cereals by fermentation. Crit. Rev. Food Sci. Nutr. 28, 349–400.

Cherbut, C., 2003. Motor effects of short-chain fatty acids and lactate in the gastrointestinal tract. Proc. Nutr. Soc. 62, 95–99.

Dordevic, T.M., Siler-Marinkovic, S.S., Dimitrijevic-Brankovic, S.I., 2010. Effect of fermentation on antioxidant properties of some cereals and pseudo cereals. Food Chem. 119, 957–963.

Ellis, P.R., Kendall, C.W., Ren, Y., Parker, C., Pacy, J.F., Waldron, K.W., Jenkins, D.J., 2004. Role of cell walls in the bioaccessibility of lipids in almond seeds. Am. J. Clin. Nutr. 80, 604–613.

Fairweather-Tait, S.J., Collings, R., Hurst, R., 2010. Selenium bioavailability: current knowledge and future research requirements. Am. J. Clin. Nutr. 91, 1484S–1491S.

Fardet, A., Chardigny, J.-M., 2013. Plant-based foods as a source of lipotropes for human nutrition: a survey of in vivo studies. Crit. Rev. Food Sci. Nutr. 53, 535–590.

Fardet, A., Rock, E., 2014a. The search for a new paradigm to study micronutrient and phytochemical bioavailability: from reductionism to holism. Med. Hypotheses 82, 181–186.

Fardet, A., Rock, E., 2014b. Toward a new philosophy of preventive nutrition: from a reductionist to a holistic paradigm to improve nutritional recommendations. Adv. Nutr. 5, 430–446.

Fardet, A., Rock, E., 2015. From a reductionist to a holistic approach in preventive nutrition to define new and more ethical paradigms. Healthcare 3, 1054–1063.

Fardet, A., Hoebler, C., Baldwin, P.M., Bouchet, B., Gallant, D.J., Barry, J.L., 1998. Involvement of the protein network in the in vitro degradation of starch from spaghetti and lasagne: a microscopic and enzymic study. J. Cereal Sci. 27, 133–145.

Fardet, A., Martin, J.-F., Chardigny, J.-M., 2011. Thermal and refining processes, not fermentation, tend to reduce lipotropic capacity of plant-based foods. Food Funct. 2, 483–504.

Fardet, A., Souchon, I., Dupont, D. (Eds.), 2013. Structure des aliments et effets nutritionnels. Quae.

Fardet, A., Morise, A., Kalonji, E., Margaritis, I., Mariotti, F., 2015a. Influence of phytosterol and phytostanol food supplementation on plasma liposoluble vitamins and provitamin A carotenoid levels in humans: an updated review of the evidence. Crit. Rev. Food Sci. Nutr.

Fardet, A., Rock, E., Bassama, J., Bohuon, P., Prabhasankar, P., Monteiro, C., Moubarac, J.-C., Achir, N., 2015b. Current food classifications in epidemiological studies do not enable solid nutritional recommendations to prevent diet-related chronic diseases: the impact of food processing. Adv. Nutr. 6, 629–638.

Fardet, A., 2010. New hypotheses for the health-protective mechanisms of whole-grain cereals: what is beyond fibre? Nutr. Res. Rev. 23, 65–134.

Fardet, A., 2014a. Editorial – are technological processes the best friends of food health potential? Adv. Nutr. Food Technol. 1, 103.

Fardet, A., 2014b. Editorial – food health potential is primarily due to its matrix structure, then nutrient composition: a new paradigm for food classification according to technological processes applied. J. Nutr. Health Food Eng. 1, 31.

Fardet, A., 2014c. Editorial – foods and health potential: is food engineering the key issue? J. Nutr. Health Food Eng. 1, 1–2.

Fardet, A., 2014d. New approaches to studying the potential health benefits of cereals: from reductionism to holism. Cereal Foods World 59, 224–229.

Fardet, A., 2015a. Complex foods versus functional foods, nutraceuticals and dietary supplements: differential health impact (Part 1). Agro Food Ind. Hi Tech 26, 20–24.

Fardet, A., 2015b. Complex foods versus functional foods, nutraceuticals and dietary supplements: differential health impact (Part 2). Agro Food Ind. Hi Tech 26, 20–22.

Fardet, A., 2015c. A shift toward a new holistic paradigm will help to preserve and better process grain product food structure for improving their health effects. Food Funct. 6, 363–382.

Ferguson, L.R., Roberton, A.M., Watson, M.E., Triggs, C.M., Harris, P.J., 1995. The effects of a soluble-fiber polysaccharide on the adsorption of carcinogens to insoluble dietary-fibers. Chemico-Biol. Interact. 95, 245–255.

Foster-Powell, K., Holt, S.H., Brand-Miller, J.C., 2002. International table of glycemic index and glycemic load values: 2002. Am. J. Clin. Nutr. 76, 5–56.

Garber, A.K., Binkley, N.C., Krueger, D.C., Suttie, J.W., 1999. Comparison of phylloquinone bioavailability from food sources or a supplement in human subjects. J. Nutr. 129, 1201–1203.

Gibson, R.S., Bailey, K.B., Gibbs, M., Ferguson, E.L., 2010. A review of phytate, iron, zinc, and calcium concentrations in plant-based complementary foods used in low-income countries and implications for bioavailability. Food Nutr. Bull. 31, S134–S146.

Gueguen, L., Pointillart, A., 2000. The bioavailability of dietary calcium. J. Am. Coll. Nutr. 19, 119S–136S.

Haber, G.B., Heaton, K.W., Murphy, D., Burroughs, L.F., 1977. Depletion and disruption of dietary fibre. Effects on satiety, plasma-glucose, and serum-insulin. Lancet 2, 679–682.

Habiba, R.A., 2002. Changes in anti-nutrients, protein solubility, digestibility, and HCl-extractability of ash and phosphorus in vegetable peas as affected by cooking methods. Food Chem. 77, 187–192.

Hambidge, K.M., Miller, L.V., Westcott, J.E., Sheng, X., Krebs, N.F., 2010. Zinc bioavailability and homeostasis. Am. J. Clin. Nutr. 91, 1478S–1483S.

Harinarayan, C.V., Ramalakshmi, T., Prasad, U.V., Sudhakar, D., Srinivasarao, P.V.L.N., Sarma, K.V.S., Kumar, E.G.T., 2007. High prevalence of low dietary calcium, high phytate consumption, and vitamin D deficiency in healthy south Indians. Am. J. Clin. Nutr. 85, 1062–1067.

Haskell, M.J., 2012. The challenge to reach nutritional adequacy for vitamin A: beta-carotene bioavailability and conversion-evidence in humans. Am. J. Clin. Nutr. 96, 1193S–1203S.

Holm, J., Lundquist, I., Bjorck, I., Eliasson, A.C., Asp, N.G., 1988. Degree of starch gelatinization, digestion rate of starch in vitro, and metabolic response in rats. Am. J. Clin. Nutr. 47, 1010–1016.

Hurrell, R., Egli, I., 2010. Iron bioavailability and dietary reference values. Am. J. Clin. Nutr. 91, 1461S–1467S.

Scrinis, G., 2015. Reformulation, fortification and functionalization: Big Food corporations' nutritional engineering and marketing strategies. J. Peasant Stud. 43, 17–37.

Singh, A.K., Rehal, J., Kaur, A., Jyot, G., 2015. Enhancement of attributes of cereals by germination and fermentation: a review. Crit. Rev. Food Sci. Nutr. 55, 1575–1589.

Srinivasan, M., Sudheer, A.R., Menon, V.P., 2007. Ferulic acid: therapeutic potential through its antioxidant property. J. Clin. Biochem. Nutr. 40, 92–100.

Surget, A., Barron, C., 2005. Histologie du grain de blé. Ind. Des. Céréales 145, 3–7.

Thompson, H.J., Heimendinger, J., Diker, A., O'Neill, C., Haegele, A., Meinecke, B., Wolfe, P., Sedlacek, S., Zhu, Z.J., Jiang, W.Q., 2006. Dietary botanical diversity affects the reduction of oxidative biomarkers in women due to high vegetable and fruit intake. J. Nutr. 136, 2207–2212.

Topping, D., Clifton, P., 2001. Short-chain fatty acids and human colonic function: roles of resistant starch and nonstarch polysaccharides. Physiol. Rev. 81, 1031–1064.

Traoret, C.J., Lokko, P., Cruz, A.C.R.F., Oliveira, C.G., Costa, N.M.B., Bressan, J., Alfenas, R.C.G., Mattes, R.D., 2008. Peanut digestion and energy balance. Int. J. Obes. 32, 322–328.

Vissers, M.C.M., Carr, A.C., Pullar, J.M., Bozonet, S.M., 2013. The bioavailability of vitamin C from kiwifruit. Adv. Food Nutr. Res. 68, 125–147.

Vitaglione, P., Napolitano, A., Fogliano, V., 2008. Cereal dietary fibre: a natural functional ingredient to deliver phenolic compounds into the gut. Trends Food Sci. Technol. 19, 451–463.

Wang, S., Meckling, K.A., Marcone, M.F., Kakuda, Y., Tsao, R., 2011. Synergistic, additive, and antagonistic effects of food mixtures on total antioxidant capacities. J. Agric. Food Chem. 59, 960–968.

Watanabe, F., 2007. Vitamin B-12 sources and bioavailability. Exp. Biol. Med. 232, 1266–1274.

The Relations Between Vegetarian Diets and Health and Disease

17

Bone Health and Vegan Diets

Kelsey M. Mangano, Katherine L. Tucker

UNIVERSITY OF MASSACHUSETTS LOWELL, LOWELL, MA, UNITED STATES

1. Introduction

Osteoporosis is a silent disease characterized by a systemic impairment of bone mass, strength, and microarchitecture, resulting in increased risk for fragility fracture. Recent prevalence data from the National Osteoporosis Foundation suggest that 9 million adults in the United States have osteoporosis, and 48 million have low bone mass, placing them at risk of fracture (Foundation, 2003). It has been estimated that one in three women and one in five men over the age of 50 years will experience a fracture in their lifetime (Melton et al., 1992, 1998). Hip fractures are associated with mortality rates of up to 24% within 1 year after fracture (Cooper et al., 1993; Leibson et al., 2002). The economic burden of incident osteoporotic fracture in the United States was estimated at nearly $17 billion in 2005, with a cumulative cost over the next 2 decades estimated at $474 billion (Burge et al., 2007). Therefore, it is imperative to identify risk factors associated with poor bone health to maximize the functional capacity of aging adults and reduce risk of fracture.

The pathogenesis of osteoporosis has been linked to tissue, cellular, and molecular processes. At the molecular level, a tightly orchestrated dance between bone resorption and bone formation comprises the essential course of bone remodeling, a process that repairs damaged bone and replaces old bone with new. Bone remodeling allows appropriate changes in bone architecture to match the current mechanical demands that occur throughout the lifespan. Excess resorption over formation leads to loss of bone mass, osteoporosis, and increased risk for fracture of the hip, spine, and wrist. Therefore, treatment and prevention of the uncoupling between bone resorption and formation is of high priority.

Prevention strategies include promoting diets that are rich in nutrients that are beneficial for bone and low in nutrients that may cause bone loss over time. Nutritional public health interventions targeting improved bone health are attractive, as they are affordable, easy to understand, and pose minimal health risks. However, dietary restrictions, due to personal preference, biological tolerance, or to religious or ethical beliefs may increase the risk of osteoporosis in certain populations, due to a lack of bone promoting nutrients in the diet. The adoption of a vegan diet has become increasingly popular in light of expert recommendations to follow plant-based diets for improved health outcomes, as discussed in many other chapters of this book. Although studies are limited, there is evidence suggesting that vegan diets may place individuals at greater risk of lower bone mineral density (BMD) and greater risk of fracture than diets that include animal based foods. This chapter will discuss the current state of research regarding vegan diets and their association with bone health, and provide suggestions as to how individuals following a vegan diet can fill the dietary gaps that may increase their risk of poor bone health.

2. Bone Status in Individuals With Vegan Diets

Although studies are sparse, there is evidence that those consuming a vegan diet may be at greater risk of lower BMD and greater risk of fracture. A 2009 meta-analysis of 9 studies, including 1880 women and 869 men aged 20–79 years, showed 4% lower BMD (95% CI: 2%, 7%) at both the femoral neck and lumbar spine in vegetarians relative to omnivores (Ho-Pham et al., 2009). Results of subgroup analysis suggested that this effect on femoral neck BMD was more pronounced among those on a vegan diet (6% lower BMD; 95% CI: 1%, 4%) than among ovolactovegetarians. A study in postmenopausal, Taiwanese women showed that long-term vegan practice was associated with almost four times the risk of low bone mass of the femoral neck relative to ovolactovegetarians or omnivores (adjusted OR: 3.9; 95% CI: 1.2, 12.8) (Chiu et al., 1997). A recent cross-sectional study among 84 young, nonobese adults found no differences in total body BMD between those following ovolactovegetarian, vegan, or omnivore diets (Knurick et al., 2015), but the small sample size may have been insufficient to see a difference.

Few studies have examined the relation between vegan diets and fracture risk. In a prospective study of 210 postmenopausal women, the 2-year incidence of fracture was not significantly different in those with vegan (5.7%) compared to omnivore diets (5.4%) (Ho-Pham et al., 2012). In a much larger analysis from the European Prospective Investigation into Cancer and Nutrition (EPIC)-Oxford cohort, with 7947 men and 26,749 women aged 20–89 years, fracture risk was higher in those with vegan diets and low calcium intake (<525 mg/day), but it did not differ between meat eaters, fish eaters, or ovolactovegetarians (Appleby et al., 2007).

The current state of research is suggestive of an increased risk of bone loss and fracture with veganism. It is important to better understand what components of a vegan diet are contributing to this general loss of bone and to elucidate dietary areas of improvement to protect the skeleton in individuals following vegan diets over time.

3. Vegan Diets and Bone Health

Our understanding of the diet–bone relationship has expanded dramatically over recent decades. We now know that individual nutrients, as well as foods and dietary patterns accounting for the synergy of nutrients in the whole diet, are involved in the mineralization and maintenance of bone health. In addition to the well-known importance of calcium and vitamin D, many nutrients and foods affect BMD and/or the risk of fracture.

Vegan diets pose particular challenges in attaining required nutrients for optimal bone health. Data from the large EPIC cohort show that vegan diets were associated with lower intakes of calcium, protein, vitamin B_{12}, vitamin D, and retinol relative to meat eaters (Davey et al., 2003). Food sources for specific nutrients also differed by diet type, with bioavailability of several key nutrients lower in vegan relative to animal-based sources. Table 17.1 outlines sources of at-risk nutrients in vegan diets (Tucker, 2014).

There are also some components of a vegan diet that may be beneficial for bone, compared to those consuming animal products. Long-term intake of a diet high in preformed vitamin A, as retinol, which is found in animal products, has been associated with increased risk of fracture in postmenopausal women (Feskanich et al., 2002). In contrast, vegan diets typically contain high amounts of previtamin A carotenoids from fruit and vegetables, and these are likely to protect bone (Sahni et al., 2009a,b). In addition to these carotenoids, vegan diets are often high in other plant-based antioxidants and antiinflammatory nutrients that protect against loss of BMD. In the EPIC study, those following vegan diets had higher intakes of folate, vitamin C, vitamin E, vitamin K, and magnesium compared to other groups (Davey et al., 2003). Further detail on food groups and nutrients specific to vegan diets that may be either detrimental or beneficial to bone health are discussed subsequently.

4. Dairy Substitutes and Their Bone Benefiting Nutrients

Dairy foods have been shown to protect against bone loss and to reduce the risk of fracture in older adults (Heaney, 2009; Rizzoli, 2014). This is likely due to the density of bone-benefiting nutrients, such as calcium, magnesium, phosphorous, vitamin D, vitamin B_{12}, and protein in these products. Vegan diets exclude dairy products making it more difficult to obtain many of these nutrients. However, dairy substitute products on the market, including soy and almond milk, are often fortified with calcium and vitamin D. A few studies have examined whether replacement of dairy with nondairy products confers the same bone benefits. Matthews et al. (2011) screened for osteoporosis among 337 postmenopausal women from the Adventist Health Study 2 (AHS-2) consuming ≥1 serving/day of soy milk or cow's milk compared to women not consuming either soy or cow's milk. Compared with women who did not drink soy or cow's milk, women drinking soy milk once a day or more had 56% lower odds of osteoporosis (OR=0.44; 95% CI: 0.20–0.98), while women consuming cow's milk had 62% reduction in the likelihood of having osteoporosis. These results suggest that consuming one or more servings of soy milk per day may confer similar protective effects against osteoporosis as cow's milk. In addition to the added calcium and vitamin D, it was once thought that soy isoflavones may protect the skeleton. However, research in this area generally does not point toward a protective effect (Lagari and Levis, 2013). Randomized controlled trials supplementing soy protein have shown no effects on BMD (Kenny et al., 2009; Kreijkamp-Kaspers et al., 2004). Overall, fortified, alternative dairy products may serve as a comparable substitute for providing some of the dairy nutrients known to protect the skeleton.

Table 17.1   Risk Nutrients for Bone Health in Vegetarian Diets and Available Food Sources

Nutrient Adult Recommended Daily Allowance/ Adequate Intake	Ovolacto Sources	Serving	Nutrient Content (Range)	Vegan Sources	Serving	Nutrient Content[a]
Calcium (1000–1200 mg)	Yogurt	244 g (1 c)	289–372	Fortified soy milk	243 g (1 c)	282–301
	Milk	244 g (1 c)	276–305	Firm calcium-set tofu	100 g (3.5 oz)	683
	Cheese	28 g (1 oz)	150–336	Fortified breakfast cereal[b]	20 g (½ c)	667
				Dark leafy greens[c]	90 g (½ c)	122
				Blackstrap molasses	20 g (1 tb)	120
Vitamin D[d] (600 IU)	Fortified milk	244 g (1 c)	115–120	Fortified soy milk	245 g (1 c)	100–105
	Fortified yogurt	245 g (1 c)	86–127	Fortified breakfast cereal[b]	20 g (½ c)	67
	Egg	1 lg	41	UV light exposed mushrooms[e]	60.5 g (½ c)	317
Vitamin B$_{12}$ (2.4 µg)	Milk	244 g (1 c)	1.1–1.2	Fortified breakfast cereal	20 g (½ c)	4.0
	Yogurt	244 g (1 c)	0.9–1.2			
	Egg	1 lg	0.4			
Zinc (8–11 mg)				Fortified breakfast cereal[b]	20 g (½ c)	10
				Pumpkin seeds	28 g (1 oz)	2.2
				Tofu, tempeh[f]	100 g (3.5 oz)	1.1
				Nuts	28 g (1 oz)	1.1
Protein (46–56 g)	Yogurt	244 g (1 c)	8.5–11.2	Dried beans, peas, cooked	89 g (½ c)	7.6
	Milk	244 g (1 c)	8.1	Soy milk	243 g (1 c)	6.0
	Egg	1 lg	6.3	Tofu, tempeh	100 g (3.5 oz)	20.3
	Cheese	28 g (1 oz)	6.6	Nuts	28 g (1 oz)	4.9
n-3 fatty acids (1.1–1.6 g)				Walnuts	28 g (1 oz)	2.6
				Walnut oil	14 g (1 tb)	1.4
				Flaxseeds	14 g (1 tb)	2.4
				Flaxseed oil	14 g (1 tb)	7.2
				Canola oil	14 g (1 tb)	1.3

c, cups; *lg*, large egg; *oz*, ounce; *RDA*, recommended daily allowance; *tb*, tablespoon.

[a]From *USDA* National Nutrient Database for Standard Reference, Release 28.

[b]Content from "Total" cereal.

[c]Content from cooked spinach.

[d]Sunlight exposure is a good source of vitamin D, depending on latitude and season.

[e]Content from cooked portabella; UV exposed mushrooms are usually labeled.

[f]Zinc in fermented products (tempeh, miso) is more bioavailable.

Reprinted from Tucker, K.L., 2014. Vegetarian diets and bone status. Am. J. Clin. Nutr. 100 (Suppl. 1), 329S–335S, American Society for Nutrition.

4.1 Calcium

Calcium is the most abundant mineral in the body, and nearly 99% of the calcium in an adult is contained in bones and teeth. Because bone undergoes constant remodeling, an adequate supply of nutrients is required to support bone health throughout the lifespan. A review of calcium trials in adults found that 50 of 52 trials demonstrated better bone balance with calcium intervention, greater bone gain during growth, less age-related bone loss, and reduced fracture risk (Heaney, 2000). However, the BMD benefits accrued from calcium supplementation were no longer evident 2 years after supplementation ceased (Dawson-Hughes et al., 2000). Data from the Women's Health Initiative of over 36,000 postmenopausal women, aged 50–79 years, supplemented with 1000 mg calcium and 400 IU vitamin D daily showed no reduced risk of hip fracture over 7 years compared to placebo (Jackson et al., 2006). In contrast, trials supplementing calcium-rich foods have shown significant protection against bone loss (Baran et al., 1990) and decreasing urinary excretion of bone turnover markers (Heaney et al., 2002).

Low calcium intake is a key area of concern with vegan diets. Although several vegetables contain calcium, such as leafy greens and legumes, the calcium from these sources is not very bioavailable (Weaver et al., 1999). Vegan populations may meet calcium requirements through consumption of calcium-set tofu, fortified orange juice, and soy and almond milk products, as these do provide adequate bioavailability. Based on available research, it may be most advantageous for vegans to attain calcium from the diet, including from fortified foods, as opposed to using calcium supplements, to maximize their bone health. Careful attention is required to ensure adequate consumption of this nutrient.

4.2 Vitamin D

Vitamin D (cholecalciferol) is critically important for bone health, as it regulates calcium absorption and stimulates bone formation. Activated vitamin D $(1,25(OH)_2D)$ stimulates bone turnover in a way that promotes overall positive bone balance. Generally, vitamin D is obtained in the diet as cholecalciferol from animal sources (fatty fish, egg yolk, and fortified diary) or in much lower quantity as ergocalciferol from plant sources [notably mushrooms exposed to ultraviolet light (Jasinghe et al., 2005)]. Many vegans are deficient in vitamin D, as their diets are limited in vitamin D–rich food sources (Dyett et al., 2013). Importantly, vitamin D can also be synthesized in the skin after sun exposure. However, synthesis of vitamin D between November and March in northern latitudes is limited, and widespread use of sunscreen, along with sun avoidance, makes food sources of vitamin D an important consideration.

Maintaining adequate serum vitamin D concentration (generally >60 nmol/L) is important in promoting BMD and reducing risk of fracture (Cummings et al., 1998; Looker and Mussolino, 2008; van Schoor et al., 2008). A meta-analysis of 9 randomized controlled trials concluded that relatively high doses of vitamin D (>400 IU/day) have been shown to decrease risk of nonvertebral fractures in adults >65 years of age (pooled RR: 0.80; 95%

CI: 0.72, 0.89) independent of calcium supplementation (Bischoff-Ferrari et al., 2009). However, a more recent meta-analysis of 23 studies in adults >20 years concluded that vitamin D supplementation did not improve BMD among adults who are not deficient (Reid et al., 2014). When evaluating vitamin D from food alone, intake >600 IU/day has been shown to reduce the odds of osteoporosis by 27%, but it was not associated with 3-year fracture risk (Nieves et al., 2008). A US study in more than 72,000 older women showed that intakes of vitamin D ≥ 500 IU/day compared with <140 IU/day were associated with 37% lower risk of hip fracture (Feskanich et al., 2003).

Vegan diets tend to be low in vitamin D, and it is important to focus on adequate intake, particularly from foods where there is the greatest support of bone-benefiting effects. Vegan food sources of vitamin D include mushrooms exposed to ultraviolet light, fortified dairy substitutes, and fortified orange juice. Regular exposure to sunlight before applying sunscreen can help to prevent vitamin D insufficiency during summer months. Supplements may be needed in northern latitudes.

5. Dietary Protein: Are Plant Sources Beneficial to Bone?

Early, short-term metabolic studies suggested that high protein intakes may be detrimental to bone health due to a calciuric effect (Kerstetter and Allen, 1990). In contrast, however, more recent studies have shown that dietary protein is beneficial to bone health, particularly under conditions of adequate calcium intake (Mangano et al., 2014). This is likely due, in part, to protein's ability to augment calcium absorption in the gut (Cao et al., 2011; Hunt et al., 2009). Other mechanisms by which protein may benefit bone structure and strength are its ability to decrease bone resorption at the cellular level (Hunt et al., 2009); to increase concentration of insulin like growth factor-1[IGF-1] (Bonjour et al., 1997), a growth hormone anabolic for bone; and its ability to improve muscle mass (Dillon et al., 2009; Sahni et al., 2015) and strength (McLean et al., 2015), which may improve BMD via increased loading of bone. Epidemiologic studies confirm the long-term benefits of a high-protein diet on BMD, including less loss of bone over time in older men and women (Hannan et al., 2000) and lower risk of fracture (Misra et al., 2011), particularly among individuals with calcium intakes greater than 800 mg/day (Sahni et al., 2010). Data from randomized controlled trials show that protein supplementation to ensure adequacy may protect against loss of bone during weight loss (Sukumar et al., 2011). However, protein supplementation in healthy adults, who are already meeting the recommended daily allowance (RDA) for protein, did not appear to improve BMD over an intervention period of 1 year (Kerstetter et al., 2015) or 2 years (Zhu et al., 2011).

Vegan sources of protein include legumes, soy, nuts and seeds, and grains. Few studies have examined whether animal or vegetable sources of protein differentially alter bone health over time. Some studies suggest that animal sources of protein (meat, eggs, fish) are most beneficial to bone health (Oh et al., 2013; Sahni et al., 2010; Promislow et al., 2002), perhaps due to their particular ability to increase circulating levels of IGF-1 (Larsson et al., 2005). However, other epidemiological studies showed that greater dietary protein was associated with higher BMD and reduced risk of fracture, regardless of whether animal or vegetable sources provides the highest amount of dietary protein (Munger et al., 1999). Overall, it appears that higher, rather than lower, dietary protein is protective against bone loss and risk of fracture. Therefore, it is imperative for vegans to attain the RDA for protein from a variety of sources to meet all essential amino acid requirements. Although randomized controlled trials supplementing soy protein have shown no beneficial effects on the skeleton, they also have shown no detrimental effects (Kenny et al., 2009; Kreijkamp-Kaspers et al., 2004). Therefore, soy protein may be one vegan protein source that could be used to augment total protein intake in effort to maximize bone health, but preferably from soy foods rather than from isolated protein supplements. Plant food servings containing 7 g of protein range from 1 oz of peanuts to approximately 2 oz of soybeans or 300 g cooked brown rice. As discussed in more detail in another chapter (Chapter 35), eating a variety of vegan protein food sources is necessary to ensure that all essential amino acid requirements are met. This is easily accomplished by pairing legumes or nuts with grains. Consuming a mixed protein diet while meeting calcium requirements may be important for vegans to protect long-term skeletal health.

6. Vitamin B_{12} Is Important for Bone Health

Vitamin B_{12} is an important risk nutrient in vegan diets, as it is almost exclusively available in animal source foods. Therefore, it is not surprising that individuals following vegan diets have been shown to have lower vitamin B_{12} concentration relative to omnivores (Elmadfa and Singer, 2009). A European study found the prevalence of poor vitamin B_{12} status (holotranscobalamin II < 35 pmol/L) was 11% in omnivores, compared with 92% of those following vegan diets (Herrmann et al., 2003). This is also discussed in detail in another chapter in this book (Chapter 43).

Early case reports identified vitamin B_{12} deficiency in patients with osteoporosis, greater fracture risk in those with pernicious anemia (an autoimmune disorder causing impaired vitamin B_{12} absorption), and improvement with vitamin B_{12} therapy (Eastell et al., 1992). A meta-analysis including more than 7000 men and women showed a 4% lower fracture risk for each 50-pmol/L increase in serum vitamin B_{12} (RR: 0.96; 95% CI: 0.92, 1.00) (van Wijngaarden et al., 2013). In a cross-sectional study of over 2000 men and women from the Framingham Osteoporosis Study, those with vitamin B_{12} concentration <148 pM had lower BMD, compared to those with vitamin B_{12} above this cutoff (Tucker et al., 2005). Data from the National Health and Nutrition Examination Survey (NHANES) also show a positive relation between serum vitamin B_{12} and BMD, in a dose–response manner up to about 200 pM (Morris et al., 2005). Further, BMD was lower and osteoporosis significantly more likely ($P < .01$) with increasing methylmalonic acid concentration (a functional marker of vitamin B_{12} status). In a study of older women in the Netherlands, low vitamin B_{12} concentration

(<210 pM) was associated with seven times the prevalence of osteoporosis, compared to those with serum concentration >320 pM (Dhonukshe-Rutten et al., 2003). A prospective study of 83 postmenopausal women from the Study of Osteoporotic Fractures found that women with vitamin B_{12} concentration at or below 207 pM lost BMD at an annual rate of −1.6% (95% CI: −2.4, −0.8%), compared with −0.2% (−0.5, 0.2%) in women with higher concentration (Stone et al., 2004). Vitamin B_{12} is a required cofactor for DNA synthesis, and thus it may be important for bone rebuilding during turnover. In support of this mechanism, lower concentrations of bone formation markers osteocalcin and alkaline phosphatase have been seen with vitamin B_{12} deficiency (Carmel et al., 1988).

One result of low vitamin B_{12} is an elevation in homocysteine, which has been independently associated with increased fracture risk, possibly by weakening collagen cross-linking. A meta-analysis with 11,511 individuals in eight studies showed a 4% greater fracture risk for each µmol/L increase in homocysteine concentration (RR: 1.04; 95% CI: 1.02, 1.07). Data from the Framingham Osteoporosis Study show that men and women in the highest quartiles of homocysteine had greater incidence of fracture, compared to those in the lowest quartile (approximately twice as high for women and four times as high for men) (McLean et al., 2004). The NHANES study also found that individuals with serum homocysteine ≥20 µmol/L had significantly lower BMD than did those with serum homocysteine <10 µmol/L (Morris et al., 2005). Therefore, attaining adequate vitamin B_{12} appears to have both direct and indirect (by lowering homocysteine) effects on bone.

Despite strong observational results, however, limited evidence from randomized controlled trials has not shown significant benefit for BMD or risk of fracture. Data from the B-PROOF study, in 1111 hyperhomocysteinemic adults aged 65 years and older, found no significant differences in femoral neck or lumbar spine BMD after 2 years of combined supplementation with 500 µg vitamin B_{12}, 400 µg of folic acid, and 600 IU of vitamin D, compared to placebo (Enneman et al., 2015). In 2919 participants from the same study, osteoporotic fracture risk did not differ significantly between groups (HR: 0.84; 95% CI: 0.58, 1.21) (van Wijngaarden et al., 2014). However, in a subset of persons aged >80 years, in per-protocol analyses, osteoporotic fracture risk was lower in the intervention group compared to placebo (HR: 0.27, 95% CI: 0.10, 0.74). It is important to note that supplementation with B_{12} and folic acid at these levels also increased the incidence of cancer in this study (HR: 1.56; 95% CI: 1.04, 2.31).

Larger and longer trials are needed to clarify the potential role of supplementation for fracture prevention. In the meantime, the evidence from epidemiological studies supports ensuring adequate vitamin B_{12} status to maintain bone health. Therefore, encouraging individuals consuming vegan diets to meet the RDA for vitamin B_{12} (2.4 mcg/day for men and women) is important. Nonanimal-based sources of vitamin B_{12} include fortified breakfast cereals, nutritional yeast, and fortified soy products. Vegans may also be advised to take a vitamin B_{12} supplement to ensure adequacy, with periodic testing of vitamin B_{12} concentration.

7. Zinc

Zinc is frequently inadequate in vegan diets, as it is largely found in animal products. Plant sources of zinc include grains, vegetables, legumes, nuts, and soy, but it is much less bioavailable in these foods than in animal sources. Deficiency in this nutrient may be detrimental to bone health. Lower serum and bone zinc have been documented in patients with osteoporosis (Atik, 1983). In a controlled trial, random assignment to supplementation with calcium, copper, and zinc for 2 years showed improvement in whole-body BMD among postmenopausal women with usual zinc intakes <8.0 mg/day, compared to those taking placebo (Nielsen et al., 2011). These effects were not seen in women consuming adequate dietary zinc. In premenarcheal girls, random assignment to daily oral zinc (9 mg elemental zinc) increased serum procollagen type 1 amino-terminal propeptide (a bone formation marker), compared to placebo, after 4 weeks (Berger et al., 2015). There were no differences between zinc supplementation and placebo in osteocalcin, bone resorption markers, or IGF-1 (a growth hormone anabolic to bone). Although research is limited, these studies suggest that zinc supplementation in prepubescent girls and women with low zinc status may improve bone status.

The Food and Nutrition Board recommends at least 50% greater zinc intake for persons consuming animal-free diets because of its low bioavailability from plant foods (Food and Nutrition Board, 2001): see also the chapter specifically on zinc in this book (Chapter 38). Plant foods rich in zinc, such as nuts, beans, and grains, also contain phytate, which is a chemical compound that chelates zinc and decreases its absorption. Soaking, heating, fermenting, and leavening foods degrades phytate and, therefore, improves bioavailability of zinc from beans and grains (Saunders et al., 2013). Fortified cereals are another important source of dietary zinc in vegan diets.

8. n-3 Fatty Acids

Investigational therapies to delay the onset and severity of bone loss include supplementation with dietary factors that possess antiinflammatory properties, including n-3 fatty acids (FA). Polyunsaturated fatty acids (PUFA) include omega 3 fatty acids (n-3 FA) and omega 6 fatty acids (n-6 FA). Two essential FA are required in the diet: the n-3 FA alpha-linolenic acid (ALA) and the n-6 FA linoleic acid (LA). Via a series of elongation and desaturation steps, these two PUFA parent compounds (ALA and LA) are converted to additional FA and various eicosanoids. Typically, downstream products of the n-3 FA family demonstrate antiinflammatory properties, while n-6 FA derivatives tend to be proinflammatory. There is competition between n-6 and n-3 FA for the desaturation enzymes during production of downstream fatty acids and for cyclooxygenase (COX) during the metabolism of various eicosanoids; therefore, greater intakes of one PUFA type over the other will determine which pathway (n-3 vs. n-6) is driven and which eicosanoids are produced. The two predominant products of ALA metabolism are the long chain n-3 FA docosahexaenoic acid (DHA) and eicosapentaenoic acid (EPA). Because the conversion from ALA is inefficient, individuals with adequate n-3 FA status tend to consume foods with DHA and EPA directly, with fish as the major source. Therefore, this is another nutrient of concern in vegan diets.

Recent research highlights the importance of n-3 FA intake or supplementation for bone health (Mangano et al., 2013). Longitudinal studies from the Framingham Osteoporosis Study have shown that both dietary (Farina et al., 2011b) and plasma fatty acids (Farina et al., 2012) are associated with less bone loss over time. Interestingly, these studies suggest an interaction between fatty acids, where arachidonic acid intake (n-6 FA) was protective of bone only in individuals with EPA and DHA intakes (n-3 FA) above the median. A randomized controlled trial in postmenopausal women showed after 6 months of supplementation, EPA + DHA significantly increased BMD at the Wards area, and it maintained BMD at the femoral neck, compared to the placebo group, who lost bone at both sites (Lappe et al., 2013). It is difficult to determine whether the protective effects of this supplementation regimen were due to n-3 FA alone or due to its combined supplementation with vitamin D, vitamin K, and genistein (a soy isoflavone). A trial in overweight boys demonstrated that supplementation with fortified bread (1.1 g/day EPA + DHA) did not affect whole-body bone mineral content, density, or bone turnover markers over 16 weeks, although there was an increase in IGF-1 in the intervention group, compared to placebo (Damsgaard et al., 2012).

Studies evaluating fracture risk have shown mixed results in relation to n-3 FA intake. Dietary n-3 FA intake appeared to be protective against hip fracture (54% lower risk in the highest vs. lowest quartile of intake) in the Framingham Osteoporosis Study (Farina et al., 2011a). The Nurses' Health Study and the Health Professionals Follow-up Study showed lower risk of hip fracture among women, but not men, with the highest intakes of total PUFA (Virtanen et al., 2012). However, an analysis in the Women's Health Initiative showed no effect of total PUFA or individual FA on risk of hip fracture in more than 137,000 postmenopausal women (Orchard et al., 2010). Overall, it appears that n-3 FA intakes are protective of bone health; however, more randomized controlled trials are needed to determine whether additional supplementation can improve bone health and reduce risk of fracture over time.

Although the most well-studied n-3 FAs in relation to bone health have been evaluated with those FAs found in fatty fish (EPA and DHA), plant sources of ALA include walnuts, flaxseeds, and canola oil. Non–fish eaters may find supplementation with n-3 FA from flaxseed and/or algae a viable option for increasing antiinflammatory n-3 FA intake.

9. Protective Nutrients in Vegan Diets

Although several nutrients, as discussed earlier, are of concern for bone health in vegan diets, these diets also tend to include higher intakes of several important nutrients that protect bone, compared to the diets of omnivores. These nutrients include magnesium, potassium, vitamin K, antioxidants, such as vitamins C and E and carotenoids, and antiinflammatory phytonutrients in fruit, vegetables, nuts, beans, tea, and herbs. Several studies have shown protective effects of dietary magnesium on bone density (New et al., 2000; Ryder et al., 2005; Tucker et al., 1999), although magnesium intake has not been associated with risk of fractures (Orchard et al., 2014). Magnesium enhances bone strength and regulates active intestinal calcium transport (Kenney et al., 1994).

Potassium, a mineral also concentrated in fruit and vegetables, may protect against bone loss by promoting renal calcium retention and neutralizing dietary acid load, thereby protecting calcium losses. In premenopausal women, a diet low in potassium was associated with 8% lower femoral neck BMD compared to women in the highest quartile of potassium intake (Macdonald et al., 2005). In perimenopausal women, potassium intake was associated with greater BMD and lower bone resorption (Sebastian et al., 1994). In the Framingham Osteoporosis Study, potassium intake was associated with greater BMD in men and women at baseline and with lower BMD loss over time in men (Tucker et al., 1999). A randomized controlled trial in men and women over the age of 50 years demonstrated that a potassium bicarbonate supplement of 1 mmol/kg over 3 months reduced bone turnover markers (Dawson-Hughes et al., 2015). Overall, greater consumption of magnesium and potassium, largely found in fruit and vegetables, may pose protective effects on bone in vegans who consume large amounts of this food group.

Vegan diets high in fruit and vegetables also tend to provide greater amounts of vitamins C and K, carotenoids, flavonoids, and other phytonutrients known to benefit health. These antioxidant and antiinflammatory nutrients have also been shown to protect bone health. Data from the Framingham Osteoporosis Study show that men with the highest intakes of vitamin C had significantly less loss of BMD over 4 years compared to those with intakes in the lowest tertile (Sahni et al., 2008). Similarly, men and women in the highest tertile of vitamin C intake had 44% lower risk of hip fracture compared to those in the lowest tertile of intake (Sahni et al., 2009c). In the same cohort, high carotenoid intakes were protective against 4 years bone loss (Sahni et al., 2009a) and lower risk of hip fracture (45% reduced risk) (Sahni et al., 2009b). Among the carotenoids, the strongest associations from the Framingham studies were with lycopene.

Vitamin K is a necessary factor for the carboxylation of osteocalcin, a bone-specific protein produced by osteoblasts that plays a role in bone mineralization. Insufficient vitamin K may lead to age-related bone loss and fracture. Several randomized controlled trials suggest that vitamin K supplementation reduces the rate of bone loss (Fang et al., 2012; Huang et al., 2015), though the effect is modest. One study showed protection against incident fracture among Japanese patients taking a vitamin K supplement, relative to controls (Cockayne et al., 2006). High consumption of fruits and vegetables are beneficial to bone health (Tucker et al., 1999), likely due to their concentration in the nutrients discussed. The higher intake of fruit and vegetables usually seen in vegan diets is a positive characteristic that may help to protect bone health.

10. Conclusions

Unless great care is taken in ensuring adequate intakes of several at-risk nutrients, individuals following a vegan diet may be at greater risk for bone loss and fracture risk over time. This may be due to insufficient intake of bone-benefiting nutrients found largely in animal products, such as calcium, vitamin D, protein, vitamin B_{12}, zinc, and n-3 fatty acids. Educating the vegan population on dietary alternatives, fortified foods, and supplements needed to meet the RDA for each of these nutrients is important for prevention of osteoporosis and age-related fracture. While many bone-promoting nutrients are lacking in the typical vegan diet, there are also many nutrients consumed in high amounts from fruit and vegetable intake that may promote bone health. With adequate knowledge and careful planning, vegan diets can be designed to ensure nutrient adequacy to build and maintain healthy bones and reduce risk of fracture.

References

Appleby, P., Roddam, A., Allen, N., Key, T., 2007. Comparative fracture risk in vegetarians and nonvegetarians in EPIC-Oxford. Eur. J. Clin. Nutr. 61, 1400–1406.

Atik, O.S., 1983. Zinc and senile osteoporosis. J. Am. Geriatr. Soc. 31, 790–791.

Baran, D., Sorensen, A., Grimes, J., Lew, R., Karellas, A., Johnson, B., Roche, J., 1990. Dietary modification with dairy products for preventing vertebral bone loss in premenopausal women: a three-year prospective study. J. Clin. Endocrinol. Metab. 70, 264–270.

Berger, P.K., Pollock, N.K., Laing, E.M., Chertin, V., Bernard, P.J., Grider, A., Shapses, S.A., Ding, K.H., Isales, C.M., Lewis, R.D., 2015. Zinc supplementation increases procollagen type 1 amino-terminal propeptide in premenarcheal girls: a randomized controlled trial. J. Nutr.

Bischoff-Ferrari, H.A., Willett, W.C., Wong, J.B., Stuck, A.E., Staehelin, H.B., Orav, E.J., Thoma, A., Kiel, D.P., Henschkowski, J., 2009. Prevention of nonvertebral fractures with oral vitamin D and dose dependency: a meta-analysis of randomized controlled trials. Arch. Intern. Med. 169, 551–561.

Bonjour, J.P., Schurch, M.A., Chevalley, T., Ammann, P., Rizzoli, R., 1997. Protein intake, IGF-1 and osteoporosis. Osteoporos. Int. 7 (Suppl. 3), S36–S42.

Burge, R., Dawson-Hughes, B., Solomon, D.H., Wong, J.B., King, A., Tosteson, A., 2007. Incidence and economic burden of osteoporosis-related fractures in the United States, 2005-2025. J. Bone Miner. Res. 22, 465–475.

Cao, J.J., Johnson, L.K., Hunt, J.R., 2011. A diet high in meat protein and potential renal acid load increases fractional calcium absorption and urinary calcium excretion without affecting markers of bone resorption or formation in postmenopausal women. J. Nutr. 141, 391–397.

Carmel, R., Lau, K.H., Baylink, D.J., Saxena, S., Singer, F.R., 1988. Cobalamin and osteoblast-specific proteins. N. Engl. J. Med. 319, 70–75.

Chiu, J.F., Lan, S.J., Yang, C.Y., Wang, P.W., Yao, W.J., Su, L.H., Hsieh, C.C., 1997. Long-term vegetarian diet and bone mineral density in postmenopausal Taiwanese women. Calcif. Tissue Int. 60, 245–249.

Cockayne, S., Adamson, J., Lanham-New, S., Shearer, M.J., Gilbody, S., Torgerson, D.J., 2006. Vitamin K and the prevention of fractures: systematic review and meta-analysis of randomized controlled trials. Arch. Intern. Med. 166, 1256–1261.

Cooper, C., Atkinson, E.J., Jacobsen, S.J., O'fallon, W.M., Melton 3rd, L.J., 1993. Population-based study of survival after osteoporotic fractures. Am. J. Epidemiol. 137, 1001–1005.

Cummings, S.R., Browner, W.S., Bauer, D., Stone, K., Ensrud, K., Jamal, S., Ettinger, B., 1998. Endogenous hormones and the risk of hip and vertebral fractures among older women. Study of Osteoporotic Fractures Research Group. N. Engl. J. Med. 339, 733–738.

Damsgaard, C.T., Molgaard, C., Matthiessen, J., Gyldenlove, S.N., Lauritzen, L., 2012. The effects of n-3 long-chain polyunsaturated fatty acids on bone formation and growth factors in adolescent boys. Pediatr. Res. 71, 713–719.

Davey, G.K., Spencer, E.A., Appleby, P.N., Allen, N.E., Knox, K.H., Key, T.J., 2003. EPIC-Oxford: lifestyle characteristics and nutrient intakes in a cohort of 33 883 meat-eaters and 31 546 non meat-eaters in the UK. Public Health Nutr. 6, 259–269.

Dawson-Hughes, B., Harris, S.S., Krall, E.A., Dallal, G.E., 2000. Effect of withdrawal of calcium and vitamin D supplements on bone mass in elderly men and women. Am. J. Clin. Nutr. 72, 745–750.

Dawson-Hughes, B., Harris, S.S., Palermo, N.J., Gilhooly, C.H., Shea, M.K., Fielding, R.A., Ceglia, L., 2015. Potassium bicarbonate supplementation lowers bone turnover and calcium excretion in older men and women: a randomized dose-finding trial. J. Bone Miner. Res. 30, 2103–2111.

Dhonukshe-Rutten, R.A., Lips, M., De Jong, N., Chin, A.P.M.J., Hiddink, G.J., Van Dusseldorp, M., De Groot, L.C., Van Staveren, W.A., 2003. Vitamin B-12 status is associated with bone mineral content and bone mineral density in frail elderly women but not in men. J. Nutr. 133, 801–807.

Dillon, E.L., Sheffield-Moore, M., Paddon-Jones, D., Gilkison, C., Sanford, A.P., Casperson, S.L., Jiang, J., Chinkes, D.L., Urban, R.J., 2009. Amino acid supplementation increases lean body mass, basal muscle protein synthesis, and insulin-like growth factor-I expression in older women. J. Clin. Endocrinol. Metab. 94, 1630–1637.

Dyett, P.A., Sabate, J., Haddad, E., Rajaram, S., Shavlik, D., 2013. Vegan lifestyle behaviors: an exploration of congruence with health-related beliefs and assessed health indices. Appetite 67, 119–124.

Eastell, R., Vieira, N.E., Yergey, A.L., Wahner, H.W., Silverstein, M.N., Kumar, R., Riggs, B.L., 1992. Pernicious anaemia as a risk factor for osteoporosis. Clin. Sci. (Lond.) 82, 681–685.

Elmadfa, I., Singer, I., 2009. Vitamin B-12 and homocysteine status among vegetarians: a global perspective. Am. J. Clin. Nutr. 89, 1693S–1698S.

Enneman, A.W., Swart, K.M., Van Wijngaarden, J.P., Van Dijk, S.C., Ham, A.C., Brouwer-Brolsma, E.M., Van Der Zwaluw, N.L., Dhonukshe-Rutten, R.A., Van Der Cammen, T.J., De Groot, L.C., Van Meurs, J., Lips, P., Uitterlinden, A.G., Zillikens, M.C., Van Schoor, N.M., Van Der Velde, N., 2015. Effect of vitamin B12 and folic acid supplementation on bone mineral density and quantitative ultrasound parameters in older people with an elevated plasma homocysteine level: B-PROOF, a randomized controlled trial. Calcif. Tissue Int. 96, 401–409.

Fang, Y., Hu, C., Tao, X., Wan, Y., Tao, F., 2012. Effect of vitamin K on bone mineral density: a meta-analysis of randomized controlled trials. J. Bone Miner. Metab. 30, 60–68.

Farina, E.K., Kiel, D.P., Roubenoff, R., Schaefer, E.J., Cupples, L.A., Tucker, K.L., 2011a. Dietary intakes of arachidonic acid and alpha-linolenic acid are associated with reduced risk of hip fracture in older adults. J. Nutr. 141, 1146–1153.

Farina, E.K., Kiel, D.P., Roubenoff, R., Schaefer, E.J., Cupples, L.A., Tucker, K.L., 2011b. Protective effects of fish intake and interactive effects of long-chain polyunsaturated fatty acid intakes on hip bone mineral density in older adults: the Framingham Osteoporosis Study. Am. J. Clin. Nutr. 93, 1142–1151.

Farina, E.K., Kiel, D.P., Roubenoff, R., Schaefer, E.J., Cupples, L.A., Tucker, K.L., 2012. Plasma phosphatidylcholine concentrations of polyunsaturated fatty acids are differentially associated with hip bone mineral density and hip fracture in older adults: the Framingham Osteoporosis Study. J. Bone Miner. Res. 27, 1222–1230.

Feskanich, D., Singh, V., Willett, W.C., Colditz, G.A., 2002. Vitamin A intake and hip fractures among postmenopausal women. JAMA 287, 47–54.

Feskanich, D., Willett, W.C., Colditz, G.A., 2003. Calcium, vitamin D, milk consumption, and hip fractures: a prospective study among postmenopausal women. Am. J. Clin. Nutr. 77, 504–511.

Food And Nutrition Board, Institute of Medicine, 2001. Dietary Reference Intakes for Vitamin A, Vitamin K, Arsenic, Boron, Chromium, Copper, Iodine, Iron, Manganese, Molybdenum, Nickel, Silicon, Vanadium, and Zinc. National Academies Press, Washington, DC.

Hannan, M.T., Tucker, K.L., Dawson-Hughes, B., Cupples, L.A., Felson, D.T., Kiel, D.P., 2000. Effect of dietary protein on bone loss in elderly men and women: the Framingham Osteoporosis Study. J. Bone Miner. Res. 15, 2504–2512.

Heaney, R.P., Rafferty, K., Dowell, M.S., 2002. Effect of yogurt on a urinary marker of bone resorption in postmenopausal women. J. Am. Diet. Assoc. 102, 1672–1674.

Heaney, R.P., 2000. Calcium, dairy products and osteoporosis. J. Am. Coll. Nutr. 19, 83S–99S.

Heaney, R.P., 2009. Dairy and bone health. J. Am. Coll. Nutr. 28 (Suppl. 1), 82S–90S.

Herrmann, W., Schorr, H., Obeid, R., Geisel, J., 2003. Vitamin B-12 status, particularly holotranscobalamin II and methylmalonic acid concentrations, and hyperhomocysteinemia in vegetarians. Am. J. Clin. Nutr. 78, 131–136.

Ho-Pham, L.T., Nguyen, N.D., Nguyen, T.V., 2009. Effect of vegetarian diets on bone mineral density: a Bayesian meta-analysis. Am. J. Clin. Nutr. 90, 943–950.

Ho-Pham, L.T., Vu, B.Q., Lai, T.Q., Nguyen, N.D., Nguyen, T.V., 2012. Vegetarianism, bone loss, fracture and vitamin D: a longitudinal study in Asian vegans and non-vegans. Eur. J. Clin. Nutr. 66, 75–82.

Huang, Z.B., Wan, S.L., Lu, Y.J., Ning, L., Liu, C., Fan, S.W., 2015. Does vitamin K2 play a role in the prevention and treatment of osteoporosis for postmenopausal women: a meta-analysis of randomized controlled trials. Osteoporos. Int. 26, 1175–1186.

Hunt, J.R., Johnson, L.K., Fariba Roughead, Z.K., 2009. Dietary protein and calcium interact to influence calcium retention: a controlled feeding study. Am. J. Clin. Nutr. 89, 1357–1365.

Jackson, R.D., Lacroix, A.Z., Gass, M., Wallace, R.B., Robbins, J., Lewis, C.E., Bassford, T., Beresford, S.A., Black, H.R., Blanchette, P., Bonds, D.E., Brunner, R.L., Brzyski, R.G., Caan, B., Cauley, J.A., Chlebowski, R.T., Cummings, S.R., Granek, I., Hays, J., Heiss, G., Hendrix, S.L., Howard, B.V., Hsia, J., Hubbell, F.A., Johnson, K.C., Judd, H., Kotchen, J.M., Kuller, L.H., Langer, R.D., Lasser, N.L., Limacher, M.C., Ludlam, S., Manson, J.E., Margolis, K.L., Mcgowan, J., Ockene, J.K., O'sullivan, M.J., Phillips, L., Prentice, R.L., Sarto, G.E., Stefanick, M.L., Van Horn, L., Wactawski-Wende, J., Whitlock, E., Anderson, G.L., Assaf, A.R., Barad, D., 2006. Calcium plus vitamin D supplementation and the risk of fractures. N. Engl. J. Med. 354, 669–683.

Jasinghe, V.J., Perera, C.O., Barlow, P.J., 2005. Bioavailability of vitamin D2 from irradiated mushrooms: an in vivo study. Br. J. Nutr. 93, 951–955.

Kenney, M.A., Mccoy, H., Williams, L., 1994. Effects of magnesium deficiency on strength, mass, and composition of rat femur. Calcif. Tissue Int. 54, 44–49.

Kenny, A.M., Mangano, K.M., Abourizk, R.H., Bruno, R.S., Anamani, D.E., Kleppinger, A., Walsh, S.J., Prestwood, K.M., Kerstetter, J.E., 2009. Soy proteins and isoflavones affect bone mineral density in older women: a randomized controlled trial. Am. J. Clin. Nutr. 90, 234–242.

Kerstetter, J.E., Allen, L.H., 1990. Dietary protein increases urinary calcium. J. Nutr. 120, 134–136.

Kerstetter, J.E., Bihuniak, J.D., Brindisi, J., Sullivan, R.R., Mangano, K.M., Larocque, S., Kotler, B.M., Simpson, C.A., Cusano, A.M., Gaffney-Stomberg, E., Kleppinger, A., Reynolds, J., Dziura, J., Kenny, A.M., Insogna, K.L., 2015. The effect of a whey protein supplement on bone mass in older Caucasian adults. J. Clin. Endocrinol. Metab. 100, 2214–2222.

Knurick, J.R., Johnston, C.S., Wherry, S.J., Aguayo, I., 2015. Comparison of correlates of bone mineral density in individuals adhering to lacto-ovo, vegan, or omnivore diets: a cross-sectional investigation. Nutrients 7, 3416–3426.

Kreijkamp-Kaspers, S., Kok, L., Grobbee, D.E., De Haan, E.H., Aleman, A., Lampe, J.W., Van Der Schouw, Y.T., 2004. Effect of soy protein containing isoflavones on cognitive function, bone mineral density, and plasma lipids in postmenopausal women: a randomized controlled trial. JAMA 292, 65–74.

Lagari, V.S., Levis, S., 2013. Phytoestrogens in the prevention of postmenopausal bone loss. J. Clin. Densitom. 16, 445–449.

Lappe, J., Kunz, I., Bendik, I., Prudence, K., Weber, P., Recker, R., Heaney, R.P., 2013. Effect of a combination of genistein, polyunsaturated fatty acids and vitamins D3 and K1 on bone mineral density in postmenopausal women: a randomized, placebo-controlled, double-blind pilot study. Eur. J. Nutr. 52, 203–215.

Larsson, S.C., Wolk, K., Brismar, K., Wolk, A., 2005. Association of diet with serum insulin-like growth factor I in middle-aged and elderly men. Am. J. Clin. Nutr. 81, 1163–1167.

Leibson, C.L., Tosteson, A.N., Gabriel, S.E., Ransom, J.E., Melton, L.J., 2002. Mortality, disability, and nursing home use for persons with and without hip fracture: a population-based study. J. Am. Geriatr. Soc. 50, 1644–1650.

Looker, A.C., Mussolino, M.E., 2008. Serum 25-hydroxyvitamin D and hip fracture risk in older U.S. white adults. J. Bone Miner. Res. 23, 143–150.

Macdonald, H.M., New, S.A., Fraser, W.D., Campbell, M.K., Reid, D.M., 2005. Low dietary potassium intakes and high dietary estimates of net endogenous acid production are associated with low bone mineral density in premenopausal women and increased markers of bone resorption in postmenopausal women. Am. J. Clin. Nutr. 81, 923–933.

Mangano, K.M., Sahni, S., Kerstetter, J.E., Kenny, A.M., Hannan, M.T., 2013. Polyunsaturated fatty acids and their relation with bone and muscle health in adults. Curr. Osteoporos. Rep.

Mangano, K.M., Sahni, S., Kerstetter, J.E., 2014. Dietary protein is beneficial to bone health under conditions of adequate calcium intake: an update on clinical research. Curr. Opin. Clin. Nutr. Metab. Care 17, 69–74.

Matthews, V.L., Knutsen, S.F., Beeson, W.L., Fraser, G.E., 2011. Soy milk and dairy consumption is independently associated with ultrasound attenuation of the heel bone among postmenopausal women: the Adventist Health Study-2. Nutr. Res. 31, 766–775.

Mclean, R.R., Jacques, P.F., Selhub, J., Tucker, K.L., Samelson, E.J., Broe, K.E., Hannan, M.T., Cupples, L.A., Kiel, D.P., 2004. Homocysteine as a predictive factor for hip fracture in older persons. N. Engl. J. Med. 350, 2042–2049.

Mclean, R.R., Mangano, K.M., Hannan, M.T., Kiel, D.P., Sahni, S., 2015. Dietary protein intake is protective against loss of grip strength among older adults in the Framingham offspring cohort. J. Gerontol. A Biol. Sci. Med. Sci.

Melton 3rd, L.J., Chrischilles, E.A., Cooper, C., Lane, A.W., Riggs, B.L., 1992. Perspective. How many women have osteoporosis? J. Bone Miner. Res. 7, 1005–1010.

Melton 3rd, L.J., Atkinson, E.J., O'connor, M.K., O'fallon, W.M., Riggs, B.L., 1998. Bone density and fracture risk in men. J. Bone Miner. Res. 13, 1915–1923.

Misra, D., Berry, S.D., Broe, K.E., Mclean, R.R., Cupples, L.A., Tucker, K.L., Kiel, D.P., Hannan, M.T., 2011. Does dietary protein reduce hip fracture risk in elders? The Framingham Osteoporosis Study. Osteoporos. Int. 22, 345–349.

Morris, M.S., Jacques, P.F., Selhub, J., 2005. Relation between homocysteine and B-vitamin status indicators and bone mineral density in older Americans. Bone 37, 234–242.

Munger, R.G., Cerhan, J.R., Chiu, B.C., 1999. Prospective study of dietary protein intake and risk of hip fracture in postmenopausal women. Am. J. Clin. Nutr. 69, 147–152.

National Osteoporosis Foundation, 2003. Osteoporosis, Disease Statistics. [Online] Available from www.nof.org.

New, S.A., Robins, S.P., Campbell, M.K., Martin, J.C., Garton, M.J., Bolton-Smith, C., Grubb, D.A., Lee, S.J., Reid, D.M., 2000. Dietary influences on bone mass and bone metabolism: further evidence of a positive link between fruit and vegetable consumption and bone health? Am. J. Clin. Nutr. 71, 142–151.

Nielsen, F.H., Lukaski, H.C., Johnson, L.K., Roughead, Z.K., 2011. Reported zinc, but not copper, intakes influence whole-body bone density, mineral content and T score responses to zinc and copper supplementation in healthy postmenopausal women. Br. J. Nutr. 106, 1872–1879.

Nieves, J.W., Barrett-Connor, E., Siris, E.S., Zion, M., Barlas, S., Chen, Y.T., 2008. Calcium and vitamin D intake influence bone mass, but not short-term fracture risk, in Caucasian postmenopausal women from the National Osteoporosis Risk Assessment (NORA) study. Osteoporos. Int. 19, 673–679.

Oh, S.M., Kim, H.C., Rhee, Y., Park, S.J., Lee, H.J., Suh, I., Feskanich, D., 2013. Dietary protein in relation to bone stiffness index and fat-free mass in a population consuming relatively low protein diets. J. Bone Miner. Metab. 31, 433–441.

Orchard, T.S., Cauley, J.A., Frank, G.C., Neuhouser, M.L., Robinson, J.G., Snetselaar, L., Tylavsky, F., Wactawski-Wende, J., Young, A.M., Lu, B., Jackson, R.D., 2010. Fatty acid consumption and risk of fracture in the Women's Health Initiative. Am. J. Clin. Nutr. 92, 1452–1460.

Orchard, T.S., Larson, J.C., Alghothani, N., Bout-Tabaku, S., Cauley, J.A., Chen, Z., Lacroix, A.Z., Wactawski-Wende, J., Jackson, R.D., 2014. Magnesium intake, bone mineral density, and fractures: results from the Women's Health Initiative Observational Study. Am. J. Clin. Nutr.

Promislow, J.H., Goodman-Gruen, D., Slymen, D.J., Barrett-Connor, E., 2002. Protein consumption and bone mineral density in the elderly: the Rancho Bernardo Study. Am. J. Epidemiol. 155, 636–644.

Reid, I.R., Bolland, M.J., Grey, A., 2014. Effects of vitamin D supplements on bone mineral density: a systematic review and meta-analysis. Lancet 383, 146–155.

Rizzoli, R., 2014. Dairy products, yogurts, and bone health. Am. J. Clin. Nutr. 99, 1256S–12562S.

Ryder, K.M., Shorr, R.I., Bush, A.J., Kritchevsky, S.B., Harris, T., Stone, K., Cauley, J., Tylavsky, F.A., 2005. Magnesium intake from food and supplements is associated with bone mineral density in healthy older white subjects. J. Am. Geriatr. Soc. 53, 1875–1880.

Sahni, S., Hannan, M.T., Gagnon, D., Blumberg, J., Cupples, L.A., Kiel, D.P., Tucker, K.L., 2008. High vitamin C intake is associated with lower 4-year bone loss in elderly men. J. Nutr. 138, 1931–1938.

Sahni, S., Hannan, M.T., Blumberg, J., Cupples, L.A., Kiel, D.P., Tucker, K.L., 2009a. Inverse association of carotenoid intakes with 4-y change in bone mineral density in elderly men and women: the Framingham Osteoporosis Study. Am. J. Clin. Nutr. 89, 416–424.

Sahni, S., Hannan, M.T., Blumberg, J., Cupples, L.A., Kiel, D.P., Tucker, K.L., 2009b. Protective effect of total carotenoid and lycopene intake on the risk of hip fracture: a 17-year follow-up from the Framingham Osteoporosis Study. J. Bone Miner. Res. 24, 1086–1094.

Sahni, S., Hannan, M.T., Gagnon, D., Blumberg, J., Cupples, L.A., Kiel, D.P., Tucker, K.L., 2009c. Protective effect of total and supplemental vitamin C intake on the risk of hip fracture–a 17-year follow-up from the Framingham Osteoporosis Study. Osteoporos. Int. 20, 1853–1861.

Sahni, S., Cupples, L.A., Mclean, R.R., Tucker, K.L., Broe, K.E., Kiel, D.P., Hannan, M.T., 2010. Protective effect of high protein and calcium intake on the risk of hip fracture in the Framingham offspring cohort. J. Bone Miner. Res.. 25, 2770–2776.

Sahni, S., Mangano, K.M., Hannan, M.T., Kiel, D.P., Mclean, R.R., 2015. Higher protein intake is associated with higher lean mass and quadriceps muscle strength in adult men and women. J. Nutr. 145, 1569–1575.

Saunders, A.V., Craig, W.J., Baines, S.K., 2013. Zinc and vegetarian diets. Med. J. Aust. 199, S17–S21.

Sebastian, A., Harris, S.T., Ottaway, J.H., Todd, K.M., Morris Jr., R.C., 1994. Improved mineral balance and skeletal metabolism in postmenopausal women treated with potassium bicarbonate. N. Engl. J. Med. 330, 1776–1781.

Stone, K.L., Bauer, D.C., Sellmeyer, D., Cummings, S.R., 2004. Low serum vitamin B-12 levels are associated with increased hip bone loss in older women: a prospective study. J. Clin. Endocrinol. Metab. 89, 1217–1221.

Sukumar, D., Ambia-Sobhan, H., Zurfluh, R., Schlussel, Y., Stahl, T.J., Gordon, C.L., Shapses, S.A., 2011. Areal and volumetric bone mineral density and geometry at two levels of protein intake during caloric restriction: a randomized, controlled trial. J. Bone Miner. Res. 26, 1339–1348.

Tucker, K.L., Hannan, M.T., Chen, H., Cupples, L.A., Wilson, P.W., Kiel, D.P., 1999. Potassium, magnesium, and fruit and vegetable intakes are associated with greater bone mineral density in elderly men and women. Am. J. Clin. Nutr. 69, 727–736.

Tucker, K.L., Hannan, M.T., Qiao, N., Jacques, P.F., Selhub, J., Cupples, L.A., Kiel, D.P., 2005. Low plasma vitamin B12 is associated with lower BMD: the Framingham Osteoporosis Study. J. Bone Miner. Res. 20, 152–158.

Tucker, K.L., 2014. Vegetarian diets and bone status. Am. J. Clin. Nutr. 100 (Suppl. 1), 329S–335S.

van Schoor, N.M., Visser, M., Pluijm, S.M., Kuchuk, N., Smit, J.H., Lips, P., 2008. Vitamin D deficiency as a risk factor for osteoporotic fractures. Bone 42, 260–266.

van Wijngaarden, J.P., Doets, E.L., Szczecinska, A., Souverein, O.W., Duffy, M.E., Dullemeijer, C., Cavelaars, A.E., Pietruszka, B., Van't Veer, P., Brzozowska, A., Dhonukshe-Rutten, R.A., De Groot, C.P., 2013. Vitamin B12, folate, homocysteine, and bone health in adults and elderly people: a systematic review with meta-analyses. J. Nutr. Metab., 486186.

van Wijngaarden, J.P., Swart, K.M., Enneman, A.W., Dhonukshe-Rutten, R.A., Van Dijk, S.C., Ham, A.C., Brouwer-Brolsma, E.M., Van Der Zwaluw, N.L., Sohl, E., Van Meurs, J.B., Zillikens, M.C., Van Schoor, N.M., Van Der Velde, N., Brug, J., Uitterlinden, A.G., Lips, P., De Groot, L.C., 2014. Effect of daily vitamin B-12 and folic acid supplementation on fracture incidence in elderly individuals with an elevated plasma homocysteine concentration: B-PROOF, a randomized controlled trial. Am. J. Clin. Nutr. 100, 1578–1586.

Virtanen, J.K., Mozaffarian, D., Willett, W.C., Feskanich, D., 2012. Dietary intake of polyunsaturated fatty acids and risk of hip fracture in men and women. Osteoporos. Int. 23, 2615–2624.

Weaver, C.M., Proulx, W.R., Heaney, R., 1999. Choices for achieving adequate dietary calcium with a vegetarian diet. Am. J. Clin. Nutr. 70, 543S–548S.

Zhu, K., Meng, X., Kerr, D.A., Devine, A., Solah, V., Binns, C.W., Prince, R.L., 2011. The effects of a two-year randomized, controlled trial of whey protein supplementation on bone structure, IGF-1, and urinary calcium excretion in older postmenopausal women. J. Bone Miner. Res. 26, 2298–2306.

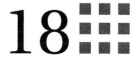

18

Weight Maintenance and Weight Loss: The Adoption of Diets Based on Predominantly Plants

Ming-Chin Yeh[1], Marian Glick-Bauer[1], David L. Katz[2]

[1]CITY UNIVERSITY OF NEW YORK, NEW YORK, NY, UNITED STATES;
[2]GRIFFIN HOSPITAL, DERBY, CT, UNITED STATES

1. Introduction

Nutritionally replete, low-fat, plant-based diets have been associated with a wide array of favorable health outcomes and are compatible with what Katz and Meller coin the "theme of optimal eating" (Katz and Meller, 2014). A 2006 literature review of weight status of vegetarians and nonvegetarians found that 38 of 40 studies reported lower body mass index (BMI) and body weight among vegetarians (Berkow and Barnard, 2006). In 2009, the American Dietetic Association (ADA) released a position statement recognizing the role of vegetarian diets in preventing chronic diseases, including obesity (Craig and Mangels, 2009). The purported role of vegetarian diets in weight management was based on several population studies (discussed subsequently) that found an association between vegetarian diets and lower BMI. In 2011 the ADA followed up with an editorial supporting the role of vegetarian diets for weight loss and long-term weight maintenance (Thedford and Raj, 2011). This chapter will explore both clinical trials and population studies to evaluate the efficacy of plant-based diets for weight loss and maintenance of a healthy BMI. Mechanisms by which plant-based diets may contribute to weight loss will be examined.

A note of caution must be sounded in equating plant-based diets with "vegetarian" diets, as there is a wide range of foods that might compose a vegetarian diet, including processed foods high in fat, sugar, refined carbohydrates, and additives. Clinical trials are easiest to compare and evaluate when the researchers are careful to specify the dietary composition of their intervention, for example, a "low-fat vegan diet" consisting of fruit, vegetables, legumes, and grains with limited high-fat avocados, nuts, and seeds (Turner-McGrievy et al., 2007). Studies that compare any weight loss diet to a "standard diet" are likely to produce unreliable results.

2. Population Studies

Population studies provide considerable insight into the relationship between plant-based diets, BMI, and weight management. A review of over 10,000 adults from the US Department of Agriculture's 1994–96 Continuing Survey of Food Intake compared vegetarian and nonvegetarian diets and found comparatively low energy intake, low fat and saturated fat intake, and low BMI associated with the vegetarian group (Kennedy et al., 2001). Analysis of the National Health and Nutrition Examination Survey (NHANES) data from 1999 to 2004 similarly indicates a lower calorie intake among participants who reported no meat consumption, further supporting the possibility that a vegetarian diet may be a strategy for weight loss (Farmer, 2014).

Perhaps the most expansive population analysis to include plant-based diets is the Adventist Health Study-2, which follows 97,000 Seventh-day Adventist church members (≥age 30) in the United States and Canada from 2002 to 2006. The study found that vegans had the lowest mean BMI ($23.6\,kg/m^2$), followed by ovolactovegetarians ($25.7\,kg/m^2$), pescetarians ($26.3\,kg/m^2$), and semivegetarians ($27.3\,kg/m^2$), while mean BMI for nonvegetarians was $28.8\,kg/m^2$ (Tonstad et al., 2009). Thus, there is an association of BMI and diet along the spectrum of vegetarian diets, with vegans showing the greatest difference from nonvegetarians; the BMI of subjects following less restrictive vegetarian diets fell somewhere in between.

This finding mirrors the results of the Oxford cohort of the European Perspective Investigation Into Cancer and Nutrition (EPIC-Oxford) study in which 57,498 participants between 1993 and 1999 completed a food frequency and lifestyle questionnaire. An analysis of BMI in this cohort found significant differences between diet groups, with highest BMI among the meat eaters and lowest among the vegans. Vegetarians and fish eaters had intermediate mean BMI (Spencer et al., 2003). Rates of obesity were significantly lower among vegans (1.9% in men and 1.8% in women) than among meat eaters (5% in men and 5.7% in women). The authors concluded that high protein and low fiber intakes were the strongest determinants of increasing BMI in this cohort.

A later study examined the association between weight gain and dietary group among 21,966 participants in the EPIC-Oxford cohort. Only small differences were found in mean annual weight gain over 5 years between all diet groups including meat eaters, fish eaters, vegetarians, and vegans. Notably, however, those who changed to a diet containing fewer animal foods during the follow-up period displayed the lowest weight gain (Rosell et al., 2006). However the authors note that those who chose to become "more vegetarian" may have been more health conscious and lower in weight before the study began. This confounding variable of lifestyle in population studies can make conclusions about diet and BMI difficult (see also Chapter 1). Another approach to deciphering the relationship between plant-based diets and weight loss is to look at clinical trials in which conflicting variables such as lifestyle can be more closely controlled.

3. Clinical Trials

With few exceptions, clinical trials indicate that plant-based diets translate into greater weight loss than omnivorous control diets. A meta-analysis of 12 randomized trails found significant weight loss benefits when subjects consumed vegetarian diets. This effect was more pronounced in the six trials that incorporated a form of energy restriction, such as a 500 kcal/day reduction (Huang et al., 2015). Another meta-analysis of 86 cross-sectional and 10 cohort prospective studies reported significantly reduced BMI in vegetarians, including vegans, versus omnivores (Dinu et al., 2016). In the short term, randomized clinical trials indicate that subjects assigned to a vegetarian diet, including vegan diet, lose from 2.5 to 7.2 kg when compared to controls (Berkow and Barnard, 2006).

Multiple clinical studies suggest that the weight loss benefits of a plant-based diet appear to be greatest for those following a vegan diet (Huang et al., 2015). An 18-week dietary intervention in a corporate setting found that 94 participants assigned to a low-fat vegan diet lost significantly more weight (−2.9 kg) than 117 controls (0.06 kg). The plant-based diet resulted in weight loss even in the absence of exercise or prescribed calorie restriction (Mishra et al., 2013).

However, weight loss benefits may be attained with less restrictive vegetarian diets as well. A study of 20 subjects assigned to change from an omnivorous diet to a lactovegetarian diet found a 2 kg weight loss after 1 year, attributed to the high fiber content of the plant-based diet (Johansson et al., 2012). A study of 50 overweight adults found that those assigned to a vegan diet lost significantly more weight than omnivore, semivegetarians, and pescetarian diet groups at 6 months. However, the percent weight loss among vegetarian subjects excluding the vegans (−6.3 ± 6.6%) was not significantly different from that of the vegan group (−7.5 ± 4.5%) (Turner-Mc-Grievy et al., 2015b). A meta-analysis of 15 clinical trials found that a prescribed vegetarian diet, or specifically a vegan diet, was associated with a mean weight reduction of 3.4–4.6 kg, but no distinction was found between ovolactovegetarian and vegan diets (Barnard et al., 2015). Again, the plant-based diets were associated with weight loss in intervention trials, regardless of whether the diet prescriptions included exercise or energy restriction.

Not all clinical trials report greater weight loss success with plant-based diets. A study of 182 subjects assigned to one of two calorie- and fat-restricted diets, either a standard or ovolactovegetarian, found comparable weight loss in both groups after 6 months, due in part to a lack of compliance among the vegetarian diet group (Burke et al., 2006). Similarly, 132 participants assigned to an omnivorous versus ovolactovegetarian diet demonstrated significant weight loss on both of these calorie- and fat-restricted diets over the course of an 18-month study (Burke et al., 2008).

Moreover, few clinical trials are sufficiently long-term (>2 years) to draw conclusions about the lasting benefits of a vegetarian diet on weight management (Dansinger et al., 2007; Huang et al., 2015; Barnard et al., 2015). One intervention found that a vegan diet resulted in greater weight loss among 59 overweight and obese women at 14 weeks than a more moderate low-fat diet, and maintenance of this weight loss continued at 1- and 2-year follow-ups (Turner-McGrievy et al., 2007). However, Burke et al. (2008) found that both omnivore and ovolactovegetarian test groups regained lost weight 6 months after the 1-year intervention had concluded. Similarly, studies supporting the weight loss benefits of a vegan diet compared to a nonvegetarian diet found that while significant weight loss was seen in the initial phases of the intervention, the benefit disappeared after 6 months (Turner-McGrievy et al., 2014), or when measured over 1 year later (Huang et al., 2015).

While many weight loss interventions do not include long-term follow-up, weight regain may be the norm. There is insufficient evidence that weight loss on plant-based diets—or any diet—contributes to long-term weight maintenance. A survey of 46 dietary counseling studies found a modest mean net treatment effect of 2 BMI units of weight loss during the first year of active counseling, yet half of this weight loss was regained after 3 years (Dansinger et al., 2007). In general, only about 20% of overweight individuals maintain their weight loss beyond 1 year (Wing and Phelan, 2005). Thus the lack of long-term benefits of plant-based diets for weight management may reflect the limits of weight loss programs in general.

4. Mechanisms

Several mechanisms may contribute to the weight loss noted with plant-based diets. Proposed factors include lower energy density, protein type and quality, fat content, and carbohydrate and fiber content. Other possible mechanisms include the interrelationship between gut microbiota, high fiber, plant-based diets, and reduced inflammation and obesity.

4.1 Energy Density

Consumption of low energy density foods is fundamental to many weight loss plans (Ornish et al., 1998; Rolls et al., 2005). Fruits and vegetables, as well as cooked grains, tend to be high in water and fiber and low in fat, resulting in low energy density. Incorporating greater amounts of fruits and vegetables in the diet, while reducing fat intake, is associated with weight loss and weight maintenance (Rolls et al., 2004; Rolls, 2009). It is important to note that there is insufficient evidence that simply adding additional fruits and vegetables to the diet translates into weight loss; there must be a compensatory reduction in total energy intake. A study of overweight adults, normal weight adults, and weight loss maintainers found that weight loss maintainers consumed a diet significantly lower in energy density. These subjects reported significantly higher intake of vegetables and whole grains and less energy from fat (Raynor et al., 2011). An analysis of randomized clinical trials evaluating diet and weight management found that the recommendation to increase intake of fruit and vegetables itself had no significant effects on body weight (Kaiser et al., 2014). Thus the overall reduced energy density of a plant-based diet, rather than fruit and vegetable intake alone, is likely the driving mechanism for weight management in these studies.

4.2 Macronutrients: Protein, Fat, and Carbohydrate

Vegetarian diets tend to be lower overall in energy intake and are typically higher in carbohydrates and fiber than other diets (Berkow and Barnard, 2006; Turner-Mc-Grievy et al., 2015b; Barnard et al., 2005). However, many clinical trials of plant-based diets for weight loss frequently manipulate one macronutrient, in an attempt to examine the role of protein, fat, or carbohydrates. Other studies explore the type and quality of macronutrient, for example, comparing plant versus animal proteins in weight loss trials.

The type of protein consumed in the course of an energy-restricted diet may not be a key factor in the resulting weight loss. A study comparing diets that vary by type and quantity of protein found that meat-based proteins do not differ from soy/legume protein sources in their effects on appetite control, thermic effect of feeding, energy expenditure, or cardio-metabolic risk factors (Li et al., 2016). The overweight and obese adults in this study lost weight regardless of the dietary protein source, indicating that energy restriction per se had the greater impact on weight loss than did the factor of animal versus plant-based protein. Similarly a study comparing meat or vegetarian (soy) high-protein weight loss diets in 20 obese men found no significant differences in weight loss or changes in body fat between the two groups after 2 weeks and no difference in subjective ratings of hunger, fullness, or desire to eat (Neacsu et al., 2014). The authors conclude that for those pursing a high-protein diet for weight loss, a vegetarian diet can be effective for losing weight and controlling appetite, while avoiding some of the disease risks of a high-meat diet.

Short-term trials have found significant weight loss among subjects following a low-fat vegan diet (Barnard et al., 2005; McDougall et al., 2014). A 7-day study of 1615 participants in a residential dietary intervention program found that the subjects following an ad libitum low-fat (≤10% of calories) vegan diet lost a median of 1.4 kg weight in 7 days (McDougall et al., 2014). Of note, this diet was also characterized as high fiber and high carbohydrate (~80% of calories). Similarly, a study of postmenopausal women assigned to an ad libitum low-fat (≤10% of calories) vegan diet lost significantly more weight (−5.8±3.2 kg) over 14 weeks than the control group (3.8±2.8 kg) following the dietary guidelines of the National Cholesterol Education Program (NCEP) (Barnard et al., 2005). Both groups reported comparable reductions in energy intake, but while the control group demonstrated a decreased carbohydrate intake, the vegan diet group reduced their fat intake while increasing carbohydrates, including fiber. Of the 59 women who completed the 14-week study, the vegan diet group lost significantly more weight than the NCEP group at 1- and 2-year follow-ups (Turner-McGrievy et al., 2007). The authors hypothesize that the vegan group were eating a greater volume of food, yet taking in fewer calories due to the high fiber content of this less energy-dense diet.

Thus the low fat component of a vegan diet may not be the sole factor that contributes to greater weight loss. It must be considered that the high fiber content of a strictly plant-based diet contributes to greater satiety and lower energy density. Fiber may also work to reduce dietary fat absorption, resulting in lower adiposity and improving insulin control

(Spencer et al., 2003). A study on subjects with type 2 diabetes supports this idea, finding that a calorie-restricted, high-carbohydrate vegetarian diet resulted in greater loss of visceral fat and subsequently improved insulin sensitivity more than a standard diabetic diet (Kahleova et al., 2011).

Several studies have attempted to isolate the role of carbohydrates in plant-based weight loss diets. One study of 23 participants who completed a 6-month reduced-calorie trial found that those who followed an ad libitum, low-carbohydrate (26% of energy) vegan diet lost modestly more weight (resulting in 7% weight reduction) than did those who followed a high-carbohydrate (58% of energy) ovolactovegetarian diet (resulting in 6% weight reduction) (Jenkins et al., 2014). However, given the differences in protein and fiber intake between the diets, it is difficult to interpret the role of carbohydrates specifically.

The low-glycemic values of most whole grain products and vegetables, and the abundance of viscous fiber in whole grain foods, are proposed as contributing factors to the weight loss observed on plant-based diets (Huang et al., 2015). For example, a study of 18 overweight women with polycystic ovary syndrome found that participants following a low-glycemic index vegan diet lost significantly more weight after 3 months than those on a low-calorie diet; however, no difference was found after 6 months (Turner-McGrievy et al., 2014). The challenge in interpreting these studies, in which protein, fat, or carbohydrates are manipulated, is that the corresponding increase or decrease in other macronutrients can confound the results.

4.3 Gut Microbiota, Inflammation, and Obesity

Diet is intricately linked with the gut bacterial profile, which in turn has implications for obesity. Obesity is characterized by an altered gut profile wherein resident bacteria may be responsible for an increased capacity for energy harvest and a state of chronic, low-grade inflammation. This inflammation, in turn, can interfere with insulin signaling and result in the metabolic dysfunction found in obesity and type 2 diabetes (Requena et al., 2013; Sanz and Moya-Pérez, 2014). The microbiota of obese subjects may be characterized by a reduced bacterial diversity, a decreased prevalence of Bacteroidetes, an increase in Firmicutes and Actinobacteria, and an increased abundance of potentially inflammatory Proteobacteria (Jeffery and O'Toole, 2013; Musso et al., 2010; Verdam et al., 2013). Low-calorie and vegetarian diets have been linked to enterotypes with a greater ratio of Bacteroidetes, while Western diets are associated with an increase in Firmicutes and Actinobacteria (Benus et al., 2010; Jin and Flavell, 2013). See Chapter 24 for an in-depth discussion of fecal microbiota and the vegetarian diet.

Matijašić et al. (2014) compared principal component analysis-based bacterial DNA profiles from fecal samples of 20 vegans, 11 lactovegetarians, and 29 omnivores who were comparable in gender, age, body mass, and height. The authors found an association between diet type and bacterial community composition in which both the vegetarian and vegan subjects were associated with a higher ratio of the *Bacteroides-Prevotella* group when compared to omnivores. Another large-scale study (Zimmer et al., 2012) set out to distinguish the fecal microbiota profile of vegans ($n = 105$) from that of less restrictive vegetarians ($n = 144$) and an equal number of controls consuming an omnivorous diet. The authors found that the gut microbiota and stool pH of (non-vegan) vegetarians fell on a continuum between that of vegans and omnivores. These results suggest that the composition of the human gut varies across the spectrum of diets, with vegan diets being the most distinct from that of omnivores, but not necessarily significantly different from that of other vegetarians (Glick-Bauer and Yeh, 2014).

The high fiber content of vegan diets may also play a significant role in regulating the inflammatory response, and this inflammation may be a critical link in the relationship between gut microbiota and obesity (Sanz and Moya-Pérez, 2014; Jin and Flavell, 2013). The microbiota of obese subjects is associated with markers of local and systemic inflammation [fecal calprotectin and plasma C-reactive protein (CRP), respectively] (Verdam et al., 2013). Dietary intake is known to influence inflammation, with vegetarians demonstrating lower levels of CRP than nonvegetarians. A 6-month weight loss intervention comparing vegan, vegetarian, pescetarian, semivegetarian, and omnivore dietary groups found significantly lower inflammatory potential (Dietary Inflammatory Index) of vegan, vegetarian, and pescetarian diets at 2 months (Turner-Mc-Grievy et al., 2015a).

A vegan diet may thus play a role in influencing obesity and inflammation (Kim et al., 2013). Six obese subjects with diabetes and/or hypertension, who followed a vegan diet for 1 month, were found to have improved blood glucose levels and reduced body weight. The vegan diet therapy induced an altered gut microbiota by reducing the abundance of Firmicutes and increasing the abundance of Bacteroidetes significantly. This alteration in the Firmicutes-to-Bacteroidetes ratio was also accompanied by a decrease in pathobionts such as Enterobacteriaceae, a family of bacteria implicated in triggering low-grade inflammation. As the subjects progressed on their vegan diets, there was a decrease in the concentrations of the inflammation markers, fecal lipocalin-2 (Lcn-2), indicating that the vegan diet directly reduced the population of pathobionts. The resulting reduction in inflammation contributed to the improved glucose tolerance and lipid metabolism of their vegan subjects (Kim et al., 2013). Thus, the increased dietary fiber of plant-based diets may be a contributing factor in reducing both inflammatory markers and obesity.

5. Conclusion

Analysis of dietary patterns of populations, including the EPIC-Oxford study, the Adventist Health Study-2, and NHANES, among others, indicates that BMI and diet type fall along a continuum, with lowest BMI and rates of obesity among vegans and greatest BMI and obesity among meat eaters (Tonstad et al., 2009; Spencer et al., 2003; Farmer, 2014). Those following a vegetarian or fish-eating diet tend to fall in between the two dietary extremes.

Multiple clinical studies have supported the efficacy of plant-based diets for weight loss, both with calorie restriction and without, though few studies have provided insight into long-term (>2 year) benefits for weight management (Huang et al., 2015; Dansinger et al., 2007; Barnard et al., 2015). Those attempting weight loss with a calorie-restricted, vegetarian diet are encouraged to seek nutrition guidance to avoid deficiencies in vitamin B_{12}, zinc, and protein (Farmer, 2014). Nonetheless, a plant-based diet may prove more effective for long-term weight management than typical weight loss diets. For example, a study of 428 college students found that those who self-identified as vegetarian had lower BMI and greater long-term diet adherence than students who followed a weight loss diet (Smith et al., 2000). Motivations for following a plant-based diet, including religion, animal welfare, health, and weight loss, likely contributed to students adhering to their diet for over 12 months. In contrast, those pursuing standard weight loss diets most often abandoned the diet in 1–3 months due to boredom and feelings of deprivation.

Compliance with plant-based diets is a potential obstacle in any weight loss trial; however, there is considerable variation among studies. A study of 74 participants with diabetes found greater adherence among subjects assigned to a vegetarian diet than to a conventional diabetic diet for 24 weeks (Kahleova et al., 2011). A study of 63 overweight and obese adults found no difference in compliance or acceptability, regardless of whether participants were assigned a vegan, vegetarian, pescetarian, semivegetarian, or omnivorous diet (Moore et al., 2015). However, some clinical trials have noted participant attrition rates as high as 50%–67% after 6 months when vegan diets are prescribed for weight loss (Jenkins et al., 2014; Turner-McGrievy et al., 2014). Huang et al. (2015) found that when diets were randomly assigned, adherence to a low-fat vegetarian diet was only 50%, while adherence to the Weight Watchers diet was 65% (Huang et al., 2015). While the US News & World Report 2016 Best Diet Ranking named both the vegan and flexitarian (semivegetarian) diets as the #7 best weight loss diets, the vegan diet received much lower scores for "easy to follow" than the more lenient flexitarian diet (health.usnews.com, 2016). Thus the prescription of a plant-based diet for weight loss may pose challenges for those unable to adhere to a comparatively restrictive eating pattern. The good news is that absolute adherence may not be necessary. One study found that subjects who were counseled to follow a plant-based diet and reduce animal product intake were more successful in weight loss, even without 100% adherence, than participants assigned to omnivorous weight loss diets (Moore et al., 2015).

While there is considerable evidence that a plant-based diet is compatible with optimal eating (Katz and Meller, 2014) and weight loss (Huang et al., 2015; Dansinger et al., 2007; Barnard et al., 2015), the appropriateness of this diet has been questioned for some segments of the population, including adolescents and athletes. While adolescents and young adults who follow a vegetarian diet may be less likely to be overweight or obese, they also report binge eating with loss of control more frequently than their nonvegetarian counterparts (Robinson-O'Brien et al., 2009): see also Chapter 4 in this book. Athletes who rely on vegetarian diets for weight control may be similarly prone to disordered eating behaviors (Barr and Rideout, 2004).

Although many vegetarians cite ethics over health as motivation for adherence to a meat-free diet (Hoffman et al., 2013), lifestyle factors such as smoking, alcohol consumption, and exercise are likely significant confounding variables in any analyses comparing vegetarian diets to a typical Western diet. For example, among 100 vegans surveyed in the United States,

47% cited health as the motive for their diet choice. This subset of vegetarians was associated with regular exercise, minimal alcohol and smoking practices, and frequent consumption of vegetables, nuts, and grains (Dyett et al., 2013). The German Vegan study similarly found that vegans tend to refrain from smoking, consume limited alcohol, and engage in higher levels of physical activity when compared to the general population (Waldmann et al., 2003). In population studies such as the Adventist Health Study-2, church members who were vegetarian were also likely to refrain from smoking and alcohol consumption as a lifestyle choice (Tonstad et al., 2009; Orlich et al., 2013). Thus population and clinical studies alike must take note of conflicting lifestyle variables when comparing vegetarians to the general population and assessing the role of plant-based diets in weight loss.

Future studies could contribute greatly to our understanding of plant-based diets for weight loss if there were follow-up beyond 6 months (Turner-Mc-Grievy et al., 2015b), or even after 1, 2, or 5 years. There is indication that those who maintain their lost weight for 2–5 years have a greater chance of ongoing, longer-term success (Wing and Phelan, 2005), and it may be that even imperfect adherence to a plant-based diet could translate into lasting benefits (Moore et al., 2015). Shifting to a long-term reliance on plant foods in our diet is more likely to succeed in a culture where a healthy lifestyle overall is encouraged. Large-scale public health measures to improve diet, such as the North Karelia Project, can have great impact on reducing obesity levels and curbing lifestyle diseases (Hyde, 2008). Public health projects to promote a healthy lifestyle should be assessed for their efficacy in promoting a plant-based diet, increasing fruit and vegetable intake, and reducing overall caloric intake.

Mechanisms by which plant-based diets contribute to weight loss deserve further exploration. Vegetarian diets are typically high in fiber and carbohydrates, though the comparative benefits of low-carbohydrate versus low-fat diets continues to be debated (Bazzano et al., 2014). Vegetarian diets likely also differ in fat content and protein quality. Teasing out the role of these macronutrients, individually and synergistically, could provide insight into the optimal plant-based diet for weight control. The role of fiber in particular deserves further study, as a contributing factor in lowering adiposity, influencing gut microbiota, and reducing the inflammation associated with obesity and metabolic disease.

References

Barnard, N.D., Levin, S.M., Yokoyama, Y., 2015. A systematic review and meta-analysis of changes in body weight in clinical trials of vegetarian diets. J. Acad. Nutr. Diet. 115 (6).

Barnard, N.D., Scialli, A.R., Turner-Mc-Grievy, G., Lanou, A.J., Glass, J., 2005. The effects of a low-fat, plant-based dietary intervention on body weight, metabolism, and insulin sensitivity. Am. J. Med. 118, 991–997.

Barr, S.I., Rideout, C.A., 2004. Nutritional considerations for vegetarian athletes. Nutrition 20, 696–703.

Bazzano, L., Hu, T., Reynolds, K., Al, E., 2014. Effects of low-carbohydrate and low-fat diets; a randomized trial. Ann. Intern. Med. 161, 309–318.

Benus, R., Van Der Werf, T.S., Welling, G.W., Judd, P.A., Taylor, M.A., Harmsen, H.J.M., Whelan, K., 2010. Association between *Faecalibacterium prausnitzii* and dietary fibre in colonic fermentation in healthy human subjects. Br. J. Nutr. 104, 693–700.

Berkow, S., Barnard, N., 2006. Vegetarian diets and weight status. Nutr. Rev. 64, 175–188.

Burke, L., Styn, M., Steenkiste, A., Music, E., Warziski, M., Choo, J., 2006. A randomized clinical trial testing treatment preference and two dietary options in behavioral weight management: preliminary results of the impact of diet at 6 months – PREFER study. Obesity 14, 2007–2017.

Burke, L., Warzoski, M., Styn, M., Music, E., Hudson, A., Sereika, S., 2008. A randomized clinical trial of a standard versus vegetarian diet for weight loss: the impact of treatment preference. Int. J. Obes. 32, 166–176.

Craig, W.J., Mangels, A.R., 2009. Position paper of the American Dietetic Association: vegetarian diets. J. Am. Diet. Assoc. 109, 1266–1282.

Dansinger, M., Tatsioni, A., Wong, J., Chung, M., Balk, E., 2007. Meta-analysis: the effect of dietary counseling for weight loss. Ann. Intern. Med. 147, 41–50.

Dinu, M., Abbate, R., Gensini, G., Casini, A., Sofi, F., 2016. Vegetarian, vegan diets and multiple health outcomes: a systematic review with meta-analysis of observational studies. Crit. Rev. Food Sci. Nutr. (Online).

Dyett, P.A., Sabaté, J., Haddad, E., Rajaram, S., Shavlik, D., 2013. Vegan lifestyle behaviors. An exploration of congruence with health-related beliefs and assessed health indices. Appetite 67, 119–124.

Farmer, B., 2014. Nutritional adequacy of plant-based diets for weight management: observations from the NHANES. Am. J. Clin. Nutr. 100, 365s–368s.

Glick-Bauer, M., Yeh, M.-C., 2014. The health advantage of a vegan diet: exploring the gut microbiota connection. Nutrients 6, 4822–4838.

Health.Usnews.Com, 2016. Best Weight-Loss Diets (Online). U.S. News & World Report L.P. Available from: http://health.usnews.com/best-diet/best-weight-loss-diets.

Hoffman, S.R., Stallings, S., Bessinger, R., Brooks, G., 2013. Differences between health and ethical vegetarians. Strength of conviction, nutrition knowledge, dietary restriction, and duration of adherence. Appetite 65, 139–144.

Huang, R.-Y., Huang, C.-C., Hu, F.B., Chavarro, J.E., 2015. Vegetarian diets and weight reduction: a meta-analysis of randomized controlled trials. J. Gen. Intern. Med. 31, 109–116.

Hyde, R., 2008. Europe battles with obesity. Lancet 371, 2160–2161.

Jeffery, I.B., O'toole, P.W., 2013. Diet-microbiota interactions and their implications for healthy living. Nutrients 5, 234–252.

Jenkins, D.J., Wong, J.M.W., Kendall, C.W.C., Esfahani, A., Ng, V.W.Y., Leong, T.C.K., Faulkner, D.A., Vidgen, E., Gregory, P., Mukherjea, R., Krul, E.S., Singer, W., 2014. Effects of a 6-month vegan low-carbohydrate ('eco-Atkins') diet on cardiovascular risk factors and body weight in hyperlipidaemic adults: a randomised controlled trial. BMJ Open 4, e003505.

Jin, C., Flavell, R.A., 2013. Innate sensors of pathogen and stress: linking inflammation to obesity. J. Allergy Clin. Immunol. 132, 287–294.

Johansson, G., Källgård, B., Öckerman, P., 2012. Effects of a shift from a mixed diet to a lacto-vegetarian diet on some coronary heart disease risk markers. Open J. Prev. Med. 2, 16–22.

Kahleova, H., Matoulek, M., Malinska, H., Oliyarnik, O., Kazdova, L., Neskudla, T., Skoch, A., Hajek, M., Hill, M., Kahle, M., Pelikanova, T., 2011. Vegetarian diet improves insulin resistance and oxidative stress markers more than conventional diet in subjects with Type 2 diabetes. Diabet. Med. 28, 549–559.

Kaiser, K., Brown, A., Brown, M., Shikany, J., Mattes, R., Allison, D., 2014. Increased fruit and vegetable intake has no discernable effect on weight loss: a systematic review and meta-analysis. Am. J. Clin. Nutr. 100, 567–576.

Katz, D.L., Meller, S., 2014. Can we say what diet is best for health? Annu. Rev. Public Health 35, 83–103.

Kennedy, E., Bowman, S., Spence, J., Freedman, M., King, J., 2001. Popular diets: correlation to health, nutrition, and obesity. J. Am. Diet. Assoc. 101, 411–420.

Kim, M.-S., Hwang, S.-S., Park, E.-J., Bae, J.-W., 2013. Strict vegetarian diet improves the risk factors associated with metabolic diseases by modulating gut microbiota and reducing intestinal inflammation. Environ. Microbiol. Rep. 5, 765–775.

Li, J., Armstrong, C.L., Campbell, W.W., 2016. Effects of dietary protein source and quantity during weight loss on appetite, energy expenditure, and cardio-metabolic responses. Nutrients 8, 63.

Matijašić, B.B., Obermajer, T., Lipoglavšek, L., Grabnar, I., Avguštin, G., Rogelj, I., 2014. Association of dietary type with fecal microbiota in vegetarians and omnivores in Slovenia. Eur. J. Nutr. 53, 1051–1064.

Mcdougall, J., Thomas, L.E., Mcdougall, C., Moloney, G., Saul, B., Finnell, J.S., Richardson, K., Petersen, K.M., 2014. Effects of 7 days on an ad libitum low-fat vegan diet: the McDougall Program cohort. Nutr. J. 13.

Mishra, S., Xu, J., Agarwal, U., Gonzales, J., Levin, S., Barnard, N., 2013. A multicenter randomized control trial of a plant-based nutrition program to reduce body weight and cardiovascular risk in the corporate setting: the GEICO study. Eur. J. Clin. Nutr. 67, 718–724.

Moore, J., Mcgrievy, M., Turner-Mcgrievy, G., 2015. Dietary adherance and acceptability of five different diets, including vegan and vegetarian diets, for weight loss: the new DIETs study. Eat. Behav. 19, 33–38.

Musso, G., Gambino, R., Cassader, M., 2010. Obesity, diabetes, and gut microbiota: the hygiene hypothesis expanded. Diabetes Care 33, 2277–2284.

Neacsu, M., Fyfe, C., Horgan, G., Johnstone, A.M., 2014. Appetite control and biomarkers of satiety with vegetarian (soy) and meat-based high-protein diets for weight loss in obese men: a randomized cross-over trial. Am. J. Clin. Nutr. 100, 548–558.

Orlich, M.J., Singh, P.N., Sabaté, J., Jaceldo-Siegl, K., Fan, J., Knutsen, S., Beeson, W.L., Fraser, G.E., 2013. Vegetarian dietary patterns and mortality in Adventist Health Study 2. JAMA Intern. Med. 173, 1230–1238.

Ornish, D., Scherwitz, L., Billings, J., Gould, L., Al, E., 1998. Intensive lifestyle changes for reversal of coronary heart disease. JAMA 280, 2001–2007.

Raynor, H., Van Walleghen, E., Bachman, J., Looney, S., Phelan, S., Wing, R., 2011. Dietary energy density and successful weight loss maintenance. Eat. Behav. 12, 119–125.

Requena, T., Cotter, P., Shahar, D.R., Kleiveland, C.R., Martínez-Cuesta, M.C., Peláez, C., Lea, T., 2013. Interactions between gut microbiota, food and the obese host. Trends Food Sci. Technol. 34, 44–53.

Robinson-O'brien, R., Perry, C.L., Wall, M.M., Story, M., Neumark-Sztainer, D., 2009. Adolescent and young adult vegetarianism: better dietary intake and weight outcomes but increased risk of disordered eating behaviors. J. Am. Diet. Assoc. 109, 648–655.

Rolls, B., 2009. The relationship between dietary energy density and energy intake. Physiol. Behav. 97, 609–615.

Rolls, B., Drewinowski, A., Ledikwe, J., 2005. Changing the energy density of the diet as a strategy for weight management. J. Am. Diet. Assoc. 105, S98–S103.

Rolls, B., Ello-Martin, J., Tohill, B., 2004. What can intervention studies tellus about the relationship between fruit and vegetable consumption and weight management? Nutr. Rev. 62, 1–17.

Rosell, M., Appleby, P., Spencer, E., Key, T., 2006. Weight gain over 5 years in 21,966 meat-eating, fish-eating, vegetarian, and vegan men and women in EPIC-Oxford. Int. J. Obes. 30, 1389–1396.

Sanz, Y., Moya-Pérez, A., 2014. Chapter 14: microbiota, inflammation and obesity. In: Lyte, M., Cryan, J.F. (Eds.), Microbial Endocrinology: The Microbiota-Gut-Brain in Health and Disease. Springer, New York.

Smith, C.F., Burke, L.E., Wing, R.R., 2000. Vegetarian and weight-loss diets among young adults. Obes. Res. 8, 123–129.

Spencer, E., Appleby, P., Davey, G., Key, T., 2003. Diets and body mass index in 38,000 EPIC-Oxford meat-eaters, fish-eaters, vegetarians and vegans. Int. J. Obes. 27, 728–734.

Thedford, K., Raj, S., 2011. A vegetarian diet for weight managment. J. Am. Diet. Assoc. 111, 816–818.

Tonstad, S., Butler, T., Yan, R., Fraser, G.E., 2009. Type of vegetarian diet, body weight, and prevalence of type 2 diabetes. Diabetes Care 32, 791–796.

Turner-Mc-Grievy, G., Wirth, M.D., Shivappa, N., Al, E., 2015a. Randomization to plant-based dietary approaches leads to larger short-term improvements in Dietary Inflammatory Index scores and macronutrient intake compared with diets that contain meat. Nutr. Res. 35, 97–106.

Turner-Mc-Grievy, G.M., Davidson, C.R., Wingard, E.E., Wilcox, S., Frongillo, E.A., 2015b. Comparative effectiveness of plant-based diets for weight loss: a randomized controlled trial of five different diets. Nutrition 31, 350–358.

Turner-Mcgrievy, G., Barnard, N.D., Scialli, A.R., 2007. A two-year randomized weight loss trial comparing a vegan diet to a more moderate low-fat diet. Obesity 15, 2276–2281.

Turner-Mcgrievy, G., Davidson, C.R., Wingard, E.E., Billings, D.L., 2014. Low glycemic index vegan or low-calorie weight loss diets for women with polycystic ovary syndrome: a randomized controlled feasibility study. Nutr. Res. 34, 552–558.

Verdam, F.J., Fuentes, S., De Jonge, C., Zoetendal, E.G., Erbil, R., Greve, J.W., Buurman, W.A., De Vos, W.M., Rensen, S.S., 2013. Human intestinal microbiota composition is associated with local and systemic inflammation in obesity. Obesity 21, E607–E615.

Waldmann, A., Koschizke, J.W., Leitzmann, C., Hahn, A., 2003. Dietary intakes and lifestyle factors of a vegan population in Germany: results from the German Vegan Study. Eur. J. Clin. Nutr. 57, 947–955.

Wing, R., Phelan, S., 2005. Long-term weight loss maintenance. Am. J. Clin. Nutr. 82 (Suppl.).

Zimmer, J., Lange, B., Frick, J.-S., Sauer, H., Zimmermann, K., Schwiertz, A., Rusch, K., Klosterhalfen, S., Enck, P., 2012. A vegan or vegetarian diet substantially alters the human colonic faecal microbiota. Eur. J. Clin. Nutr. 66, 53–60.

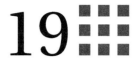

19

Cancer Risk and Vegetarian Diets

Timothy J. Key

UNIVERSITY OF OXFORD, OXFORD, OXFORDSHIRE, UNITED KINGDOM

1. Introduction

Cancer is defined as a disease in which the normal control of cell division is lost, so that an individual cell multiplies inappropriately to form a tumor. The tumor may eventually spread through the body and overwhelm it, thus causing death (Stewart and Kleihues, 2003). Cancer can arise from the cells of different tissues and organs in the body; therefore there are many different types of cancer. Cancer incidence rates vary markedly between different populations around the world (Torre et al., 2015). Furthermore, cancer incidence rates vary within populations with time, and they usually change in migrants from one population to another. These observations show that the majority of cancer cases are due to environmental and lifestyle factors rather than to inherited genetic factors and are therefore, in principle, preventable (Swerdlow et al., 2010). The variations in cancer rates between populations could be due to a wide range of environmental and lifestyle factors, and smoking is the single most important cause of cancer. Dietary factors are also of particular interest because diets vary dramatically between populations and because there are many plausible mechanisms by which diet might affect cancer risk (Stewart and Wild, 2014). Forty years ago, it was pointed out that, for many common types of cancer such as colorectal cancer and breast cancer, the incidence rates were much higher in Western countries, which had a high consumption of meat and dairy products, than in poor countries with low intakes of these foods (Armstrong and Doll, 1975), and this observation underlies the hypothesis that high intakes of meat and other animal products might increase the risk for some types of cancer.

Vegetarian diets exclude all meat and fish, and vegan diets further exclude dairy products and eggs. Compared to meat eaters, vegetarians usually eat more cereals, vegetables, fruits, and nuts. It is possible that vegetarian diets would affect cancer risk because of the absence of foods such as meat or fish or because of relatively high intakes of foods such as cereals, fruit, vegetables, and associated nutrients and nutritional factors such as dietary fiber.

2. How Can Diet Affect Cancer?

Most factors that are well-established determinants of cancer risk are factors that increase risk. For example, cigarette smoke contains many mutagenic chemicals and therefore causes damage to DNA and a large increase in the risk of many cancers, such as lung cancer;

other factors cause cancer because they are mutagenic, include ionizing radiation and some oncogenic viruses. There are also factors that cause cancer by altering the rate of cell division; for example, some hormones such as estrogens and insulin-like growth factor-1 (IGF-1) increase mitosis and reduce apoptosis and can therefore increase the chance of mutations occurring and being replicated, as well as promoting the growth of early tumors.

For diet there are a few factors that are known to increase risk by causing mutations; this is probably the mechanism by which Cantonese-style salted fish increases the risk of nasopharyngeal cancer, and this may be part of the mechanism linking foods such as processed meat and salt-preserved foods with the risk for some cancers of the gastrointestinal tract. Diet may also have other effects on cancer by supplying protective factors, such as dietary fiber, fruit, and vegetables; it has long been thought that antioxidant vitamins and other antioxidant nonnutrients in plants might reduce cancer risk, but despite many years of research the importance of this mechanism remains uncertain. Diet may also affect cancer risk by affecting metabolism and thus the level of key hormones such as estrogens and IGF-1. In the context of vegetarian diets, the main potential mechanisms for an effect of cancer are the absence of putative adverse effects due to meat and other animal products, and perhaps to a lesser extent the presence of higher intakes of putative protective factors in some plant foods. The potential relevance of such factors varies between cancers at different sites, and it is discussed further subsequently.

3. Established Associations of Diet With Cancer Risk

Few dietary factors have been convincingly shown to affect the risk of cancer (Table 19.1). The most important are obesity and alcohol, both of which increase the risk for several types of cancer. In terms of dietary composition, the only relationships that have been judged by expert advisory groups to be convincing are for meat and fiber in relation to the risk for colorectal cancer; high intakes of both red meat and processed meat increase the risk for colorectal cancer, whereas high intakes of dietary fiber reduce the risk for colorectal cancer (WCRF, 2007).

4. The Evidence Available on Cancer Risk and Vegetarian Diets

There is relatively little direct evidence on the risk of cancer in people following vegetarian diets, and so far very little evidence for vegan diets. Most of the evidence comes from a handful of prospective cohort studies conducted in the United Kingdom (UK) and among Seventh-day Adventists in the United States. These studies set out to recruit a large proportion of vegetarians; their prospective design means that their results should not be seriously affected by recall bias or participation bias, but like all observational studies, their results can be affected by confounding due to other dietary and nondietary factors that may affect the risk of cancer.

The early cohort studies of vegetarians have mainly published results on cancer mortality. A summary of these data is provided by a pooled analysis of individual participant

Table 19.1   Dietary Risk Factors, Dietary Protective Factors, and Other Major Risk Factors for Common Cancers

Cancer	Dietary and Diet-Related Risk Factors	Dietary Protective Factors	Major Nondietary Risk Factors
Oral cavity, pharynx, and larynx	Alcohol	Probably fruits and vegetables	Smoking
Nasopharynx	Cantonese-style salted fish		Epstein–Barr virus
Esophagus	Alcohol	Probably fruits and vegetables	Smoking
	Obesity (adenocarcinoma of the esophagus)		
Stomach	Probably high intake of salt and salt-preserved foods	Probably fruits and vegetables	Infection by *Helicobacter pylori*
			Smoking
Colorectum	Alcohol	Dietary fiber	Sedentary lifestyle
	Obesity	Probably fruits and vegetables	Smoking
	Processed meat		
	Probably red meat		
Liver	Alcohol	None established	Hepatitis viruses
	Obesity		Smoking
	Foods contaminated with aflatoxin		
Pancreas	Obesity	None established	Smoking
Lung	None established	None established	Smoking
Breast	Alcohol	None established	Reproductive and hormonal factors
	Obesity (postmenopausal)		
Cervix	None established	None established	Human papillomavirus
			Smoking
Endometrium	Obesity	None established	Reproductive and hormonal factors
Ovary	Obesity	None established	Reproductive and hormonal factors
Prostate	Probably obesity for aggressive disease	None established	None established
Kidney	Obesity	None established	Smoking
Bladder	None established	None established	Smoking
			Occupational risk factors
Non-Hodgkin lymphoma	Obesity	None established	None established

data from five prospective studies (Key et al., 1999). Some data on cancer incidence have also been published from some of these early studies, such as the first Adventist Health Study (AHS; Fraser, 1999), but most of the data now available on cancer incidence in vegetarians comes from EPIC-Oxford in the UK (Key et al., 2014; this publication includes data from EPIC-Oxford and also from the earlier Oxford Vegetarian Study) and from the Adventist Health Study-2 (AHS-2) in the United States (AHS-2; Tantamango-Bartley et al., 2013; Orlich et al., 2015; Tantamango-Bartley et al., 2016).

I have not reviewed here the data on cancer risk for vegetarians in non-Western populations. Few such data are available, and they are largely from case–control studies. More data should become available over the next few years, particularly from India where the proportion of vegetarians in the population is high. The characteristics of vegetarian diets differ between Western and non-Western populations, and effects on cancer risk are also likely to differ; therefore it cannot be assumed that the conclusions reached in this chapter would also apply to vegetarians in non-Western populations.

4.1 The Role of Body Mass Index and Obesity

As discussed earlier and in Table 19.1, obesity increases the risk for several types of cancer. Vegetarians in Western populations have been consistently shown to have a lower body mass index than vegetarians, with a correspondingly lower prevalence of obesity (Davey et al., 2003). The lower body mass index of vegetarians almost certainly causes a corresponding reduction in the risk for the cancers caused by obesity, but the size of the difference in body mass index [e.g., 1–2 units (kg/m^2) of body mass index in EPIC-Oxford] is not large enough to cause a large reduction in cancer risk. In the following sections on individual cancer sites, the relative risks reported are those that have been adjusted for relevant risk factors and for body mass index (with the exception of endometrial cancer, where the impact of adjusting for body mass index is described); thus the relative risks reported should be interpreted as the evidence for an impact of vegetarian diet on cancer risk *after allowing for* the lower body mass index of vegetarians.

5. Cancers of the Upper Gastrointestinal Tract and Stomach

For cancers of the lip, oral cavity, pharynx, and esophagus, the main risk factors in Western countries are alcohol and tobacco, as well as obesity for one type of cancer of the esophagus (adenocarcinoma). The evidence available does not suggest that the risk for these cancers differs substantially between vegetarians and nonvegetarians (Key et al., 2014).

Stomach cancer risk is associated with chronic infection with the bacterium *Helicobacter pylori* and with high intakes of salt-preserved and pickled foods such as meat, fish, and vegetables. There is also some evidence that the risk for stomach cancer is inversely associated with the intake of fresh fruit and vegetables. In the pooled analysis of cancer mortality in five prospective studies, there was no difference in the risk of death from stomach cancer between vegetarians and nonvegetarians [relative risk 1.02 (0.64–1.62)], whereas in the UK prospective studies the risk of stomach cancer was approximately 60% lower in vegetarians than in meat eaters [Table 19.2: relative risk 0.38 (0.20–0.71)]. Both these analyses were based on small numbers of cases of stomach cancer; therefore no firm conclusion can be drawn.

6. Colorectal Cancer

Early "ecological" studies that compared diets and cancer rates in different populations showed a strong positive correlation between estimates of meat intake at a national level

Table 19.2 Vegetarians: Relative Risks for Stomach, Colorectal, Breast, Prostate, and Hematological Cancers, and All Cancers Combined, Compared to Meat Eaters

Cancer Site	Results From UK Cohorts[a]	Results From AHS[b]	Results From AHS-2[c]
Stomach	0.38 (0.20–0.71)	–	–
Colorectum	1.04 (0.84–1.28)	0.53 (0.35–0.81)[d]	0.83 (0.66–1.05)
Breast	0.96 (0.83–1.10)	0.80 (0.56–1.15)	–
Prostate	0.83 (0.64–1.06)	0.65 (0.44–0.95)	0.96 (0.83–1.12)
Lymphatic and hematopoietic tissue	0.64 (0.48–0.84)	–	–
All cancers	0.90 (0.93–0.96)	–	0.93 (0.85–1.02)

[a]All vegetarians including vegans compared to meat eaters.
[b]Adventist Health Study; all vegetarians including vegans compared to nonvegetarians.
[c]Adventist Health Study-2; lactovegetarians compared to regular meat eaters.
[d]Colon cancer.

and the incidence of colorectal cancer (Armstrong and Doll, 1975). The results of subsequent population-based prospective studies have varied somewhat, but overall they show that, on average, people with relatively high intakes of red meat and processed meat have a higher risk for this type of cancer; for example, in a meta-analysis of prospective studies, Chan et al. (2011) showed that the relative risk for colorectal cancer was 1.17 (1.05–1.31) for an increase in intake of red meat of 100 g/day and 1.18 (1.10–1.28) for an increase in intake of processed meat of 50 g/day. Together with the results of laboratory-based research, these findings led the International Agency for Research on Cancer (part of the World Health Organization) to classify red meat as probably carcinogenic and processed meat as certainly carcinogenic (Bouvard et al., 2015). For a more detailed examination of the relationship between meat intake and cancer risk, the reader is referred to another chapter of this book (Chapter 12).

In view of these conclusions, it would be expected that vegetarians would have a relatively low risk for colorectal cancer, but the direct findings on this have not been consistent. In a pooled analysis of the five early prospective studies, the relative risk for death from colorectal cancer in vegetarians compared to nonvegetarians was 0.99 (0.77–1.27), providing no evidence for a reduction in risk. In subsequent studies reporting on the incidence of colorectal cancer, the relative risk in vegetarians compared to nonvegetarians in the UK studies was 1.04 (0.84–1.28), again showing no evidence of a reduction in risk (Table 19.2); there was a reduction in risk for people who did not eat meat but did eat fish [relative risk compared to meat eaters=0.67 (0.48–0.98)]. In the AHS, the risk was not reported for colorectal cancer, but the relative risk for colon cancer in nonmeat eaters compared to meat eaters was 0.53 (0.35–0.81) (Table 19.2). In the AHS-2, the risk for colorectal cancer in comparison to regular meat eaters was 0.79 (0.64–0.97) for all "vegetarians," but this broad category included people with a low intake of meat and people who did not eat meat but did eat fish, as well as true vegetarians; the relative risks were 0.83 (0.66–1.05) in lactovegetarians (Table 19.2) and 0.58 (0.40–0.84) in people who did not eat meat but did eat fish. A recent analysis in a cohort in the Netherlands that included a moderate number of vegetarians found no significant difference in risk of colorectal cancer between vegetarians and regular meat eaters (Gilsing et al., 2015). Thus, neither the

Table 19.3 Vegans: Relative Risks for Colorectal, Breast, and Prostate Cancer and All Cancers Combined, Compared to Meat Eaters

Cancer Site	Results From UK Cohorts[a]	Results From AHS-2[b]
Colorectum	1.31 (0.82–2.11)	0.86 (0.59–1.24)
Breast	0.91 (0.61–1.34)	–
Prostate	0.61 (0.31–1.20)	0.66 (0.50–0.87)
All cancers	0.82 (0.68–1.00)	0.84 (0.72–0.99)

[a]Vegans compared to meat eaters.
[b]Adventist Health Study-2; vegans compared to regular meat eaters.

older data on mortality nor the recent data on incidence show a consistently reduced risk in vegetarians; two recent studies do suggest a reduced risk in people who do not eat meat but do eat fish (Key et al., 2014; Orlich et al., 2015), but the observations on fish eaters are based on only 78 cases overall and should be regarded as tentative. For the vegetarians, the absence of a clear reduction in risk in the UK studies appears inconsistent with the conclusions reached by the International Agency for Research on Cancer, but this may be partly because average meat intake in the meat eaters in these studies was not high enough to give a detectable difference in risk.

For vegans, the UK cohorts reported a relative risk of 1.31 (0.82–2.11) compared to meat eaters, and the AHS-2 reported a relative risk of 0.86 (0.59–1.24) compared to regular meat eaters (Table 19.3); the total number of cases among vegans in these two studies was only 59; therefore more data are needed before any firm conclusion can be drawn.

7. Cancer of the Pancreas

The main established risk factor for cancer of the pancreas is smoking, and obesity also causes a moderate increase in risk. There is little evidence on the risk of cancer of the pancreas in vegetarians. In the UK cohorts the relative risk in comparison with meat eaters was 0.70 (0.42–1.17); further analyses of mortality from this cancer were reported in relation to regular meat eaters and showed a significant reduction in risk [hazard ratio 0.44 (0.26–0.76); Appleby et al., 2016].

8. Lung Cancer

Heavy smoking increases the risk of lung cancer by around 40-fold, and smoking causes over 80% of lung cancers in Western countries. Some observational studies have found that lung cancer patients report a relatively lower intake of fruits, vegetables, and related nutrients (such as β-carotene) than controls, but these findings may be due to residual confounding by smoking because smokers usually eat less fruit and vegetables than nonsmokers. There is no evidence suggesting that, after allowing for smoking, there is any difference in the risk of lung cancer between vegetarians and nonvegetarians. For example, in the UK cohort studies the relative risk of lung cancer in vegetarians compared to meat eaters was 1.09 (0.78–1.53).

9. Breast Cancer

Breast cancer is strongly related to reproductive and hormonal factors; a higher risk is associated with early menarche (age at first menstrual period) and late menopause, while risk is lower in women who have children at a young age, with risk decreasing with a greater number of children and with longer breastfeeding. Obesity after menopause increases risk, probably because it causes an increase in circulating estrogens. Studies of major foods, food groups, macronutrients, and micronutrients have not shown any definite associations with breast cancer risk, and studies of vegetarians have not shown any difference in breast cancer risk compared to nonvegetarians; for example, the UK studies of vegetarians reported a relative risk of 0.96 (0.83–1.10) in vegetarians compared to meat eaters (Table 19.2), and another population-based cohort study in the UK also reported no difference in risk of breast cancer between vegetarians and red meat eaters (Cade et al., 2010).

Circulating IGF-1 is positively associated with the risk of breast cancer (Endogenous Hormones and Breast Cancer Collaborative Group, 2010), and vegans (but not lactovegetarians) have relatively low circulating IGF-1; it is therefore possible that vegans might have a relatively low risk of breast cancer, but data published so far show no significant difference in breast cancer risk between vegans and meat eaters [in the UK cohorts the relative risk was 0.87 (0.59–1.28); Table 19.3].

10. Cancer of the Endometrium

The risk for endometrial cancer is strongly related to hormonal factors. Risk is increased by obesity, which raises circulating concentrations of estrogens. Exposure to progesterone during pregnancy, or progestogens in oral contraceptives, both cause a decrease in risk. There is little evidence that dietary composition affects risk independently of any association with obesity. In the UK cohorts, the risk for endometrial cancer in vegetarians compared to meat eaters was 0.91 (0.62–1.33), and this was attenuated to the null by adjustment for body mass index, which was lower in vegetarians than in meat eaters [adjusted relative risk=0.99 (0.67–1.45)].

11. Cancer of the Cervix

The major cause of cervical cancer is infection with certain subtypes of the human papillomavirus. Fruits, vegetables, and related nutrients such as carotenoids and folate have been inversely related with risk in some observational studies, but these associations may be due to confounding by papillomavirus infections, smoking, and other factors, and overall there is little evidence that dietary factors influence the risk of this cancer. In the UK studies the risk for cervical cancer in vegetarians compared to meat eaters was 1.90 (1.00–3.60); this borderline statistically significant large increase in risk in vegetarians was unexpected and requires further investigation, for example, to examine whether it might be related to less uptake of cervical cancer screening in vegetarians.

12. Cancer of the Ovary

Risk for cancer of the ovary is reduced by high parity and by long-term use of combined oral contraceptives. Adult height is weakly associated with risk, and obesity is associated with risk in postmenopausal women who have not used hormonal therapy for menopause. Some studies have suggested that risk might be increased by high intakes of fat or dairy products and reduced by high intakes of vegetables, but the data are not consistent and overall are inconclusive. In the UK cohorts the relative risk for vegetarians in comparison with meat eaters was 0.87 (0.61–1.22).

13. Prostate Cancer

Little is known about the etiology of prostate cancer, and the only well-established risk factors are increasing age, family history, black ethnic background, and genetic factors. Ecological studies suggest that risk may be positively associated with a Western-style diet, and diets high in red meat, dairy products, and animal fat have been implicated in the development of prostate cancer, but the data are not consistent and overall are inconclusive. For vegetarians, the UK cohorts report a relative risk for prostate cancer in lactovegetarians compared to meat eaters of 0.86 (0.61–1.11), the AHS reports a relative risk of 0.65 (0.44–0.95), and AHS-2 reports a relative risk of 0.96 (0.66–1.24) (Table 19.2).

Prostate cancer risk is positively associated with circulating levels of IGF-1, and vegans have relatively low circulating concentrations of this hormone. The UK cohorts report a relative risk for prostate cancer in vegans compared to meat eaters of 0.61 (0.31–1.20), and AHS-2 reports a relative risk of 0.66 (0.50–0.87) (Table 19.3); these findings are consistent with the hypothesis that vegans may have a reduced risk of prostate cancer, but they are based on only 68 cases in vegans, and more research is needed on this topic.

14. Cancers of the Lymphatic and Hematopoietic Tissue

This is a rather heterogeneous group of cancers. Some studies have suggested that an increased risk may be associated with consumption of meat and/or exposure to live animals and raw meat among farmers and butchers. For vegetarians, the UK cohorts reported that the relative risk for this group of cancers, compared to meat eaters, was 0.64 (0.48–0.84); potential mechanisms could include mutagenic compounds and/or viruses in meat, and more research on the risk for these cancers in vegetarians is needed.

15. Other Types of Cancer

There are many different types of cancer, and for most of these, there is little or no direct evidence as to whether risk differs between vegetarians and nonvegetarians. In addition to the cancer sites discussed earlier, the report from the UK cohorts covered four other cancer sites (melanoma, kidney, bladder, and brain), and for none of these was there evidence that risk differed between vegetarians and meat eaters. However, the numbers of cases for each cancer site were small, and therefore more research is needed to determine whether there is any influence of a vegetarian diet on the risk for these cancers.

16. All Cancers Combined

The reports from both the UK cohorts and from AHS-2 included the relative risks for all cancers combined in lactovegetarians compared with meat eaters; the risks were 0.90 (0.84–0.97) and 0.93 (0.85–1.02), respectively (Table 19.2). For vegans the relative risks for all cancers combined in these cohorts were 0.82 (0.68–1.00) and 0.84 (0.72–0.99), respectively (Table 19.3). Thus the results from these studies appear broadly consistent, suggesting that risk for all cancers combined may be ~10% lower in lactovegetarians than in meat eaters, and the risk in vegans might be nearly 20% lower. However, these findings need to be interpreted very cautiously. They are so far based on only two studies, and further research may differ. Furthermore, risk for all cancers combined is influenced not only by the cancer sites that may be affected by diet, but also by other cancer sites for which diet may have little or no impact but for which confounding factors may still differ between dietary groups.

17. Conclusions

Overall, there is relatively little evidence on whether the risk of cancer differs between Western vegetarians and nonvegetarians, and no firm conclusions can be reached. Some studies have shown a lower risk for stomach cancer and colorectal cancer in vegetarians, but the data are not consistent. The evidence does not suggest any substantial differences between vegetarians and nonvegetarians in risk for breast cancer or prostate cancer. One study has shown that vegetarians may have a lower risk for cancers of the lymphatic and hematopoietic tissue than nonvegetarians. Few data are available for vegans, but these suggest that they might have a reduced risk for prostate cancer and perhaps of all cancers combined. For many types of cancer, there is little evidence, and much more research is needed both in Western vegetarians and in other populations.

References

Appleby, P.N., Crowe, F.L., Bradbury, K.E., Travis, R.C., Key, T.J., 2016. Mortality in vegetarians and comparable nonvegetarians in the United Kingdom. Am. J. Clin. Nutr. 103, 218–230.

Armstrong, B., Doll, R., 1975. Environmental factors and cancer incidence and mortality in different countries, with special reference to dietary practices. Int. J. Cancer 15, 617–631.

Bouvard, V., Loomis, D., Guyton, K.Z., Grosse, Y., Ghissassi, F.E., Benbrahim-Tallaa, L., Guha, N., Mattock, H., Straif, K., International Agency for Research on Cancer Monograph Working Group, 2015. Carcinogenicity of consumption of red and processed meat. Lancet Oncol. 16. pii:S1470-2045(15) 00444-1.

Cade, J.E., Taylor, E.F., Burley, V.J., Greenwood, D.C., 2010. Common dietary patterns and risk of breast cancer: analysis from the United Kingdom Women's Cohort Study. Nutr. Cancer 62, 300–306.

Chan, D.S., Lau, R., Aune, D., Vieira, R., Greenwood, D.C., Kampman, E., Norat, T., 2011. Red and processed meat and colorectal cancer incidence: meta-analysis of prospective studies. PLoS One 6, e20456.

Davey, G.K., Spencer, E.A., Appleby, P.N., Allen, N.E., Knox, K.H., Key, T.J., 2003. EPIC-Oxford: lifestyle characteristics and nutrient intakes in a cohort of 33 883 meat-eaters and 31 546 non meat-eaters in the UK. Public Health Nutr. 6, 259–269.

Endogenous Hormones and Breast Cancer Collaborative Group, Key, T.J., Appleby, P.N., Reeves, G.K., Roddam, A.W., 2010. Insulin-like growth factor 1 (IGF1), IGF binding protein 3 (IGFBP3), and breast cancer risk: pooled individual data analysis of 17 prospective studies. Lancet Oncol. 11, 530–542.

Fraser, G.E., 1999. Associations between diet and cancer, ischemic heart disease, and all-cause mortality in non-Hispanic white California Seventh-day Adventists. Am. J. Clin. Nutr. 70, 532s–538s.

Gilsing, A.M., Schouten, L.J., Goldbohm, R.A., Dagnelie, P.C., van den Brandt, P.A., Weijenberg, M.P., 2015. Vegetarianism, low meat consumption and the risk of colorectal cancer in a population based cohort study. Sci. Rep. 5, 13484.

Key, T.J., Fraser, G.E., Thorogood, M., Appleby, P.N., Beral, V., Reeves, G., Burr, M.L., Chang-Claude, J., Frentzel-Beyme, R., Kuzma, J.W., Mann, J., McPherson, K., 1999. Mortality in vegetarians and nonvegetarians: detailed findings from a collaborative analysis of 5 prospective studies. Am. J. Clin. Nutr. 70, 516S–524S.

Key, T.J., Appleby, P.N., Crowe, F.L., Bradbury, K.E., Schmidt, J.A., Travis, R.C., 2014. Cancer in British vegetarians: updated analyses of 4998 incident cancers in a cohort of 32,491 meat eaters, 8612 fish eaters, 18,298 vegetarians, and 2246 vegans. Am. J. Clin. Nutr. 100, 378S–385S.

Orlich, M.J., Singh, P.N., Sabaté, J., Fan, J., Sveen, L., Bennett, H., Knutsen, S.F., Beeson, W.L., Jaceldo-Siegl, K., Butler, T.L., Herring, R.P., Fraser, G.E., 2015. Vegetarian dietary patterns and the risk of colorectal cancers. JAMA Intern. Med. 175, 767–776.

Stewart, B.W., Kleihues, P. (Eds.), 2003. World Cancer Report. World Health Organization, Lyon.

Stewart, B.W., Wild, C.P. (Eds.), 2014. World Cancer Report. World Health Organization, Lyon.

Swerdlow, A.J., Doll, R.S., Peto, R., 2010. Epidemiology of cancer. In: Warrell, D.A., Cox, T.M., Firth, J.D. (Eds.), Oxford Textbook of Medicine, fifth ed. Oxford University Press, Oxford, pp. 193–218.

Tantamango-Bartley, Y., Jaceldo-Siegl, K., Fan, J., Fraser, G., 2013. Vegetarian diets and the incidence of cancer in a low-risk population. Cancer Epidemiol. Biomarkers Prev. 22, 286–294.

Tantamango-Bartley, Y., Knutsen, S.F., Knutsen, R., Jacobsen, B.K., Fan, J., Beeson, W.L., Sabate, J., Hadley, D., Jaceldo-Siegl, K., Penniecook, J., Herring, P., Butler, T., Bennett, H., Fraser, G., 2016. Are strict vegetarians protected against prostate cancer? Am. J. Clin. Nutr. 103, 153–160.

Torre, L.A., Siegel, R.L., Ward, E.M., Jemal, A., 2015. Global cancer incidence and mortality rates and trends—an update. Cancer Epidemiol. Biomarkers Prev. http://dx.doi.org/10.1158/1055-9965.EPI-15-0578.

World Cancer Research Fund/American Institute for Cancer Research, 2007. Food, Nutrition, Physical Activity, and the Prevention of Cancer: A Global Perspective. AICR, Washington, DC.

Further Reading

World Cancer Research Fund International. Continuous Update Project. Available online: http://www.wcrf.org/int/research-we-fund/continuous-update-project-cup.

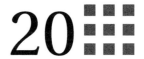

20

Vegetarian Diets and the Risk of Type 2 Diabetes

Serena Tonstad[1,2], Peter Clifton[3,4]

[1]OSLO UNIVERSITY HOSPITAL, OSLO, NORWAY; [2]LOMA LINDA UNIVERSITY, LOMA LINDA, CA, UNITED STATES; [3]UNIVERSITY OF SOUTH AUSTRALIA, ADELAIDE, SA, AUSTRALIA; [4]SCHOOL OF HEALTH SCIENCES FLINDERS UNIVERSITY, ADELAIDE, SA, AUSTRALIA

1. Introduction

Lifestyles characterized by excessive energy intake and inadequate physical activity contribute to the incidence of chronic diseases, particularly obesity and type 2 diabetes. The current "diabesity" epidemic is posed to consume healthcare resources globally and reverse some of the gains in cardiovascular longevity that have been achieved during the past decades. Global policy solutions have been called for to counter this epidemic (Hu et al., 2015). Public health recommendations focus on energy balance, asking populations to eat less and move more. Indeed, among subjects with glucose intolerance an energy-reduced, low-fat, high-fiber diet combined with 150 min/week of physical activity lowered the incidence of diabetes similarly in Finnish and US studies (Tuomilehto et al., 2001; Diabetes Prevention Program Research group, 2002). This type of lifestyle intervention appears superior to pharmacological approaches (Hopper et al., 2011). Conversely, a low-fat diet high in fruit, vegetables, and grains that did not incorporate increased physical activity or target weight reduction did not reduce incidence of diabetes in the Women's Health Initiative (Tinker et al., 2008). Yet, some evidence suggests that specific dietary and macronutrient patterns including low glycemic index or load diets (Bhupathiraju et al., 2014) and Mediterranean diets without energy restriction (Salas-Salvadó et al., 2014) may reduce the risk of type 2 diabetes beyond weight loss.

Given the paucity of randomized controlled trials comparing dietary patterns, consensus regarding the best protective diet against type 2 diabetes has not been achieved. However, the healthiest diets are generally food based and include lots of fruit, vegetables, legumes, whole grains, plant oils, and fish but are low in meat, sugar, and many processed foods (Jacobs and Orlich, 2014; Fardet and Boirie, 2014). These characteristics are typical of a plant-based diet and close to vegetarian diets. Furthermore, vegetarians are slimmer than nonvegetarians (Dinu et al., 2016) and on this basis alone are expected to carry a lower risk of type 2 diabetes than their omnivorous counterparts. This notion is bolstered by initial observations made in 1985 indicating that Seventh-day Adventist vegetarians incurred one-half the risk of diabetes as cause of death compared to the general population of US Whites (Snowdon and Phillips, 1985). Further evidence reviewed herein has accumulated from cross-sectional and prospective studies in a range of populations, as well as suggestions that vegetarianism is associated with lower insulin resistance and lesser risk of metabolic syndrome, a precursor of type 2 diabetes.

2. Diabetes Prevalence in Vegetarians

2.1 Seventh-Day Adventist Populations

Studies of Seventh-day Adventist vegetarians were initiated in 1960 with what became known as the "Adventist Mortality Study," conducted among church members residing in California (Snowdon and Phillips, 1985). Participants completed questionnaires regarding dietary habits and were asked if they "ever had diabetes" (without distinguishing between noninsulin or insulin-dependent diabetes). Nonvegetarians had a higher prevalence ratio of diabetes compared to vegetarians, a risk that was more pronounced in the underweight group (Snowdon and Phillips, 1985). Nearly two decades later, a small study of Seventh-day Adventists in Barbados likewise found that those who identified as vegetarian were leaner than nonvegetarians and had a lower prevalence of diabetes (Brathwaite et al., 2003).

The Adventist Health Study-2 was initiated in 2002 among churchgoers in North America. In an analysis among 60,903 participants, vegetarians exhibited a lower prevalence of type 2 diabetes than nonvegetarians (Fraser, 2009). Furthermore, an incremental reduction in prevalence of diabetes was observed with increasing exclusion of animal foods (Tonstad et al., 2009). Compared to nonvegetarians, semivegetarians (who ate red meat or poultry at least once a month but less than once a week) and pescetarians (who ate fish at least once a month, but not red meat or poultry) had risk reductions of one-third to one-quarter, while ovolactovegetarians and vegans had nearly a halving of risk after adjustment for BMI and other known risk factors for diabetes. Without adjustment for BMI risk, reductions were larger, ranging from 31% for semivegetarians to 68% for vegans. The diagnosis of diabetes was based on validated self-report, as blood analyses for glucose or HbA1C concentrations were not feasible in this large cohort. In a subset of 592 Black participants where blood test results were conducted, odds of diabetes in vegetarians/vegans were one-half the risk of nonvegetarians (Fraser et al., 2015), reductions that were similar to those observed in the large cohort.

2.2 Other Western Populations

The EPIC-Oxford cohort study has studied health outcomes among men and women living in England and Scotland, of whom 34% reported consuming a vegetarian diet (Crowe et al., 2013). A very small percentage of this cohort (0.4%–1.9%) reported a diabetes diagnosis. While this proportion was numerically lower in vegetarians than nonvegetarians, this may be due to the lower age of the vegetarians (Crowe et al., 2013). Further analyses from this cohort have not been reported to date.

2.3 Asian Populations

Lower BMI and prevalence of diabetes have been observed in Asian vegetarians, though not all studies are consistent. In a cross-sectional study of Taiwanese Buddhists, the prevalence of diabetes in vegetarians was lower than in nonvegetarians (Chiu et al., 2014). In contrast, the Indian Migration Study found no difference in the prevalence of diabetes between vegetarians and nonvegetarians (Shridhar et al., 2014). However, a large, nationally representative sample of Indian adults found that lacto-, ovolacto- and semivegetarian diets were associated with a lower likelihood of diabetes (Agrawal et al., 2014). BMI differences between vegetarians and nonvegetarians in this study were small, and BMI was low (~21 kg/m^2) in all groups.

3. Diabetes Incidence in Vegetarians

Only data from Seventh-day Adventist populations appears to be available. Snowdon and Phillips (1985) reported that diabetes as an underlying cause of death was halved in vegetarians compared to nonvegetarians in the Adventist Mortality Study cohort of 25,698 White church members followed for 21 years. Men who were vegetarians had a substantially lower risk of diabetes as an underlying or contributing cause of death. Among 8401 persons who participated in both the Adventist Mortality Study and Adventist Health Study (started in 1976, the precursor of the Adventist Health Study-2) and who were nondiabetic at baseline, 543 incident cases of diabetes were identified during 17 years of follow-up between the studies (Vang et al., 2008). After control for baseline body weight and change in weight, weekly meat intake was a significant risk factor for diabetes (odds ratio (OR) 1.38; 95% CI 1.06–1.80) compared to long-term vegetarianism. Preliminary data combining data from these two Adventist follow-up studies further suggested that changing from a vegetarian to a nonvegetarian dietary pattern over the 17-year interval was associated with significant increases in the likelihood of diabetes (Singh et al., 2014).

In the Adventist Health Study-2, 41,387 participants who did not report diabetes (type 1 or 2) at baseline responded to a self-report follow-up questionnaire administered 2 years later (Tonstad et al., 2013). In multivariate analysis adjusted for age, sex, education, income, television watching, physical activity, sleep, alcohol, smoking, and BMI, ORs for developing diabetes compared with nonvegetarians were 0.38 (95% CI 0.24–0.62) for vegans, 0.62 (95% CI 0.50–0.76) for ovolactovegetarians, 0.79 (95% CI 0.58–1.09) for pescetarians, and 0.49 (95% CI 0.31, 0.76) for semivegetarians (Tonstad et al., 2013). In the subset of Blacks in this study, only vegan and ovolactovegetarian diets were protective. These associations were strengthened when BMI was removed from the analyses.

4. Meat Intake and Risk of Diabetes

An accumulating body of data suggests a link between consumption of red or processed meat and diabetes. In meta-analysis of seven studies, consumption of processed meat was associated with a 19% (95% CI 11%–27%) higher incidence of diabetes, but red meat intake showed no association (Micha et al., 2010). In a subsequent meta-analysis the risk of type 2 diabetes was shown to increase by 51% (95% CI 25%–83%) per 50 g per person per day of processed red meat intake (Pan et al., 2011). The increase in risk was lower but statistically significant for consumption of unprocessed red meat (19%; 95% CI 4%–37% per 100 g per person per day). There was significant heterogeneity between studies. After adjustment to exclude publication bias, the risk was still increased for consumption of processed red meat (23%; 95% CI 1.01–1.52). The latest meta-analysis identified data for total meat from 14 separate cohorts and resulted in a pooled relative risk of 1.15 for each 100 g of total meat consumed with some heterogeneity (Feskens et al., 2013). For red meat (14 studies), the overall relative risk was 1.13 per 100 g (95% CI 1.03–1.23), and for processed meat the summary estimate of 21 separate cohorts was 1.32 per 50 g/day (95% CI 1.19–1.48) with high heterogeneity. Further analyses looked at changes in meat consumption over the course of 4 years in three large prospective US studies. A significant relation was found between an increase in the consumption of red meat and the incidence of type 2 diabetes over the course of 4 years of follow-up (Feskens et al., 2013). An increase of >1.5 oz (~42 g) per day compared to no change was associated with a 48% (95% CI 1.37–1.59) increase in risk of diabetes (Pan et al., 2013). The increase in risk was only modestly attenuated after adjustment for initial BMI and concurrent weight gain, and it was observed both for processed and unprocessed red meat. Notably, a statistically significant interaction was observed between initial BMI and changes in red meat intake and the risk of diabetes. The risk associated with eating more red meat was more pronounced in nonobese individuals, but statistically significant also in the obese. Changing from high to low intakes of red meat showed a long-term benefit on incidence of diabetes. Thus, a reduction of >1.5 oz (~42 g) per day was associated with a 10% (95% CI 0.83–0.97) lower risk after adjustment for initial BMI and concurrent weight gain.

Readers can also refer to Chapter 12 for a review of meat intake and health, including diabetes risk.

5. Metabolic Syndrome and Components

5.1 Vegetarian Diets and Metabolic Syndrome

Metabolic syndrome, a constellation of cardiovascular disease risk factors including abdominal obesity, dyslipidemia, hypertension, and impaired fasting glucose, often precedes development of type 2 diabetes and is associated with insulin resistance. A number of studies have found protective associations between vegetarianism and metabolic syndrome or some of its components.

5.1.1 Lipids, Body Weight, and Glucose

In a meta-analysis of observational studies, vegetarian diets were associated with a lower BMI and several specific components of metabolic syndrome including fasting glucose and triglyceride concentrations (Dinu et al., 2016). On the other hand, vegetarian diets were associated with lower HDL cholesterol. A vegan diet was associated with lower BMI and glucose levels but not lower triglycerides (Dinu et al., 2016). In a mechanistic study, vegans exhibited rapid removal of remnant triglyceride-containing atherogenic lipoproteins from the circulation compared to omnivores but not lower triglyceride concentrations (Vinagre et al., 2013). In line with this, a meta-analysis of randomized controlled trials of the effects of vegetarian diets on blood lipids did not find that vegetarian diets lowered triglyceride concentrations, though LDL cholesterol concentrations were improved (Wang et al., 2015). Confounding in observational studies by unmeasured differences between vegetarians and nonvegetarians may explain inconsistencies with randomized controlled trials. Furthermore, vegetarianism includes a wide spectrum of food patterns. Diets completely excluding animal foods are generally very low in fat, explaining low HDL cholesterol levels often observed in vegans. Other lifestyle characteristics of traditional vegans may further explain this observation including low alcohol consumption. The relation between HDL and cardiovascular disease is complex, and low HDL levels induced by low-fat diets are unlikely to present a risk for disease (Voight et al., 2012).

A meta-analysis of 14 studies that included genetic data concluded that consumption of meat was associated with higher fasting glucose and insulin concentrations regardless of glucose and insulin genetic risk scores (Fretts et al., 2015). However, the associations were attenuated and no longer statistically significant after control for BMI.

5.1.2 Blood Pressure
A meta-analysis found that consumption of a vegetarian diet is associated with lower systolic and diastolic blood pressure compared to omnivorous diets (Yokoyama et al., 2014). This difference is not only due to lower BMIs in vegetarians. Studies controlling for body weight have demonstrated a blood pressure–lowering effect of vegetarian diets (Yokoyama et al., 2014). This subject is presented in a dedicated chapter of this book.

5.1.3 Metabolic Syndrome
Cross-sectional and case control studies as well as one retrospective cohort study examining the risk of metabolic syndrome according to vegetarian diet published between 2006 and 2013 were identified in a review (Sabate and Wien, 2015). The studies were performed both in Asian and Western populations. Generally, the prevalence of metabolic syndrome was lower in vegetarians than nonvegetarians (Sabate and Wien, 2015), though a large study from Taiwan found a higher prevalence of metabolic syndrome in vegans than nonvegetarians (attributable to lower HDL cholesterol levels), while ovolactovegetarians and pescetarians had a lower risk in this study (Shang et al., 2011).

In a subset of subjects that participated in the Adventist Health Study-2, a vegetarian dietary pattern was associated with a 56% lower risk of metabolic syndrome compared with a nonvegetarian pattern (OR 0.44; 95% CI 0.30–0.64) (Rizzo et al., 2011). Individual components of metabolic syndrome that were less prevalent in vegetarians included waist circumference, triglycerides, blood glucose, and blood pressure. These findings persisted after adjustment for other characteristics. Nuts may be one of the components of vegetarian diets that may be protective against metabolic syndrome. In the same study, the odds of metabolic syndrome was inversely related to the amount, frequency, and pattern of nuts consumed (Jaceldo-Siegl et al., 2014).

5.2 Meat Consumption and Metabolic Syndrome

In addition to evidence that suggested a protective association between vegetarian diets and metabolic syndrome, meat consumption appears to increase the risk of metabolic syndrome. Among participants in the PREDIMED study, those in the upper quartile of red meat consumption were more likely to meet criteria for metabolic syndrome than those in the reference quartile at baseline, even after adjustment for potential confounders (Babio et al., 2012). In a longitudinal analysis conducted among those without metabolic syndrome at baseline, the odds of developing metabolic syndrome were increased after 1 year of follow-up (OR 2.7; 95% CI 1.1–6.8). At least two other prospective studies have found an association between red meat intake and metabolic syndrome (Lutsey et al., 2008; Damião et al., 2006).

6. Insulin Resistance and Sensitivity

6.1 Vegetarian Diets and Insulin Resistance and Sensitivity

6.1.1 Observational Studies

Type 2 diabetes results from insulin insufficiency superimposed on long-term insulin resistance. Some evidence indicates lower insulin resistance (Huang et al., 2015; Chiang et al., 2013; Valachovicova et al., 2006) and higher insulin sensitivity in vegetarians compared to nonvegetarians (Kuo et al., 2004; Gojda et al., 2013). In a case control study involving nondiabetic female Buddhist health fair attendees in Taiwan, vegetarians had a significantly lower Homeostasis Model Assessment–Insulin Resistance index (HOMA-IR) and reduced risk for insulin resistance of borderline significance compared to the nonvegetarian group after adjusting for age, menopause, waist, glucose, and triglyceride and activity (Chiang et al., 2013). In normal weight adults residing in Bratslava, HOMA-IR values were lower among ovolactovegetarians compared with nonvegetarians (Valachovicova et al., 2006). Among a group of Chinese volunteers, ovolactovegetarians and omnivores had similar BMIs, but the vegetarians were more insulin sensitive than their omnivorous counterparts (Kuo et al., 2004). In a study of vegans and omnivores matched for BMI and other relevant characteristics, vegans had higher insulin sensitivity but comparable mitochondrial density and intramyocellular lipid content as omnivores (Gojda et al., 2013).

6.1.2 Intervention Studies

In the New Nordic dietary intervention study, 166 volunteers with features of metabolic syndrome completed an 18–24 week dietary period that included whole-grain products, berries, fruits and vegetables, rapeseed oil, three fish meals per week, and low-fat dairy products and white meat instead of red meat. An average Nordic diet served as a control diet. Body weight remained stable in both groups. No effects of the intervention diet were seen on insulin sensitivity or blood pressure (Uusitupa et al., 2013). A randomized study among people at high risk of cardiovascular disease compared the intakes of one to two, four, or seven portions per day of fruit and vegetables for 12 weeks on insulin resistance measured by the two-step euglycemic-hyperinsulinemic clamp after a washout period of one to two portions per day for 4 weeks. Body weight remained stable in all the groups. No significant difference was found between groups in regard to measures of whole-body, peripheral, or hepatic insulin resistance (Wallace et al., 2013).

6.2 Meat Consumption and Insulin Resistance

Evidence supporting an association between meat consumption and glucose and insulin concentrations has appeared in cross-sectional and cohort studies. A cross-sectional study of 292 nondiabetic US women found that moderate and high meat intakes were associated with insulin resistance, but differences in body fat contributed significantly to the association (Tucker et al., 2015). In those with low meat intake, odds of insulin resistance were lower than their counterparts with moderate or high meat intake (OR 0.34; 95% CI 0.14–0.83), also after control for body fat. A study that enrolled men and women resident in the Attica area of Greece without diabetes or cardiovascular disease found that red meat consumption was associated with hyperglycemia, hyperinsulinemia, and HOMA levels even after adjustment for BMI and other potential confounders (Panagiotakos et al., 2005). In a meta-analysis of 14 cohort studies conducted among 50,345 Caucasians, processed meat intake was associated with higher fasting glucose, while unprocessed red meat was associated with both higher fasting glucose and insulin concentrations after adjustment for potential confounders (but not BMI). After additional adjustment for BMI the observed associations were attenuated and no longer statistically significant (Fretts et al., 2015). Notably, the associations of meat consumption with higher fasting glucose and insulin concentrations were not modified by an index of glucose- and insulin-related single-nucleotide polymorphisms.

Interventional data is sparse. In a randomized crossover intervention study, high consumption of dairy reduced insulin sensitivity compared to a diet high in lean red meat in overweight and obese subjects (Turner et al., 2015). This finding was in line with the observation that very lean red meat consumption was not associated with insulin resistance in the study among US women (Tucker et al., 2015). These findings suggest that any influence of red meat on insulin resistance may be due to its nonheme contents, though this notion requires further study. Specifically studies comparing the effects of plant protein and nonlean red meat on insulin resistance would be of interest.

7. Discussion

The lower BMI of vegans and vegetarians is readily postulated as the most pertinent factor explaining the lower risks of diabetes in these groups (Dinu et al., 2016; Wang et al., 2015;

Huang et al., 2015). Other confounders may be present as well, as vegetarians tend to be more health conscious than nonvegetarians. Variables associated both with meat consumption and risk of diabetes may explain the associations observed in observational studies (Joost, 2013). Indeed, red meat consumption is associated with smoking, high BMI, and male sex, all risk factors for diabetes. In many, but not all studies, associations between meat intake and incident diabetes remain after control for major confounders, including BMI. On the other hand, it may be argued that control for BMI, which is likely to be a major intermediate factor on the pathway between meat consumption and incident type 2 diabetes, leads to an inappropriate attenuation of risk estimates. In observational studies, total meat consumption is associated with weight gain (Vergnaud et al., 2010). Overall, randomized controlled trials show that vegetarian diets result in greater weight loss than nonvegetarian diets of 2–3 kg (Wang et al., 2015; Huang et al., 2015), buttressing the idea that lower BMI is an important contributor to the protection afforded vegetarian diets.

In the absence of data from randomized controlled studies, studies showing change in consumption that lead to either increased or decreased risk are helpful in establishing causality (Singh et al., 2014; Feskens et al., 2013; Pan et al., 2013). Yet, it remains possible that unmeasured or incompletely controlled confounders remain. More health conscious individuals may remove meat from their diets, while conversely less health conscious persons may increase their intake: in either case, these and other characteristics may explain changes in risk rather than meat consumption.

An elucidation of underlying mechanisms provides a strong underpinning of the causal role of red meat consumption in increasing risk of type 2 diabetes. Both the absence of meat and the presence of plant foods in the diet may influence the risk of diabetes in vegetarians and are discussed in turn. The most consistent difference between vegetarian and other diets is the absence of red meat.

As summarized in a review, the putative etiologies of the association between red meat consumption and type 2 diabetes include the role of saturated fatty acids, sodium, advanced glycation end products, nitrates/nitrites, heme iron, trimethylamine *N*-oxide, branched amino acids, and endocrine disruptor chemicals (Kim et al., 2015). Processed and unprocessed meats are a major source of saturated fatty acids in the diet. Given the inconsistent results of intervention studies regarding saturated fats and insulin sensitivity, it remains unclear what role saturated fats play in increasing risk of incident diabetes. Likewise, it is unclear whether the sodium content of processed meats leads to insulin resistance and other risk factors for type 2 diabetes (Kim et al., 2015). Advanced glycation end products are present in meat exposed to dry heat, high temperature during food preparation. Some evidence suggests that restricting advanced glycation end products ameliorates insulin resistance, but the quality of the evidence is low (Kellow and Savige, 2013). Nitrates and nitrites used in the preservation of processed meat have long been postulated to promote diabetes. These compounds may be converted to nitrosamines by binding to amino compounds. Nitrosamines are toxic to pancreatic beta cells and impair insulin responses in animal studies (Kim et al., 2015). Relationships between consumption of processed meat and type 2 diabetes appear stronger than those between nonprocessed red meat and type 2 diabetes (Micha et al., 2010; Pan et al., 2011), giving some credence to an etiologic role of nitrogen-containing compounds. Red meat provides an oversupply of heme iron, leading to higher ferritin concentrations among meat eaters than vegetarians. High body iron stores are associated with an increased risk of type 2 diabetes, possibly by increasing oxidative stress and inflammation (Rajpathak et al., 2009; White and Collinson, 2013). Furthermore, some evidence suggests that phlebotomy may increase insulin sensitivity, but appropriately performed and controlled studies have not been done (Kim et al., 2015). Products produced by bacterial degradation of phosphatidylcholine and carnitine from red meat by intestinal bacteria may have deleterious effects. Choline and L-carnitine are metabolized to trimethylamine *N*-oxide by the microbiota, a substance shown to produce impaired glucose tolerance in high-fat diet–fed mice. Vegans or vegetarians have lower fasting levels of L-carnitine and produce less trimethylamine *N*-oxide from dietary L-carnitine compared with omnivorous subjects (Koeth et al., 2013). Other deleterious substances in red meat include branched-chain amino acids, which have been suspected to influence insulin secretion and resistance (Vergnaud et al., 2010). In animal studies, branch-chain amino acid supplementation requires the background of a high-fat diet to promote insulin resistance (Newgard, 2012). A red meat–derived glycan appears to promote inflammation and cancer progression and potentially incite the development of type 2 diabetes (Samraj et al., 2015).

Vegetarian dietary patterns rich in fruits, vegetables, whole grains, and other plant foods provide a rich and synergistic combination of antioxidants and phytochemicals that may protect against type 2 diabetes and have been discussed in detail (Jenkins et al., 2003). Whole grains (Aune et al., 2013) and green leafy vegetables (Cooper et al., 2012) appear to afford such protection in observational studies. Nuts or extra virgin olive oil added to a Mediterranean diet lowered risk of diabetes in nondiabetic participants in the PREDIMED study without weight loss compared to a control group following a low-fat diet (Salas-Salvado et al., 2011). Dairy products, which are high in ovolactovegetarian diets, may contribute to reduce type 2 diabetes, though the evidence is not conclusive (Salas-Salvado et al., 2011; Tong et al., 2011; Gao et al., 2013; Chen et al., 2014). However, to date, high fruit and vegetable interventions have had no effect on insulin sensitivity in studies where body weight remained stable (Uusitupa et al., 2013; Wallace et al., 2013).

8. Conclusions

A number of plausible mechanisms support the biological plausibility of epidemiological observations of the diabetes-promoting effects of red meat. However, direct evidence that red meat consumption impairs insulin sensitivity or increases insulin resistance is lacking. The most convincing explanation of the lower risk of type 2 diabetes in vegetarians is the totality of lower BMI and benefits of generally healthier diets than those consumed by omnivores, in addition to the absence of processed and perhaps also unprocessed meat in the diet.

References

Agrawal, S., Millett, C.J., Dhillon, P.K., Subramanian, S., Ebrahim, S., 2014. Type of vegetarian diet, obesity and diabetes in adult Indian population. Nutr. J. 13, 89.

Aune, D., Norat, T., Romundstad, P., Vatten, L.J., 2013. Whole grain and refined grain consumption and the risk of type 2 diabetes: a systematic review and dose-reponse meta-analysis of cohort studies. Eur. J. Epidemiol. 28, 845–858.

Babio, N., Sorli, M., Bulló, M., Basora, J., Ibarrola-Jurado, N., Fernández-Ballart, J., et al., 2012. Association between red meat consumption and metabolic syndrome in a Mediterranean population at high cardiovascular risk: cross-sectional and 1-year follow-up assessment. Nutr. Metab. Cardiovasc. Dis. 22, 200–207.

Bhupathiraju, S.N., Tobias, D.K., Malik, V.S., Pan, A., Hurby, A., Manson, J.E., et al., 2014. Glycemic index, glycemic load, and risk of type 2 diabetes: results from 3 large US cohorts and an updated meta-analysis. Am. J. Clin. Nutr. 100, 218–232.

Brathwaite, N., Fraser, H.S., Modeste, N., Broome, H., King, R., 2003. Obesity, diabetes, hypertension, and vegetarian status among Seventh-day Adventists in Barbados: preliminary results. Ehtn Dis. 13, 34–39.

Chen, M., Sun, Q., Giovannucci, E., Mozaffarian, D., Manson, J.E., Willett, W.C., et al., 2014. Dairy consumption and risk of type 2 diabetes: 3 cohorts of US adults and an updated meta-analysis. BMC Med. 12, 215.

Chiang, J.-K., Lin, Y.-L., Chen, C.-L., Ouyang, C.-M., Wu, Y.-T., Chi, Y.-C., et al., 2013. Reduced risk for metabolic syndrome and insulin resistance associated with ovo-lacto-vegetarian behavior in female Buddhists: a case-control study. PLoS One 8, e71799.

Chiu, T.H.T., Huang, H.-Y., Chiu, Y.-F., et al., 2014. Taiwanese vegetarians and omnivores: dietary composition, prevalence of diabetes and IFG. PLoS One 9, e88547.

Cooper, A.J., Forouhi, N.G., Ye, Z., Buijsse, B., Arriola, L., Balkau, B., et al., 2012. Fruit and vegetable intake and type 2 diabetes: EPIC-InterAct prospective study and meta-analysis. Eur. J. Clin. Nutr. 66, 1082–1092.

Crowe, F.L., Appleby, P.N., Travis, R.C., Key, T.J., 2013. Risk of hospitalization or death from ischemic heart disease among British vegetarians and nonvegetarians: results from the EPIC-Oxford cohort study. Am. J. Clin. Nutr. 97, 1–7.

Damião, R., Castro, T.G., Cardoso, M.A., Gmeno, S.G., 2006. Ferrerira ST for the Japanese-Brazilian Diabetes Study Group. Dietary intakes associated with metabolic syndrome in a cohort of Japanese ancestry. Br. J. Nutr. 96, 532–538.

Diabetes Prevention Program Research group, 2002. Reduction in the incidence of type 2 diabetes with lifestyle intervention or metformin. N. Engl. J. Med. 346, 393–403.

Dinu, M., Abbate, R., Gensini, G.F., Casini, A., Sofi, F., 2016. Vegetarian, vegan diets and multiple health outcomes: a systematic review with meta-analysis of observational studies. Crit. Rev. Food Sci. Nutr. Epub Ahead of Print.

Fardet, A., Boirie, Y., 2014. Associations between food and beverage groups and major diet-related chronic disease: an exhaustive review of pooled/meta-analyses and systematic reviews. Nutr. Rev. 72, 741–762.

Feskens, E.J.M., Sluik, D., van Woudenbergh, G.J., 2013. Meat consumption, diabetes, and ist complications. Curr. Diabetes Rep. 13, 298–306.

Fraser, G.E., 2009. Vegetarian diets: what do we know of their effects of common chronic diseases? Am. J. Clin. Nutr. 89 (Suppl.), 1607S–1612S.

Fraser, G., Katuli, S., Anousheh, R., Knutsen, S., Herring, P., Fan, J., 2015. Vegetarian diets and cardiovascular risk factors in black members of the Adventist Health Study-2. Public Health Nutr. 18, 537–545.

Fretts, A.M., Follis, J.L., Nettleton, J.A., Lemaitre, R.N., Ngwa, J.S., Wojczynski, M.K., et al., 2015. Consukption of meat is associated with higher fasting glucose and insulin concentrations regardless of glucose and insulin genetic risk scores: a meta-analysis of 50,345 Caucasians. Am. J. Clin. Nutr. 102, 1266–1278.

Gao, D., Ning, N., Wang, C., Wang, Y., Li, Q., Meng, Z., et al., 2013. Dairy products consumption and risk of type 2 diabetes: systematic review and dose-response meta-analysis. PLoS One 8, e73965.

Gojda, J., Patkova, J., Jacek, M., Ptochkova, J., Trnka, A., Kraml, P., Andel, M., 2013. Higher insulin sensitivity in vegans is not associated with higher mitochondrial density. Eur. J. Clin. Nutr. 67, 1310–1315.

Hopper, I., Billah, B., Skiba, M., Krum, H., 2011. Prevention of diabetes and reduction in major cardiovascular events in studies of subjects with prediabetes: meta-analysis of randomised controlled clinical trials. Eur. J. Cardiovasc. Prev. Rehabil. 18, 813–823.

Hu, F.B., Satija, A., Manson, J.E., 2015. Curbing the diabetes pandemic: the need for global policy solutions. JAMA 313, 2319–2320.

Huang, R.-Y., Huang, C.-C., Hu, F.B., Chavarro, J.E., 2015. Vegetarian diets and weight reduction: a meta-analysis of randomized controlled trials. J. Gen. Intern. Med.

Jaceldo-Siegl, K., Haddad, E., Oda, K., et al., 2014. Tree nuts are inversely associated with metabolic syndrome and obesity: the Adventist Health Study-2. PLoS One 9, e85133.

Jacobs Jr., D.R., Orlich, M.J., 2014. Diet pattern and longevity: do simple rules suffice? A commentary. Am. J. Clin. Nutr. 100 (Suppl.), 313S–319S.

Jenkins, D.J.A., Kendall, C.W.C., Marchie, A., Jenkins, A.L., Augustin, L.S.A., Ludwig, D.S., et al., 2003. Type 2 diabetes and the vegetarian diet. Am. J. Clin. Nutr. 78 (Suppl.), 610S–616S.

Joost, H.-G., 2013. Red meat and T2DM – the difficult path to a proof of causality. Nat. Rev. Endocrinol. 9, 509–511.

Kellow, N.J., Savige, G.S., 2013. Dietary advanced glycation end-product restriction for the attenuation of insulin resistance, oxidative stress and endothelial dysfunction: a systematic review. Eur. J. Clin. Nutr. 67, 239–248.

Kim, Y., Keogh, J., Clifton, P.M., 2015. A review of potential metabolic etiologies of the observed association between red meat consumption and development of type 2 diabetes mellitus. Metabolism 64, 768–779.

Koeth, R.A., Wang, Z., Levison, B.S., Buffa, J.A., Org, E., Sheehy, B.T., et al., 2013. Intestinal microbiota metabolism of L-carnitine, a nutrient in red meat, promotes atherosclerosis. Nat. Med. 19, 576–585.

Kuo, C.-S., Lai, N.-S., Ho, L.-T., Lin, C.-L., 2004. Insulin sensitivity in chinese ovo-lactovegetarians compared with omnivores. Eur. J. Clin. Nutr. 58, 312–316.

Lutsey, P.L., Steffen, L.M., Stevens, J., 2008. Dietary intake and the development of the metabolic syndrome: the Atherosclerosis Risk in Communities study. Circulation 117, 754–761.

Micha, R., Wallace, S.K., Mozaffarian, D., 2010. Red and processed meat consumption and risk of incident coronary heart disease, stroke, and diabetes mellitus: a systematic review and meta-analysis. Circulation 121, 2271–2283.

Newgard, C.B., 2012. Interplay between lipids and branched-chain amino acids in development of insulin resistance. Cell Metab. 15, 606–614.

Pan, A., Sun, Q., Bernstein, A.M., et al., 2011. Red meat consumption and risk of type 2 diabetes: 3 cohorts of US adults and an updated meta-analysis. Am. J. Clin. Nutr. 94, 1088–1096.

Pan, A., Sun, Q., Bernstein, A.M., et al., 2013. Changes in red meat consumption and subsequent risk of type 2 diabetes mellitus: three cohorts of US men and women. JAMA Intern. Med. 173, 1328–1335.

Panagiotakos, D.B., Tzima, N., Pitsavos, C., Chrysohoou, C., Papakonstantinou, E., Zampelas, A., et al., 2005. The relationship between dietary habits, blood glucose and insulin levels among people without cardiovascular disease and type 2 diabetes; the ATTICA study. Rev. Diabet. Stud. 2, 208–215.

Rajpathak, S.N., Crandall, J.P., Wylie-Rosett, J., Kabat, G.C., Rohan, T.E., Hu, F.B., 2009. The role of iron in type 2 diabetes in humans. Biochim. Biophys. Acta 1790, 671–681.

Rizzo, N.S., Sabate, J., Jaceldo-Siegl, K., Fraser, G.E., 2011. Vegetarian dietary patterns are associated with a lower risk of metabolic syndrome: the Adventist Health Study 2. Diabetes Care 34, 1225–1227.

Sabate, J., Wien, M., 2015. A perspective on vegetarian dietary patterns and risk of metabolic syndrome. Br. J. Nutr. 113, S136–S143.

Salas-Salvado, J., Bullo, M., Babio, N., Martinez-Gonzalez, M.A., Ibarrola-Jurado, N., Basora, J., et al., 2011. Reduction in the incidence of type 2 diabetes with the Mediterranean diet: results of the PREDIMED-Reus nutrition intervention randomized trial. Diabetes Care 34, 14–19.

Salas-Salvadó, J., Bulló, M., Estruch, R., Ros, E., Covas, M.I., Ibarrola-Jurado, N., et al., 2014. Prevention of diabetes with Mediterranean diets: a subgroup analysis of a randomized trial. Ann. Intern. Med. 160, 1–10.

Samraj, A.N., Pearce, O.M., Laubli, H., Crittenden, A.N., Bergfeld, A.K., Banda, K., et al., 2015. A red meat-derived glycan promotes inflammation and cancer progression. Proc. Natl. Acad. Sci. U.S.A. 112, 542–547.

Shang, P., Shu, Z., Wang, Y., et al., 2011. Veganism does not reduce the risk of the metabolic syndrome in a Taiwanese cohort. Asia Pac. J. Clin. Nutr. 20, 404–410.

Shridhar, K., Dhillon, P.K., Bower, L., et al., 2014. The association between a vegetarian diet and cardiovascular disease (CVD) risk factors in India: the Indian migration study. PLoS One 9, e110586.

Singh, P.N., Arthur, K.N., Orlich, M.J., James, W., Purty, A., Jayakaran, S.J., Rajaram, S., Sabate, J., 2014. Global epidemiology of obesity, vegetarian dietary patterns, and noncommunicable disease in Asian Indians. Am. J. Clin. Nutr. 100 (Suppl.), 359S–364S.

Snowdon, D.A., Phillips, R.L., 1985. Does a vegetarian diet reduce the occurrence of diabetes? Am. J. Public Health 75, 507–512.

Tinker, L.F., Bonds, D.E., Margolis, K.L., Manson, J.E., Howard, B.V., Larson, J., et al., 2008. Low-fat dietary pattern and risk of treated diabetes mellitus in postmenopausal women: the Women's Health Initiative randomized controlled dietary modification trial. Arch. Intern. Med. 168, 1500–1511.

Tong, X., Dong, J.-Y., Wu, Z.-W., Li, W., Qin, L.-Q., 2011. Dairy consumption and risk of type 2 diabetes mellitus: a meta-analysis of cohort studies. Eur. J. Clin. Nutr. 65, 1027–1031.

Tonstad, S., Butler, T., Yan, R., Fraser, G.E., 2009. Type of vegetarian diet, body weight and prevalence of type 2 diabetes. Diabetes Care 32, 791–796.

Tonstad, S., Stewart, K., Oda, K., Batech, M., Herring, R.P., Fraser, G.E., 2013. Vegetarian diets and incidence of type 2 diabetes. Nutr. Metab. Cardiovasc. Dis. 23, 292–299.

Tucker, L.A., LeCheminant, J.D., Bailey, B.W., 2015. Meat intake and insulin resistance in women without type 2 diabetes. J. Diabetes Res. 174742. http://dx.doi.org/10.1155/2015/174742. Epub 2015.

Tuomilehto, J., Lindström, J., Eriksson, J.G., Valle, T.T., Hämäläinen, H., Ilanne-Parikka, P., et al., 2001. Prevention of type 2 diabetes mellitus by changes in lifestyle among subjects with impaired glucose tolerance. N. Engl. J. Med. 344, 1343–1350.

Turner, K.M., Keogh, J.B., Clifton, P.M., 2015. Red meat, dairy and insulin sensitivity: a randomized cross-over intervention study. Am. J. Clin. Nutr. 101, 1173–1179.

Uusitupa, M., Hermansen, K., Savolainen, M.J., et al., 2013. Effects of an isocaloric healthy Nordic diet on insulin sensitivity, lipid profile and inflammation markers in metabolic syndrome – a randomized study (SYSDIET). J. Intern. Med. 274, 52–66.

Valachovicova, M., Krajcovicova-Kudlackova, M., Blazicek, P., Babinska, K., 2006. No evidence of insulin resistance in normal weight vegetarians. A case control study. Eur. J. Nutr. 45, 52–54.

Vang, A., Singh, P.N., Lee, J.W., Haddad, E.H., Brinegar, C.H., 2008. Meats, processed meats, obesity, weight gain and occurrence of diabetes among adults: findings from Adventist Health Studies. Ann. Nutr. Metab. 52, 96–104.

Vergnaud, A.-C., Norat, T., Romaguera, D., Mouw, T., May, A.M., Travier, N., et al., 2010. Meat consumption and prospective weight change in participants of the EPIC-PANACEA study. Am. J. Clin. Nutr. 92, 398–407.

Vinagre, J.C., Vinagre, C.G., Pozzi, F.S., Slywitch, E., Maranhao, R.C., 2013. Metabolism of triglyceride-rich lipoproteins and transfer of lipids to high-density lipoproteins (HDL) in vegan and omnivore subjects. Nutr. Metab. Cardiovasc. Dis. 23, 61–67.

Voight, B.G., Peloso, G.M., Orho-Melander, M., Frikke-Schmidt, R., Barbalic, M., Jensen, M.K., et al., 2012. Plasma HDL cholesterol and risk of myocardial infarction: a mendelian randomisation study. Lancet 380, 572–580.

Wallace, I.R., McEvoy, C.T., Hunter, S.J., et al., 2013. Dose-response effect of fruit and vegetables on insulin resistance in people at high risk of cardiovascular disease: a randomized controlled trial. Diabetes Care 36, 3888–3896.

Wang, F., Zheng, J., Yang, B., Jiang, J., Fu, Y., Li, D., 2015. Effects of vegetarian diets on blood lipids: a systematic review and meta-analysis of randomized controlled trials. J. Am. Heart Assoc. 4, e002408.

White, D.L., Collinson, A., 2013. Red meat, dietary heme iron, and risk of type 2 diabetes: the involvement of advanced lipoxidation endproducts. Adv. Nutr. 4, 403–411.

Yokoyama, Y., Nishimura, K., Barnard, N.D., Takegami, M., Watanabe, M., Sekikawa, A., et al., 2014. Vegetarian diets and blood pressure: a meta-analysis. JAMA Intern. Med. 174, 577–587.

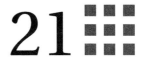

21

Vegetarian Diets in People With Type 2 Diabetes

Hana Kahleova, Terezie Pelikanova

INSTITUTE FOR CLINICAL AND EXPERIMENTAL MEDICINE, PRAGUE, CZECH REPUBLIC

1. Introduction

The prevalence of type 2 diabetes (T2D) has been increasing worldwide. Among adults (20–79 years of age), 382 million people worldwide had diabetes in 2013; this number is expected to rise to 592 million by 2035 (Guariguata et al., 2014). The economic burden associated with diabetes (both diagnosed and undiagnosed) exceeded $322 billion in 2012 in the United States (Dall et al., 2014). Therefore, interventions to effectively manage T2D and its complications are desirable.

Treatment of diabetes is not only about glycemic control, but it also includes control of other cardiovascular risk factors (such as blood lipids, blood pressure, and body weight) and preventing or at least delaying of diabetes complications. A reduced energy diet, together with physical activity, is crucial for the treatment of T2D (Evert et al., 2014). The goals of nutritional treatment in diabetes are to (1) attain individualized glycemic, blood pressure, and lipid target values; (2) achieve and maintain body weight goals; (3) delay or prevent complications of diabetes; (4) address nutritional needs of the individuals, taking into account personal and cultural preferences and willingness to change; (5) maintain the pleasure of eating by providing positive messages about food choices while limiting food choices only when indicated by scientific evidence; and (6) increase the quality of life (Evert et al., 2014).

Conventional dietary recommendations for people with T2D typically stress caloric restriction, especially reduced intake of saturated and trans-fatty acids, cholesterol, and carbohydrates (particularly simple sugars). Evidence suggests that there is not an ideal percentage of calories from carbohydrate, protein, and fat for all people with diabetes; therefore, energy and macronutrient distribution should be based on individualized assessment of current dietary patterns, eating preferences, and metabolic goals (Evert et al., 2014). Reducing the intake of fat and added sugars while increasing the intake of fiber and complex carbohydrates seems to be a reasonable approach (Vitale et al., 2016). Both the American Diabetes Association and the European Association for the Study of Diabetes recommend that diets may be individualized to meet the patient's needs (Evert et al., 2014; Mann et al., 2004). However, the major limitation of conventional reduced energy diets is the poor long-term adherence.

Vegetarian diets may be an effective strategy to increase consumption of foods with a lower energy density. Vegetarian diets are characterized by elimination of all flesh foods from the diet (including fish and white meat) and are typically based on the consumption of whole grains, legumes, vegetables, fruits, and nuts. Vegan diets contain only plant foods, while ovolactovegetarian diets include also dairy and/or egg products (see Chapter 1 of this book for details). Unfortunately, there is not enough data to be able to compare directly the effects of vegan and ovolactovegetarian diets in the treatment of T2D, but the randomized clinical trials indicate clear benefits for both of them in the treatment of T2D compared with a conventional hypocaloric diet due to greater weight loss (Berkow and Barnard, 2006), improved glycemic control (Barnard et al., 2006), increased insulin sensitivity (Kahleova et al., 2011; Kuo et al., 2004; Hung et al., 2006), and reduced cardiovascular risk factors (Barnard et al., 2006; Kahleova et al., 2011) compared to conventional diabetic diets. In this chapter, we summarize the most recent findings on the effect of vegetarian diets on people with type 2 diabetes: on cardiovascular risk factors, microvascular complications, and quality of life. We also discuss the practical aspects of the use of vegetarian diets, their healthy components, possible mechanisms of the positive effects, and their nutritional adequacy.

2. Vegetarian Diets in the Treatment of Type 2 Diabetes

Vegetarian diets proved to be effective in the treatment of T2D in several clinical trials. Early studies reported a dramatic reduction in antidiabetic medication and in plasma glucose levels in response to a plant-based diet combined with exercise (Anderson and Ward, 1979; Barnard et al., 1994).

Even without exercise, beneficial effects of vegetarian diets included reduced body weight, better glycemic control, and lower blood lipids compared to a conventional diabetic diet in treatment of T2D: vegetarian diets being almost twice as effective (Barnard et al., 2006; Kahleova et al., 2011; Nicholson et al., 1999).

Interestingly, the positive effects of a vegetarian diet compared to a conventional reduced energy diet were partially preserved 1 year after the end of the intervention, although the patients did not continue with their originally assigned diets and consumed a comparable diet during that year (Kahleova et al., 2014).

2.1 Cardiovascular Risk Factors

2.1.1 Glycemic Control and Insulin Sensitivity

Management of glycemic control is one of the cornerstones of diabetes care (American Diabetes Association, 2014). It has been well established that improved glycemic control reduces the risk of microvascular complications, whereas the role of glycemic control in reducing macrovascular complications is less clear.

Most observational studies have demonstrated a positive association between glucose control and the risk of cardiovascular disease (Avogaro et al., 2007; Gerstein et al., 2005;

Turner et al., 1998; Elley et al., 2008; Duckworth et al., 2001; Khaw et al., 2004; Kirkman et al., 2006). Patients with HbA1c concentrations of 6.0%–6.9% had 20% lower relative risk of fatal/nonfatal coronary heart disease than patients with HbA1c concentrations of 7.0%–7.9%. Limited data from four large, randomized, controlled trials and their follow-ups also suggests that chronic hyperglycemia is associated with an increased risk for cardiovascular disease in patients with diabetes (Selvin et al., 2004; Intensive blood-glucose, 1998; Effect of intensive blood-glucose, 1998; Group et al., 2009; Duckworth et al., 2009; ADVANCE Collaborative Group et al., 2008; Action to Control Cardiovascular Risk in Diabetes Study Group et al., 2008; Gerstein et al., 2014; Zoungas et al., 2014; Hayward et al., 2015). However, caution must be taken to avoid hypoglycemia, especially in high-risk patients with T2D (Action to Control Cardiovascular Risk in Diabetes Study Group et al., 2008). Meta-analyses of these trials demonstrated significantly reduced risks of fatal/nonfatal myocardial infarction (15%) and cardiovascular disease (11%–15%) with around 1% HbA1c reduction, as well as no significant risk increase with regard to fatal CVD or total mortality (Group et al., 2009; Ray et al., 2009; Mannucci et al., 2009).

A meta-analysis of six randomized controlled trials showed that consumption of vegetarian diets led to a significant reduction in HbA1c by 0.4% compared with conventional diets in patients with T2D (Yokoyama et al., 2014a). This reduction in HbA1c alone (i.e., independently from the association with the decrease in body weight, improvement in blood lipids, blood pressure, platelet aggregation, and others) might (according to educated estimates based on data from large prospective studies) decrease risks of myocardial infarction and cardiovascular disease by about 6% and 4.4%–6%, respectively. Other factors may add further reduction of this risk.

One of the major possible mechanisms responsible for improved glycemic control is increased insulin sensitivity in response to vegetarian diets compared with a conventional diabetic diet (Kahleova et al., 2011). Also, partial replacement of meat with soy products increased insulin sensitivity in a randomized crossover trial (van Nielen et al., 2014b), which makes the findings applicable in everyday practice.

Another potential mechanism responsible for improved glycemic control is improved gastrointestinal hormone response. Gastrointestinal hormones, especially the incretins, play an important role in postprandial increase in plasma insulin (Nauck et al., 1986a). In patients with T2D, the incretin effect is diminished (Nauck et al., 1986b), and it seems to be impacted by diet composition. It has been demonstrated that consumption of processed meat leads to impaired release of gastrointestinal hormones including the incretins both in a fasting state and after the meal compared with an isocaloric vegan meal (Belinova et al., 2014). These results suggest that vegetarian diets may be beneficial for improvement in gastrointestinal hormone release in patients with T2D.

2.1.2 Body Weight and Metabolic Syndrome

Vegetarians, both men and women, have lower BMI values compared to nonvegetarians (Berkow and Barnard, 2006). BMI values tend to increase with increasing frequency of meat consumption in the general population (Fraser, 1999; Appleby et al., 1999). Among vegetarians, vegans have the lowest values of BMI (Brathwaite et al., 2003). It takes about 5 years for all the benefits of a vegetarian diet to become fully manifested (Brathwaite et al., 2003). The average individual yearly weight gain is reduced when people limit consumption of animal foods (Rosell et al., 2006). Vegetarian diet might increase resting energy expenditure (Montalcini et al., 2015), which may be partly responsible for the lower BMI values in vegetarians. Vegetarian diets have been shown to be a most effective dietary approach for weight loss (Moore et al., 2015; Barnard et al., 2015). The reader may refer to Chapter 18 for a review of weight loss and plant-based diets.

Introducing vegetarian diets to patients with T2D leads to reduction in body weight almost twice as effectively as a conventional diabetic diet (Barnard et al., 2006; Nicholson et al., 1999), due especially to reduction in volume of visceral (Kahleova et al., 2011) and ectopic fat, like intramyocellular lipids (Goff et al., 2005), which may be responsible for a substantial portion of the positive effect of vegetarian diets on insulin sensitivity. The mean weight loss after initiating a vegetarian diet is around 4 kg. Greater weight loss was reported in trials with higher baseline body weights, fewer female participants, in studies with older participants or longer durations, and in trials where weight loss was a goal (Barnard et al., 2015).

Vegetarian diets reduce the risk of developing metabolic syndrome, with an estimate of one-half reduction (Rizzo et al., 2011). They reduce the risk of individual components of the metabolic syndrome (except for HDL cholesterol) and are associated with lower waist circumference (Rizzo et al., 2011), lower concentrations of triglycerides, total and LDL cholesterol (Rizzo et al., 2011; Teixeira et al., 2007; De Biase et al., 2007), blood sugar, and blood pressure (Rizzo et al., 2011; Teixeira et al., 2007).

2.1.3 Blood Pressure

Hypertension is a major cardiovascular risk factor, especially in people with T2D who are at higher risk for cardiovascular disease (Preis et al., 2009). Each 20-mm Hg increase in systolic blood pressure and each 10-mm Hg increase in diastolic blood pressure double the risk of death from ischemic heart disease or stroke (Lewington et al., 2002). A tight control in blood pressure is important for general population but even more for patients with diabetes.

Blood pressure has been shown to be increased by increased animal protein intake, especially meat consumption (Mattos et al., 2015). On the other hand, consumption of potassium-rich plant foods decreases blood pressure in people with hypertension (Aburto et al., 2013), and their consumption during childhood may prevent the increase in blood pressure later in life (Buendia et al., 2015). A recent meta-analysis of seven randomized controlled trials and 32 observational studies concluded that consumption of a vegetarian diet is associated with lower blood pressure (both systolic and diastolic) compared to omnivorous diets. The overall difference in systolic blood pressure was –4.8 mm Hg in controlled trials and –6.9 mm Hg in observational studies. For diastolic blood pressure, the differences were –2.2 mm Hg in controlled trials and –4.7 mm Hg in observational studies (Yokoyama et al., 2014b). The reduction in systolic blood pressure by 5 mm Hg is estimated to result in a reduction in mortality by 7% due to all causes, by 9% due to coronary heart disease, and by 14% due to stroke (Yokoyama et al., 2014b; Whelton et al., 2002). The reader may refer to Chapter 22 for a review of blood pressure and vegetarian diets.

2.1.4 Blood Lipids

Data from clinical studies indicate that for every 1% reduction in serum LDL cholesterol, there is a corresponding 1% drop in the chance of suffering a heart attack, stroke, or some other type of cardiac event (Grundy et al., 2004). This is significant given that the proper lifestyle changes (especially diet and exercise) can help lower LDL levels by 30%–40% in people at risk for heart disease (including patients with T2D), creating a corresponding drop in the risk for cardiac events. In individuals with type 2 diabetes, reducing LDL cholesterol to lower targets than in general population results in even more marked benefits (Howard et al., 2008).

A meta-analysis demonstrated that dietary cholesterol increases serum lipids, both total and LDL cholesterol (Berger et al., 2015). Vegetarian diets, especially vegan diets (minimizing the dietary cholesterol intake), improve both fasting and postprandial blood lipids compared with conventional diabetic diets (Barnard et al., 2006; Kahleova et al., 2011; Riccardi et al., 2004; Bradbury et al., 2014), with an effect comparable to a statin therapy (Jenkins et al., 2005). If combined with moderate physical exercise, smoking cessation, and stress management, the reduction of blood lipids can be even higher (Ornish et al., 1990).

Plant foods are a rich source of n-6 polyunsaturated fatty acids, including linoleic acid. Studies have shown that people with T2D and also people with metabolic syndrome have a low proportion of linoleic acid in serum phospholipids (Li et al., 2009b; Vessby et al., 1994; Feskens, 2001). Vegetarian diet-induced increase in linoleic acid (18:2n-6) in serum phospholipids was associated with improved insulin sensitivity in subjects with T2D (Kahleova et al., 2013b). This suggests increased content of linoleic acid as a potential mechanism of the insulin-sensitizing effect of vegetarian diets. Limited data also suggest that supplementation of α-linolenic acid may have insulin-sensitizing potential in patients with T2D (Gomes et al., 2015).

2.1.5 Platelet Aggregation

Vegetarian diets have been shown to reduce platelet aggregation and thus reduce the cardiovascular risk (McEwen, 2014). Plant foods with low glycemic index (whole grains, vegetables, nuts, legumes), garlic, ginger, onion, purple grape juice, tomatoes, berries, and dark chocolate are particularly efficient in reducing platelet aggregation. In contrast, energy drinks have been shown to increase platelet aggregation and caffeine increases platelet microparticle formation (McEwen, 2014).

2.1.6 Atherosclerosis

To the best of our knowledge, a low-fat vegetarian diet is the only diet with documented angiographic evidence of coronary atherosclerosis regression (Ornish et al., 1990, 1998) and arrest of coronary artery disease (Esselstyn et al., 1995), especially when combined with exercise and stress management (Daubenmier et al., 2007; Frattaroli et al., 2008).

2.1.7 Oxidative Stress

Oxidative stress is supposed to be the link between hyperglycemia and cardiovascular disease in patients with T2D (Ceriello, 2012). Both enzymatic and nonenzymatic antioxidant defense mechanisms work in synergy against different types of free radicals (Maritim et al., 2003); this plays a major role in the development, progression, and complications of diabetes (Forbes et al., 2008).

It has been demonstrated that a vegetarian diet improved both enzymatic and nonenzymatic oxidative stress markers in patients with T2D more than a conventional diabetic diet (Kahleova et al., 2011). The observed positive changes in oxidative stress markers in response to a vegetarian diet in patients with T2D reflect the improved capacity to combat the pathophysiologic mechanisms of the disease and the potential to reduce the risk of both macro- and microvascular diabetes complications.

2.2 Microvascular Complications

2.2.1 Diabetic Nephropathy

The Western dietary pattern characterized by a high consumption of industrially processed and refined foods, especially sugar, salt, fat, and protein from red meat is one of the major risk factors for deterioration of renal function and development of chronic renal insufficiency (Odermatt, 2011). Consumption of plant-based rather than animal protein can slow the process of deterioration and loss of renal function. The Nurses' Health Study showed that in women with some degree of renal impairment at baseline, the consumption of animal protein (especially from meat) resulted in further deterioration of renal function (Knight et al., 2003). Mild impairment of renal function is present in about 40% of patients with diabetes (Soroka et al., 1998). Several studies have reported a reduction of microalbuminuria and proteinuria in patients with nephropathy when consuming a vegetarian or a reduced–red-meat diet (de Mello et al., 2006; Barsotti et al., 1988; Jibani et al., 1991). One study showed a 54% decrease of microalbuminuria in patients with type 1 diabetes after 8 weeks of a vegetarian diet (Jibani et al., 1991). Reduction in microalbuminuria with a vegetarian diet has also been reported in patients with T2D (Barnard et al., 2006).

In patients with nephrotic syndrome, a vegetarian diet proved to have positive effects on renal hemodynamic response to protein, progressive renal insufficiency, proteinuria, glomerulosclerosis, blood pressure, and hyperlipoproteinemia (Segasothy and Phillips, 1999). However, the evidence for the role of protein in chronic kidney disease is now considered to be inconclusive, and there is need for further studies before clear recommendations for patients with diabetes can be given (Evert et al., 2014).

2.2.2 Diabetic Neuropathy

More than 50% of diabetic patients suffer from diabetic neuropathy (Deli et al., 2013). The most common clinical manifestations of diabetic neuropathy include pain, insensitivity to trauma, orthostatic hypotension, cardiac autonomic neuropathy, gastroparesis, and erectile dysfunction (Boulton et al., 2005). Diabetic neuropathy has a negative impact on the patients' quality of life, and it is associated with increased risk of sleep disturbances, depression, and anxiety (Alleman et al., 2015). Diabetic neuropathy also increases the risk of amputations and cardiovascular disease (Lam et al., 2015).

A 20-week controlled pilot study demonstrated an improvement in diabetic neuropathy in response to a low-fat plant-based diet: Electrochemical skin conductance in the foot and perceived pain improved compared with the control group (Bunner et al., 2015). These results are consistent with those of previous, smaller studies showing improvements in neuropathy in response to a plant-based diet combined with exercise (Crane, 1994; Smith et al., 2006), probably due to improved endoneurial microcirculatory perfusion (McCarty, 2002).

2.2.3 Diabetic Retinopathy and Macular Degeneration

To the best of our knowledge, the influence of vegetarian diets on diabetic retinopathy has not yet been studied. However, dietary factors important for slowing down the process of macular degeneration have been described. Macular concentrations of the carotenoids lutein and zeaxanthin decrease with age. These carotenoids are potent antioxidants that neutralize free radicals formed by light, act as a filter for blue light, and protect photoreceptors from its harmful effects. Plant foods are their only dietary source. Macular lutein and zeaxanthin concentrations are dependent on the degree of consumption (Szostak and Szostak-Wegierek, 2008); high consumption acts protectively against macular degeneration (Szostak and Szostak-Wegierek, 2008; Guggenbühl, 2006). Therefore, we suppose that diversiform plant-based diets may be an effective way how to slow down the process of macular degeneration.

2.3 Quality of Life, Mood, and Eating Behavior

Studies show that vegetarian diets improve quality of life compared with a conventional diabetic diet in people with T2D (Kahleova et al., 2013a; Katcher et al., 2010). It has been demonstrated that restriction in meat intake may improve mood (Beezhold and Johnston, 2012), and vegetarians have fewer negative emotions than omnivores (Kahleova et al., 2013a; Beezhold et al., 2010). The reader may refer to Chapter 28 on vegetarian diets and mood. The mechanism by which a vegetarian diet improves mood may partly be explained by differences in the rate of neurotransmitter synthesis and receptor dynamics reported in earlier studies (Maher, 2000).

Two interventional studies revealed that dietary restraint (voluntary control over food intake with the aim to lower body weight) increased less with a vegetarian than with a conventional diabetic diet, suggesting that the vegetarian-group participants felt less constrained by their prescribed diet (Kahleova, 2013a; Barnard et al., 2009a), while disinhibition (overeating, e.g., in stressful situations) and feelings of hunger decreased more with a vegetarian diet compared with a conventional diabetic diet (Kahleova et al., 2013a), suggesting that for patients with T2D a vegetarian diet is sustainable in the long run and may elicit desired improvements in not only physical but also in mental health.

3. Healthy Components of a Vegetarian Diet Related to Diabetes

Vegetarian diets are characterized by removal of all flesh foods from the diet. This, together with increased consumption of whole plant foods, such as whole grains, legumes, vegetables, fruits, and nuts, seem to have positive health effects in patients with type 2 diabetes.

Consumption of whole grains and legumes modulates the genetic effect of the APOA5-113C variant on changes in triglyceride concentrations in patients with impaired fasting glucose or newly diagnosed T2D (Kang et al., 2014), suggesting potential cardioprotective effects in these patients. A meta-analysis of randomized controlled trials demonstrated the potential of legumes in lowering fasting plasma glucose and improving glycemic control in people both with and without diabetes (Sievenpiper et al., 2009). Substitution of red meat with legumes also improves cardiometabolic risk factors in patients with T2D (Hosseinpour-Niazi et al., 2015). Eating vegetables seems to be an effective strategy to decrease glucose excursions in response to a meal and to improve glycemic control in patients with T2D (Imai et al., 2014). Increased fruit intake was associated with lower carotid intima-media thickness and prevalence of carotid plaque (Chan et al., 2013), as well as reduced incident diabetic retinopathy among patients with T2D (Tanaka et al., 2013). Regular consumption of nuts is associated with a lower risk of cardiovascular disease in women with T2D: 5 servings (1 serving is 28 g) of nuts per week was associated with a 44% lower risk of cardiovascular disease and a more favorable plasma lipid profile (Li et al., 2009a). Acute feeding studies have demonstrated the ability of nuts, when eaten with a carbohydrate (bread), to depress postprandial plasma glucose concentrations. Furthermore, there was evidence of reduced postprandial oxidative stress associated with nut consumption (Jenkins et al., 2008). Limited data suggests that dairy consumption may increase insulin sensitivity in patients with type 2 diabetes, but there is a clear need for larger and longer term studies (Pasin and Comerford, 2015).

3.1 Possible Mechanisms of Positive Effects of Vegetarian Diets on Diabetes

Several possible mechanisms may explain the beneficial effects of vegetarian diets for diabetes management (Barnard et al., 2009b): energy restriction, reduced intake of saturated fatty acids, high intake of polyunsaturated and monounsaturated fatty acids, low glycemic index, increased intake of fiber, higher intake of nonheme-iron and reduction in iron stores, increased intake of antioxidants, vitamins, and micronutrients, high intake of vegetable instead of animal protein, and high intake of plant sterols and prebiotics. All of these have been cited as positive independent factors in the prevention and treatment of T2D.

3.1.1 Energy Restriction

Energy restriction is the number one recommendation for losing weight and improving glycemic control and insulin sensitivity. A reduction in energy intake can have profound effects on glucose control, insulin secretion, and insulin resistance even before any changes in body weight occur (Hughes et al., 1984; Numata et al., 1993). Vegetarian diets may reduce total energy intake by consumption of foods with a lower energy density (Trapp and Barnard, 2010).

3.1.2 Reduced Intake of Saturated Fatty Acids

Several studies have demonstrated that dietary saturated fat can impair insulin sensitivity (Vessby et al., 2001; Xiao et al., 2006; Lichtenstein and Schwab, 2000). Decreased saturated fat intake may increase insulin sensitivity, independently of changes in body weight (Lovejoy, 2002; Defronzo, 2009). On the other hand, increased intake of saturated fat increases risk of cardiovascular disease and mortality in patients with diabetes (Tanasescu et al., 2004; Trichopoulou et al., 2006).

3.1.3 High Intake of Polyunsaturated Fatty Acids

Polyunsaturated fatty acids seem to be cardioprotective (Karlström et al., 2011) and reno-protective, especially in patients with diabetic nephropathy (Shapiro et al., 2011) although the cardioprotective effects have not been convincingly proven (Chowdhury et al., 2014). Their potential beneficial effects are explained mainly by activation of the peroxisome proliferator–activator receptors (PPAR) (Jump, 2002) and affecting mitochondrial function (Rohrbach, 2009). Because the n-6 fatty acids are precursors of proinflammatory eicosanoids, it was assumed that their higher intake might be harmful. Thus it used to be advised to reduce their intake (Hamazaki and Okuyama, 2003; Ailhaud, 2008), and the importance of the n-3:n-6 ratio was discussed (Simopoulos, 2008). However, this hypothesis is not well established. In humans, consumption of even large amounts of n-6 fatty acids is not associated with increased concentrations of inflammatory markers (Willett, 2007). Beneficial effects of n-6 fatty acids on total and LDL cholesterol (Nichaman et al., 1967; Shepherd et al., 1980) and blood pressure (Hall, 2009) have been known for a long time, and increased intake of n-6 fatty acids has been shown to reduce cardiovascular risk, mostly when substituted for saturated fatty acids (Turpeinen et al., 1979; Miettinen et al., 1983; Harris et al., 2009).

The main n-6 dietary fatty acid is linoleic acid (18:2n-6), found in vegetable oils (especially soybean, sunflower, corn, and rapeseed oil). Linoleic acid is one of the essential fatty acids, and food is its only source for humans and other mammals (Holman, 1961).

The Nurses' Health Study showed that higher intake of linoleic acid (about 8% of total energy intake) was strongly associated with a lower incidence of myocardial infarction (relative risk 0.55) and total cardiovascular mortality (relative risk 0.85) (Hu et al., 1999). Since n-3 fatty acids were also associated with a lower incidence of cardiovascular disease, the ratio of n-3 to n-6 did not play any role in cardiovascular risk (Willett, 2007). In men, high intake of linoleic acid reduced the risk of death from cardiovascular disease by 40% compared to men with low intake (Laaksonen et al., 2005).

The n-6 fatty acids seem to improve insulin resistance (Risérus, 2008; Summers et al., 2002), probably by activating PPARγ receptors (peroxisome proliferator–activator receptors γ) (Trichopoulou et al., 2006), and their consumption is protective against developing

T2D (Salmerón et al., 2001). Adequate intake of both n-6 and n-3 fatty acids is important for good health and lower risk of cardiovascular disease and T2D; their ratio does not seem to be important (Griffin, 2008). Reduction of the intake of linoleic acid, which would lead to "improvement" of this ratio is likely to increase the risk of cardiovascular disease and T2D (Willett, 2007). n-6 fatty acids should comprise at least 5%, preferably 10%, of total energy intake (Harris et al., 2009; Czernichow et al., 2010).

3.1.4 High Intake of Monounsaturated Fatty Acids

Monounsaturated fatty acids improve insulin resistance by influencing the composition of cell membranes, which at least partially reflects the composition of dietary fats (Palomer et al., 2008). A multicenter study KANWU showed that the transition from a diet rich in saturated fats to a diet rich in monounsaturated fatty acids improves insulin sensitivity (Vessby et al., 2001).

Oleic acid (18:1n-9c) has antiatherogenic and antithrombotic effects, increases HDL/LDL cholesterol ratio and reduces platelet aggregation (Holman, 1961). Replacing saturated fats with oleic acid (approximately 7% of total energy intake with fat intake up to 30% of energy intake) reduced the plasma levels of triglycerides and LDL cholesterol while increasing HDL cholesterol, and it improved insulin sensitivity (Palomer et al., 2008). Olive oil, the main dietary source of oleic acid, seems to have protective anticancer effects according to experimental studies (Costa et al., 2011), and it modulates the inflammatory response (Rodrigues et al., 2010).

3.1.5 Low Glycemic Index

Consumption of foods with low glycemic index is associated with good health, especially in regard to chronic diseases associated with aging, including T2D (Chiu et al., 2011). In contrast, a diet with a high glycemic index increases the risk of T2D by 40% compared to a low glycemic index diet (Barclay et al., 2008). Low glycemic index diets have been shown to reduce HbA1c in patients with diabetes (Brand-Miller et al., 2003) and are important in diabetes management.

3.1.6 High Intake of Fiber

A diet rich in fiber (50 g/day) reduces glucose and insulin concentrations in people with T2D (Chandalia et al., 2000). Dietary fiber may help to improve glycemic control in diabetic patients (Jenkins et al., 1978; Weickert and Pfeiffer, 2008). Its consumption should be encouraged, especially in people with T2D.

3.1.7 High Intake of Antioxidants, Vitamins, and Micronutrients

People with diabetes need to consume adequate amounts of vitamins and minerals from natural plant foods, especially fruits, nuts, and vegetables (Wheeler et al., 2012; Benzie and Choi, 2014). Foods rich in antioxidants (tocopherols, carotenoids, vitamin C, and flavonoids) are especially encouraged. Consumption of foods rich in folate (e.g., citrus fruits and legumes) may help to reduce risk of coronary heart disease (Mann et al., 2004; Wheeler et al., 2012), particularly in people with T2D.

3.1.8 Reductions in Heme-Iron Intake

Observational studies indicate that serum ferritin concentrations are positively associated with insulin resistance (Tsimihodimos et al., 2006; Jehn et al., 2004) and predict the development of hyperglycemia (Fumeron et al., 2006) and T2D (Jiang et al., 2004). Vegetarians are more insulin sensitive and have lower serum ferritin concentrations compared with nonvegetarians. Serum ferritin and insulin resistance are strongly positively correlated (Hua et al., 2001).

Reduction in iron status enhances insulin-mediated glucose disposal (Hua et al., 2001). Heme-iron intake from meat is positively, while nonheme-iron intake from plants is negatively, associated with diabetes (Lee et al., 2004). Vegetarian diets are rich in nonheme-iron and may reduce iron stores (Cook, 1990).

3.1.9 High Intake of Vegetable Proteins Instead of Animal Proteins

Amino acids influence the secretion of insulin and glucagon. The composition of dietary proteins may therefore play a role in the balance between insulin and glucagon. Vegetable proteins (especially soy) contain more nonessential amino acids than animal proteins and thus may affect glucagon secretion positively (Hubbard et al., 1989). Some dietary plant proteins have also been reported to reduce the levels of blood lipids (Anderson et al., 1995, 1998; Jenkins et al., 1989; Ruiz et al., 2014), may have antiinflammatory effects, and reduce the risk of obesity and cardiovascular disease (McCarty, 1999; Anderson et al., 1999; Liu et al., 2014; Bodai and Tuso, 2015).

Consumption of animal protein leads to a higher risk of obesity and T2D (even after adjustment for other factors, including intake of saturated fat), while consumption of vegetable protein reduces this risk (Bujnowski et al., 2011; van Nielen et al., 2014a).

Plant proteins seem to have a renoprotective effect (Anderson et al., 1999). It has been demonstrated that renal blood flow increases in response to a meal high in animal protein, especially red meat. This hyperfiltration and subsequent glomerular hypertension leads to progressive deterioration of renal function. On the other hand, omitting red meat from the diet may decrease microalbuminuria in people with T2D (de Mello et al., 2006).

Consumption of vegetable instead of animal protein seems to protect against the development of diabetic nephropathy and slows down the progression of this disease in patients with preexisting chronic renal insufficiency (Jibani et al., 1991; Anderson et al., 1998; Kontessis et al., 1990; Brenner et al., 1982).

3.1.10 High Intake of Plant Sterols

Plant sterols are substances with a structure similar to cholesterol that are naturally present in plant foods. Their function is to maintain the structure and function of plant cell membranes. After ingestion (from sterols-enriched foods), they reduce intestinal absorption of cholesterol into the blood. Unabsorbed cholesterol is then eliminated from the body, thus its concentration in the blood decreases. Plant sterols are present naturally in plants and in vegetable oils. Sitosterol and campesterol are markers of cholesterol absorption (Smahelová et al., 2004). Plant sterols decrease the levels of blood lipids (LDL cholesterol and triglycerides), have a positive effect on HDL cholesterol and the ratio of apo B/apo AI, and might reduce cardiovascular risk (Derdemezis et al., 2010).

Higher serum concentrations of plant sterols (upper tertile) were associated with only half the mortality (follow-up 22 years) in middle-aged men with high cardiovascular risks, compared with men in the bottom tertile (Strandberg et al., 2009). Plant sterols also have antiinflammatory effects (Othman and Moghadasian, 2011) and positively affect coagulation and platelet function. There is also some evidence of beneficial effects on oxidative stress, but this effect is no greater than can be expected from the reduction in LDL cholesterol (Derdemezis et al., 2010). Serum levels of plant sterols have also been shown to correlate negatively with glycemic control (HbA1c) in diabetic patients (Smahelová et al., 2004).

3.2 Meal Suggestions

After explaining the science behind following a vegetarian diet, we need to translate the knowledge into everyday eating habits. Here are a few suggestions of whole plant–based meals, high in fiber and all other beneficial constituents described earlier, providing the promised positive effects on glycemic control and cardiovascular risk factors in patients with T2D.

> Breakfast:
> traditional oatmeal with strawberries and banana,
> whole rye bread with beans spread and vegetables, and
> cooked millet with plums and almonds.
> Lunch:
> lentil soup with carrots and cabbage,
> bean burrito and green leaf salad, and
> buckwheat pasta, tomato chunks, fresh basil.
> Dinner:
> whole wheat pita bread, hummus, tomato salad with green onions,
> brown rice with marinated tofu and bean sprouts, and
> red quinoa with champignons.
> Snacks
> vegetables,
> fruits, and
> rice puffs (no added salt or sugar).

3.3 Seven Most Common Mistakes When Starting a Vegetarian Diet in Diabetes

1. A mere omission of meat from the diet, one-sided diet
   Ditching meat does not automatically mean that the patients will eat healthy. "Junk food (or donut) vegetarians," who consume cheese, chips, French fries, donuts, and sugar-containing soft drinks every day, definitely do not eat healthy and are likely to gain weight and make their diabetes control even worse. A healthy vegetarian diet is

a plant-based diet, based on little processed food. It must include fresh vegetables, fruits, whole grains, legumes, nuts, and seeds.

2. Assumption that all vegetarian products are healthy

Not all products that are vegetarian are also healthy. Many processed vegetarian foods frequently contain an excess of fat, salt, or refined sugars. Therefore, it is good to read the labels, check the ingredient list, and favor the less processed food items.

3. Excessive consumption of good things

The fact that something is healthy does not mean that it is healthy to overeat. It is important to eat and drink even healthy foods in moderation.

4. Condemnation of carbohydrates

Consumption of excess simple carbohydrates, especially sugar and high-fructose corn syrup, in the form of sweetened beverages, biscuits, wafers, products made from white flour, chocolate, and other sweets, is considered as one of the leading causes of obesity epidemics. A low consumption is necessary, especially for patients with diabetes. However, while counting and cutting down simple carbohydrates, many people condemn carbohydrates altogether, which is not only unnecessary but also a disadvantage because foods rich in complex carbohydrates contain a considerable amount of fiber, which slows down the absorption of carbohydrates, which is very helpful for glucose control. As a source of carbohydrates, we should prioritize natural foods rich in fiber, with a low glycemic index, as brown rice, millet, buckwheat, barley, oatmeal, or whole grain bread.

5. Underestimating the power of a vegetarian diet and its reducing effect on plasma glucose levels

A vegetarian diet can produce big results. It is very effective in reducing plasma glucose levels. Both patients with diabetes and their physicians need to be aware that there is a risk that low blood sugar can occur if diabetes medications are not lowered accordingly. It usually takes a few days or weeks to make all necessary adjustments to avoid hypoglycemia.

6. Vegetarianism as martyrdom

Some people feel that they do something for their health only if they eat foods that are healthy but not tasty. This is perhaps partly because they cannot imagine that vegetarian food can be tasty, and they do not know how many diverse tastes can be achieved within a vegetarian diet. The important principle is that the food we eat should be both healthy and tasty. To combine both is a culinary art.

7. Vegetarianism as a religion and insufficient attention to problematic vitamins and minerals

Adopting a vegetarian diet is a healthy choice. However, please do not cherish a false sense of confidence that you know all the best and you cannot learn anything new anymore. Vegetarian diets should be well-planned, with simple principles, and vegans need to pay a great attention to the risk of deficiency, in particular because of low intakes of some nutrients such as vitamin B_{12} and calcium, as it will be discussed for the general population in several chapters of this book.

3.4 Practical Aspects of Changing a Diet in Patients With Diabetes

It is one thing to prove scientifically that a diet is effective in the treatment of diabetes, but it is another thing to put it into practice in the real world. Here are the important principles for this task:

1. **Information first**
   Teach the patients the basic principles of the plant-based diet first, equipping them with all the information they need to know before they start.
2. **Planning and preparing meals**
   The dietary change involves also changes in selection of foods, buying the needed ingredients, charting restaurants near work or home and the healthy choices there, and eventually, preparing lunches to work, and charting options to purchase healthy foods at nearby stores and supermarkets.
3. **Avoiding problematic foods may be easier than trying to consume them in moderation.**
   For people who are addicted to some problematic foods that lead to weight gain (mostly chocolate, but also other sweets and fatty foods), food addictions can be overcome by excluding the problematic foods from the diet more easily and effectively. A period of 3–4 weeks usually represents sufficient time to establish new habits and combat addiction to unhealthy foods. It is also enough time to see the positive health effects, which also motivates the patients to continue to stick to the prescribed diet. However, if there is no food addiction, people may benefit from simply eating these foods only occasionally and in moderation.
4. **A bigger diet change is more effective than small gradual steps**
   Recommending significant changes in eating habits increases the chances that the patients really change something. After a few days or weeks of major diet changes, it is likely that the patients will see improvements in their health, which will encourage them to stick to these changes.
5. **Anticipate hypoglycemia**
   A plant-based diet reduces plasma glucose levels. The patients need to be informed on how to recognize hypoglycemia and how to solve it. It is good to equip them with a glucometer to be able to perform self-monitoring. If hypoglycemia occurs repeatedly, it is necessary to inform the doctor, who will consider reducing the doses of insulin and hypoglycemic medication accordingly.
6. **Schedule regular appointments, motivate, and encourage**
   During the time of a big change the patient is about to make, he or she will appreciate your support, motivation, and encouragement. Regularly scheduled checks of food records help the patients see their progress, and they also allow nutritional therapists and physicians to provide further suggestions for improvement. Schedule regular appointments (once a week at the beginning and once every 2 or 3 weeks later on). Discuss the patient's challenges and how to face them.

7. Social support

It is good to also involve family members in education, especially those who are involved in food purchasing and preparation. And it is important to explain the benefits of a plant-based diet even for them. Equip them with printed materials. It is great to set up group sessions where the patients can not only learn new information and gain new cooking skills, but where they can also share and form new friendships.

4. Official Position Statements on Vegetarian Diets

The position of the American Dietetic Association on vegetarian diets is as follows. "Appropriately planned vegetarian diets, including total vegetarian or vegan diets, are healthful, nutritionally adequate, and may provide health benefits in the prevention and treatment of certain diseases" (Craig and Mangels, 2009). We suggest that T2D is one of them. "A vegetarian diet can meet current recommendations for all nutrients including protein, n-3 fatty acids, iron, zinc, iodine, calcium, and vitamins D and B_{12}" (Craig and Mangels, 2009; Craig, 2010). The American Diabetes Association states in the 2014 Clinical Practice Guidelines that plant-based diets improve metabolic control in diabetic subjects (American Diabetes Association, 2014).

5. Conclusions

Vegetarian diets represent a promising alternative to conventional dietary treatments of T2D. According to official position statements, transition to vegetarian diets should be done under supervision of a qualified physician and a skillful registered dietician. Properly planned vegetarian diets are healthy and nutritionally adequate, are effective for weight and glycemic control, bestow metabolic and cardiovascular benefits, and reduce diabetes complications. They are sustainable in the long-term and may elicit desirable improvements not only in physical but also in mental health. Larger clinical trials are needed to confirm the effectiveness of vegetarian diets and to promote their use in dietary guidelines for the prevention and treatment of T2D.

References

Aburto, N.J., Hanson, S., Gutierrez, H., Hooper, L., Elliott, P., Cappuccio, F.P., 2013. Effect of increased potassium intake on cardiovascular risk factors and disease: systematic review and meta-analyses. BMJ 346, f1378.

Action to Control Cardiovascular Risk in Diabetes Study Group, Gerstein, H.C., Miller, M.E., Byington, R.P., Goff, D.C., Bigger, J.T., et al., June 12, 2008. Effects of intensive glucose lowering in type 2 diabetes. N. Engl. J. Med. 358 (24), 2545–2559.

ADVANCE Collaborative Group, Patel, A., MacMahon, S., Chalmers, J., Neal, B., Billot, L., et al., June 12, 2008. Intensive blood glucose control and vascular outcomes in patients with type 2 diabetes. N. Engl. J. Med. 358 (24), 2560–2572.

Ailhaud, G., 2008. Omega-6 fatty acids and excessive adipose tissue development. World Rev. Nutr. Diet. 98, 51–61.

Alleman, C.J.M., Westerhout, K.Y., Hensen, M., Chambers, C., Stoker, M., Long, S., et al., August 2015. Humanistic and economic burden of painful diabetic peripheral neuropathy in Europe: a review of the literature. Diabetes Res. Clin. Pract 109 (2), 215–225. http://dx.doi.org/10.1016/j.diabres.2015.04.031.

American Diabetes Association, January 2014. Standards of medical care in diabetes–2014. Diabetes Care 37 (Suppl. 1), S14–S80.

Anderson, J.W., Ward, K., November 1979. High-carbohydrate, high-fiber diets for insulin-treated men with diabetes mellitus. Am. J. Clin. Nutr. 32 (11), 2312–2321.

Anderson, J.W., Johnstone, B.M., Cook-Newell, M.E., August 3, 1995. Meta-analysis of the effects of soy protein intake on serum lipids. N. Engl. J. Med. 333 (5), 276–282.

Anderson, J.W., Blake, J.E., Turner, J., Smith, B.M., December 1998. Effects of soy protein on renal function and proteinuria in patients with type 2 diabetes. Am. J. Clin. Nutr. 68 (6 Suppl.), 1347S–1353S.

Anderson, J.W., Smith, B.M., Washnock, C.S., September 1999. Cardiovascular and renal benefits of dry bean and soybean intake. Am. J. Clin. Nutr. 70 (3 Suppl.), 464S–474S.

Appleby, P.N., Thorogood, M., Mann, J.I., Key, T.J., September 1999. The Oxford vegetarian study: an overview. Am. J. Clin. Nutr. 70 (3 Suppl.), 525S–531S.

Avogaro, A., Giorda, C., Maggini, M., Mannucci, E., Raschetti, R., Lombardo, F., et al., May 2007. Incidence of coronary heart disease in type 2 diabetic men and women: impact of microvascular complications, treatment, and geographic location. Diabetes Care 30 (5), 1241–1247.

Barclay, A.W., Petocz, P., McMillan-Price, J., Flood, V.M., Prvan, T., Mitchell, P., et al., March 2008. Glycemic index, glycemic load, and chronic disease risk–a meta-analysis of observational studies. Am. J. Clin. Nutr. 87 (3), 627–637.

Barnard, R.J., Jung, T., Inkeles, S.B., December 1994. Diet and exercise in the treatment of NIDDM. The need for early emphasis. Diabetes Care 17 (12), 1469–1472.

Barnard, N.D., Cohen, J., Jenkins, D.J.A., Turner-McGrievy, G., Gloede, L., Jaster, B., et al., August 2006. A low-fat vegan diet improves glycemic control and cardiovascular risk factors in a randomized clinical trial in individuals with type 2 diabetes. Diabetes Care 29 (8), 1777–1783.

Barnard, N.D., Gloede, L., Cohen, J., Jenkins, D.J.A., Turner-McGrievy, G., Green, A.A., et al., February 2009a. A low-fat vegan diet elicits greater macronutrient changes, but is comparable in adherence and acceptability, compared with a more conventional diabetes diet among individuals with type 2 diabetes. J. Am. Diet. Assoc. 109 (2), 263–272.

Barnard, N.D., Katcher, H.I., Jenkins, D.J., Cohen, J., Turner-McGrievy, G., 2009b. Vegetarian and vegan diets in type 2 diabetes management. Nutr. Rev. 67 (5), 255–263.

Barnard, N.D., Levin, S.M., Yokoyama, Y., June 2015. A systematic review and meta-analysis of changes in body weight in clinical trials of vegetarian diets. J. Acad. Nutr. Diet 115 (6), 954–969.

Barsotti, G., Navalesi, R., Giampietro, O., Ciardella, F., Morelli, E., Cupisti, A., et al., 1988. Effects of a vegetarian, supplemented diet on renal function, proteinuria, and glucose metabolism in patients with "overt" diabetic nephropathy and renal insufficiency. Contrib. Nephrol. 65, 87–94.

Beezhold, B.L., Johnston, C.S., 2012. Restriction of meat, fish, and poultry in omnivores improves mood: a pilot randomized controlled trial. Nutr. J. 11, 9.

Beezhold, B.L., Johnston, C.S., Daigle, D.R., 2010. Vegetarian diets are associated with healthy mood states: a cross-sectional study in Seventh day Adventist adults. Nutr. J. 9, 26.

Belinova, L., Kahleova, H., Malinska, H., Topolcan, O., Vrzalova, J., Oliyarnyk, O., et al., 2014. Differential acute postprandial effects of processed meat and isocaloric vegan meals on the gastrointestinal hormone response in subjects suffering from type 2 diabetes and healthy controls: a randomized crossover study. PLoS One 9 (9), e107561.

Benzie, I.F.F., Choi, S.-W., 2014. Antioxidants in food: content, measurement, significance, action, cautions, caveats, and research needs. Adv. Food Nutr. Res. 71, 1–53.

Berger, S., Raman, G., Vishwanathan, R., Jacques, P.F., Johnson, E.J., August 2015. Dietary cholesterol and cardiovascular disease: a systematic review and meta-analysis. Am. J. Clin. Nutr. 102 (2), 276–294.

Berkow, S.E., Barnard, N., April 2006. Vegetarian diets and weight status. Nutr. Rev. 64 (4), 175–188.

Bodai, B.I., Tuso, P., 2015. Breast cancer survivorship: a comprehensive review of long-term medical issues and lifestyle recommendations. Perm. J. 19 (2), 48–79.

Boulton, A.J.M., Vinik, A.I., Arezzo, J.C., Bril, V., Feldman, E.L., Freeman, R., et al., April 2005. Diabetic neuropathies: a statement by the American Diabetes Association. Diabetes Care 28 (4), 956–962.

Bradbury, K.E., Crowe, F.L., Appleby, P.N., Schmidt, J.A., Travis, R.C., Key, T.J., February 2014. Serum concentrations of cholesterol, apolipoprotein A-I and apolipoprotein B in a total of 1694 meat-eaters, fish-eaters, vegetarians and vegans. Eur. J. Clin. Nutr. 68 (2), 178–183.

Brand-Miller, J., Hayne, S., Petocz, P., Colagiuri, S., August 2003. Low-glycemic index diets in the management of diabetes: a meta-analysis of randomized controlled trials. Diabetes Care 26 (8), 2261–2267.

Brathwaite, N., Fraser, H.S., Modeste, N., Broome, H., King, R., 2003. Obesity, diabetes, hypertension, and vegetarian status among Seventh-Day Adventists in Barbados: preliminary results. Ethn. Dis. 13 (1), 34–39.

Brenner, B.M., Meyer, T.W., Hostetter, T.H., September 9, 1982. Dietary protein intake and the progressive nature of kidney disease: the role of hemodynamically mediated glomerular injury in the pathogenesis of progressive glomerular sclerosis in aging, renal ablation, and intrinsic renal disease. N. Engl. J. Med. 307 (11), 652–659.

Buendia, J.R., Bradlee, M.L., Daniels, S.R., Singer, M.R., Moore, L.L., June 2015. Longitudinal effects of dietary sodium and potassium on blood pressure in adolescent girls. JAMA Pediatr. 169 (6), 560–568.

Bujnowski, D., Xun, P., Daviglus, M.L., Van Horn, L., He, K., Stamler, J., August 2011. Longitudinal association between animal and vegetable protein intake and obesity among men in the United States: the Chicago Western Electric Study. J. Am. Diet. Assoc. 111 (8) 1150.e1–1155.e1.

Bunner, A.E., Wells, C.L., Gonzales, J., Agarwal, U., Bayat, E., Barnard, N.D., May 2015. A dietary intervention for chronic diabetic neuropathy pain: a randomized controlled pilot study. Nutr. Diabetes 5 (5), e158.

Ceriello, A., December 2012. The emerging challenge in diabetes: the "metabolic memory". Vascul. Pharmacol. 57 (5–6), 133–138.

Chan, H.-T., Yiu, K.-H., Wong, C.-Y., Li, S.-W., Tam, S., Tse, H.-F., January 2013. Increased dietary fruit intake was associated with lower burden of carotid atherosclerosis in Chinese patients with type 2 diabetes mellitus. Diabet. Med. 30 (1), 100–108.

Chandalia, M., Garg, A., Lutjohann, D., von Bergmann, K., Grundy, S.M., Brinkley, L.J., May 11, 2000. Beneficial effects of high dietary fiber intake in patients with type 2 diabetes mellitus. N. Engl. J. Med. 342 (19), 1392–1398.

Chiu, C.-J., Liu, S., Willett, W.C., Wolever, T.M., Brand-Miller, J.C., Barclay, A.W., et al., April 2011. Informing food choices and health outcomes by use of the dietary glycemic index. Nutr. Rev. 69 (4), 231–242.

Chowdhury, R., Warnakula, S., Kunutsor, S., Crowe, F., Ward, H.A., Johnson, L., et al., March 18, 2014. Association of dietary, circulating, and supplement fatty acids with coronary risk: a systematic review and meta-analysis. Ann. Intern. Med. 160 (6), 398–406.

Cook, J.D., February 1990. Adaptation in iron metabolism. Am. J. Clin. Nutr. 51 (2), 301–308.

Costa, I., Moral, R., Solanas, M., Andreu, F.J., Ruiz de Villa, M.C., Escrich, E., February 2011. High corn oil and extra virgin olive oil diets and experimental mammary carcinogenesis: clinicopathological and immunohistochemical p21Ha-Ras expression study. Virchows Arch. 458 (2), 141–151.

Craig, W.J., Mangels, A.R., July 2009. Position of the American Dietetic Association: vegetarian diets. J. Am. Diet. Assoc. 109 (7), 1266–1282.

Craig, W.J., December 2010. Nutrition concerns and health effects of vegetarian diets. Nutr. Clin. Pract. 25 (6), 613–620.

Crane, M.G., 1994. Regression of diabetic neuropathy with total vegetarian (vegan) diet. J. Nutr. Med. 4, 431–439.

Czernichow, S., Thomas, D., Bruckert, E., September 2010. n-6 Fatty acids and cardiovascular health: a review of the evidence for dietary intake recommendations. Br. J. Nutr. 104 (6), 788–796.

Dall, T.M., Yang, W., Halder, P., Pang, B., Massoudi, M., Wintfeld, N., et al., December 2014. The economic burden of elevated blood glucose levels in 2012: diagnosed and undiagnosed diabetes, gestational diabetes mellitus, and prediabetes. Diabetes Care 37 (12), 3172–3179.

Daubenmier, J.J., Weidner, G., Sumner, M.D., Mendell, N., Merritt-Worden, T., Studley, J., et al., February 2007. The contribution of changes in diet, exercise, and stress management to changes in coronary risk in women and men in the multisite cardiac lifestyle intervention program. Ann. Behav. Med. 33 (1), 57–68.

De Biase, S.G., Fernandes, S.F.C., Gianini, R.J., Duarte, J.L.G., January 2007. Vegetarian diet and cholesterol and triglycerides levels. Arq. Bras. Cardiol. 88 (1), 35–39.

de Mello, V.D.F., Zelmanovitz, T., Perassolo, M.S., Azevedo, M.J., Gross, J.L., May 2006. Withdrawal of red meat from the usual diet reduces albuminuria and improves serum fatty acid profile in type 2 diabetes patients with macroalbuminuria. Am. J. Clin. Nutr. 83 (5), 1032–1038.

Defronzo, R.A., April 2009. Banting Lecture. From the triumvirate to the ominous octet: a new paradigm for the treatment of type 2 diabetes mellitus. Diabetes 58 (4), 773–795.

Deli, G., Bosnyak, E., Pusch, G., Komoly, S., Feher, G., 2013. Diabetic neuropathies: diagnosis and management. Neuroendocrinology 98 (4), 267–280.

Derdemezis, C.S., Filippatos, T.D., Mikhailidis, D.P., Elisaf, M.S., June 2010. Review article: effects of plant sterols and stanols beyond low-density lipoprotein cholesterol lowering. J. Cardiovasc. Pharmacol. Ther. 15 (2), 120–134.

Duckworth, W.C., McCarren, M., Abraira, C., VA Diabetes Trial, May 2001. Glucose control and cardiovascular complications: the VA diabetes trial. Diabetes Care 24 (5), 942–945.

Duckworth, W., Abraira, C., Moritz, T., Reda, D., Emanuele, N., Reaven, P.D., et al., January 8, 2009. Glucose control and vascular complications in veterans with type 2 diabetes. N. Engl. J. Med. 360 (2), 129–139.

Effect of intensive blood-glucose control with metformin on complications in overweight patients with type 2 diabetes (UKPDS 34). UK Prospective Diabetes Study (UKPDS) Group. Lancet 352 (9131), September 12, 1998, 854–865.

Elley, C.R., Kenealy, T., Robinson, E., Drury, P.L., November 2008. Glycated haemoglobin and cardiovascular outcomes in people with Type 2 diabetes: a large prospective cohort study. Diabet. Med. 25 (11), 1295–1301.

Esselstyn Jr., C.B., Ellis, S.G., Medendorp, S.V., Crowe, T.D., December 1995. A strategy to arrest and reverse coronary artery disease: a 5-year longitudinal study of a single physician's practice. J. Fam. Pract. 41 (6), 560–568.

Evert, A.B., Boucher, J.L., Cypress, M., Dunbar, S.A., Franz, M.J., Mayer-Davis, E.J., et al., January 2014. Nutrition therapy recommendations for the management of adults with diabetes. Diabetes Care 37 (Suppl. 1), S120–S143.

Feskens, E.J., September 2001. Can diabetes be prevented by vegetable fat? Diabetes Care 24 (9), 1517–1518.

Forbes, J.M., Coughlan, M.T., Cooper, M.E., June 2008. Oxidative stress as a major culprit in kidney disease in diabetes. Diabetes 57 (6), 1446–1454.

Fraser, G.E., September 1999. Associations between diet and cancer, ischemic heart disease, and all-cause mortality in non-Hispanic white California Seventh-day Adventists. Am. J. Clin. Nutr. 70 (3 Suppl), 532S–538S.

Frattaroli, J., Weidner, G., Merritt-Worden, T.A., Frenda, S., Ornish, D., April 1, 2008. Angina pectoris and atherosclerotic risk factors in the multisite cardiac lifestyle intervention program. Am. J. Cardiol. 101 (7), 911–918.

Fumeron, F., Péan, F., Driss, F., Balkau, B., Tichet, J., Marre, M., et al., September 2006. Ferritin and transferrin are both predictive of the onset of hyperglycemia in men and women over 3 years: the data from an epidemiological study on the Insulin Resistance Syndrome (DESIR) study. Diabetes Care 29 (9), 2090–2094.

Gerstein, H.C., Pogue, J., Mann, J.F.E., Lonn, E., Dagenais, G.R., McQueen, M., et al., September 2005. The relationship between dysglycaemia and cardiovascular and renal risk in diabetic and non-diabetic participants in the HOPE study: a prospective epidemiological analysis. Diabetologia 48 (9), 1749–1755.

Gerstein, H.C., Miller, M.E., Ismail-Beigi, F., Largay, J., McDonald, C., Lochnan, H.A., et al., November 29, 2014. Effects of intensive glycaemic control on ischaemic heart disease: analysis of data from the randomised, controlled ACCORD trial. Lancet 384 (9958), 1936–1941.

Goff, L.M., Bell, J.D., So, P.-W., Dornhorst, A., Frost, G.S., February 2005. Veganism and its relationship with insulin resistance and intramyocellular lipid. Eur. J. Clin. Nutr. 59 (2), 291–298.

Gomes, P.M., Hollanda-Miranda, W.R., Beraldo, R.A., Castro, A.V.B., Geloneze, B., Foss, M.C., et al., June 2015. Supplementation of α-linolenic acid improves serum adiponectin levels and insulin sensitivity in patients with type 2 diabetes. Nutrition 31 (6), 853–857.

Griffin, B.A., February 2008. How relevant is the ratio of dietary n-6 to n-3 polyunsaturated fatty acids to cardiovascular disease risk? Evidence from the OPTILIP study. Curr. Opin. Lipidol. 19 (1), 57–62.

Control Group, Turnbull, F.M., Abraira, C., Anderson, R.J., Byington, R.P., Chalmers, J.P., et al., November 2009. Intensive glucose control and macrovascular outcomes in type 2 diabetes. Diabetologia 52 (11), 2288–2298.

Grundy, S.M., Cleeman, J.I., Merz, C.N.B., Brewer, H.B., Clark, L.T., Hunninghake, D.B., et al., August 4, 2004. Implications of recent clinical trials for the National Cholesterol Education Program Adult Treatment Panel III Guidelines. J. Am. Coll. Cardiol. 44 (3), 720–732.

Guariguata, L., Whiting, D.R., Hambleton, I., Beagley, J., Linnenkamp, U., Shaw, J.E., February 2014. Global estimates of diabetes prevalence for 2013 and projections for 2035. Diabetes Res. Clin. Pract. 103 (2), 137–149.

Guggenbühl, N., 2006. The source of antioxidants. Bull. Soc. Belge Ophtalmol. 301, 41–45.

Hall, W.L., June 2009. Dietary saturated and unsaturated fats as determinants of blood pressure and vascular function. Nutr. Res. Rev. 22 (1), 18–38.

Hamazaki, T., Okuyama, H., 2003. The Japan Society for Lipid Nutrition recommends to reduce the intake of linoleic acid. A review and critique of the scientific evidence. World Rev. Nutr. Diet. 92, 109–132.

Harris, W.S., Mozaffarian, D., Rimm, E., Kris-Etherton, P., Rudel, L.L., Appel, L.J., et al., February 17, 2009. Omega-6 fatty acids and risk for cardiovascular disease: a science advisory from the American Heart Association Nutrition Subcommittee of the Council on Nutrition, Physical Activity, and Metabolism; Council on Cardiovascular Nursing; and Council on Epidemiology and Prevention. Circulation 119 (6), 902–907.

Hayward, R.A., Reaven, P.D., Emanuele, N.V., VADT Investigators, September 3, 2015. Follow-up of glycemic control and cardiovascular outcomes in type 2 diabetes. N. Engl. J. Med. 373 (10), 978.

Holman, R.T., December 2, 1961. How essential are fatty acids? JAMA 178, 930–933.

Hosseinpour-Niazi, S., Mirmiran, P., Hedayati, M., Azizi, F., May 2015. Substitution of red meat with legumes in the therapeutic lifestyle change diet based on dietary advice improves cardiometabolic risk factors in overweight type 2 diabetes patients: a cross-over randomized clinical trial. Eur. J. Clin. Nutr. 69 (5), 592–597.

Howard, B.V., Roman, M.J., Devereux, R.B., Fleg, J.L., Galloway, J.M., Henderson, J.A., et al., April 9, 2008. Effect of lower targets for blood pressure and LDL cholesterol on atherosclerosis in diabetes: the SANDS randomized trial. JAMA 299 (14), 1678–1689.

Hu, F.B., Stampfer, M.J., Manson, J.E., Rimm, E.B., Wolk, A., Colditz, G.A., et al., May 1999. Dietary intake of alpha-linolenic acid and risk of fatal ischemic heart disease among women. Am. J. Clin. Nutr. 69 (5), 890–897.

Hua, N.W., Stoohs, R.A., Facchini, F.S., October 2001. Low iron status and enhanced insulin sensitivity in lacto-ovo vegetarians. Br. J. Nutr. 86 (4), 515–519.

Hubbard, R., Kosch, C.L., Sanchez, A., Sabate, J., Berk, L., Shavlik, G., March 1989. Effect of dietary protein on serum insulin and glucagon levels in hyper- and normocholesterolemic men. Atherosclerosis 76 (1), 55–61.

Hughes, T.A., Gwynne, J.T., Switzer, B.R., Herbst, C., White, G., July 1984. Effects of caloric restriction and weight loss on glycemic control, insulin release and resistance, and atherosclerotic risk in obese patients with type II diabetes mellitus. Am. J. Med. 77 (1), 7–17.

Hung, C.-J., Huang, P.-C., Li, Y.-H., Lu, S.-C., Ho, L.-T., Chou, H.-F., January 2006. Taiwanese vegetarians have higher insulin sensitivity than omnivores. Br. J. Nutr. 95 (1), 129–135.

Imai, S., Fukui, M., Kajiyama, S., January 2014. Effect of eating vegetables before carbohydrates on glucose excursions in patients with type 2 diabetes. J. Clin. Biochem. Nutr. 54 (1), 7–11.

Intensive blood-glucose control with sulphonylureas or insulin compared with conventional treatment and risk of complications in patients with type 2 diabetes (UKPDS 33). UK Prospective Diabetes Study (UKPDS) Group. Lancet 352 (9131), September 12, 1998, 837–853.

Jehn, M., Clark, J.M., Guallar, E., October 2004. Serum ferritin and risk of the metabolic syndrome in U.S. adults. Diabetes Care 27 (10), 2422–2428.

Jenkins, D.J., Wolever, T.M., Leeds, A.R., Gassull, M.A., Haisman, P., Dilawari, J., et al., May 27, 1978. Dietary fibres, fibre analogues, and glucose tolerance: importance of viscosity. Br. Med. J. 1 (6124), 1392–1394.

Jenkins, D.J., Wolever, T.M., Spiller, G., Buckley, G., Lam, Y., Jenkins, A.L., et al., August 1989. Hypocholesterolemic effect of vegetable protein in a hypocaloric diet. Atherosclerosis 78 (2–3), 99–107.

Jenkins, D.J.A., Kendall, C.W.C., Marchie, A., Faulkner, D.A., Wong, J.M.W., de Souza, R., et al., February 2005. Direct comparison of a dietary portfolio of cholesterol-lowering foods with a statin in hypercholesterolemic participants. Am. J. Clin. Nutr. 81 (2), 380–387.

Jenkins, D.J.A., Hu, F.B., Tapsell, L.C., Josse, A.R., Kendall, C.W.C., September 2008. Possible benefit of nuts in type 2 diabetes. J. Nutr. 138 (9), 1752S–1756S.

Jiang, R., Manson, J.E., Meigs, J.B., Ma, J., Rifai, N., Hu, F.B., February 11, 2004. Body iron stores in relation to risk of type 2 diabetes in apparently healthy women. JAMA 291 (6), 711–717.

Jibani, M.M., Bloodworth, L.L., Foden, E., Griffiths, K.D., Galpin, O.P., December 1991. Predominantly vegetarian diet in patients with incipient and early clinical diabetic nephropathy: effects on albumin excretion rate and nutritional status. Diabet. Med. 8 (10), 949–953.

Jump, D.B., April 2002. Dietary polyunsaturated fatty acids and regulation of gene transcription. Curr. Opin. Lipidol. 13 (2), 155–164.

Kahleova, H., Matoulek, M., Malinska, H., Oliyarnik, O., Kazdova, L., Neskudla, T., et al., May 2011. Vegetarian diet improves insulin resistance and oxidative stress markers more than conventional diet in subjects with type 2 diabetes. Diabet. Med. 28 (5), 549–559.

Kahleova, H., Hrachovinova, T., Hill, M., Pelikanova, T., January 2013a. Vegetarian diet in type 2 diabetes–improvement in quality of life, mood and eating behaviour. Diabet. Med. 30 (1), 127–129.

Kahleova, H., Matoulek, M., Bratova, M., Malinska, H., Kazdova, L., Hill, M., et al., 2013b. Vegetarian diet-induced increase in linoleic acid in serum phospholipids is associated with improved insulin sensitivity in subjects with type 2 diabetes. Nutr. Diabetes 3, e75.

Kahleova, H., Hill, M., Terezie, P., et al., 2014. Vegetarian vs. conventional diabetic diet – a 1-year-follow-up. Cor Vasa, e140–e144.

Kang, R., Kim, M., Chae, J.S., Lee, S.-H., Lee, J.H., 2014. Consumption of whole grains and legumes modulates the genetic effect of the APOA5 -1131C variant on changes in triglyceride and apolipoprotein A-V concentrations in patients with impaired fasting glucose or newly diagnosed type 2 diabetes. Trials 15, 100.

Karlström, B.E., Järvi, A.E., Byberg, L., Berglund, L.G., Vessby, B.O.H., July 2011. Fatty fish in the diet of patients with type 2 diabetes: comparison of the metabolic effects of foods rich in n-3 and n-6 fatty acids. Am. J. Clin. Nutr. 94 (1), 26–33.

Katcher, H.I., Ferdowsian, H.R., Hoover, V.J., Cohen, J.L., Barnard, N.D., 2010. A worksite vegan nutrition program is well-accepted and improves health-related quality of life and work productivity. Ann. Nutr. Metab. 56 (4), 245–252.

Khaw, K.-T., Wareham, N., Bingham, S., Luben, R., Welch, A., Day, N., September 21, 2004. Association of hemoglobin A1c with cardiovascular disease and mortality in adults: the European prospective investigation into cancer in Norfolk. Ann. Intern. Med. 141 (6), 413–420.

Kirkman, M.S., McCarren, M., Shah, J., Duckworth, W., Abraira, C., VADT Study Group, April 2006. The association between metabolic control and prevalent macrovascular disease in type 2 diabetes: the VA Cooperative Study in diabetes. J. Diabetes Complications 20 (2), 75–80.

Knight, E.L., Stampfer, M.J., Hankinson, S.E., Spiegelman, D., Curhan, G.C., March 18, 2003. The impact of protein intake on renal function decline in women with normal renal function or mild renal insufficiency. Ann. Intern. Med. 138 (6), 460–467.

Kontessis, P., Jones, S., Dodds, R., Trevisan, R., Nosadini, R., Fioretto, P., et al., July 1990. Renal, metabolic and hormonal responses to ingestion of animal and vegetable proteins. Kidney Int. 38 (1), 136–144.

Kuo, C.-S., Lai, N.-S., Ho, L.-T., Lin, C.-L., February 2004. Insulin sensitivity in Chinese ovo-lactovegetarians compared with omnivores. Eur. J. Clin. Nutr. 58 (2), 312–316.

Laaksonen, D.E., Nyyssönen, K., Niskanen, L., Rissanen, T.H., Salonen, J.T., January 24, 2005. Prediction of cardiovascular mortality in middle-aged men by dietary and serum linoleic and polyunsaturated fatty acids. Arch. Intern. Med. 165 (2), 193–199.

Lam, T., Burns, K., Dennis, M., Cheung, N.W., Gunton, J.E., May 15, 2015. Assessment of cardiovascular risk in diabetes: risk scores and provocative testing. World J. Diabetes 6 (4), 634–641.

Lee, D.-H., Folsom, A.R., Jacobs, D.R., February 2004. Dietary iron intake and Type 2 diabetes incidence in postmenopausal women: the Iowa Women's Health Study. Diabetologia 47 (2), 185–194.

Lewington, S., Clarke, R., Qizilbash, N., Peto, R., Collins, R., Prospective Studies Collaboration, December 14, 2002. Age-specific relevance of usual blood pressure to vascular mortality: a meta-analysis of individual data for one million adults in 61 prospective studies. Lancet 360 (9349), 1903–1913.

Li, T.Y., Brennan, A.M., Wedick, N.M., Mantzoros, C., Rifai, N., Hu, F.B., July 2009a. Regular consumption of nuts is associated with a lower risk of cardiovascular disease in women with type 2 diabetes. J. Nutr. 139 (7), 1333–1338.

Li, X., Xu, Z., Lu, X., Yang, X., Yin, P., Kong, H., et al., February 9, 2009b. Comprehensive two-dimensional gas chromatography/time-of-flight mass spectrometry for metabonomics: biomarker discovery for diabetes mellitus. Anal. Chim. Acta 633 (2), 257–262.

Lichtenstein, A.H., Schwab, U.S., June 2000. Relationship of dietary fat to glucose metabolism. Atherosclerosis 150 (2), 227–243.

Liu, Y., Colditz, G.A., Cotterchio, M., Boucher, B.A., Kreiger, N., June 2014. Adolescent dietary fiber, vegetable fat, vegetable protein, and nut intakes and breast cancer risk. Breast Cancer Res. Treat. 145 (2), 461–470.

Lovejoy, J.C., October 2002. The influence of dietary fat on insulin resistance. Curr. Diab. Rep. 2 (5), 435–440.

Maher, T.J., 2000. Effects of nutrients on brain function. Prog. Brain Res. 122, 187–194.

Mann, J.I., De Leeuw, I., Hermansen, K., Karamanos, B., Karlström, B., Katsilambros, N., et al., December 2004. Evidence-based nutritional approaches to the treatment and prevention of diabetes mellitus. Nutr. Metab. Cardiovasc. Dis. 14 (6), 373–394.

Mannucci, E., Monami, M., Lamanna, C., Gori, F., Marchionni, N., November 2009. Prevention of cardiovascular disease through glycemic control in type 2 diabetes: a meta-analysis of randomized clinical trials. Nutr. Metab. Cardiovasc. Dis. 19 (9), 604–612.

Maritim, A.C., Sanders, R.A., Watkins, J.B., 2003. Diabetes, oxidative stress, and antioxidants: a review. J. Biochem. Mol. Toxicol. 17 (1), 24–38.

Mattos, C.B., Viana, L.V., Paula, T.P., Sarmento, R.A., Almeida, J.C., Gross, J.L., et al., 2015. Increased protein intake is associated with uncontrolled blood pressure by 24-hour ambulatory blood pressure monitoring in patients with type 2 diabetes. J. Am. Coll. Nutr. 34 (3), 232–239.

McCarty, M.F., December 1999. Vegan proteins may reduce risk of cancer, obesity, and cardiovascular disease by promoting increased glucagon activity. Med. Hypotheses 53 (6), 459–485.

McCarty, M.F., June 2002. Favorable impact of a vegan diet with exercise on hemorheology: implications for control of diabetic neuropathy. Med. Hypotheses 58 (6), 476–486.

McEwen, B.J., March 2014. The influence of diet and nutrients on platelet function. Semin. Thromb. Hemost. 40 (2), 214–226.

Miettinen, M., Turpeinen, O., Karvonen, M.J., Pekkarinen, M., Paavilainen, E., Elosuo, R., March 1983. Dietary prevention of coronary heart disease in women: the Finnish Mental Hospital Study. Int. J. Epidemiol. 12 (1), 17–25.

Montalcini, T., De Bonis, D., Ferro, Y., Carè, I., Mazza, E., Accattato, F., et al., July 2015. High vegetable fats intake is associated with high resting energy expenditure in vegetarians. Nutrients 7 (7), 5933–5947.

Moore, W.J., McGrievy, M.E., Turner-McGrievy, G.M., July 2, 2015. Dietary adherence and acceptability of five different diets, including vegan and vegetarian diets, for weight loss: the New DIETs study. Eat. Behav. 19, 33–38.

Nauck, M., Stöckmann, F., Ebert, R., Creutzfeldt, W., January 1986a. Reduced incretin effect in type 2 (non-insulin-dependent) diabetes. Diabetologia 29 (1), 46–52.

Nauck, M.A., Homberger, E., Siegel, E.G., Allen, R.C., Eaton, R.P., Ebert, R., et al., August 1986b. Incretin effects of increasing glucose loads in man calculated from venous insulin and C-peptide responses. J. Clin. Endocrinol. Metab. 63 (2), 492–498.

Nichaman, M.Z., Sweeley, C.C., Olson, R.E., October 1967. Plasma fatty acids in normolipemic and hyperlipemic subjects during fasting and after linoleate feeding. Am. J. Clin. Nutr. 20 (10), 1057–1069.

Nicholson, A.S., Sklar, M., Barnard, N.D., Gore, S., Sullivan, R., Browning, S., August 1999. Toward improved management of NIDDM: a randomized, controlled, pilot intervention using a lowfat, vegetarian diet. Prev. Med. 29 (2), 87–91.

Numata, K., Tanaka, K., Saito, M., Shishido, T., Inoue, S., February 1993. Very low calorie diet-induced weight loss reverses exaggerated insulin secretion in response to glucose, arginine and glucagon in obesity. Int. J. Obes. Relat. Metab. Disord. 17 (2), 103–108.

Odermatt, A., November 2011. The Western-style diet: a major risk factor for impaired kidney function and chronic kidney disease. Am. J. Physiol. Renal Physiol. 301 (5), F919–F931.

Ornish, D., Brown, S.E., Scherwitz, L.W., Billings, J.H., Armstrong, W.T., Ports, T.A., et al., July 21, 1990. Can lifestyle changes reverse coronary heart disease? The Lifestyle Heart Trial. Lancet 336 (8708), 129–133.

Ornish, D., Scherwitz, L.W., Billings, J.H., Brown, S.E., Gould, K.L., Merritt, T.A., et al., December 16, 1998. Intensive lifestyle changes for reversal of coronary heart disease. JAMA 280 (23), 2001–2007.

Othman, R.A., Moghadasian, M.H., July 2011. Beyond cholesterol-lowering effects of plant sterols: clinical and experimental evidence of anti-inflammatory properties. Nutr. Rev. 69 (7), 371–382.

Palomer, X., González-Clemente, J.M., Blanco-Vaca, F., Mauricio, D., March 2008. Role of vitamin D in the pathogenesis of type 2 diabetes mellitus. Diabetes Obes. Metab. 10 (3), 185–197.

Pasin, G., Comerford, K.B., May 2015. Dairy foods and dairy proteins in the management of type 2 diabetes: a systematic review of the clinical evidence. Adv. Nutr. 6 (3), 245–259.

Preis, S.R., Pencina, M.J., Hwang, S.-J., D'Agostino, R.B., Savage, P.J., Levy, D., et al., July 21, 2009. Trends in cardiovascular disease risk factors in individuals with and without diabetes mellitus in the Framingham Heart Study. Circulation 120 (3), 212–220.

Ray, K.K., Seshasai, S.R.K., Wijesuriya, S., Sivakumaran, R., Nethercott, S., Preiss, D., et al., May 23, 2009. Effect of intensive control of glucose on cardiovascular outcomes and death in patients with diabetes mellitus: a meta-analysis of randomised controlled trials. Lancet 373 (9677), 1765–1772.

Riccardi, G., Giacco, R., Rivellese, A.A., August 2004. Dietary fat, insulin sensitivity and the metabolic syndrome. Clin. Nutr. 23 (4), 447–456.

Risérus, U., March 2008. Fatty acids and insulin sensitivity. Curr. Opin. Clin. Nutr. Metab. Care 11 (2), 100–105.

Rizzo, N.S., Sabaté, J., Jaceldo-Siegl, K., Fraser, G.E., May 2011. Vegetarian dietary patterns are associated with a lower risk of metabolic syndrome: the adventist health study 2. Diabetes Care 34 (5), 1225–1227.

Rodrigues, H.G., Vinolo, M.A.R., Magdalon, J., Fujiwara, H., Cavalcanti, D.M.H., Farsky, S.H.P., et al., September 2010. Dietary free oleic and linoleic acid enhances neutrophil function and modulates the inflammatory response in rats. Lipids 45 (9), 809–819.

Rohrbach, S., 2009. Effects of dietary polyunsaturated fatty acids on mitochondria. Curr. Pharm. Des. 15 (36), 4103–4116.

Rosell, M., Appleby, P., Spencer, E., Key, T., September 2006. Weight gain over 5 years in 21,966 meat-eating, fish-eating, vegetarian, and vegan men and women in EPIC-Oxford. Int. J. Obes. 30 (9), 1389–1396.

Ruiz Ruiz, J.C., Betancur Ancona, D.A., Segura Campos, M.R., 2014. Bioactive vegetable proteins and peptides in lipid-lowering; nutraceutical potential. Nutr. Hosp. 29 (4), 776–784.

Salmerón, J., Hu, F.B., Manson, J.E., Stampfer, M.J., Colditz, G.A., Rimm, E.B., et al., June 2001. Dietary fat intake and risk of type 2 diabetes in women. Am. J. Clin. Nutr. 73 (6), 1019–1026.

Segasothy, M., Phillips, P.A., September 1999. Vegetarian diet: panacea for modern lifestyle diseases? QJM 92 (9), 531–544.

Selvin, E., Marinopoulos, S., Berkenblit, G., Rami, T., Brancati, F.L., Powe, N.R., et al., September 21, 2004. Meta-analysis: glycosylated hemoglobin and cardiovascular disease in diabetes mellitus. Ann. Intern. Med. 141 (6), 421–431.

Shapiro, H., Theilla, M., Attal-Singer, J., Singer, P., February 2011. Effects of polyunsaturated fatty acid consumption in diabetic nephropathy. Nat. Rev. Nephrol. 7 (2), 110–121.

Shepherd, J., Packard, C.J., Grundy, S.M., Yeshurun, D., Gotto Jr., A.M., Taunton, O.D., January 1980. Effects of saturated and polyunsaturated fat diets on the chemical composition and metabolism of low density lipoproteins in man. J. Lipid Res. 21 (1), 91–99.

Sievenpiper, J., Kendall, C., Esfahani, A., Wong, J., Carleton, A., Jiang, H., et al., June 13, 2009. Effect of non-oil-seed pulses on glycaemic control: a systematic review and meta-analysis of randomised controlled experimental trials in people with and without diabetes. Diabetologia. Available from: http://www.ncbi.nlm.nih.gov/pubmed/19526214.

Simopoulos, A.P., June 2008. The importance of the omega-6/omega-3 fatty acid ratio in cardiovascular disease and other chronic diseases. Exp. Biol. Med. Maywood 233 (6), 674–688.

Smahelová, A., Zadák, Z., Hyspler, R., Haas, T., February 2004. Significance of plant sterols in diabetes. Vnitr. Lek. 50 (2), 147–152.

Smith, A.G., Russell, J., Feldman, E.L., Goldstein, J., Peltier, A., Smith, S., et al., June 2006. Lifestyle intervention for pre-diabetic neuropathy. Diabetes Care 29 (6), 1294–1299.

Soroka, N., Silverberg, D.S., Greemland, M., Birk, Y., Blum, M., Peer, G., et al., 1998. Comparison of a vegetable-based (soya) and an animal-based low-protein diet in predialysis chronic renal failure patients. Nephron 79 (2), 173–180.

Strandberg, T.E., Gylling, H., Tilvis, R.S., Miettinen, T.A., November 13, 2009. Serum plant and other noncholesterol sterols, cholesterol metabolism and 22-year mortality among middle-aged men. Atherosclerosis. Available from: http://www.ncbi.nlm.nih.gov/pubmed/19962145.

Summers, L.K.M., Fielding, B.A., Bradshaw, H.A., Ilic, V., Beysen, C., Clark, M.L., et al., March 2002. Substituting dietary saturated fat with polyunsaturated fat changes abdominal fat distribution and improves insulin sensitivity. Diabetologia 45 (3), 369–377.

Szostak, W.B., Szostak-Wegierek, D., 2008. Nutrition in prevention of age-related macular degeneration. Przegl. Lek. 65 (6), 308–311.

Tanaka, S., Yoshimura, Y., Kawasaki, R., Kamada, C., Tanaka, S., Horikawa, C., et al., March 2013. Fruit intake and incident diabetic retinopathy with type 2 diabetes. Epidemiology 24 (2), 204–211.

Tanasescu, M., Cho, E., Manson, J.E., Hu, F.B., June 2004. Dietary fat and cholesterol and the risk of cardiovascular disease among women with type 2 diabetes. Am. J. Clin. Nutr. 79 (6), 999–1005.

Teixeira, R., de, C.M., de, A., Molina, M., del, C.B., Zandonade, E., Mill, J.G., October 2007. Cardiovascular risk in vegetarians and omnivores: a comparative study. Arq. Bras. Cardiol. 89 (4), 237–244.

Trapp, C.B., Barnard, N.D., April 2010. Usefulness of vegetarian and vegan diets for treating type 2 diabetes. Curr. Diab. Rep. 10 (2), 152–158.

Trichopoulou, A., Psaltopoulou, T., Orfanos, P., Trichopoulos, D., June 2006. Diet and physical activity in relation to overall mortality amongst adult diabetics in a general population cohort. J. Intern. Med. 259 (6), 583–591.

Tsimihodimos, V., Gazi, I., Kalaitzidis, R., Elisaf, M., Siamopoulos, K.C., 2006. Increased serum ferritin concentrations and liver enzyme activities in patients with metabolic syndrome. Metab. Syndr. Relat. Disord. 4 (3), 196–203.

Turner, R.C., Millns, H., Neil, H.A., Stratton, I.M., Manley, S.E., Matthews, D.R., et al., March 14, 1998. Risk factors for coronary artery disease in non-insulin dependent diabetes mellitus: United Kingdom Prospective Diabetes Study (UKPDS: 23). BMJ 316 (7134), 823–828.

Turpeinen, O., Karvonen, M.J., Pekkarinen, M., Miettinen, M., Elosuo, R., Paavilainen, E., June 1979. Dietary prevention of coronary heart disease: the Finnish Mental Hospital study. Int. J. Epidemiol. 8 (2), 99–118.

van Nielen, M., Feskens, E.J.M., Mensink, M., Sluijs, I., Molina, E., Amiano, P., et al., July 2014b. Dietary protein intake and incidence of type 2 diabetes in Europe: the EPIC-InterAct Case-Cohort Study. Diabetes Care 37 (7), 1854–1862.

van Nielen, M., Feskens, E.J.M., Rietman, A., Siebelink, E., Mensink, M., September 2014b. Partly replacing meat protein with soy protein alters insulin resistance and blood lipids in postmenopausal women with abdominal obesity. J. Nutr. 144 (9), 1423–1429.

Vessby, B., Aro, A., Skarfors, E., Berglund, L., Salminen, I., Lithell, H., November 1994. The risk to develop NIDDM is related to the fatty acid composition of the serum cholesterol esters. Diabetes 43 (11), 1353–1357.

Vessby, B., Uusitupa, M., Hermansen, K., Riccardi, G., Rivellese, A.A., Tapsell, L.C., et al., March 2001. Substituting dietary saturated for monounsaturated fat impairs insulin sensitivity in healthy men and women: the KANWU Study. Diabetologia 44 (3), 312–319.

Vitale, M., Masulli, M., Rivellese, A.A., Babini, A.C., Boemi, M., Bonora, E., et al., June 2016. Influence of dietary fat and carbohydrates proportions on plasma lipids, glucose control and low-grade inflammation in patients with type 2 diabetes – The TOSCA.IT Study. Eur. J. Nutr. 55 (4), 1645–1651. http://dx.doi.org/10.1007/s00394-015-0983-1.

Weickert, M.O., Pfeiffer, A.F.H., March 2008. Metabolic effects of dietary fiber consumption and prevention of diabetes. J. Nutr. 138 (3), 439–442.

Wheeler, M.L., Dunbar, S.A., Jaacks, L.M., Karmally, W., Mayer-Davis, E.J., Wylie-Rosett, J., et al., February 2012. Macronutrients, food groups, and eating patterns in the management of diabetes: a systematic review of the literature, 2010. Diabetes Care 35 (2), 434–445.

Whelton, P.K., He, J., Appel, L.J., Cutler, J.A., Havas, S., Kotchen, T.A., et al., October 16, 2002. Primary prevention of hypertension: clinical and public health advisory from The National High Blood Pressure Education Program. JAMA 288 (15), 1882–1888.

Willett, W.C., September 2007. The role of dietary n-6 fatty acids in the prevention of cardiovascular disease. J. Cardiovasc. Med. Hagerstown 8 (Suppl. 1), S42–S45.

Xiao, C., Giacca, A., Carpentier, A., Lewis, G.F., June 2006. Differential effects of monounsaturated, polyunsaturated and saturated fat ingestion on glucose-stimulated insulin secretion, sensitivity and clearance in overweight and obese, non-diabetic humans. Diabetologia 49 (6), 1371–1379.

Yokoyama, Y., Barnard, N.D., Levin, S.M., Watanabe, M., October 2014a. Vegetarian diets and glycemic control in diabetes: a systematic review and meta-analysis. Cardiovasc. Diagn. Ther. 4 (5), 373–382.

Yokoyama, Y., Nishimura, K., Barnard, N.D., Takegami, M., Watanabe, M., Sekikawa, A., et al., April 2014b. Vegetarian diets and blood pressure: a meta-analysis. JAMA Intern. Med. 174 (4), 577–587. http://dx.doi.org/10.1001/jamainternmed.2013.14547.

Zoungas, S., Chalmers, J., Neal, B., Billot, L., Li, Q., Hirakawa, Y., et al., October 9, 2014. Follow-up of blood-pressure lowering and glucose control in type 2 diabetes. N. Engl. J. Med. 371 (15), 1392–1406.

Further Reading

Tonstad, S., Butler, T., Yan, R., Fraser, G.E., May 2009. Type of vegetarian diet, body weight, and prevalence of type 2 diabetes. Diabetes Care 32 (5), 791–796.

Tvrzicka, E., Kremmyda, L.-S., Stankova, B., Zak, A., June 2011. Fatty acids as biocompounds: their role in human metabolism, health and disease – a review. Part 1: classification, dietary sources and biological functions. Biomed. Pap. Med. Fac. Univ. Palacký Olomouc Czech Republic 155 (2), 117–130.

22

Blood Pressure and Vegetarian Diets

Yoko Yokoyama[1], Kunihiro Nishimura[2],
Neal D. Barnard[3,4], Yoshihiro Miyamoto[2]

[1]KEIO UNIVERSITY, KANAGAWA, JAPAN; [2]NATIONAL CEREBRAL AND CARDIOVASCULAR
CENTER, OSAKA, JAPAN; [3]PHYSICIANS COMMITTEE FOR RESPONSIBLE MEDICINE,
WASHINGTON, DC, UNITED STATES; [4]GEORGE WASHINGTON UNIVERSITY SCHOOL OF
MEDICINE AND HEALTH SCIENCES, WASHINGTON, DC, UNITED STATES

1. Epidemiology of Blood Pressure

Hypertension is a major independent risk factor for coronary artery diseases, irrespective of age, race, or sex (Rosendorff et al., 2015). The World Health Organization reports that hypertension underlies at least 45% of deaths due to heart disease and 51% of deaths due to stroke (World Health Organization, 2011a). In addition, a study demonstrated that hypertension increased lifetime risk of stroke, regardless of age and sex (Turin et al., 2016). The number of people with hypertension has increased over the years, from 600 million in 1980 to 1 billion in 2008 (World Health Organization, 2011b), and the Centers for Disease Control and Prevention estimate that 32.5% of adults aged ≥20 years have hypertension (National Center for Health Statistics, 2015). This high prevalence demands implementation of public health approaches to preventing hypertension.

Identification and targeting of modifiable factors is a potentially useful approach to reducing the hypertension prevalence. Substantial evidence has implicated diet, body weight, physical activity, and alcohol intake in the development of hypertension, and dietary modification has been shown to be particularly effective in preventing and managing hypertension (James et al., 2014).

Nutritional epidemiology often examines disease incidence with consideration of only a single or few nutrients or foods (Hu, 2002). However, the results of such nutrient analyses can be difficult to interpret, as individuals do not consume nutrients in isolation (Hu, 2002). To remedy this problem, dietary pattern analysis has become popular in nutritional epidemiology. Results of dietary interventions may be easier to implement and more comprehensive when they are initiated as changes in the overall dietary pattern.

2. Vegetarian Diets and Blood Pressure

The US Department of Health and Human Services defines dietary patterns as, "the quantities, proportions, variety, or combinations of different foods and beverages in diets, and the frequency with which they are habitually consumed" (Hu, 2002). A position statement issued by the Academy of Nutrition and Dietetics, defines a vegetarian diet as, "[a diet] that does not include meat (including fowl) or seafood, or products containing those foods" (Craig and Mangels, 2009). However, researchers vary in their definitions when reporting outcomes related to vegetarian diets. An overview of the vegetarian diets is provided in Chapter 1 of this book.

2.1 Cross-Sectional Studies With High Percentages of Vegetarian Participants

The information in this section is based on three cross-sectional studies with substantial numbers of vegetarian participants (Appleby and Key, 2015): the Adventist Health Study-2 (AHS-2) (Pettersen et al., 2012) (36%), the European Prospective Investigation into Cancer and Nutrition-Oxford (EPIC-Oxford) (Appleby et al., 2002) (33%), and the UK Women's Cohort Study (Cade et al., 2004) (29%) (Table 22.1).

In all three studies, nonvegetarians were recruited as a comparison group drawn from the same population and with a similar socioeconomic status to that of the targeted vegetarians, thereby reducing the likelihood that any observed health differences were due to nondietary rather than dietary factors.

The AHS-2 cohort comprised more than 96,000 Seventh-day Adventist members recruited from the United States and Canada between 2002 and 2007. Blood pressure (BP) data were analyzed from the AHS-2 calibration study, which was primarily designed to evaluate the accuracy of data collection and reporting. AHS-2 calibration study participants were chosen randomly from the parent cohort (AHS-2 cohort). The EPIC-Oxford cohort comprised 57,500 British men and women recruited between 1993 and 1999. The UK Women's Study examined the relationships between diet and cancer incidence and mortality among middle-aged (35–69 years) women in the United Kingdom. A total of 35,372 women answered the baseline questionnaire. Nutrient intake by dietary pattern, such as vegetarian and omnivore, is shown in Table 22.1.

In the AHS-2 calibration cohort, BP values were compared by dietary pattern among 500 nonblack participants. Their mean age was 62.7 years, and 36% were men. Dietary patterns were determined using a validated food frequency questionnaire (FFQ) that inquired about participants' typical or average diet over the past year. Individuals consuming a vegan diet (meat, fish, and dairy products less than once a month) had a lower prevalence of hypertension (defined as systolic BP > 139 mm Hg, diastolic BP > 89 mm Hg, or taking prescribed antihypertensive medications) than omnivorous individuals (odds ratio [OR] = 0.37, 95% confidence interval [CI] 0.19–0.74). Further, ovolactovegetarians (consume meat or fish less than once a month but dairy products or eggs more than once a month) also had a lower estimated odds of hypertension (OR = 0.57, 95% CI 0.36–0.92) than omnivores (Pettersen et al., 2012). However, after adjusting for body mass index (BMI), the ORs were no longer statistically significant, suggesting that the effect of vegetarian diets on BP was partly mediated by the effect of diet on BMI.

Table 22.1 Dietary Pattern and Nutritional Components

Reference Dietary Pattern	Adventist Health Study-2 (Pettersen et al., 2012)[b]		EPIC-Oxford (Appleby et al., 2002)		UK Women's Cohort (Cade et al., 2004)		NHANES (2011–12) (Reese et al., 1960; Smit et al., 1999)
	Omnivore	Vegetarian	Omnivore	Vegetarian	Total	Vegetarian	Omnivore
Energy	1773 kcal	1791 kcal	2180 kcal	1926 kcal	2361 kcal	2303 kcal	2191 kcal
Carbohydrate	53.4 %E	61.7 %E	47.6 %E	54.7 %E	52.6 %E	55.7 %E	49 %E
Protein	14.9 %E	14.1 %E	16.1%	12.8 %E	15.1 %E	13.1 %E	16 %E
Fat	34.5 %E	29.4 %E	31.5 %E	28.7 %E	32.4 %E	32 %E	33 %E
Fiber[a]	33.6 g	51.8 g	NR	NR	22.0 g	25.2 g	16.5 g
Sodium[a]	3.7 g	3.4 g	2.7 g	2.9 g	NR	NR	3.3 g

[a] Per 2000 kcal.
[b] Results from AHS-2 (n = 71,751) (Rizzo et al., 2013).

In the EPIC-Oxford study, BP was evaluated in 1790 men and 6873 women. Participants were allocated to four diet groups based on answers to questions regarding their dietary intake of meat, fish, dairy products, and eggs. Systolic and diastolic BPs were significantly lower in the vegan group (did not eat any meat, fish, eggs, and dairy products) than in all other groups (omnivores, pescetarians, ovolactovegetarians) after adjustment for age. However, the relationship lost significance after adjustment for both age and BMI (Appleby et al., 2002). Other dietary factors, including saturated fat intake and ratio of polyunsaturated fat to unsaturated fat, were associated with BP in both sexes; alcohol and carbohydrate intake were associated with BP in men only, while calcium intake was associated with BP in women only.

In the UK Women's Cohort Study, prevalence of hypertension was compared between vegetarians and omnivores in a population of 35,372 women living in England, Wales, and Scotland. In this study, vegetarians were defined as participants who ate meat or fish less than once a week, as determined using an FFQ. Overall, those identifying as vegetarians tended to be younger and were less likely to drink alcohol more than once a week than omnivorous participants. Nutrient intake analysis showed that vegetarians had lower total energy intake and higher percentage energy from carbohydrates, whereas omnivores had lower intake of carbohydrates and percentage energy from carbohydrates, fiber, vitamin C, folate iron, and calcium but higher intake of vitamin A and zinc. Vegetarians also had lower absolute protein, fat, and saturated fat intake and a lower prevalence of hypertension than omnivores (11.4% vs. 19.6%) (Cade et al., 2004) as well as lower mean BMI (23.3 vs. 25.0 kg/m^2) and lower likelihood of consuming alcohol more than once a week (45% vs. 54%).

Findings from these three cross-sectional studies with high percentages of vegetarian participants showed that vegetarian diets were associated not only with reduced BP and prevalence of hypertension but also lower BMI, compared with omnivorous diets, and the relationship between a vegetarian diet and BP lost significance after adjustment for BMI in two studies. BMI may therefore be a major factor in the relationship between a vegetarian diet and BP. Although causality cannot be inferred from cross-sectional studies, these findings do suggest relatively long-term effects of vegetarian diets.

2.2 Meta-analysis of Observational Studies

A meta-analysis included 32 observational studies (Yokoyama et al., 2014). The 32 studies included 21,604 participants (median sample size 152, range 20 to 9242) with a mean age of 46.6 years (range 28.8–68.4 years). Each of the 32 observational studies used cross-sectional designs (Pettersen et al., 2012; Appleby et al., 2002; Armstrong et al., 1979; Haines et al., 1980; Burr et al., 1981; Rouse et al., 1983a; Ophir et al., 1983; Wiseman et al., 1987; Sanders and Key, 1987; Melby et al., 1989, 1994; Orlov et al., 1994; Wyatt et al., 1995; Williams, 1997; Harman and Parnell, 1998; Famodu et al., 1998; Lu et al., 2000; Goff et al., 2005; Su et al., 2006; Sebekova et al., 2006; Teixeira Rde et al., 2007; Fontana et al., 2007; Slavicek et al., 2008; Nakamoto et al., 2008; Pitla and Nagalla, 2009; Lin et al., 2010; Yang et al., 2011; Rodenas et al., 2011; Fernandes Dourado et al., 2011; Chen et al., 2011; Yang et al., 2012; Kim and Bae, 2012).

In 22 of these studies, participants had been following vegetarian diets for >1 year (Pettersen et al., 2012; Burr et al., 1981; Ophir et al., 1983; Wiseman et al., 1987; Sanders and Key, 1987; Melby et al., 1989; Orlov et al., 1994; Wyatt et al., 1995; Lu et al., 2000; Goff et al., 2005; Su et al., 2006; Sebekova et al., 2006; Teixeira Rde et al., 2007; Fontana et al., 2007; Slavicek et al., 2008; Pitla and Nagalla, 2009; Lin et al., 2010; Yang et al., 2011; Fernandes Dourado et al., 2011; Chen et al., 2011; Yang et al., 2012; Kim and Bae, 2012). Five studies focused on vegan diets (Sanders and Key, 1987; Orlov et al., 1994; Goff et al., 2005; Fontana et al., 2007; Lin et al., 2010), 2 on lactovegetarian diets (Pitla and Nagalla, 2009; Yang et al., 2012), 10 on ovolacto-vegetarian diets (Armstrong et al., 1979; Rouse et al., 1983a; Ophir et al., 1983; Wyatt et al., 1995; Sebekova et al., 2006; Slavicek et al., 2008; Yang et al., 2011; Fernandes Dourado et al., 2011; Chen et al., 2011; Kim and Bae, 2012), and 15 on mixed diet types (vegan, lactovegetar-ian, ovolactovegetarian, pescetarian, and/or semivegetarian) (Pettersen et al., 2012; Appleby et al., 2002; Haines et al., 1980; Burr et al., 1981; Wiseman et al., 1987; Melby et al., 1989, 1994; Williams, 1997; Harman and Parnell, 1998; Famodu et al., 1998; Lu et al., 2000; Su et al., 2006; Teixeira Rde et al., 2007; Nakamoto et al., 2008; Rodenas et al., 2011).

In this meta-analysis, the consumption of a vegetarian diet was associated with a reduced mean systolic BP (−6.9 mm Hg; 95% CI, −9.1 to −4.7) (Yokoyama et al., 2014). Given the statistically significant heterogeneity in this meta-analysis of 32 observational studies, the heterogeneous factors were examined using metaregression. The number of men, baseline systolic and diastolic BP, and BMI were found to be significant, indicating that the association between a vegetarian diet and BP was stronger among men and in participants with higher baseline systolic and diastolic BPs or higher BMIs.

2.3 Meta-analysis of Clinical Trials

A meta-analysis (Yokoyama et al., 2014) included seven trials (Rouse et al., 1983b; Margetts et al., 1986; Hakala and Karvetti, 1989; Kestin et al., 1989; Sciarrone et al., 1993; Nicholson et al., 1999; Ferdowsian et al., 2010) with a total of 311 participants (mean age, 44.5 years). All were open (nonmasked) controlled trials conducted for 6–52 weeks (mean, 15.7 weeks). Vegan diets were examined in two trials (Nicholson et al., 1999; Ferdowsian et al., 2010), a lactovegetarian diet in one (Hakala and Karvetti, 1989), and an ovolactovegetarian diet in four (Rouse et al., 1983b; Margetts et al., 1986; Kestin et al., 1989; Sciarrone et al., 1993). Intervention methods differed across trials; for example, Hakala and Karvetti (1989) sim-ply counseled participants to follow a specific dietary pattern, whereas in other trials, food was at least partly provided for participants (Pettersen et al., 2012; Appleby et al., 2002; Armstrong et al., 1979; Haines et al., 1980; Burr et al., 1981; Rouse et al., 1983a; Ophir et al., 1983; Wiseman et al., 1987; Sanders and Key, 1987; Melby et al., 1989, 1994; Orlov et al., 1994; Wyatt et al., 1995; Williams, 1997; Harman and Parnell, 1998; Famodu et al., 1998; Lu et al., 2000; Goff et al., 2005; Su et al., 2006; Sebekova et al., 2006; Teixeira Rde et al., 2007; Fontana et al., 2007; Slavicek et al., 2008; Nakamoto et al., 2008; Pitla and Nagalla, 2009; Lin et al., 2010; Yang et al., 2011; Rodenas et al., 2011; Fernandes Dourado et al., 2011; Chen et al., 2011; Yang et al., 2012; Kim and Bae, 2012).

In these seven trials, a vegetarian diet was associated with a reduction in mean systolic BP (–4.8 mm Hg; 95% CI: –6.6 to –3.1; *P* < .001) and diastolic BP (–2.2 mm Hg; 95% CI: –3.5 to –1.0; *P* < .001), compared with an omnivorous diet (Yokoyama et al., 2014). Whelton et al. (2005) reported that a 5 mm Hg reduction in systolic BP resulted in a 14% overall reduction in mortality due to stroke, 9% reduction in mortality due to cardiovascular heart disease, and 7% decrease in all-cause mortality.

However, visual examination of funnel plots for the seven clinical trials suggested that smaller trials reporting small reductions in systolic BP may have been overrepresented. In the absence of publication bias, study results would be symmetrically represented about the mean effect size; our findings suggest that a few studies were missing in the bottom left side. This visual impression was confirmed by the Egger test (*P* = .04). Results obtained using the trim-and-fill method suggested that three trials may have been missing, the addition of which would change the overall effect on systolic BP to a 5.2 mm Hg reduction (95% CI: –6.9 to –3.5) (Yokoyama et al., 2014).

Notably, the studies available did not involve large sample sizes. However, the findings from cross-sectional studies and meta-analyses are consistent with those of a previous review of observational studies that found that the systolic BP of vegetarians was 3–14 mm Hg lower and diastolic BP 5–6 mm Hg lower than in omnivores (Berkow and Barnard, 2005). In addition, randomized controlled trials (RCTs) have shown that BP is lower when animal products are replaced with plant-based products in both normotensive and hypertensive participants (Berkow and Barnard, 2005). The Dietary Approaches to Stop Hypertension (DASH) study showed that a diet rich in fruits and vegetables reduced systolic BP by 5.5 mm Hg (*P* < .001) and diastolic BP by 3 mm Hg (*P* < .001) (Appel et al., 1997). The DASH study was based in part on the observation that vegetarian diets are associated with a significantly reduced risk of hypertension compared with omnivorous diets (Sacks et al., 1995).

2.4 Update Search After Meta-analysis

Since the meta-analysis was published in 2014 (and with a research date from November 2013), we performed another bibliographic research, and 44 studies were published through August 2016. Of these, one prospective cohort study and two cross-sectional studies met the inclusion and exclusion criteria we used in the meta-analysis. The matched cohort study was from the 1994–2008 MJ Health Screening Database and included 4109 nonsmokers (3423 omnivores and 686 vegetarians) (Chuang et al., 2016). Vegetarians had lower systolic BP (–2.4 mm Hg, *P* < .05) and diastolic BP (–1.1 mm Hg, *P* < .05) adjusting for age, sex, C-reactive protein, waist circumstance, and fasting glucose. A cross-sectional study conducted in India included 6555 participants (4407 omnivorous and 2148 lactovegetarians). After adjustment for age, sex, sibling clusters, BMI, smoking, alcohol, site, migration status, energy, physical activity, and sibling pair, lactovegetarians had lower diastolic BP (β = –0.7 mm Hg, *P* = .02) but not significantly lower in systolic BP (β = –0.9 mm Hg, *P* = .07) (Shridhar et al., 2014). A cross-sectional study conducted in Taiwan included 2397 premenopausal (2285 omnivores, 36 vegans, and 76 ovolactovegetarians) and 1154 post-menopausal women (1040 omnivores, 63 vegans, and 51 ovolactovegetarians) (Huang et al., 2014). Results showed that baseline systolic BP and diastolic BP were not different between vegans or ovolactovegetarians and omnivores. However, this analysis did not adjust for any potential confounders except sex and menopausal status.

In our meta-analysis, calculating the failsafe number revealed that 1498 additional negative studies that would be needed to increase the *P*-value over .05. Therefore, addition of these three studies would not change our meta-analysis results.

3. Possible Mechanisms

3.1 Nutrition-Related Factors Affecting Vegetarians

Results from the aforementioned three cohort studies showed that both BMI and the proportion of obese subjects tended to be lower among vegetarians than nonvegetarians (Key et al., 1999). According to a meta-analysis of clinical trials, a vegetarian diet helps reduce body weight (Barnard et al., 2015). The lower energy intake among vegetarians might be attributable to the reduced energy density of the diet, owing to the higher fiber and lower fat content than found in omnivorous diets. Given that obesity is a major diet-related risk factor for hypertension (Appleby and Key, 2015), a reduction in body weight might represent an important intervening variable explaining the effect of vegetarian diets on BP. Previous studies in various populations revealed that BMI is nearly linearly related with systolic and diastolic BP (Hall, 2003; Jones et al., 1994). Part of the reason may be increased renal tubular sodium reabsorption, impairing natruresis (Hall et al., 2015). The possible mechanisms that could explain development of obesity-related hypertension include physical compression of the kidneys by fat in and around the kidneys, mineralocorticoid receptor activation, activation of the renin–angiotensin–aldosterone system, and increased sympathetic nervous system activity (Hall et al., 2015). Although an estimated 78% of cases of primary hypertension in men and 65% of cases in women can be assigned to overweight, not all obese patients develop hypertension (Garrison et al., 1987). In addition, most studies have shown that vegetarian diets retain their association with reduced BP even after controlling for body weight; as such, weight differences alone do not fully explain the observed BP differences between vegetarians and nonvegetarians (Rizzo et al., 2013).

Other lifestyle modifications recommended for lowering hypertension include moderating alcohol consumption and increasing physical activity (National Heart, Lung, and Blood Institute, 2003). Previous cohort studies have shown that vegetarians tend to drink less alcohol than nonvegetarians (Appleby et al., 2002; Rizzo et al., 2013), suggesting that low alcohol intake may be another factor partially explaining the apparent effects of vegetarian diets on BP. In addition, consumption of vegetarian diets has been associated with reduced blood viscosity, which may affect BP (Ernst et al., 1986). The next section will discuss potential foods and nutrients in a vegetarian dietary pattern that may be responsible for the BP-lowering effects of the diet.

3.2 Key Foods and Nutrients for Vegetarians

The Academy of Nutrition and Dietetics describes vegetarians as consuming primarily foods of plant origin, particularly vegetables, grains, legumes, and fruits (Table 22.2) (Craig and Mangels, 2009).

A previous study examined the food consumption patterns of vegetarians in the AHS-2 cohort (Orlich et al., 2014). Dietary intake was measured using an FFQ, and vegetarian dietary patterns were categorized according to the reported intake of animal-based foods. Vegetarians were defined as people who consumed dairy products, fish, and all other meats <1 time/month.

Foods were categorized into 58 food groups, and adjusted mean consumption of each food group for vegetarian dietary patterns was compared with that for the nonvegetarian dietary pattern. Mean consumption differed significantly across dietary patterns for all food groups. For example, increased consumption of many plant foods, including fruits, vegetables, avocados, nonfried potatoes, whole grains, legumes, soya foods, nuts, and seeds was observed among vegetarians, along with reduced consumption of meats, dairy products, eggs, refined grains, added fats, sweets, snack foods, and nonwater beverages (Orlich et al., 2014).

A nutrient level intake study was additionally conducted in this same AHS-2 cohort. Caloric intake and percentages of energy from carbohydrates, protein, and fat were similar across vegetarian and omnivorous individuals. Intake of plant protein, total fiber, beta-carotene, and magnesium was significantly higher, after adjustments for sex, age, and race, in vegetarians than in nonvegetarians (Rizzo et al., 2013). In contrast, intake of animal protein, saturated fatty acid, trans-fatty acid, arachidonic acid, DHA, and vitamin D was significantly lower in vegetarians. Sodium intake was similar between both groups (3.5 mg for vegetarians vs. 3.8 mg for nonvegetarians) (Rizzo et al., 2013). In the EPIC-Oxford study, energy intake and percentages of energy from protein, total fat, and saturated fat were higher, while percentages of energy from carbohydrates and polyunsaturated fat were lower in omnivores than in vegetarians. Intake of calcium was lower and that of magnesium higher in vegetarians than in omnivores (Appleby et al., 2002). In the UK Women's Study, vegetarians had lower protein, fat, saturated fat, vitamin A, and zinc intake but higher carbohydrate, fiber, vitamin C, folate, iron, and calcium intake than nonvegetarians (Cade et al., 2004). Compared with NHANES data, energy intake was lower in the AHS-2 cohort but comparable in the EPIC-Oxford and UK Women's studies (Table 22.1). Overall, the vegetarian dietary pattern was characterized

Table 22.2 Characteristics of Vegetarian Diets (Craig and Mangels, 2009)

	Higher in Vegetarians	Lower in Vegetarians
Food	Grains, vegetables, fruits, legumes, seeds, nuts	Meat (including fowl) or seafood or products containing those foods
Nutrient	Dietary fiber, magnesium, potassium, vitamins C and E, folate, carotenoids, flavonoids, other phytochemicals	Saturated fat, cholesterol, vitamins D and B_{12}, calcium, zinc, long-chain n-3 fatty acids

by greater energy intake from carbohydrates and less from protein and fat than nonvegetarian patterns.

3.3 Key Foods and Nutrients Effective in Lowering Blood Pressure

3.3.1 Fruits and Vegetables

Fruits and vegetables are rich in minerals such as magnesium, vitamin C, folic acid, flavonoids, and carotenoids, all of which are believed to lower BP by improving endothelial function (Whelton et al., 1997; Toh et al., 2013; Juraschek et al., 2012; Aburto et al., 2013). A meta-analysis of 25 observational studies found that consumption of fruits and vegetables was associated with a reduced prevalence of hypertension. On comparing the highest and lowest consumption groups, the pooled relative risks of hypertension were 0.81 (95% CI: 0.74–0.89) for fruits and 0.7 (95% CI: 0.62–0.86) for vegetables (Li et al., 2016).

3.3.2 Legumes

While soy products have been consumed in Asia for centuries, they are relatively new foods among US consumers (Messina and Messina, 2010). Soy intake among vegetarians is generally higher than in nonvegetarians; however, Western vegans typically consume about 10–12 g/day of soy protein, an intake level similar to that of nonvegetarian Japanese and Shanghai Chinese, and nonvegan Western vegetarians consume only about half this amount (Messina et al., 2006). Analysis of AHS-2 participants suggested that age-, sex-, and race-adjusted legume intake was 84.4 g/day for vegetarian and 52.5 g/day for nonvegetarians. In particular, a marked difference was noted in intake of soy foods and meat analogs between these groups (202.9 g/day for vegans and 88.1 g/day for nonvegetarians) (Orlich et al., 2014). Meta-analysis of 27 RCTs suggested that subjects having a soy protein dietary intervention experienced a 2.21 mm Hg (95% CI: –4.10 to –0.33, $P = .021$) reduction in systolic BP and a 1.44 mm Hg (95% CI: –2.56 to –0.31, $P = .012$) reduction in diastolic BP, compared with the control group (nonsoy protein) (Dong et al., 2011a). Metaregression analysis revealed that the observed heterogeneity ($I^2 = 65.7\%$ for systolic BP and 61.5% for diastolic BP) was most likely due to pretreatment BP and the diet consumed by control subjects (Dong et al., 2011a; Messina et al., 2006; Messina and Messina, 2010; Orlich et al., 2014).

While the underlying mechanism by which soy protein influences BP remains unclear, soy food products contain isoflavones and high amounts of arginine. Given that isoflavones may stimulate the synthesis or improve the bioavailability of the potent vasodilator nitrous oxide (NO) (Squadrito et al., 2002; Chin-Dusting et al., 2004) and arginine is a precursor of NO (Luiking et al., 2010; Urschel et al., 2007), these compounds might reduce BP when consumed through soy foods (Dong et al., 2011b).

3.3.3 Nuts

Vegetarians tend to consume greater amounts of nuts than omnivores (Orlich et al., 2014). In the AHS-2 study, adjusted daily mean consumption of nuts and seeds was 36 g/day for vegans and 18.8 g/day for omnivores (Orlich et al., 2014). A meta-analysis of 21 RCTs examined the effect of consumption of nuts (including walnuts, almonds, pistachios, cashews, hazelnuts, macadamia nuts, pecans, peanuts, and soy nuts) on systolic and diastolic BP. The pooled effect size was −1.29 mm Hg (95% CI: −2.35 to −0.22, $P = .02$) for systolic BP in participants without type 2 diabetes, but no marked effect was observed in the total population (Mohammadifard et al., 2015). The antihypertensive effect of nuts might come from components such as dietary fiber, plant proteins, antioxidants, bioactive substances such as flavonoids or phytosterols, vitamins, and minerals such as potassium and magnesium (Allen, 2008). However, the reasons why an antihypertensive effect of nuts only appeared in participants without type 2 diabetes is unknown.

3.3.4 Minerals

Sodium intake in vegetarians compared with omnivores is not consistent among studies. While some studies have revealed that vegetarian diets might be lower in sodium than omnivorous diets (Larsson and Johansson, 2002; Clarys et al., 2014), other studies reported no clear differences (Rizzo et al., 2013), and some studies have reported that, on average, some vegetarians may consume *more* sodium than omnivores (Woo et al., 1998). Sodium intake in participants in three cohort studies referenced in this paper is shown in Table 22.1. Overall, sodium content does not appear to be substantially different between vegetarian diets and in omnivore diets.

A meta-analysis of 107 RCTs found a strong dose–response relationship between reduced sodium intake and BP (Mozaffarian et al., 2014); indeed, a 2.3-g reduction in sodium per day was associated with a 3.82 mm Hg reduction in BP (95% CI; 3.08–4.55) (Mozaffarian et al., 2014). Efforts have been made to capitalize on this relationship. For example, the DASH dietary pattern focuses on vegetable and fruit consumption, and in trials that controlled sodium intake, the DASH diet had a greater BP-lowering effect than a non-DASH diet with sodium reduction alone (Appel et al., 1997; Sacks et al., 2001). Further studies are needed to clarify the effects of vegetarian diets with controlled sodium intake on BP.

Potassium is abundant in vegetarian diets (Rizzo et al., 2013), and a meta-analysis of RCTs found that potassium supplementation to omnivorous diets decreases BP (Rizzo et al., 2013; Whelton et al., 1997; Aburto et al., 2013). Further, high potassium intake increases vasodilation and glomerular filtration rate while decreasing renin levels, renal sodium reabsorption, reactive oxygen species production, and platelet aggregation (McDonough and Nguyen, 2012; Elliott et al., 2008; Kass et al., 2012).

3.3.5 Protein Source

The source of consumed protein—plant- or animal-based—seems to influence BP. For example, findings from the INTERMAP study suggested that plant protein intake (2.8% energy) was associated with a 2.1 mm Hg reduction in systolic BP (Elliott et al., 2006). Other prospective cohort studies have similarly indicated that higher plant protein intake is associated with BP reduction (Wang et al., 2008) or a reduced risk of incident hypertension (Alonso et al., 2006). While a meta-analysis of trials with subjects stratified by type of protein consumed found no marked differences in effects on BP between protein from plant or animal sources (Tielemans et al., 2013), the sample size of the meta-analysis was small (3 trials, $N = 327$ for plant protein; and 4 trials, $N = 574$ for animal protein), and the effects of plant or animal protein were not directly compared. Further intervention studies and meta-analyses are therefore needed to understand the influence of protein source on BP.

3.3.6 Specific Amino Acids

Previous studies have suggested that plasma concentrations and intake of amino acids differ between vegetarians and omnivores (Abdulla et al., 1981; Krajcovicova-Kudlackova et al., 2000). In the INTERMAP study, glutamic acid intake was higher among those consuming predominantly plant-based protein than in those consuming predominantly animal-based protein (Stamler et al., 2009). A 2-standard-deviation-higher intake of glutamic acid (4.7% of total protein) was associated with a 1.5 mm Hg reduction in systolic BP (Stamler et al., 2009). Glutamic acid is a precursor of arginine, which is itself a precursor for the vasodilator NO (Luiking et al., 2010; Urschel et al., 2007) and may contribute to BP reduction.

In the EPIC-Oxford cohort, plasma amino acid concentrations were compared between vegetarians and omnivores for 392 men, aged 30–49 years. Levels of lysine, methionine, tryptophan, and tyrosine were significantly lower in vegans than in omnivores, while those of alanine and glycine were significantly higher (Schmidt et al., 2016). Lysine competes with arginine for transport into the cell (Luiking and Deutz, 2007; Li et al., 2009), and arginine deficiency is associated with endothelial activation and immune dysfunction in humans (Lorin et al., 2014; Luiking and Deutz, 2007; Li et al., 2009). Therefore, the lysine/arginine ratio may strongly influence the BP-lowering effect of a vegetarian diet. Plant-based proteins tend to contain lower lysine levels and a lower lysine/arginine ratio than animal-based proteins (Vega-Lopez et al., 2010). Plant-based proteins may therefore reduce BP by stimulating NO production. A small ($N=30$), randomized crossover trial attempted to clarify the effect of changing the dietary lysine/arginine ratio on cardiovascular risk factors (Vega-Lopez et al., 2010) by providing 30 healthy adults with a low- (0.7) or high- (1.4) lysine/arginine ratio diet. While no marked difference was observed in BP between groups after 35 days of intervention in this instance (Vega-Lopez et al., 2010), the longer-term effects of consuming a low-lysine/arginine ratio diet remain unclear.

A 2-year prospective cohort study ($N=92$) showed that increased dietary intake of methionine and alanine is associated with increased BP (Tuttle et al., 2012). Methionine is a homocysteine precursor that increases BP by increasing levels of asymmetric dimethylarginine, a competitive inhibitor of NO (Stuhlinger et al., 2003). Methionine is abundant in animal protein and scarce in plant protein (McCarty et al., 2009); therefore, a predominantly plant-based protein diet will typically have a lower methionine content than a diet rich in animal-based proteins. However, the relationships between dietary methionine intake and plasma homocysteinemia are still obscure. Metabolic phenotyping analysis conducted as part of the INTERMAP study showed that urinary alanine excretion was associated with elevated BP (Holmes et al., 2008). In the same study, dietary alanine was higher in people consuming a predominantly omnivorous diet than in those consuming a predominantly vegetarian diet (Elliott et al., 2006).

3.3.7 Vitamin C

Fruits and vegetables are rich in vitamin C. A meta-analysis of 29 clinical trials with a median vitamin C dose of 500 mg/day and median intervention duration of 8 weeks showed pooled changes of −3.84 mm Hg (95% CI: −5.29 to −2.38, $P < .01$) in systolic BP and −1.48 mm Hg (95% CI: −2.86 to −0.10 mm Hg, $P = .04$) in diastolic BP (Juraschek et al., 2012). Heterogeneity was significant for both systolic and diastolic BP and may have been due in part to the age of participants and methods of intervention (Juraschek et al., 2012). The effects of vitamin C on improving NO bioavailability may underlie its influence on BP (Juraschek et al., 2012; Huang et al., 2000; Suematsu et al., 2010).

3.3.8 Vitamin B_{12}

Some vegetarians tend to have lower intake of vitamin B_{12} than omnivores (Craig and Mangels, 2009), and B_{12} deficiency can occur in vegans who do not proactively consume vitamin B_{12}-fortified foods or take supplements (Woo et al., 2014). While vegan diets have been found in some studies to have protective effects on cardiovascular-related risk, Woo et al. (2014) found in their study of Chinese vegetarians with suboptimal vitamin B_{12} levels and normal or high salt intake that vegan diets can adversely affect arterial endothelial function and carotid intima-media thickness. In addition to the classical, important manifestation of vitamin B_{12} deficiency (see Chapter 43), Vitamin B_{12} deficiency results in increased homocysteine levels (please also see Chapter 41), which are associated with arterial endothelial dysfunction and are an independent risk factor for cardiovascular disease (Homocysteine Studies Collaboration, 2002). Pawlak (2015) similarly suggested that vitamin B_{12} deficiency may reduce the benefits of a vegetarian diet on preventing cardiovascular disease. Vegetarians should therefore make an effort to consume nutrients that are often deficient in their diet.

3.3.9 Antioxidants

Fruits and vegetables are rich in antioxidants. A 6-month RCT found that increased consumption of fruits and vegetables was associated with increased intake of antioxidants, such as alpha-carotene, beta-carotene, lutein, β-cryptoxanthin, and ascorbic acid (John et al., 2002). In addition, when compared with a lower consumption group, subjects consuming more fruits and vegetables had significantly greater reductions in systolic (−4.0 mm Hg; $P < .0001$) and diastolic (−1.5 mm Hg; $P = .02$) BP (John et al., 2002).

3.3.10 Fiber

Fiber is common in plant-based foods, and vegetarian diets contain a greater amount of fiber than an omnivore diet. A meta-analysis of 24 RCTs revealed that dietary fiber supplementation (average dose: 11.5 g/day) nonsignificantly reduced systolic BP by −1.13 mm Hg (95% CI: −2.49 to 0.23) and significantly reduced diastolic BP by −1.26 mm Hg (95% CI: −2.04 to −0.48) (Streppel et al., 2005). Another meta-analysis of 25 RCTs indicated that dietary fiber intake was associated with a nonsignificant −1.15 mm Hg (95% CI: −2.68 to 0.39) reduction in systolic BP and a −1.65 mm Hg (95% CI: −2.70 to −0.61) reduction in diastolic BP (Whelton et al., 2005). Effects of dietary fiber supplementation on both systolic and diastolic BP were stronger and more significant in hypertensive subjects than in normotensive ones (Whelton et al., 2005). Although these data are insufficient to determine the effectiveness of dietary fiber supplementation for reducing BP, dietary fiber consumption may indeed influence the effectiveness of dietary pattern intervention.

3.3.11 Microbiome

The microbiota may influence the development of cardiovascular disease, including arteriosclerosis and hypertension (Jose and Raj, 2015), and the composition of human gut microbiota can change rapidly with diet alterations, such as dietary fiber supplementation (Holscher et al., 2015) or exclusion of animal-based foods (David et al., 2014). This topic is presented in detail in Chapter 24. Toxic metabolites, such as p-cresol sulfate, indoxyl sulfate, and trimethylamine N-oxide (TMAO), are produced by gut microbiota through fermentation of proteins (Ramezani and Raj, 2014; Wang et al., 2011; Tuso et al., 2015). Previous trials have shown that average excretion of p-cresol sulfate and indoxyl sulfate, two compounds associated with vascular disease and mortality in patients with chronic kidney disease (CKD) (Barreto et al., 2009; Liabeuf et al., 2010), was 62% and 58% lower, respectively, in participants consuming a vegetarian diet than in those consuming an omnivorous diet (Patel et al., 2012). Plasma TMAO concentration in patients with CKD was significantly higher than in those without CKD and was associated with a 2.8-fold increased risk of mortality with highest quartile compared with lowest quartile of plasma TMAO. TMAO is produced by metabolism of dietary choline, phosphatidylcholine, and L-carnitine by microbiota (Wang et al., 2011; Koeth et al., 2013; Tang et al., 2013, 2015), and elevated plasma TMAO levels are primarily due to gut microbial action, as genes play only a minor role in determining TMAO levels in humans (Hartiala et al., 2014). However, no studies have yet investigated a direct association between TMAO level and BP (Ufnal et al., 2014).

4. Conclusion

Results from meta-analyses of clinical trials show that a vegetarian dietary pattern is associated with reduced BP compared with an omnivorous diet. This effect appears to be due in part to the weight reduction that often accompanies vegetarian diets, as well as to the specific effects of certain nutrients. Further studies should be conducted in non-Western populations involving subjects with higher intakes of sodium or animal products, along with controlled studies examining potential mechanisms of BP reduction by typical nutrients in vegetarian diets as well as their synergetic effects.

References

Abdulla, M., Andersson, I., Asp, N.G., et al., 1981. Nutrient intake and health status of vegans. Chemical analyses of diets using the duplicate portion sampling technique. Am. J. Clin. Nutr. 34 (11), 2464–2477.

Aburto, N.J., Hanson, S., Gutierrez, H., Hooper, L., Elliott, P., Cappuccio, F.P., 2013. Effect of increased potassium intake on cardiovascular risk factors and disease: systematic review and meta-analyses. BMJ 346, f1378.

Allen, L.H., 2008. Priority areas for research on the intake, composition, and health effects of tree nuts and peanuts. J. Nutr. 138 (9), 1763S–1765S.

Alonso, A., Beunza, J.J., Bes-Rastrollo, M., Pajares, R.M., Martinez-Gonzalez, M.A., 2006. Vegetable protein and fiber from cereal are inversely associated with the risk of hypertension in a Spanish cohort. Arch. Med. Res. 37 (6), 778–786.

Appel, L.J., Moore, T.J., Obarzanek, E., et al., 1997. A clinical trial of the effects of dietary patterns on blood pressure. DASH Collaborative Research Group. N. Engl. J. Med. 336 (16), 1117–1124.

Appleby, P.N., Key, T.J., 2015. The long-term health of vegetarians and vegans. Proc. Nutr. Soc. 1–7.

Appleby, P.N., Davey, G.K., Key, T.J., 2002. Hypertension and blood pressure among meat eaters, fish eaters, vegetarians and vegans in EPIC-Oxford. Public Health Nutr. 5 (5), 645–654.

Armstrong, B., Clarke, H., Martin, C., Ward, W., Norman, N., Masarei, J., 1979. Urinary sodium and blood pressure in vegetarians. Am. J. Clin. Nutr. 32 (12), 2472–2476.

Barnard, N.D., Levin, S.M., Yokoyama, Y., 2015. A systematic review and meta-analysis of changes in body weight in clinical trials of vegetarian diets. J. Acad. Nutr. Diet 115 (6), 954–969.

Barreto, F.C., Barreto, D.V., Liabeuf, S., et al., 2009. Serum indoxyl sulfate is associated with vascular disease and mortality in chronic kidney disease patients. Clin. J. Am. Soc. Nephrol. 4 (10), 1551–1558.

Berkow, S.E., Barnard, N.D., 2005. Blood pressure regulation and vegetarian diets. Nutr. Rev. 63 (1), 1–8.

Burr, M.L., Bates, C.J., Fehily, A.M., St Leger, A.S., 1981. Plasma cholesterol and blood pressure in vegetarians. J. Hum. Nutr. 35 (6), 437–441.

Cade, J.E., Burley, V.J., Greenwood, D.C., 2004. Group UK Women's cohort study sterring group. The UK Women's cohort study: comparison of vegetarians, fish-eaters and meat-eaters. Public Health Nutr. 7 (7), 871–878.

Chen, C.W., Lin, C.T., Lin, Y.L., Lin, T.K., Lin, C.L., 2011. Taiwanese female vegetarians have lower lipoprotein-associated phospholipase A2 compared with omnivores. Yonsei Med. J. 52 (1), 13–19.

Chin-Dusting, J.P., Boak, L., Husband, A., Nestel, P.J., 2004. The isoflavone metabolite dehydroequol produces vasodilatation in human resistance arteries via a nitric oxide-dependent mechanism. Atherosclerosis 176 (1), 45–48.

Chuang, S.Y., Chiu, T.H., Lee, C.Y., et al., 2016. Vegetarian diet reduces the risk of hypertension independent of abdominal obesity and inflammation: a prospective study. J. Hypertens. 34 (11), 2164–2171.

Clarys, P., Deliens, T., Huybrechts, I., et al., 2014. Comparison of nutritional quality of the vegan, vegetarian, semi-vegetarian, pesco-vegetarian and omnivorous diet. Nutrients 6 (3), 1318–1332.

Craig, W.J., Mangels, A.R., 2009. American Dietetic A. Position of the American Dietetic association: vegetarian diets. J. Am. Diet. Assoc. 109 (7), 1266–1282.

David, L.A., Maurice, C.F., Carmody, R.N., et al., 2014. Diet rapidly and reproducibly alters the human gut microbiome. Nature 505 (7484), 559–563.

Dong, J.Y., Tong, X., Wu, Z.W., Xun, P.C., He, K., Qin, L.Q., 2011a. Effect of soya protein on blood pressure: a meta-analysis of randomised controlled trials. Br. J. Nutr. 106 (3), 317–326.

Dong, J.Y., Qin, L.Q., Zhang, Z., et al., 2011b. Effect of oral L-arginine supplementation on blood pressure: a meta-analysis of randomized, double-blind, placebo-controlled trials. Am. Heart J. 162 (6), 959–965.

Elliott, P., Stamler, J., Dyer, A.R., et al., 2006. Association between protein intake and blood pressure: the INTERMAP Study. Arch. Intern. Med. 166 (1), 79–87.

Elliott, P., Kesteloot, H., Appel, L.J., et al., 2008. Dietary phosphorus and blood pressure: international study of macro- and micro-nutrients and blood pressure. Hypertension 51 (3), 669–675.

Ernst, E., Pietsch, L., Matrai, A., Eisenberg, J., 1986. Blood rheology in vegetarians. Br. J. Nutr. 56 (3), 555–560.

Famodu, A.A., Osilesi, O., Makinde, Y.O., Osonuga, O.A., 1998. Blood pressure and blood lipid levels among vegetarian, semi-vegetarian, and non-vegetarian native Africans. Clin. Biochem. 31 (7), 545–549.

Ferdowsian, H.R., Barnard, N.D., Hoover, V.J., et al., 2010. A multicomponent intervention reduces body weight and cardiovascular risk at a GEICO corporate site. Am. J. Health Promot. AJHP 24 (6), 384–387.

Fernandes Dourado, K., de Arruda Camara, E.S.C.F., Sakugava Shinohara, N.K., 2011. Relation between dietary and circulating lipids in lacto-ovo vegetarians. Nutr. Hosp. 26 (5), 959–964.

Fontana, L., Meyer, T.E., Klein, S., Holloszy, J.O., 2007. Long-term low-calorie low-protein vegan diet and endurance exercise are associated with low cardiometabolic risk. Rejuvenation Res. 10 (2), 225–234.

Garrison, R.J., Kannel, W.B., Stokes 3rd, J., Castelli, W.P., 1987. Incidence and precursors of hypertension in young adults: the Framingham Offspring Study. Prev. Med. 16 (2), 235–251.

Goff, L.M., Bell, J.D., So, P.W., Dornhorst, A., Frost, G.S., 2005. Veganism and its relationship with insulin resistance and intramyocellular lipid. Eur. J. Clin. Nutr. 59 (2), 291–298.

Haines, A.P., Chakrabarti, R., Fisher, D., Meade, T.W., North, W.R., Stirling, Y., 1980. Haemostatic variables in vegetarians and non-vegetarians. Thromb. Res. 19 (1–2), 139–148.

Hakala, P., Karvetti, R.L., 1989. Weight reduction on lactovegetarian and mixed diets. Changes in weight, nutrient intake, skinfold thicknesses and blood pressure. Eur. J. Clin. Nutr. 43 (6), 421–430.

Hall, J.E., 2003. The kidney, hypertension, and obesity. Hypertension 41 (3 Pt. 2), 625–633.

Hall, J.E., do Carmo, J.M., da Silva, A.A., Wang, Z., Hall, M.E., 2015. Obesity-induced hypertension: interaction of neurohumoral and renal mechanisms. Circ. Res. 116 (6), 991–1006.

Harman, S.K., Parnell, W.R., 1998. The nutritional health of New Zealand vegetarian and non-vegetarian Seventh-day Adventists: selected vitamin, mineral and lipid levels. N. Z. Med. J. 111 (1062), 91–94.

Hartiala, J., Bennett, B.J., Tang, W.H., et al., 2014. Comparative genome-wide association studies in mice and humans for trimethylamine N-oxide, a proatherogenic metabolite of choline and L-carnitine. Arterioscler. Thromb. Vasc. Biol. 34 (6), 1307–1313.

Holmes, E., Loo, R.L., Stamler, J., et al., 2008. Human metabolic phenotype diversity and its association with diet and blood pressure. Nature 453 (7193), 396–400.

Holscher, H.D., Caporaso, J.G., Hooda, S., Brulc, J.M., Fahey Jr., G.C., Swanson, K.S., 2015. Fiber supplementation influences phylogenetic structure and functional capacity of the human intestinal microbiome: follow-up of a randomized controlled trial. Am. J. Clin. Nutr. 101 (1), 55–64.

Homocysteine Studies Collaboration, 2002. Homocysteine and risk of ischemic heart disease and stroke: a meta-analysis. JAMA 288 (16), 2015–2022.

Hu, F.B., 2002. Dietary pattern analysis: a new direction in nutritional epidemiology. Curr. Opin. Lipidol. 13 (1), 3–9.

Huang, A., Vita, J.A., Venema, R.C., Keaney Jr., J.F., 2000. Ascorbic acid enhances endothelial nitric-oxide synthase activity by increasing intracellular tetrahydrobiopterin. J. Biol. Chem. 275 (23), 17399–17406.

Huang, Y.W., Jian, Z.H., Chang, H.C., et al., 2014. Vegan diet and blood lipid profiles: a cross-sectional study of pre and postmenopausal women. BMC Womens Health 14, 55.

James, P.A., Oparil, S., Carter, B.L., et al., 2014. 2014 evidence-based guideline for the management of high blood pressure in adults: report from the panel members appointed to the Eighth Joint National Committee (JNC 8). JAMA 311 (5), 507–520.

John, J.H., Ziebland, S., Yudkin, P., et al., 2002. Effects of fruit and vegetable consumption on plasma antioxidant concentrations and blood pressure: a randomised controlled trial. Lancet 359 (9322), 1969–1974.

Jones, D.W., Kim, J.S., Andrew, M.E., Kim, S.J., Hong, Y.P., 1994. Body mass index and blood pressure in Korean men and women: the Korean National blood pressure Survey. J. Hypertens. 12 (12), 1433–1437.

Jose, P.A., Raj, D., 2015. Gut microbiota in hypertension. Curr. Opin. Nephrol. Hypertens. 24 (5), 403–409.

Juraschek, S.P., Guallar, E., Appel, L.J., Miller 3rd, E.R., 2012. Effects of vitamin C supplementation on blood pressure: a meta-analysis of randomized controlled trials. Am. J. Clin. Nutr. 95 (5), 1079–1088.

Kass, L., Weekes, J., Carpenter, L., 2012. Effect of magnesium supplementation on blood pressure: a meta-analysis. Eur. J. Clin. Nutr. 66 (4), 411–418.

Kestin, M., Rouse, I.L., Correll, R.A., Nestel, P.J., 1989. Cardiovascular disease risk factors in free-living men: comparison of two prudent diets, one based on lactoovovegetarianism and the other allowing lean meat. Am. J. Clin. Nutr. 50 (2), 280–287.

Key, T.J., Fraser, G.E., Thorogood, M., et al., 1999. Mortality in vegetarians and nonvegetarians: detailed findings from a collaborative analysis of 5 prospective studies. Am. J. Clin. Nutr. 70 (Suppl. 3), 516S–524S.

Kim, M.H., Bae, Y.J., 2012. Postmenopausal vegetarians' low serum ferritin level may reduce the risk for metabolic syndrome. Biol. Trace Elem. Res. 149 (1), 34–41.

Koeth, R.A., Wang, Z., Levison, B.S., et al., 2013. Intestinal microbiota metabolism of L-carnitine, a nutrient in red meat, promotes atherosclerosis. Nat. Med. 19 (5), 576–585.

Krajcovicova-Kudlackova, M., Simoncic, R., Bederova, A., Babinska, K., Beder, I., 2000. Correlation of carnitine levels to methionine and lysine intake. Physiol. Res. 49 (3), 399–402.

Larsson, C.L., Johansson, G.K., 2002. Dietary intake and nutritional status of young vegans and omnivores in Sweden. Am. J. Clin. Nutr. 76 (1), 100–106.

Li, X., Bazer, F.W., Gao, H., et al., 2009. Amino acids and gaseous signaling. Amino Acids 37 (1), 65–78.

Li, B., Li, F., Wang, L., Zhang, D., 2016. Fruit and vegetables consumption and risk of hypertension: a meta-analysis. J. Clin. Hypertens. 18 (5), 468–476 (Greenwich).

Liabeuf, S., Barreto, D.V., Barreto, F.C., et al., 2010. Free p-cresylsulphate is a predictor of mortality in patients at different stages of chronic kidney disease. Nephrol. Dial. Transpl. 25 (4), 1183–1191.

Lin, C.K., Lin, D.J., Yen, C.H., et al., 2010. Comparison of renal function and other health outcomes in vegetarians versus omnivores in Taiwan. J. Health Popul. Nutr. 28 (5), 470–475.

Lorin, J., Zeller, M., Guilland, J.C., Cottin, Y., Vergely, C., Rochette, L., 2014. Arginine and nitric oxide synthase: regulatory mechanisms and cardiovascular aspects. Mol. Nutr. Food Res. 58 (1), 101–116.

Lu, S.C., Wu, W.H., Lee, C.A., Chou, H.F., Lee, H.R., Huang, P.C., 2000. LDL of Taiwanese vegetarians are less oxidizable than those of omnivores. J. Nutr. 130 (6), 1591–1596.

Luiking, Y.C., Deutz, N.E., 2007. Biomarkers of arginine and lysine excess. J. Nutr. 137 (6 Suppl. 2), 1662S–1668S.

Luiking, Y.C., Engelen, M.P., Deutz, N.E., 2010. Regulation of nitric oxide production in health and disease. Curr. Opin. Clin. Nutr. Metab. Care 13 (1), 97–104.

Margetts, B.M., Beilin, L.J., Vandongen, R., Armstrong, B.K., 1986. Vegetarian diet in mild hypertension: a randomised controlled trial. Br. Med. J. (Clin. Res. Ed.) 293 (6560), 1468–1471.

McCarty, M.F., Barroso-Aranda, J., Contreras, F., 2009. The low-methionine content of vegan diets may make methionine restriction feasible as a life extension strategy. Med. Hypotheses 72 (2), 125–128.

McDonough, A.A., Nguyen, M.T., 2012. How does potassium supplementation lower blood pressure? Am. J. Physiol. Ren. Physiol. 302 (9), F1224–F1225.

Melby, C.L., Goldflies, D.G., Hyner, G.C., Lyle, R.M., 1989. Relation between vegetarian/nonvegetarian diets and blood pressure in black and white adults. Am. J. Public Health 79 (9), 1283–1288.

Melby, C.L., Toohey, M.L., Cebrick, J., 1994. Blood pressure and blood lipids among vegetarian, semivegetarian, and nonvegetarian African Americans. Am. J. Clin. Nutr. 59 (1), 103–109.

Messina, M., Messina, V., 2010. The role of soy in vegetarian diets. Nutrients 2 (8), 855–888.

Messina, M., Nagata, C., Wu, A.H., 2006. Estimated Asian adult soy protein and isoflavone intakes. Nutr. Cancer 55 (1), 1–12.

Mohammadifard, N., Salehi-Abargouei, A., Salas-Salvado, J., Guasch-Ferre, M., Humphries, K., Sarrafzadegan, N., 2015. The effect of tree nut, peanut, and soy nut consumption on blood pressure: a systematic review and meta-analysis of randomized controlled clinical trials. Am. J. Clin. Nutr. 101 (5), 966–982.

Mozaffarian, D., Fahimi, S., Singh, G.M., et al., 2014. Global sodium consumption and death from cardiovascular causes. N. Engl. J. Med. 371 (7), 624–634.

Nakamoto, K., Watanabe, S., Kudo, H., Tanaka, A., 2008. Nutritional characteristics of middle-aged Japanese vegetarians. J. Atheroscler. Thromb. 15 (3), 122–129.

National Center for Health Statistics, 2015. Health, United States, 2014: With Special Feature on Adults Aged 55–64. Hyattsville, MD.

National Heart, Lung, and Blood Institute, 2003. National Institutes of Health, Your Guide to Lowering Blood Pressure. NHLBI produced publications.

Nicholson, A.S., Sklar, M., Barnard, N.D., Gore, S., Sullivan, R., Browning, S., 1999. Toward improved management of NIDDM: a randomized, controlled, pilot intervention using a lowfat, vegetarian diet. Prev. Med. 29 (2), 87–91.

Ophir, O., Peer, G., Gilad, J., Blum, M., Aviram, A., 1983. Low blood pressure in vegetarians: the possible role of potassium. Am. J. Clin. Nutr. 37 (5), 755–762.

Orlich, M.J., Jaceldo-Siegl, K., Sabate, J., Fan, J., Singh, P.N., Fraser, G.E., 2014. Patterns of food consumption among vegetarians and non-vegetarians. Br. J. Nutr. 112 (10), 1644–1653.

Orlov, S.N., Agren, J.J., Hanninen, O.O., et al., 1994. Univalent cation fluxes in human erythrocytes from individuals with low or normal sodium intake. J. Cardiovasc. Risk 1 (3), 249–254.

Patel, K.P., Luo, F.J., Plummer, N.S., Hostetter, T.H., Meyer, T.W., 2012. The production of p-cresol sulfate and indoxyl sulfate in vegetarians versus omnivores. Clin. J. Am. Soc. Nephrol. 7 (6), 982–988.

Pawlak, R., 2015. Is vitamin B12 deficiency a risk factor for cardiovascular disease in vegetarians? Am. J. Prev. Med. 48 (6), e11–26.

Pettersen, B.J., Anousheh, R., Fan, J., Jaceldo-Siegl, K., Fraser, G.E., 2012. Vegetarian diets and blood pressure among white subjects: results from the Adventist Health Study-2 (AHS-2). Public Health Nutr. 15 (10), 1909–1916.

Pitla, S., Nagalla, B., 2009. Gender-related differences in the relationship between plasma homocysteine, anthropometric and conventional biochemical coronary heart disease risk factors in middle-aged Indians. Ann. Nutr. Metab. 54 (1), 1–6.

Ramezani, A., Raj, D.S., 2014. The gut microbiome, kidney disease, and targeted interventions. J. Am. Soc. Nephrol. 25 (4), 657–670.

Reese, D.R., Chong, C.W., Swintosky, J.V., 1960. Physical properties of lipids used in pharmacy. 1. Screening raw materials via photomicrography. J. Am. Pharm. Assoc. 49 (2), 85–89.

Rizzo, N.S., Jaceldo-Siegl, K., Sabate, J., Fraser, G.E., 2013. Nutrient profiles of vegetarian and nonvegetarian dietary patterns. J. Acad. Nutr. Diet 113 (12), 1610–1619.

Rodenas, S., Sanchez-Muniz, F.J., Bastida, S., Sevillano, M.I., Larrea Marin, T., Gonzalez-Munoz, M.J., 2011. Blood pressure of omnivorous and semi-vegetarian postmenopausal women and their relationship with dietary and hair concentrations of essential and toxic metals. Nutr. Hosp. 26 (4), 874–883.

Rosendorff, C., Lackland, D.T., Allison, M., et al., 2015. Treatment of hypertension in patients with coronary artery disease: a scientific statement from the American Heart Association, American College of Cardiology, and American Society of Hypertension. J. Am. Coll. Cardiol. 65 (18), 1998–2038.

Rouse, I.L., Armstrong, B.K., Beilin, L.J., 1983a. The relationship of blood pressure to diet and lifestyle in two religious populations. J. Hypertens. 1 (1), 65–71.

Rouse, I.L., Beilin, L.J., Armstrong, B.K., Vandongen, R., 1983b. Blood-pressure-lowering effect of a vegetarian diet: controlled trial in normotensive subjects. Lancet 1 (8314–5), 5–10.

Sacks, F.M., Obarzanek, E., Windhauser, M.M., et al., 1995. Rationale and design of the Dietary Approaches to Stop Hypertension trial (DASH). A multicenter controlled-feeding study of dietary patterns to lower blood pressure. Ann. Epidemiol. 5 (2), 108–118.

Sacks, F.M., Svetkey, L.P., Vollmer, W.M., et al., 2001. Effects on blood pressure of reduced dietary sodium and the dietary approaches to Stop hypertension (DASH) diet. DASH-sodium collaborative research group. N. Engl. J. Med. 344 (1), 3–10.

Sanders, T.A., Key, T.J., 1987. Blood pressure, plasma renin activity and aldosterone concentrations in vegans and omnivore controls. Hum. Nutr. Appl. Nutr. 41 (3), 204–211.

Schmidt, J.A., Rinaldi, S., Scalbert, A., et al., 2016. Plasma concentrations and intakes of amino acids in male meat-eaters, fish-eaters, vegetarians and vegans: a cross-sectional analysis in the EPIC-Oxford cohort. Eur. J. Clin. Nutr. 70 (3), 306–312.

Sciarrone, S.E., Strahan, M.T., Beilin, L.J., Burke, V., Rogers, P., Rouse, I.L., 1993. Biochemical and neurohormonal responses to the introduction of a lacto-ovovegetarian diet. J. Hypertens. 11 (8), 849–860.

Sebekova, K., Boor, P., Valachovicova, M., et al., 2006. Association of metabolic syndrome risk factors with selected markers of oxidative status and microinflammation in healthy omnivores and vegetarians. Mol. Nutr. Food Res. 50 (9), 858–868.

Shridhar, K., Dhillon, P.K., Bowen, L., et al., 2014. The association between a vegetarian diet and cardiovascular disease (CVD) risk factors in India: the Indian Migration Study. PLoS One 9 (10), e110586.

Slavicek, J., Kittnar, O., Fraser, G.E., et al., 2008. Lifestyle decreases risk factors for cardiovascular diseases. Cent. Eur. J. Public Health 16 (4), 161–164.

Smit, E., Nieto, F.J., Crespo, C.J., Mitchell, P., 1999. Estimates of animal and plant protein intake in US adults: results from the Third National Health and Nutrition Examination Survey, 1988-1991. J. Am. Diet. Assoc. 99 (7), 813–820.

Squadrito, F., Altavilla, D., Morabito, N., et al., 2002. The effect of the phytoestrogen genistein on plasma nitric oxide concentrations, endothelin-1 levels and endothelium dependent vasodilation in postmenopausal women. Atherosclerosis 163 (2), 339–347.

Stamler, J., Brown, I.J., Daviglus, M.L., et al., 2009. Glutamic acid, the main dietary amino acid, and blood pressure: the INTERMAP study (International Collaborative Study of Macronutrients, Micronutrients and Blood Pressure). Circulation 120 (3), 221–228.

Streppel, M.T., Arends, L.R., van 't Veer, P., Grobbee, D.E., Geleijnse, J.M., 2005. Dietary fiber and blood pressure: a meta-analysis of randomized placebo-controlled trials. Arch. Intern. Med. 165 (2), 150–156.

Stuhlinger, M.C., Oka, R.K., Graf, E.E., et al., 2003. Endothelial dysfunction induced by hyperhomocyst(e)inemia: role of asymmetric dimethylarginine. Circulation 108 (8), 933–938.

Su, T.C., Jeng, J.S., Wang, J.D., et al., 2006. Homocysteine, circulating vascular cell adhesion molecule and carotid atherosclerosis in postmenopausal vegetarian women and omnivores. Atherosclerosis 184 (2), 356–362.

Suematsu, N., Ojaimi, C., Recchia, F.A., et al., 2010. Potential mechanisms of low-sodium diet-induced cardiac disease: superoxide-NO in the heart. Circ. Res. 106 (3), 593–600.

Tang, W.H., Wang, Z., Levison, B.S., et al., 2013. Intestinal microbial metabolism of phosphatidylcholine and cardiovascular risk. N. Engl. J. Med. 368 (17), 1575–1584.

Tang, W.H., Wang, Z., Kennedy, D.J., et al., 2015. Gut microbiota-dependent trimethylamine N-oxide (TMAO) pathway contributes to both development of renal insufficiency and mortality risk in chronic kidney disease. Circ. Res. 116 (3), 448–455.

Teixeira Rde, C., Molina Mdel, C., Zandonade, E., Mill, J.G., 2007. Cardiovascular risk in vegetarians and omnivores: a comparative study. Arq. Bras. Cardiol. 89 (4), 237–244.

Tielemans, S.M., Altorf-van der Kuil, W., Engberink, M.F., et al., 2013. Intake of total protein, plant protein and animal protein in relation to blood pressure: a meta-analysis of observational and intervention studies. J. Hum. Hypertens. 27 (9), 564–571.

Toh, J.Y., Tan, V.M., Lim, P.C., Lim, S.T., Chong, M.F., 2013. Flavonoids from fruit and vegetables: a focus on cardiovascular risk factors. Curr. Atheroscler. Rep. 15 (12), 368.

Turin, T.C., Okamura, T., Afzal, A.R., et al., 2016. Hypertension and lifetime risk of stroke. J. Hypertens. 34 (1), 116–122.

Tuso, P., Stoll, S.R., Li, W.W., 2015. A plant-based diet, atherogenesis, and coronary artery disease prevention. Perm. J. 19 (1), 62–67.

Tuttle, K.R., Milton, J.E., Packard, D.P., Shuler, L.A., Short, R.A., 2012. Dietary amino acids and blood pressure: a cohort study of patients with cardiovascular disease. Am. J. Kidney Dis. 59 (6), 803–809.

Ufnal, M., Jazwiec, R., Dadlez, M., Drapala, A., Sikora, M., Skrzypecki, J., 2014. Trimethylamine-N-oxide: a carnitine-derived metabolite that prolongs the hypertensive effect of angiotensin II in rats. Can. J. Cardiol. 30 (12), 1700–1705.

Urschel, K.L., Rafii, M., Pencharz, P.B., Ball, R.O., 2007. A multitracer stable isotope quantification of the effects of arginine intake on whole body arginine metabolism in neonatal piglets. Am. J. Physiol. Endocrinol. Metab. 293 (3), E811–E818.

Vega-Lopez, S., Matthan, N.R., Ausman, L.M., et al., 2010. Altering dietary lysine:arginine ratio has little effect on cardiovascular risk factors and vascular reactivity in moderately hypercholesterolemic adults. Atherosclerosis 210 (2), 555–562.

Wang, Y.F., Yancy Jr., W.S., Yu, D., Champagne, C., Appel, L.J., Lin, P.H., 2008. The relationship between dietary protein intake and blood pressure: results from the PREMIER study. J. Hum. Hypertens. 22 (11), 745–754.

Wang, Z., Klipfell, E., Bennett, B.J., et al., 2011. Gut flora metabolism of phosphatidylcholine promotes cardiovascular disease. Nature 472 (7341), 57–63.

Whelton, P.K., He, J., Culter, J.A., et al., 1997. Effects of oral potassium on blood pressure. Meta-analysis of randomized controlled clinical trials. JAMA 277 (20), 1624–1632.

Whelton, S.P., Hyre, A.D., Pedersen, B., Yi, Y., Whelton, P.K., He, J., 2005. Effect of dietary fiber intake on blood pressure: a meta-analysis of randomized, controlled clinical trials. J. Hypertens. 23 (3), 475–481.

Williams, P.T., 1997. Interactive effects of exercise, alcohol, and vegetarian diet on coronary artery disease risk factors in 9242 runners: the National Runners' Health Study. Am. J. Clin. Nutr. 66 (5), 1197–1206.

Wiseman, M.J., Hunt, R., Goodwin, A., Gross, J.L., Keen, H., Viberti, G.C., 1987. Dietary composition and renal function in healthy subjects. Nephron 46 (1), 37–42.

Woo, J., Kwok, T., Ho, S.C., Sham, A., Lau, E., 1998. Nutritional status of elderly Chinese vegetarians. Age Ageing 27 (4), 455–461.

Woo, K.S., Kwok, T.C., Celermajer, D.S., 2014. Vegan diet, subnormal vitamin B-12 status and cardiovascular health. Nutrients 6 (8), 3259–3273.

World Health Organization, 2011a. Cause of Death 2008. Geneva. Available from: http://www.who.int/healthinfo/global_burden_disease/cod_2008_sources_methods.pdf.

World Health Organization, 2011b. Global Status Report on Noncommunicable Diseases 2010. World Health Organization, Geneva.

Wyatt, C.J., Velazquez, C., Grijalva, I., Valencia, M.E., 1995. Dietary-intake of sodium, potassium and blood-pressure in lacto-ovo-vegetarians. Nutr. Res. 15 (6), 819–830.

Yang, S.Y., Zhang, H.J., Sun, S.Y., et al., 2011. Relationship of carotid intima-media thickness and duration of vegetarian diet in Chinese male vegetarians. Nutr. Metab. (Lond) 8 (1), 63.

Yang, S.Y., Li, X.J., Zhang, W., et al., 2012. Chinese lacto-vegetarian diet exerts favorable effects on metabolic parameters, intima-media thickness, and cardiovascular risks in healthy men. Nutr. Clin. Pract. 27 (3), 392–398.

Yokoyama, Y., Nishimura, K., Barnard, N.D., et al., 2014. Vegetarian diets and blood pressure: a meta-analysis. JAMA Intern. Med. 174 (4), 577–587.

23

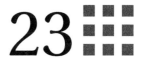

Ischemic Heart Disease in Vegetarians and Those Consuming a Predominantly Plant-Based Diet

Jim Mann

UNIVERSITY OF OTAGO, DUNEDIN, NEW ZEALAND

1. Introduction

Cardiovascular disease (comprising ischemic heart disease, IHD) and cerebrovascular disease (stroke) account for a substantial proportion of premature mortality and serious morbidity worldwide. While IHD death rates are decreasing in many relatively affluent Western countries since peaking in the 1960s and 1970s, this disease continues to account for a high proportion of total mortality as a result of aging populations. While lifestyle changes, improved medical care and drug treatment of raised blood pressure and cholesterol, in particular, undoubtedly explain to some extent the reduction of IHD in some countries, it is noteworthy that IHD death rates had declined appreciably in some of these countries before the widespread introduction of statins. In some Eastern European countries the increase in IHD death rates started much later, and mortality in some of them remain very much higher than in the West. The Czech and Slavic Republics and Hungary now have the highest IHD mortality rates in the world.

In recent years, as case fatality rates have declined and diagnostic facilities and information systems have improved, there has been increasing interest in the overall burden of disease. This is reported in *Disability Adjusted Life Years* (DALYs), a measure of years of life lost due to ill health, disability, or death. In 2010, cardiovascular heart disease was the leading cause of DALYs in the world. This is largely a result of increasing mortality from IHD in low- and middle-income countries. In these countries, IHD events and deaths have increased due to a number of factors, including population growth, aging populations, and changing patterns of risk factors, which may differ among countries. In many of these countries, the average age of onset of IHD is lower than in high-income countries, resulting in an increasing burden of disease as IHD increases. The situation is particularly concerning in countries where affluence and poverty coexist and which are said to be in a state of nutrition transition. In such countries (e.g., India and South Africa), IHD rates are high among the relatively affluent and those accumulating wealth, whereas diseases of undernutrition remain prevalent among the poor and underprivileged. The situation is the reverse of what is observed in most high-income countries where the socioeconomically disadvantaged have higher IHD rates than better educated, more affluent groups in the community.

The striking geographic variation, rapidly changing trends, and experience of migrants who tend to acquire the characteristics of the host nation over a relatively short period suggest the importance of environmental factors in the etiology of IHD. Dietary factors have long been accepted as playing a pivotal role in IHD. Early attention was focused almost entirely on the role of saturated fat. While there is little doubt that fat intake does play an important role in the etiology of IHD, there is increasing evidence that other foods and nutrients may have a deleterious effect and that a range of plant foods and dietary patterns that are largely plant-based may be protective. This chapter examines the evidence suggesting that plant-based dietary patterns and meat avoidance protect against IHD.

1.1 Epidemiological Evidence

Populations following traditional diets that are largely plant-based or are rich in plant-based foods tend to have low rates of cardiovascular heart disease. This observation applies to dietary patterns as diverse as the maize-based diets followed in many parts of rural Africa, the rice-based diets in many countries in Asia, and the several Mediterranean dietary patterns characterized by a range of plant-based foods.

The earliest attempt to quantify the effects of a vegetarian dietary pattern in a Western society were based on Seventh-day Adventists living in California (Snowdon et al., 1984). Many adherents to this faith are vegetarian, and as a group, they were found to have appreciably lower IHD mortality rates than the population at large. Similar results were reported from the experience of a relatively small group of German vegetarians (Chang-Claude et al., 1992; Chang-Claude and Frentzel-Beyme, 1993) and people in the United Kingdom (UK) identified as vegetarian, who when visiting health food shops were compared with meat eaters also visiting these stores (Burr and Butland, 1988). Subsequent analyses of the Adventist data that involved comparisons of those who were vegetarians and those who were not confirmed the lower mortality rates among vegetarians (Snowdon, 1988). The inability to disentangle the benefit conferred by the vegetarian dietary pattern from confounding healthy lifestyle-related variables potentially associated with vegetarianism and lower risk of IHD (e.g., not smoking, regular physical activity) were the stimulus to the setting up of the Oxford Vegetarian Study (Appleby et al., 1999). Vegetarians were recruited from among the members of the Vegetarian Society of the UK and more widely through the news media, word of mouth, and advertisements. To identify a comparable group of nonvegetarians, vegetarians were asked to recruit nonvegetarian relatives and friends. Over 11,000 participants were identified, and the vegetarian and meat eating cohorts were reasonably well matched for the major nondietary lifestyle-related determinants of IHD. Follow-up of the two cohorts revealed a significantly lower standardized mortality ratio for IHD mortality among the vegetarians compared with meat eaters, but after adjustment for smoking, body mass index (BMI), and social class, the 28% reduction in IHD did not achieve conventional levels of statistical significance (adjusted death rate ratio 0.72, 95% CI: 0.47, 1.10) (Thorogood et al., 1994).

Key et al. (1999) combined the data from the two studies of Seventh-day Adventists, the UK Health Food Shoppers Study, German Vegetarians, and the Oxford Vegetarian Study.

There were 8330 deaths after a mean of 10.6 years of follow-up of 76,172 men and women. After adjustment for age, sex, and smoking status, mortality from IHD was 24% lower in vegetarians than nonvegetarians (death rate ratio 0.75, 95% CI: 0.62, 0.94, $P<$ .01). The difference in mortality was greater at younger ages and was restricted to those who had followed their diet for more than 5 years. In this aggregation of the data, BMI data were not available for all subjects, so the ratios could not be adjusted for this potential confounder as had been done in the Oxford Vegetarian Study. However, it could be argued that this was more appropriate since body fatness could be involved in the causal chain linking a dietary attribute and IHD. This is further discussed subsequently.

Two important cohort studies have been published. They have involved a large number of participants and obtained more detailed data regarding dietary intake and potentially confounding variables than had been the case in previous studies. The Adventist Health Study 2 reported a 5.8-year follow-up of 73,308 participants in the United States and Canada; 48% were nonvegetarians, 29% ovolactovegetarians, 10% pescetarians, 8% vegans, and 5% semivegetarians. Vegetarians had lower risk of all-cause mortality compared with nonvegetarians (HR: 0.88, 95% CI: 0.72, 0.94) with comparable reductions in the various "vegetarian" subgroups. IHD mortality was also lower in the "vegetarian" groups, but the reduction did not achieve conventional levels of statistical significance (e.g., among ovolactovegetarians HR: 0.82, 95% CI: 0.62, 1.06) (Orlich et al., 2013).

The EPIC-Oxford Study, a successor to the Oxford Vegetarian Study, involved 57,446 participants who were vegetarians, vegans, or others representative of the UK general population. They were recruited through General Practices in Oxfordshire, Buckinghamshire, and Greater Manchester between 1993 and 1999 and followed for an average of 11.6 years. Approximately one-third of the participants reported consuming a vegetarian diet. Through linkage with both hospital records and death certificates, it was possible to identify incident cases of IHD in addition to mortality. Detailed dietary data were obtained from a validated semiqualitative food frequency questionnaire that estimated intake of 130 food items over the past 12 months. Information was also obtained relating to a range of lifestyle-related variables, medical history, weight, and height. Blood pressure and lipid measurements were obtained at the time of recruitment. Vegetarians had a 32% lower risk of IHD than nonvegetarians after adjustment for age, smoking, alcohol intake, physical activity, educational level, deprivation index, and in women, use of oral contraceptives or hormone treatment (HR: 0.68, 95% CI: 0.58, 0.81) (Crowe et al., 2013).

The most recent report relating to mortality among vegetarians has combined data from the Oxford Vegetarian Study and EPIC-Oxford (Appleby et al., 2016). The finding of no difference in cardiovascular mortality between vegetarians and nonvegetarians, a somewhat surprising finding in the light of earlier findings, may be explained by at least two observations. Nonvegetarians may have been more likely than vegetarians to have commenced treatment with statins, and there is some evidence that this is the case (Key, 2016). EPIC-Oxford included participants up to age 90 years, and many of the deaths will, of course, have occurred in the oldest members of the cohort. At this age, it is conceivable that individual risk and protective factors including those associated with vegetarianism are likely to be less influential.

2. Effects of Vegetarianism and Plant-Based Diets on Major Cardiovascular Risk Factors

2.1 Body Fatness

Increasing body fatness, most often measured by the BMI, has been consistently shown to be an important cardiovascular risk factor, especially when centrally distributed, as demonstrated by increasing waist circumference or waist/hip ratio. Vegetarians, and even more strikingly vegans, are appreciably less likely to be overweight or obese than comparable (their relatives and friends) meat eaters (see Fig 23.1) (Appleby et al., 2002). However, it is impossible to disentangle the extent to which attributes of a generally healthy lifestyle (e.g., regular physical activity, low consumption of energy dense foods) or any specific features of vegetarianism or a largely plant-based diet contribute to a lower risk of this important determinant of cardiovascular health. The satiety enhancing effect of dietary fiber, typically high in vegetarian and other plant-based dietary patterns, seems a likely candidate, but so do the nondietary environmental factors that characterize the lives of many who choose a vegetarian or largely plant-based diet. Lower rates of overweight and obesity may exert a cardioprotective effect by favorably influencing other risk factors.

2.2 Blood Pressure

A clear linear relationship exists between increasing levels of blood pressure and increasing risk of CHD and stroke. Meta-analysis of 7 controlled dietary intervention studies and 32 observational studies has shown that vegetarian diets are consistently associated with lower levels of blood pressure than diets including meat (Yokoyama et al., 2014). These data and a further analysis are presented in detail in Chapter 22. In brief, in the clinical trials, systolic and diastolic pressures were, respectively, 4.8 and 2.2 mm Hg lower in the vegetarians. More striking differences (6.9 and 4.7 mm Hg) for systolic and diastolic were apparent in the meta-analysis of the observational studies. Such an effect is approximately half that which might be associated with the use of a blood pressure–lowering drug. Reductions in blood pressure of this size might be expected to translate into a reduction of approximately 9% in IHD mortality and 14% in stroke mortality. Overweight and obesity and high intakes of alcohol are clearly established causes of increasing blood pressure and may have confounded the findings in the observational studies but not in the controlled trials. Dietary sodium is probably the most clearly described dietary determinant of blood pressure, but (World Health Organisation, 2012) vegetarian diets are not consistently low in sodium, nor is a difference in sodium intake likely to explain the findings of the randomized trials. On the other hand, vegetarian diets are typically characterized by high intakes of potassium, which have been shown to be associated with blood pressure lowering and a range of effects on renal function that could explain this finding (Whelton et al., 1997). The extent to which plant protein may be associated with lower blood pressure levels has also been extensively studied. The INTERMAP Study (International Collaborative Study of Macronutrients, Micronutrients and Blood pressure) suggested that plant protein is

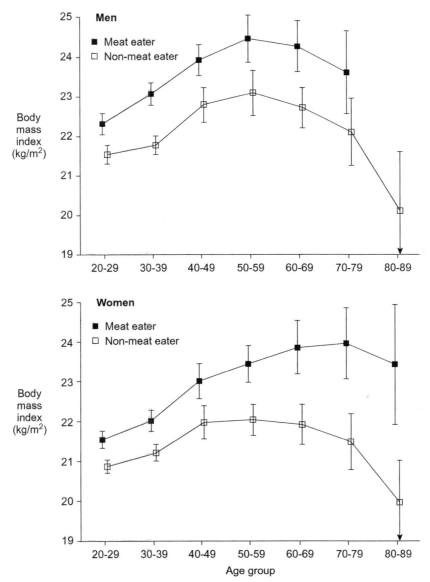

FIGURE 23.1 Mean body mass index by diet and age group (showing 95% confidence intervals). There were no male meat eaters aged 80–89. *Courtesy of Macmillan Publishers Ltd; Appleby, P.N., Thorogood, M., Mann, J.I., Key, T.J., 1998. Low body mass index in nonmeat eaters: the possible roles of animal fat, dietary fiber and alcohol. Int. J. Obes. Relat. Metab. Disord. 22, 454–460.*

associated with a modest reduction in blood pressure (2.1 mm Hg) and that the higher levels of glutamic acid (a precursor of arginine) seen in those eating a predominantly plant-based diet may explain the blood pressure lowering effect (Elliott et al., 2006). Amino acid profiles in vegetarians, vegans, and meat eaters have been studied in the EPIC-Oxford cohort and unsurprisingly showed expected differences between vegans and meat eaters

(Schmidt et al., 2016). A low lysine/arginine ratio may contribute to the lower blood pressure of nonmeat eaters by stimulating nitric oxide (NO) production (Lorin et al., 2014). The readers can refer to Chapter 36 for a discussion on the relation between cardiovascular health and protein and amino acids in plant-based diet. The extent to which other nutrients may contribute to the lower blood pressure levels of those consuming largely plant-based diets is unclear.

2.3 Lipids and Lipoproteins

The Oxford Vegetarian Study clearly demonstrated lower levels of total and LDL cholesterol in vegetarians compared with meat eaters and even lower levels in vegans. Triglyceride levels did not differ among the groups (Thorogood et al., 1987). Meta-analysis of 10 randomized controlled trials confirmed these findings, with total, LDL, and non-HDL cholesterol being 0.36, 0.31, and 0.30 mmol/L lower on the vegetarian diets (see Fig 23.2) (Wang et al., 2015). Vegetarian diets were also associated with lower (−0.10 mmol/L) levels of HDL cholesterol, but it is noteworthy that the reduction in LDL was appreciably greater than the reduction in HDL. Furthermore, a meta-analysis of observational studies has not confirmed lower HDL cholesterol among vegetarians. Unsurprisingly a greater cholesterol lowering effect was seen in trials analyzed on a per protocol basis than in those analyzed on an intention to treat basis. The effect was most striking in those with BMI in the normal range. Given the importance of total and LDL cholesterol as determinants of cardiovascular disease, it seems highly likely that the lower cardiovascular risk associated with a vegetarian or plant-based diet is to an important extent explained by the effect on lipids and lipoproteins. Given that a 1 mmol/L reduction in total cholesterol results in a nearly 30% decrease in risk of a cardiovascular event and that a vegetarian diet produces a reduction in cholesterol of approximately 0.35 mmol/L, the cholesterol reduction may by itself reduce CVD by 10% in vegetarians (Schwingshackl and Hoffmann, 2013).

The lower intake of saturated fatty acids, relatively higher intakes of *cis*-unsaturated fatty acids, dietary fiber (especially the soluble forms), and soy-based products are all features of plant-based diets that have been clearly shown to be associated with low levels of total and LDL cholesterol. In addition a wide range of dietary phytochemicals that are prevalent in vegetarian diets may influence lipid metabolism (Mann and McLean, 2017).

2.4 Diabetes and Insulin Sensitivity

People with diabetes and prediabetes are at appreciably increased risk of cardiovascular disease. Meat intake has been linked to an increased risk of diabetes (Pan et al., 2011), though the effect has not been entirely consistent. However, dietary fiber (especially the soluble forms) reduces blood glucose levels in people with diabetes and prediabetes (Mann et al., 2004), and the KANWU Study has shown that replacing saturated with *cis*-unsaturated fatty acids increases insulin sensitivity when total fat consumption is within the usual range of intakes (Riserus et al., 2009). The readers may refer to Chapter 20 for a full review.

(A)   **Effect of vegetarian diets on TC concentrations**

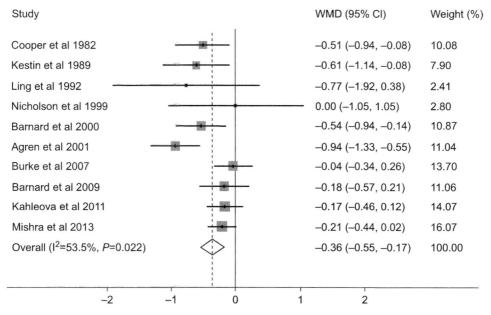

(B)   **Effect of vegetarian diets on LDL–C concentrations**

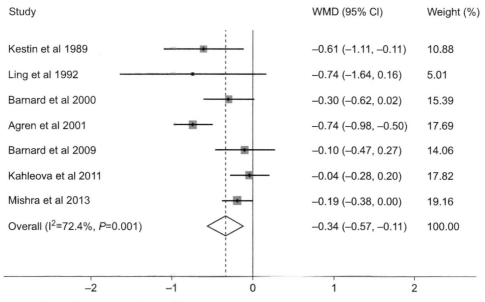

FIGURE 23.2 Effects of vegetarian diets on (A) total cholesterol and (B) LDL cholesterol concentrations. *From open access article under the terms of the Creative Commons Attribution-NonCommercial Licence, Published on behalf of the American Heart Assocation, Inc., by Wiley Blackwell; Wang, F., Zheng, J., Yang, B., Jiang, J., Fu, Y., Li, D., 2015. Effects of vegetarian diets on blood lipids: a systematic review and metaanalysis of randomized controlled trials. J. Am. Heart Assoc. 4, e002408.*

2.5 Other Risk Determinants

In addition to the major risk factors, many other pathophysiological processes contribute to cardiovascular risk. An increased tendency to thrombosis may result from increased hemostatic factors and enhanced platelet aggregation. Platelet linoleic acid is higher in vegetarians and vegans than in meat eaters, and polyunsaturated fatty acids of the $\omega 6$ series (such as linoleic acid) may reduce platelet aggregation by providing the Series 1 prostanoid PGE_1, which is antiaggregatory (Fisher et al., 1986). High levels of CRP (and possibly other makers of inflammation) are indictors of cardiovascular risk, which has been shown to be reduced by adherence to a plant-based diet. Oxidizability of LDL may be reduced by the relatively large amounts of antioxidants present in plant-based diets (Jenkins et al., 2015).

3. Effects of Individual Plant-Based Foods and Dietary Patterns on Cardiovascular Risk

A number of individual plant-based foods, food groups, and predominantly plant-based dietary patterns, though not exclusively vegetarian or vegan, have been associated with protection against IHD or stroke or lower levels of risk factors. A consideration of these foods and eating patterns may further help to understand the mechanisms by which plant-based diets confer their protective effect as well as provide information that can usefully inform food-based dietary guidelines.

3.1 Nuts

Several prospective cohort studies have shown a clear cardioprotective effect of nut consumption since this was first observed in the Adventist Health Study (Fraser et al., 1992). In the Nurses' Health Study, consuming nuts, five or more times per week, was associated with a nearly 40% reduction in risk of total CHO when compared with never or infrequent consumption of nuts. The effect appeared to be independent of most known risk factors for IHD and applies to peanuts as well as other nuts (Hu and Stampfer, 1999). An appreciable number of intervention studies has shown that a range of nuts (including walnuts, almonds, hazelnuts, and peanuts) have the potential to lower total and LDL cholesterol and the ratio of total cholesterol or LDL cholesterol to HDL ratio, presumably as a result of the relatively high content of $\omega 6$ and $\omega 9$ *cis*-unsaturated fatty acids (Kris-Etherton et al., 2001). Their $\omega 3$ unsaturated fatty acid content (α-linolenic acid) may have antithrombotic and antidysrhythmic effects (Hu et al., 2001). Nuts are also high in arginine, a precursor of NO, which plays a central role in vascular health (Cooke et al., 1993). The readers may refer to Chapter 15 for further review.

3.2 Whole Grains

Whole grain foods derived from wheat, rye, oats, and barley have been shown in several cohort studies to be protective against IHD (see Fig 23.3). Whole grain products, which

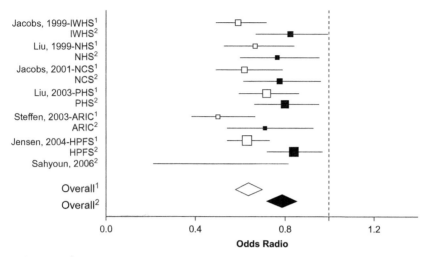

FIGURE 23.3 Odds ratios of incident cardiovascular disease, comparing high versus low whole grain intake. *Courtesy of Elsevier; Mellen, P.B., Walsh, T.F., Herrington, D.M., 2008. Whole grain intake and cardiovascular disease: a meta-analysis. Nutr. Metab. Cardiovasc. Dis. 18, 283–290.*

include the outer bran layer of the grain, contain a range of potentially cardioprotective nutrients including dietary fiber, unsaturated fatty acids, and vitamins and phytochemicals with antioxidant properties. However, it is noteworthy that the Nurses' Health Study has shown that the protective effect persists after adjusting for the effects of some of these nutrients, suggesting that some other attribute of whole grains may be involved (Liu et al., 1999). An explanation may lie in the milling process. Retaining at least to some extent the structure of the grain, as this is done in milling whole grain, will result in the starch content being more slowly digested, hence a lower glycemic response than would be expected following a meal containing highly refined grain. It should be noted that the definition of "whole grain" refers principally to the composition of the product (i.e., it is required to contain a high proportion of the nutrients present in the whole grain) but does not refer to the structure (i.e., the extent to which it is milled), so a product marketed as whole grain might be highly refined. Such products are becoming increasingly available and may not confer the same health benefits as more lightly milled foods. The readers may refer to Chapter 14 for further review.

3.3 Fruit and Vegetables

Those who choose predominantly plant-based diets typically have high intakes of fruit and vegetables. Many cohort studies have demonstrated a protective effect of total fruit and vegetable intake against IHD (Gaziano et al., 1995; Joshipura et al., 1999, 2001; Liu et al., 2000; Knekt et al., 1994). The readers may refer to Chapter 13 for further review. A range of individual fruits and vegetables have been identified as protective in different studies. In the Nordic countries, berries have been shown to be protective (Knekt et al., 1994).

In the Nurses' Health Study and the Health Professionals' Follow-Up Study, green leafy and cruciferous vegetables were the main contributors to the reduction in IHD risk. It is not possible to disentangle which of the protective nutrients in fruits and vegetables (antioxidant vitamins, flavonoids, potassium, dietary fiber) are especially important in explaining the reduction in risk.

3.4 Dietary Patterns

A number of very different traditional dietary patterns that are largely plant-based or at least rich in plant-based foods, though not necessarily vegetarian, are associated with a low risk of IHD. These range from the high-carbohydrate, relatively low-fat rice-based diets of Japan, China, and other Asian countries and the maize-based diets of Africa to the varied Mediterranean diets that are rich in pulses and a wide range of fruits and vegetables. Mediterranean diets are not low in fat, but olive oil (rich in *cis*-monounsaturated fatty acids) predominates, so the overall dietary pattern tends to be appreciably different from that in many other Western countries where more of the dietary fat is saturated. The DASH diet has been widely recommended for blood pressure lowering and prevention of cardiovascular disease. This diet is high in fresh fruit and vegetables and low-fat dairy products, so it is low in saturated fat and high in potassium, calcium, and fiber. Nuts, whole grains, fish, and poultry are encouraged, and red meat and sugary foods are limited. The blood pressure lowering effect of the DASH diet is even more striking when combined with sodium restriction (Sacks et al., 2001). A dietary "portfolio" developed in Toronto including soy protein foods, foods rich in viscous fiber, nuts, and plant sterol margarine has been shown to have similar blood pressure lowering properties and a beneficial effect on a range of other cardiovascular risk factors (Jenkins et al., 2015). In the Nurses' Health Study and the Health Professionals' Study, it was possible to identify a "prudent" dietary pattern that was associated with an appreciably lower risk of cardiovascular disease other than the "Western" dietary pattern. The "prudent" pattern was associated with higher intakes of vegetables, fruits, legumes, fish, poultry, and whole grains and the "Western" pattern with higher intakes of red and processed meats, butter, and other high fat dairy products, refined grains, and potatoes (Hu, 2002).

4. Conclusion

Vegetarians, vegans, and those who choose to eat a predominantly plant-based diet appear to have a relatively favorably risk factor profile and lower risk of IHD. There are many nutritional attributes of plant-based diets that are cardioprotective. The most clearly established of these are relatively high intakes of dietary fiber, naturally occurring unsaturated vegetable oils, antioxidant nutrients, potassium, and low intakes of saturated fat. There is no convincing evidence that total avoidance of meat and meat products confers cardio-protection per se.

References

Appleby, P.N., Thorogood, M., Mann, J.I., Key, T.J., 1999. The Oxford vegetarian study: an overview. Am. J. Clin. Nutr. 70, 525S–531S.

Appleby, P.N., Davey, G.K., Key, T.J., 2002. Hypertension and blood pressure among meat eaters, fish eaters, vegetarians and vegans in EPIC-Oxford. Public Health Nutr. 5, 645–654.

Appleby, P.N., Crowe, F.L., Bradbury, K.E., Travis, R.C., Key, T.J., 2016. Mortality in vegetarians and comparable nonvegetarians in the United Kingdom. Am. J. Clin. Nutr. 103, 218–230.

Burr, M.L., Butland, B.K., 1988. Heart disease in British vegetarians. Am. J. Clin. Nutr. 48, 830–832.

Chang-Claude, J., Frentzel-Beyme, R., 1993. Dietary and lifestyle determinants of mortality among German vegetarians. Int. J. Epidemiol. 22, 228–236.

Chang-Claude, J., Frentzel-Beyme, R., Eilber, U., 1992. Mortality pattern of German vegetarians after 11 years of follow-up. Epidemiology 3, 395–401.

Cooke, J.P., Tsao, P., Singer, A., Wang, B.Y., Kosek, J., Drexler, H., 1993. Anti-atherogenic effect of nuts: is the answer NO? Arch. Intern. Med. 153 896, 899, 902.

Crowe, F.L., Appleby, P.N., Travis, R.C., Key, T.J., 2013. Risk of hospitalization or death from ischemic heart disease among British vegetarians and nonvegetarians: results from the EPIC-Oxford cohort study. Am. J. Clin. Nutr. 97, 597–603.

Elliott, P., Stamler, J., Dyer, A.R., Appel, L., Dennis, B., Kesteloot, H., Ueshima, H., Okayama, A., Chan, Q., Garside, D.B., Zhou, B., 2006. Association between protein intake and blood pressure: the INTERMAP Study. Arch. Intern. Med. 166, 79–87.

Fisher, M., Levine, P.H., Weiner, B., Ockene, I.S., Johnson, B., Johnson, M.H., Natale, A.M., Vaudreuil, C.H., Hoogasian, J., 1986. The effect of vegetarian diets on plasma lipid and platelet levels. Arch. Intern. Med. 146, 1193–1197.

Fraser, G.E., Sabate, J., Beeson, W.L., Strahan, T.M., 1992. A possible protective effect of nut consumption on risk of coronary heart disease. The Adventist Health Study. Arch. Intern. Med. 152, 1416–1424.

Gaziano, J.M., Manson, J.E., Branch, L.G., Colditz, G.A., Willett, W.C., Buring, J.E., 1995. A prospective study of consumption of carotenoids in fruits and vegetables and decreased cardiovascular mortality in the elderly. Ann. Epidemiol. 5, 255–260.

Hu, F.B., 2002. Dietary pattern analysis: a new direction in nutritional epidemiology. Curr. Opin. Lipidol. 13, 3–9.

Hu, F.B., Stampfer, M.J., 1999. Nut consumption and risk of coronary heart disease: a review of epidemiologic evidence. Curr. Atheroscler. Rep. 1, 204–209.

Hu, F.B., Manson, J.E., Willett, W.C., 2001. Types of dietary fat and risk of coronary heart disease: a critical review. J. Am. Coll. Nutr. 20, 5–19.

Jenkins, D.J., Jones, P.J., Frohlich, J., Lamarche, B., Ireland, C., Nishi, S.K., Srichaikul, K., Galange, P., Pellini, C., Faulkner, D., De Souza, R.J., Sievenpiper, J.L., Mirrahimi, A., Jayalath, V.H., Augustin, L.S., Bashyam, B., Leiter, L.A., Josse, R., Couture, P., Ramprasath, V., Kendall, C.W., 2015. The effect of a dietary portfolio compared to a DASH-type diet on blood pressure. Nutr. Metab. Cardiovasc. Dis. 25, 1132–1139.

Joshipura, K.J., Ascherio, A., Manson, J.E., Stampfer, M.J., Rimm, E.B., Speizer, F.E., Hennekens, C.H., Spiegelman, D., Willett, W.C., 1999. Fruit and vegetable intake in relation to risk of ischemic stroke. JAMA 282, 1233–1239.

Joshipura, K.J., Hu, F.B., Manson, J.E., Stampfer, M.J., Rimm, E.B., Speizer, F.E., Colditz, G., Ascherio, A., Rosner, B., Spiegelman, D., Willett, W.C., 2001. The effect of fruit and vegetable intake on risk for coronary heart disease. Ann. Intern. Med. 134, 1106–1114.

Key, T., August 2, 2016. RE: Personal Communication.

Key, T.J., Fraser, G.E., Thorogood, M., Appleby, P.N., Beral, V., Reeves, G., Burr, M.L., Chang-Claude, J., Frentzel-Beyme, R., Kuzma, J.W., Mann, J., Mcpherson, K., 1999. Mortality in vegetarians and nonveg-etarians: detailed findings from a collaborative analysis of 5 prospective studies. Am. J. Clin. Nutr. 70, 516S–524S.

Knekt, P., Reunanen, A., Jarvinen, R., Seppanen, R., Heliovaara, M., Aromaa, A., 1994. Antioxidant vitamin intake and coronary mortality in a longitudinal population study. Am. J. Epidemiol. 139, 1180–1189.

Kris-Etherton, P.M., Zhao, G., Binkoski, A.E., Coval, S.M., Etherton, T.D., 2001. The effects of nuts on coro-nary heart disease risk. Nutr. Rev. 59, 103–111.

Liu, S., Stampfer, M.J., Hu, F.B., Giovannucci, E., Rimm, E., Manson, J.E., Hennekens, C.H., Willett, W.C., 1999. Whole-grain consumption and risk of coronary heart disease: results from the Nurses' Health Study. Am. J. Clin. Nutr. 70, 412–419.

Liu, S., Manson, J.E., Lee, I.M., Cole, S.R., Hennekens, C.H., Willett, W.C., Buring, J.E., 2000. Fruit and vegetable intake and risk of cardiovascular disease: the Women's Health Study. Am. J. Clin. Nutr. 72, 922–928.

Lorin, J., Zeller, M., Guilland, J.C., Cottin, Y., Vergely, C., Rochette, L., 2014. Arginine and nitric oxide syn-thase: regulatory mechanisms and cardiovascular aspects. Mol. Nutr. Food Res. 58, 101–116.

Mann, J.I., De Leeuw, I., Hermansen, K., Karamanos, B., Karlstrom, B., Katsilambros, N., Riccardi, G., Rivellese, A.A., Rizkalla, S., Slama, G., Toeller, M., Uusitupa, M., Vessby, B., 2004. Evidence-based nutri-tional approaches to the treatment and prevention of diabetes mellitus. Nutr. Metab. Cardiovasc. Dis. 14, 373–394.

Mann, J., McLean, R., 2017. Cardiovascular diseases. In: Mann, J., Truswell, S. (Eds.), Essentials of Human Nutrition, fifth ed. Oxford University Press, Oxford, UK.

Orlich, M.J., Singh, P.N., Sabate, J., Jaceldo-Siegl, K., Fan, J., Knutsen, S., Beeson, W.L., Fraser, G.E., 2013. Vegetarian dietary patterns and mortality in Adventist Health Study 2. JAMA Intern. Med. 173, 1230–1238.

Pan, A., Sun, Q., Bernstein, A.M., Schulze, M.B., Manson, J.E., Willett, W.C., Hu, F.B., 2011. Red meat con-sumption and risk of type 2 diabetes: 3 cohorts of US adults and an updated meta-analysis. Am. J. Clin. Nutr. 94, 1088–1096.

Riserus, U., Willett, W.C., Hu, F.B., 2009. Dietary fats and prevention of type 2 diabetes. Prog. Lipid Res. 48, 44–51.

Sacks, F.M., Svetkey, L.P., Vollmer, W.M., Appel, L.J., Bray, G.A., Harsha, D., Obarzanek, E., Conlin, P.R., Miller 3rd, E.R., Simons-Morton, D.G., Karanja, N., Lin, P.H., 2001. Effects on blood pressure of reduced dietary sodium and the Dietary Approaches to Stop Hypertension (DASH) diet. DASH-Sodium Collaborative Research Group. N. Engl. J. Med. 344, 3–10.

Schmidt, J.A., Rinaldi, S., Scalbert, A., Ferrari, P., Achaintre, D., Gunter, M.J., Appleby, P.N., Key, T.J., Travis, R.C., 2016. Plasma concentrations and intakes of amino acids in male meat-eaters, fish-eaters, vege-tarians and vegans: a cross-sectional analysis in the EPIC-Oxford cohort. Eur. J. Clin. Nutr. 70, 306–312.

Schwingshackl, L., Hoffmann, G., 2013. Comparison of effects of long-term low-fat vs high-fat diets on blood lipid levels in overweight or obese patients: a systematic review and meta-analysis. J. Acad. Nutr. Diet. 113, 1640–1661.

Snowdon, D.A., 1988. Animal product consumption and mortality because of all causes combined, cor-onary heart disease, stroke, diabetes, and cancer in Seventh-day Adventists. Am. J. Clin. Nutr. 48, 739–748.

Snowdon, D.A., Phillips, R.L., Fraser, G.E., 1984. Meat consumption and fatal ischemic heart disease. Prev. Med. 13, 490–500.

Thorogood, M., Carter, R., Benfield, L., Mcpherson, K., Mann, J.I., 1987. Plasma lipids and lipoprotein cho-lesterol concentrations in people with different diets in Britain. Br. Med. J. (Clin. Res. Ed.) 295, 351–353.

Thorogood, M., Mann, J., Appleby, P., Mcpherson, K., 1994. Risk of death from cancer and ischaemic heart disease in meat and non-meat eaters. BMJ 308, 1667–1670.

Wang, F., Zheng, J., Yang, B., Jiang, J., Fu, Y., Li, D., 2015. Effects of vegetarian diets on blood lipids: a systematic review and meta-analysis of randomized controlled trials. J. Am. Heart Assoc. 4, e002408.

Whelton, P.K., He, J., Cutler, J.A., Brancati, F.L., Appel, L.J., Follmann, D., Klag, M.J., 1997. Effects of oral potassium on blood pressure. Meta-analysis of randomized controlled clinical trials. JAMA 277, 1624–1632.

World Health Organisation, 2012. Guideline: Sodium Intake for Adults and Children. World Health Organisation (WHO), Geneva.

Yokoyama, Y., Nishimura, K., Barnard, N.D., Takegami, M., Watanabe, M., Sekikawa, A., Okamura, T., Miyamoto, Y., 2014. Vegetarian diets and blood pressure: a meta-analysis. JAMA Intern. Med. 174, 577–587.

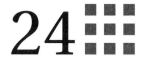

24

Vegetarian Diets and the Microbiome

Michael J. Orlich, Gina Siapco, Sarah Jung
LOMA LINDA UNIVERSITY, LOMA LINDA, CA, UNITED STATES

1. Introduction

The microbiome has become a hot topic. In the scientific community, it is viewed as an area of great promise for new understandings of human health and disease. In medicine, the use of fecal transplants (Manichanh et al., 2010) has recently suggested the potential for novel, effective therapies targeting the microbiome. The health-oriented public is being promised many benefits through microbiome-focused supplements, fortified foods, and books. Likewise, the topic has been prominently featured in popular media outlets such as the New York Times and National Public Radio. In this mix of well-founded scientific interest, commercial interests, and hype, we seek to review what we know about the microbiome, its potential relevance to human health, and specifically its relationship to vegetarian diets. We will begin with introductory information on the microbiome as a concept and field of study, including the important technologies that have brought it to the fore. We will then review some of what has been learned about the relevance of the microbiome to human health and disease: this will of necessity be illustrative, rather than comprehensive. Subsequently, we will examine the connections between diet—that highly complex and important set of exposures—and the microbiome. Specifically, we will focus on what is known regarding the relationship of vegetarian diets to the microbiome. We will end with some thoughts and questions regarding the future of this interesting field.

2. Background

We begin with terminology. The *microbiota* is the collection of all microbes in a certain location or environment, which can be thought of as forming a microbial community; this can include all microorganisms (such as viruses, microscopic fungi, protozoa, etc.), but the major focus is often on bacteria. It has also been described as the microbial flora, borrowing a term from the plant world, but microbiota has become the standard term. A closely related term is the *microbiome*, which refers to the collective genetic material of the community of microorganisms in a particular location or environment. Since genomic methods have become the primary tools for investigating the microbiota, the term microbiome has become the more predominant of the two and is often used synonymously with microbiota. For simplicity, we will generally use microbiome throughout this chapter, unless a particular distinction is called for.

Various animals, plants, locations, and other environmental niches all have their own microbiomes. Here we focus on human microbiomes. In humans, we can conceive and speak of the microbiome at different levels. We can refer to an individual's total microbiome being the collection of all microbes from all body sites. More expansively, we could conceive of a community microbiome, combining the microbiomes of related individuals. However, we usually focus on individuals and their unique microbiomes and then focus on site-specific microbiomes defined by a particular location, organ, or environment, such as the skin microbiome. Due to the focus of this book on diet and health, we will mostly be concerned about the microbiome of the digestive tract, or gut, from the mouth to the anus. More specifically, because of the large quantity and variety of microbes in the large intestine, or colon and rectum, the colorectal microbiome is a major focus of attention. The most common approach in humans to study the gut microbiome is through fecal samples, and so much relevant scientific evidence relates to the fecal microbiome. Thus, unless otherwise specified, reference to the microbiome in this chapter is to the human gut microbiome generally, as reflected in fecal microbiome samples.

Microbes thought to be beneficial to the human host (or at least not harmful) and which constitute a normal part of the human microbiome are often referred to as *commensals*. In contrast, microbes thought to be harmful or disease-causing are called pathogens; the term *pathobionts* is used when microbes sometimes cause disease as opportunistic pathogens, when they predominate, or through indirect mechanisms. When the microbiota is altered in a way thought to be detrimental to health or to promote disease, this is sometimes labeled *dysbiosis*. It should be borne in mind that these labels may be attempts to oversimplify complex relationships that are often not yet well understood, so the categorical judgements they imply must be interpreted cautiously.

Interest in the microbes that inhabit humans, their link to diet, and their impact upon health is not new. Antonie van Leeuwenhoek's lenses revealed an amazing world of microscopic organisms in the 17th century. The early triumphs of the germ theory of disease by Pasteur, Koch, and others in the late 19th and early 20th centuries heralded a revolution in medical science and practice. At this time, Ilya Ilyich Mechnikov theorized that toxic gut bacteria might contribute to aging and disease and advocated consumption of yogurt and lactobacillus. Similar theories of colonic putrefaction and autointoxication were popularized by John Harvey Kellogg at his famous Battle Creek Sanitarium. Such early theories and related therapies persist today in the use of so-called probiotics (microorganisms that have health benefits when ingested) and in some alternative medicine practices such as colon "cleanses" and colonics. For more than a 100 years, scientists, physicians, and others have hypothesized links between healthy and unhealthy colonic microbial communities and health, chronic disease, and aging. Why then has the microbiome recently become such a strong area of scientific interest? What has changed to cause such a renaissance of interest in the microbial flora of the gut? The answer lies in the technical and scientific revolution that is genomics.

2.1 Microbiome Methodologies

The last quarter century witnessed an exponential increase in our ability to sequence DNA. It took years for many laboratories around the United States, working together in a Manhattan-project-style effort, to sequence the complete human genome for the first time. Now, automated, "next-generation" sequencing machines that employ mass parallel ("shotgun") sequencing approaches and use bioinformatics algorithms to sort and assemble the sequence data are able to sequence an entire human genome in a matter of hours. These developments in genomics have led to a revolution in microbiology. Classical microbiology relied on staining and microscopy methods on the one hand and culture methods on the other. Unfortunately, many bacteria were very difficult to isolate and identify using these traditional methods, which were also laborious and thus costly. As a result, our knowledge of microbes inhabiting the human gut (and other environments) was quite limited, usually to more easily cultured species. While classical microbiology methods continue to be important, genomics methods have become powerful tools in microbiology. It is now possible to simultaneously sequence DNA from all of the microbes in a particular environment and use bioinformatics methods to identify which microbes are present, in what relative abundances, and what are some of their functional capabilities, all without growing any of these organisms in culture.

We now briefly review the principal genomics methodologies currently used to study the microbiome, considering their relative advantages. These approaches are referred to as metagenomics methods, because they involve sequencing DNA from the whole community of microorganisms together, rather than from isolated individual organisms. The first major approach relies on targeted sequencing of a particular gene or DNA region. For bacteria, this usually involves sequencing the gene encoding the RNA that forms the bacterial 16S ribosomal subunit (Inglis et al., 2012; Weinstock, 2012). This 16S ribosomal subunit is not present in eukaryotic cells, so it is specific to bacteria. It is shared by all bacteria and has nine variable regions (Inglis et al., 2012; Kuczynski et al., 2012) where sequence differences have gradually accumulated over the course of evolutionary time. Thus, by comparing sequence similarities of the 16S ribosomal subunit RNA gene, a phylogenetic, or evolutionary, tree can be reconstructed, and species and strains can be identified by their location in this taxonomic framework. In addition, libraries have been constructed of 16S sequences for known species and strains, so many of these can be identified precisely by name based upon the 16S sequence. So the 16S ribosomal subunit sequencing method can be used for broad and comprehensive taxonomic classification of a microbiome, that is, the identification of which microbes are present. It can also give information regarding the relative abundance of the various microbial taxa, though such relative abundance estimates may be somewhat biased due to systematically different polymerase chain reaction (PCR) amplification (Inglis et al., 2012). Accuracy of relative abundance at the species level has been demonstrated for certain bacteria in particular projects (Conlan et al., 2012). While sequencing of the entire 16S RNA gene including all nine variable regions yields good species-level specificity, current high-throughput sequencing methods typically can only sequence smaller lengths of DNA. Consequently, only three variable regions are often covered, yielding somewhat less accuracy at the species level, but good accuracy at higher taxonomic levels (Inglis et al., 2012; Weinstock, 2012). Careful strategies may maximize the taxonomic information for a given sequencing method (Kuczynski et al., 2012). In general, targeted sequencing methods have the advantage of being relatively fast, easy, and inexpensive, given that only a single gene need to be amplified and sequenced.

However, though targeted sequencing methods provide important information about the taxonomic distribution and relative abundances, they do not directly give information about the genes present in the microbiome and the functions coded for by those genes. This distinction is magnified by the phenomenon of lateral gene transfer, by which bacteria commonly obtain genes from neighboring bacteria of other species. Thus, the phylogeny of a bacterium may not correlate very well with its genetic composition. Gene-frequency information can be obtained by a broader sequencing strategy, referred to as whole-genome shotgun (WGS) sequencing. In WGS, a collective random sample of the complete genomes of all organisms in the microbiome is sequenced, rather than a single gene (Weinstock, 2012). The advantages and costs of this approach are obvious. This approach requires much more DNA to be sequenced, and is thus more time-intensive and costly. However, it yields far more information than the 16S method. It not only allows for taxonomic identification and relative abundances, but also provides functional data. Two taxonomically distinct bacteria may share certain genes that relate to a specific physiologic function, which may be of interest. WGS is able to identify the presence of particular functional genes in the microbiome and the abundances of these genes, thus providing a gene profile of the collective microbial community, which may reveal some of the collective metabolic or physiologic functional capacity of the microbiome.

2.2 The Human Microbiome

The application of these genomics methods to the study of the human microbiome has received much attention recently. Several major projects have begun to provide a foundational knowledge regarding the human microbiome. Among the most important of these has been the Human Microbiome Project (HMP) of the US National Institutes of Health (NIH) (Turnbaugh et al., 2007; Group et al., 2009). The HMP was established in 2008, funded by the NIH, as a coordinated effort of several sequencing centers. The project has included efforts at sequencing the complete genomes of many individual microbes, developing tools and technologies for the study of the microbiome and analysis of microbiomic data (Gevers et al., 2012), and the application metagenomics approaches to microbiome analysis in a reference population of healthy adults at several body regions (Group et al., 2009) including the nasal passages, oral cavity, skin, gastrointestinal tract, and vagina, with multiple sampling sites in some regions (Aagaard et al., 2013; Proctor, 2011) (http://hmp-dacc.org/overview/about.php).

The HMP has now included repeated sampling of multiple body sites in hundreds of healthy adults, yielding a large and valuable reference dataset for the range of variation in the normal human microbiome (Human Microbiome Project, 2012a). A new phase of the HMP is seeking to analyze changes in the microbiome and host functional properties over time (Integrative, 2014). Another important human microbiome reference project is the Metagenomics of the Human Intestinal Tract (MetaHIT) project, financed by the European Commission, which focuses on a WGS approach to the intestinal microbiome, seeking to provide a large microbiome gene database that might be relevant to a disease risk (Qin et al., 2010) (http://www.metahit.eu/). The International Human Microbiome Consortium (http://www.human-microbiome.org/) seeks to promote cooperation and data sharing among human microbiome projects.

The human gut microbiome composition dynamically changes based on feeding and other environmental exposures from birth onward. In the adult microbiome, the majority of bacteria typically belong to two phyla: the Firmicutes (which includes *Clostridium*, *Enterococcus*, *Lactobacillus*, and *Ruminococcus*) and the Bacteroidetes (which includes the *Bacteroides* and *Prevotella*) (Arumugam et al., 2011; Eckburg et al., 2005). One interesting finding has been the identification of "enterotypes," or distinct clusters of individuals with similar patterns of species abundance in the gut. Three enterotypes have been described, with three genera of bacteria, *Bacteroides*, *Prevotella*, and *Ruminococcus*, each being the predominant genus of its respective enterotype (Arumugam et al., 2011). However, analysis of HMP and MetaHIT data by others have revealed more continuous gradations of relative abundance, rather than supporting distinct enterotypes, suggesting possible dependence on analytic techniques (Koren et al., 2013).

3. The Microbiome in Health and Disease

The human gut microbiome plays many important roles in human physiology and development and thus in health. Examples are its role in nutrition and metabolism, its involvement in the development and proper function of both the gut mucosa and the immune system, and the protection it provides against pathogens. The genetic diversity of the microorganisms in the gut makes available various enzymes and biochemical pathways distinct from those of the host. For example, the nutrients vitamin K and biotin are both produced in the gut by bacteria. Gut bacteria can also produce the mood-regulating neurotransmitter serotonin, as well as enzymes to metabolize drugs, toxins, and hormones. But what constitutes a healthy microbiome? What relative abundances of various bacterial species and strains (or of related microbial genes) are associated with optimal health (and under what environmental or dietary conditions)? And which changes in the balance and composition of the microbiome might lead to the development or worsening of diseases, and thus to ill health? These are important and interesting questions and are the subject of much ongoing research.

The study of the human microbiome is still relatively new, with survey projects such as HMP and MetaHIT seeking to provide a better understanding of the characteristics and variation of the "normal" microbiome in healthy humans (Human Microbiome Project, 2012b). Such efforts will help to provide context for microbiome findings in the setting of disease. Certain concepts that might define a healthy microbiome have been proposed, including ecologic stability (or resilience) and a favorable functional profile, which might provide benefits to the host (Backhed et al., 2012). Preliminary associations of microbiome patterns with disease states should be interpreted with caution, given the current limited state of knowledge. Nonetheless, there is great interest in the role that alterations in the microbiome may play in the pathogenesis of diseases. Considerable research efforts have begun to explore such connections.

We will now examine a few interesting findings linking the microbiome to several important diseases in humans. Many of the initial findings are from cross-sectional comparisons, where the direction of association is particularly difficult to discern; prospective studies of such associations are needed (Mai and Morris, 2013).

3.1 Infectious Diseases

A link between infectious diseases and the human microbiome might be expected, but the nature of such a link could be complex and variable. There are indicators that commensal bacteria, or bacteria indigenous to the host, provide protection against enteric pathogens, for instance by competing for sites of colonization and nutrient uptake. Commensal bacteria also activate the production of barrier immunity factors that prevent pathogen contact with host mucosa and augment the immune response against invading pathogens (Khosravi and Mazmanian, 2013). The microbiome may impact the virulence and pathogenesis of infectious pathogens. For example, in a mouse model for human infections, competition with the normal microbiome reduced pathogen infectivity and required the expression of virulence factors in the pathogen, which were not needed for virulence in germ-free hosts (Kamada et al., 2012). Such concepts of competitive defense by commensals in the microbiome have led to hypotheses about the role of probiotics in the prevention of important infections, such as pneumococcal disease (Licciardi et al., 2012). Infectious diseases may alter the microbiome by reducing diversity and by increasing harmful while decreasing beneficial microbe populations as a part of the pathogenic process (Zhang et al., 2015b). For example, early research suggests that alterations in the gut microbiome may play a role in HIV pathogenesis (Gori et al., 2008).

3.2 Inflammation and Inflammatory Diseases

A primary role of the immune system is to monitor for and defend against potential harm by external agents such as microbes. There must then be substantial interactions between the host immune system and the microbiome. These are likely to be complex and bidirectional, with the immune system regulating the microbiome, and the microbiome stimulating, suppressing, or modulating the immune system. Given that activation of components of the immune system is central to inflammatory conditions and autoimmune disorders, it has been proposed that factors affecting the microbiome may contribute to the pathogenesis of these disorders (Belkaid and Hand, 2014). Evidence also exists, both in humans (Blekhman et al., 2015) and in animals

(Schokker et al., 2015), that host genetic variation is associated with microbiome composition. Interactions of host genetic factors with the environment, specifically the microbial environment, would often modulate the extent and direction of inflammatory response (Mclean and El-Omar, 2009).

A breakdown of the protective intestinal mucosal barrier may be an important step in the pathogenesis of inflammatory conditions. In an animal model, it has been demonstrated that the colon is protected from its resident microbes by two-layers of structure of the protein mucin 2 (Johansson et al., 2008), where the inner layer is firmly attached to the epithelium and free from bacteria, while the outer layer is movable and colonized by bacteria. Disruption of this mucosal barrier structure by chemicals ingested or due to altered bacterial composition can result in the translocation of bacteria to the inner mucus layer and damage to the epithelial wall (Johansson et al., 2008), which eventually leads to a mucosal inflammatory response. Such mucosal barrier breakdown, along with alterations in epithelial cell junctions, can lead to abnormal intestinal permeability (sometimes referred to as "leaky gut"), which may be relevant to systemic inflammatory conditions. Increased intestinal permeability allows the translocation of bacterial or microbiome-derived lipopolysaccharides (LPS), also known as lipoglycans or endotoxins, into the bloodstream. If plasma LPS levels increase two to three times the normal level (which is 10–50 times lower than found in septicemia or infections), a threshold defined as metabolic endotoxemia is reached (Cani et al., 2007). Metabolic endotoxemia may set off toll-like receptor 4–mediated inflammatory activation that can precipitate low-grade inflammation and oxidative stress (Cani et al., 2008; Neves et al., 2013), both of which are associated with obesity (Boutagy et al., 2016; Neves et al., 2013), metabolic (Luche et al., 2013), and cardiovascular (Neves et al., 2013) diseases.

Specific microbiome patterns, often with substantial alterations in composition and complexity, have been associated with inflammatory bowel disease (IBD) (Kostic et al., 2014). In fact, such associations have led to the development of microbiome-based diagnostic methods for IBD (Papa et al., 2012). It is suspected that dietary factors may impact IBD through microbiome alterations (Lee et al., 2015). For example, the reduction in commensal bacteria that use fermentable substrates for energy may lead to increased inflammation since the short-chain fatty acids (SCFAs) they produce can inhibit gastrointestinal inflammation (Belkaid and Hand, 2014). The microbiome may be a factor in nongastrointestinal inflammatory conditions as well. Dysbiosis has been associated with rheumatoid arthritis (RA), and the resolution of dysbiosis might help in the treatment of RA (Zhang et al., 2015a).

3.3 Obesity

Much attention has been given in the last 10 years to a potential link between the microbiome and obesity. It appears that the microbiome is essential for maximal caloric extraction from food. Germ-free mice are much leaner than those with a normal microbiome, despite similar or greater food intake (Backhed et al., 2004). In addition to caloric extraction, the microbiome may affect eating behaviors, generating either food cravings or dysphoria

(Alcock et al., 2014). One characteristic of the microbiome that may be relevant to obesity is bacterial gene richness (as measured by the number of microbial genes), with low richness associated with obesity (Le Chatelier et al., 2013). Relative abundances may also be important. Obese people have been found to have relatively fewer Bacteroidetes compared to lean people (Ley et al., 2006). A reduced ratio of Bacteroidetes to Firmicutes has been shown to correlate with obesity and metabolic diseases (Arora and Sharma, 2011). Other bacterial biomarkers are still emerging.

3.4 Diabetes Mellitus

Diabetes mellitus may be related to the microbiome in more than one way. Type 1 diabetes is an autoimmune disease. It has been hypothesized that dysbiosis and increased gut permeability may lead to autoimmunity in this condition (Davis-Richardson and Triplett, 2015). Type II diabetes is characterized by insulin resistance, and it is strongly correlated to obesity. Thus, an obesogenic microbiome may increase diabetes risk. Insulin-resistant women with previous gestational diabetes have been found to have higher proportions of Pevotellaceae and lower abundances of Firmicutes than women who had normoglycemic pregnancies (Fugmann et al., 2015).

3.5 Cardiovascular Disease

A rather specific link between the gut microbiome and atherosclerotic cardiovascular disease (CVD) has been proposed. Hazen et al. have found that serum trimethylamine-*N*-oxide (TMAO) is correlated with CVD risk in humans and can promote atherogenesis in animal models (Brown and Hazen, 2014). TMAO has also been associated with disease severity, poor clinical outcomes, and survival in congestive heart failure (Tang et al., 2015; Troseid et al., 2015). TMAO can be produced by the metabolism of dietary L-carnitine, abundant in red meat, by the intestinal microbiome (Koeth et al., 2013). TMAO can similarly be produced by the microbiome-mediated metabolism of phosphatidylcholine (lecithin), abundant in egg yolks (Tang et al., 2013; Wang et al., 2011). This diet-microbiome-TMAO-CVD pathway has been described as "a new direction in cardiovascular research" (Lim, 2013), offering a novel mechanism by which red meat and egg yolks may promote atherosclerosis, and pointing to the gut microbiome as an environmental risk factor for CVD (Stock, 2013).

3.6 Cancer

Emerging microbiome tools and data sources may play an important role in cancer epidemiology (Lampe, 2008). A number of microbe–cancer connections are well established, such as that between *Helicobacter pylori* and gastric cancer; in fact 15% of cancer cases are estimated to be attributable to infectious agents (Abreu and Peek, 2014). However, beyond such well-established connections between particular microbes (e.g., *H. pylori*, Epstein–Barr virus, human papillomavirus, etc.) and specific cancers, there is much interest in the potential role of more complex or varied changes in the microbiome affecting the risk of cancers (e.g., does fecal microbiome composition affect colorectal cancer risk?). The microbiome may affect cancer risk by modulating inflammation or host gene expression (even epigenetically) (Bultman, 2014; Gagliani et al., 2014). Gut microbial metabolites may have procarcinogenic effects (e.g., secondary bile acids) or protective effects (e.g., SCFAs like butyrate) (Louis et al., 2014; Ou et al., 2013). In animal models, fecal transplantation has been able to modify cancer risk, with an effect remaining across generations (Poutahidis et al., 2015). In humans, case–control studies examining the microbiome and colorectal cancer (CRC) have been conducted. In one, CRC was associated with a reduced microbiome diversity (Ahn et al., 2013). CRC cases also had lower relative abundances of *Clostridium* and higher abundances of *Fusobacterium* and *Porphyromonas* (Ahn et al., 2013). In one study comparing CRC patients with healthy volunteers, CRC patients had more opportunistic pathogens and a reduced number of butyrate-producing bacteria (Wang et al., 2012).

4. Diet and the Microbiome

Having introduced the microbiome as a subject of study and having surveyed some early evidence of the relationship of the microbiome to health and disease, we now turn our attention to the relationship between diet and the microbiome. As one of the major environmental factors that affect the microbiome, diet plays an important role in shaping its diversity and functionality (Maukonen and Saarela, 2015; Moschen et al., 2012). Before examining the evidence specific to vegetarian diets and the microbiome, we will first consider a number of dietary factors, such as nutrients. Several of these dietary aspects may be relevant to an understanding of vegetarian diets and the microbiome.

4.1 Probiotics and Fermented Foods

When considering the effects of diet on the microbiome, perhaps the most obvious place to start is with foods rich in live microorganisms. Many traditional fermented foods have live bacteria or yeasts. These include yogurt, buttermilk, certain cheeses, kefir, sauerkraut, kimchi, kombucha, and miso. Originally, such foods likely became popular primarily because the fermentation lowered their sugar content and/or increased their acidity, helping to preserve the foods from spoiling and extend their "shelf life." In addition to these, there are now many commercial food products with live bacterial cultures added as well as bacterial culture supplements. The live microorganisms in these foods and/or supplements are generally referred to as *probiotics*, based on the concept that consumption of these is likely to be beneficial to the host, often due to their effects on the microbiome. However, not all bacterial strains have probiotic properties, and the purported health effects of probiotics have been demonstrated to be strain-specific (Luyer et al., 2005; Kekkonen, 2008). The World Health Organization defines probiotics as "live microorganisms which when administered in adequate amounts confer a health benefit on the host" and has a set of guidelines to determine if a bacterial strain can be correctly classified as a probiotic (WHO, 2002). But does the consumption of probiotics truly benefit the gut microbiome? What are the impacts? Research is now exploring these questions.

In general, the benefits of probiotics may include "antipathogenic effects, immunomodulatory features, regulation of cell proliferation, the ability to promote normal physiologic development of the mucosal epithelium, and enhancement of human nutrition" (Hsieh and Versalovic, 2008). Strains from lactobacilli (Giraffa, 2012), enterococci (Wang et al., 2014), and bifidobacteria (Di Gioia et al., 2014) are the most studied and commonly used probiotics. *Bifidobacterium* species are predominant in the gut of breastfed infants, and they may help to prevent infections with gram-negative pathogens (Lievin et al., 2000). Probiotics can enhance certain metabolic pathways, such as the conversion of prebiotic oligosaccharides to SCFAs. In a mouse model, *Bifidobacterium longum* supplementation increased production of biotin and butyrate (Sugahara et al., 2015). Consumption of a fermented milk product that included *Bifidobacterium animalis* was demonstrated to enhance SCFA production (Veiga et al., 2014). In addition, it led to a decreased abundance of a pathological bacterial strain (Veiga et al., 2014), illustrating the possible protection from pathogens through probiotic strain competition or inhibition.

It appears that ingested probiotics may interact with resident commensal strains in complex ways, including gene expression regulation and alteration of the metabolic activity of the host strains (Arora et al., 2013). Importantly, probiotics may help to prevent or control certain diseases. Milk fermented with *Lactobacillus casei* (Shirota strain) appeared to reduce both the incidence and duration of upper respiratory infections in adult men (Shida et al., 2015). Probiotics may play a role in the prevention and treatment of obesity (Arora et al., 2013). Probiotic lactic acid bacteria and bifidobacteria may be helpful in the treatment of ulcerative colitis and synbiotics in the treatment of Crohn's disease (Saez-Lara et al., 2015). In celiac disease, probiotics seem to reduce inflammation as they restore the balance of beneficial bacteria in the gastrointestinal tract (Marasco et al., 2016). It has been argued that probiotics may even contribute to mental health (Selhub et al., 2014) including the prevention of depression (Logan and Katzman, 2005).

4.2 Carbohydrates and Prebiotics

Carbohydrates, including sugars and starches, are major sources of energy in the human diet. However, there are also many carbohydrates not catabolized by human digestive enzymes, which thus remain intact until they reach the large intestine. These include certain short-chain carbohydrates, or oligosaccharides, such as fructooligosaccharides (e.g., from certain vegetables) and galactooligosaccharides (e.g., from human milk), and longer chain polysaccharides that include resistant starches and nonstarch polysaccharides. These components of dietary fiber have been traditionally valued for their physical property of adding to fecal bulk and decreasing transit time. However, many of the beneficial effects attributed to these humanly indigestible carbohydrates may also be a result of their fermentation and digestion by the colonic microbiota. As an energy source, many microbial species are able enzymatically to break down the dietary fiber molecules because of genes that encode carbohydrate-active enzymes (El Kaoutari et al., 2013). As these indigestible carbohydrates reach the colon, they are fermented by commensal bacteria, so they are designated *prebiotics*. The types and amounts of carbohydrates available are probably the factors that most shape the composition of the microbiome (Cantarel et al., 2012).

One possible consequence of the microbial digestion of such carbohydrates is the increased energy extraction from food. This relates to the discussion in the previous section of the microbiome and obesity. In this case, the enhanced energy extraction from humanly indigestible carbohydrates by bacteria may be beneficial to the human host in food-scarcity situations, but obesogenic in many modern, food-rich environments.

Another consequence of microbial carbohydrate digestion is the production of chemical compounds. In particular, bacterial metabolism of oligosaccharides leads to the production of short-chain fatty acids (SCFAs) such as acetate, propionate, and butyrate. Such SCFAs, particularly butyrate, seem to be important substrates for the healthy maintenance of the colonic epithelium. In the normal colon, butyrate promotes the integrity of the mucosal barrier by regulating colonic motility, cell growth, and differentiation, and it modulates the immune and inflammatory response (Fung et al., 2012). In colorectal tumor cells, butyrate induces apoptosis by activating the intrinsic and extrinsic apoptosis pathways and inducing autophagic cell death; inhibits histone deacetylation that arrests tumorigenesis; and reduces inflammation by regulating inflammatory factors including nuclear factor NF-κB (Fung et al., 2012). An adequate supply of SCFAs may be relevant for the prevention of conditions such as inflammatory bowel diseases or colorectal cancer (Zampa et al., 2004; Toden et al., 2007b). For example, SCFAs produced from the microbial fermentation of undigested bean components inhibited the growth of a human colon cancer cell line (HT-29), and they induced morphological changes and modulated expression of proteins related to apoptosis (Campos-Vega et al., 2012). On the other hand, diets low in carbohydrates (including fiber), may impact gut health by leading to a reduced production of SCFAs (Duncan et al., 2007). These SCFAs also serve as substrate for synthesis of long-chain fatty acids, cholesterol, and other substances (Den Besten et al., 2013).

Whatever the mechanisms by which they may affect human physiology, saccharides seem to be important in shaping the gut microbiome. Fructooligosaccharides (FOS) and β-galactooligosaccharides (GOS), two of the currently established prebiotics, stimulate the gram-positive, strictly fermentative saccharolytic microorganisms, *Bifidobacteria* and *Lactobacilli* (Goh and Klaenhammer, 2015). Some of the natural food sources of FOS are Jerusalem artichoke tubers, chicory roots, onions, bananas, garlic, asparagus, jícama, leeks, yacón, and blue agave. Lentils are a good source of GOS and resistant starches, which also serve as prebiotics (Johnson et al., 2013). In an early study in rats colonized with human microbiota, consumption of resistant starch led to a 10- to 100-fold increase in *Lactobacilli* and *Bifidobacteria* and decreases in enterobacteria when compared to consumption of sucrose (Silvi et al., 1999). In a more recent human feeding study, a 60-g daily dose of whole grains resulted in increased microbial diversity and a higher ratio of Firmicutes to Bacteroidetes, while also leading to lower levels of plasma IL-6 and peak postprandial glucose (Martinez et al., 2013).

Human milk contains prebiotic oligosaccharides that confer immuno-protective effects, among many others, on the breastfed infant. Prebiotic supplementation of infant formula shows some evidence of improvement in intestinal microbiota, metabolic activity, stool consistency and frequency, and development of some immune markers (Vandenplas et al., 2015); however, despite efforts to mimic human milk, evidence is insufficient to equate the benefits of prebiotic-supplemented infant formula to those of human milk (Vandenplas et al., 2014). During infancy, the period when brain cholesterol synthesis is highest coincides with increased production of acetate in the gut during breastfeeding (Edwards et al., 1994; Mischke and Plosch, 2013), which indicates the possible role of human milk prebiotics in the brain development of breastfed infants.

Prebiotics may also reduce serum triglycerides (Causey et al., 2000), improve treatment of *Clostridium difficile*-associated diarrhea in adult patients (Lewis et al., 2005), and reduce the incidence of atopic dermatitis (Baquerizo Nole et al., 2014), and eczema (Moro et al., 2006; Osborn and Sinn, 2013). Intentional combination of probiotics with prebiotics (i.e., synbiotics) seems to favor the colonization and growth of beneficial bacteria in the gut. Adhesion of the live bacteria to prebiotic granules in some synbiotic products may help ensure the viability of the ingested probiotic when it reaches the large intestine (Topping et al., 2003). In children, synbiotics improved the survival and proliferation of both the beneficial allochthonous (i.e., probiotic) and autochthonous (i.e., commensals) bacteria in the intestinal tract compared to probiotics alone (Piirainen et al., 2008). In an elderly population, the ingestion of a probiotic followed by a prebiotic resulted in an increase of beneficial types of bacteria and organic acid production compared to the probiotic alone (Nyangale et al., 2014).

4.3 Fats

The quantity and types of dietary fat consumed appear to impact the gut microbiome. In a mouse model, a high-saturated-fat diet resulted in reduced diversity of the microbiome and an increased ratio of Firmicutes to Bacteroidetes as well as weight gain and liver fat accumulation, compared to a low-fat diet or to diets high in monounsaturated or polyunsaturated fats (De Wit et al., 2012). Changes in the fecal microbiome from high-fat diets may be linked to cancer risk. One explanation is the reduction in the integrity of the intestinal mucosa due to an increase in gut microbes that secrete pro-inflammatory compounds (Moreira et al., 2012; Shen et al., 2014). This can result in the diffusion of lipopolysaccharides or endotoxins from the gut to the circulatory system, which can trigger an inflammatory response (Moreira et al., 2012). Diets high in long-chain saturated fatty acids may lead to obesity due to a decrease in mucin-producing bacteria shown (in a mouse model) to inhibit the development of diet-induced obesity and to the production of proinflammatory compounds that can enhance energy harvest (Shen et al., 2014). On the other hand, evidence from cell culture models suggests mechanisms by which diets rich in n-3 polyunsaturated fatty acids may protect colonocytes from proinflammatory insults by reducing proinflammatory eicosanoid production, inhibiting the activation of proinflammatory mitogen-activated protein kinases (MAPKs) and oxidative stress pathways, and increasing peroxisome proliferator-activated receptor gamma (PPARγ) or G protein–coupled receptor 120 (GRP120) (Shen et al., 2014). In mice susceptible to intestinal cancer due to a K-ras mutation, a high-fat diet led to changes in microbiome composition, immune system modification, and tumor progression (Schulz et al., 2014). However, when butyrate was also administered, some of the immune system function was restored and tumor progression attenuated (Schulz et al., 2014). This suggests that diets high in fiber, leading to the production of butyrate, may be partially protective against the possible cancer risks of high-fat diets, with both the risk and protective factors being mediated through changes in the microbiome. In this same model, fecal samples from mice fed high-fat diets were able to transmit the carcinogenic effect to mice not fed high-fat diets, and antibiotic administration blocked the tumor formation associated with high-fat diets, both of these facts underscoring the key role of the microbiome in carcinogenesis in this model (Schulz et al., 2014). While high-fat diets cause important and consequential changes in the microbiome, these changes appear to be reversible over a period of weeks in mice, when the dietary fats are returned to normal levels (Zhang et al., 2012).

4.4 Proteins

Dietary proteins provide colonic bacteria with the nitrogen needed for growth. Dietary protein that escapes digestion in the small intestines increases the amount of nitrogenous substrate in the colon, which can increase putrefactive fermentation, particularly if fermentable carbohydrate levels are low (Silvester and Cummings, 1995). The concentration of a number of chemicals shown in animal and in vivo studies to be cytotoxic, genotoxic, and carcinogenic—ammonia, phenols, hydrogen sulfide, amines, thiols, and indoles—subsequently increases (Hughes et al., 2000). A high-protein, low-carbohydrate diet may favor the growth of harmful proinflammatory bacteria that, combined with increased amounts of putrefactive fermentation products, can lead to colonic epithelial damage and mucosal inflammation (Yao et al., 2016). Excessive colonic protein fermentation—often in the context of protein supplementation or high-protein diets with carbohydrate restriction—is associated with irritable bowel syndrome, ulcerative colitis, and colorectal carcinogenesis (Yao et al., 2016). High-protein, low-carbohydrate diets are also associated with greater DNA damage in colonic mucosa (Russell et al., 2011). Both animal (Conlon et al., 2009; Toden et al., 2007a) and human studies (Humphreys et al., 2014) show that resistant starch, a fermentable carbohydrate, attenuates colonic damage brought about by high-protein intake. These studies also indicate that different types of protein differ in their effects on colonocyte DNA.

4.5 Phytochemicals

Phytochemicals are a wide variety of nonnutritive chemical compounds found in plant foods, which may have health effects. A few examples of well-known phytochemicals are the flavonoids, phenolic acids, isoflavones, curcumin, isothiocyanates, and carotenoids. The many phytochemicals in common plant foods, herbs, and spices represent a broad range of chemical compounds. Most phytochemicals have low bioavailability; thus, many reach the large intestines and are acted upon by the gut microbiota. Given the diverse and robust metabolic capabilities of microbes, we would expect that microbial metabolism of phytochemicals would be complex, and potentially important. Microbial phytochemical metabolism would be of interest in elucidating the health effects of phytochemicals.

Isoflavones and lignans are phytoestrogens found in soy and other foods, which may affect breast cancer risk. In germ-free rats fed a diet high in soy isoflavones, both daidzein and genistein (both soy isoflavones) are well absorbed. However, the lignan enterolactone and the isoflavone metabolites O-desmethylangolensin and equol were not detected in urine (not absorbed) in germ-free mice but were in mice with a human fecal microbiome, thus illustrating the essential role of the microbial metabolism in the absorption of these phytoestrogens (Bowey et al., 2003). Polyphenols have some degree of antimicrobial effect, which may help to modulate microbiome composition (Cueva et al., 2015), though the inhibitory effect appears to vary greatly with the specific polyphenol and the type of intestinal bacteria (Duda-Chodak, 2012). Conversely, the microbiome appears to play an important role in the metabolism of polyphenols (Duda-Chodak et al., 2015). Glucosinolates in cruciferous vegetables are converted to more active isothiocyanates by enzymes that coexist in the plant but which are inactivated by heat; in that case, conversion of glucosinolates to isothiocyanates is dependent on the gut microbiome, and this conversion is blocked by antibiotics and varies largely among individuals (Fahey et al., 2012). The microbiome composition thus seems important in determining the effective exposure to isothiocyanates. As with polyphenols, the glucosinolate–microbiome relationship appears to be bidirectional. In human-microbiota-associated rats, consumption of Brussels sprouts (a glucosinolate-containing crucifer) was shown to increase the production of acetate by gut microbes (Humblot et al., 2005). In a human crossover feeding study, a high cruciferous vegetable diet appeared to alter microbiome composition compared to a control diet, but the nature of that alteration was individual specific (Li et al., 2009).

4.6 Artificial Compounds and Food Additives

Modern diets often contain a variety of food additives and artificial compounds. Microbial metabolism of such compounds or the impact of such compounds on gut microbes may be important in mediating any health effects. A potentially important example of the latter is that of dietary emulsifiers. These are detergent-like compounds added to many processed foods. There is concern that such emulsifying agents might disrupt the protective intestinal mucus layers. In mice, common emulsifiers led to altered microbiome composition along with inflammation, obesity, and the metabolic syndrome (Chassaing et al., 2015). In susceptible mice, the emulsifiers led to overt colitis (Chassaing et al., 2015).

Another class of artificial compounds common in modern diets is that of the non-sugar sweeteners. These have seemed to be attractive alternatives to sugar, particularly in the control of obesity and diabetes, since they cannot be catabolized by humans and thus have no caloric value. Surprisingly, however, in some epidemiologic studies, diet soft drinks made with artificial sweeteners are associated with obesity and diabetes to a similar degree as sugar-sweetened soft drinks. How can this be the case? The microbiome may provide part of the answer. In mouse models, consumption of artificial sweeteners caused changes in the composition and functions of the gut microbiome and led to glucose intolerance (Suez et al., 2014). The glucose intolerance was transferrable by fecal transplantation. In a small number of healthy human subjects, artificial sweeteners also led to microbiome changes and glucose intolerance (Suez et al., 2014). Again, the glucose intolerance was transferrable to mice by fecal transplantation from the affected human subjects. It thus appears that artificial sweeteners, despite having no calories, may not provide a "free lunch," and may in fact have adverse metabolic effects mediated by alterations to the gut microbiome. Chronic exposure to artificial sweeteners "may cause dysbiosis with loss of microbial genetic and phylogenetic diversity"(Payne et al., 2012).

4.7 Dietary Patterns

Along with the specific nutrients, foods, and food additives already discussed, another way to consider the impact of diet on the microbiome is at the level of broader dietary patterns. Such dietary patterns can vary in their classification and definitions. Some are traditional, such as the Mediterranean diet and the vegetarian diet. Some have been theoretically constructed, such as the DASH diet. Others have been derived with data-driven methods. In the next section, we will explore the relationship of vegetarian dietary patterns to the microbiome.

The Mediterranean diet is patterned after certain traditional eating patterns of southern European countries like Greece. It has been associated with numerous health benefits and is often characterized by high amounts of olive oil, fruits, nuts, vegetables, and cereals; moderate amounts of fish and poultry; low amounts of dairy, red and processed meats, and sweets; and moderate intake of red wine. In one observational study, greater adherence to a Mediterranean diet pattern was associated with lower levels of urinary TMAO, a microbially derived compound linked with cardiovascular disease (De Filippis et al., 2015).

5. Vegetarian Diets and the Microbiome

We now turn our attention specifically to the relationship of vegetarian diets and the gut microbiome. The scientific literature specific to this relationship remains quite small, though growing. What is known about how vegetarian diets may affect the gut microbiome is therefore much less than the questions that remain.

5.1 International Comparisons

Studies of geographically and culturally distinct populations with widely differing dietary habits suggest the potential for large differences. De Filippo et al. (2010) compared the fecal microbiome of children in Europe (EU) with children in rural Burkina Faso (BF) and found quite different microbiome patterns. Compared to the European diet, the BF diet was described as "predominantly vegetarian" and "low in fat and animal protein and rich in starch, fiber, and plant polysaccharides" (De Filippo et al., 2010). The BF children had a much greater predominance of the phylum Bacteroidetes and far fewer bacteria of the phylum Firmicutes. BF children had substantial amounts of *Prevotella* and *Xylanibacter*, which were absent in EU children, whereas EU children had more Enterobacteriaceae (*Shigella* and *Escherichia*). BF children had more SCFA than EU children (De Filippo et al., 2010). Given the predominantly plant-based diets of the BF children, this study suggests that such dietary differences could lead to pronounced differences in the gut microbiome. Similar studies have also noted major differences between typical "Western" populations and those of rural African and South American populations. One compared healthy child and adult populations in an urban US environment, in rural Malawi, and in rural Venezuelan Guahibo Amerindians. Among adults, the US population was again distinguished by a lower ratio of Bacteroidetes to Firmicutes and by a reduction in bacteria from the genus *Prevotella* (Yatsunenko et al., 2012). Another group of Amerindians, the Yanomami, was found to have a low abundance of *Bacteroides* and a high abundance of *Prevotella* species compared to Western populations (Clemente et al., 2015). These studies demonstrate notable fecal microbiome differences between populations consuming a typical modern Western diet and those consuming more traditional hunter-gather or subsistence agrarian diets, which could be referred to as plant-based diets. However, many other environmental factors differ between such populations. While they may give an indication of the potential for diet-induced microbiome variation, they do not necessarily predict what is likely to be the result of the voluntary adoption of a plant-based or vegetarian diet in a modern Western context.

5.2 Feeding Studies

Another line of evidence relevant to vegetarian diets and the microbiome comes from studies looking at the effect of short-term changes in diet along an animal-food to plant-food spectrum. These suggest that the gut microbiome can be changed rapidly by diet, though perhaps not in fundamental ways. David et al. (2014) examined the ability of short-term changes in diet to alter the fecal microbiome. In 10 American volunteers, 5 days of ad libitum intake of an almost completely animal-based diet yielded a significant change in microbial diversity compared to baseline. Twenty-two bacterial clusters were noted to have changed significantly. Notably, the abundance of bile-tolerant organisms increased, such as *Alistipes*, *Bacteroides*, and *Bilophila* including *Bilophila wadsworthia*, which animal models suggest may be linked to IBD. When the volunteers were placed on 5 days of ad libitum intake of an exclusively plant-based diet, changes were seen in only three bacterial clusters compared to baseline. One subject, identified as a lifelong vegetarian, had a decrease in *Prevotella* abundance on the animal-based diet (David et al., 2014). Similarly, Wu et al. (2011) conducted a controlled feeding study in 10 subjects randomized to 10 days of either a high-fat/low-fiber or low-fat/high-fiber diet, which showed that microbiome abundances shifted significant and rapidly (within 24 h) in response to dietary alternation, but these changes were modest and did not alter the enterotypes.

5.3 Early Studies of Vegetarians

The earliest scientific comparisons of fecal microbial composition in those consuming vegetarian and nonvegetarian diets date back to the 1975 study by Reddy et al. This short-term crossover-design compared a high-meat, high-fat diet and a vegetarian diet in eight volunteers. Using traditional culture-based methods, they found lower levels of total anaerobes, *Bacteroides*, *Bifidobacterium*, *Peptococcus*, *Bacillus*, and anaerobic *Lactobacillus* but higher amounts of *Streptococcus* and *Staphylococcus* on the vegetarian diet compared to the high-meat diet (Reddy et al., 1975). In a 1987 crossover feeding study comparing a mixed Western (nonvegetarian), ovolactovegetarian, and vegan diet for 20 days each in 12 healthy males, van Faassen found reductions in bile acid concentrations in the ovolactovegetarians and vegans and also found the vegans to have lower amounts of fecal *Lactobacilli* and *Enterococci*. No significant difference was found in the amount of total anaerobes, *Clostridia*, *Bifidobacterium*, *Bacteroides*, total aerobes, or enterobacteriaceae (Van faassen et al., 1987).

In the 1990s, Peltonen used chromatography of bacterial fatty acids as a global marker of fecal microbial change in 53 patients with RA treated with a 1-year vegetarian diet and found significant alteration of the fecal flora between the different diets (Peltonen et al., 1994). Using the same chromatography method in 43 RA patients randomized to usual omnivore diet or a raw vegan diet rich in lactobacilli, he again saw evidence of change of the fecal microbial fatty acids on the vegan diet (Peltonen et al., 1997). He found a similar change among 18 healthy volunteers on a raw vegan diet (Peltonen et al., 1992).

5.4 Recent Studies of Vegetarians

Some more recent descriptive or intervention studies have examined the microbiome of vegetarians. These are briefly described next, and their methods and findings are also summarized in Table 24.1 for easy reference. In a small intervention in six obese subjects with either hypertension or diabetes mellitus type II who were placed on a vegan diet for 1 month, Kim et al. (2013) reported no change in microbial diversity or enterotype. A reduction in the Firmicutes-to-Bacteroidetes ratio was observed, as was a reduction in pathobionts such as Enterobacteriaceae and an increase in some commensals such as *Bacteroides fragilis* and *Clostridium* clusters XIVa and IV. There was a reduction in SCFA levels (Kim et al., 2013). In a study of the fecal microbial diversity of a vegan woman in

Table 24.1 Summary of Recent Studies on Vegetarian Diets and the Gut Microbiome

Author/Year	Population	Purpose	Methods	Findings	Authors' Conclusions
Hayashi et al. (2002)	1 vegan Japanese woman	Determine fecal microbial diversity of a vegan	16S ribosomal deoxyribonucleic acid (rDNA) library method, terminal restriction fragment length polymorphism (t-RLFP) analysis, and culture-based method	• 29% of the 183 clones obtained were from 13 known species, while 71% were from novel phylotypes • isolates included *Bacteroides*, *Bifidobacterium*, and predominately, *Clostridium* clusters IV, XIVa, XVI, and XVIII (*C. ramosum*)	Unidentified bacteria reside in the intestinal tract of a vegan. Certain phylotypes may be associated with vegan intestinal tract ecology
Liszt et al. (2009)	15 vegetarians (3 vegans + 12 ovolactovegetarians) and 14 omnivores	Compare the fecal microbiota of vegetarian and nonvegetarian groups	Quantitative polymerase chain reaction (PCR); PCR-DGGE (denaturing gradient gel electrophoresis) fingerprinting	• vegetarians had significantly higher counts (12%) of bacterial DNA, significantly lower *Clostridium* cluster IV, and nonsignificantly higher abundance of *Bacteroides* than nonvegetarians	A vegetarian diet affects the gut microbiota by decreasing the amount of *Clostridium* cluster IV
Wu et al. (2011)	98 healthy volunteers for a cross-sectional study; 10 individuals in a short-term controlled feeding study for low-fat/high-fiber and high-fat/low-fiber diets	Investigate association between short-term and long-term dietary factors and the gut microbiota	DNA samples analyzed by 454/Roche pyrosequencing of 16s ribosomal ribonucleic acid (rRNA) gene segments (for calculating pairwise UniFrac distances); shotgun metagenomics for selected samples	• cross-sectional analysis: *Bacteroides* enterotype associated with protein/animal fat, while *Prevotella* enterotype with carbohydrates • controlled feeding study: changes in microbiome composition were detected within 24 h, but no steady change in enterotypes happened during the diets	Enterotype clustering is associated with long-term diet only. Extreme dietary changes result in rapid alterations in microbial composition but not in a different enterotype
Kabeerdoss et al. (2012)	32 ovolactovegetarians and 24 nonvegetarian 18–27-year-old Indian women	Compare ovolactovegetarians and nonvegetarian fecal microbiota	Quantitative PCR (using primers targeted at 16S rDNA of several butyrate-producing bacterial species)	• compared to ovolactovegetarians, nonvegetarians had higher levels of *Clostridium* cluster XIVa (*C. coccoides-E. rectale* group) with increases in *Roseburia-E. rectale* but not *R. productus*, *C. coccoides*, and *Butyrivibrio*	*Clostridium* cluster XIVa and butyrate-producing bacteria are significantly more abundant in nonvegetarians than in ovolactovegetarians
Zimmer et al. (2012)	144 ovolactovegetarians and 105 vegans versus same number of age-and-gender-matched existing fecal samples of nonvegetarians and 46 volunteer nonvegetarians	Compare fecal bacterial counts of ovolactovegetarians, vegans, and nonvegetarians	Gram staining and colony morphologies, and API and VITEK systems (automated measurements of metabolism, enzymatic activities, and antibiotic resistance)	• compared with nonvegetarians, vegans had significantly lower counts of *Bacteroides*, *Bifidobacterium*, *E. coli*, and Enterobacteriaceae spp., while ovolactovegetarians had significantly lower counts of *Bacteroides* and *Bifidobacterium* • vegans and ovolactovegetarians had lower stool pH compared to nonvegetarians	Although total microbial counts remain the same, maintaining a vegan or ovolactovegetarian diet significantly changes microbiota composition

Reference	Subjects	Objective	Methods	Results	Conclusion
Kim et al. (2013)	6 obese subjects assigned to a vegan diet for 1 month	Modulation of microbial composition with change in diet	454-Pyrosequencing of V1-V2 region amplicons of 16S rRNA genes. Operational taxonomic units (OTUs) determined with sequence clustering, and UniFrac distances were calculated to assess OTUs differences	• vegan diet nonsignificantly decreased Firmicutes and significantly increased Bacteroidetes; however, there was no change in enterotypes • vegan diet-related decreases in Enterobacteriaceae and other pathobionts and increases of commensals (*Bacteroides fragilis*, *Clostridium* clusters XIVa and IV, Lachnospiraceae, Ruminococcaceae)	Increased dietary fiber intake with vegan diet altered the gut microbiota composition to one that could reduce gut inflammation. This in turn may reduce metabolic risk
Matijasic et al. (2014)	31 vegetarian versus 29 nonvegetarians in Slovenia ages 1.5–67 years old	Compare fecal bacterial composition of vegetarians and nonvegetarians who adhered to that diet for ≥1 year	Relative quantification by real-time PCR; PCR-DGGE fingerprinting of the V3 16S rRNA gene region	• vegetarians had significantly higher ratios of *Bacteroides-Prevotella*, *Bacteroides thetaiotaomicron*, *Clostridium clostridioforme*, and *Faecalibacterium prausnitzii* but a lower ratio of *Clostridium* cluster XIVa than nonvegetarians • DGGE bands for *Bifidobacterium*, *Streptococcus*, *Collinsella*, and Lachnospiraceae were higher in nonvegetarians, while *Subdoligranulum* was higher in vegetarians	Shifts in the quantity and diversity of fecal microbiota composition are associated with differences in intake of foods of animal origin regardless of age, gender, BMI, or social status
Ruengsomwong et al. (2014)	6 nonvegetarian and 7 vegetarian (ovolactovegetarians and lactovegetarians) Thais ages 42–78 years	Compare gut microbiota of healthy vegetarian and nonvegetarian seniors	PCR-DGGE using HDA1-GC and HDA2 to amplify 16S rRNA gene and real-time PCR analysis	• vegetarian microbiota was characterized by *Clostridium colicanis*, *Eubacterium rectale*, *F. prausnitzii*, *M. funiformis*, *P. copri*, and *R. intestinalis* • nonvegetarians had different combinations of *Bacteroides uniformis*, *Bacteroides vulgatus*, *Bacteroides ovatus*, and *Bacteroides thetaiotaomicron*, and *F. prausnitzii*. • vegetarians had significantly higher *Prevotella* but significantly lower *Bacteroides* compared to nonvegetarians. No differences in *Bifidobacterium*, Enterobacteriaceae, *C. coccoides*–*E. rectale*, *C. leptum*, and *Lactobacillus*	The microbiota composition of the subjects in this study may reflect other healthy Asians with similar diets

Continued

Table 24.1 Summary of Recent Studies on Vegetarian Diets and the Gut Microbiome—cont'd

Author/Year	Population	Purpose	Methods	Findings	Authors' Conclusions
David et al. (2014)	6 males and 4 females aged 21–33 years with BMI of 19–32 kg/m^2 subjected to crossover feeding on both animal-based and plant-based diets	Determine if short-term exposure to animal- or plant-based diet alters gut microbiota	Feeding trial (crossover-design); 16S rRNA gene sequencing used on daily distal gut microbiota samples	• distal gut microbiota had changes within 1 day after animal-based diet ingestion and returned to original structure 2 days after the diet ended • animal-based diet had greater impact on gut microbiota than plant-based diet. • animal-based diet increased the abundance of bile-tolerant microbes (*Alitipes, Bilophila, Bacteroides*), decreased levels of polysaccharide-metabolizing Firmicutes (*Roseburia, Eubacterium rectale, Ruminococcus bromii*), and increased the abundance and activity of *Bilophila wardsworthia*. • fecal samples during animal diet reflected bacteria associated with cheese and cured meats (*L. lactis, P. acidilactici,* and *Staphylococcus*) • In 1 long-term vegetarian subject, *Prevotella* significantly decreased during animal-based diet	Gut microbiome can rapidly respond to dietary changes
Ferrocino et al. (2015)	153 healthy vegan, ovolactovegetarian, or nonvegetarian men and women aged 18–55 years old from 4 locations in Italy	Investigate differences in the fecal microbiota of vegans, ovolactovegetarians, and nonvegetarians	PCR and rRNA-DGGE; amplification at the V3 and V9 regions of the 16S rRNA genes	• Viable counts comparisons: *Pseudomonas* sp. and *Aeromonas* sp. significantly higher for ovolactovegetarians; coliforms and *Bifidobacterium* significantly lower for vegans; *Bacteroides* and *Prevotella* significantly lower but *B. fragilis* significantly higher in nonvegetarians. • V3 region shows *Bacteroides salanitronis, B. coprocola,* and *Prevotella copri* as characteristic bands for nonvegetarians; *Prevotella micans* and *Bacteroides vulgatus* for the ovolactovegetarians, and *Bacteroides salyersiae* for the vegan group. • characteristic bands in the V9 region identified *Veillonella parvula* for the vegan group, *Faecalibacterium prausnitzii* for the vegetarian group, and *E. coli* for the nonvegetarian group	Vegans, ovolactovegetarians, and nonvegetarians have differences in fecal microbiota; the type of foods consumed have a greater impact on fecal microbiota than geography

| Wu et al. (2016) | 15 vegans and 6 nonvegetarians in urban US | Investigate the effect of diet on the gut microbiota and host metabolome | 16S rRNA-tagged sequencing and plasma and urinary metabolomics | • gut microbiota between vegans and nonvegetarians were not significantly different.
• higher fecal short-chain fatty acid level was not associated with increased intake of fermentable substrate in vegans.
• plasma and urinary metabolome significantly differed between vegans and nonvegetarians. Plasma metabolome of vegans was higher in bacterial but lower in lipid and amino acid metabolites compared to nonvegetarians | Diet influences the bacterial metabolome more than gut microbiota composition. Gut microbial community membership may be affected more by place of residence than by diet alone |

Japan, common isolates included the *Bifidobacterium* group, the *Bacteroides* group, and *Clostridium* clusters IV, XIVa, XVI, and XVIII (Hayashi et al., 2002).

A number of more recent studies have compared the gut microbiome of vegetarians and nonvegetarians within similar geographic and cultural contexts. In a comparison of 15 vegetarians (3 vegans + 12 ovolactovegetarians) and 14 nonvegetarians in Austria, vegetarians were found to have reduced quantities of *Clostridium* cluster IV but a higher abundance of *Bacteroides* (Liszt et al., 2009).

A small study compared seven ovolactovegetarian and lactovegetarian and six nonvegetarian volunteers in Thailand. Vegetarians had higher abundances of the genus *Prevotella*, whereas nonvegetarians had higher abundances of the genus *Bacteroides* (Ruengsomwong et al., 2014). Significant differences were not found for *Bifidobacterium*, Enterobacteriaceae, the *Clostridium coccoides-Eubacterium rectale* group, the *Clostridium leptum* group, or *Lactobacillus* (Ruengsomwong et al., 2014). Notably, yogurt consumption was much higher among the ovolactovegetarians and lactovegetarians in this study (Ruengsomwong et al., 2014).

A study among young women in southern India compared 32 ovolactovegetarians with 24 nonvegetarians, matched for age, socioeconomic status, and anthropometric measures (Kabeerdoss et al., 2012). Notably, total energy, calcium, and complex carbohydrate dietary intake was significantly higher among the nonvegetarians. Compared to the ovolactovegetarians, nonvegetarians had higher abundances of *Clostridium* cluster XIVa, and *Roseburia Eubacterium rectale* in particular. Other microbial abundances did not differ. A gene associated with butyrate production was higher among the nonvegetarians (Kabeerdoss et al., 2012).

In a Slovenian population, 31 vegetarians (11 ovolactovegetarians and 20 vegans) were compared with 29 nonvegetarians. Vegetarians (combined) had a higher abundance of a group containing *Bacteroides* and *Prevotella* genera, of *Bacteroides thetaiotaomicron*, of *Clostridium clostidioforme*, and of *Faecalibacterium prausnitzii*, but a lower abundance of *Clostridium* cluster XIVa (Matijasic et al., 2014). *F. prausnitzii* is an important butyrate producer, and it may be linked to reduced inflammatory reactions (Matijasic et al., 2014). Because the PCR technique used in this study did not quantify *Bacteroides* and *Prevotella* separately, the ratio of *Bacteroides* to *Prevotella* was not determined.

Wu et al. studied 98 individuals in a cross-sectional observational comparison of diet and fecal microbiome. In this study, the *Prevotella* enterotype was associated with higher carbohydrate intake, whereas the *Bacteroides* enterotype was associated with animal protein and saturated fats. Eleven self-reported vegetarians were more likely to be in the *Prevotella* enterotype than the *Bacteroides* enterotype, and the only self-reported vegan was in the *Prevotella* enterotype (Wu et al., 2011). In a more recent study, Wu et al. compared both the fecal microbiome and plasma metabolome of 15 vegans and 16 nonvegetarians. They found statistically significant differences in the microbiome between the two dietary patterns only in a few low-prevalence taxa and not in *Prevotella*. They also did not find a difference in fecal SCFA concentrations between vegans and nonvegetarians. In contrast, they did detect substantial differences in the plasma metabolome, with

28 metabolites significantly more abundant in vegans, a third of which were products of microbial metabolism in the gut. Of note, 40% of vegans had detectable equol levels (see prior section on phytochemicals) in the blood, which while more than the nonvegetarians (none had detectable equol), who consumed little equol precursors, is less than in the Asian populations (Wu et al., 2016).

In a somewhat larger study from 4 locations in Italy, 51 ovolactovegetarians and 51 vegans were compared to 51 nonvegetarians. Subjects were recruited though advertisements. They had to have adhered to their respective dietary patterns for at least 1 year. Using traditional bacterial culture methods, little overall distinction was found between the diet groups, but instead a high level of similarity. Ovolactovegetarians had more *Pseudomonas* and *Aeromonas* than vegans or nonvegetarians; vegans had fewer coliforms and *Bidiobacteria* than the other two groups; and nonvegetarians had higher counts of *B. fragilis* (Ferrocino et al., 2015). When nucleic acids were studied (rDNA denaturing gel gradient electrophoresis), again there was a high degree of similarity, with only a few bands differing between the diet groups. Notably, *F. prausnitzii* was characteristic of the ovolactovegetarian group (Ferrocino et al., 2015).

Zimmer et al. (2012) conducted a still larger study of vegetarian diets and the microbiome. They recruited 144 ovolactovegetarians and 105 vegans at the World Vegetarian and Vegan Congress in 2008, in Dresden, Germany. They compared these with two control populations, one a random sample of equal size from samples routinely analyzed by the Institute of Microecology in Herborn, Germany. A second control group was comprised of 46 persons attending a German Gastroenterology Society meeting; in this second instance, the controls were compared with a random sample of 46 of the 144 ovolactovegetarians and 46 of the 105 vegans. Analysis was by traditional culture-based techniques. Ovolactovegetarians had lower counts of *Bacteroides* and *Bifidobacterium* compared to nonvegetarian controls; vegans had lower counts of *Bacteroides*, *Bifidobacterium*, *E. coli*, and Enterobacteriaceae than nonvegetarian controls; there were no statistically significant differences between the vegans and the ovolactovegetarians (Zimmer et al., 2012). Vegans had a lower stool pH (6.3) than did nonvegetarian controls (6.8); ovolactovegetarians had an intermediate stool pH (6.6), which was not statistically significantly different from the nonvegetarians (Zimmer et al., 2012). This lower stool pH is thought to result from SCFA production from the degradation of dietary fibers; it may in turn cause an inhibition of certain bacteria such as *E. coli* and Enterobacteriaceae (Zimmer et al., 2012).

5.5 Summary

It is evident from this review of the literature that the relationship between vegetarian diets and the nature of the gut microbiome is not yet well understood. There is evidence that the fecal microbiome varies greatly between typical Western populations and certain tribal populations that are more plant-based. However, the environments and diets of these populations differ in many ways and generally to a much greater extent than the differences between vegetarians and nonvegetarians within the same culture and geographic setting. There is also evidence that the human fecal microbiome can be rapidly altered—even within 24 h—in response to marked changes in dietary consumption. However, such rapid, notable changes in the relative abundance of taxa may not indicate a change in the structure of the gut microbiota that is likely to be persistent. Such short-term changes do not seem to affect enterotype, and appear to be quickly reversible. However, little is known about the consequences of long-term dietary intervention on the gut microbiota.

The studies of long-term vegetarians compared to nonvegetarians have mostly had small sample sizes. Even some of the moderately larger and more recent studies have relied on older culture-based methods, which have limitations. The results thus have been variable. There is some evidence that vegetarian diets tend to be associated with a lower ratio of Firmicutes to Bacteroidetes. They may be more likely to be associated with *Prevotella* and the *Prevotella* enterotype. They may promote certain commensals such as *F. prausnitzii* while inhibiting certain pathobionts such as *E. coli* and other Enterobacteriaceae. There is some evidence that vegetarian diets may lead to higher production of SCFAs like butyrate. They appear also to result in higher levels of certain bacterial metabolites of phytochemicals. However, these findings are not consistent in the existing literature, with some of the existing small-sample studies having contradictory findings.

6. Conclusions and Future Directions

The human microbiome is a fascinating area of inquiry, and the study of the microbiome has seen marked growth, enabled by developments in genomic sequencing technology and bioinformatics analysis. There is growing evidence that the gastrointestinal microbiome in particular is an important contributor to human physiology and likely has effects on human health. Obesity, cardiovascular disease, IBD, certain cancers, and other conditions are likely affected by the gut microbiome. Diet is a complex, major environmental exposure that clearly can be quite influential in the taxonomic and functional composition of the gut microbiome. Probiotics, prebiotic carbohydrates, and many other dietary nutrients and other components may affect the microbiome and thus impact health and disease risk. Overall dietary patterns, combining differences in many dietary factors, may substantially affect the microbiome. This is reflected in comparisons of geographically distinct populations with substantially different diets and quite different microbiome compositions. It seems entirely plausible that vegetarian diets may lead to significantly different microbiome compositions, compared to omnivore diets. However, the published literature examining this question is thus far quite limited and somewhat inconsistent.

Thus, much remains to be done in the study of vegetarian diets and the microbiome. Larger comparison studies of geographically similar vegetarians and nonvegetarians are needed. In particular, it would be helpful to have microbiome comparison studies among well-studied populations of vegetarians and nonvegetarians, such as the EPIC-Oxford cohort and the Adventist Health Study - 2. Much of the research examining the microbiome and disease is cross-sectional or from animal models. There is a need for established prospective observational cohort studies to develop biorepositories of samples suitable for fecal microbiome analysis. This would allow for prospective studies of the microbiome and disease risk; for example, a nested case–control analysis of fecal microbiome patterns and incident CRC. Many of the studies of vegetarians and the microbiome have used culture-based methods, often targeting a limited number of culturable bacterial taxa. Future studies, while possibly using culture methods for validation or for other specific purposes or detailed investigations of particular microbial species and strains, should take advantage of newer metagenomics methods, which can identify the full range of microbes present. 16-S ribosomal subunit sequencing should increasingly take the place of culture-based methods as a basic tool for microbiome study. Where possible, WGS methods should be used because of the much richer data they provide, including the ability to study gene prevalence and related metabolic and functional capacities. The study of vegetarian diets and the microbiome is in its infancy. We await with interest the important scientific knowledge that may be gained by further developments in this field.

References

Aagaard, K., Petrosino, J., Keitel, W., Watson, M., Katancik, J., Garcia, N., Patel, S., Cutting, M., Madden, T., Hamilton, H., Harris, E., Gevers, D., Simone, G., Mcinnes, P., Versalovic, J., 2013. The Human Microbiome Project strategy for comprehensive sampling of the human microbiome and why it matters. FASEB J. 27, 1012–1022.

Abreu, M.T., Peek Jr., R.M., 2014. Gastrointestinal malignancy and the microbiome. Gastroenterology 146, 1534e3–1546e3.

Ahn, J., Sinha, R., Pei, Z., Dominianni, C., Wu, J., Shi, J., Goedert, J.J., Hayes, R.B., Yang, L., 2013. Human gut microbiome and risk for colorectal cancer. J. Natl. Cancer Inst. 105, 1907–1911.

Alcock, J., Maley, C.C., Aktipis, C.A., 2014. Is eating behavior manipulated by the gastrointestinal microbiota? Evolutionary pressures and potential mechanisms. Bioessays 36, 940–949.

Arora, T., Sharma, R., 2011. Fermentation potential of the gut microbiome: implications for energy homeostasis and weight management. Nutr. Rev. 69, 99–106.

Arora, T., Singh, S., Sharma, R.K., 2013. Probiotics: interaction with gut microbiome and antiobesity potential. Nutrition 29, 591–596.

Arumugam, M., Raes, J., Pelletier, E., Le Paslier, D., Yamada, T., Mende, D.R., Fernandes, G.R., Tap, J., Bruls, T., Batto, J.M., Bertalan, M., Borruel, N., Casellas, F., Fernandez, L., Gautier, L., Hansen, T., Hattori, M., Hayashi, T., Kleerebezem, M., Kurokawa, K., Leclerc, M., Levenez, F., Manichanh, C., Nielsen, H.B., Nielsen, T., Pons, N., Poulain, J., Qin, J., Sicheritz-Ponten, T., Tims, S., Torrents, D., Ugarte, E., Zoetendal, E.G., Wang, J., Guarner, F., Pedersen, O., De Vos, W.M., Brunak, S., Dore, J., Meta, H.I.T.C., Antolin, M., Artiguenave, F., Blottiere, H.M., Almeida, M., Brechot, C., Cara, C., Chervaux, C., Cultrone, A., Delorme, C., Denariaz, G., Dervyn, R., Foerstner, K.U., Friss, C., Van De Guchte, M., Guedon, E., Haimet, F., Huber, W., Van Hylckama-Vlieg, J., Jamet, A., Juste, C., Kaci, G., Knol, J., Lakhdari, O., Layec, S., Le Roux, K., Maguin, E., Merieux, A., Melo Minardi, R., M'rini, C., Muller, J., Oozeer, R., Parkhill, J., Renault, P., Rescigno, M., Sanchez, N., Sunagawa, S., Torrejon, A., Turner, K., Vandemeulebrouck, G., Varela, E., Winogradsky, Y., Zeller, G., Weissenbach, J., Ehrlich, S.D., Bork, P., 2011. Enterotypes of the human gut microbiome. Nature 473, 174–180.

Backhed, F., Ding, H., Wang, T., Hooper, L.V., Koh, G.Y., Nagy, A., Semenkovich, C.F., Gordon, J.I., 2004. The gut microbiota as an environmental factor that regulates fat storage. Proc. Natl. Acad. Sci. U.S.A. 101, 15718–15723.

Backhed, F., Fraser, C.M., Ringel, Y., Sanders, M.E., Sartor, R.B., Sherman, P.M., Versalovic, J., Young, V., Finlay, B.B., 2012. Defining a healthy human gut microbiome: current concepts, future directions, and clinical applications. Cell Host Microbe 12, 611–622.

Baquerizo Nole, K.L., Yim, E., Keri, J.E., 2014. Probiotics and prebiotics in dermatology. J. Am. Acad. Dermatol. 71, 814–821.

Belkaid, Y., Hand, T.W., 2014. Role of the microbiota in immunity and inflammation. Cell 157, 121–141.

Blekhman, R., Goodrich, J.K., Huang, K., Sun, Q., Bukowski, R., Bell, J.T., Spector, T.D., Keinan, A., Ley, R.E., Gevers, D., Clark, A.G., 2015. Host genetic variation impacts microbiome composition across human body sites. Genome Biol. 16.

Bowey, E., Adlercreutz, H., Rowland, I., 2003. Metabolism of isoflavones and lignans by the gut microflora: a study in germ-free and human flora associated rats. Food Chem. Toxicol. 41, 631–636.

Boutagy, N.E., Mcmillan, R.P., Frisard, M.I., Hulver, M.W., 2016. Metabolic endotoxemia with obesity: is it real and is it relevant? Biochimie 124, 11–20.

Brown, J.M., Hazen, S.L., 2014. Metaorganismal nutrient metabolism as a basis of cardiovascular disease. Curr. Opin. Lipidol. 25, 48–53.

Bultman, S.J., 2014. Emerging roles of the microbiome in cancer. Carcinogenesis 35, 249–255.

Campos-Vega, R., Garcia-Gasca, T., Guevara-Gonzalez, R., Ramos-Gomez, M., Oomah, B.D., Loarca-Pina, G., 2012. Human gut flora-fermented nondigestible fraction from cooked bean (*Phaseolus vulgaris* L.) modifies protein expression associated with apoptosis, cell cycle arrest, and proliferation in human adenocarcinoma colon cancer cells. J. Agric. Food Chem. 60, 12443–12450.

Cani, P.D., Amar, J., Iglesias, M.A., Poggi, M., Knauf, C., Bastelica, D., Neyrinck, A.M., Fava, F., Tuohy, K.M., Chabo, C., Waget, A., Delmee, E., Cousin, B., Sulpice, T., Chamontin, B., Ferrieres, J., Tanti, J.F., Gibson, G.R., Casteilla, L., Delzenne, N.M., Alessi, M.C., Burcelin, R., 2007. Metabolic endotoxemia initiates obesity and insulin resistance. Diabetes 56, 1761–1772.

Cani, P.D., Bibiloni, R., Knauf, C., Waget, A., Neyrinck, A.M., Delzenne, N.M., Burcelin, R., 2008. Changes in gut microbiota control metabolic endotoxemia-induced inflammation in high-fat diet-induced obesity and diabetes in mice. Diabetes 57, 1470–1481.

Cantarel, B.L., Lombard, V., Henrissat, B., 2012. Complex carbohydrate utilization by the healthy human microbiome. PLos One 7, e28742.

Causey, J.L., Feirtag, J.M., Gallaher, D.D., Tungland, B.C., Slavin, J.L., 2000. Effects of dietary inulin on serum lipids, blood glucose and the gastrointestinal, environment in hypercholesterolemic men. Nutr. Res. 20, 191–201.

Chassaing, B., Koren, O., Goodrich, J.K., Poole, A.C., Srinivasan, S., Ley, R.E., Gewirtz, A.T., 2015. Dietary emulsifiers impact the mouse gut microbiota promoting colitis and metabolic syndrome. Nature 519, 92–96.

Clemente, J.C., Pehrsson, E.C., Blaser, M.J., Sandhu, K., Gao, Z., Wang, B., Magris, M., Hidalgo, G., Contreras, M., Noya-Alarcon, O., Lander, O., Mcdonald, J., Cox, M., Walter, J., Oh, P.L., Ruiz, J.F., Rodriguez, S., Shen, N., Song, S.J., Metcalf, J., Knight, R., Dantas, G., Dominguez-Bello, M.G., 2015. The microbiome of uncontacted Amerindians. Sci. Adv. 1.

Conlan, S., Kong, H.H., Segre, J.A., 2012. Species-level analysis of DNA sequence data from the NIH Human Microbiome Project. PLos One 7, e47075.

Conlon, M.A., Topping, D.L., Toden, S., Bird, A.R., 2009. Resistant starch opposes colonic DNA damage induced by dairy and non-dairy dietary protein. Aust. J. Dairy Technol. 64, 110–112.

Cueva, C., Bartolome, B., Moreno-Arribas, M.V., Bustos, I., Requena, T., Gonzalez-Manzano, S., Santos-Buelga, C., Turrientes, M.C., Del Campo, R., 2015. Susceptibility and tolerance of human gut culturable aerobic microbiota to wine polyphenols. Microb. Drug Resist. 21, 17–24.

David, L.A., Maurice, C.F., Carmody, R.N., Gootenberg, D.B., Button, J.E., Wolfe, B.E., Ling, A.V., Devlin, A.S., Varma, Y., Fischbach, M.A., Biddinger, S.B., Dutton, R.J., Turnbaugh, P.J., 2014. Diet rapidly and reproducibly alters the human gut microbiome. Nature 505, 559–563.

Davis-Richardson, A.G., Triplett, E.W., 2015. On the role of gut bacteria and infant diet in the development of autoimmunity for type 1 diabetes. Reply to Hanninen Alm and Toivonen Rk [letter]. Diabetologia 58, 2197–2198.

De Filippis, F., Pellegrini, N., Vannini, L., Jeffery, I.B., La Storia, A., Laghi, L., Serrazanetti, D.I., Di Cagno, R., Ferrocino, I., Lazzi, C., Turroni, S., Cocolin, L., Brigidi, P., Neviani, E., Gobbetti, M., O'toole, P.W., Ercolini, D., 2015. High-level adherence to a Mediterranean diet beneficially impacts the gut microbiota and associated metabolome. Gut.

De Filippo, C., Cavalieri, D., Di Paola, M., Ramazzotti, M., Poullet, J.B., Massart, S., Collini, S., Pieraccini, G., Lionetti, P., 2010. Impact of diet in shaping gut microbiota revealed by a comparative study in children from Europe and rural Africa. Proc. Natl. Acad. Sci. U.S.A. 107, 14691–14696.

De Wit, N., Derrien, M., Bosch-Vermeulen, H., Oosterink, E., Keshtkar, S., Duval, C., De Vogel-Van Den Bosch, J., Kleerebezem, M., Muller, M., Van Der Meer, R., 2012. Saturated fat stimulates obesity and hepatic steatosis and affects gut microbiota composition by an enhanced overflow of dietary fat to the distal intestine. Am. J. Physiol. Gastrointest. Liver Physiol. 303, G589–G599.

Den Besten, G., Van Eunen, K., Groen, A.K., Venema, K., Reijngoud, D.J., Bakker, B.M., 2013. The role of short-chain fatty acids in the interplay between diet, gut microbiota, and host energy metabolism. J. Lipid Res. 54, 2325–2340.

Di Gioia, D., Aloisio, I., Mazzola, G., Biavati, B., 2014. Bifidobacteria: their impact on gut microbiota composition and their applications as probiotics in infants. Appl. Microbiol. Biotechnol. 98, 563–577.

Duda-Chodak, A., 2012. The inhibitory effect of polyphenols on human gut microbiota. J. Physiol. Pharmacol. 63, 497–503.

Duda-Chodak, A., Tarko, T., Satora, P., Sroka, P., 2015. Interaction of dietary compounds, especially polyphenols, with the intestinal microbiota: a review. Eur. J. Nutr. 54, 325–341.

Duncan, S.H., Belenguer, A., Holtrop, G., Johnstone, A.M., Flint, H.J., Lobley, G.E., 2007. Reduced dietary intake of carbohydrates by obese subjects results in decreased concentrations of butyrate and butyrate-producing bacteria in feces. Appl. Environ. Microbiol. 73, 1073–1078.

Eckburg, P.B., Bik, E.M., Bernstein, C.N., Purdom, E., Dethlefsen, L., Sargent, M., Gill, S.R., Nelson, K.E., Relman, D.A., 2005. Diversity of the human intestinal microbial flora. Science 308, 1635–1638.

Edwards, C.A., Parrett, A.M., Balmer, S.E., Wharton, B.A., 1994. Fecal short-chain fatty-acids in breast-fed and formula-fed babies. Acta Paediatr. 83, 459–462.

El Kaoutari, A., Armougom, F., Gordon, J.I., Raoult, D., Henrissat, B., 2013. The abundance and variety of carbohydrate-active enzymes in the human gut microbiota. Nat. Rev. Microbiol. 11, 497–504.

Fahey, J.W., Wehage, S.L., Holtzclaw, W.D., Kensler, T.W., Egner, P.A., Shapiro, T.A., Talalay, P., 2012. Protection of humans by plant glucosinolates: efficiency of conversion of glucosinolates to isothiocyanates by the gastrointestinal microflora. Cancer Prev. Res. (Phila.) 5, 603–611.

Ferrocino, I., Di Cagno, R., De Angelis, M., Turroni, S., Vannini, L., Bancalari, E., Rantsiou, K., Cardinali, G., Neviani, E., Cocolin, L., 2015. Fecal microbiota in healthy subjects following omnivore, vegetarian and vegan diets: culturable populations and rRNA DGGE profiling. PLos One 10, e0128669.

Fugmann, M., Breier, M., Rottenkolber, M., Banning, F., Ferrari, U., Sacco, V., Grallert, H., Parhofer, K.G., Seissler, J., Clavel, T., Lechner, A., 2015. The stool microbiota of insulin resistant women with recent gestational diabetes, a high risk group for type 2 diabetes. Sci. Rep. 5, 13212.

Fung, K.Y.C., Cosgrove, L., Lockett, T., Head, R., Topping, D.L., 2012. A review of the potential mechanisms for the lowering of colorectal oncogenesis by butyrate. Br. J. Nutr. 108, 820–831.

Gagliani, N., Hu, B., Huber, S., Elinav, E., Flavell, R.A., 2014. The fire within: microbes inflame tumors. Cell 157, 776–783.

Gevers, D., Pop, M., Schloss, P.D., Huttenhower, C., 2012. Bioinformatics for the Human Microbiome Project. PLos Comput. Biol. 8, e1002779.

Giraffa, G., 2012. Selection and design of lactic acid bacteria probiotic cultures. Eng. Life Sci. 12, 391–398.

Goh, Y.J., Klaenhammer, T.R., 2015. Genetic mechanisms of prebiotic oligosaccharide metabolism in probiotic microbes. Annu. Rev. Food Sci. Technol. 6, 137–156.

Gori, A., Tincati, C., Rizzardini, G., Torti, C., Quirino, T., Haarman, M., Ben Amor, K., Van Schaik, J., Vriesema, A., Knol, J., Marchetti, G., Welling, G., Clerici, M., 2008. Early impairment of gut function and gut flora supporting a role for alteration of gastrointestinal mucosa in human immunodeficiency virus pathogenesis. J. Clin. Microbiol. 46, 757–758.

Group, N.H.W., Peterson, J., Garges, S., Giovanni, M., Mcinnes, P., Wang, L., Schloss, J.A., Bonazzi, V., Mcewen, J.E., Wetterstrand, K.A., Deal, C., Baker, C.C., Di Francesco, V., Howcroft, T.K., Karp, R.W., Lunsford, R.D., Wellington, C.R., Belachew, T., Wright, M., Giblin, C., David, H., Mills, M., Salomon, R., Mullins, C., Akolkar, B., Begg, L., Davis, C., Grandison, L., Humble, M., Khalsa, J., Little, A.R., Peavy, H., Pontzer, C., Portnoy, M., Sayre, M.H., Starke-Reed, P., Zakhari, S., Read, J., Watson, B., Guyer, M., 2009. The NIH human microbiome project. Genome Res. 19, 2317–2323.

Hayashi, H., Sakamoto, M., Benno, Y., 2002. Fecal microbial diversity in a strict vegetarian as determined by molecular analysis and cultivation. Microbiol. Immunol. 46, 819–831.

Hsieh, M.H., Versalovic, J., 2008. The human microbiome and probiotics: implications for pediatrics. Curr. Probl. Pediatr. Adolesc. Health Care 38, 309–327.

Hughes, R., Magee, E.A., Bingham, S., 2000. Protein degradation in the large intestine: relevance to colorectal cancer. Curr. Issues Intest. Microbiol. 1, 51–58.

Human Microbiome Project Consortium, 2012a. A framework for human microbiome research. Nature 486, 215–221.

Human Microbiome Project Consortium, 2012b. Structure, function and diversity of the healthy human microbiome. Nature 486, 207–214.

Humblot, C., Bruneau, A., Sutren, M., Lhoste, E.F., Dore, J., Andrieux, C., Rabot, S., 2005. Brussels sprouts, inulin and fermented milk alter the faecal microbiota of human microbiota-associated rats as shown by PCR-temporal temperature gradient gel electrophoresis using universal, *Lactobacillus* and *Bifidobacterium* 16S rRNA gene primers. Br. J. Nutr. 93, 677–684.

Humphreys, K.J., Conlon, M.A., Young, G.P., Topping, D.L., Hu, Y., Winter, J.M., Bird, A.R., Cobiac, L., Kennedy, N.A., Michael, M.Z., Le Leu, R.K., 2014. Dietary manipulation of oncogenic microrna expression in human rectal mucosa: a randomized trial. Cancer Prev. Res. 7, 786–795.

Inglis, G.D., Thomas, M.C., Thomas, D.K., Kalmokoff, M.L., Brooks, S.P., Selinger, L.B., 2012. Molecular methods to measure intestinal bacteria: a review. J. AOAC Int. 95, 5–23.

Integrative HMP Research Network Consortium, 2014. The Integrative Human Microbiome Project: dynamic analysis of microbiome-host omics profiles during periods of human health and disease. Cell Host Microbe 16, 276–289.

Johansson, M.E., Phillipson, M., Petersson, J., Velcich, A., Holm, L., Hansson, G.C., 2008. The inner of the two Muc2 mucin-dependent mucus layers in colon is devoid of bacteria. Proc. Natl. Acad. Sci. U.S.A. 105, 15064–15069.

Johnson, C.R., Thavarajah, D., Combs, G.F., Thavarajah, P., 2013. Lentil (*Lens culinaris* L.): a prebiotic-rich whole food legume. Food Res. Int. 51, 107–113.

Joint FAO/WHO Working Group Report on Drafting Guidelines for the Evaluation of Probiotics in Food London, Ontario, Canada, April 30 and May 1, 2002.

Kabeerdoss, J., Devi, R.S., Mary, R.R., Ramakrishna, B.S., 2012. Faecal microbiota composition in vegetarians: comparison with omnivores in a cohort of young women in southern India. Br. J. Nutr. 108, 953–957.

Kamada, N., Kim, Y.G., Sham, H.P., Vallance, B.A., Puente, J.L., Martens, E.C., Nunez, G., 2012. Regulated virulence controls the ability of a pathogen to compete with the gut microbiota. Science 336, 1325–1329.

Kekkonen, R.-A., 2008. Probiotic intervention has strain-specific anti-inflammatory effects in healthy adults. World J. Gastroenterol. 14, 2029.

Khosravi, A., Mazmanian, S.K., 2013. Disruption of the gut microbiome as a risk factor for microbial infections. Curr. Opin. Microbiol. 16, 221–227.

Kim, M.S., Hwang, S.S., Park, E.J., Bae, J.W., 2013. Strict vegetarian diet improves the risk factors associated with metabolic diseases by modulating gut microbiota and reducing intestinal inflammation. Environ. Microbiol. Rep. 5, 765–775.

Koeth, R.A., Wang, Z., Levison, B.S., Buffa, J.A., Org, E., Sheehy, B.T., Britt, E.B., Fu, X., Wu, Y., Li, L., Smith, J.D., Didonato, J.A., Chen, J., Li, H., Wu, G.D., Lewis, J.D., Warrier, M., Brown, J.M., Krauss, R.M., Tang, W.H., Bushman, F.D., Lusis, A.J., Hazen, S.L., 2013. Intestinal microbiota metabolism of L-carnitine, a nutrient in red meat, promotes atherosclerosis. Nat. Med. 19, 576–585.

Koren, O., Knights, D., Gonzalez, A., Waldron, L., Segata, N., Knight, R., Huttenhower, C., Ley, R.E., 2013. A guide to enterotypes across the human body: meta-analysis of microbial community structures in human microbiome datasets. PLoS Comput. Biol. 9, e1002863.

Kostic, A.D., Xavier, R.J., Gevers, D., 2014. The microbiome in inflammatory bowel disease: current status and the future ahead. Gastroenterology 146, 1489–1499.

Kuczynski, J., Lauber, C.L., Walters, W.A., Parfrey, L.W., Clemente, J.C., Gevers, D., Knight, R., 2012. Experimental and analytical tools for studying the human microbiome. Nat. Rev. Genet. 13, 47–58.

Lampe, J.W., 2008. The Human Microbiome Project: getting to the guts of the matter in cancer epidemiology. Cancer Epidemiol. Biomarkers Prev. 17, 2523–2524.

Le Chatelier, E., Nielsen, T., Qin, J., Prifti, E., Hildebrand, F., Falony, G., Almeida, M., Arumugam, M., Batto, J.M., Kennedy, S., Leonard, P., Li, J., Burgdorf, K., Grarup, N., Jorgensen, T., Brandslund, I., Nielsen, H.B., Juncker, A.S., Bertalan, M., Levenez, F., Pons, N., Rasmussen, S., Sunagawa, S., Tap, J., Tims, S., Zoetendal, E.G., Brunak, S., Clement, K., Dore, J., Kleerebezem, M., Kristiansen, K., Renault, P., Sicheritz-Ponten, T., De Vos, W.M., Zucker, J.D., Raes, J., Hansen, T., Meta, H.I.T.C., Bork, P., Wang, J., Ehrlich, S.D., Pedersen, O., 2013. Richness of human gut microbiome correlates with metabolic markers. Nature 500, 541–546.

Lee, D., Albenberg, L., Compher, C., Baldassano, R., Piccoli, D., Lewis, J.D., Wu, G.D., 2015. Diet in the pathogenesis and treatment of inflammatory bowel diseases. Gastroenterology 148, 1087–1106.

Lewis, S., Burmeister, S., Brazier, J., 2005. Effect of the prebiotic oligofructose on relapse of Clostridium difficile-associated diarrhea: a randomized, controlled study. Clin. Gastroenterol. Hepatol. Off. Clin. Pract. J. Am. Gastroenterol. Assoc. 3, 442–448.

Ley, R.E., Turnbaugh, P.J., Klein, S., Gordon, J.I., 2006. Microbial ecology: human gut microbes associated with obesity. Nature 444, 1022–1023.

Li, F., Hullar, M.A., Schwarz, Y., Lampe, J.W., 2009. Human gut bacterial communities are altered by addition of cruciferous vegetables to a controlled fruit- and vegetable-free diet. J. Nutr. 139, 1685–1691.

Licciardi, P.V., Toh, Z.Q., Dunne, E., Wong, S.S., Mulholland, E.K., Tang, M., Robins-Browne, R.M., Satzke, C., 2012. Protecting against pneumococcal disease: critical interactions between probiotics and the airway microbiome. PLoS Pathog. 8, e1002652.

Lievin, V., Peiffer, I., Hudault, S., Rochat, F., Brassart, D., Neeser, J.R., Servin, A.L., 2000. Bifidobacterium strains from resident infant human gastrointestinal microflora exert antimicrobial activity. Gut 47, 646–652.

Lim, G.B., 2013. Risk factors: intestinal microbiota: "a new direction in cardiovascular research". Nat. Rev. Cardiol. 10, 363.

Liszt, K., Zwielehner, J., Handschur, M., Hippe, B., Thaler, R., Haslberger, A.G., 2009. Characterization of bacteria, clostridia and Bacteroides in faeces of vegetarians using qPCR and PCR-DGGE fingerprinting. Ann. Nutr. Metab. 54, 253–257.

Logan, A.C., Katzman, M., 2005. Major depressive disorder: probiotics may be an adjuvant therapy. Med. Hypotheses 64, 533–538.

Louis, P., Hold, G.L., Flint, H.J., 2014. The gut microbiota, bacterial metabolites and colorectal cancer. Nat. Rev. Microbiol. 12, 661–672.

Luche, E., Cousin, B., Garidou, L., Serino, M., Waget, A., Barreau, C., Andre, M., Valet, P., Courtney, M., Casteilla, L., Burcelin, R., 2013. Metabolic endotoxemia directly increases the proliferation of adipocyte precursors at the onset of metabolic diseases through a CD14-dependent mechanism. Mol. Metab. 2, 281–291.

Luyer, M.D., Buurman, W.A., Hadfoune, M., Speelmans, G., Knol, J., Jacobs, J.A., Dejong, C.H., Vriesema, A.J., Greve, J.W., 2005. Strain-specific effects of probiotics on gut barrier integrity following hemorrhagic shock. Infect. Immun. 73, 3686–3692.

Mai, V., Morris, J.G.J.R., 2013. Need for prospective cohort studies to establish human gut microbiome contributions to disease risk. J. Natl. Cancer Inst. 105, 1850–1851.

Manichanh, C., Reeder, J., Gibert, P., Varela, E., Llopis, M., Antolin, M., Guigo, R., Knight, R., Guarner, F., 2010. Reshaping the gut microbiome with bacterial transplantation and antibiotic intake. Genome Res. 20, 1411–1419.

Marasco, G., Di Biase, A.R., Schiumerini, R., Eusebi, L.H., Iughetti, L., Ravaioli, F., Scaioli, E., Colecchia, A., Festi, D., 2016. Gut microbiota and celiac disease. Dig. Dis. Sci.

Martinez, I., Lattimer, J.M., Hubach, K.L., Case, J.A., Yang, J., Weber, C.G., Louk, J.A., Rose, D.J., Kyureghian, G., Peterson, D.A., Haub, M.D., Walter, J., 2013. Gut microbiome composition is linked to whole grain-induced immunological improvements. ISME J. 7, 269–280.

Matijasic, B.B., Obermajer, T., Lipoglavsek, L., Grabnar, I., Avgustin, G., Rogelj, I., 2014. Association of dietary type with fecal microbiota in vegetarians and omnivores in Slovenia. Eur. J. Nutr. 53, 1051–1064.

Maukonen, J., Saarela, M., 2015. Human gut microbiota: does diet matter? Proc. Nutr. Soc. 74, 23–36.

Mclean, M.H., El-Omar, E.M., 2009. Genetic aspects of inflammation. Curr. Opin. Pharmacol. 9, 370–374.

Mischke, M., Plosch, T., 2013. More than just a gut instinct-the potential interplay between a baby's nutrition, its gut microbiome, and the epigenome. Am. J. Physiol. Regul. Integr. Comp. Physiol. 304, R1065–R1069.

Moreira, A.P.B., Texeira, T.F.S., Ferreira, A.B., Peluzio, M.D.G., Alfenas, R.D.G., 2012. Influence of a high-fat diet on gut microbiota, intestinal permeability and metabolic endotoxaemia. Br. J. Nutr. 108, 801–809.

Moro, G., Arslanoglu, S., Stahl, B., Jelinek, J., Wahn, U., Boehm, G., 2006. A mixture of prebiotic oligosaccharides reduces the incidence of atopic dermatitis during the first six months of age. Arch. Dis. Child. 91, 814–819.

Moschen, A.R., Wieser, V., Tilg, H., 2012. Dietary factors: major regulators of the Gut's microbiota. Gut Liver 6, 411–416.

Neves, A.L., Coelho, J., Couto, L., Leite-Moreira, A., Roncon-Albuquerque, R.J.R., 2013. Metabolic endotoxemia: a molecular link between obesity and cardiovascular risk. J. Mol. Endocrinol. 51, R51–R64.

Nyangale, E.P., Farmer, S., Keller, D., Chernoff, D., Gibson, G.R., 2014. Effect of prebiotics on the fecal microbiota of elderly volunteers after dietary supplementation of *Bacillus coagulans* GBI-30, 6086. Anaerobe 30, 75–81.

Osborn, D.A., Sinn, J.K.H., 2013. Prebiotics in infants for prevention of allergy. Cochrane Database Syst. Rev. 3, CD006474.

Ou, J.H., Carbonero, F., Zoetendal, E.G., Delany, J.P., Wang, M., Newton, K., Gaskins, H.R., O'keefe, S.J.D., 2013. Diet, microbiota, and microbial metabolites in colon cancer risk in rural Africans and African Americans. Am. J. Clin. Nutr. 98, 111–120.

Papa, E., Docktor, M., Smillie, C., Weber, S., Preheim, S.P., Gevers, D., Giannoukos, G., Ciulla, D., Tabbaa, D., Ingram, J., Schauer, D.B., Ward, D.V., Korzenik, J.R., Xavier, R.J., Bousvaros, A., Alm, E.J., 2012. Non-invasive mapping of the gastrointestinal microbiota identifies children with inflammatory bowel disease. PLoS One 7, e39242.

Payne, A.N., Chassard, C., Lacroix, C., 2012. Gut microbial adaptation to dietary consumption of fructose, artificial sweeteners and sugar alcohols: implications for host-microbe interactions contributing to obesity. Obes. Rev. 13, 799–809.

Peltonen, R., Kjeldsen-Kragh, J., Haugen, M., Tuominen, J., Toivanen, P., Forre, O., Eerola, E., 1994. Changes of faecal flora in rheumatoid arthritis during fasting and one-year vegetarian diet. Br. J. Rheumatol. 33, 638–643.

Peltonen, R., Ling, W.H., Hanninen, O., Eerola, E., 1992. An uncooked vegan diet shifts the profile of human fecal microflora: computerized analysis of direct stool sample gas-liquid chromatography profiles of bacterial cellular fatty acids. Appl. Environ. Microbiol. 58, 3660–3666.

Peltonen, R., Nenonen, M., Helve, T., Hanninen, O., Toivanen, P., Eerola, E., 1997. Faecal microbial flora and disease activity in rheumatoid arthritis during a vegan diet. Br. J. Rheumatol. 36, 64–68.

Piirainen, L., Kekkonen, R.A., Kajander, K., Ahlroos, T., Tynkkynen, S., Nevala, R., Korpela, R., 2008. In school-aged children a combination of galacto-oligosaccharides and *Lactobacillus* GG increases bifidobacteria more than *Lactobacillus* GG on its own. Ann. Nutr. Metabolism 52, 204–208.

Poutahidis, T., Varian, B.J., Levkovich, T., Lakritz, J.R., Mirabal, S., Kwok, C., Ibrahim, Y.M., Kearney, S.M., Chatzigiagkos, A., Alm, E.J., Erdman, S.E., 2015. Dietary microbes modulate transgenerational cancer risk. Cancer Res. 75, 1197–1204.

Proctor, L.M., 2011. The human microbiome project in 2011 and beyond. Cell Host Microbe 10, 287–291.

Qin, J., Li, R., Raes, J., Arumugam, M., Burgdorf, K.S., Manichanh, C., Nielsen, T., Pons, N., Levenez, F., Yamada, T., Mende, D.R., Li, J., Xu, J., Li, S., Li, D., Cao, J., Wang, B., Liang, H., Zheng, H., Xie, Y., Tap, J., Lepage, P., Bertalan, M., Batto, J.M., Hansen, T., Le Paslier, D., Linneberg, A., Nielsen, H.B., Pelletier, E., Renault, P., Sicheritz-Ponten, T., Turner, K., Zhu, H., Yu, C., Li, S., Jian, M., Zhou, Y., Li, Y., Zhang, X., Li, S., Qin, N., Yang, H., Wang, J., Brunak, S., Dore, J., Guarner, F., Kristiansen, K., Pedersen, O., Parkhill, J., Weissenbach, J., Meta, H.I.T.C., Bork, P., Ehrlich, S.D., Wang, J., 2010. A human gut microbial gene catalogue established by metagenomic sequencing. Nature 464, 59–65.

Reddy, B.S., Weisburger, J.H., Wynder, E.L., 1975. Effects of high risk and low risk diets for colon carcinogenesis on fecal microflora and steroids in man. J. Nutr. 105, 878–884.

Ruengsomwong, S., Korenori, Y., Sakamoto, N., Wannissorn, B., Nakayama, J., Nitisinprasert, S., 2014. Senior Thai fecal microbiota comparison between vegetarians and non-vegetarians using PCR-DGGE and real-time PCR. J. Microbiol. Biotechnol. 24, 1026–1033.

Russell, W.R., Gratz, S.W., Duncan, S.H., Holtrop, G., Ince, J., Scobbie, L., Duncan, G., Johnstone, A.M., Lobley, G.E., Wallace, R.J., Duthie, G.G., Flint, H.J., 2011. High-protein, reduced-carbohydrate weight-loss diets promote metabolite profiles likely to be detrimental to colonic health. Am. J. Clin. Nutr. 93, 1062–1072.

Saez-Lara, M.J., Gomez-Llorente, C., Plaza-Diaz, J., Gil, A., 2015. The role of probiotic lactic acid bacteria and bifidobacteria in the prevention and treatment of inflammatory bowel disease and other related diseases: a systematic review of randomized human clinical trials. Biomed. Res. Int. 2015, 505878.

Schokker, D., Veninga, G., Vastenhouw, S.A., Bossers, A., De Bree, F.M., Kaal-Lansbergen, L.M.T.E., Rebel, J.M.J., Smits, M.A., 2015. Early life microbial colonization of the gut and intestinal development differ between genetically divergent broiler lines. BMC Genom. 16.

Schulz, M.D., Atay, C., Heringer, J., Romrig, F.K., Schwitalla, S., Aydin, B., Ziegler, P.K., Varga, J., Reindl, W., Pommerenke, C., Salinas-Riester, G., Bock, A., Alpert, C., Blaut, M., Polson, S.C., Brandl, L., Kirchner, T., Greten, F.R., Polson, S.W., Arkan, M.C., 2014. High-fat-diet-mediated dysbiosis promotes intestinal carcinogenesis independently of obesity. Nature 514, 508–512.

Selhub, E.M., Logan, A.C., Bested, A.C., 2014. Fermented foods, microbiota, and mental health: ancient practice meets nutritional psychiatry. J. Physiol. Anthropol. 33, 2.

Shen, W., Gaskins, H.R., Mcintosh, M.K., 2014. Influence of dietary fat on intestinal microbes, inflammation, barrier function and metabolic outcomes. J. Nutr. Biochem. 25, 270–280.

Shida, K., Sato, T., Iizuka, R., Hoshi, R., Watanabe, O., Igarashi, T., Miyazaki, K., Nanno, M., Ishikawa, F., 2015. Daily intake of fermented milk with *Lactobacillus casei* strain Shirota reduces the incidence and duration of upper respiratory tract infections in healthy middle-aged office workers. Eur. J. Nutr.

Silvester, K.R., Cummings, J.H., 1995. Does digestibility of meat protein help explain large-bowel cancer risk. Nutr. Cancer 24, 279–288.

Silvi, S., Rumney, C.J., Cresci, A., Rowland, I.R., 1999. Resistant starch modifies gut microflora and microbial metabolism in human flora-associated rats inoculated with faeces from Italian and UK donors. J. Appl. Microbiol. 86, 521–530.

Stock, J., 2013. Gut microbiota: an environmental risk factor for cardiovascular disease. Atherosclerosis 229, 440–442.

Suez, J., Korem, T., Zeevi, D., Zilberman-Schapira, G., Thaiss, C.A., Maza, O., Israeli, D., Zmora, N., Gilad, S., Weinberger, A., Kuperman, Y., Harmelin, A., Kolodkin-Gal, I., Shapiro, H., Halpern, Z., Segal, E., Elinav, E., 2014. Artificial sweeteners induce glucose intolerance by altering the gut microbiota. Nature 514, 181–186.

Sugahara, H., Odamaki, T., Fukuda, S., Kato, T., Xiao, J.Z., Abe, F., Kikuchi, J., Ohno, H., 2015. Probiotic Bifidobacterium longum alters gut luminal metabolism through modification of the gut microbial community. Sci. Rep. 5, 13548.

Tang, W.H., Wang, Z., Levison, B.S., Koeth, R.A., Britt, E.B., Fu, X., Wu, Y., Hazen, S.L., 2013. Intestinal microbial metabolism of phosphatidylcholine and cardiovascular risk. N. Engl. J. Med. 368, 1575–1584.

Tang, W.H., Wang, Z., Shrestha, K., Borowski, A.G., Wu, Y., Troughton, R.W., Klein, A.L., Hazen, S.L., 2015. Intestinal microbiota-dependent phosphatidylcholine metabolites, diastolic dysfunction, and adverse clinical outcomes in chronic systolic heart failure. J. Card. Fail 21, 91–96.

Toden, S., Bird, A.R., Topping, D.L., Conlon, M.A., 2007a. Differential effects of dietary whey, casein and soya on colonic DNA damage and large bowel SCFA in rats fed diets low and high in resistant starch. Br. J. Nutr. 97, 535–543.

Toden, S., Bird, A.R., Topping, D.L., Conlon, M.A., 2007b. Dose-dependent reduction of dietary protein-induced colonocyte DNA damage by resistant starch in rats correlates more highly with caecal butyrate than with other short chain fatty acids. Cancer Biol. Ther. 6, 253–258.

Topping, D.L., Fukushima, M., Bird, A.R., 2003. Resistant starch as a prebiotic and synbiotic: state of the art. Proc. Nutr. Soc. 62, 171–176.

Troseid, M., Ueland, T., Hov, J.R., Svardal, A., Gregersen, I., Dahl, C.P., Aakhus, S., Gude, E., Bjorndal, B., Halvorsen, B., Karlsen, T.H., Aukrust, P., Gullestad, L., Berge, R.K., Yndestad, A., 2015. Microbiota-dependent metabolite trimethylamine-N-oxide is associated with disease severity and survival of patients with chronic heart failure. J. Intern. Med. 277, 717–726.

Turnbaugh, P.J., Ley, R.E., Hamady, M., Fraser-Liggett, C.M., Knight, R., Gordon, J.I., 2007. The human microbiome project. Nature 449, 804–810.

Van faassen, A., Bol, J., Van dokkum, W., Pikaar, N.A., Ockhuizen, T., Hermus, R.J., 1987. Bile acids, neutral steroids, and bacteria in feces as affected by a mixed, a lacto-ovovegetarian, and a vegan diet. Am. J. Clin. Nutr. 46, 962–967.

Vandenplas, Y., De greef, E., Veereman, G., 2014. Prebiotics in infant formula. Gut Microbes 5, 681–687.

Vandenplas, Y., Zakharova, I., Dmitrieva, Y., 2015. Oligosaccharides in infant formula: more evidence to validate the role of prebiotics. Br. J. Nutr. 113, 1339–1344.

Veiga, P., Pons, N., Agrawal, A., Oozeer, R., Guyonnet, D., Brazeilles, R., Faurie, J.M., Van hylckama Vlieg, J.E., Houghton, L.A., Whorwell, P.J., Ehrlich, S.D., Kennedy, S.P., 2014. Changes of the human gut microbiome induced by a fermented milk product. Sci. Rep. 4, 6328.

Wang, S.G., Hibberd, M.L., Pettersson, S., Lee, Y.K., 2014. *Enterococcus faecalis* from healthy infants modulates inflammation through MAPK signaling pathways. PLoS One 9.

Wang, T., Cai, G., Qiu, Y., Fei, N., Zhang, M., Pang, X., Jia, W., Cai, S., Zhao, L., 2012. Structural segregation of gut microbiota between colorectal cancer patients and healthy volunteers. ISME J. 6, 320–329.

Wang, Z., Klipfell, E., Bennett, B.J., Koeth, R., Levison, B.S., Dugar, B., Feldstein, A.E., Britt, E.B., Fu, X., Chung, Y.M., Wu, Y., Schauer, P., Smith, J.D., Allayee, H., Tang, W.H., Didonato, J.A., Lusis, A.J., Hazen, S.L., 2011. Gut flora metabolism of phosphatidylcholine promotes cardiovascular disease. Nature 472, 57–63.

Weinstock, G.M., 2012. Genomic approaches to studying the human microbiota. Nature 489, 250–256.

Wu, G.D., Chen, J., Hoffmann, C., Bittinger, K., Chen, Y.Y., Keilbaugh, S.A., Bewtra, M., Knights, D., Walters, W.A., Knight, R., Sinha, R., Gilroy, E., Gupta, K., Baldassano, R., Nessel, L., Li, H., Bushman, F.D., Lewis, J.D., 2011. Linking long-term dietary patterns with gut microbial enterotypes. Science 334, 105–108.

Wu, G.D., Compher, C., Chen, E.Z., Smith, S.A., Shah, R.D., Bittinger, K., Chehoud, C., Albenberg, L.G., Nessel, L., Gilroy, E., Star, J., Weljie, A.M., Flint, H.J., Metz, D.C., Bennett, M.J., li, H., Bushman, F.D., Lewis, J.D., 2016. Comparative metabolomics in vegans and omnivores reveal constraints on diet-dependent gut microbiota metabolite production. Gut 65, 63–72.

Yao, C.K., Muir, J.G., Gibson, P.R., 2016. Review article: insights into colonic protein fermentation, its modulation and potential health implications. Aliment. Pharmacol. Ther. 43, 181–196.

Yatsunenko, T., Rey, F.E., Manary, M.J., Trehan, I., Dominguez-bello, M.G., Contreras, M., Magris, M., Hidalgo, G., Baldassano, R.N., Anokhin, A.P., Heath, A.C., Warner, B., Reeder, J., Kuczynski, J., Caporaso, J.G., Lozupone, C.A., Lauber, C., Clemente, J.C., Knights, D., Knight, R., Gordon, J.I., 2012. Human gut microbiome viewed across age and geography. Nature 486, 222–227.

Zampa, A., Silvi, S., Fabiani, R., Morozzi, G., Orpianesi, C., Cresci, A., 2004. Effects of different digestible carbohydrates on bile acid metabolism and SCFA production by human gut micro-flora grown in an in vitro semi-continuous culture. Anaerobe 10, 19–26.

Zhang, C., Zhang, M., Pang, X., Zhao, Y., Wang, L., Zhao, L., 2012. Structural resilience of the gut microbiota in adult mice under high-fat dietary perturbations. ISME J. 6, 1848–1857.

Zhang, X., Zhang, D., Jia, H., Feng, Q., Wang, D., Liang, D., Wu, X., Li, J., Tang, L., Li, Y., Lan, Z., Chen, B., Li, Y., Zhong, H., Xie, H., Jie, Z., Chen, W., Tang, S., Xu, X., Wang, X., Cai, X., Liu, S., Xia, Y., Li, J., Qiao, X., Al-Aama, J.Y., Chen, H., Wang, L., Wu, Q.J., Zhang, F., Zheng, W., Li, Y., Zhang, M., Luo, G., Xue, W., Xiao, L., Li, J., Chen, W., Xu, X., Yin, Y., Yang, H., Wang, J., Kristiansen, K., Liu, L., Li, T., Huang, Q., Li, Y., Wang, J., 2015a. The oral and gut microbiomes are perturbed in rheumatoid arthritis and partly normalized after treatment. Nat. Med. 21, 895–905.

Zhang, Y.F., Lun, C.Y., Tsui, S.K.W., 2015b. Metagenomics: a new way to illustrate the crosstalk between infectious diseases and host microbiome. Int. J. Mol. Sci. 16, 26263–26279.

Zimmer, J., Lange, B., Frick, J.S., Sauer, H., Zimmermann, K., Schwiertz, A., Rusch, K., Klosterhalfen, S., Enck, P., 2012. A vegan or vegetarian diet substantially alters the human colonic faecal microbiota. Eur. J. Clin. Nutr. 66, 53–60.

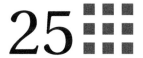

25

Vegetarianism and the Risk of Gastroesophageal Reflux Disease

Jae G. Jung[1,2], Hyoun W. Kang[1]

[1]DONGGUK UNIVERSITY ILSAN HOSPITAL, GOYANG, KOREA; [2]INCHEON SARANG HOSPITAL, INCHEON, KOREA

1. Introduction

Gastroesophageal reflux disease (GERD) is a condition that develops when the reflux of stomach content causes troublesome symptoms and/or complications (Vakil et al., 2006). GERD is one of the most common gastrointestinal diseases in Western countries, where its symptoms such as heartburn and acid regurgitation affect up to 20%–30% of people at least weekly and about 60% of people at some time during the course of a year. Reflux esophagitis is the most common sign of GERD on endoscopy. Its medical, personal, social, and economic burdens are enormous and will be increasing. Additionally, it tends to relapse frequently and may develop complications, such as hemorrhage, stricture, Barrett esophagus, and adenocarcinoma (Vakil et al., 2007).

The prevalence of GERD and related disorders has been increasing worldwide. When defined as at least weekly heartburn or acid regurgitation, the prevalence in Western populations generally ranges between 10% and 20%. The prevalence in North America has been shown to be higher than in Europe (Vakil, 2010). In Japan, the overall prevalence of reflux esophagitis among the adult population is around 10%–15% (Fujiwara and Arakawa, 2009). In Taiwan, the prevalence of reflux esophagitis in subjects evaluated for upper gastrointestinal symptoms is 15% (Yeh et al., 1997). The prevalence of reflux esophagitis in Korean subjects undergoing health check-ups was reported at approximately 2%–5% in the 1990s, 8% in 2006, and 11% in 2009 (Shim et al., 2009; Song et al., 2009; Inamori et al., 2003). Widespread health check-ups, developments in endoscopic examination, Westernized diet, and lifestyle may have contributed to the increased prevalence of reflux esophagitis in Korea (Song et al., 2009).

2. Obesity and GERD Development

Risk factors for GERD include older age (Lee et al., 2011; Mold et al., 1991), male sex (Sonnenberg and El-Serag, 1999), obesity (El-Serag, 2008a; El-Serag and Johanson, 2002; Corley and Kubo, 2006), metabolic syndrome (Song et al., 2009; Chung et al., 2008), hiatal hernia (Wilson et al., 1999; Iovino et al., 2006), cigarette smoking, and alcohol consumption

(Stanciu and Bennett, 1972; Kaufman and Kaye, 1978). Obesity, typically defined as a body mass index (BMI) >30 kg/m^2, has risen to epidemic proportions in Western populations. The prevalence of obesity has increased to 34% for adults in the United States, where 68% of the population is considered to be either overweight or obese (Flegal et al., 2010). Moreover, a severe increase in overweight and obesity prevalence has also been reported in children and adolescents over the last four decades (Ogden et al., 2010). Increased food availability, larger serving sizes, higher energy density, and decreased physical activity are the main causes responsible for the observed trends (Eusebi et al., 2012).

The mainstay of treatment in GERD is the proton pump inhibitor (PPI). But recently, many adverse drug reactions of long-term PPI use have been identified, including B$_{12}$ deficiency, iron deficiency, increased susceptibility to pneumonia, enteric infections, fractures, and hypergastrinemia (Sheen and Triadafilopoulos, 2011). So, it is important to find correctable risk factors and correct them. Known correctable risk factors of reflux esophagitis are obesity, metabolic syndrome, cigarette smoking, and alcohol consumption (El-Serag, 2008a; El-Serag and Johanson, 2002; Corley and Kubo, 2006; Song et al., 2009; Chung et al., 2008; Stanciu and Bennett, 1972; Kaufman and Kaye, 1978).

Reflux esophagitis might be a part of the disease spectrum of the metabolic syndrome showing significant relationship of reflux esophagitis to obesity, low HDL cholesterol, high triglyceride, high blood pressure, and elevated fasting glucose (Song et al., 2009). Another study reported that metabolic syndrome and abdominal obesity, especially visceral obesity, were important risk factors for reflux esophagitis (Nam et al., 2010; Chung et al., 2008). It appears that a dietary pattern characterized by high fat and low fiber consumption and lack of other beneficial elements is related to the metabolic syndrome, thus having the potential to increase the risk for reflux. A study found a relative association between uninvestigated reflux and adherence to a pattern of consuming fast food, suggesting that this contributes to the risk for developing reflux (Khodarahmi et al., 2016).

Since the incidence of obesity and GERD is increasing in parallel, it has been reasonably suggested that elevated BMI could be a contributing factor for development of GERD and related disorders.

A large meta-analysis and systematic review of epidemiological studies mostly conducted in North America or Western Europe countries showed a statistically significant association between obesity and an increased risk of GERD and related complications among both men and women (Hampel et al., 2005). In particular, the increase in developing GERD symptoms and esophagitis was 1.43 [95% confidence interval (CI), 1.158–1.774] for individuals with BMI from 25 to 30 and 1.94 (95% CI, 1.468–2.566) for BMI >30, as compared to individuals with normal BMI (Hampel et al., 2005).

The direct correlation between weight gain and the risk for GERD and its complications has also been evaluated in a large population-based case–control study showing that a BMI increase of >3.5 was associated with a 2.7-fold (95% CI, 2.3- to 3.2-fold) increase in risk of developing reflux symptoms (Nilsson et al., 2003).

Similar results were reported in a large cohort of women by Jacobson et al. (2006) who observed that the risk of developing GERD symptoms rises progressively with increasing

BMI, not only in overweight or obese but also in normal-weight people. Interestingly, the authors showed that even moderate amounts of weight gain may result in the development or exacerbation of GERD symptoms, although the efficacy of weight loss as a therapeutic measure in reflux disease showed conflicting results (Jacobson et al., 2006). Nevertheless, avoiding weight gain in the first place has been associated with a lower risk of GERD symptoms (El-Serag, 2008b).

By performing a 24-h pH-metry in their patients, El-Serag et al. (2007) found that both high waist circumference and BMI >30 were associated with a significant increase in short and/or long reflux episodes. Similarly, Jacobson et al. (2006), who performed a study on a cohort of more than 10,000 women, reported that both BMI and the waist-to-hip ratio were associated with frequent GERD symptoms. However, when analyzing both factors simultaneously, BMI appeared to have a more significant role in this association.

Especially, abdominal obesity seems to be more important than general obesity as expressed by an elevated BMI (El-Serag et al., 2007; Kang et al., 2007). Several mechanisms by which obesity may cause GERD-related disorders have been suggested, starting from the role of abdominal obesity. A number of studies have indicated that the abdominal diameter and/or the waist circumference represent important risk factors for developing GERD symptoms, independent of BMI (El-Serag, 2008b). This is mainly due to a mechanical pathogenesis related to the extrinsic gastric compression caused by the abdominal adipose tissue. It may affect esophageal reflux through increased intraabdominal pressures, impaired gastric emptying, decreased lower esophageal sphincter pressure, and increased frequency of transient lower esophageal sphincter relaxation (Hampel et al., 2005). Moreover, abdominal obesity promotes gastroesophageal reflux through the anatomical disruption of the gastroesophageal junction causing an increased reflux across the lower esophageal sphincter with subsequent increased esophageal exposure to gastroduodenal contents (El-Serag, 2008b).

Together with the mechanical hypothesis, it has also been suggested that adipose tissue might contribute to the pathogenesis of GERD also through its hormonal, endocrine, and paracrine activity. Indeed, the adipose tissue, apart from being cellular fat deposit, is known to be an endocrine organ, producing several hormones and, in particular, estrogens. Two large population-based case–control studies indicated that the association of obesity and GERD might be mediated by the effects of circulating estrogens since the results showed that severely obese women had a higher risk (OR=6.3; 95% CI, 4.9–8.0) of GERD symptoms compared with obese men (OR=3.3; 95% CI, 2.4–4.7). Such risk was highest among premenopausal women and postmenopausal women on estrogen therapy (Nilsson et al., 2003). The same studies showed a significant association between obesity and esophagitis in women, an effect that was furthermore potentiated if the overweight postmenopausal women underwent estrogen treatment. However, the estrogen hypothesis is in contrast with most of the epidemiological studies that generally report no significant association between gender and GERD development (Vakil, 2010).

Last, the metabolic activity of the adipose tissue has also been strongly associated with increased release of several proinflammatory cytokines such as interleukin-1β, interleukin-6, and tumor necrosis factor-α, as well as with low serum levels of adiponectin, an antiapoptotic and antiproliferative molecule. Therefore, abdominal obesity might be a contributing factor that induces the increased inflammation and malignant transformation often reported in patients with GERD (El-Serag, 2008b).

3. Vegetarian Diet and GERD Prevention

A vegetarian diet typically excludes meat from all sources. It is characterized by the inclusion of grains, legumes, fruit, vegetables, and oils and may or may not include dairy products or eggs. A vegan diet excludes all animal products, including eggs, milk, and cheese. There are variations to the vegetarian dietary pattern including lactovegetarian, ovovegetarian, ovolactovegetarian, and pescetarian, and there are also semivegetarian diets: see Chapter 1 of this book for details. Individual reasons for following a vegetarian/vegan diet vary (Craig et al., 2009).

Data document that individuals following a vegetarian dietary pattern typically have lower cholesterol levels (Ferdowsian and Barnard, 2009), blood pressure (Appleby et al., 2002), and lower BMI (Alewaeters et al., 2005). This places them at a lower risk for many disease states including heart disease, diabetes, cancer, and hypertension (Fraser, 1999; Orlich et al., 2015; Tonstad et al., 2009). Because of the strength of the relationship between obesity and GERD, a lower BMI and a lower prevalence of obesity with vegetarian diet is an important factor lowering the risk of GERD in people consuming a vegetarian or plant-based diet.

Several studies comparing vegetarian diets to other weight loss approaches have reported success with the vegetarian diet (Burke et al., 2007; Barnard et al., 2006; Jenkins et al., 2009; Dansinger et al., 2005), as it is reviewed in full in Chapter 18 of this book. It appears that the vegetarian dietary pattern can naturally induce weight loss and also maintain healthy weight status long term. A study showed that weight loss of at least 10% is recommended in all patients with GERD to boost the effect of PPI on reflux symptom relief and to reduce chronic medication use (De Bortoli et al., 2016). So, the patients who lost weight using vegetarian diets could get a great improvement in typical GERD-related symptoms; yet it is unknown to what extent this simply reflects the decrease in body weight or if it could also be in part related to the vegetarian diet, if this diet is kept after weight loss and the weight control period. If there is a specific interest in vegetarian diet beyond weight control and the risk of overweight/obesity is the question at issue, which we will analyze here.

Physiologically, GERD is caused by the abnormal reflux of the gastric contents into the esophagus. Decreased lower esophageal sphincter, transient lower esophageal sphincter relaxation, esophageal acid clearance, and delayed gastric emptying have been implicated in the pathogenesis of GERD (Castell et al., 2004). In addition, oxidative stress caused by free radicals may be an important factor in the pathogenesis of esophageal mucosal damage in GERD (Olyaee et al., 1995; Oh et al., 2001). Oxygen free radicals can cause oxidative injury to cells by damaging proteins, cell membranes, or DNA. Vegetarian diets are characterized by greater consumption of fruit and vegetables containing innumerable phytochemicals, dietary fiber, and antioxidants than omnivores, while restricting their consumption of animal-sources of food (Rauma and Mykkanen, 2000; Blomhoff, 2005). This type of diet helps improve antioxidant status, lowers oxidative stress, and reduces blood lipid levels (Szeto et al., 2004). Moreover, fatty meals decrease lower esophageal sphincter pressure, which may aggravate gastroesophageal reflux. Vegetarian diet has lower fat components compared with most conventional diet (Clarys et al., 2014). Several studies showed that consumption of nonvegetarian foods was an independent predictor of GERD (Jung et al., 2013; Bhatia et al., 2011; Ramu et al., 2011).

Jung et al. (2013) found that nonvegetarianism was significantly associated with reflux esophagitis after adjusting for multiple confounding factors including smoking, alcohol consumption, and waist circumference (OR = 2.08; 95% CI, 1.09–3.97). This study showed that male sex and negative *H. pylori* IgG antibody were also associated with the presence of reflux esophagitis. Lifestyle factors, such as smoking and alcohol consumption, were significantly associated with reflux esophagitis. However, in a multivariate analysis adjusting for multiple potential confounding factors including diet, lifestyle factors were not associated with reflux esophagitis (Table 25.1). This suggests that nonvegetarian diet may be a more important risk factor for reflux esophagitis than other risk factors, such as smoking, alcohol consumption, obesity, or metabolic syndrome. In this study, they could not identify any significant relationship between reflux esophagitis and obesity indexes,

Table 25.1 Risk Factors of Reflux Esophagitis

	Univariate Analysis		Multivariate Analysis[a]	
	OR (95% CI)	*P* Value	OR (95% CI)	*P* Value
H. pylori IgG Antibody				
Negative	1.89 (1.02–3.49)	.04	1.96 (1.04–3.71)	.04
Sex				
Male	3.33 (1.66–6.67)	<.001	3.44 (1.70–6.97)	.01
Diet				
Vegetarianism	1		1	
Regular diet	1.99 (1.06–3.74)	.03	2.08 (1.09–3.97)	.03
Waist Circumference (cm)				
Male ≤90 cm, female ≤80 cm	1		1	
Male >90 cm, female >80 cm	1.99 (1.06–3.74)	.03	1.23 (0.63–2.41)	.55
Lifestyle Factors				
Current smoking	3.37 (1.44–7.88)	.01	1.82 (0.69–4.79)	.23
Alcohol consumption	2.75 (1.38–5.48)	.01	1.36 (0.56–3.31)	.50

CI, confidence interval; *OR*, odds ratio.
[a]Adjusted for *H. pylori* IgG antibody, sex, diet, waist circumference, HbA1c, smoking, and alcohol.
From Jung, J.G., Kang, H.W., Hahn, S.J., Kim, J.H., Lee, J.K., Lim, Y.J., Koh, M.S., Lee, J.H., 2013. Vegetarianism as a protective factor for reflux esophagitis: a retrospective, cross-sectional study between Buddhist priests and general population. Dig. Dis. Sci. 58, 2244–2252 in *n* = 246, normal versus *n* = 50, reflux esophagitis.

Table 25.2 Effect of Variables on Reflux Esophagitis

	Univariate Analysis	
	OR (95% CI)	P Value
Body Mass Index (kg/m²)		
<25	1	
≥25	0.97 (0.53–1.78)	.92
Waist-to-Hip Ratio		
<0.90	1	
≥0.90	1.25 (0.65–2.39)	.50
Visceral Adipose Tissue Area (cm²)		
Quartile I	1	
Quartile II	0.89 (0.37–2.16)	.79
Quartile III	1.10 (0.47–2.60)	.83
Quartile IV	1.23 (0.52–2.87)	.64
Subcutaneous Adipose Tissue Area (cm²)		
Quartile I	1	
Quartile II	1.60 (0.75–3.43)	.22
Quartile III	1.86 (0.76–4.55)	.17
Quartile IV	2.09 (0.70–6.27)	.18
Metabolic Syndrome		
Yes	1.00 (0.49–2.04)	.99

CI, confidence interval; OR, odds ratio.
From Jung, J.G., Kang, H.W., Hahn, S.J., Kim, J.H., Lee, J.K., Lim, Y.J., Koh, M.S., Lee, J.H., 2013. Vegetarianism as a protective factor for reflux esophagitis: a retrospective, cross-sectional study between Buddhist priests and general population. Dig. Dis. Sci. 58, 2244–2252 in n = 246, normal versus n = 50, reflux esophagitis.

including BMI (a marker of body fat percentage), waist-to-hip ratio, and abdominal adipose tissue area (a marker of visceral obesity), apart from waist circumference (a marker of central obesity). Also, they failed to detect any association between reflux esophagitis and metabolic syndrome (Table 25.2).

Another study also demonstrated that consumption of nonvegetarian foods was an independent predictor of GERD (OR = 0.34; 95% CI, 0.21–0.55) (Bhatia et al., 2011). They showed that frequent consumption of meat, fried food, and spices was higher among subjects with GERD on univariate analysis. Tea/coffee consumption was more frequent among subjects with GERD. There was no relationship between tobacco use or alcohol consumption and GERD. However, on multivariate analysis, only intake of nonvegetarian food was positively associated with GERD (Table 25.3).

Therefore, vegetarian diets may offer protective effect for reflux esophagitis. It is uncertain whether established health benefits for vegetarians are attributable to the absence of meat in the diet, the increased consumption of particular food components, the pattern of foods taken within the vegetarian diet, or other healthy lifestyle components often associated with vegetarianism (Mcevoy et al., 2012).

Table 25.3   Factors Independently Associated With GERD on Multivariate Analysis

	Multivariate Analysis	
	Adjusted OR (95% CI)	P Value (LR-Test)
Age >40 versus age ≤40 years	1.05 (0.75–1.47)	.79
Female versus male	0.76 (0.53–1.08)	.12
Nonspicy food versus spicy food	0.90 (0.60–1.36)	.62
Nonfried food versus fried food	1.15 (0.80–1.64)	.45
Nonaerated drink versus aerated drink	2.02 (0.84–4.89)	.12
Tea/coffee: no versus yes	0.66 (0.29–1.50)	.31
Vegetarian food versus nonvegetarian food	0.34 (0.21–0.55)	<.001

CI, confidence interval; *GERD*, gastroesophageal reflux disease; *LR-test*: likelihood ratio test; *OR*, odds ratio.
From Bhatia, S.J., Reddy, D.N., Ghoshal, U.C., Jayanthi, V., Abraham, P., Choudhuri, G., Broor, S.L., Ahuja, V., Augustine, P., Balakrishnan, V., Bhasin, D.K., Bhat, N., Chacko, A., Dadhich, S., Dhali, G.K., Dhawan, P.S., Dwivedi, M., Goenka, M.K., Koshy, A., Kumar, A., Misra, S.P., Mukewar, S., Raju, E.P., Shenoy, K.T., Singh, S.P., Sood, A., Srinivasan, R., 2011. Epidemiology and symptom profile of gastroesophageal reflux in the Indian population: report of the Indian Society of Gastroenterology Task Force. Indian J. Gastroenterol. 30, 118–127 in 245 (7.6%) GERD patients of 3224 subjects.

4. Conclusion

The association between obesity and the increase in GERD has been confirmed by both epidemiological data and a large amount of evidence explaining the mechanisms of their association. Abdominal obesity causing increased intragastric pressures and disruption of the gastroesophageal junction, the hormonal release related to adipose tissue, and the visceral fat metabolic activity linked to the release of proinflammatory molecules have been suggested as the main mechanisms linking obesity and GERD-related symptoms.

Weight gain rather than obesity itself seems to be the cause of the increase in GERD and its related symptoms. Vegetarian dietary pattern can induce weight control and be helpful for weight loss program, being favorable to maintaining a healthy weight status for a long time.

Oxidative stress to esophageal mucosa may also play a key role in the pathogenesis of GERD. Vegetarian diets are enriched in antioxidants, which may reduce oxidative stress. Antioxidant defense mechanisms work against different types of free radicals, which may play a role in the development of reflux esophagitis. Therefore, vegetarian diet may reduce the risk of GERD and its complications. Further study would be needed to confirm this important effect and to decipher the underlying mechanisms.

References

Alewaeters, K., Clarys, P., Hebbelinck, M., Deriemaeker, P., Clarys, J.P., 2005. Cross-sectional analysis of BMI and some lifestyle variables in Flemish vegetarians compared with non-vegetarians. Ergonomics 48, 1433–1444.

Appleby, P.N., Davey, G.K., Key, T.J., 2002. Hypertension and blood pressure among meat eaters, fish eaters, vegetarians and vegans in EPIC-Oxford. Public Health Nutr. 5, 645–654.

Barnard, N.D., Cohen, J., Jenkins, D.J., Turner-Mcgrievy, G., Gloede, L., Jaster, B., Seidl, K., Green, A.A., Talpers, S., 2006. A low-fat vegan diet improves glycemic control and cardiovascular risk factors in a randomized clinical trial in individuals with type 2 diabetes. Diabetes Care 29, 1777–1783.

Bhatia, S.J., Reddy, D.N., Ghoshal, U.C., Jayanthi, V., Abraham, P., Choudhuri, G., Broor, S.L., Ahuja, V., Augustine, P., Balakrishnan, V., Bhasin, D.K., Bhat, N., Chacko, A., Dadhich, S., Dhali, G.K., Dhawan, P.S., Dwivedi, M., Goenka, M.K., Koshy, A., Kumar, A., Misra, S.P., Mukewar, S., Raju, E.P., Shenoy, K.T., Singh, S.P., Sood, A., Srinivasan, R., 2011. Epidemiology and symptom profile of gastroesophageal reflux in the Indian population: report of the Indian Society of Gastroenterology Task Force. Indian J. Gastroenterol. 30, 118–127.

Blomhoff, R., 2005. Dietary antioxidants and cardiovascular disease. Curr. Opin. Lipidol. 16, 47–54.

Burke, L.E., Hudson, A.G., Warziski, M.T., Styn, M.A., Music, E., Elci, O.U., Sereika, S.M., 2007. Effects of a vegetarian diet and treatment preference on biochemical and dietary variables in overweight and obese adults: a randomized clinical trial. Am. J. Clin. Nutr. 86, 588–596.

Castell, D.O., Murray, J.A., Tutuian, R., Orlando, R.C., Arnold, R., 2004. Review article: the pathophysiology of gastro-oesophageal reflux disease – oesophageal manifestations. Aliment. Pharmacol. Ther. 20 (Suppl. 9), 14–25.

Chung, S.J., Kim, D., Park, M.J., Kim, Y.S., Kim, J.S., Jung, H.C., Song, I.S., 2008. Metabolic syndrome and visceral obesity as risk factors for reflux oesophagitis: a cross-sectional case-control study of 7078 Koreans undergoing health check-ups. Gut 57, 1360–1365.

Clarys, P., Deliens, T., Huybrechts, I., Deriemaeker, P., Vanaelst, B., De Keyzer, W., Hebbelinck, M., Mullie, P., 2014. Comparison of nutritional quality of the vegan, vegetarian, semi-vegetarian, pesco-vegetarian and omnivorous diet. Nutrients 6, 1318–1332.

Corley, D.A., Kubo, A., 2006. Body mass index and gastroesophageal reflux disease: a systematic review and meta-analysis. Am. J. Gastroenterol. 101, 2619–2628.

Craig, W.J., Mangels, A.R., American Dietetic, A., 2009. Position of the American Dietetic Association: vegetarian diets. J. Am. Diet. Assoc. 109, 1266–1282.

Dansinger, M.L., Gleason, J.A., Griffith, J.L., Selker, H.P., Schaefer, E.J., 2005. Comparison of the Atkins, Ornish, Weight Watchers, and Zone diets for weight loss and heart disease risk reduction: a randomized trial. JAMA 293, 43–53.

De Bortoli, N., Guidi, G., Martinucci, I., Savarino, E., Imam, H., Bertani, L., Russo, S., Franchi, R., Macchia, L., Furnari, M., Ceccarelli, L., Savarino, V., Marchi, S., 2016. Voluntary and controlled weight loss can reduce symptoms and proton pump inhibitor use and dosage in patients with gastroesophageal reflux disease: a comparative study. Dis. Esophagus. 29 (2), 197–204. http://dx.doi.org/10.1111/dote.12319.

El-Serag, H., 2008a. The association between obesity and GERD: a review of the epidemiological evidence. Dig. Dis. Sci. 53, 2307–2312.

El-Serag, H., 2008b. Role of obesity in GORD-related disorders. Gut 57, 281–284.

El-Serag, H.B., Ergun, G.A., Pandolfino, J., Fitzgerald, S., Tran, T., Kramer, J.R., 2007. Obesity increases oesophageal acid exposure. Gut 56, 749–755.

El-Serag, H.B., Johanson, J.F., 2002. Risk factors for the severity of erosive esophagitis in *Helicobacter pylori*-negative patients with gastroesophageal reflux disease. Scand. J. Gastroenterol. 37, 899–904.

Eusebi, L.H., Fuccio, L., Bazzoli, F., 2012. The role of obesity in gastroesophageal reflux disease and Barrett's esophagus. Dig. Dis. 30, 154–157.

Ferdowsian, H.R., Barnard, N.D., 2009. Effects of plant-based diets on plasma lipids. Am. J. Cardiol. 104, 947–956.

Flegal, K.M., Carroll, M.D., Ogden, C.L., Curtin, L.R., 2010. Prevalence and trends in obesity among US adults, 1999-2008. JAMA 303, 235–241.

Fraser, G.E., 1999. Associations between diet and cancer, ischemic heart disease, and all-cause mortality in non-Hispanic white California Seventh-day Adventists. Am. J. Clin. Nutr. 70, 532S–538S.

Fujiwara, Y., Arakawa, T., 2009. Epidemiology and clinical characteristics of GERD in the Japanese population. J. Gastroenterol. 44, 518–534.

Hampel, H., Abraham, N.S., El-Serag, H.B., 2005. Meta-analysis: obesity and the risk for gastroesophageal reflux disease and its complications. Ann. Intern. Med. 143, 199–211.

Inamori, M., Togawa, J., Nagase, H., Abe, Y., Umezawa, T., Nakajima, A., Saito, T., Ueno, N., Tanaka, K., Sekihara, H., Kaifu, H., Tsuboi, H., Kayama, H., Tominaga, S., Nagura, H., 2003. Clinical characteristics of Japanese reflux esophagitis patients as determined by Los Angeles classification. J. Gastroenterol. Hepatol. 18, 172–176.

Iovino, P., Angrisani, L., Galloro, G., Consalvo, D., Tremolaterra, F., Pascariello, A., Ciacci, C., 2006. Proximal stomach function in obesity with normal or abnormal oesophageal acid exposure. Neurogastroenterol. Motil. 18, 425–432.

Jacobson, B.C., Somers, S.C., Fuchs, C.S., Kelly, C.P., Camargo Jr., C.A., 2006. Body-mass index and symptoms of gastroesophageal reflux in women. N. Engl. J. Med. 354, 2340–2348.

Jenkins, D.J., Wong, J.M., Kendall, C.W., Esfahani, A., Ng, V.W., Leong, T.C., Faulkner, D.A., Vidgen, E., Greaves, K.A., Paul, G., Singer, W., 2009. The effect of a plant-based low-carbohydrate ("Eco-Atkins") diet on body weight and blood lipid concentrations in hyperlipidemic subjects. Arch. Intern. Med. 169, 1046–1054.

Jung, J.G., Kang, H.W., Hahn, S.J., Kim, J.H., Lee, J.K., Lim, Y.J., Koh, M.S., Lee, J.H., 2013. Vegetarianism as a protective factor for reflux esophagitis: a retrospective, cross-sectional study between Buddhist priests and general population. Dig. Dis. Sci. 58, 2244–2252.

Kang, M.S., Park, D.I., Oh, S.Y., Yoo, T.W., Ryu, S.H., Park, J.H., Kim, H.J., Cho, Y.K., Sohn, C.I., Jeon, W.K., Kim, B.I., 2007. Abdominal obesity is an independent risk factor for erosive esophagitis in a Korean population. J. Gastroenterol. Hepatol. 22, 1656–1661.

Kaufman, S.E., Kaye, M.D., 1978. Induction of gastro-oesophageal reflux by alcohol. Gut 19, 336–338.

Khodarahmi, M., Azadbakht, L., Daghaghzadeh, H., Feinle-Bisset, C., Keshteli, A.H., Afshar, H., Feizi, A., Esmaillzadeh, A., Adibi, P., 2016. Evaluation of the relationship between major dietary patterns and uninvestigated reflux among Iranian adults. Nutrition 32, 573–583.

Lee, S.W., Chang, C.M., Chang, C.S., Kao, A.W., Chou, M.C., 2011. Comparison of presentation and impact on quality of life of gastroesophageal reflux disease between young and old adults in a Chinese population. World J. Gastroenterol. 17, 4614–4618.

Mcevoy, C.T., Temple, N., Woodside, J.V., 2012. Vegetarian diets, low-meat diets and health: a review. Public Health Nutr. 1–8.

Mold, J.W., Reed, L.E., Davis, A.B., Allen, M.L., Decktor, D.L., Robinson, M., 1991. Prevalence of gastro-esophageal reflux in elderly patients in a primary care setting. Am. J. Gastroenterol. 86, 965–970.

Nam, S.Y., Choi, I.J., Ryu, K.H., Park, B.J., Kim, H.B., Nam, B.H., 2010. Abdominal visceral adipose tissue volume is associated with increased risk of erosive esophagitis in men and women. Gastroenterology 139 1902–1911.e2.

Nilsson, M., Johnsen, R., Ye, W., Hveem, K., Lagergren, J., 2003. Obesity and estrogen as risk factors for gastroesophageal reflux symptoms. JAMA 290, 66–72.

Ogden, C.L., Carroll, M.D., Curtin, L.R., Lamb, M.M., Flegal, K.M., 2010. Prevalence of high body mass index in US children and adolescents, 2007-2008. JAMA 303, 242–249.

Oh, T.Y., Lee, J.S., Ahn, B.O., Cho, H., Kim, W.B., Kim, Y.B., Surh, Y.J., Cho, S.W., Hahm, K.B., 2001. Oxidative damages are critical in pathogenesis of reflux esophagitis: implication of antioxidants in its treatment. Free Radic. Biol. Med. 30, 905–915.

Olyaee, M., Sontag, S., Salman, W., Schnell, T., Mobarhan, S., Eiznhamer, D., Keshavarzian, A., 1995. Mucosal reactive oxygen species production in oesophagitis and Barrett's oesophagus. Gut 37, 168–173.

Orlich, M.J., Singh, P.N., Sabate, J., Fan, J., Sveen, L., Bennett, H., Knutsen, S.F., Beeson, W.L., Jaceldo-Siegl, K., Butler, T.L., Herring, R.P., Fraser, G.E., 2015. Vegetarian dietary patterns and the risk of colorectal cancers. JAMA Intern. Med. 175, 767–776.

Ramu, B., Mohan, P., Rajasekaran, M.S., Jayanthi, V., 2011. Prevalence and risk factors for gastroesophageal reflux in pregnancy. Indian J. Gastroenterol. 30, 144–147.

Rauma, A.L., Mykkanen, H., 2000. Antioxidant status in vegetarians versus omnivores. Nutrition 16, 111–119.

Sheen, E., Triadafilopoulos, G., 2011. Adverse effects of long-term proton pump inhibitor therapy. Dig. Dis. Sci. 56, 931–950.

Shim, K.N., Hong, S.J., Sung, J.K., Park, K.S., Kim, S.E., Park, H.S., Kim, Y.S., Lim, S.H., Kim, C.H., Park, M.J., Yim, J.Y., Cho, K.R., Kim, D., Park, S.J., Jee, S.R., Kim, J.I., Park, J.Y., Song, G.A., Jung, H.Y., Lee, Y.C., Kim, J.G., Kim, J.J., Kim, N., Park, S.H., Jung, H.C., Chung, I.S., H. pylori and GERD Study Group of Korean College of Helicobacter and Upper Gastrointestinal Research, 2009. Clinical spectrum of reflux esophagitis among 25,536 Koreans who underwent a health check-up: a nationwide multicenter prospective, endoscopy-based study. J. Clin. Gastroenterol. 43, 632–638.

Song, H.J., Shim, K.N., Yoon, S.J., Kim, S.E., Oh, H.J., Ryu, K.H., Ha, C.Y., Yeom, H.J., Song, J.H., Jung, S.A., Yoo, K., 2009. The prevalence and clinical characteristics of reflux esophagitis in koreans and its possible relation to metabolic syndrome. J. Korean Med. Sci. 24, 197–202.

Sonnenberg, A., El-Serag, H.B., 1999. Clinical epidemiology and natural history of gastroesophageal reflux disease. Yale J. Biol. Med. 72, 81–92.

Stanciu, C., Bennett, J.R., 1972. Smoking and gastro-oesophageal reflux. Br. Med. J. 3, 793–795.

Szeto, Y.T., Kwok, T.C., Benzie, I.F., 2004. Effects of a long-term vegetarian diet on biomarkers of antioxidant status and cardiovascular disease risk. Nutrition 20, 863–866.

Tonstad, S., Butler, T., Yan, R., Fraser, G.E., 2009. Type of vegetarian diet, body weight, and prevalence of type 2 diabetes. Diabetes Care 32, 791–796.

Vakil, N., 2010. Disease definition, clinical manifestations, epidemiology and natural history of GERD. Best Pract. Res. Clin. Gastroenterol. 24, 759–764.

Vakil, N., Van Zanten, S.V., Kahrilas, P., Dent, J., Jones, R., Global Consensus, G., 2006. The Montreal definition and classification of gastroesophageal reflux disease: a global evidence-based consensus. Am. J. Gastroenterol. 101, 1900–1920 quiz 1943.

Vakil, N., Van Zanten, S.V., Kahrilas, P., Dent, J., Jones, R., Globale, K., 2007. The Montreal definition and classification of gastroesophageal reflux disease: a global, evidence-based consensus paper. Z. Gastroenterol. 45, 1125–1140.

Wilson, L.J., Ma, W., Hirschowitz, B.I., 1999. Association of obesity with hiatal hernia and esophagitis. Am. J. Gastroenterol. 94, 2840–2844.

Yeh, C., Hsu, C.T., Ho, A.S., Sampliner, R.E., Fass, R., 1997. Erosive esophagitis and Barrett's esophagus in Taiwan: a higher frequency than expected. Dig. Dis. Sci. 42, 702–706.

26

Defecation and Stools in Vegetarians: Implications in Health and Disease

Preetam Nath, Shivaram Prasad Singh

S.C.B. MEDICAL COLLEGE, CUTTACK, INDIA

1. Introduction

Defecation is defined as the final act of digestion, by which organisms eliminate their undigested waste material from the digestive tract via the anus. Bowel habits and stool types vary considerably between different populations. Even individuals of a single community have different defecation profiles. Both genetic and environmental factors influence the pattern of defecation in a person. Among the environmental factors, diet is the most important one. Today, there is a growing awareness and curiosity about the health implications of vegetarian and vegan diet, and it is fast gaining recognition as a healthy and potentially therapeutic dietary choice (Craig, 2009). Vegetarian diet does have effects on each and every organ and system of the human body, and vegetarian diets have been accepted as a dietary treatment strategy for good health. It also helps in managing several diseases and conditions ranging from cardiovascular diseases to malignancies (Craig, 2009). Vegetarian diets have also been proposed as medical nutrition therapy for treatment of conditions like metabolic syndrome, including obesity, diabetes, nonalcoholic fatty liver disease, and cardiovascular diseases (Le and Sabaté, 2014; Tonstad et al., 2013; Jenkins et al., 2014; Kahleova et al., 2011). Some researchers have proposed that it may confer protection against chronic inflammatory conditions such as rheumatoid arthritis (Kjeldsen-Kragh, 1999; Peltonen et al., 1997). The gastrointestinal tract happens to be the largest organ system of our body, and there is a definite difference in motility of gut and the composition of human gut microbiota between people consuming plant-based vegetarian and ovolactovegetarian diets and those taking a nonvegetarian diet (Kabeerdoss et al., 2012). Defecation, being an important part of digestion, is also affected by the type of diet we consume. In this chapter, we will discuss the defecation and stool patterns in vegetarians as compared to nonvegetarians.

2. Frequency of Bowel Movements

A plant-based vegetarian diet contains higher amounts of complex starch and dietary fibers than a nonvegetarian diet. People who consume a vegetarian diet have usually a higher number of average bowel movements per day than others (see Table 26.1). The mean transit time is lower in individuals consuming a vegetarian diet. Vegetarian and vegan diet consumers are less prone to develop constipation both in terms of bowel frequency and stool consistency. A study from coastal eastern India has shown that nonvegetarianism was associated with lesser daily bowel movements and harder stool forms; however, on multivariate analysis, only female gender and older age (>35 years) were found to be independent predictors of constipation (≤3 stools per week). In the same study, vegetarians and occasional nonvegetarians had higher daily stool frequency than nonvegetarians (11.8±4.5 and 12.8±4.7 vs. 11.3±4.7, respectively) (Panigrahi et al., 2013). Davies et al. (1986) too had observed that people of Kingston, Surrey, who adhered to vegan diet had higher daily stool frequency (1.7±0.9) than ovolactovegetarians (1.2±0.5) followed by nonvegetarians (1.0±0.2). Similarly, in the Prospective Netherlands Cohort Study on diet by Gilsing et al. (2013), 7% of vegetarians had more than two stools per day, which was higher than pescetarians (5%), followed by meat consumers (3%). The proportions of individuals with stool frequency fewer than three per week in the three groups were 2%, 3%, and 6%, respectively. This study clearly demonstrated an inverse dose relationship between the amount of meat in the diet and frequency of defecation. Sanjoaquin et al. (2003), in a large prospective study, had investigated the relationships between nutritional and lifestyle factors and bowel movement frequency. They also observed that the odds of having daily bowel movements for vegans compared with meat eaters were 2.49 (95% CI: 1.33–4.64) for men and 3.59 (95% CI: 2.50–5.16) for women.

3. Form and Consistency of Stool

Stool form and caliber is an important part of assessment of defecatory disorder in any patient, and the Bristol stool chart (Fig. 26.1) is the most widely accepted scale for

Table 26.1 Comparison of Stool Defecation Frequency (per Week) Among Different Dietary Categories

Study	Nonvegetarian	Ovolactovegetarian	Vegans	P Value
Davies et al. (1986)	7.0±1.4	8.4±3.5	11.9±6.3	<0.001
Panigrahi et al. (2013)	11.3±4.7	12.8±4.7[a]		<0.05
Sanjoaquin et al. (2003)	9.5 (men)	–	11.6 (men)	–
	8.2 (women)		10.5 (women)	

Ovolactovegetarian: taking dairy and eggs, but no meat, fish and seafood.

Vegans: taking no animal products at all. They also avoid the use of honey and animal-related products.

[a]In the study by Panigrahi et al., the ovolactovegetarians and vegans were clubbed onto a single group (i.e., vegetarians).

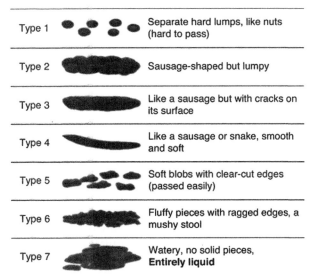

FIGURE 26.1 Bristol stool form scale.

assessment of stool form and consistency (Heaton et al., 1991). This stool scale has been validated and has been found to correlate with transit time of the whole gut (O'Donnell et al., 1988). Stool form is directly related to the amount of fiber and water in stool. Decreased intake of dietary fluids and low fibers lead to hard stools. The resultant stool often assumes the shape of a wide sausage with large cracks on the surface (Bristol score 2–3). On the contrary, a diet rich in high fiber and fluids helps in making the stool look like a sausage or snake with smooth surface and soft consistency, sometimes as soft blobs with clear-cut edges (Bristol score 4–5). Vegetarian diet is rich in dietary fiber. Davies et al. (1986), in a group of 17 subjects (10 females and 7 males), assessed the amount of dietary fiber in nonvegetarian, ovolactovegetarian, and vegan diets, and they found that the mean fiber intake was 23, 37, and 47 g, respectively, in the three types of diet. They also observed that there is a significant correlation between amount of dietary fiber intake and various stool parameters. They used a linear scale to objectively assess the stool form and consistency in the study subjects. The scale had scores ranging from 1 to 8. A score of 1 represented the loose and watery stools. As the score advanced, the form of the stool became harder. A score of 8 was used when stool took the shape of fragmented segments or pellets like sheep droppings or corrugated formations and button-like discs. They observed that the mean stool form in nonvegetarians, plant-based vegetarians, and ovolactovegetarians was 5.7 ± 1.3, 5.0 ± 1.5, and 4.5 ± 1.2, respectively. This study reaffirmed that vegetarians differ a lot from their nonvegetarian counterparts in terms of stool form, shape, and consistency. Besides, as vegetarian diet contains a higher amount of fiber, this leads to increased daily fecal wet weight. In vegetarians, the shape of the stool veers toward the lower end of the fecal form scale (Davies et al., 1986); people who consume vegetarian diets tend to have softer stools with fewer superficial cracks.

4. Vegetarian Diet and Constipation

Studies by Panigrahi et al. (2013) and Davies et al. (1986) have shown that people who consume a vegan or vegetarian diet have higher frequency of bowel movements, as mentioned earlier. Similarly, Gilsing et al. (2013) and Sanjoaquin et al. (2003) observed that average bowel movement frequency is significantly higher in vegetarians, and they have higher odds of having bowel movement daily. Besides, the consistency of stool is softer than in nonvegetarians, with increased mean fecal weight (Davies et al., 1986). Intestinal transit time is also comparatively faster in vegetarians than nonvegetarians. As a result, vegetarians are less prone to suffer from straining during defecation.

4.1 Fecal Microbiota Composition in Vegetarians

After the newer molecular characterization of intestinal microbiota, there is growing interest in the relationship between diet, microbiota, nutrition, and human health. A study has demonstrated that people consuming a vegan diet had decreased levels of *Bacteroides* spp., *Bifidobacterium* spp., *Escherichia coli*, and *Enterobacteriaceae* spp. as compared to controls (nonvegetarians), with vegetarians lying in between them (Zimmer et al., 2012). Another study also observed that the animal-based diets increased the abundance of bile-tolerant organisms such as *Alistipes*, *Bilophila*, and *Bacteroides*, and decreased the level of Firmicutes that helps in metabolizing dietary plant polysaccharides like *Roseburia*, *Eubacterium rectale*, and *Ruminoccus bromii* (David et al., 2013). The interaction between diet and gut microbiota and their relation to health and disease have been discussed in detail in Chapter 24.

5. Vegetarian Diet and Gastrointestinal Diseases

5.1 Effect of Vegetarian Diet on Irritable Bowel Syndrome

Irritable bowel syndrome (IBS) is a common chronic gastrointestinal disorder that affects about 5%–20% of the general population (Agréus et al., 1995; Hungin et al., 2003). This condition impairs the quality of life considerably, though it is not known to progress into any serious disease or to cause death (Whitehead et al., 1996; Gralnek et al., 2000). IBS patients typically suffer from intermittent abdominal pain/discomfort, altered bowel habits, and/or abdominal bloating/distension (El-Salhy et al., 2012; Thompson, 2002).

To date, vegan and vegetarian diets as a whole have not been definitely linked to IBS. However, certain vegetarian foods have been identified as predictors of symptoms of IBS. In a study conducted in China, Guo et al. (2014) observed that people who consume fruits (OR=3.08), vegetables (OR=3.78), and legumes (OR=2.11) at least once weekly have higher risk of having IBS symptoms than those who consumed less than once a week. For the rest of the food items, i.e., noodles, canned foods, pickled foods, pastries (cakes, ice cream, and cream), milk, coffee, and carbonated drinks, there were no significant statistical differences in food preference between the two groups.

In other studies also, food items commonly implicated for IBS symptoms are wheat, milk, dairy products, fructose, caffeine, certain meats, fatty foods, alcohol, spices, and grains (Simrén et al., 2001; Williams et al., 2011; Nanda et al., 1989; Hayes et al., 2014). However, data on the impact of different dietary practices on IBS is inadequate, and more robust data is needed to establish a definite relationship between particular foods and IBS symptoms.

From the previous studies, it has been seen that diets rich in FODMAPs (fermentable oligosaccharides, disaccharides, monosaccharides, and polyols) result in symptoms of IBS, whereas a low-FODMAP diet helps in relieving the symptoms. Both retrospective and prospective open studies have shown that symptoms reduce after introduction of a low-FODMAP diet in IBS patients with suspected or proven fructose or lactose malabsorption (Shepherd and Gibson, 2006; Roest et al., 2013). These findings have also been confirmed by randomized controlled trials, which showed a significant improvement of overall symptoms, including abdominal pain and bloating in patients with bloating and/or diarrhea (Staudacher et al., 2012).

We need more well-designed studies on the effect of food intake on symptom generation. The potential benefit of a low-FODMAP diet seems promising but requires further study. However, dietary guidance is essential due to the complexity of the regimens and risks of inadequate nutrient intake.

6. Impact of Vegetarian Diet in Inflammatory Bowel Disease

Inflammatory bowel disease (IBD) is a chronic immune-mediated disease of the intestinal mucosa occurring in genetically predisposed individuals activated by environmental triggers. Ulcerative colitis (UC) and Crohn disease (CD) are the two major types of IBD. Among the environmental triggers, diet plays an important role. Our bowel lumen is continually exposed to numerous antigens, including the food that we consume and the enormous population of microorganisms that compose the gut microbiome. There are several proposed mechanisms by which diet could influence the incidence and course of IBD; the dietary antigens may alter the gut microbiome, and they may also affect gastrointestinal permeability (Chapman-Kiddell et al., 2010). IBD patients frequently seek advice for food and diet that can improve, or even cure, their disease. However, there is insufficient data on the impact of diet on IBD.

There are a very few observational studies on the association of diet with the natural history of IBD. In the prospective study by Jowett et al. (2004) on patients with ulcerative colitis, it was observed that while patients with higher intake of meat, eggs, protein, and alcohol consumption were more likely to have a relapse of UC, higher intake of fruits and vegetables did not have any significant influence on disease relapse. The explanation given by the authors was that these foods have increased risk of relapse because of higher content of sulfur and sulfate, which increase the concentration of fecal hydrogen sulfide that is toxic to the colonocytes. Subsequently, Magee et al. (2005) too demonstrated a correlation between dietary sulfite consumption and endoscopic disease activity in UC.

They calculated a food sigmoidoscopy score for each food by amount of concerned food consumed and sigmoidoscopic findings, and from the results the authors concluded that sulfite and caffeine were harmful, while thiamin and resistant starch were potentially beneficial in patients of UC. This suggests that IBD patients on a vegetarian or vegan diet may have an advantage over patients on a nonvegetarian diet with regard to the natural course and relapses.

In a dietary interventional uncontrolled trial, food-specific IgG4 levels were used to select which foods to exclude (Rajendran and Kumar 2011). Among all foods, eggs and beef were found to be the most common foods with high IgG4 antibody levels and were excluded in most of the patients. Patients on the exclusion diet had a significant reduction in IBD symptoms and ESR as compared to pretreatment levels. The absence of a control group for comparison was a major drawback of the study. In another study by Chiba et al. (2010), a semivegetarian diet demonstrated superiority over a nonvegetarian diet in maintaining clinical remission over 2 years (94% vs. 33%). In a prospective cohort study, Jantchou et al. (2010) observed that there is a strong association of high animal protein intake with the development of IBD (HR 3.01). However, large randomized controlled trials are needed to prove these associations.

7. Vegetarian Diet and Diverticular Diseases

According to the hypothesis by Painter and Burkitt (1971), diverticular disease is a fiber-deficiency disease caused by a refined carbohydrate diet with low dietary fiber. In a study on health professionals, Aldoori et al. (1994) observed an inverse relationship between dietary fiber intake and risk of symptomatic diverticular disease. They also suggested that certain dietary factors like a high intake of meat might increase the risk of developing diverticular disease. Lower rates of diverticular disease among vegetarians compared with meat eaters have been reported in some cross-sectional studies (Gear et al., 1979; Crowe et al., 2011). In these studies, a vegetarian diet with a relatively high intake of dietary fiber (>25 g/day) was associated with a reduced risk of hospital admission and death from diverticular disease. Vegans experienced even lower risk of diverticular disease, but the size of the population was very small.

It has been observed that both a vegetarian diet and a high intake of dietary fiber were positively correlated with rapid bowel transit time (Gear et al., 1981) and increased daily frequency of bowel movements (Sanjoaquin et al., 2004). This could be the biological mechanism by which people with vegetarian diet and a high intake of dietary fiber have an advantage over nonvegetarians in terms of reduced risk of diverticular disease. A reduced transit time implies that lesser amount of water gets reabsorbed from the lower gastrointestinal tract, especially in the colon, which results in larger, softer stools that are easier to pass. The resultant lower intraluminal bowel pressure offers a benefit by reduced likelihood of formation of the pouches or bulges through the weakened intestinal wall leading to decreased incidence of diverticula (Stollman and Raskin, 2004).

8. Impact of Vegetarian Diet on Colorectal Carcinoma

It has been estimated that nutrition probably accounts for more than one-third of deaths due to malignancies (Doll and Peto, 1981), and people consuming a vegetarian diet may have lower incidence of colonic malignancies. This may be due to the fact that a vegetarian diet leads to softer stools with rapid colonic transit, which helps in decreased exposure of the colonic epithelium to intestinal carcinogens in the gut (Cummings et al., 1992). The relationship between diet and colorectal carcinoma has been discussed in a separate dedicated chapter (Chapter 19).

9. Conclusions

The hope of impacting health through diet is one of the oldest concepts in medicine. The recent developments in medical science have paved the way for a better understanding of human physiology and how it is impacted by individual dietary components and practices. Vegetarian and vegan diets offer a lot of health benefits, including those involving the gastrointestinal tract. Vegetarians have lower incidence of constipation, hard stools, and various gut disorders like irritable bowel disorders, IBD, diverticular diseases, and colorectal malignancies.

In the light of the available data, it would be reasonable to surmise that awareness about the beneficial effects of vegetarian diet could have a beneficial impact on the incidence and burden of these different gastrointestinal disorders, as well as the overall quality of life in the general population. Large-scale interventional studies are necessary to further validate and reinforce these conclusions and to justify promotion of adoption of a vegetarian diet.

References

Agréus, L., Svärdsudd, K., Nyrén, O., Tibblin, G., 1995. Irritable bowel syndrome and dyspepsia in the general population: overlap and lack of stability over time. Gastroenterology 109 (3), 671–680.

Aldoori, W.H., Giovannucci, E.L., Rimm, E.B., Wing, A.L., Trichopoulos, D.V., Willett, W.C., 1994. A prospective study of diet and the risk of symptomatic diverticular disease in men. Am. J. Clin. Nutr. 60, 757–764.

Chapman-Kiddell, C.A., Davies, P.S., Gillen, L., Radford-Smith, G.L., 2010. Role of diet in the development of inflammatory bowel disease. Inflamm. Bowel Dis. 16, 137–151.

Chiba, M., Abe, T., Tsuda, H., Sugawara, T., Tsuda, S., Tozawa, H., Fujiwara, K., Imai, H., 2010. Lifestyle-related disease in Crohn's disease: relapse prevention by a semi-vegetarian diet. World J. Gastroenterol. 16 (20), 2484.

Craig, W.J., 2009. Health effects of vegan diets. Am. J. Clin. Nutr. 89, 1627S–1633S.

Crowe, F.L., Appleby, P.N., Allen, N.E., Key, T.J., 2011. Diet and risk of diverticular disease in Oxford cohort of European Prospective Investigation into Cancer and Nutrition (EPIC): prospective study of British vegetarians and non-vegetarians. BMJ 343, d4131.

Cummings, J.H., Bingham, S.A., Heaton, K.W., Eastwood, M.A., 1992. Fecal weight, colon cancer risk, and dietary intake of nonstarch polysaccharides (dietary fiber). Gastroenterology 103, 1783–1789.

David, L.A., Maurice, C.F., Carmody, R.N., Gootenberg, D.B., Button, J.E., Wolfe, B.E., et al., 2013. Diet rapidly and reproducibly alters the human gut microbiome. Nature 505 (7484), 559–563.

Davies, G.J., Crowder, M., Reid, B., Dickerson, J.W.T., 1986. Bowel function measurements of individuals with different eating patterns. Gut 27, 164–169.

Doll, R., Peto, R., 1981. The causes of cancer: quantitative estimates of avoidable risks of cancer in the United States today. J. Natl. Cancer Inst. 66, 1191–1308.

El-Salhy, M., Gundersen, D., Hatlebakk, J.G., Hausken, T., 2012. Irritable Bowel Syndrome: Diagnosis, Pathogenesis and Treatment Options. Nova Science Publishers, Inc., New York.

Gear, J.S.S., Fursdon, P., Nolan, D.J., Ware, A., Mann, J.I., Brodribb, A.J.M., Vessey, M.P., 1979. Symptomless diverticular disease and intake of dietary fibre. Lancet 313 (8115), 511–514.

Gear, J.S.S., Brodribb, A.J.M., Ware, A., Mann, J.I., 1981. Fibre and bowel transit times. Br. J. Nutr. 45, 77–82.

Gilsing, A.M.J., Weijenberg, M.P., Goldbohm, R.A., Dagnelie, P.C., van den Brandt, P., Schouten, L.J., 2013. The Netherlands Cohort Study – meat Investigation Cohort; a population-based cohort over-represented with vegetarians, pescetarians and low meat consumers. Nutr. J. 12, 156.

Gralnek, I.M., Hays, R.D., Kilbourne, A., Naliboff, B., Mayer, E.A., 2000. The impact of irritable bowel syndrome on health-related quality of life. Gastroenterology 119 (3), 654–660.

Guo, Y.B., Zhuang, K.M., Kuang, L., Zhan, Q., Wang, X.F., Liu, S.D., 2014. Association between diet and lifestyle habits and irritable bowel syndrome: a case-control study. Gut Liver 9, 649–656.

Hayes, P., Corish, C., O'mahony, E., Quigley, E.M.M., 2014. A dietary survey of patients with irritable bowel syndrome. J. Hum. Nutr. Diet. 27 (s2), 36–47.

Heaton, K.W., Ghosh, S., Braddon, F.E., 1991. How bad are the symptoms and bowel dysfunction of patients with the irritable bowel syndrome? A prospective, controlled study with emphasis on stool form. Gut 32, 73–79.

Hungin, A.P.S., Whorwell, P.J., Tack, J., Mearin, F., 2003. The prevalence, patterns and impact of irritable bowel syndrome: an international survey of 40 000 subjects. Aliment. Pharmacol. Ther. 17 (5), 643–650.

Jantchou, P., Morois, S., Clavel-Chapelon, F., Boutron-Ruault, M.C., Carbonnel, F., 2010. Animal protein intake and risk of inflammatory bowel disease: the E3N prospective study. Am. J. Gastroenterol. 105 (10), 2195–2201.

Jenkins, D.J.A., Wong, J.M.W., Kendall, C.W.C., Esfahani, A., Ng, V.W.Y., Leong, T.C.K., Faulkner, D.A., Vidgen, E., Paul, G., Mukherjea, R., et al., 2014. Effect of a 6-month vegan low-carbohydrate ("eco-atkins") diet on cardiovascular risk factors and body weight in hyperlipidaemic adults: a randomised controlled trial. BMJ Open 4, e003505.

Jowett, S.L., Seal, C.J., Pearce, M.S., Phillips, E., Gregory, W., Barton, J.R., Welfare, M.R., 2004. Influence of dietary factors on the clinical course of ulcerative colitis: a prospective cohort study. Gut 53 (10), 1479–1484.

Kabeerdoss, J., Devi, R.S., Mary, R.R., Ramakrishna, B.S., 2012. Faecal microbiota composition in vegetarians: comparison with omnivores in a cohort of young women in southern India. Br. J. Nutr. 108, 953–957.

Kahleova, H., Matoulek, M., Malinska, H., Oliyarnik, O., Kazdova, L., Neskudla, T., Skoch, A., et al., 2011. Vegetarian diet improves insulin resistance and oxidative stress markers more than conventional diet in subjects with type 2 diabetes. Diabet. Med. 28, 549–559.

Kjeldsen-Kragh, J., 1999. Rheumatoid arthritis treated with vegetarian diets. Am. J. Clin. Nutr. 70, 594S–600S.

Le, L.T., Sabaté, J., 2014. Beyond meatless, the health effects of vegan diets: findings from the adventist cohorts. Nutrients 6, 2131–2147.

Magee, E.A., Edmond, L.M., Tasker, S.M., Kong, S.C., Curno, R., Cummings, J.H., 2005. Associations between diet and disease activity in ulcerative colitis patients using a novel method of data analysis. Nutr. J. 4 (7).

Nanda, R., James, R., Smith, H., Dudley, C.R., Jewell, D.P., 1989. Food intolerance and the irritable bowel syndrome. Gut 30 (8), 1099–1104.

O'Donnell, L.J.D., Virjee, J., Heaton, K.W., 1988. Pseudo-diarrhoea in the irritable bowel syndrome: patients' records of stool form reflect transit time while stool frequency does not. Gut 29, A1455 [Abstract].

Painter, N.S., Burkitt, D.P., 1971. Diverticular disease of the colon: a deficiency disease of Western civilization. BMJ 2, 450–454.

Panigrahi, M.K., Kar, S.K., Singh, S.P., Ghoshal, U.C., 2013. Defecation frequency and stool form in a coastal eastern indian population. J. Neurogastroenterol. Motil. 19 (3), 374–380.

Peltonen, R., Nenonen, M., Helve, T., Hänninen, O., Toivanen, P., Eerola, E., 1997. Faecal microbial flora and disease activity in rheumatoid arthritis during a vegan diet. Br. J. Rheumatol. 36, 64–68.

Rajendran, N., Kumar, D., 2011. Food-specific IgG4-guided exclusion diets improve symptoms in Crohn's disease: a pilot study. Colorectal Dis. 13, 1009–1013.

Roest, R.D., Dobbs, B.R., Chapman, B.A., Batman, B., O'Brien, L.A., Leeper, J.A., Hebblethwaite, C.R., Gearry, R.B., 2013. The low FODMAP diet improves gastrointestinal symptoms in patients with irritable bowel syndrome: a prospective study. Int. J. Clin. Pract. 67, 895–903.

Sanjoaquin, M.A., Appleby, P.N., Spencer, E.A., Key, T.J., 2004. Nutrition and lifestyle in relation to bowel movement frequency: a cross-sectional study of 20 630 men and women in EPIC–Oxford. Public Health Nutr. 7, 77–83.

Sanjoaquin, M.A., Appleby, P.N., Spencer, E.A., Key, T.J., 2003. Nutrition and lifestyle in relation to bowel movement frequency: a cross-sectional study of 20 630 men and women in EPIC–Oxford. Public Health Nutr. 7 (1), 77–83.

Shepherd, S.J., Gibson, P.R., 2006. Fructose malabsorption and symptoms of irritable bowel syndrome: guidelines for effective dietary management. J. Am. Diet. Assoc. 106, 1631–1639.

Simrén, M., Månsson, A., Langkilde, A.M., Svedlund, J., Abrahamsson, H., Bengtsson, U., Björnsson, E.S., 2001. Food-related gastrointestinal symptoms in the irritable bowel syndrome. Digestion 63 (2), 108–115.

Staudacher, H.M., Lomer, M.C., Anderson, J.L., Barrett, J.S., Muir, J.G., Irving, P.M., Whelan, K., 2012. Fermentable carbohydrate restriction reduces luminal bifidobacteria and gastrointestinal symptoms in patients with irritable bowel syndrome. J. Nutr. 142, 1510–1518.

Stollman, N., Raskin, J.B., 2004. Diverticular disease of the colon. Lancet 363, 631–639.

Thompson, W.G., 2002. A World View of IBS. Irritable Bowel Syndrome: Diagnosis and Treatment. Saunders, Philadelphia and London. 1726.

Tonstad, S., Stewart, K., Oda, K., Batech, M., Herring, R.P., Fraser, G.E., 2013. Vegetarian diets and the incidence of diabetes in the Adventist Health Study-2. Nutr. Metab. Cardiovasc. Dis. 23, 292–299.

Whitehead, W.E., Burnett, C.K., Cook III, E.W., Taub, E., 1996. Impact of irritable bowel syndrome on quality of life. Dig. Dis. Sci. 41 (11), 2248–2253.

Williams, E.A., Nai, X., Corfe, B.M., 2011. Dietary intakes in people with irritable bowel syndrome. BMC Gastroenterol. 11 (1), 9.

Zimmer, J., Lange, B., Frick, J.S., Sauer, H., Zimmermann, K., Schwiertz, A., et al., 2012. A vegan or vegetarian diet substantially alters the human colonic faecal microbiota. Eur. J. Clin. Nutr. 66 (1), 53–60.

27

Plant-Based Diets and Asthma

Motoyasu Iikura

NATIONAL CENTER FOR GLOBAL HEALTH AND MEDICINE, TOKYO, JAPAN

1. Introduction

Asthma attacks are induced by several factors, including allergen inhalation, viral infection, smoking, alcohol drinking, exercise, and the use of nonsteroidal antiinflammatory drugs. Many investigators have reported relationships between various lifestyle factors and asthma (Bakirtas, 2009; Frode, 2005; Hartert, 2001; Iikura, 2013; Radon, 2002; Rodríguez-Rodríguez, 2010; Rönmark, 2005; Westermann, 2008; Young, 2001). Among many lifestyle factors, changes in diet have been suggested to be responsible for the increase in allergies (Devereux, 2005). Dietary patterns appear to be the most important of several lifestyle factors for disease modification (Barros, 2015). Dietary patterns are associated with asthma prevalence, incidence, control, pulmonary function, and exacerbation. The intake of raw vegetables is particularly important among several healthy diets.

2. Asthma Prevalence and Diet

Several observational studies have investigated the effects of dietary intake on asthma. Frode (2005) reported that daily intakes of fresh fruit and vegetables in infancy was associated with a lower risk of asthma in school-age children. Rodríguez-Rodríguez (2010) found that increased intakes of saturated fatty acids, myristic and palmitic acids, and butter appeared to be related to the risk of current asthma in children. Nagel (2010) reported that more frequent consumption of fruit, vegetables, and fish was associated with a lower lifetime prevalence of asthma, whereas high burger consumption was associated with higher lifetime asthma prevalence. A survey of 32,644 Portuguese adults found that a "high fat, sugar, and salt" dietary pattern was associated with high prevalence of asthma [odds ratio (OR) = 1.13; 95% confidence interval (CI) = 1.03–1.24] (Barros, 2015). Data from the International Study of Asthma and Allergies in Childhood revealed that an increased risk of severe asthma in adolescents and children was associated with the consumption of fast food more than three times per week (Ellwood, 2013). A study of French schoolchildren reported an inverse association between the consumption of fruit juice, meat, and fish and the prevalence of asthma symptoms among children aged 9–11 years, while fast food consumption and butter intake were associated with an increased prevalence of asthma symptoms among atopic children (Saadeh, 2015). On the other hand, a study of children aged 2–9 years in the United States reported that excessive intake of free fructose beverages, such as apple juice, fruit drinks, and soda, was significantly associated with asthma (DeChristopher, 2016). An investigation of Brazilian adolescents reported that consumption of stuffed biscuits and fried snacks three or more times a week was independently associated with asthma prevalence, while consumption of fruit three or more times a week was associated with asthma as a protective factor (Gomes, 2015). Wong (2004) reported that the consumption of fruit and raw vegetables was associated with high asthma prevalence using data from 10,902 Chinese schoolchildren. Han (2015a,b) reported that frequent consumption of vegetables and grains and low consumption of dairy products and sweets were associated with 36% decreased odds of childhood asthma in Puerto Ricans with lower plasma levels of interleukin-17F. A study of Japanese preschool children revealed that high intakes of vitamin C and E were associated with a reduced prevalence of asthma (Nakamura, 2013). A meta-analysis revealed that the total intake of fruit and vegetables had an inverse association with risk of asthma in adults and children [relative risk (RR) = 0.54; 95% CI 0.41–0.69] (Seyedrezazadeh, 2014). Among fruit, high intake of apples or citrus was associated with lower asthma prevalence. In subgroup analysis, high raw vegetable consumption was inversely associated with risk of asthma (RR = 0.87; 95% CI 0.81–0.94). Consuming fruit and vegetables during pregnancy showed no association with risk of asthma in offspring (Seyedrezazadeh, 2014). Backer (2016) reported that dietary changes may be important for the development of asthma regardless of genetically homogeneous background. Two Inuit populations were recruited: one living in Greenland, and the other in Denmark. Consumption of whale, seal, and wild meat was higher among Greenlandic Inuit, while the consumption of fruit and vegetables was higher among Denmark Inuit. Asthma prevalence was higher in Denmark (9%) compared to Greenland (3.6%, $P < .0001$) and associated with increased expression of the IL-6 gene in adipose tissue and increased BMI, possibly as a result of a differential dietary exposure (Backer, 2016). One of the mechanisms underlying the association between asthma and diet is the change in airway gene expression in asthmatics (Li, 2016). This study reported differences in inflammatory gene expression that may contribute to increased airway neutrophilia following a high-fat meal in subjects with asthma (Li, 2016).

On the other hand, other investigators found no clear relationships between dietary patterns and asthma incidence (Bakolis, 2010; Varraso, 2009). Varraso (2009) reported that no association between dietary patterns and asthma prevalence was observed in 54,672 French females. Lv (2014) reported from a meta-analysis that no association between dietary patterns and asthma prevalence in adults or between maternal diet and childhood asthma was evident.

Concerning the maternal diet and asthma in children, pooling of the four randomized controlled trials (Fälth-Magnusson, 1987; Lilja, 1989; Zeiger, 1989; Arshad, 1992) found no significant differences between maternal restricted and unrestricted diets (RR, 0.95; 95% CI, 0.70–1.30; $n = 619$ children) on the development of asthma in children (Netting, 2014). Eighteen prospective studies reported wheeze or asthma in children as an outcome of maternal diet. Few associations between maternal diet and development of asthma were seen in children in these studies (Netting, 2014). Maternal consumption of olive oil, vitamin D, apples, and oily fish or use of a Western dietary pattern was associated with lower risk of asthma in children from some studies (Netting, 2014).

Garcia-Larson (2016) summarized high-quality systematic reviews of dietary habit and asthma. They used AMSTAR as a validated instrument to assess in detail the methodological quality of included reviews. Allen reported an increased overall risk of asthma with decreasing intakes of vitamin C in 10 observational studies (OR = 1.12; 95% CI = 1.04–1.21) and wheeze (OR = 1.10; 95% CI = 1.00–1.20) (Allen, 2009). No evidence was seen of any effect of maternal vitamin C intake and infant wheeze (OR = 1.30; 95% CI = 0.47–3.62) (Garcia-Larsen, 2016). Maternal intake of vitamin D was inversely associated with risk of recurrent wheeze or wheeze in the last 12 months in children (OR = 0.56; 95% CI = 0.42–0.73) in four cohort studies included in a meta-analysis (Nurmatov, 2011). Four cross-sectional studies included in a meta-analysis showed that dietary intake of fruit (but not vegetables) correlated inversely with wheeze in children aged 10–14 years (OR = 0.75; 95% CI = 0.61–0.94), with high evidence of heterogeneity (Nurmatov, 2011). Adherence to a Mediterranean diet was related to a lower risk of current wheeze in children in a meta-analysis of nine cross-sectional studies (OR = 0.85; 95% CI = 0.75–0.98) (Garcia-Marcos, 2013).

3. Asthma Control and Diet

Few reports have examined the relationship between asthma control and daily lifestyle (Barros, 2011; Iikura, 2013). Barros reported that dietary intake of fruit (>300 g) was associated with better asthma control (Barros, 2011). They also reported that a dietary pattern of "fish, fruit, and vegetables" was inversely associated with current asthma symptoms (OR = 0.84; 95% CI = 0.72–0.98). Ellwood reported that fruit intake (more than three times per week) had a protective effect against severe asthma in children and adolescents.

In our study of 437 stable Japanese asthmatic patients, younger age (<65 years old), periodic exercise (>3 metabolic equivalent hours per week), and raw vegetable intake (>5 units per week) were significantly associated with good asthma control in multiple linear regression analysis (Iikura, 2013). Asthma control test (ACT) score was significantly higher among patients who consumed >5 units of raw vegetables per week compared to that among patients consuming ≤5 units of raw vegetables per week (Iikura, 2013). Additional subgroup analyses stratified by sex and age group demonstrated that the association between ACT and raw vegetable diet was present only in men (P = .001) and in patients >64 years old (P = .005). Similarly, median ACT score was significantly higher among patients who consumed more than one unit of vegetable juice per week compared to that in patients consuming less than or equal to one unit of vegetable juice per week (P = .02), but only in patients ≤64 years old. No association was seen between asthma control and cooked vegetables, fresh fruit, or fruit juice intake in our study. In multiple linear regression analysis, raw fresh vegetable intake remained significantly associated with higher levels of asthma control (P = .005) (Table 27.1). From the perspective of patient characteristics in our study, patients were relatively old (mean age, 64 years), with relatively severe treatment steps [asthma treatment steps as measured by Global Initiative for Asthma (GINA) 2007 in step

Table 27.1   Association Between Asthma Control Test and Vegetable, Fruit or Juice Intake

	β	S.E	t	P
Cooked vegetables	−0.051	0.027	−1.027	0.31
Raw vegetables	0.133	0.031	2.794	0.005
Citrus fruits	0.025	0.033	0.495	0.62
Other fruits	0.004	0.036	0.092	0.93
Mixed juice	−0.032	0.063	−0.671	0.50
Vegetable juice	0.036	0.063	0.763	0.45
100% fruit juice	−0.027	0.084	−0.568	0.57

Multiple linear regression adjusted for gender, age, exercise, smoking status, second-hand smoke, alcohol drinking, and asthma treatment steps (observational study, $n=437$, Iikura, 2013).

1 (5.5%), step 2 (17.4%), step 3 (7.6%), step 4 (60.2%), and step 5 (9.4%)] compared to other previous asthma studies. The conclusion of our study was that a raw vegetable diet plays the most potent protective role in current asthma control among several plant-based diets despite older age or severe treatment steps.

One Australian study demonstrated that increased consumption of antioxidant-rich foods (>5 servings of vegetables per day, >2 servings of fruit per day, >8$^{1/2}$ servings of grains (mostly whole grains) per day, and 3–4 servings of lean meat per week) for 12 weeks improved maternal asthma control, compared to standard dietary intake during pregnancy (Grieger, 2014).

4. Asthma Lung Function and Diet

Asthma is characterized by air flow limitation. Romieu (2001) reported that the impact of nutrition on obstructive lung disease was most evident for antioxidant vitamins, particularly vitamin C and, to a lesser extent, vitamin E or ω-3 fatty acids. Daily intake of vitamin C at levels slightly exceeding the current recommended dietary allowance (60 mg/day among nonsmokers, 100 mg/day among smokers) may have protective effects against decrements in lung function. An increase of 40 mg/day in vitamin C intake led to an approximate 20-mL increase in forced expiratory volume in 1 s (FEV1) (Romieu, 2001). A paper reported that high dietary intake of vegetables as well as intake of arctic marine mammals had independent positive associations with FEV1 in the cohort of Greenlandic Inuit (Baines, 2015). Ng (2013) reported that daily supplementation with vitamins A/C/E, daily fish intake at least thrice weekly, and daily supplementary n-3 polyunsaturated fatty acids (PUFA) were individually associated with FEV1. Supplemental n-3 PUFA was also positively associated with forced vital capacity. No significant associations with daily dairy product intake, vitamin D, or Se supplements were observed (Ng, 2013). Asthmatic patients consuming a diet high in antioxidants (five serving of vegetables and two servings of fruit per day) for 14 days had a higher percentage predicted FEV1 and forced vital capacity (FVC) than those consuming a low-antioxidant diet (Wood, 2012).

5. Asthma Exacerbation and Diet

The "high fat, sugar and salt" dietary pattern was associated with a higher risk of emergency room visits for asthma attack within the previous 12 months from a Portuguese survey (OR = 1.23; 95% CI = 1.03–1.48), while a "fish, fruit, and vegetables" dietary pattern may play a protective role against asthma independent of the level of physical activity (Barros, 2015). The Western dietary pattern (pizza/salty pies, dessert, and cured meats) was associated with an increased risk of frequent asthma attacks in French females (OR = 1.79; 95% CI = 1.11–3.73), while a nuts and wine dietary pattern was associated with a lower risk of asthma attacks (OR = 0.65; 95% CI = 0.31–0.96) (Varraso, 2009). The low-antioxidant diet intervention group was 2.26 times (95% CI 1.04–4.91; P = .039) as likely to show exacerbation compared to the high-antioxidant diet group (Wood, 2012).

6. Relationship Between Plant-Based Diets and Asthma

Plant-based diets had a beneficial effect on asthma according to several studies, including our own (Iikura, 2013). Raw vegetable intake was associated with low asthma prevalence, good asthma control, and low asthma exacerbation (Barros, 2015; Iikura, 2013; Nagel, 2010; Wong, 2004). Nutrients from raw vegetable diets may exert effects involving antioxidant, antiinflammatory, and immunomodulatory mechanisms against asthma (Ng, 2013; Han, 2015a,b). Fresh vegetables contain large amounts of the supplementary vitamins A/C/E and n-3 PUFA, all of which have been positively associated with obstructive pulmonary dysfunction (Ng, 2013). Intake of α-linolenic acid and a low ratio of n-6:n-3 PUFA were associated with lower exhaled NO and better asthma control (Barros, 2011). A high n-6 PUFA diet may increase prostaglandin (PG) E2 and leukotriene B4 synthesis and favor allergic inflammation, which may have led to the increase in asthma (James, 2000). A decrease in the consumption of diets containing n-3 PUFA, EPA, and DHA, which inhibit the production of PGE2, may lead to an increase in the prevalence of asthma (Black, 1997). In general, flavonoids and related polyphenolic compounds in vegetables are lost with heating, and flavonoids and related polyphenolic compounds reportedly exert significant antiinflammatory activity (González, 2011), including free radical scavenging, modulation of enzymatic activity, inhibition of cellular proliferation, and inhibition of Th2 type cytokine release (Tanaka, 2013). In addition, flavonoids may enhance the activities of endogenous antioxidants (Middleton, 2000), which may decrease airway inflammation by protecting the airways against oxidants from both endogenous and exogenous sources. Recent reports mentioned the importance of antioxidant intake from vegetables for asthma (Wood, 2012; Ng, 2013). In addition, raw vegetables are sources of dietary fiber, which affect the gut microbiota balance, including propionate, which potentially reduces airway hyperresponsiveness and the severity of allergic airway inflammation (Trompette, 2014). In general, citrus fruits contain higher levels of vitamin C than other fruits. Previous studies have reported the relationship between consumption of citrus fruits and incidence of asthma (Forastiere, 2000; Patel, 2006), implying that ingestion of citrus fruit has an anti-inflammatory effect (Hirota, 2010).

Based on several epidemiological and preliminary studies, several food intervention studies in asthmatic subjects have been reported. Wood (2012) reported that increasing antioxidant intake maintained good lung function and reduced exacerbation. Adult asthma patients were randomly assigned to a high-antioxidant diet (5 servings of vegetables and 2 servings of fruit daily) or low-antioxidant diet (≤3 servings of vegetables and 1 serving of fruit daily) for 14 days. Decreases in predicted FEV1 and predicted FVC from baseline were observed at day 14 compared with baseline in the low-antioxidant diet group, and these values were significantly different from those in the high-antioxidant diet group, in which no change between baseline and day 14 was observed. Subjects consuming a low-antioxidant diet displayed increased plasma levels of C-reactive protein (CRP) on day 14. No change in CRP was found in the high-antioxidant group. In addition, time to exacerbation was greater in the high-antioxidant diet than in the low-antioxidant diet group, and the low-antioxidant diet group was 2.26 times as likely to experience an exacerbation at any time compared with the high-antioxidant diet group. A small but significant decrease in scores from the Asthma Control Questionnaire was seen in the high-antioxidant diet group compared with the low-antioxidant group (Wood, 2012). In pregnant women, an intervention with a Mediterranean diet is currently underway to test whether a net increase in dietary antioxidants can reduce the risk of asthma in offspring (Sewell, 2013). Garcia-Larsen (2014) reported the feasibility of undertaking a fresh fruit intervention to test for changes in asthma-related symptoms in a pilot study of asthmatic children at 6–10 years old. Further interventional randomized control studies are required to elucidate the effects of plant-based diets on asthma.

7. Conclusion

Comparisons of dietary patterns between studies is somewhat complicated given the different methodological approaches to assessing dietary intake, characterizing food patterns, and the different socio-geographic characteristics of the studied populations. However, a large amount of evidence supports the concept that plant-based diets, and raw vegetable diets in particular, have beneficial effects on asthma.

References

Allen, S., 2009. Association between antioxidant vitamins and asthma outcome measures: systematic review and meta-analysis. Thorax 64 (7), 610–619.

Arshad, S.H., 1992. Effect of allergen avoidance on development of allergic disorders in infancy. Lancet 339 (8808), 1493–1497.

Baines, K.J., 2015. Investigating the effects of arctic dietary intake on lung health. Eur. J. Clin. Nutr. 69 (11), 1262–1266.

Backer, V., 2016. Increased asthma and adipose tissue inflammatory gene expression with obesity and Inuit migration to a western country. Respir. Med. 111, 8–15.

Bakirtas, A., 2009. Acute effects of passive smoking on asthma in childhood. Inflamm. Allergy Drug Targets 8 (5), 353–358.

Bakolis, I., 2010. Dietary patterns and adult asthma: population-based case-control study. Allergy 65 (5), 606–615.

Barros, R., 2011. Dietary intake of α-linolenic acid and low ratio of n-6:n-3 PUFA are associated with decreased exhaled NO and improved asthma control. Br. J. Nutr. 106 (3), 441–450.

Barros, R., 2015. Dietary patterns and asthma prevalence, incidence and control. Clin. Exp. Allergy 45 (11), 1673–1680.

Black, P.N., 1997. Dietary fat and asthma: is there a connection? Eur. Respir. J. 10 (1), 6–12.

DeChristopher, L.R., 2016. Intakes of apple juice, fruit drinks and soda are associated with prevalent asthma in US children aged 2–9 years. Public Health Nutr. 19 (1), 123–130.

Devereux, G., 2005. Diet as a risk factor for atopy and asthma. J. Allergy Clin. Immunol. 115 (6), 1109–1117.

Ellwood, P., 2013. Do fast foods cause asthma, rhinoconjunctivitis and eczema? Global findings from the International Study of Asthma and Allergies in Childhood (ISAAC) phase three. Thorax 68 (4), 351–360.

Fälth-Magnusson, K., 1987. Maternal abstention from cow milk and egg in allergy risk pregnancies. Effect on antibody production in the mother and the newborn. Allergy 42 (1), 64–73.

Forastiere, F., 2000. Consumption of fresh fruit rich in vitamin C and wheezing symptoms in children. Thorax 55 (4), 283–288.

Frode, N.J.A., 2005. Effects of early intake of fruit or vegetables in relation to later asthma and allergic sensitization in school-age children. Acta Pædiatrica 94 (2), 147–154.

Garcia-Larsen, V., 2014. The Chelsea, asthma and fresh fruit intake in children (CHAFFINCH) trial – pilot study. Clin. Transl. Allergy 4, O6.

Garcia-Larsen, V., 2016. Asthma and dietary intake: an overview of systematic reviews. Allergy 71 (4), 433–442.

Garcia-Marcos, L., 2013. Influence of Mediterranean diet on asthma in children: a systematic review and meta-analysis. Pediatr. Allergy Immunol. 24 (4), 330–338.

Gomes de Luna Mde, F., 2015. Factors associated with asthma in adolescents in the city of Fortaleza. Braz. J. Asthma 52 (5), 485–491.

González, R., 2011. Effects of flavonoids and other polyphenols on inflammation. Crit. Rev. Food Sci. Nutr. 51 (4), 331–362.

Grieger, J.A., 2014. Antioxidant-rich dietary intervention for improving asthma control in pregnancies complicated by asthma: study protocol for a randomized controlled trial. Trials 15, 108. http://dx.doi.org/10.1186/1745-6215-15-108.

Han, Y.Y., 2015a. Diet, interleukin-17, and childhood asthma in Puerto Ricans. Ann. Allergy Asthma Immunol. 115 (4), 288–293.

Han, Y.Y., 2015b. Diet and asthma: an update. Curr. Opin. Allergy Clin. Immunol. 15 (4), 369–374.

Hartert, T.V., 2001. Dietary antioxidants and adult asthma. Curr. Opin. Allergy Clin. Immunol. 1 (5), 421–429.

Hirota, R., 2010. Anti-inflammatory effects of limonene from yuzu (*Citrus junos* Tanaka) essential oil on eosinophils. J. Food Sci. 75 (3), H87–H92.

Iikura, M., 2013. Effect of lifestyle on asthma control in Japanese patients: importance of periodical exercise and raw vegetable diet. PLos One 8 (7), e68290.

James, M.J., 2000. Dietary polyunsaturated fatty acids and inflammatory mediator production. Am. J. Clin. Nutr. 71, 343S–348S.

Li, Q., 2016. Changes in expression of genes regulating airway inflammation following a high-fat mixed meal in asthmatics. Nutrients 8 (1). http://dx.doi.org/10.3390/nu8010030. pii:E30.

Lilja, G., 1989. Effects of maternal diet during late pregnancy and lactation on the development of atopic diseases in infants up to 18 months of age–in-vivo results. Clin. Exp. Allergy 19 (4), 473–479.

Lv, N., 2014. Dietary pattern and asthma: a systematic review and meta-analysis. J. Asthma Allergy 7, 105–121.

Middleton Jr., E., 2000. The effects of plant flavonoids on mammalian cells: implications for inflammation, heart disease, and cancer. Pharmacol. Rev. 52 (4), 673–751.

Nagel, G., 2010. Effect of diet on asthma and allergic sensitisation in the International Study on Allergies and Asthma in Childhood (ISAAC) Phase Two. Thorax 65 (6), 516–522.

Nakamura, K., 2013. Associations of intake of antioxidant vitamins and fatty acids with asthma in preschool children. Public Health Nutr. 16 (11), 2040–2045.

Netting, M.J., 2014. Does maternal diet during pregnancy and lactation affect outcomes in offspring? A systematic review of food-based approaches. Nutrition 30 (11–12), 1225–1241.

Ng, T.P., 2013. Dietary and supplemental antioxidant and anti-inflammatory nutrient intakes and pulmonary function. Public Health Nutr. 17 (9), 2081–2086.

Nurmatov, U., 2011. Nutrients and foods for the primary prevention of asthma and allergy: systematic review and meta-analysis. J. Allergy Clin. Immunol. 127 (3), 724–733.

Patel, B.D., 2006. Dietary antioxidants and asthma in adults. Thorax 61 (5), 388–393.

Radon, K., 2002. Passive smoking exposure: a risk factor for chronic bronchitis and asthma in adults? Chest 122 (3), 1086–1090.

Rodríguez-Rodríguez, E., 2010. Fat intake and asthma in Spanish schoolchildren. Eur. J. Clin. Nutr. 64 (10), 1065–1071.

Romieu, I., 2001. Diet and obstructive lung diseases. Epidemiol. Rev. 23 (2), 268–287.

Rönmark, E., 2005. Obesity increases the risk of incident asthma among adults. Eur. Respir. J. 25 (2), 282–288.

Saadeh, D., 2015. Prevalence and association of asthma and allergic sensitization with dietary factors in schoolchildren: data from the french six cities study. BMC Public Health 15, 993. http://dx.doi.org/10.1186/s12889-015-2320-2.

Sewell, D.A., 2013. Investigating the effectiveness of the Mediterranean diet in pregnant women for the primary prevention of asthma and allergy in high-risk infants: protocol for a pilot randomised controlled trial. Trials 14, 173. http://dx.doi.org/10.1186/1745-6215-14-173.

Seyedrezazadeh, E., 2014. Fruit and vegetable intake and risk of wheezing and asthma: a systematic review and meta-analysis. Nutr. Rev. 72 (7), 411–428.

Tanaka, T., 2013. Flavonoids and asthma. Nutrients 5 (6), 2128–2143.

Trompette, A., 2014. Gut microbiota metabolism of dietary fiber influences allergic airway disease and hematopoiesis. Nat. Med. 20 (2), 159–166.

Varraso, R., 2009. Dietary patterns and asthma in the E3N study. Eur. Respir. J. 33, 33–41.

Westermann, H., 2008. Obesity and exercise habits of asthmatic patients. Ann. Allergy Asthma Immunol. 101 (5), 488–494.

Wong, G.W., 2004. Factors associated with difference in prevalence of asthma in children from three cities in China: multicentre epidemiological survey. BMJ 329 (7464), 486.

Wood, L.G., 2012. Manipulating antioxidant intake in asthma: a randomized controlled trial. Am. J. Clin. Nutr. 96 (3), 534–543.

Young, S.Y., 2001. Body mass index and asthma in the military population of the northwestern United States. Arch. Intern. Med. 161 (13), 1605–1611.

Zeiger, R.S., 1989. Effect of combined maternal and infant food-allergen avoidance on development of atopy in early infancy: a randomized study. J. Allergy Clin. Immunol. 84 (1), 72–89.

Further Reading

Grieger, J.A., 2016. Asthma control in pregnancy is associated with pre-conception dietary patterns. Public Health Nutr. 19 (2), 332–338.

28

Vegetarian Diet and Possible Mechanisms for Impact on Mood

Carol S. Johnston

ARIZONA STATE UNIVERSITY, PHOENIX, AZ, UNITED STATES

1. Overview

The *Merriam-Webster Dictionary* defines mood as the predominant emotion. Mood and cognitive processes are regulated by the action of the neurotransmitters serotonin and norepinephrine and by neuroplasticity (Wohleb et al., 2015; Poon et al., 2015; Rosenblat et al., 2014). Factors that disrupt these signaling pathways or that hinder the brain's restructuring capacity can worsen mood states. Mood disturbance can manifest as lethargy, apathy, sleepiness, anxiety, and/or depression. Causes of mood disturbance include chronic disease, diet, inactivity, and genetic susceptibility, many of which are linked to inflammatory states. Hence, much attention has focused on the role of proinflammatory mediators in mood, specifically the inflammatory cytokines (e.g., IL-1β, TNF-α, IL-6, and IL-2), prostaglandins [mainly prostaglandin E_2 (PGE_2)], and the hormone cortisol (Myint and Kim, 2014; Su, 2008). These mediators play critical roles in times of fight-or-flight by eliminating infectious agents, clearing tissue debris, and maintaining physiologic homeostasis, but their actions spawn a neuro-vegetative state. This "sickness" behavior has physiological relevance during acute illness and injury as it focuses resources on survival and resolves once the threat is eliminated (Hart, 1988), but in the modern world where inflammatory states are often long-lasting in association with chronic disease, poor lifestyles, and mental stress, mood disturbance is a disruptive force that jeopardizes health.

This chapter will focus on the aspects of vegetarian diets that would theoretically promote healthful mood states by minimizing the impact of proinflammatory mediators and by promoting neurotransmitter action.

2. Evidences That Vegetarian Diets May Favorably Impact Mood

Indeed, several controlled randomized trials have demonstrated that the adoption of a vegetarian diet improved mood significantly based on well-validated measures of mood states. Kahleova et al. (2013) randomized 74 adult omnivores with type 2 diabetes to one of two calorie-restricted diets (−500 kcal/day): a lactovegetarian diet ($n=37$) or a standard diabetic diet (*n*=37). All foods were provided to participants, and the study extended 24 weeks. The vegetarian diet was composed of vegetables, grains, legumes, fruits, and nuts, and one serving of low-fat yogurt was allowed daily. The macronutrient distribution was 25% energy from protein, 15% energy from fat, and 60% energy from carbohydrates. The diabetic diet followed the guidelines established by the Diabetes and Nutrition Study Group of the European Association for the Study of Diabetes and was low fat (<30% energy) with 20% energy from protein. At study week 24, mood (assessed using the Beck Depression Inventory) was significantly improved for participants in the vegetarian diet group (scores improved approximately 54% from baseline) compared to those following the standard diabetic diet (scores improved approximately 12% from baseline) (Kahleova et al., 2013).

In the second study, 39 healthy adult omnivores were randomized to one of three diet groups for 2 weeks: omnivore diet (meat and/or poultry consumed daily), pescetarian diet (fish consumed three to four times per week while restricting all meat and poultry from diet), or lactovegetarian diet (all animal products restricted from diet with the exception of dairy) (Beezhold and Johnston, 2012). Food frequency questionnaires administered at baseline and at study week 2 indicated good compliance to diet instruction based on the change in the dietary levels of the long-chain fatty acids, arachidonic acid, and eicosapentaenoic acid, over the course of the study. Mood was assessed at baseline and at week 2 using the Depression Anxiety Stress Scales and the Profile of Mood States questionnaire. Mental stress decreased significantly from baseline only for the vegetarian group (within group comparison, $P<.05$), and confusion scores improved significantly from baseline only for the vegetarian group (within group comparison, $P<.01$) (Beezhold and Johnston, 2012).

Although these data are intriguing and suggest that vegetarian diets improve mood states in both the short- and long-term, biomarkers associated with mood and cognitive processes were not measured in either trial, and it is still not clear whether the adoption of a vegetarian diet can lower the concentrations of the proinflammatory mediators that adversely impact mood and/or improve the concentrations of the neurotransmitters that control mood and cognition.

3. Antiinflammatory Properties of Vegetarian Diets

There is some evidence that vegetarian diets possess "antiinflammatory" properties. Patients with chronic inflammatory conditions, rheumatoid arthritis or fibromyalgia, reported significantly reduced pain and other disease symptoms when adhering to vegetarian diets (Adam et al., 2003; Kjeldsen-Kragh, 1999; Kaartinen et al., 2000). The proinflammatory mediators associated with chronic diseases or other common environmental stressors can induce brain inflammation as well as produce pain since they enter the brain via humoral and neural routes (Poon et al., 2015). In the brain, these mediators may lead to mood disturbance by disrupting serotonin production and altering brain structure. The evidence for lowered circulating levels of the proinflammatory mediators in vegetarians is outlined next.

3.1 The Proinflammatory Cytokines

The proinflammatory cytokines (IL-1β, TNF-α, and IL-6) are released from systemic macrophages as well as from brain microglia in response to chronic stress including unresolved disease states, obesity, smoking, and environmental pressures (Guarner and Rubio-Ruiz, 2015; Shi et al., 2010). These cytokines disrupt serotonin production by upregulating the enzyme indoleamine-2,3-dioxygenase that catabolizes tryptophan, the sole substrate for serotonin biosynthesis (Capuron et al., 2011). IL-6 has been shown to increase serotonin catabolism as well (Wang and Dunn, 1998). The proinflammatory cytokines also stimulate the hypothalamic-pituitary-adrenal axis, and they release cortisol, which blocks the biosynthesis of serotonin (Oxenkrug, 2013). Furthermore, these cytokines inhibit neurogenesis in the hippocampus by reducing the production, migration, and survival of new neurons (Zonis et al., 2015). Oxidative stress is a major stimulus for immune system activation, which is a major source of the proinflammatory cytokines. Hence, antioxidant therapies may reduce the levels of these cytokines and have shown some promise for improving mood states (Siwek et al., 2013; Scapagnini et al., 2012).

Vegetarian diets are primarily plant-based and rich in the antioxidant phytochemicals, including phenolic acids, flavonoids, and carotenoids, and the antioxidant vitamins C and E. As would be expected, biochemical assessments in vegetarian populations consistently show high antioxidant concentrations in blood in comparison to matched omnivore controls (Rauma and Mykkänen, 2000; Haldar et al., 2007). In particular, vitamin C concentrations in blood are often reported to be 50% higher in vegetarians compared to meat eaters (Kazimírová et al., 2006; Szeto et al., 2004), and carotenoids are consistently raised as well (Haldar et al., 2007; Kazimírová et al., 2006). However, certain antioxidants are low in the blood of vegetarians compared to meat eaters (e.g., selenium, Judd et al., 1997); hence, it is important to measure the total antioxidant capacity of blood as opposed to single nutrient concentrations. The total antioxidant capacity (TAC) of plasma can be measured using multiple methods, each focused on quantifying resistance to oxidation. Wang et al. (2012) compared the commonly used TAC methods, vitamin C equivalent antioxidant capacity (VCEAC), ferric-reducing ability of plasma (FRAP), and oxygen radical absorbance capacity, and they concluded that VCEAC best correlated with plasma antioxidant status as well as with dietary antioxidant levels.

Several reports have examined the ex vivo antioxidant potential of vegetarians in comparison to omnivores with conflicting results, perhaps a reflection of the assay system used to measure antioxidant status. Lim et al. (2012) reported a 25% higher plasma TAC score in Malaysian vegetarians compared to their omnivorous counterpart using a modified VCEAC assay, and the significance was retained in both obese and nonobese subsets. Yet, most investigators utilized FRAP to measure TAC and concluded that adherence to vegetarian diets is not associated with a higher plasma TAC as compared to that of omnivores (Haldar et al., 2007; Kazimírová et al., 2006; Szeto et al., 2004; Kim et al., 2012). It is important to note that high uric acid concentrations in blood influence TAC, particularly when the FRAP system is used (Wang et al., 2012). Omnivores tend to have higher blood uric acid concentrations compared to vegetarians since dietary meat contributes to uric acid formation due to its high purine content. However, Schmidt et al. (2013) reported that strict vegans have higher blood uric acid concentrations than either meat eaters or vegetarians, which may relate to the absence of dairy in the diet since dairy products reduce uric acid concentrations in vivo. The relevance of uric acid to health is disputed since, although a strong antioxidant, it has been implicated in heart disease, hypertension, and insulin resistance (Benzie and Strain, 1996). The data concerning the overall plasma antioxidant status in vegetarians remains therefore not very conclusive.

Since antioxidants combat free radicals and oxidative stress, reactive oxygen compounds can be measured in addition to TAC to assess overall oxidative balance. Utilizing a population of Korean Seventh-day Adventists, Kim et al., 2012 reported that the levels of free radicals in blood were significantly lower in 45 long-term vegetarians (diet followed for a minimum of 15 years) compared to 30 omnivores. Additionally, lipid peroxidation products, representing cellular damage due to oxidative stress, are commonly measured to assess free radical damage in vivo. In separate cross-sectional analyses in South Indian populations, investigators reported that the lipid peroxidation product, malondialdehyde (MDA), was significantly lower in the blood of vegetarians compared to omnivores (Somannavar and Kodliwadmath, 2012; Manjari et al., 2001). In a Bratislava population, Krajcovicová-Kudláčková et al. (2008) observed significantly lower concentrations of oxidative damage products (oxidized purines and pyrimidines) in the plasma of older vegetarians (aged 60–70 years) compared to age-matched nonvegetarians, and concomitantly, concentrations of vitamin C and β-carotene were raised 40% and 130%, respectively, in these vegetarians compared to the nonvegetarians. In a short intervention trial, Ji et al. (2010) reported that adherence to a vegetarian diet resulted in 40%–50% reduction lipid peroxidation products in urine after 5 days.

Several studies have assessed the concentrations of the inflammatory cytokines IL-2, IL-6, and TNF-α, and the antiinflammatory cytokine IL-10, in vegetarians versus omnivores. In a cross-sectional investigation of male Chinese vegetarians ($n = 89$, minimum diet adherence, 6 months) and nonvegetarians ($n = 106$), Yu et al. (2014) found no differences between groups for blood concentrations of IL-1, TNF-α, or IL-10; however, IL-6 was significantly elevated in the vegetarians versus the nonvegetarians (+10%). In a separate study, IL-6 did not differ between Italian vegetarians ($n = 25$, minimum diet adherence 3 years) and nonvegetarians, yet IL-1 was significantly higher for the vegetarians compared to the nonvegetarians (Montalcini et al., 2015).

Although the proinflammatory cytokines are strongly associated with brain inflammation and depressive disorders in the general population (Myint and Kim, 2014; Su, 2008), the total antioxidant status and the cytokine profile of vegetarians do not appear to vary significantly from omnivores and would not be expected to contribute to the improved mood states or antiinflammatory properties attributed to vegetarian diets. However, markers of oxidative stress are generally lower in vegetarians and may contribute to the improved mood states noted for individuals adhering to vegetarian diet; but this reduction in oxidative stress is not likely a function of an improved TAC or a consequence of lower concentrations of circulating proinflammatory cytokines.

3.2 The Proinflammatory Prostaglandin PGE$_2$

The proinflammatory prostaglandins are derived from the fatty acid arachidonic acid that is released from membrane phospholipids. The release of arachidonic acid is triggered by the phospholipase A$_2$ enzyme, activated by inflammatory signals or by free radical per-oxidation of membrane lipids (Poon et al., 2015). The freed arachidonic acid is converted to a series of prostaglandins including PGE$_2$ by the cyclooxygenase-2 (COX-2) enzyme, which is constitutively expressed in brain and also upregulated by inflammatory signals in the brain and in endothelial and immune cells (Park et al., 2006). Elevations in PGE$_2$ are implicated in neuronal pathology and memory disruption (Yui et al., 2015; Hein and O'Banion, 2009), and COX-2 inhibitors are proven therapies for depression (Müller et al., 2006; Na et al., 2014). Interestingly, PGE$_2$ levels, as well as COX-2 levels, are lower in healthy vegetarians compared to omnivores.

In the Yu et al. (2014) study mentioned earlier, PGE$_2$ and COX-2 values were 13%–28% lower in the vegetarians compared to the omnivores. Yet, plasma arachidonic acid (reported as percent of total fatty acids) was 36% higher in the vegetarians compared to the omnivores. These data suggest that the high portion of arachidonic acid in plasma fatty acids did not translate to higher PGE$_2$ concentrations in this vegetarian population. In fact, the correlation between the arachidonic acid percentage and PGE$_2$ concentration in plasma was low for the vegetarians and for omnivores, $r=0.106$ and $r=0.163$, respectively. Using a single-group design in a 2-month feeding trial conducted at a private hospital in patients with atopic dermatitis, the adoption of a vegetarian diet reduced PGE$_2$ concentrations in peripheral blood mononuclear cells by over 50% (Tanaka et al., 2001). Although only a few reports have provided PGE$_2$ data for vegetarian populations, the data suggest that a portion of the antiinflammatory properties attributed to vegetarian diets may relate to lower PGE$_2$ concentrations.

The mechanisms for lowered PGE$_2$ concentrations in vegetarians are not known. Several investigators have demonstrated that fecal water from vegetarians possessed COX-2-inhibiting activity (Karlsson et al., 2005; Pettersson et al., 2008); however, neither study included a meat eating control group to assess differences between diet plans. Fecal water contains many metabolites, reflecting dietary intakes, and these results suggest that components of vegetarian diets may contribute to COX-2 inhibition and lower PGE$_2$ concentrations in vivo. B-carotene and the carotenoids are dietary constituents known to possess COX-2 inhibitory action (Palozza et al., 2005; Hadad and Levy, 2012) and are consistently elevated in the blood of vegetarians (Rauma and Mykkänen, 2000; Haldar et al., 2007; Kazimírová et al., 2006; Markussen et al., 2015). Vitamin C is another nutrient consistently raised in the blood of vegetarians (Rauma and Mykkänen, 2000; Kazimírová et al., 2006; Szeto et al., 2004) that inhibits COX-2 (Liang et al., 2014; Lee et al., 2008).

The COX-2 inhibitory action of the carotenoids and vitamin C is likely a result of the strong reducing potentials of these compounds. COX-2 expression is controlled by the nuclear factor kappa-light-chain-enhancer of activated B cells (NF-κB), a key cell signaling pathway for inflammatory processes. The activation of NF-κB is via oxidation and is thus dependent on the redox status of cells (Flohé et al., 1997). Reactive oxygen species are generated during normal metabolism (e.g., the superoxide anion radical or the hydroxyl radical) and during immune cell activation (e.g., singlet oxygen) as well as during other metabolic processes. If the production of these radicals is not balanced by quenching by reducing agents, either due to low antioxidant status or to accelerated production due to stressful stimuli, oxidative stress predominates, NF-κB is activated, and inflammation ensues. The carotenoids are considered the most efficient singlet oxygen quenchers in vivo (Edge et al., 1997), whereas vitamin C is the premier water-soluble antioxidant in vivo, a potent quencher of both the superoxide anion and hydroxyl radicals and capable of regenerating vitamin E (Buettner and Jurkiewicz, 1993; May, 1998). Moreover, the strong reduction potential of vitamin C regenerates the parent carotenoids further reducing the oxidation state in tissue (Böhm et al., 2012). Vitamin C also inhibited cytokine stimulation of NF-κB via a nonantioxidant pathway (Bowie and O'Neill, 2000). Hence, it is likely that the high carotenoid and vitamin C statuses typical among vegetarian populations confer a particularly robust protective shield to oxidative stress and, thus, the inhibition of COX-2 and an attenuated PGE_2 response. Interestingly, vitamin C therapy (1000 mg/day) in acutely hospitalized patients with hypovitaminosis C decreased total mood disturbance by 71% (Wang et al., 2013). Although the specific mechanisms for this improvement in mood were not identified, vitamin C is a known COX-2 inhibitor, and since COX-2 inhibition by manufactured drugs is currently under investigation as a therapy for mood disturbance, future investigations should assess the therapeutic effects of vitamin C supplementation, if any. If such effects are achievable at nutritional doses should also be studied.

Aside from the inhibition of COX-2 enzyme, the reductions in PGE_2 concentrations noted in vegetarians may also relate to reductions in lipid peroxidation. Both the carotenoids and vitamin C effectively reduce lipid peroxidation (Buettner, 1993), and as previously discussed, adoption of a vegetarian diet resulted in 40%–50% reduction of lipid peroxidation products in urine after 5 days (Ji et al., 2010). The inhibition of lipid peroxidation will reduce the amount of arachidonic acid freed from membrane lipids, thus reducing the substrate for PGE_2. The high levels of these antioxidants in vegetarian diets and the blood of vegetarians may indeed help to explain the better mood states of vegetarians in comparison to omnivores. In nonvegetarians, cross-sectional investigations have demonstrated strong inverse associations between dietary B-carotene and vitamin C and mood disturbance in community-dwelling elderly and in male college students (Oishi et al., 2009; Prohan et al., 2014).

In the Yu et al. (2014) trial discussed earlier, Chinese vegetarians displayed a significantly higher proportion of plasma total fatty acids as arachidonic acid compared to omnivores. However, trials in the United States and Australia show that the portion of total fatty acids as arachidonic acid in serum or in platelets was markedly lower in vegetarians versus omnivores (−22% to −25%) (Li et al., 1999; Fisher et al., 1986). Low concentrations of arachidonic acid in vegetarian blood samples might be expected since meat, fish, and poultry are the main dietary sources of arachidonic acid. The only arachidonic acid in vegetarian diets is that from eggs; consequently, vegan diets do not contain arachidonic acid. In vivo, arachidonic acid is synthesized from linoleic acid at very low rates (<0.1% of total body linoleic acid is converted to arachidonic acid) (Plourde and Cunnane, 2007). (Note that, generally, the linoleic acid content of vegetarian diets surpasses that of omnivore diets.) Since preformed arachidonic acid is low in the diets of vegetarians, it is not surprising that tissue concentrations are also low in this population. Low concentrations of arachidonic acid in cell membranes may contribute to the low PGE_2 concentrations noted in vegetarians complementing the antioxidant-induced COX-2 inhibition and the lower lipid peroxidation rates of vegetarian diets as discussed earlier. Hence, there are plausible mechanisms to explain the 50% reduction in PGE_2 concentrations noted by Tanaka et al. (2001) in a patient population following the adoption of a vegetarian diet for 2 months and to propose why positive mood states are noted in vegetarian populations. Much work is needed to fully understand the impact of vegetarian diets on key proinflammatory mediators; however, the evidence to date warrants further investigations to examine the efficacy of vegetarian diets for reducing neuroinflammation via reductions in PGE_2.

4. Neurotransmitter Action and Vegetarian Diets

Mood and cognitive processes are regulated by the action of the neurotransmitters serotonin and norepinephrine, and almost all drug therapies currently available for mood disturbance seek to enhance the activity of these neurotransmitters. A reduction in serotonin is linked to anxiety, obsessions, and compulsions, whereas reduced norepinephrine is linked to decreased alertness, inattention, poor concentration, and reduced cognitive ability (Nutt, 2008). The remainder of this chapter will focus on the attributes of vegetarian diets that can increase serotonin and norepinephrine concentrations in brain.

4.1 Serotonin

The amino acid tryptophan is the substrate for serotonin synthesis; however, this process is negatively impacted by (1) the activation of indoleamine 2,3-deoxygenase that catabolizes tryptophan in various tissues including the brain and (2) the reduced passage of tryptophan through the blood–brain barrier. The inflammatory cytokines and PGE_2 are key activators of indoleamine 2,3-deoxygenase, and they contribute to impaired mood and cognition states via reduced serotonin concentrations in brain. Thus, as outlined earlier, adherence to vegetarian diets lowers PGE_2 concentrations in vivo, likely by several mechanisms. Lower PGE_2 concentrations have been associated with high levels of tryptophan (Iachininoto et al., 2013). As outlined next, there is much evidence demonstrating the influence of diet on the ability of tryptophan to pass the blood–brain barrier and thereby potentially allowing for enhanced serotonin synthesis and improved mood states.

4.1.1 Dietary Tryptophan

A diet rich in tryptophan contributes to higher circulating concentrations of tryptophan in blood and to the greater likelihood of tryptophan passing into the brain to promote serotonin synthesis (Nishizawa et al., 1997). Schmidt et al. (2015) demonstrated a significant relationship between tryptophan intakes and blood concentrations in 392 men representing meat eaters, fish eaters, vegetarians, and vegans ($r=0.16$, $P<.001$). Interestingly, although tryptophan intake was slightly lower in vegetarians compared to omnivores (−12%), plasma concentrations of tryptophan were significantly higher in the vegetarians compared to omnivores (+4%). Foods particularly rich in tryptophan include nuts, seeds, cheese, legumes, fish, and chicken. A vegetarian meal plan that includes 6 ounces of cheese, 1 cup legumes, 2 ounces seeds, and 6 servings of whole grain would contain approximately 2 g tryptophan at minimum. In healthy adults, ingestion of a tryptophan-rich egg white protein hydrolysate (4 g) increased blood tryptophan concentrations 33%–45% after 90 min (Mitchell et al., 2011; Gibson et al., 2014). A smaller dosage (2 g) increased blood tryptophan concentrations 12% (Gibson et al., 2014). Furthermore, wellbeing and fatigue (measured using a validated computer-based mental and physical sensations rating system) were significantly improved at 90 min following ingestion of the egg white protein hydrolysate compared to the control treatment (casein hydrolysate) in elderly women (Gibson et al., 2014). These data suggest that vegetarian diets are good sources of tryptophan, particularly with careful planning, and are associated with high circulating concentrations of tryptophan. The data are limited, however, and more investigation is required to validate these results. It is important to note that vegan diets are lower in tryptophan than ovolactovegetarian diets, and blood concentrations of tryptophan in vegans have been reported to be lower than those of omnivores (Schmidt et al., 2015).

Other dietary constituents can impact the passage of tryptophan to the brain. High circulating levels of the large neutral amino acids (LNAA), which include tryptophan, compete for entry into the brain as they utilize the same transporter. Due to this competition among amino acids, the blood tryptophan to LNAA ratio (Trp:LNAA) impacts the transport of tryptophan into the brain more so than the absolute blood tryptophan concentration, with higher ratios favoring tryptophan passage into brain. Dietary carbohydrates have a direct impact on insulin concentrations, and insulin promotes the uptake of the LNAA into muscle cells in the postprandial period, particularly the amino acids leucine, isoleucine, and valine, collectively termed the branched-chain amino acids (BCAA), as well as tyrosine and phenylalanine, thereby effectively raising the Trp:LNAA ratio (De Montis et al., 1978; Adeva et al., 2012). Thus, high carbohydrate diets favor a high Trp:LNAA ratio, which encourages tryptophan transport into the brain. Teff et al. (1989) fed healthy participants an isocaloric carbohydrate beverage containing either 0%, 4%, 8%, or 12% protein on different occasions and observed that only the 0% protein drink raised the plasma Trp:LNAA ratio (+26%). In women diagnosed with premenstrual syndrome, Sayegh et al. (1995) demonstrated that a glucose-rich drink (dextrose + maltodextrin) significantly improved mood scores on days during the late luteal phase of the menstrual cycle when premenstrual symptoms were apparent in comparison to a casein + dextrose drink or a galactose + dextrose drink. Furthermore, of the three drinks, only the glucose-rich drink raised the Trp:LNAA ratio, as it elicited the greatest insulin response and did not increase amino acid concentrations in serum.

Theoretically, a vegetarian diet (rich in tryptophan and generally characterized by a high carbohydrate-to-protein ratio in comparison to meat-based diets) should promote a greater brain uptake of tryptophan. To date, this possibility has not been examined. However, an animal-protein-rich meal elicits a surge in BCAA concentrations in blood (+90%), reflecting the high levels of BCAA in animal proteins (Aoki et al., 1976). Plant-based proteins have lower concentrations of the BCAA, and expectantly, the plasma Trp:BCAA ratio was significantly elevated for vegetarians compared to meat eaters (Schweiger et al., 1986). In addition, the plasma Trp:BCAA ratio was significantly related to dietary protein ($r = -0.44$, $P < .05$) not to dietary energy ($r = -0.22$) (Anderson and Blendis, 1981). In an early report, Schweiger et al. (1986) observed a significant correlation between the plasma Trp:LNAA ratio and global mood ($r = -0.52$) and that the mood state of the trial vegetarians only improved significantly. These data suggest that adherence to a vegetarian diet, in comparison to the typical omnivorous diet, creates a blood amino acid pattern that favors tryptophan passage into the brain.

Yet, marked differences in brain tryptophan concentrations as well as brain serotonin synthesis rates were noted following the ingestion of proteins common to vegetarian diets. Choi et al. (2009) fed fasted rats controlled meals differing only in protein content, casein, lactalbumin (a whey protein), soy protein isolate, zein (a corn protein), or wheat gluten, and at 2.5h postmeal, rats were euthanized for blood and tissue analyses. The meals containing the lactalbumin or the soy protein isolate raised brain tryptophan concentrations 84% and 25%, respectively, relative to fasting levels, whereas the other proteins did not raise brain tryptophan concentrations (Choi et al., 2009). Similar trends were noted for brain serotonin synthesis rates (+58% and +20%, respectively, for lactalbumin and soy protein isolate vs. fasting levels) with no increase reported for the remaining proteins. Control diets that substituted carbohydrate for the test protein also increased brain tryptophan concentrations (+40% vs. fasting level) and brain serotonin synthesis rates (+41% vs. fasting level) (Choi et al., 2009). These data suggest that although vegetarian diets in general appear to favor tryptophan passage into the brain, a specially formulated vegetarian diet may maximize serotonin production in the brain. Specifically, adoption of a vegetarian diet containing tryptophan-rich foods (nuts, seeds, and legumes), cow's milk, tempeh, and edamame may particularly improve mood states. Such a designer diet for improving mood state is an intriguing concept, particularly considering the improvements in health and longevity already attributed to vegetarian diets.

4.1.2 Vitamin B_6

The biosynthesis of serotonin is a two-step process: the conversion of tryptophan to 5-hydroxytryptophan (required enzyme: tryptophan hydroxylase) followed by the conversion of 5-hydroxytryptophan to 5-hydroxytryptamine, also known as serotonin (required enzyme: aromatic L-amino acid decarboxylase). Pyridoxal-6-phosphate, the cofactor form of vitamin B_6, is required for optimal activity of the decarboxylase enzyme, and plasma vitamin B_6 concentrations impact the serotonin synthesis rates in vivo (Kang and Joh, 1990; Hartvig et al., 1995). Once again, the importance of diet in the promotion of mental health is highlighted. Excellent sources of vitamin B_6 include chickpeas, tuna, chicken, turkey, potatoes, banana, and beef, while bulgur, nuts, spinach, and avocado represent good sources. A survey of vegetarians and vegans in Switzerland showed that B_6 deficiency, based on plasma concentrations, was the most pronounced nutrient deficiency among vegetarians (excluding iodine): the prevalences of vitamin B_6 deficiency were 59%, 25%, and 29% for the vegetarians ($n=53$), vegans ($n=53$), and omnivores ($n=100$), respectively (Schüpbach et al., 2015). Importantly, diet analyses did not reveal differences in vitamin B_6 intake between the vegetarians and omnivores (2.0 and 1.9 mg/day, respectively) (average requirement = 1.1–1.3 mg/day), whereas the vegans did report significantly higher intakes compared to the other diet groups (2.9 mg/day) (Schüpbach et al., 2015). These data illustrate the importance of biochemical assessment for determining vitamin B_6 status compared to reliance on dietary data.

Majchrzak et al. (2006) also reported better vitamin B_6 status among Austrian vegetarians and vegans compared to other diet groups, yet vitamin B_6 deficiency was surprisingly high for all diet groups; roughly 30% of individuals displayed vitamin B_6 deficiency based on a functional measure of enzyme activity, the glutamic oxaloacetic transaminase activation coefficient. However, Huang et al. (2003) reported that the plasma vitamin B_6 concentration was 32% lower among Taiwanese vegetarians compared to meat eaters although dietary intakes were similar (0.94 and 1.05 mg/day, respectively). The investigators did not report the prevalence of vitamin B_6 deficiency, but a functional measure, the mean erythrocyte aspartate aminotransaminase activity coefficient (EAST-AC; a measure of vitamin B_6 activity with higher values indicating lower in vivo activity), indicated poor vitamin B_6 status in both diet groups, with the vegetarians displaying a worse vitamin B_6 status compared to the meat eaters. Vudhivai et al. (1991) also observed a higher level of vitamin B_6 deficiency among a cohort of Thailand vegetarians compared to meat eaters, 29% versus 4% based on EAST-AC values. In a German vegetarian cohort, participants were classified as "strict vegans" (vegans) or "moderate vegans" (ovolactovegetarians with modest intake of dairy and/or eggs), and the prevalence of vitamin B_6 deficiency, determined as EAST-AC >1.85, was 18% in the "strict vegans" and 12% in the "moderate vegans" (Waldmann et al., 2006). For comparison, the investigators cite others who report a 4% vitamin B_6 deficiency in the German population at large. For the entire cohort, EAST-AC was not related to dietary vitamin B_6 intake ($r=0.007$), verifying the importance of biochemical assessment for determining vitamin B_6 status.

In the United States, based on the *Second National Report on Biochemical Indicators of Diet and Nutrition in the U.S. Population*, vitamin B_6 was the most common nutrient deficiency, with nearly 11% of the Americans at risk for deficiency (Pfeiffer et al., 2013). These data may seem perplexing since vitamin B_6 is well distributed across food groups with certain meats, vegetables, fruits, and nuts representing rich sources. Both meat eaters and vegetarians should be able to obtain adequate amounts of vitamin B_6 from diet. However, vitamin B_6 bioavailability is dependent on a number of factors including degree of thermal processing, fiber content, and the presence of pyridoxine glycosides. Although vitamin B_6 bioavailability is highest for animal products, the heating of meat can reduce vitamin bioavailability by 30% (Reynolds, 1988). In plant foods, fiber may reduce vitamin B_6 bioavailability up to 17% (Reynolds, 1988); moreover, in many plants, vitamin B_6 may be in a conjugated form known as pyridoxine glucoside, which reduces the bioavailability of the vitamin by 10%–15% (Hansen et al., 1996). Broccoli, cabbage, carrots, orange juice, cabbage, and soybeans are particularly high in pyridoxine glucosides (>40% of the vitamin B_6) whereas avocados, bananas, peas, and nuts have low levels of vitamin B_6 as pyridoxine glucosides (<15%) (Reynolds, 1988). Shredded-wheat cereal and wheat bran contain moderate amounts of vitamin B_6 as pyridoxine glucosides (17%–36%) (Reynolds, 1988). Thus, the high rates of vitamin B_6 deficiency noted in many populations around the globe, both omnivores and vegetarians, likely reflects thermal processing and the presence of pyridoxine glucosides. In their survey of German vegetarians, Waldmann et al. (2006) reported that vitamin B_6 inadequacy, measured using EAST-AC, was directly related to cereal intake ($r=0.252$) and inversely related to fruit intake ($r=-0.236$). These data provide insight regarding the bioavailability of dietary vitamin B_6 in foods commonly consumed by vegetarians.

Cross-sectional trials have demonstrated a strong correlation between plasma vitamin B_6 concentrations and depression in adults and the elderly (Hvas et al., 2004; Merete et al., 2008; Pan et al., 2012). In a systematic review of vitamin B_6 trials that examined the effect of vitamin B_6 supplementation on depressive symptoms, four met the quality criteria, and three of the four trials demonstrated significant benefits of vitamin B_6 supplementation on symptoms of depression (Williams et al., 2005). Since some investigations have reported a higher vitamin B_6 status among vegans compared to omnivores (Schüpbach et al., 2015; Majchrzak et al., 2006), serotonin synthesis rates may be high in vegans and contribute to improved mood states. However, reports from different countries are revealing a high prevalence of deficiency in vegetarians and nonvegetarians alike, as high as 60%. Given that marginal or deficient vitamin B_6 status may adversely impact mood, this connection warrants investigation in the general population.

4.2 Norepinephrine

The role of norepinephrine in mood disturbances has not been studied to the same extent as serotonin; yet, the noradrenergic pathways project into many regions of the brain, including the amygdala, hippocampus, and hypothalamus, and they regulate emotion and cognition (Moret and Briley, 2011). Although selective serotonin reuptake inhibitors represent the primary antidepressant therapy in the United States, norepinephrine-specific reuptake inhibitors provided added benefits in some situations (Bradley and Lenox-Smith, 2013). Ingestion of carbohydrate, notably sucrose and glucose, stimulates the sympathetic nervous system (Rappaport et al., 1982). In a cross-sectional investigation, Toth and Poehlman (1994) reported a higher fasting plasma concentration of norepinephrine in a sample of vegetarian and nonvegetarian adults (216±33 and 165±18 pg/mL, respectively), which they attributed to differences in carbohydrate intakes between the groups. However, Sciarrone et al. (1993) did not observe a difference in fasting plasma norepinephrine concentrations in male subjects following a 6-week intervention that compared effects of a vegetarian diet against an omnivore diet. Moreover, both of these trials reported significantly lower systolic blood pressures in the vegetarian groups compared to the nonvegetarians, an observation that does not support increased sympathetic activity in vegetarians. In fact, Fu et al. (2006) demonstrated that vegetarian diets are associated with higher levels of vagal activity compared to omnivorous diets, whereas sympathetic activity was similar between diet groups.

5. Conclusion

Several randomized controlled intervention trials have reported improvements in mood following the adoption of vegetarian diets. However, mechanisms contributing to this improvement have not been investigated. Mood is regulated by the action of the neurotransmitters serotonin and norepinephrine, and the proinflammatory cytokines (e.g., IL-1β, TNF-α, IL-6, and IL-2) and eicosanoids (e.g., PGE_2), as well as oxidative stress, are known to inhibit these neurotransmitters. Moreover, food choices can impact the levels of serotonin and norepinephrine and likely contribute importantly to mood states. This chapter has outlined characteristics of vegetarian diets that may possibly improve mood states. These diets, inherently rich in antioxidants, particularly vitamin C and β-carotene, are associated with lower oxidative stress and PGE_2 concentrations compared to meat-based diets. The high carbohydrate-to-protein ratio of vegetarian diets should facilitate tryptophan entry into the brain and the production of serotonin. Given the health and wellness impact of improving mood state, research examining the possible mechanisms of vegetarian diet-induced mood improvement is warranted. Vegetarian diets are already associated with healthful outcomes in terms of weight management, cardiovascular disease, and certain cancers, and these diets are sustainable with a low environmental impact. It is fun to speculate that vegetarian diets may make us happy as well as healthy.

References

Adam, O., Beringer, C., Kless, T., Lemmen, C., Adam, A., Wiseman, M., Adam, P., Klimmek, R., Forth, W., 2003. Anti-inflammatory effects of a low arachidonic acid diet and fish oil in patients with rheumatoid arthritis. Rheumatol. Int. 23, 27–36.

Adeva, M.M., Calviño, J., Souto, G., Donapetry, C., 2012. Insulin resistance and the metabolism of branched-chain amino acids in humans. Amino Acids 43, 171–181.

Anderson, G.H., Blendis, L.M., 1981. Plasma neutral amino acid ratios in normal man and in patients with hepatic encephalopathy: correlations with self-selected protein and energy consumption. Am. J. Clin. Nutr. 34, 377–385.

Aoki, T.T., Brennan, M.F., Müller, W.A., Soeldner, J.S., Alpert, J.S., Saltz, S.B., Kaufmann, R.L., Tan, M.H., Cahill Jr., G.F., 1976. Amino acid levels across normal forearm muscle and splanchnic bed after a protein meal. Am. J. Clin. Nutr. 29, 340–350.

Beezhold, B.L., Johnston, C.S., 2012. Restriction of meat, fish, and poultry in omnivores improves mood: a pilot randomized controlled trial. Nutr. J. 11, 9.

Benzie, I.F.F., Strain, J.J., 1996. Uric acid: friend or foe? Redox Rep. 2, 231–234.

Böhm, F., Edge, R., Truscott, T.G., 2012. Interactions of dietary carotenoids with singlet oxygen ($1O_2$) and free radicals: potential effects for human health. Acta Biochim. Pol. 59, 27–30.

Bowie, A.G., O'Neill, L.A., 2000. Vitamin C inhibits NF-kappa B activation by TNF via the activation of p38mitogen-activated protein kinase. J. Immunol. 165, 7180–7188.

Bradley, A.J., Lenox-Smith, A.J., 2013. Does adding noradrenaline reuptake inhibition to selective serotonin reuptake inhibition improve efficacy in patients with depression? A systematic review of meta-analyses and large randomised pragmatic trials. J. Psychopharmacol. 27, 740–758.

Buettner, G.R., 1993. The pecking order of free radicals and antioxidants: lipid peroxidation, alpha-tocopherol, and ascorbate. Arch. Biochem. Biophys. 300, 535–543.

Buettner, G.R., Jurkiewicz, B.A., 1993. Ascorbate free radical as a marker of oxidative stress: an EPR study. Free Radic. Biol. Med. 14, 49–55.

Capuron, L., Schroecksnadel, S., Féart, C., Aubert, A., Higueret, D., Barberger-Gateau, P., Layé, S., Fuchs, D., 2011. Chronic low-grade inflammation in elderly persons is associated with altered tryptophan and tyrosine metabolism: role in neuropsychiatric symptoms. Biol. Psychiatry 70, 175–182.

Choi, S., Disilvio, B., Fernstrom, M.H., Fernstrom, J.D., 2009. Meal ingestion, amino acids and brain neurotransmitters: effects of dietary protein source on serotonin and catecholamine synthesis rates. Physiol. Behav. 98, 156–162.

De Montis, M.G., Olianas, M.C., Haber, B., Tagliamonte, A., 1978. Increase in large neutral amino acid transport into brain by insulin. J. Neurochem. 30, 121–124.

Edge, R., McGarvey, D.J., Truscott, T.G., 1997. The carotenoids as anti-oxidants–a review. J. Photochem. Photobiol. B 41, 189–200.

Fisher, M., Levine, P.H., Weiner, B., Ockene, I.S., Johnson, B., Johnson, M.H., Natale, A.M., Vaudreuil, C.H., Hoogasian, J., 1986. The effect of vegetarian diets on plasma lipid and platelet levels. Arch. Intern. Med. 146, 1193–1197.

Flohé, L., Brigelius-Flohé, R., Saliou, C., Traber, M.G., Packer, L., 1997. Redox regulation of NF-kappa B activation. Free Radic. Biol. Med. 22, 1115–1126.

Fu, C.H., Yang, C.C., Lin, C.L., Kuo, T.B., 2006. Effects of long-term vegetarian diets on cardiovascular autonomic functions in healthy postmenopausal women. Am. J. Cardiol. 97, 380–383.

Gibson, E.L., Vargas, K., Hogan, E., Holmes, A., Rogers, P.J., Wittwer, J., Kloek, J., Goralczyk, R., Mohajeri, M.H., 2014. Effects of acute treatment with a tryptophan-rich protein hydrolysate on plasma amino acids, mood and emotional functioning in older women. Psychopharmacol. Berl. 231, 4595–4610.

Guarner, V., Rubio-Ruiz, M.E., 2015. Low-grade systemic inflammation connects aging, metabolic syndrome and cardiovascular disease. Interdiscip. Top. Gerontol. 40, 99–106.

Hadad, N., Levy, R., 2012. The synergistic anti-inflammatory effects of lycopene, lutein, β-carotene, and carnosic acid combinations via redox-based inhibition of NF-κB signaling. Free Radic. Biol. Med. 53, 1381–1391.

Haldar, S., Rowland, I.R., Barnett, Y.A., Bradbury, I., Robson, P.J., Powell, J., Fletcher, J., 2007. Influence of habitual diet on antioxidant status: a study in a population of vegetarians and omnivores. Eur. J. Clin. Nutr. 61, 1011–1022.

Hansen, C.M., Leklem, J.E., Miller, L.T., 1996. Vitamin B-6 status indicators decrease in women consuming a diet high in pyridoxine glucoside. J. Nutr. 126, 2512–2518.

Hart, B.L., 1988. Biological basis of the behavior of sick animals. Neurosci. Biobehav. Rev. 12, 123–137.

Hartvig, P., Lindner, K.J., Bjurling, P., Laengstrom, B., Tedroff, J., 1995. Pyridoxine effect on synthesis rate of serotonin in the monkey brain measured with positron emission tomography. J. Neural Transm. Gen. Sect. 102, 91–97.

Hein, A.M., O'Banion, M.K., 2009. Neuroinflammation and memory: the role of prostaglandins. Mol. Neurobiol. 40, 15–32.

Huang, Y.C., Chang, S.J., Chiu, Y.T., Chang, H.H., Cheng, C.H., 2003. The status of plasma homocysteine and related B-vitamins in healthy young vegetarians and nonvegetarians. Eur. J. Nutr. 42, 84–90.

Hvas, A.M., Juul, S., Bech, P., Nexø, E., 2004. Vitamin B_6 level is associated with symptoms of depression. Psychother. Psychosom. 73, 340–343.

Iachininoto, M.G., Nuzzolo, E.R., Bonanno, G., Mariotti, A., Procoli, A., Locatelli, F., De Cristofaro, R., Rutella, S., 2013. Cyclooxygenase-2 (COX-2) inhibition constrains indoleamine 2,3-dioxygenase 1 (IDO1) activity in acute myeloid leukaemia cells. Molecules 18, 10132–10145.

Ji, K., Lim Kho, Y., Park, Y., Choi, K., 2010. Influence of a five-day vegetarian diet on urinary levels of antibiotics and phthalate metabolites: a pilot study with "Temple Stay" participants. Environ. Res. 110, 375–382.

Judd, P.A., Long, A., Butcher, M., Caygill, C.P., Diplock, A.T., 1997. Vegetarians and vegans may be most at risk from low selenium intakes. BMJ 314, 1834.

Kaartinen, K., et al., 2000. Vegan diet alleviates fibromyalgia symptoms. Scand. J. Rheumatol. 29, 308.

Kahleova, H., Hrachovinova, T., Hill, M., Pelikanova, T., 2013. Vegetarian diet in type 2 diabetes–improvement in quality of life, mood and eating behaviour. Diabet. Med. 30, 127–129.

Kang, U.J., Joh, T.H., 1990. Deduced amino acid sequence of bovine aromatic L-amino acid decarboxylase: homology to other decarboxylases. Brain Res. Mol. Brain Res. 8, 83–87.

Karlsson, P.C., Huss, U., Jenner, A., Halliwell, B., Bohlin, L., Rafter, J.J., 2005. Human fecal water inhibits COX-2 in colonic HT-29 cells: role of phenolic compounds. J. Nutr. 135, 2343–2349.

Kazimírová, A., Barancokova, M., Krajcovicová-Kudláčková, M., Volkovová, K., Staruchová, M., Valachovicová, M., Pauková, V., Blazícek, P., Wsólová, L., Dusinská, M., 2006. The relationship between micronuclei in human lymphocytes and selected micronutrients in vegetarians and non-vegetarians. Mutat. Res. 611, 64–70.

Kim, M.K., Cho, S.W., Park, Y.K., 2012. Long-term vegetarians have low oxidative stress, body fat, and cholesterol levels. Nutr. Res. Pract. 6, 155–161.

Kjeldsen-Kragh, J., 1999. Rheumatoid arthritis treated with vegetarian diets. Am. J. Clin. Nutr. 70 (3 Suppl.), 594S–600S.

Krajcovicová-Kudláčková, M., Valachovicová, M., Pauková, V., Dusinská, M., 2008. Effects of diet and age on oxidative damage products in healthy subjects. Physiol. Res. 57, 647–651.

Lee, S.K., Kang, J.S., Jung da, J., Hur, D.Y., Kim, J.E., Hahm, E., Bae, S., Kim, H.W., Kim, D., Cho, B.J., Cho, D., Shin, D.H., Hwang, Y.I., Lee, W.J., 2008. Vitamin C suppresses proliferation of the human melanoma cell SK-MEL-2 through the inhibition of cyclooxygenase-2 (COX-2) expression and the modulation of insulin-like growth factor II (IGF-II) production. J. Cell Physiol. 216, 180–188.

Li, D., Ball, M., Bartlett, M., Sinclair, A., 1999. Lipoprotein(a), essential fatty acid status and lipoprotein lipids in female Australian vegetarians. Clin. Sci. (Lond.) 97, 175–181.

Liang, T., Chen, X., Su, M., Chen, H., Lu, G., Liang, K., 2014. Vitamin C exerts beneficial hepatoprotection against Concanavalin A-induced immunological hepatic injury in mice through inhibition of NF-κB signal pathway. Food Funct. 5, 2175–2182.

Lim, S.H., Fan, S.H., Say, Y.H., 2012. Plasma total antioxidant capacity (TAC) in obese Malaysian subjects. Malays J. Nutr. 18, 345–354.

Majchrzak, D., Singer, I., Männer, M., Rust, P., Genser, D., Wagner, K.H., Elmadfa, I., 2006. B-vitamin status and concentrations of homocysteine in Austrian omnivores, vegetarians and vegans. Ann. Nutr. Metab. 50, 485–491.

Manjari, V., Suresh, Y., Sailaja Devi, M.M., Das, U.N., 2001. Oxidant stress, anti-oxidants and essential fatty acids in south Indian vegetarians and non-vegetarians. Prostagl. Leukot. Essent. Fat. Acids 64, 53–59.

Markussen, M.S., Veierød, M.B., Sakhi, A.K., Ellingjord-Dale, M., Blomhoff, R., Ursin, G., Andersen, L.F., 2015. Evaluation of dietary patterns among Norwegian postmenopausal women using plasma carotenoids as biomarkers. Br. J. Nutr. 113, 672–682.

May, J.M., 1998. Ascorbate function and metabolism in the human erythrocyte. Front. Biosci. 3, d1–10.

Merete, C., Falcon, L.M., Tucker, K.L., 2008. Vitamin B_6 is associated with depressive symptomatology in Massachusetts elders. J. Am. Coll. Nutr. 27, 421–427.

Mitchell, E.S., Slettenaar, M., Quadt, F., Giesbrecht, T., Kloek, J., Gerhardt, C., Bot, A., Eilander, A., Wiseman, S., 2011. Effect of hydrolysed egg protein on brain tryptophan availability. Br. J. Nutr. 105, 611–617.

Montalcini, T., De Bonis, D., Ferro, Y., Carè, I., Mazza, E., Accattato, F., Greco, M., Foti, D., Romeo, S., Gulletta, E., Pujia, A., 2015. High vegetable fats intake is associated with high resting energy expenditure in vegetarians. Nutrients 7, 5933–5947.

Moret, C., Briley, M., 2011. The importance of norepinephrine in depression. Neuropsychiatr. Dis. Treat. 7 (Suppl. 1), 9–13.

Müller, N., Schwarz, M.J., Dehning, S., Douhe, A., Cerovecki, A., Goldstein-Müller, B., Spellmann, I., Hetzel, G., Maino, K., Kleindienst, N., Möller, H.J., Arolt, V., Riedel, M., 2006. The cyclooxygenase-2 inhibitor celecoxib has therapeutic effects in major depression: results of a double-blind, randomized, placebo controlled, add-on pilot study to reboxetine. Mol. Psychiatry 11, 680–684.

Myint, A.M., Kim, Y.K., 2014. Network beyond IDO in psychiatric disorders: revisiting eurodegeneration hypothesis. Prog. Neuropsychopharmacol. Biol. Psychiatry 48, 304–313.

Na, K.S., Lee, K.J., Lee, J.S., Cho, Y.S., Jung, H.Y., 2014. Efficacy of adjunctive celecoxib treatment for patients with major depressive disorder: a meta-analysis. Prog. Neuropsychopharmacol. Biol. Psychiatry 48, 79–85.

Nishizawa, S., Benkelfat, C., Young, S.N., Leyton, M., Mzengeza, S., de Montigny, C., Blier, P., Diksic, M., 1997. Differences between males and females in rates of serotonin synthesis in human brain. Proc. Natl. Acad. Sci. U.S.A. 94, 5308–5313.

Nutt, D.J., 2008. Relationship of neurotransmitters to the symptoms of major depressive disorder. J. Clin. Psychiatry 69 (Suppl. E1), 4–7.

Oishi, J., Doi, H., Kawakami, N., 2009. Nutrition and depressive symptoms in community-dwelling elderly persons in Japan. Acta Med. Okayama 63, 9–17.

Oxenkrug, G., 2013. Serotonin-kynurenine hypothesis of depression: historical overview and recent developments. Curr. Drug Targets 14, 514–521.

Palozza, P., Serini, S., Maggiano, N., Tringali, G., Navarra, P., Ranelletti, F.O., Calviello, G., 2005. beta-Carotene downregulates the steady-state and heregulin-alpha-induced COX-2 pathways in colon cancer cells. J. Nutr. 135, 129–136.

Pan, W.H., Chang, Y.P., Yeh, W.T., Guei, Y.S., Lin, B.F., Wei, I.L., Yang, F.L., Liaw, Y.P., Chen, K.J., Chen, W.J., 2012. Co-occurrence of anemia, marginal vitamin B_6, and folate status and depressive symptoms in older adults. J. Geriatr. Psychiatry Neurol. 25, 170–178.

Park, J.Y., Pillinger, M.H., Abramson, S.B., 2006. Prostaglandin E2 synthesis and secretion: the role of PGE2 synthases. Clin. Immunol. 119, 229–240.

Pettersson, J., Karlsson, P.C., Choi, Y.H., Verpoorte, R., Rafter, J.J., Bohlin, L., 2008. NMR metabolomic analysis of fecal water from subjects on a vegetarian diet. Biol. Pharm. Bull. 31, 1192–1198.

Pfeiffer, C.M., Sternberg, M.R., Schleicher, R.L., Haynes, B.M., Rybak, M.E., Pirkle, J.L., 2013. The CDC's Second National Report on Biochemical Indicators of Diet and Nutrition in the U.S. Population is a valuable tool for researchers and policy makers. J. Nutr. 143, 938S–947S.

Plourde, M., Cunnane, S.C., 2007. Extremely limited synthesis of long chain polyunsaturates in adults: implications for their dietary essentiality and use as supplements. Appl. Physiol. Nutr. Metab. 32, 619–634.

Poon, D.C., Ho, Y.S., Chiu, K., Wong, H.L., Chang, R.C., 2015. Sickness: from the focus on cytokines, prostaglandins, and complement factors to the perspectives of neurons. Neurosci. Biobehav. Rev. 57, 30–45.

Prohan, M., Amani, R., Nematpour, S., Jomehzadeh, N., Haghighizadeh, M.H., 2014. Total antioxidant capacity of diet and serum, dietary antioxidant vitamins intake, and serum hs-CRP levels in relation to depression scales in university male students. Redox Rep. 19, 133–139.

Rappaport, E.B., Young, J.B., Landsberg, L., February 1982. Initiation, duration and dissipation of diet-induced changes in sympathetic nervous system activity in the rat. Metabolism 31 (2), 143–146.

Rauma, A.L., Mykkänen, H., 2000. Antioxidant status in vegetarians versus omnivores. Nutrition 16, 111–119.

Reynolds, R.D., 1988. Bioavailability of vitamin B-6 from plant foods. Am. J. Clin. Nutr. 48 (Suppl. 3), 863–867.

Rosenblat, J.D., Cha, D.S., Mansur, R.B., McIntyre, R.S., 2014. Inflamed moods: a review of the interactions between inflammation and mood disorders. Prog. Neuropsychopharmacol. Biol. Psychiatry 53, 23–34.

Sayegh, R., Schiff, I., Wurtman, J., Spiers, P., McDermott, J., Wurtman, R., 1995. The effect of a carbohydrate-rich beverage on mood, appetite, and cognitive function in women with premenstrual syndrome. Obstet. Gynecol. 86 (4 Pt. 1), 520–528.

Scapagnini, G., Davinelli, S., Drago, F., De Lorenzo, A., Oriani, G., 2012. Antioxidants as antidepressants: fact or fiction? CNS Drugs 26, 477–490.

Schmidt, J.A., Crowe, F.L., Appleby, P.N., Key, T.J., Travis, R.C., 2013. Serum uric acid concentrations in meat eaters, fish eaters, vegetarians and vegans: a cross-sectional analysis in the EPIC-Oxford cohort. PLoS One 8, e56339.

Schmidt, J.A., Rinaldi, S., Scalbert, A., Ferrari, P., Achaintre, D., Gunter, M.J., Appleby, P.N., Key, T.J., Travis, R.C., September 23, 2015. Plasma concentrations and intakes of amino acids in male meat-eaters, fish-eaters, vegetarians and vegans: a cross-sectional analysis in the EPIC-Oxford cohort. Eur. J. Clin. Nutr. [Epub ahead of print].

Schüpbach, R., Wegmüller, R., Berguerand, C., Bui, M., Herter-Aeberli, I., October 26, 2015. Micronutrient status and intake in omnivores, vegetarians and vegans in Switzerland. Eur. J. Nutr. [Epub ahead of print].

Schweiger, U., Laessle, R., Kittl, S., Dickhaut, B., Schweiger, M., Pirke, K.M., 1986. Macronutrient intake, plasma large neutral amino acids and mood during weight-reducing diets. J. Neural Transm. 67, 77–86.

Sciarrone, S.E., Strahan, M.T., Beilin, L.J., Burke, V., Rogers, P., Rouse, I.R., 1993. Ambulatory blood pressure and heart rate responses to vegetarian meals. J. Hypertens. 11, 277–285.

Shi, P., Raizada, M.K., Sumners, C., 2010. Brain cytokines as neuromodulators in cardiovascular control. Clin. Exp. Pharmacol. Physiol. 37, e52–e57.

Siwek, M., Sowa-Kućma, M., Dudek, D., Styczeń, K., Szewczyk, B., Kotarska, K., Misztakk, P., Pilc, A., Wolak, M., Nowak, G., 2013. Oxidative stress markers in affective disorders. Pharmacol. Rep. 65, 1558–1571.

Somannavar, M.S., Kodliwadmath, M.V., 2012. Correlation between oxidative stress and antioxidant defence in south Indian urban vegetarians and non-vegetarians. Eur. Rev. Med. Pharmacol. Sci. 16, 351–354.

Su, K.P., 2008. Mind-body interface: the role of n-3 fatty acids in psychoneuroimmunology, somatic presentation, and medical illness comorbidity of depression. Asia Pac. J. Clin. Nutr. 17 (Suppl. 1), 151–157.

Szeto, Y.T., Kwok, T.C., Benzie, I.F., 2004. Effects of a long-term vegetarian diet on biomarkers of antioxidant status and cardiovascular disease risk. Nutrition 20, 863–866.

Tanaka, T., Kouda, K., Kotani, M., Takeuchi, A., Tabei, T., Masamoto, Y., Nakamura, H., Takigawa, M., Suemura, M., Takeuchi, H., Kouda, M., 2001. Vegetarian diet ameliorates symptoms of atopic dermatitis through reduction of the number of peripheral eosinophils and of PGE2 synthesis by monocytes. J. Physiol. Anthropol. Appl. Hum. Sci. 20, 353–361.

Teff, K.L., Young, S.N., Blundell, J.E., 1989. The effect of protein or carbohydrate breakfasts on subsequent plasma amino acid levels, satiety and nutrient selection in normal males. Pharmacol. Biochem. Behav. 34, 829–837.

Toth, M.J., Poehlman, E.T., 1994. Sympathetic nervous system activity and resting metabolic rate in vegetarians. Metabolism 43, 621–625.

Vudhivai, N., Ali, A., Pongpaew, P., Changbumrung, S., Vorasanta, S., Kwanbujan, K., Charoenlarp, P., Migasena, P., Schelp, F.P., 1991. Vitamin B_1, B_2 and B_6 status of vegetarians. J. Med. Assoc. Thai. 74, 465–470.

Waldmann, A., Dörr, B., Koschizke, J.W., Leitzmann, C., Hahn, A., 2006. Dietary intake of vitamin B_6 and concentration of vitamin B_6 in blood samples of German vegans. Public Health Nutr. 9, 779–784.

Wang, J., Dunn, A.J., 1998. Mouse interleukin-6 stimulates the HPA axis and increases brain tryptophan and serotonin metabolism. Neurochem. Int. 33, 143–154.

Wang, Y., Yang, M., Lee, S.G., Davis, C.G., Kenny, A., Koo, S.I., Chun, O.K., 2012. Plasma total antioxidant capacity is associated with dietary intake and plasma level of antioxidants in postmenopausal women. J. Nutr. Biochem. 23, 1725–1731.

Wang, Y., Liu, X.J., Robitaille, L., Eintracht, S., MacNamara, E., Hoffer, L.J., 2013. Effects of vitamin C and vitamin D administration on mood and distress in acutely hospitalized patients. Am. J. Clin. Nutr. 98, 705–711.

Williams, A.L., Cotter, A., Sabina, A., Girard, C., Goodman, J., Katz, D.L., 2005. The role for vitamin B-6 as treatment for depression: a systematic review. Fam. Pract. 22, 532–537.

Wohleb, E.S., McKim, D.B., Sheridan, J.F., Godbout, J.P., 2015. Monocyte trafficking to the brain with stress and inflammation: a novel axis of immune-to-brain communication that influences mood and behavior. Front. Neurosci. 8, 447.

Yu, X., Huang, T., Weng, X., Shou, T., Wang, Q., Zhou, X., Hu, Q., Li, D., 2014. Plasma n-3 and n-6 fatty acids and inflammatory markers in Chinese vegetarians. Lipids Health Dis. 13, 151.

Yui, K., Imataka, G., Nakamura, H., Ohara, N., Naito, Y., 2015. Eicosanoids derived from arachidonic acid and their family prostaglandins and cyclooxygenase in psychiatric disorders. Curr. Neuropharmacol. 13, 776–785.

Zonis, S., Pechnick, R.N., Ljubimov, V.A., Mahgerefteh, M., Wawrowsky, K., Michelsen, K.S., Chesnokova, V., 2015. Chronic intestinal inflammation alters hippocampal neurogenesis. J. Neuroinflammation 12, 65.

Life Events

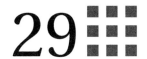
Vegetarian Infants and Complementary Feeding

Silvia Scaglioni[1], Valentina De Cosmi[1,2], Alessandra Mazzocchi[1,2], Silvia Bettocchi[1,3], Carlo Agostoni[1,2]

[1]FONDAZIONE IRCCS CÀ GRANDA OSPEDALE MAGGIORE POLICLINICO, MILAN, ITALY; [2]UNIVERSITY OF MILAN, MILAN, ITALY; [3]UNIVERSITÀ CATTOLICA DEL SACRO CUORE, MILAN, ITALY

1. Introduction

Complementary feeding is the period of time when infants are introduced to food different from milk in their diet, together with a gradual reduction of the intake of milk (either breast milk or formula), to finally and gradually acquire their family's diet model (Alvisi et al., 2015). This definition is based on the one proposed by the European Food Safety Authority (EFSA, 2009) and by the European Society for Pediatric Gastroenterology, Hepatology, and Nutrition (ESPGHAN) (ESPGHAN Committee on Nutrition, 2015). The World Health Organization (WHO) has described the complementary feeding period as "the period during which other foods or liquids are provided along with breast milk" and states that "any nutrient-containing foods or liquids other than breast milk given to young children during the period of complementary feeding are defined as complementary foods."

The ESPGHAN Committee on Nutrition, the American Academy of Pediatrics (AAP), and the WHO consider that exclusive or full breast-feeding for 6 months is a desirable goal (ESPGHAN Committee on Nutrition, 2015; Kleinman, 2000; WHO, 2003). The introduction of complementary foods should not be before 17 weeks but should not be delayed beyond 26 weeks. Around the sixth month of life, breast milk becomes insufficient to meet requirements for macronutrients and micronutrients, as the infant's age and weight both increase. Infants gradually lose the extrusion reflex, and they develop the ability to swallow solids and start to show an interest in adult family foods. A balanced number of factors let them gain a good relationship with food and the achievement of nutritional requirements (Alvisi et al., 2015):

- acquisition of fundamental milestones in neuromotor development
- development of taste and personal inclinations
- maturation of renal and gastrointestinal functionality
- qualitative and quantitative implementation of nutritional intake
- interaction of cultural and socioeconomic factors with local and family traditions

Enough attention should be paid to all these aspects: nutritional and developmental reasons drive this transition, which will influence later health. The AAP recommends that breast milk should be continued for at least 12 months along with appropriate supplementary foods (American Academy of Pediatrics, 2005). Important data point out that breast milk has a favoring role in psychological and nutritional aspects and in the development of tolerance; thus, it might reduce the onset of allergies (Grimshaw et al., 2013). Exclusive breast-feeding by well-nourished mothers for 6 months can meet a healthy infant's requirements for water, energy, protein, calcium, and most vitamins and minerals (EFSA, 2013). The breast milk of ovolactovegetarian women is similar in composition to that of nonvegetarians, and it is nutritionally adequate too (Craig et al., 2009). For that reason, there are no evidences that timing of solid foods introduction in vegetarian weaning should differ from nonvegetarians.

In the first year of life, if breast-feeding is not possible, the only alternative is infant formula, or soy formula for vegan infants. The introduction of cow milk should not be before the 12th month of life, due to its high protein content, low iron concentration, and the risk of iron deficiency (Domellöf et al., 2014). Fortified soy milk can be used as a primary beverage starting at age of 1 year or older, too (Mangels and Messina, 2001). Other preparations including soy milk, rice milk, and homemade formulas should not be used to replace breast milk or commercial infant formula, due to their poor nutritional quality. Different weaning practices have characterized this stage of life according to traditions, ethnical origins, and scientific beliefs. Actually, there are not rigid schemes on timing of food introduction, especially fruits and vegetables (Alvisi et al., 2015). In the latest suggestions issued by AAP, ESPGHAN, and European Academy of Allergy and Clinical Immunology (De Silva et al., 2014), it is recognized that there is no scientific evidence to justify the delayed introduction of solid foods (after 6 months of age), even those recognized as more allergenic, to prevent allergic diseases (Agostoni and Laicini, 2014). Vegetarian complementary feeding is widespread because vegetarian families are increasing and they want their children to share their nutritional habits starting from complementary feeding: vegetarians and vegans have been estimated to constitute 5% and 2%, respectively, of the US population, and in Italy, vegetarians are 7.1% of the total population (EURISPES survey; Appleby et al., 2016). Literature informs that well-planned vegetarian diets are appropriate for individuals during all stages of the life cycle, including pregnancy, lactation, infancy, childhood, and adolescence, and for athletes (Craig et al., 2009). A vegetarian diet is characterized by the choice of a wide variety of foods of vegetal origin and by the exclusion of animal foods (meat, fish, and their derivatives). The reader may read Chapter 1 of this book for a full characterization of the different diets. The two main categories of vegetarian complementary feeding that will be discussed in this chapter are ovolactovegetarian, which includes dairy and egg products, and vegan weaning, which is characterized by the absence of any type of animal foods.

The period from birth to 1 year is a time of nutritional vulnerability when attention to proper nutrition is critical to support the extremely rapid growth, including brain growth. In this phase, particular attention should be paid because a regular growth and neurodevelopment are relevant goals. Ovolactovegetarian weaning can be adopted, but it must be correctly designed, to favor a healthy diet and to prevent nutritional deficiencies that are a real risk of vegetarian diet. Foods in the vegan diet repertoire cannot alone cover energy, macronutrients, and micronutrients requirements of the infant; consequently supplementations are needed (Amit, 2010; Chalouhi et al., 2008; Kaganov et al., 2015).

2. Vegetarian Complementary Solid Food, Macronutrients, and Micronutrients Requirements

Differences between vegetarian solid foods and nonvegetarian ones are limited to replacement of meat with mashed or pureed tofu, legumes (pureed and strained if necessary), soy or dairy yogurt, cooked egg yolk, and cottage cheese. Later, around 7–10 months, foods such as cubed tofu, cheese or soy cheese, and small pieces of veggie burgers can be started. A balanced use of foods out of the following alimentary groups—fruits, vegetables, cereals, dried fruits, legumes, water, and oilseeds—permit one to conduct a good vegetarian complementary feeding (Craig et al., 2009).

In the second half of the first year of life, breast milk alone is not enough to supply a sufficient amount of calories, proteins, zinc, iron, and fat-soluble vitamins (vitamins A, D, K) that are necessary to guarantee an adequate growth to the infant (ESPGHAN Committee on Nutrition, 2015; EFSA, 2009). Complementary feeding is an important phase in the growth of a child, and it can play a major role in a child's future health and in its future feeding behavior.

Early feeding contributes to prevent noncommunicable adult diseases (United Nations System Standard Committee on Nutrition, 2006). The recommended intakes suggested subsequently for infants in the second semester of life have been extracted from EFSA Scientific Opinions on Dietary Reference Values for energy, micronutrients, and macronutrients and from a position paper by the American Dietetic Association (ADA) about vegetarian diets (Craig et al., 2009).

2.1 Energy in Infants (7–12 Months)

EFSA: The recommended intake of energy is 76–79 kcal/Kg/day (EFSA, 2013).

The recommended energy intake should be correctly distributed among the various macronutrients, both in terms of quantity and quality (Alvisi et al., 2015). It is known that the energy content of human milk varies within a meal, with lactational stage, and between individuals. Assuming an average energy content of human milk of 0.67 kcal/g, mean energy requirements are met by exclusive breast-feeding during the first 6 months of life and possibly longer (Butte, 2007). Also, the protein content of human milk changes with lactational stage and is on average 13 g/L in the second week, 9 g/L in the second month, and 8 g/L in the fourth month until weaning. In mature milk, there is a low content of iron (0.2–0.4 mg/L) and zinc (about 0.5 mg/L at 6 months), and both decrease with the length of lactation (EFSA, 2013).

The energy density of many vegetarian foods (cereals, fruits, vegetables) is low, due to low fat and high fiber content, and infants may have difficulty consuming the necessary volume of diet to achieve adequate energy intake (British Paediatric Association, 1988). Their stomach capacity is limited, and children from 1–3 years of age are able to take 200–300 mL at each meal. Fiber and complex carbohydrates have a higher water content, and this results in a lower energy density of the foods and favors early satiation (Jacobs and JT, 1988).

Energy is needed to maintain physiological activities and deposition of tissues. Growing is a dynamic and energy-consuming process that should be adequately supported: it is about 5 kcal/g of new tissue (3.5 kcal energy "stored" and 1.5 kcal for cost of synthesis). In the first month of life, energy requirements for growth are 40%, and they decrease to about 3% at the age of 12 months, due to the decrease of growth rate (Butte, 2007).

Growth during complementary feeding should continue to be monitored and plotted on standard centile charts as part of health surveillance by the pediatrician, and mothers should be advised appropriately if growth deviates from the expected. It is important that vegetarian parents know how to ensure an adequate intake of energy by their infants. Doctors, dieticians, and nurses should give them practical tips on how to increase energy density of foods (Mangels and Messina, 2001). The first practical trick is to feed their baby at least four times a day, including energy-dense complementary foods at each meal. Ripe bananas have 15%–20% carbohydrate, and avocados are rich in fat; thus both of them are good sources of energy. Cereals and pulses are usually more energy-dense than fruits. Adding fats such as extra virgin olive oil to cereal meals or peanut butter to bread improve the energy density of the meal itself. Parents should promote water consumption, avoiding allowing the infant to drink any kind of energy-providing liquids.

Key point: Energy is needed to support growth. High-fiber and high-complex-carbohydrate diets lower the caloric density of the foods and favor an early satiety.

2.2 Protein in Infants (7–12 Months)

EFSA: The recommended intake is about 10% of total calories (1.1 g/Kg/day, average recommended intake 11 g/day for 6 months of age) (EFSA, 2012). *ADA: Precautional protein increase of 10%–15% of the recommended intake for age* (Craig et al., 2009).

Recommended protein intake has been reduced in the past few years, due to the alignment on human milk content (EFSA, 2014a,b), falling in line with the hypothesis that hyperproteic diets in early life may favor the onset of obesity (Alvisi et al., 2015). An excess of proteins would stimulate the secretion of insulin and IGF1, both responsible for adipogenesis and the differentiation of adipocytes. Data available in literature suggest that between 6 and 24 months of age, a protein intake of more than 15% of total energy can lead, in some subjects, to early adiposity rebound phenomena, thus favoring the development of future obesity (Agostoni et al., 2005; Rolland-Cachera et al., 2006). No association has been found between a high intake of fats with complementary feeding and obesity in the following ages; on the contrary, Rolland-Cachera et al. identified in a high-protein and low-fat dietary pattern a hyperproteic and hypolipidic pattern of infants living in developed countries as a possible contributing factor of early adiposity rebound and, later in life, of body fat and leptin resistance (Rolland-Cachera et al., 2013; Alvisi et al., 2015; Escribano et al., 2012). The diet of infants in the general population is characterized by high protein and low fat intakes (Michaelsen and Greer, 2014). Together with the attention to protein and fat intake, energy has to be taken into account, since it represents the main determinant of fat deposition. Nevertheless, the relation between protein intake during complementary feeding and later risk of noncommunicable diseases is still unclear. Not only the quantity, but also the quality of proteins seems to play a role in the association between early intakes and later fatness. The longitudinal DONALD study reported that the protein sources that may be mostly responsible for the association with adiposity at 7 years old are animal protein, and more specifically dairy products at 12 months (Günther et al., 2007). However, in vegetarian infants the risk is rather to fail reaching the recommended protein intake, and this risk can be reduced by continuing the intake of breast milk or formula.

It has to be taken into account that many vegetable proteins are low in one or more essential amino acids, and the total indispensable amino acid content in vegetable foods is low when compared to animal protein sources (Craig et al., 2009). Because vegetable foods have not the same quantity and quality of proteins, vegetarians' dietary choices are crucial to achieve the adequate protein intake. Plant proteins can meet protein requirements when a variety of plant foods are consumed and energy needs are met (Mangels and Messina, 2001). Eating a huge variety of plant foods over the course of a day can provide all essential amino acids and adequate nitrogen retention (American Academy of Pediatrics Committee on Nutrition, 1998). Encouraging infants to continue to take about 500 mL/day of breast milk or formula reduces the needs for other proteins sources. Mixing breast milk or formula intake, which provides proteins rich in indispensable amino acids, with vegetable protein foods enhances the amino acid composition of the meal and improves net protein utilization. Legumes and soy beans have a high proportion of proteins (over 20% and about 36%, respectively), but a low biological value. Based on the protein digestibility-corrected amino acid score, which is the standard method for determining protein quality, a combination of legumes and wheat proteins enhances the nitrogen utilization efficiency (Craig et al., 2009), and the choice of shelled beans minimizes the phytic acid intake. In vegetarian infant diet, a precautionary increase of proteins is suggested, around 10%–15% of the recommended energy intake for age. Attention should be paid to not to exceed the 15% and to avoid the risk of protein excess (Joint WHO/FAO/UNU Expert Consultation, 2007).

Key point: Proteins are crucial for growth. In not well-balanced vegetarian diets, there is a consistent risk to not reach protein requirements.

2.3 Lipids in Infants (7–12 Months)

EFSA: Lipids: recommended intake is 40% of total calories (EFSA, 2010a,b).

Lipids are the main energy source in the infant diet and are necessary for normal growth and physical activity. Lipids are also important structural components of neural and other body tissues (Uauy and Dangour, 2009; Butte et al., 2010). The selection of dietary fat and fatty acid sources during the first years of life is now considered to be of critical importance (Uauy and Dangour, 2009).

Consumption of n-3 PUFAs eicosapentaenoic acid (EPA) and docosahexaenoic acid (DHA) have demonstrated physiological benefits on blood pressure, heart rate, triglycerides, and likely inflammation, endothelial function, and cardiac diastolic function (Aranceta and Perez-Rodrigo, 2012). DHA plays a major role in development of the brain and retina during fetal development and the first 2 years of life (Uauy and Dangour, 2009). When DHA-rich products are excluded, the recommended intake of total lipids and of ω-3 series cannot be achieved, and there is the risk of low DHA blood level and relative deficiency (Rosell et al., 2005).

The proposal that dietary DHA enhances neurocognitive functioning in term infants is controversial. Theoretical evidence, laboratory research, and human epidemiological studies have convincingly demonstrated that DHA deficiency can negatively impact neurocognitive development (Schwartz et al., 2009).

DHA deficiency may be the cause of many disorders, such as depression, inability to concentrate, excessive mood swings, anxiety, cardiac disease, type 2 diabetes, and dry skin (De Mel and Suphioglu, 2014). Nutrient deficiency during development may have long-lasting consequences for the central nervous system that range from devastating malformations to subtle effects on neural functioning. DHA is enriched in brain and retina membranes, where it functions in early development events, such as neurogenesis, neurite outgrowth, synaptic plasticity, axonal elimination, and gene expression (Mulder et al., 2014).

One of the main considerations when trying to meet current recommendations for n-3 fatty acids is that current intake of PUFAs consists primarily of n-6 fatty acids. The competition for desaturases and elongases in n-3 and n-6 PUFA metabolism results in inverse effects on tissue concentrations of these fatty acids. This is of even greater concern in vegetarians and vegans, who have relatively high intakes of linoleic acid (LA) combined with low intakes of EPA and DHA (Aranceta and Perez-Rodrigo, 2012).

Vegetarians tend to consume a lot of n-6 but marginal amounts of n-3 fatty acids. To restore n6/n3 balance, regular consumption of micro-algae (rich in DHA) and of walnuts, canola oil, flaxseed oil, enriched dairy products, seeds, peanut butter, soy beans, and derivatives (rich in alfa-linolenic fatty acid, ALA) is recommended (Van Winckel et al., 2011).

EFSA has not established recommended intakes for n3-PUFAs but for specific n-3 fatty acids, namely ALA, EPA, and DHA. EFSA proposed not to set specific values for the n-3/n-6 ratio and to set an average intake of 100mg DHA for infants (>6months) and young children. In older infants, DHA intakes at levels of 50–100mg per day have been found effective for visual function in the complementary feeding period and are considered to be adequate for that period. EFSA has set the adequate intake value of 0.5% of total energy for ALA in all population groups (EFSA, 2010a,b).

The FAO/WHO 2008 report defines 15% of total energy as upper AMRD (acceptable macronutrients distribution rate) for infants 6–12months old (Aranceta and Perez-Rodrigo, 2012).

An increased intake of ALA, the precursor of endogenous DHA synthesis, has been supposed to be an (alternative) strategy to support infant DHA status. Few studies have tested the effect of replacing LA-rich corn oil with ALA-rapeseed oil in complementary food. It still seems to be a promising strategy, but it remains to be confirmed how this approach affects the DHA status (Libuda et al., 2016).

Key point. Lipids are the main energy source (40% of total energy) for the infant, and they are essential for growth and for neural tissue structure. Polyunsaturated and mono-unsaturated fats have to be preferred. A regular intake of DHA-rich foods is recommended for both vegetarians and vegans.

2.4 Carbohydrates in Infants (7–12 Months)

Dietary carbohydrates are the major macronutrients for humans. Both adults and children in the Western countries obtain approximately half their daily caloric requirements from dietary carbohydrates. In other countries, carbohydrate has been the major source of energy, at least until the more recent introduction of "Western foods," with higher proportions of fat and protein, to many developing countries.

There are not current recommendations for infants; EFSA has proposed 45%–60% of total energy as the reference intake range for carbohydrates applicable to both adults and children older than 1 year of age (EFSA, 2010a,b).

To decrease the risk of overweight, obesity, and tooth decay, a WHO guideline recommends adults and children reduce their daily intake of free sugars to less than 10% of their total energy intake. A further reduction to below 5% would provide additional health benefits (WHO, 2015).

Based on the available evidence on bowel function, EFSA has considered dietary fiber intakes of 25 g/day to be adequate in adults and of 2 g/MJ to be adequate in children from the age of 1 year (EFSA, 2010a,b).

It is advisable to prefer starchy alimentary sources, if possible with a low glycemic index, and above all, it is strongly recommended to limit the intake of simple sugars (such as fruit juices, sugar, and sweeteners in general). Carbohydrates in foods with a low glycemic index are more slowly digested and absorbed; consequently, diets with a low glycemic index are beneficial in controlling postprandial plasma glucose excursions. Diets with a low glycemic index and glycemic load, but not low in total carbohydrates, are associated with lower type 2 diabetes mellitus risk, cardiovascular disease risk, and levels of proinflammatory markers and fasting insulin (Blaak, 2016; Rouhani et al., 2016).

Recent literature failed to confirm that introducing gluten between week 17 and 26, while the infant is still being breast-fed, would have a protective role on the onset of celiac disease, type 1 diabetes, and wheat allergy (Vriezinga et al., 2014; Beyerlein et al., 2014).

Cereals are rich in starch, proteins, minerals, vitamins, and insoluble fibers. Amaranth, quinoa, buckwheat, soy, and lupine have all the indispensable amino acids in sufficient amounts. Other cereals are low in lysine but rich in methionine, whereas this is the opposite in legumes; therefore these protein sources are well known to complement each other. Adding legumes to cereals is possible to obtain adequate biological protein value.

Choosing refined and lower fiber cereals allows a reduction of phytic acid content, which usually lowers the absorption of minerals (namely, iron, zinc, calcium, and magnesium). ESPGHAN Committee on Nutrition recommends that iron-rich complementary foods (iron-fortified cereals) should be given to all infants from 6 months of age (ESPGHAN Committee on Nutrition, 2015). Both vegetarian and nonvegetarian infants should be introduced to whole grains before the end of the second year of life.

Key point. Carbohydrates in starchy alimentary sources are preferred. Reducing free sugars to less than 10% of their total energy intake is recommended.

2.5 Iron in Infants (7–12 Months)

EFSA: Iron: a daily intake of 11 mg is recommended (EFSA, 2015a,b,c). *ADA: 1.8 times that of nonvegetarians* (Craig et al., 2009).

Iron is critical for normal growth, hematopoiesis, and neurologic development during infancy.

When complementary feeding is not introduced in exclusive breast-fed infants, they are at risk of developing an iron deficit in the second semester (Alvisi et al., 2015). Prevalence of iron deficiency anemia among vegetarians is similar to that of nonvegetarians, and it is approximately 2%–3% at 6–9 months and 3%–9% at 1–3 years of life (Domellöf et al., 2014). Complementary foods have the important role to provide more than 90% of the iron requirements in breast-fed infants (Domellöf et al., 2014). Between 6 and 24 months of age, the infant becomes dependent on additional dietary iron, and because of rapid growth, iron requirements per kilogram body weight are higher than during any other period of life. It has been shown that infants have the ability to upregulate iron absorption when iron requirements increase (Domellöf et al., 2002). This ability of each individual to be able to adapt iron absorption to iron status is likely to make infants more resistant to iron deficiency.

The ESPGHAN Committee on Nutrition states that meat products and iron-fortified foods are the major dietary source of iron. Therefore an early introduction of iron-rich complementary foods is highly recommended for preventing iron deficiency anemia in infants (ESPGHAN Committee on Nutrition, 2015).

Foods containing iron are meat and fish (bovine: 1.9 mg/100 g; cod 0.7 mg/100 g) and some vegetables (legumes, endive, green chicory, spinach). EFSA assumes a mean value of 10% of iron absorption in healthy and nonanemic infants; however, absorption depends on iron bioavailability of different foods and on the infant's iron storage. Iron found in fish and meat (heme iron) is absorbed for about 25%, while the percentage of iron absorbed from vegetables (nonheme) varies from 2% to 13% (EFSA, 2015a,b,c). Because of lower bioavailability of iron from a vegetarian diet, the recommended iron intakes for vegetarians are 1.8 times that of nonvegetarians (Craig et al., 2009) (Trumbo et al., 2001).

The iron in plant foods is nonheme iron, which is sensitive to both inhibitors and enhancers of iron absorption. Inhibitors of iron absorption include phytates, calcium, and the polyphenolics compounds in tea, coffee, herb teas, and cocoa. Fiber only slightly inhibits iron absorption (Coudray et al., 1997). Some food preparation techniques such as soaking and sprouting of beans, grains, and seeds, and the leavening of bread, can diminish phytate levels. Other fermentation processes, such as those used to make miso and tempeh, may also improve iron bioavailability. Vegetable foods with high iron content are dark green leafy vegetables, lentils, chickpeas, peas, and curry powder (it is still unclear how efficiently the iron in curry powder is absorbed). Vitamin C and other organic acids found in fruits and vegetables can substantially enhance iron absorption and reduce the inhibitory effects of phytate and thereby improve iron status (Hallberg and Hulthén, 2000).

Key point. Iron bioavailability of plant foods is low. Some food preparation techniques diminish phytate levels. Vitamin C enhances iron absorption. Iron-fortified cereals are recommended to all vegetarian and nonvegetarian infants from the sixth month of life.

2.6 Zinc in Infants (7–12 Months)

EFSA: Zinc: a daily intake of 2.9 mg is recommended (EFSA, 2015a,b).

The bioavailability of zinc from vegetarian diets is lower than from nonvegetarian diets, mainly due to the higher phytic acid content of vegetarian diets (Hunt, 2003). Zinc sources include soy products, legumes, grains, cheese, and nuts. Food preparation techniques are the same used for increasing iron bioavailability, which can reduce binding of zinc by phytic acid and increase zinc bioavailability, too (Lönnerdal, 2000). Organic acids, such as citric acid, can also enhance zinc absorption to some extent (Lönnerdal, 2000). The reader may read the specific chapter about zinc intake and status in vegetarians to further develop the question. Zinc is important for growth and the maintenance and development of immune cells of both the innate and adaptive immune system (Maares and Haase, 2016). Breast milk provides sufficient zinc for the first 4–6 months of life but does not provide recommended amounts of zinc for infants aged 7–12 months, who need 2.9 mg/day. Thus, foods with zinc (fortified or natural) should be introduced at 7 months. Vegetarian infants who grow slowly should be assessed for zinc intake and status.

Key point. Zinc bioavailability of plant foods is low. As for iron, food preparation techniques and organic acids can enhance zinc absorption.

2.7 Calcium in Infants (7–12 Months)

EFSA: Average intake is estimated to be 280 mg/day. This is close to the value derived using the factorial approach, 241 mg/day (EFSA, 2015a,b).

Calcium intakes of ovolactovegetarians are similar to those of nonvegetarians, whereas intakes of vegans tend to be lower and may fall below recommended intakes (Craig et al., 2009). Breast milk and infant formula both provide an adequate amount of calcium. The bioavailability of calcium from soy infant formula fortified with calcium carbonate is equivalent to infant formula (Messina et al., 2003). Ovolactovegetarian babies can get calcium from low-oxalate greens (broccoli, cabbage, collards, and kale) that are sources of highly bioavailable calcium, and from calcium-set tofu and sesame seeds, almonds, and dried beans that have a lower bioavailability (Weaver et al., 1999). Many vegans meet their calcium requirements by using calcium-fortified foods (e.g., calcium-fortified cereals) or dietary supplements (Weaver et al., 1999). Factors present in plant-based diets such as oxalic acid and phytic acid can potentially interfere with absorption and retention of calcium and thereby have a negative effect on bone mineral density. As mentioned before, some food preparation techniques can diminish phytate level. Approximately 30% of calcium is absorbed from dairy products and fortified food; almost twice as much is absorbed from some vegetables such as broccoli and kale (Mangels, 2014). Another important source of calcium is mineral water that contributes to reach the requirements. The daily recommended intake of liquids is 100 mL/Kg (Alvisi et al., 2015). It is advisable to consume water and to avoid energy-providing liquids, which present a high content of free sugars.

Key point. Dairy products and calcium-rich vegetables and fruits are recommended. Water is a fundamental calcium source.

2.8 Sodium in Infants (7–12 Months)

EFSA: Data are not sufficient to establish an upper level from dietary sources; a reduction in the sodium consumed in the diet is recommended for the whole population (EFSA, 2005).

Nonspecific recommendations are needed for vegetarian complementary feeding. For the general infant population, it is advisable not to add salt to food until 1 year of age, as the sodium content of some foods is enough to cover the daily requirement (EFSA, 2005).

Key point. It is advisable not to add salt to food until 1 year of age.

2.9 Vitamin B_{12} in Infants (7–12 Months)

EFSA: Average intake is 1.5 µg/day in infants aged 7–11 months (EFSA, 2015a,b).

Plant foods do not contain a significant amount of active vitamin B_{12}, thus the status of vegetarians is less than adequate (Herrmann et al., 2001). Vitamin B_{12} must be obtained from regular use of vitamin B_{12}-fortified foods; otherwise a daily supplement is needed (Craig et al., 2009). Ovolactovegetarian infants usually have sufficient levels of vitamin B_{12} from a regular consumption of dairy foods, eggs, and vitamin B_{12}-fortified foods (fortified soy formula and some cereals). Vegans are thus at great risk of B_{12} deficiency, and the infant born to a vegan mother may be already deficient in B_{12} and may present neural defects at birth (Peker et al., 2015). Breast-fed infants of nonsupplemented vegan mothers need to take vitamin B_{12} supplementation. Infants should be given supplements as prescribed by the health care provider (Craig et al., 2009).

Key point. Plant foods are not a source of vitamin B_{12}. B_{12}-fortified foods (for example, cereals) have to be preferred. Supplements are needed both for vegan infants and vegan breast-feeding mothers.

3. Conclusion

Plant-based milk substitutes (such as soy, rice, or almond milk), homemade formulas, cow's milk, and goat's milk should not be used to replace breast milk or infant formula during the first year of life. These foods do not have the right amounts and quality of protein, fat, and carbohydrate. They do not have enough of many vitamins and minerals that the infant requires.

A well-planned ovolactovegetarian diet can be completely adequate during infancy, and complementary feeding should follow the same timing and principles as for nonvegetarian infants. As concerning growth and development, some descriptive cohort studies have demonstrated an identical growth and weight evolution in ovolactovegetarian children and adolescents compared to their omnivorous peers, whereas vegan children tend to be leaner and smaller (Van Winckel et al., 2011).

On the contrary, careful dietary planning is needed for infants who are weaned onto vegan diet, who have to be supplemented with vitamin B_{12}, with special attention to adequate intakes of calcium and zinc and energy-dense foods containing enough high-quality protein. Vegetarian diets can be as diverse as omnivorous ones, but it is important to remember that the more restricted the diet and the younger the child, the greater the risk for deficiencies (Yen et al., 2008) and the risk of later feeding behavior difficulties. Parents and caregivers should be knowledgeable to provide an adequate vegetarian nutrition. The best advice for parents who want their children to follow a vegetarian regimen is to ask informed pediatricians or dieticians, to find out how to create an optimal dietary menu for their infants. As in the infant general population, monitoring weight changes, growth, and psychomotor evolution is indicated and part of the nutritional evaluation of vegetarian infants, too.

The period of life between birth and 2 years is important for the development of eating habits and to shape infants' preferences. The most important phase may be the beginning of complementary feeding, when infants discover the sensory (texture, taste, and flavor) aspect of the foods that will be part of their adult diet. In this period, eating preferences emerge, and they depend on the foods offered and on the context of feeding (Nicklaus, 2015). Offering food variety is the best rule to ensure the achievement of both nutritional requirements and the goal of teaching infants the different tastings of foods. If early experience includes exposure to a variety of foods and flavors, then a wider range of foods and flavors will be accepted. Caregivers have the responsibility for making the decisions about their infant's feeding, and they may serve as a model for an infant's eating, because much of the early learning about food occurs in the family (Birch and Doub, 2014). Doctors, nurses, and dieticians can play a key role in helping parents provide varied vegetarian diets for their infants that contain adequate amounts of nutrients and energy and to identify the characteristics of the eating experience that will contribute to drive an infant's eating behavior.

Further studies are needed to assess the bioavailability of micronutrients in vegetarian infants and relative supplementations and to tailor specific recommendations.

4. Nutritional Advices in Vegetarian Infants (0–12 Months)

- Exclusive breast-feeding for 6 months is a desirable goal.
- The introduction of complementary foods should not be before 17 weeks or delayed beyond 26 weeks.
- Vegetarian complementary feeding should be carefully planned by a pediatrician or dietician. Infant growth, neurological development, and nutritional habits should be all monitored.
- Continued breast-feeding or at least 500 mL of infant formula during complementary feeding ensures reaching calcium requirements.
- Rice, almond, and soy "milk" are not suitable milk substitutes, even if supplemented with calcium. Infant formula or soy formula are indicated.
- The introduction of cow or soy milk should not be before 12 months of life.
- Timing of solid foods introduction is the same as in nonvegetarians.
- Particular attention should be given to reach adequate energy, protein, and lipids requirements.
- Iron-rich complementary foods should be given to avoid iron deficiency.
- Vitamin B_{12} supplements are recommended to ovolactovegetarians, and especially vegans, to ensure adequate vitamin B_{12} intake to prevent deficiency.
- Caregivers should offer their infants a variety of foods to teach them different flavors.

References

Agostoni, C., Laicini, E., 2014. Early exposure to allergens: a new window of opportunity for noncommunicable disease prevention in complementary feeding? Int. J. Food Sci. Nutr. 65 (1), 1–2.

Agostoni, C., et al., 2005. How much protein is safe? Int. J. Obes. 29 (Suppl. 2), S8–S13.

Alvisi, P., et al., 2015. Recommendations on complementary feeding for healthy, full-term infants. Ital. J. Pediatr. 41, 36.

American Academy of Pediatrics Committee on Nutrition, 1998. Soy protein-based formulas: recommendations for use in infant feeding. Pediatrics 101 (1 Pt 1), 148–153.

American Academy of Pediatrics, 2005. Breastfeeding and the use of human milk. Pediatrics 115 (2), 496–506.

Amit, M., May 2010. Vegetarian diets in children and adolescents. Paediatr. Child Health 15 (5), 303–314.

Appleby, P.N., Crowe, F.L., Bradbury, K.E., et al., January 2016. Mortality in vegetarians and comparable nonvegetarians in the United Kingdom. Am. J. Clin. Nutr. 103 (1), 218–230.

Aranceta, J., Perez-Rodrigo, C., 2012. Recommended dietary reference intakes, nutritional goals and dietary guidelines for fat and fatty acids: a systematic review. Br. J. Nutr. 107, S8–S22.

Association, N.S.C.O.T.B.P., 1988. Vegetarian weaning. Arch. Dis. Child. 63, 1286–1292 1–7.

Beyerlein, A., et al., 2014. Timing of gluten introduction and islet autoimmunity in young children: updated results from the BABYDIET study. Diabetes Care 37 (9), e194–e195.

Birch, L.L., Doub, A.E., 2014. Learning to eat: birth to age 2 y. Am. J. Clin. Nutr. 99 (3), 723S–728S.

Blaak, E.E., 2016. Carbohydrate quantity and quality and cardio-metabolic risk. Curr. Opin. Clin. Nutr. Metab. Care 19 (4), 289–293.

Butte, N.F., 2007. Energy requirements of infants. Public Health Nutr. 8 (7a).

Butte, N.F., et al., 2010. Nutrient intakes of US infants, toddlers, and preschoolers meet or exceed dietary reference intakes. J. Am. Diet. Assoc. 110 (Suppl. 12), S27–S37.

Chalouhi, C., Faesch, S., Anthoine-Milhomme, M.C., et al., August 2008. Neurological consequences of vitamin B12 deficiency and its treatment. Pediatr. Emerg. Care 24 (8), 538–541.

Coudray, C., et al., 1997. Effect of soluble or partly soluble dietary fibres supplementation on absorption and balance of calcium, magnesium, iron and zinc in healthy young men. Eur. J. Clin. Nutr. 51 (6), 375–380.

Craig, W.J., Mangels, A.R., American Dietetic Association, 2009. Position of the American Dietetic Association: vegetarian diets. J. Am. Diet. Assoc. 109 (7), 1266–1282.

De Mel, D., Suphioglu, C., August 15, 2014. Fishy business: effect of omega-3 fatty acids on zinc transporters and free zinc availability in human neuronal cells. Nutrients 6 (8), 3245–3258.

De Silva, D., et al., 2014. Primary prevention of food allergy in children and adults: systematic review. Allergy 69 (5), 581–589.

Domellöf, M., et al., 2002. Iron absorption in breast-fed infants: effects of age, iron status, iron supplements, and complementary foods. Am. J. Clin. Nutr. 76 (1), 198–204.

Domellöf, M., et al., 2014. Iron requirements of infants and toddlers. J. Pediatr. Gastroenterol. Nutr. 58 (1), 119–129.

EFSA Panel on Dietetic Products, Nutrition, and Allergies (NDA), 2005. Opinion of the scientific panel on dietetic products, nutrition and allergies on a request from the commission related to the tolerable upper intake level of sodium. EFSA J. 209, 1–26.

EFSA Panel on Dietetic Products, Nutrition, and Allergies (NDA), 2009. Scientific opinion on the appropriate age for introduction of complementary feeding of infants. EFSA J. 7 (12), 1423.

EFSA Panel on Dietetic Products, Nutrition, and Allergies (NDA), 2010a. Scientific opinion on dietary reference values for carbohydrates and dietary fibre. EFSA J. 8 (3), 1462.

EFSA Panel on Dietetic Products, Nutrition, and Allergies (NDA), 2010b. Scientific opinion on dietary reference values for fats, including saturated fatty acids, polyunsaturated fatty acids, monounsaturated fatty acids, trans fatty acids, and cholesterol. EFSA J. 8 (3), 1461.

EFSA Panel on Dietetic Products, Nutrition, and Allergies (NDA), 2012. Scientific opinion on dietary reference values for protein. EFSA J. 10 (2), 2557, 66 pp. http://dx.doi.org/10.2903/j.efsa.2012.255.

EFSA Panel on Dietetic Products, Nutrition, and Allergies (NDA), 2013. Scientific opinion on dietary reference values for energy. EFSA J. 11 (1), 3005.

EFSA Panel on Dietetic Products, Nutrition, and Allergies (NDA), 2014a. Scientific opinion on dietary reference values for zinc. EFSA J. 12 (10), 3844.

EFSA Panel on Dietetic Products, Nutrition and Allergies (NDA), 2014b. Scientific opinion on the essential composition of infant and follow-on formulae. EFSA J. 12 (7), 3760 106.

EFSA Panel on Dietetic Products, Nutrition, and Allergies (NDA), 2015a. Scientific opinion on dietary reference values for calcium. EFSA J. 13 (5), 4101 82.

EFSA Panel on Dietetic Products, Nutrition and Allergies (NDA), 2015b. Scientific opinion on dietary reference values for cobalamin (vitamin B_{12}). EFSA J. 13 (7), 4150.

EFSA Panel on Dietetic Products, Nutrition, and Allergies (NDA), 2015c. Scientific opinion on dietary reference values for iron. EFSA J. 13 (10), 4254, 115 pp. http://dx.doi.org/10.2903/j.efsa.2015.4254.

Escribano, J., et al., 2012. Effect of protein intake and weight gain velocity on body fat mass at 6 months of age: the EU Childhood Obesity Programme. Int. J. Obes. (2005) 36 (4), 548–553.

ESPGHAN Committee on Nutrition, 2015. Complementary Feeding: A Commentary by the ESPGHAN Committee on Nutrition, pp. 1–12.

Grimshaw, K.E.C., et al., 2013. Introduction of complementary foods and the relationship to food allergy. Pediatrics 132 (6), e1529–e1538.

Guideline: Sugars Intake for Adults and Children, 2015. World Health Organization, Geneva.

Günther, A.L.B., et al., 2007. Early protein intake and later obesity risk: which protein sources at which time points throughout infancy and childhood are important for body mass index and body fat percentage at 7 y of age? Am. J. Clin. Nutr. 86 (6), 1765–1772.

Hallberg, L., Hulthén, L., 2000. Prediction of dietary iron absorption: an algorithm for calculating absorption and bioavailability of dietary iron. Am. J. Clin. Nutr. 71 (5), 1147–1160.

Herrmann, W., et al., 2001. Total homocysteine, vitamin B12, and total antioxidant status in vegetarians. Clin. Chem. 47 (6), 1094–1101 pp. 1–8.

Hunt, J.R., 2003. Bioavailability of iron, zinc, and other trace minerals from vegetarian diets. Am. J. Clin. Nutr. 78 (Suppl. 3), 633S–639S.

Jacobs, C., JT, D., 1988. Vegetraina infants: appropriate and inappropriate diets. Am. J. Clin. Nutr. 1–8.

Joint WHO/FAO/UNU Expert Consultation, 2007. Protein and Amino Acid Requirements in Human Nutrition. World Health Organization technical report series, (935), pp. 1–265.

Kaganov, B., Caroli, M., Mazur, A., et al., May 13, 2015. Suboptimal micronutrient intake among children in Europe. Nutrients 7 (5), 3524–3535.

Kleinman, R.E., 2000. American Academy of Pediatrics recommendations for complementary feeding. Pediatrics 106 (5), 1274.

Libuda, L., Mesch, C., Stimming, M., Demmelmair, H., Koletzko, B., Warschburger, P., et al., 2016. Fatty acid supply with complementary foods and LC-PUFA status in healthy infants: results of a randomised controlled trial. Eur. J. Nutr. 55 (4), 1633–1644.

Lönnerdal, B., 2000. Dietary factors influencing zinc absorption. J. Nutr. 130 (5S Suppl.), 1378S–1383S.

Mangels, A.R., Messina, V., 2001. Considerations in planning vegan diets: infants. J. Am. Diet. Assoc. 101 (6), 670–677.

Maares, M., Haase, H., 2016. Zinc and immunity: an essential interrelation. Arch. Biochem. Biophys. 611 (Epub ahead of print).

Mangels, A.R., July 2014. Bone nutrients for vegetarians. Am. J. Clin. Nutr. 100 (Suppl. 1), 469S–475S.

Messina, V., Melina, V., Mangels, A.R., 2003. A new food guide for North American vegetarians. J. Am. Diet. Assoc. 103 (6), 771–775.

Michaelsen, K.F., Greer, F.R., 2014. Protein needs early in life and long-term health. Am. J. Clin. Nutr. 99 (3), 718S–722S.

Mulder, K.A., King, D.J., Innis, S.M., 2014. Omega-3 fatty acid deficiency in infants before birth identified using a randomized trial of maternal DHA supplementation in pregnancy. PLoS One 9 (1), e83764.

Nicklaus, S., 2015. The role of food experiences during early childhood in food pleasure learning. Appetite 104, 3–9.

Peker, E., Demir, N., Tuncer, O., et al., November 2015. The levels of vitamin B12, folate and homocysteine in mothers and their babies with neural tube defects. J. Matern. Fetal Neonatal Med. 23, 1–5 (Epub ahead of print).

Rolland-Cachera, M.F., et al., 2006. Early adiposity rebound: causes and consequences for obesity in children and adults. Int. J. Obes. 30, S11–S17.

Rolland-Cachera, M.F., et al., 2013. Association of nutrition in early life with body fat and serum leptin at adult age. Int. J. Obes. (Lond.) 37, 1116–1122.

Rosell, M.S., et al., 2005. Long-chain n-3 polyunsaturated fatty acids in plasma in British meat-eating, vegetarian, and vegan men. Am. J. Clin. Nutr. 82 (2), 327–334.

Rouhani, M.H., Kelishadi, R., Hashemipour, M., et al., April 2016. The impact of a low glycemic index diet on inflammatory markers and serum adiponectin concentration in adolescent overweight and obese girls: a randomized clinical trial. Horm. Metab. Res. 48 (4), 251–256.

Schwartz, J., Dube, K., Sichert-Hellert, W., et al., 2009. Modification of dietary polyunsaturated fatty acids via complementary food enhances n-3 long-chain polyunsaturated fatty acid synthesis in healthy infants: a double blinded randomized controlled trial. Arch. Dis. Child. 94 (11), 876–882.

Trumbo, P., Yates, A.A., Schlicker, S., Poos, M., March 2001. Dietary reference intakes: vitamin A, vitamin K, arsenic, boron, chromium, copper, iodine, iron, manganese, molybdenum, nickel, silicon, vanadium, and zinc. J. Am. Diet. Assoc. 101 (3), 294–301.

Uauy, R., Dangour, A.D., 2009. Fat and fatty acid requirements and recommendations for infants of 0–2 years and children of 2-18 years. Ann. Nutr. Metab. 55 (1–3), 76–96.

United Nations System Standard Committee on Nutrition, 2006. Report of the Standing Committee on Nutrition at its Thirty-Third Session. 1–27.

Van Winckel, M., et al., 2011. Clinical practice: vegetarian infant and child nutrition. Eur. J. Pediatr. 170 (12), 1489–1494.

Vriezinga, S.L., et al., 2014. Randomized feeding intervention in infants at high risk for celiac disease. N. Engl. J. Med. 371 (14), 1304–1315.

Weaver, C.M., Proulx, W.R., Heaney, R., 1999. Choices for achieving adequate dietary calcium with a vegetarian diet. Am. J. Clin. Nutr. 70 (Suppl. 3), 543S–548S.

WHO, 2003. Guiding Principles for Complementary Feeding of the Breastfed Child. 1–40.

Yen, C.E., et al., 2008. Dietary intake and nutritional status of vegetarian and omnivorous preschool children and their parents in Taiwan. Nutr. Res. 28 (7), 430–436.

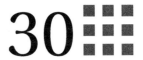
Nutritional Status of Vegetarian Children

Daiva Gorczyca
WROCLAW MEDICAL UNIVERSITY, WROCLAW, POLAND

There are societies in which a vegetarian diet has always been a natural part of everyday life due to their geographical location, economic status, or because of certain philosophical-religious beliefs (e.g., Buddhists and Seventh-day Adventists). However, for several decades, there has been an increase in interest of potential health outcomes associated with plant-based diets, thus increasing the number of supporters of organic and natural foods, and increasing the number of vegetarians in the adult and pediatric population. In the United States and England, 2%–4% of both adults and children reported that they were vegetarian. Less than 1% reported following a vegan diet (Stahler, 2012; The Vegetarian Society, 2000). There is no data recorded about how many children have been vegetarian since their birth. Among young people aged 15–17 years, the percentage following a vegetarian diet is as high as 12% (Povey et al., 2001).

According to the position of the American Dietetic Association and Dietitians of Canada on vegetarian diets, well-planned vegetarian diets are appropriate for individuals during all stages of life, including childhood and adolescence (Craig and Mangels, 2009; Mangels et al., 2003). Therefore, it can be assumed that a vegetarian diet can be considered a conventional type of diet. As a major positive implication on children's health with a vegetarian diet, it is essential to point out its protective effect against obesity. Studies show that as developing countries consume more meat in combination with refined foods high in sugar and fat, they may find themselves having to deal with obesity before they have overcome undernutrition, leading to an increase in healthcare costs that could otherwise be used to alleviate poverty (Godfray et al., 2010). However, the consumption of plant foods (cereals, legumes, and nuts) is associated with a lower risk of overweight children (Fig. 30.1).

There are a variety of reasons why people choose a vegetarian diet, as is reviewed in Section 1 of this book. In contrast, vegetarianism in children is a decision of the parents to implicate a vegetarian diet from birth or infancy. Consequently, nutritional status of vegetarian children largely depends on the level of education and level of knowledge about the diet of a parent or parents. For example, studies show higher scores for vegetarian patterns observed in children whose mothers had higher levels of education (Bhandari et al., 2002; Northstone et al., 2014). Depending on whether the parents themselves were raised as vegetarians or nonvegetarians, a different approach to a vegetarian diet in a child can be observed. If the parents are "new" vegetarians, their fear of any nutritional deficiency in

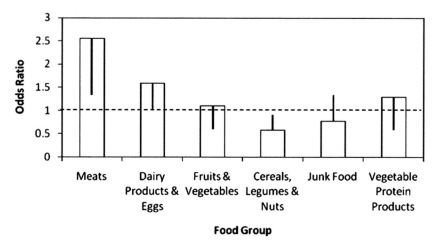

FIGURE 30.1 Odds ratios (with 95% CIs) of risk of overweight in school-aged children in the six food groups. *From Lousuebsakul, V., Sabate, J., 2009. The association between childhood obesity and dietary intake. Available from: http://www.vegetariannutrition.org/5icvn_program.pdf (cited 20 August 2009).*

eliminating animal products is higher; consequently, their children are at a relatively low risk of inadequate dietary intake and inadequate nutritional status. In contrast, parents who have been vegetarians since there were born are more experienced and may have better knowledge of how to compose meals and when to use enriched products. Without a doubt, knowledge of the rules of well-planned vegetarian diets is helpful for a parent when his/her child is avoiding foods of animal origin because of sensory and taste preferences or a specific food allergy.

Particularly noteworthy is vegetarianism in adolescents. Adolescents often are not prepared to follow a vegetarian diet. Their knowledge of a vegetarian diet is often limited only to the decision to use food products that are not of animal origin. In line with their wish to be self-reliant and independent, they rarely read professional information sources, and they are not interested in planning vegetarian meals. Studies show that vegetarian patterns are of better quality in girls than in boys (Northstone et al., 2014). Despite the fact that adolescent vegetarians may experience the health benefits associated with increased fruit and vegetable intake and benefit of decreased risk for overweight and obesity, in vegetarian teenagers, lower weight and body mass index (BMI) is more frequent than in non-vegetarians (Perry et al., 2001; Robinson-O'Brien et al., 2009; Smith et al., 2000). The very decision to switch to a vegetarian diet does not mean that a teenager has an eating disorder. Although in vegetarian adolescents an increased risk for extreme unhealthful weight-control behaviors may be observed (Perry et al., 2001; Robinson-O'Brien et al., 2009), so far there is no firm evidence that a vegetarian diet increases the risk of eating disorders. Nevertheless, a young vegetarian who suddenly and greatly limits food choices requires attention by healthcare and nutrition professionals.

A shared feature of many nutrients is that their deficiency results primarily in growth disorders. Therefore, a balanced diet should result into a normal growth rate, which is extremely important in children. Carbohydrates, fats, and proteins are the most important sources of energy. Proteins, vitamins, minerals, and trace elements are crucial for growth and development of tissues. When foods of animal origin are excluded from diet, nutrients contained in them should be provided from other sources that are naturally rich in those nutrients, or are fortified.

To evaluate nutritional status requires anthropometric measurements: body weight and height. If you examine research data concerning growth and weight of vegetarian children, some of the results from the 1980s showed low growth velocities of "new" vegetarians, vegans, or macrobiotic children (Dwyer et al., 1983; Shull et al., 1977). But since the 1990s, studies have demonstrated an identical growth and weight evolution in ovolacto-vegetarian children and adolescents compared to their omnivorous peers, whereas vegan and macrobiotic children tend to be leaner and smaller (Dagnelie and van Staveren, 1994; Nathan et al., 1997; Sabaté et al., 1990; Yen et al., 2008). Growth retardation was most commonly associated with deficiencies of energy, protein, vitamin B_{12}, vitamin D, calcium, and riboflavin. Now in supermarkets and vegetarian and natural foods stores, there is an array of widely available fortified foods such as soy-based milks, meat analogs, juice, and breakfast cereals. Also via the Internet and in cookbooks, one can find an abundance of information on vegetarianism. The nutritional status of present-day vegetarians varies considerably from that of a vegetarian one to two decades ago.

1. Energy

The basis of physical development and health is to maintain a sustainable balance between the amount of energy ingested with food and that used for basal metabolism, physical activity, and food-induced thermogenesis. A human body needs energy to operate, and a child's organism also needs energy to grow. Therefore, in children a negative energy balance leads to weight loss and development disorders.

Because studies show that the physical development (as assessed by body weight, height, and BMI) of vegetarian children is not significantly different from their omnivores peers, it can be concluded that energy intake in vegetarian children is mostly adequate (Yen et al., 2008). Analysis of the dietary intake also shows that the supply of energy in vegetarian children is not different from the omnivores (Donovan and Gibson, 1996; Nathan et al., 1996). This may be related to the fact that the diet of vegetarians and vegans contains large quantities of high-energy products often added to various meals, including vegetable oils, nuts, seeds, oil-baked cakes, and pastries. However, vegan diets, macrobiotic, and raw-food vegetarian diets have lower energy intakes as compared to other diets.

2. Proteins

Proteins are a major structural component of all tissues and many biologically active compounds (e.g., enzymes and hormones) that regulate metabolism and many body functions. Antibodies of an immune system are proteins, which are responsible for defending an organism against bacteria and viruses.

The quality of proteins depends on the number of indispensable and dispensable amino acids relative to the proportions of particular indispensable amino acids and the protein digestibility. Good sources of protein include eggs, milk and dairy products, meat, and fish. Among vegetable products, important sources of protein are cereal products and legumes. Whereas animal proteins are rich in all indispensable amino acids, the plant-derived proteins are relatively lower in indispensable amino acids, and some may have a slightly lower digestibility. In addition, lysine is the limiting amino acid for cereals such as wheat, corn, and rice, and sulfur amino acid for legumes as in soy and lentils (van Winckel et al., 2011). This will be discussed further in a dedicated chapter of this book (Chapter 35).

Protein deficiency in children is manifested in fatigue, abdominal bloating, swelling, a decrease in the level of plasma proteins, and in severe cases, kwashiorkor and marasmus (protein and energy deficiency). Because infants have a higher annual body weight gain, they are most likely to be affected by insufficient protein intake. In developed countries, different sources of vegetable protein are available; therefore protein deficiency is rare, and only presents with extremely inappropriate eating habits.

Vegetarian diets contain adequate protein to support nitrogen balance, provided that a variety of foods are consumed. The most diverse, in terms of proteins, is a ovolactovegetarian diet, and the poorest is a vegan diet. A full range of amino acids will be consumed if starches (e.g., rice, corn, potatoes) are eaten with legumes, such as lentils or beans, with the addition of vegetables and fruits. The different types of plant proteins should be eaten during the same day, but not necessarily within the same meal (Messina and Messina, 1996). However, we must remember that infants on a vegan diet, if not breastfed, are at risk for protein malnutrition (Kirby and Danner, 2009).

3. Fats

Fats are one of the essential nutrients and are a concentrated source of energy. They are required in building the structure of cell membranes and are also acquired for absorption of fat soluble vitamins A, D, E, F, and K. Essential fatty acids are not produced by the body and are acquired via diet. They are needed for cellular membrane functions (especially retina and central nervous system cells) and the production of eicosanoids, which act in inflammation processes, platelet aggregation, and blood pressure control.

The source of fats in diet are vegetable oils (received from seeds, fruits, oilseeds, and cereals), fish and fish oils, butter and dairy products, eggs, and nuts. A significant amount of essential fatty acids is provided by the consumption of plant products and fish. Many linoleic acids (LA, C18:2n-6) are found in corn oil, sunflower oil, soybean oil, and rapeseed oil. α-Linolenic acid (ALA, C18:3n-3) is generally present in membranes of chloroplasts of plants and in smaller quantities in seeds, canola oil, and flaxseed oil. A good source of eicosapentaenoic acid (EPA, C20:5n-3) and docosahexaenoic acid (DHA, C22:6n-3) is marine fish fats. It is believed that at least one to two servings of marine fish per week ensure adequate amount of EPA and DHA in the diet. The ability to synthetize long-chain polyunsaturated fatty acids in sufficient amounts from the parent fatty acids (linoleic acid, α-linolenic acid) or from one track to the other remains a matter of debate.

Significant inadequate intake of fats leads to a lack of satiety (fatty hunger) and weight deficiency. Skin disorders are associated with low levels of linoleic acid deficiency. Also, n-3 fatty acid deficiency is associated with abnormalities in visual and brain function. For children, very restrictive diets that include little fat (20%–25% of energy) may lead to delayed growth and development (Dagnelie and van Staveren, 1994). The dietary intake of fat depends on the degrees of vegetarianism. Most commonly, a vegetarian diet results in lower intake of saturated fatty acids, higher intake of n-6 fatty acids, and marginal intake of n-3 fatty acids (Gorczyca et al., 2011). A similar lipid profile was found in omnivores who consume little or no fish. Eggs and milk products contain a small amount of AA, EPA, and DHA; hence, ovolactovegetarians receive a sufficient amount of saturated fatty acids as well as essential polyunsaturated fatty acids. Intakes of α-linolenic acid and linoleic acid of vegans and vegetarian children are often greater than those in omnivores, but the ratio of ALA to LA is lower in vegetarians, and it is particularly low in vegans. To have an appropriate n-6/n-3 balance, regular consumption of micro-algae (rich in DHA) and of walnuts, canola oil, or flaxseed oil is recommended (van Winckel et al., 2011).

4. Carbohydrates and Dietary Fiber

Carbohydrates are the main source of easily digestible energy for a human body. In developed countries, carbohydrates provide 45%–60% of the energy requirements, and in developing countries, it is 60%–85%.

The richest sources of monosaccharides are fruits, honey, refined sugar, and candy. Lactose is the main carbohydrate of milk, which is the main source of nutrients for infants. Cereal products (flour, cereal, pastas, bread, and cereals) are rich in carbohydrates, which contain 50%–80% of starch. Many carbohydrates are found in pastries, cakes, processed fruit products, and dry seed pulses. As for fiber, the largest quantities comprise nuts and dry seeds of legumes. In the daily diet of an average European child, the largest amounts of carbohydrates and fiber come from cereal products.

It is believed that if the diet covers the recommended allowance for protein and fat, then carbohydrates should meet the remaining energy requirement. The intake of carbohydrates and the proportion of energy from carbohydrates in vegetarian children is similar or higher than that of omnivores (Ambroszkiewicz et al., 2011; Yen et al., 2008). Insufficient intake of carbohydrates in children may lead to a shortage of body weight. It is worth noting that if the diet provides less than 15% of carbohydrate products or if there is fasting, a nondiabetic ketoacidosis develops. These situations can happen in adolescent vegetarians, who often have too little knowledge on food intake patterns or have disordered eating behaviors.

Excessive intake of sucrose and monosaccharides together with low physical activity lead to being overweight and an increase in cardiometabolic risk. Plant-based diets are low in energy density and high in complex carbohydrates, fiber, and water, which may increase satiety and resting energy expenditure. This may explain why vegetarian diets are associated with a lower BMI and a lower prevalence of obesity in children (Sabaté and Wien, 2010). Moreover, plant foods (cereals, legumes, and nuts) are associated with a lower risk of obesity. Excessive consumption of sweets between meals also causes tooth decay: one of the most common oral diseases in children. Children eating a vegetarian diet had significantly higher mean number of decayed teeth than children on mixed diets (Herman et al., 2011; Shailee et al., 2012).

A high intake of fiber tends to reduce the absorption of minerals and increases the risk of diarrhea. Because vegetarian and particularly vegan diets include a very high intake of fiber, the nutritional status of some micronutrients such as zinc is a question at issue in vegetarian children.

5. Sodium and Potassium

Sodium is responsible for osmotic pressure, acid–base balance, and water balance; it is responsible for muscle contraction and nerve conduction. Potassium is responsible for extracellular osmotic pressure and fluid balance, muscle contraction, heart rhythm, and conduction of nerve impulses.

On average, one-third of dietary sodium comes from salt, the rest from bread, milk, eggs, vegetables, and meat.

A rich source of potassium and sodium are legumes, nuts, potatoes, fish, tomatoes, currants, and bananas. All of these products are frequently and regularly consumed by vegetarians.

To maintain proper blood pressure the ratio of sodium to potassium is very important. Because vegetarians and vegans, in particular, consume a lot of plant-based products, which are poor in sodium, they use a variety of spices and not salt to enhance the taste of food, so their supply of sodium intake is decreased (Clarys et al., 2014). Consequently, vegetarian diets were associated with lower systolic blood pressure and lower diastolic blood pressure both in children and in adults.

6. Calcium

Calcium is the main building structure of bones and teeth (up to 99% of the envelope of this element is designed to perform this function). In addition, calcium is involved in muscle contraction, cell membrane permeability, and regulation of blood clotting; it is also a cofactor of many enzymes. The status of calcium in a human body is regulated by vitamin D, parathyroid hormone, and calcitonin.

The main sources of dietary calcium are milk and milk products (yogurt, cheese, ice cream). Others include canned, bone-in sardines, salmon, and oysters. A good plant source of calcium is kale, beans, green leafy vegetables, broccoli, Chinese cabbage, and collard greens.

A short-term insufficient intake of calcium is asymptomatic since complex homeostatic mechanisms maintain its concentration. In the longer term, insufficient supply of calcium and its absorption from the gastrointestinal tract as a result of vitamin D deficiency in children, especially in infants and toddlers, leads to rickets, growth disorders, and abnormal calcification of growing bones. Unfortunately, calcium status is impossible to assess in routine laboratory testing because the serum level is controlled by different mechanisms.

Vegetarian and omnivorous children generally have a similar intake of calcium, but differences emerge depending on the type of vegetarian diet. Greater calcium intake is observed in ovolactovegetarians, whereas in vegans and in children following macrobiotic diets, calcium intake is often lower than recommended (Larsson and Johansson, 2002). Also, the intake of calcium varies with the child's age: the older the child is, the fewer milk and dairy products he/she eats (Wallace et al., 2013). To increase the intake of calcium in many countries, calcium carbonate is added to flour, pasta, breads, and rice. An alternative source of calcium in children's vegetarian diets may be soy drinks, almond milk, rice drinks (milk), and orange juice with added calcium. However, while ensuring the proper supply of calcium, it is necessary to remember that calcium tends to reduce the absorption of iron, zinc, and magnesium from the gastrointestinal tract (Kambalia and Zlotkin, 2008).

7. Phosphorus

Phosphorus is an essential component of bones and teeth, nucleoid acids, and brain tissue, and it forms part of the structure of cell membranes. It is a major intracellular anion and activator of many enzymes.

Sources of phosphorus are milk, dairy products, egg yolk, legumes (beans and peas), nuts, and whole grains. Indeed, phosphorus is one of the most ubiquitous nutrients in foods, so the supply of phosphorus from the vegetarian or nonvegetarian diets complies with the recommendations, and deficiency is not observed.

8. Magnesium

Magnesium creates part of the structure of bones and teeth, participates in the metabolism of carbohydrates, and is responsible for muscle contraction and nerve conduction, as well as activating a number of enzymes. It is an important intracellular cation.

The greatest sources of magnesium include cereals (e.g., buckwheat, oatmeal, and brown rice), legumes, nuts, and milk.

Prevalence of inadequacy between vegetarian and nonvegetarian children for magnesium is similar (Craig and Mangels, 2009). Vegetarian diets are often richer in magnesium than nonvegetarian diets (Farmer et al., 2011). Magnesium deficiency in children occurs with poor absorption from the small intestine (mostly associated with diarrhea).

9. Iron

Iron is an essential nutrient for all living organisms. It is present in hemoglobin and myoglobin, oxidative enzymes, cytochromes, desaturation of fatty acids, and iodination of tyrosine.

Heme iron and nonheme iron sources can be distinguished in diet. Heme iron sources include liver, kidney, mussels, red meat, chicken, processed meat, and fish. In contrast, nonheme forms are found in legumes, egg yolk, green vegetables, whole grains, legumes, and nuts.

Iron deficiency is associated with iron deficiency anemia, loss of appetite, pallor, general lassitude and apathy, increased susceptibility for infection, and psychomotor and cognitive development disorders. This will be discussed and reviewed in a specific chapter for adults in this book (Chapter 39). The prevalence of iron deficiency and iron deficiency anemia is high, especially in infants and young children (Borgna-Pignatti and Marsella, 2008). The increased use of iron-fortified infant formulas has lowered the iron deficiency prevalence in infants to 2% (Eussen et al., 2015), but breastfeeding for an extended period of time and early introduction to cow's milk still pose a risk for developing iron deficiency.

Iron deficiency mostly occurs when iron requirements cannot be met by iron absorption from the diet. It has been suggested that vegetarians could be at greater risk of iron deficiency, although some research shows that eliminating meat leads to a higher intake of whole grain and fortified cereals, legumes, nuts, seeds, and dried fruit, so total iron intake is often greater than that of omnivores (Alexander et al., 1994; Nathan et al., 1996). However, poorer iron status observed in vegetarian children is more common than in omnivores, at least partly due to lower iron bioavailability since nonheme iron is not absorbed as well as heme iron (Hurrell and Egli, 2010). This is presented in a dedicated chapter in this book (Chapter 39). Many plant foods contain substances that positively influence nonheme iron absorption (mainly vitamin C, and to a lesser extent β-carotene and organic acids) but also substances that considerably lower nonheme iron absorption, among them phytates and polyphenols, as you can see in Table 30.1.

Our own research showed that the main source of iron in vegetarian children is cereal products, which usually form the base of the food pyramid in vegetarian diets in different populations, as demonstrated in Fig. 30.2. Cereals, especially whole grain foods, can provide considerable amounts of iron, and this product type is allowed to be fortified with iron, which increases the contribution of cereals to the iron supply. Published data reveals that vegetarians eat fruits that are richer in vitamin C than omnivores, which enhances nonheme absorption. However, the insufficient iron intake in vegetarians can lead to iron deficiency despite a high intake of vitamin C (Gorczyca et al., 2013b). It can be connected to both high consumption of phytate-rich foods such as cereal products and legumes. The other inhibitors of iron absorption such as polyphenols from black tea and milk proteins in lactovegetarian diets should also be taken into account.

As iron metabolism is very complex, the cover of demand may be provided even if there is low supply for a long time, or there is the supply of iron with poor bioavailability. Therefore,

Table 30.1   Dietary Factors Affecting Nonheme Dietary Iron Absorption

Enhancers	Inhibitors
Fish and other seafood	Polyphenols (list see Pérez-Jiménez et al., 2010)
Sugars	Oxalic acid (e.g., rhubarb and spinach)
Fermented vegetables	Phytates/phytic acid (e.g., cereals, legumes, oil seeds, nuts)
Soy sauces	Iron-binding phenolic compounds
Vitamin C	Calcium, calcium phosphate salts
Retinol	Zinc, manganese, and nickel
Carotenes	Soy protein
	Phosvitin (e.g., egg yolk)
	Tannins (e.g., tea and red wine)
	Coffee, cocoa, and some spices slightly impair absorption

Adapted from reference Hurrell, R., Egli, I., 2010. Iron bioavailability and dietary reference values. Am. J. Clin. Nutr. 91 (5), 1461S–1467S.

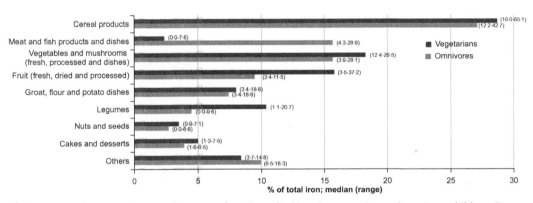

FIGURE 30.2 Food sources of iron and percent of total supplied iron in vegetarian and omnivore children. *From reference Gorczyca, D., Paściak, M., Szponar, B., Gamian, A., Jankowski, A., 2011. An impact of the diet on serum fatty acid and lipid profiles in Polish vegetarian children and children with allergy. Eur. J. Clin. Nutr. 65 (2), 191–195.*

periodically, specific laboratory measurements should be used to monitor the status of iron in vegetarian children (Zimmermann and Hurrell, 2007). Unfortunately, no single measurement is currently available that will characterize the iron status of a child. An accessible and relatively cheap way to diagnose iron deficiency is to measure serum ferritin in combination with C-reactive protein to eliminate false negative cases in the course of inflammation.

10. Zinc

Zinc is a constituent for more than 300 enzymes. It is essential for the synthesis of protein and nucleic fats, gene expression, protection against free radicals, humoral and cellular immunity, and many other features.

The highest concentration of zinc is found generally in animal products, especially meats. Dairy products, bread and cereal, nuts, and legumes are nonmeat sources of zinc.

Table 30.2   Dietary Factors Affecting Dietary
Zinc Absorption

Enhancers	Inhibitors
Animal protein	Phytates/phytic acid
Citric acid	Nonheme iron
Some amino acids	Copper
	Calcium at presence of phytates
	Oxalic acid
	Fiber

However, the bioavailability of zinc in the diet also depends on its composition. Zinc from many plant-derived foods is less likely to be bioavailable owing to phytic acid, an inhibitor of zinc absorption, as demonstrated in Table 30.2.

Symptoms of zinc deficiency in infants and children are skin lesions, diarrhea, loss of appetite, alopecia, hypogonadism and sexual retardation in boys, and growth stunting, as well as abnormal sense of taste and decreased immunity. In vegetarian children, IgG concentration correlates positively with energy, zinc, copper, and vitamin B_6 intake (Gorczyca et al., 2013a). Zinc deficiency is hard to define solely by serum levels because concentrations are markedly depressed in the severe states of deficiency, and moderate hypozincemia occurs in more moderate zinc deficiency states.

Existing data indicate no differences in serum zinc or growth between vegetarian and omnivorous young children, although there is some evidence of low serum zinc concentrations in vegetarian adolescents (Gibson et al., 2014). Low zinc intake is unlikely to be a problem for ovolactovegetarian children who consume dairy products and several ready-to-eat breakfast cereals fortified with zinc. But vegans should be considered as children at high risk for zinc deficiency. Additionally, some vegetarian immigrants from underprivileged households may be predisposed to zinc deficiency because of nondietary factors including chronic inflammation, parasitic infections, and being overweight. To confirm the diagnosis of zinc deficiency, clinicians should utilize a combination of serum zinc levels, presenting signs and symptoms (stunting, respiratory infections, diarrhea, and dermatitis), and dietary assessment (Willoughby and Bowen, 2014).

11. Selenium

Selenium is an essential component of glutathione peroxidase (involved in the body's defense against damaging impact of reactive oxygen species), is involved in thyroid hormone synthesis, and participates in immune function.

Concentrations of selenium in food varies with geographic region and soil content. Also, concentrations depend on specific methods of food processing. Generally, seafood, kidney, liver, and meat are the best sources of selenium. Whole grains are also good sources of selenium, provided that soils in which they are grown are not low in the nutrient. Milk and dairy products provide 11% of dietary selenium. Vegetables and fruits, with the exception of garlic, provide little quantity.

Milder degrees of selenium insufficiency have not been associated with adverse clinical consequences. Selenium has a protective effect on some illnesses and regulates the inflammatory mediators in asthma. Insufficient selenium intake in vegetarian children is rare and depends on whether vegetarians consume eggs and milk products or other specific dietary selenium sources (Hoeflich et al., 2010).

12. Iodine

Iodine is necessary to produce thyroid hormones and is involved in normal mental and physical growth and development.

Iodized salt, fish, and other marine products and cow's milk are the main sources of iodine in the diet.

Too little iodine and excessive intake leads to thyroid dysfunction. Goiter may occur in children, as well as mental development disorders and growth stunting.

Ovolactovegetarian and semivegetarian children usually have adequate intakes of iodine. However, vegans do not consume iodine-rich seafood and milk; therefore, their intake of iodine is frequently lower (Craig and Mangels, 2009; Leung et al., 2011). Iodine deficiency in pregnant vegan women may be dangerous for their unborn children's health. There have been case reports describing transient neonatal hypothyroiditis as a consequence of maternal diet (Shaikh et al., 2003).

It is believed that consumption of small amounts of iodized salt or seaweed in a vegan diet prevents iodine deficiency. Iodine supplementation may be required in areas where dietary fortification is not feasible.

13. Vitamin A

Vitamin A (retinol) is required for growth and normal development of tissues (bones, teeth, and epithelium), vision, healthy skin, and in immunity.

The main sources of vitamin A are milk and dairy products, eggs, and fish (especially herring, sardines, and tuna). In plant products, vitamin A is found mainly in the form of provitamin A (carotenoids). The sources of carotene are green leafy vegetables and yellow/orange vegetables or fruits. Red palm oil produced in several countries worldwide is especially rich in provitamin A. In contrast, grains are low in carotenes, but adequate levels are found in fortified breakfast cereals. Quantity and quality of proteins and vegetable fats in diet influence the bioavailability of vitamin A and carotenoids. A small quantity and poor quality of protein reduces the intestinal absorption of vitamin A.

Insufficient supply of vitamin A in diet after a longer time leads to deficiency and manifests in poor adaptation to see in darkness, blindness, xerophthalmia, conjunctivitis, abnormal formation of epiphyses, damage to tooth enamel, actinic mucous membranes, lowering body's resistance to infections, and inhibition of linear growth in children. Vitamin

A deficiency is a risk factor for iron deficiency anemia. Vitamin A-deficient children were shown to have an increased risk of developing respiratory disease and an increased severity of diarrheal disease.

Excessive intake of dietary vitamin A, depending on individual sensitivity, can lead to anorexia, slow growth, xeroderma pigmentosum, hepatosplenomegaly, long bone pain, and even bone fracture.

Intakes of vitamin A in vegetarian children is generally adequate, and there is no significant difference when compared with omnivores (Thane and Bates, 2000). Vegetarian and vegan diets are typically noted to be higher in carotenoids. Vegans receive retinol only from fortified foods.

14. Vitamin B_1

Vitamin B_1 (thiamine) participates in various energy processes, oxidative decarboxylation, and in neurophysiological processes.

The richest source of vitamin B_1 are cereals, seeds, legumes (peas, beans), yeast, pork, milk, and nuts.

Long-term deficiency of vitamin B_1 can lead to beriberi disease, fatigue, irritability, anorexia, constipation, headaches, insomnia, tachycardia, and neuritis. Today, beriberi occurs only in regions of the world where diet is based on unenriched rice or white flour or fish containing thiaminase is eaten in large amounts.

A vegetarian diet usually contains more grains and legumes, resulting in an intake of thiamine that is higher in vegetarians than in nonvegetarians (Farmer et al., 2011; Majchrzak et al., 2006).

15. Vitamin B_2

Vitamin B_2 (riboflavin) is a part of flavoproteins, which protects tissues against lipid peroxidation and plays a key role in energy production and in metabolism of lipids and amino acids.

The main sources of dietary riboflavin are milk, cheeses, eggs, meat, fish, whole grain products, leafy green vegetables, almonds, and enriched products.

The symptoms associated with riboflavin deficiency are stomatitis, dermatitis, keratitis, anemia, and neurological dysfunction.

Currently, data shows that intakes of riboflavin in Western vegetarians is higher than for nonvegetarians (Farmer et al., 2011; Majchrzak et al., 2006). However, vegans must add riboflavin-fortified foods to their diet (e.g., breakfast cereals and fortified drinks).

16. Vitamin B_6

Vitamin B_6 is a coenzyme in more than 100 enzymes that takes part in various metabolic processes of the body.

There are no particularly rich sources of vitamin B_6. It is present in meat, liver, kidney, whole grains, peanuts, and soybeans.

Continued vitamin B_6 deficiency in children leads to excitability, convulsions, and hypochromic anemia.

Intake of vitamin B_6 in vegetarian children is comparable with omnivores (Huang et al., 2003). In vegans, it is advised to include foods with high pyridoxine bioavailability, such as beans, lentils, and bananas, daily.

17. Vitamin B_{12}

Vitamin B_{12} is an essential cofactor in DNA and RNA synthesis, and it is involved in synthesis and maintenance of myelin sheaths.

Foods of animal origin are the only reliable dietary source of vitamin B_{12} or cobalamin, e.g., meat and offal, fish, eggs, milk, and cheeses. Cobalamin present in algae and seaweeds has been shown to be a nonactive analog of vitamin B_{12} (Watanabe, 2007). The daily requirement for vitamin B_{12} is $2\,\mu g$.

Vitamin B_{12} deficiency results in hematological (megaloblastic anemia) and neurological disorders (neurodevelopmental delay and regression, neuropsychiatric disorders).

The prevalence of B_{12} deficiency was estimated to be 55% among US children (67% among children who followed a vegetarian diet all their life vs. 25% among other vegetarian children) and 50% among children of Asian Indian origin (macrobiotic diet) (Miller et al., 1991; Rush et al., 2009). It is considered that people consuming fish or meat less than once a week are at risk of vitamin B_{12} deficiency (van Winckel et al., 2011). Infants breastfed by vegan or macrobiotic mothers can develop serious vitamin B_{12} deficiency manifested by megaloblastic anemia and neurodevelopmental regression, especially between the age of 2 and 12 months (Dagnelie et al., 1989; Rasmussen et al., 2001).

Vegetarian children, regardless of the type of vegetarian diet they adhere to, should be screened for vitamin B_{12} deficiency. Vitamin B_{12} status is best determined by measurement of serum B_{12} level. See Chapter 43 for more information regarding general B_{12} deficiency in vegetarians.

18. Vitamin C

Vitamin C integrates and maintains intracellular structure in all tissues, helps absorption of iron and folic acid metabolism, is involved in lipid metabolism, is a strong antioxidant, and is related to several aspects of immune function.

Vitamin C is found in plant foods, mainly in raw vegetables and fruits: citrus fruits, tomatoes, berries (fruit of wild rose, black currant, strawberry), peppers, brussels sprouts, and broccoli.

Vitamin C deficiency among infants manifests in the form of bone abnormalities, hemorrhagic symptoms, and anemia.

Since vegetarian children consume copious amounts of vegetables and fruits rich in vitamin C, vitamin C intakes in vegetarian children are higher than in omnivorous children (Gorczyca et al., 2013b; Yen et al., 2008).

19. Vitamin D

The most important effect of vitamin D is in its participation in calcium and bone metabolism. In addition, the biologically active metabolite 1,25-dihydroxycholecalciferol $(1,25(OH)_2D_3)$ is involved in normal function of the immune system.

Vitamin D is present in most animal products and oily fish as well as eggs. From vegetable products, it is found in yeast and mushrooms. Other sources of vitamin D are fortified products: breakfast cereals, soya drinks, all margarines, fat spreads, and milk.

Vitamin D deficiency in children is associated primarily with the development of rickets. In addition, current research shows that vitamin D insufficiency could be associated with respiratory tract infections, diabetes, autoimmune diseases, hypertension, and even cancer development.

Deficiency in vitamin D is frequent in all age groups, regardless of diet (Kaganov et al., 2015). This may be related to the fact that foods rich in vitamin D are not very popular in usual diets. Sunlight exposure provides vitamin D synthesis in the skin, but using creams with ultraviolet filters to decrease risk of skin cancer reduces the synthesis of vitamin D to zero. Therefore, studies show that a vegetarian diet does not directly lead to deficiency in vitamin D (Wallace et al., 2013). Since vegans usually avoid consumption of foods fortified with animal-derived vitamin D_3, the risk of inadequate intake of vitamin D is high in vegan infants and young children. Macrobiotic diets are also very low in vitamin D, and studies of children under 6 years of age have shown high prevalence of rickets as the result of vitamin D deficiency.

Numerous studies have used plasma 25-OH-vitamin D as a measure of vitamin D status. It is believed that the plasma 25-OH-vitamin D levels above 27 nmol/L indicates normal bone health (WHO and FAO, 2004).

Because suboptimal vitamin D status in children is widespread all around the world, it is recommended that children take 10–20 mg (doses varying between countries) of vitamin D supplement in tablet form per day, regardless whether they are vegetarians or omnivores. Measurement of serum 25-OH-vitamin D concentration helps to assess vitamin D status.

20. Vitamin E

Vitamin E is a natural antioxidant that reduces oxidation of carotene, vitamin A, polyunsaturated fatty acids, and protects against tissue damage caused by lipid peroxidation.

Vegetable oils, whole grain products, nuts, and legumes are rich sources of vitamin E, whereas vegetables and fruits supply only a moderate quantity.

Vitamin E deficiency is more common among premature infants and is characterized by hemolytic anemia and neurological alterations.

Intakes of vitamin E are generally adequate and are frequently higher in vegetarians than in omnivores (Farmer et al., 2011; Thane and Bates, 2000; Yean et al., 2008).

21. Vitamin K

The main role of vitamin K is to participate in the formation of clotting factors. Vitamin K is important for bone health and is also a cofactor for the synthesis of osteocalcin.

Vitamin K is commonly found in leafy green vegetables, which contain the largest amounts (the more chlorophyll, the more vitamin K), as well as pig's liver.

Vitamin K deficiency leads to bleeding and abnormal bone status.

Ovolactovegetarians and vegans generally consume more leafy green vegetables, such as broccoli, spinach, brussels sprouts, and green tea; therefore, there is no risk of inadequate intake. It is worth mentioning that an adequate amount of vitamin K can contribute to bone health or stronger bones in children (van Summeren et al., 2007).

22. Conclusion

According to long-term experience and opinions of expert nutritionists and pediatricians from all over the world, well-planned vegetarian diets are appropriate for all stages of childhood and adolescence, and they are comparable in this regard to conventional diets.

Assessment of nutritional status, regardless of whether the child is vegetarian or an omnivore, first consists of monitoring physical, psychomotor, and puberty development. When vegetarian children are fed a well-balanced diet, they develop well. It is often observed that vegetarian children have better nutritional status, and their diet appears more aligned with guidelines than is the case observed in omnivores.

Dietary deficiencies are possible in any unbalanced diet. Parents of vegetarian children face many of the same challenges as their omnivore peers in providing healthful foods. However, some foods that play important roles in vegetarian diets are unpopular with many children, posing more difficulties for parents of vegetarian children to compose an appropriate diet.

Vegetarian diets in children may raise concern for inadequate intake of calcium, zinc, iron, vitamin B_{12}, vitamin D, fiber, calories, protein, and omega 3 fatty acids. That is why all parents should be aware of the importance of identifying good sources of these nutrients in their children's diet. All children following a vegan diet should have a reliable source of vitamin B_{12} and vitamin D (i.e., they should receive fortified foods or supplements). Indications for vitamin D supplements for other types of vegetarian diets do not differ from the guidelines for omnivore children.

To detect suboptimal iron, vitamin D, and vitamin B_{12} deficiency, a regular determination of serum ferritin, 25-OH-vitamin D, and vitamin B_{12} concentrations is recommended.

Healthcare and nutrition professionals can be helpful for parents to plan appropriate vegetarian diets. Young vegetarians, especially, may require professional help to ensure proper nutrition. Moreover, there is a need to educate parents and adolescents specifically on how to enrich their diet with good sources of macro- and micronutrients allowed in a vegetarian diet and to increase absorption from the diet by adjusting food preparation techniques, food selection, and food combinations.

Further investigation is required to assess the interaction of vitamin A, vitamin E, vitamin D, vitamin C, and iron with immune response in children. Further studies would also interestingly investigate the association between biological markers of the status of some particular nutrients in children and the risk of disease.

References

Alexander, D., Ball, M.J., Mann, J., 1994. Nutrient intake and haematological status of vegetarians and age-sex matched omnivores. Eur. J. Clin. Nutr. 48 (8), 538–546.

Ambroszkiewicz, J., Klemarczyk, W., Gajewska, J., Chełchowska, M., Rowicka, G., Ołtarzewski, M., Laskowska-Klita, T., 2011. Serum concentration of adipocytokines in prepubertal vegetarian and omnivorous children. Med. Wieku Rozwoj. 15 (3), 326–334.

Bhandari, N., Bahl, R., Taneja, S., de Onis, M., Bhan, M.K., 2002. Growth performance of affluent Indian children is similar to that in developed countries. Bull. World Health Organ. 80 (3), 189–195.

Borgna-Pignatti, C., Marsella, M., 2008. Iron deficiency in infancy and childhood. Pediatr. Ann. 37 (5), 329–337.

Clarys, P., Deliens, T., Huybrechts, I., Deriemaeker, P., Vanaelst, B., De Keyzer, W., Hebbelinck, M., Mullie, P., 2014. Comparison of nutritional quality of the vegan, vegetarian, semi-vegetarian, pesco-vegetarian and omnivorous diet. Nutrients 6 (3), 1318–1332.

Craig, W.J., Mangels, A.R., American Dietetic Association, 2009. Position of the American Dietetic Association: vegetarian diets. J. Am. Diet. Assoc. 109 (7), 1266–1282.

Dagnelie, P.C., van Staveren, W.A., 1994. Macrobiotic nutrition and child health: results of a population-based, mixed-longitudinal cohort study in The Netherlands. Am. J. Clin. Nutr. 59 (Suppl. 5), S1187–S1196.

Dagnelie, P.C., van Staveren, W.A., Vergote, F.J., Dingjan, P.G., van den Berg, H., Hautvast, J.G., 1989. Increased risk of vitamin B-12 and iron deficiency in infants on macrobiotic diets. Am. J. Clin. Nutr. 50 (4), 818–824.

Donovan, U.M., Gibson, R.S., 1996. Dietary intakes of adolescent females consuming vegetarian, semi-vegetarian, and omnivorous diets. J. Adolesc. Health 18, 292–300.

Dwyer, J.T., Andrew, E.M., Berkey, C., Valadian, I., Reed, R.B., 1983. Growth in "new" vegetarian preschool children using the Jenss-Bayley curve fitting technique. Am. J. Clin. Nutr. 37 (5), 815–827.

Eussen, S., Alles, M., Uijterschout, L., Brus, F., van der Horst-Graat, J., 2015. Iron intake and status of children aged 6-36 months in Europe: a systematic review. Ann. Nutr. Metab. 66 (2–3), 80–92.

Farmer, B., Larson, B.T., Fulgoni 3rd, V.L., Rainville, A.J., Liepa, G.U., 2011. A vegetarian dietary pattern as a nutrient-dense approach to weight management: an analysis of the national health and nutrition examination survey 1999-2004. J. Am. Diet. Assoc. 111 (6), 819–827.

Gibson, R.S., Heath, A.L., Szymlek-Gay, E.A., 2014. Is iron and zinc nutrition a concern for vegetarian infants and young children in industrialized countries? Am. J. Clin. Nutr. 100 (Suppl. 1), S459–S468.

Godfray, H.C., Beddington, J.R., Crute, I.R., Haddad, L., Lawrence, D., Muir, J.F., Pretty, J., Robinson, S., Thomas, S.M., Toulmin, C., 2010. Food security: the challenge of feeding 9 billion people. Science 327 (5967), 812–818.

Gorczyca, D., Paściak, M., Szponar, B., Gamian, A., Jankowski, A., 2011. An impact of the diet on serum fatty acid and lipid profiles in Polish vegetarian children and children with allergy. Eur. J. Clin. Nutr. 65 (2), 191–195.

Gorczyca, D., Prescha, A., Szeremeta, K., 2013a. Impact of vegetarian diet on serum immunoglobulin levels in children. Clin. Pediatr. (Phila.) 52 (3), 241–246.

Gorczyca, D., Prescha, A., Szeremeta, K., Jankowski, A., 2013b. Iron status and dietary iron intake of vegetarian children from Poland. Ann. Nutr. Metab. 62 (4), 291–297.

Herman, K., Czajczyńska-Waszkiewicz, A., Kowalczyk-Zając, M., Dobrzyński, M., 2011. Assessment of the influence of vegetarian diet on the occurrence of erosive and abrasive cavities in hard tooth tissues. Postepy Hig. Med. Dosw. 65, 764–769.

Hoeflich, J., Hollenbach, B., Behrends, T., Hoeg, A., Stosnach, H., Schomburg, L., 2010. The choice of biomarkers determines the selenium status in young German vegans and vegetarians. Br. J. Nutr. 104 (11), 1601–1604.

Huang, Y.C., Chang, S.J., Chiu, Y.T., Chang, H.H., Cheng, C.H., 2003. The status of plasma homocysteine and related B-vitamins in healthy young vegetarians and nonvegetarians. Eur. J. Nutr. 42 (2), 84–90.

Hurrell, R., Egli, I., 2010. Iron bioavailability and dietary reference values. Am. J. Clin. Nutr. 91 (5), 1461S–1467S.

Kaganov, B., Caroli, M., Mazur, A., Singhal, A., Vania, A., 2015. Suboptimal micronutrient intake among children in Europe. Nutrients 7 (5), 3524–3535.

Kambalia, A.Z., Zlotkin, S.H., 2008. Iron. In: Duggan, C., Watkins, J., Walker, W.A. (Eds.), Nutrition in Pediatrics: Basic Science, Clinical Applications, fourth ed. BC Decker Inc Hamilton, Ontario, pp. 83–98 (Chapter 9).

Kirby, M., Danner, E., 2009. Nutritional deficiencies in children on restricted diets. Pediatr. Clin. North Am. 56 (5), 1085–1103.

Larsson, C.L., Johansson, G.K., 2002. Dietary intake and nutritional status of young vegans and omnivores in Sweden. Am. J. Clin. Nutr. 76 (1), 100–106.

Leung, A.M., Lamar, A., He, X., Braverman, L.E., Pearce, E.N., 2011. Iodine status and thyroid function of Boston-area vegetarians and vegans. J. Clin. Endocrinol. Metab. 96 (8), E1303–E1307. http://dx.doi.org/10.1210/jc.2011-0256. Available from:.

Lousuebsakul, V., Sabate, J., 2009. The association between childhood obesity and dietary intake. Available from: http://www.vegetariannutrition.org/5icvn_program.pdf (cited 20 August 2009).

Majchrzak, D., Singer, I., Männer, M., Rust, P., Genser, D., Wagner, K.H., Elmadfa, I., 2006. B-vitamin status and concentrations of homocysteine in Austrian omnivores, vegetarians and vegans. Ann. Nutr. Metab. 50 (6), 485–491.

Mangels, A.R., Messina, V., Melina, V., 2003. Position of the American Dietetic Association and dietitians of Canada: vegetarian diets. J. Am. Diet. Assoc. 103, 748–765.

Messina, M., Messina, V., 1996. The Dietitian's Guide to Vegetarian Diets: Issues and Applications. Aspen, Gaithersburg.

Miller, D.R., Specker, B.L., Ho, M.L., Norman, E.J., 1991. Vitamin B-12 status in a macrobiotic community. Am. J. Clin. Nutr. 53 (2), 524–529.

Nathan, I., Hackett, A.F., Kirby, S., 1996. The dietary intake of a group of vegetarian children aged 7-11 years compared with matched omnivores. Br. J. Nutr. 75 (4), 533–544.

Nathan, I., Hackett, A.F., Kirby, S., 1997. A longitudinal study of the growth of matched pairs of vegetarian and omnivorous children, aged 7-11 years, in the north-west of England. Eur. J. Clin. Nutr. 51 (1), 20–25.

Northstone, K., Smith, A.D., Cribb, V.L., Emmett, P.M., 2014. Dietary patterns in UK adolescents obtained from a dual-source FFQ and their associations with socio-economic position, nutrient intake and modes of eating. Public Health Nutr. 17 (7), 1476–1485.

Pérez-Jiménez, J., Neveu, V., Vos, F., Scalbert, A., 2010. Identification of the 100 richest dietary sources of polyphenols: an application of the Phenol-Explorer database. Eur. J. Clin. Nutr. 64 (Suppl. 3), S112–S120.

Perry, C.L., Mcguire, M.T., Neumark-Sztainer, D., Story, M., 2001. Characteristics of vegetarian adolescents in a multiethnic urban population. J. Adolesc. Health 29 (6), 406–416.

Povey, R., Wellens, B., Conner, M., 2001. Attitudes towards following meat, vegetarian and vegan diets: an examination of the role of ambivalence. Appetite 37 (1), 15–26.

Rasmussen, S.A., Fernhoff, P.M., Scanlon, K.S., 2001. Vitamin B_{12} deficiency in children and adolescents. J. Pediatr. 138 (1), 10–17.

Robinson-O'Brien, R., Perry, C.L., Wall, M.M., Story, M., Neumark-Sztainer, D., 2009. Adolescent and young adult vegetarianism: better dietary intake and weight outcomes but increased risk of disordered eating behaviors. J. Am. Diet. Assoc. 109 (4), 648–655.

Rush, E.C., Chhichhia, P., Hinckson, E., Nabiryo, C., 2009. Dietary patterns and vitamin B_{12} status of migrant Indian preadolescent girls. Eur. J. Clin. Nutr. 63 (4), 585–587.

Sabaté, J., Wien, M., 2010. Vegetarian diets and childhood obesity prevention. Am. J. Clin. Nutr. 91 (5), 1525S–1529S.

Sabaté, J., Lindsted, K.D., Harris, R.D., Johnston, P.K., 1990. Anthropometric parameters of schoolchildren with different life-styles. Am. J. Dis. Child. 144 (10), 1159–1163.

Shaikh, M.G., Anderson, J.M., Hall, S.K., Jackson, M.A., 2003. Transient neonatal hypothyroidism due to a maternal vegan diet. J. Pediatr. Endocrinol. Metab. 16 (1), 111–113.

Shailee, F., Sogi, G.M., Sharma, K.R., Nidhi, P., 2012. Dental caries prevalence and treatment needs among 12- and 15- year old schoolchildren in Shimla city, Himachal Pradesh, India. Indian J. Dent. Res. 23 (5), 579–584.

Shull, M.W., Reed, R.B., Valadian, I., Palombo, R., Thorne, H., Dwyer, J.T., 1977. Velocities of growth in vegetarian preschool children. Pediatrics 60 (4), 410–417.

Smith, C.F., Burke, L.E., Wing, R.R., 2000. Vegetarian and weight-loss diets among young adults. Obes. Res. 8 (2), 123–129.

Stahler, C., 2012. How Often Do Americans Eat Vegetarian Meals? And How Many Adults in the U.S. Are Vegetarian? The Vegetarian Resource Group Asks in a 2012 National Harris Poll. (Online). Available from: http://www.vrg.org/blog/2012/05/18/how-often-do-americans-eat-vegetarian-meals-and-how-many-adults-in-the-u-s-are-vegetarian/#sthash.xRqV0BuS.dpuf.

Thane, C.W., Bates, C.J., 2000. Dietary intakes and nutrient status of vegetarian preschool children from a British national survey. J. Hum. Nutr. Diet. 13 (3), 149–162.

The Vegetarian Society, 2000. The Vegetarian Society U.K.: 21st Century Vegetarian. (Online) Available from: https://www.vegsoc.org/sslpage.aspx?pid=753.

van Summeren, M., Braam, L., Noirt, F., Kuis, W., Vermeer, C., 2007. Pronounced elevation of undercarboxylated osteocalcin in healthy children. Pediatr. Res. 61 (3), 366–370.

van Winckel, M., Vande Velde, S., De Bruyne, R., Van Biervliet, S., 2011. Clinical practice: vegetarian infant and child nutrition. Eur. J. Pediatr. 170 (12), 1489–1494.

Wallace, T.C., Reider, C., Fulgoni 3rd, V.L., 2013. Calcium and vitamin D disparities are related to gender, age, race, household income level, and weight classification but not vegetarian status in the United States: analysis of the NHANES 2001-2008 data set. J. Am. Coll. Nutr. 32 (5), 321–330.

Watanabe, F., 2007. Vitamin B_{12} sources and bioavailability. Exp. Biol. Med. (Maywood) 232 (10), 1266–1274.

Willoughby, J.L., Bowen, C.N., 2014. Zinc deficiency and toxicity in pediatric practice. Curr. Opin. Pediatr. 26 (5), 579–584.

World Health Organization, Food and Agricultural Organization of the United Nations, 2004. Vitamin and Mineral Requirements in Human Nutrition, second ed. (Online) Available from: http://apps.who.int/iris/bitstream/10665/42716/1/9241546123.pdf?ua=1.

Yen, C.E., Yen, C.H., Huang, M.C., Cheng, C.H., Huang, Y.C., 2008. Dietary intake and nutritional status of vegetarian and omnivorous preschool children and their parents in Taiwan. Nutr. Res. 28 (7), 430–436.

Zimmermann, M.B., Hurrell, R.F., 2007. Nutritional iron deficiency. Lancet 370 (9586), 511–520.

Further Reading

Farmer, B., 2014. Nutritional adequacy of plant-based diets for weight management: observations from the NHANES. Am. J. Clin. Nutr. 100 (Suppl. 1), S365–S368.

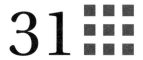

31

Food and Meals in Vegetarian Children and Adolescents

Ute Alexy[1], Nicole Janz[2], Mathilde Kersting[2]

[1]UNIVERSITY OF BONN, BONN, GERMANY; [2]UNIVERSITY CLINIC BOCHUM, BOCHUM, GERMANY

1. Introduction

Little is known about food intake pattern in current vegetarian diets in children and adolescents in Western societies, like in Europe. In adults, dietary surveys show that the dietary intake patterns of individuals describing themselves as vegetarian are diverse and quite distinct from the general population. On average, vegetarians consume more grains, legumes, vegetables and fruits (Haddad and Tanzman, 2003; Elorinne et al., 2016), nuts and seeds, potatoes, and avocados (Orlich et al., 2014), but less added fats, sweets, snack foods, and nonwater beverages (Orlich et al., 2014), resulting in overall better dietary eating pattern, e.g., measured by the Healthy Eating Index (Clarys et al., 2013, 2014). In the subgroup of vegans, the consumption of dairy and meat substitutes is common, e.g., soy milk, soy yogurt, and soy groats, wheat protein seitan, and falafel (Orlich et al., 2014; Elorinne et al., 2016).

A systematic review on vegetarian diets in infants, children, and adolescents in Western countries analyzed 24 publications with sufficient information to define dietary habits from 16 studies (not including studies on Seventh-day Adventists). Most of them were from the 1980s and 1990s and covered small samples (Schürmann et al., 2017). Nowadays, the food market is more diversified, including more and more special products for vegetarians. In Germany, foods of plant origin, which were uncommon during earlier decades, e.g., pseudo-cereals as amaranth, quinoa, chia seeds, are easily available today. In addition, dairy substitutes based on soy, grain, or almonds, as well as meat substitutes based on soy, wheat products, eggs, or milk protein have been developed by the food industry. Fortified foods became increasingly popular and contribute significantly to nutrient intake in children and adolescents (Sichert-Hellert et al., 1999). Additionally, supplements (Sichert-Hellert et al., 2006) are in use for these age groups. Last but not least, the Internet yields novel opportunities for dietary information. A poll in Germany showed the World Wide Web being the most important source of information about potential critical nutrients in vegans (Epp, 2016). However, it remains difficult for families to evaluate the background and the correctness of such information as well as to evaluate the relevance of food labeling information.

2. Food-Based Dietary Guidelines for Vegetarian Children and Adolescents

2.1 Principles

In public health nutrition, it is recommended that food-based dietary guidelines (FBDG) should be developed to translate nutrient-based dietary recommendations into food-based guidelines, so they are understandable for the population (Scientific Opinion on Establishing Food-Based Dietary Guidelines, 2010).

Existing dietary habits and health problems should be taken into account. FBDG should cover the total diet, not only single foods. For Germany, the Research Institute of Child Nutrition has developed FBDG for an omnivorous diet for children and adolescents aged 1–18 years based on optimized 7-day menus (Kersting et al., 2005). In this so-called *Optimized Mixed Diet*, three key messages guide food selection: consume plenty of plant-based foods, moderate amounts of food of animal origin, and sparingly of high-fat, high-sugar food. By use of common, nonfortified food (except iodized salt) the current German dietary reference intakes for energy and nutrients (Referenzwerte für die Nährstoffzufuhr, 2015) were achieved except for vitamin D.

2.2 Sample Menus for Vegetarian Diets

Some general guidelines for planning vegetarian diets have been given for the general population (Haddad et al., 1999; Messina and Mangels, 2001) or children and adolescents (Messina and Mangels, 2001).

In Germany, the principles of the omnivorous Optimized Mixed Diet (consideration of existing dietary habits, total diet, conventional nonfortified food) were used to develop 7-day vegetarian sample menus for children and adolescents starting with an ovolactovegetarian diet (Table 31.1; Fig. 31.1), which was afterward modified and optimized similarly into a vegan diet. The sample menus were calculated for the reference age group of 4- to 6-year-old children assuming low physical activity [energy requirement: 1350 kcal/day (Referenzwerte für die Nährstoffzufuhr, 2015)]. Subsequently, reference food group intakes for ovolactovegetarian and vegan children and adolescents were calculated, and nutrient intake was checked. Principles of food selection and food proportions can be transferred to other age groups between 1 and 18 years, while total food amount differs depending on individual energy requirements.

In the ovolactovegetarian diet, beverages account for 40% of daily dietary intake, followed by vegetables and legumes (16%), dairy (15%), fruit (10%), and the bread/grain/potatoes/rice/pasta group (12%). The food groups fat/oil (1.3%), eggs (1%), and nuts/seed (0.5%) and sweets (<2%) should be consumed in small amounts due to their high energy content. Special vegetarian products such as soy tofu make up 1% of total dietary intake.

In the vegan diet (Fig. 31.2), the exclusion of dairy and eggs is made up by an almost similar proportion of special vegan products, mainly plant-based milk alternatives in the form of soy drinks. Therefore, the proportions of the other food groups remain almost the same as in the ovolactovegetarian diet.

Table 31.1 Seven-Day Sample Menus[a] of an Ovolactovegetarian or Vegan[b] Diet for Children and Adolescents in Germany

	Day 1	Day 2	Day 3	Day 4	Day 5	Day 6	Day 7
Breakfast	Muesli, pear, cow's milk	Bircher muesli, fruit, cow's milk	Toast, jam, orange juice	Bun with jam, nectarine, hot chocolate	Oat flakes gruel, fruit, hot chocolate	Muesli, apple, cow's milk	Bread with hazelnut spread, apricot
Snack	Bread with cheese, carrot	Bread, lentil spread, capsicum	Vegetable sticks, crispbread	Pretzel, orange	Bread, camembert, grapes	Vegetable muffins	Tea cake, carrot salad
Lunch	Bulgur vegetable cassercle, salad	Pasta with lentil Bolognese	Fried potatoes, egg, salad	Chili con tofu	Millet burger, vegetables	Carrot stew, bread	Eggs, rice, broccoli
Snack	Cake, kiwi fruit	Shortbread, yogurt, wine gums	Fruit salad, ice cream	Orange, crisps	Fruit, nuts, chocolate	Pudding, raspberries	Yogurt, nectarine
Dinner	Quinoa salad with capsicum	Cucumber sandwich, grapes	Cheese sandwich, pear, lingonberry	Bread, tomato, mozzarella	Bread with cream cheese, turnip cabbage	Minestrone	Tortilla, vegetables, mozzarella

[a]Additionally water as beverage at meals.
[b]For the vegan sample menu, cow milk was replaced by soy drink (fortified with calcium, vitamin B_1, and vitamin B_{12}), cream was replaced by soy-based cream substitute, yogurt by a vegan soy-based yogurt substitute, cheese was replaced by vegan bread spread, egg was replaced by textured soy flakes.

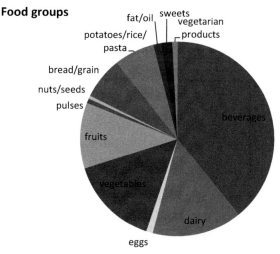

FIGURE 31.1 Reference food group intake in 7-day sample menus for an ovolactovegetarian diet for children and adolescents.

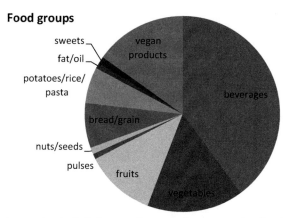

FIGURE 31.2 Reference food group intake in 7-day sample menus for a vegan diet for children and adolescents.

2.3 Analysis of Nutrient Intake

In the ovolactovegetarian sample menus, the construction of the menus resulted in the following macronutrient proportions that were in line with the German references: carbohydrates yields about 50% of energy intake (%E), fat 37%E, and protein 13%E; proportion of polyunsaturated fatty acids is high (9%E) and of saturated fatty acids low (10%E). The portion of added sugars is 6.5%E. Reference values for most vitamins and minerals are reached or exceeded (Fig. 31.3).

The vegan sample menus provide similar levels of macro- and micronutrients as the ovolactovegetarian menus with the exception of vitamin B_{12}, which is absent in the vegan diet (Fig. 31.4). In both menus, the iodine intake from food alone (without

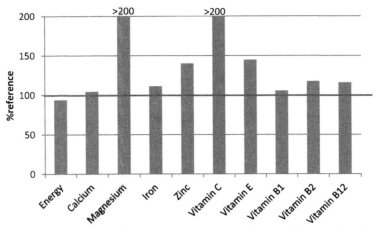

FIGURE 31.3 Energy and nutrient intake with the **ovolactovegetarian** sample menus (%reference values).

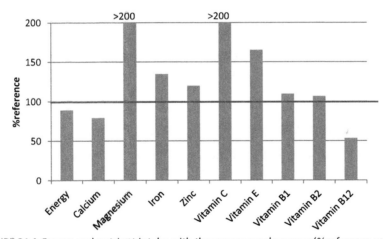

FIGURE 31.4 Energy and nutrient intake with the **vegan** sample menus (%reference values).

use of iodized salt) is well below the reference. Vitamin D intake was not examined here, as it is well-known to be far below the reference even in omnivorous children and adolescents, and vitamin D status in insufficient in large sectors of children and adolescents in Germany (Hintzpeter et al., 2008). In optimized omnivorous and even more in ovolactovegetarian and vegan diets in children and adolescents in Germany, which consider all nutrients at the same time, it is not possible to achieve the reference dietary intake level of vitamin D by food alone, including the use of fortified food available today.

The relatively low calcium intake in the vegan menus is a compromise to dietary practice in children and adolescents. For a further increase in dietary calcium, more specific plant food that is not common in Germany, like sesame or amaranth, would be needed.

3. Food Groups in Detail

3.1 Beverages

Water is the most essential nutrient (Manz et al., 2002). Mild dehydration can impair physical and cognitive performance (Popkin et al., 2010). Since body surface in relation to body weight is higher in children than in adults, high intake of beverages is of particular importance during childhood (Popkin et al., 2010). In the sample menus, beverages account for almost half of total daily intake. Children, regardless of vegetarian or omnivorous diet, should be encouraged to drink regularly at meals and in between. Water is the optimal beverage since it is free of energy. Tap water in industrialized countries is easily available and cheap. For vegans who avoid dairy, which is otherwise the major dietary source of calcium, mineral water rich in calcium (at least 150 mg/L) can increase calcium intake. There are indications that low water consumption seems to be associated with higher weight status in children and adolescents, and longitudinal studies suggest a weight-reducing effect of water consumption (Muckelbauer et al., 2014). In contrast, sugar-sweetened beverages may contribute to the development of obesity, since compensation for energy consumed in liquid form is suggested to be incomplete (Libuda et al., 2008). This applies not only to soft drinks or fruit juice drinks but also to 100% fruit juices, which all contain about 10 g sugar/100 mL. Therefore, at most one serving of fruit juice per day should replace one serving of natural fruit.

3.2 Vegetables and Fruit

Vegetables and fruit provide plenty of vitamins and bioactive compounds, and they could also be a source of iron and calcium in vegetarian diets. Iron-rich vegetables, e.g., spinach (3.4 mg/100 g), chard (2.7 mg/100 g), or curly kale (1.9 mg/100 g), are often not liked by children due to their bitter taste. Vegetables and fruit can also indirectly contribute to iron supply, since ascorbic acid and organic acids can significantly enhance the low absorption of nonheme iron from plant foods in particular in iron deficiency (Domellöf et al., 2014). Suitable meals are these, for example:

- muesli from oat flakes (4.4 mg iron/100 g) and orange juice (40 mg vitamin C/100 g)
- casserole from whole grain pasta (3.9 mg iron/100 g) and broccoli (70 mg vitamin C/100 g)

Vegetables relatively rich in calcium are, e.g., savoy cabbage (64 mg/100 g), broccoli (58 mg/100 g), and fennel (38 mg/100 g).

In spite of health advantages of a high consumption of vegetables and fruit, in real-life conditions the level of consumption of this food group is low in children and adolescents in Germany. This is mainly due to a low consumption of vegetables of no more than half of the amounts as recommended in the Optimized Mixed Diet (Richter et al., 2008). Several promising strategies can help to increase acceptance: early introduction of a variety of vegetables during complementary feeding (Foterek et al., 2015; Maier et al., 2008), repeated exposure to get familiar with the taste (Maier et al., 2007), flavor-flavor learning by combining familiar with novel tastes (Birch and Doub, 2014), increasing availability of vegetables and fruits in the family and school environment (Blanchette and Brug, 2005), avoiding pressure to eat vegetables and fruits (Galloway et al., 2006), and role model of parents and other caretakers (Pearson et al., 2009).

3.3 Nuts and Seeds

Nuts are energy-dense foods, rich in total fat, unsaturated fatty acids, and bioactive compounds, e.g., polyphenols (Ros, 2009). There is evidence that dietary pattern including nuts and seeds (e.g., almonds, walnuts, cashews, sunflower seeds, sesame seeds) have positive health effects (Mozaffarian, 2016). In spite of their high energy density, they appear to protect against chronic weight gain (Mozaffarian, 2016). The readers may refer to Chapter 18 for a detailed review. In vegan diets, these foods are suggested as alternatives of other high protein foods (½ ounce of nuts or seeds can be considered as a 1-ounce equivalent from the Protein Foods Group) (United States Department of Agriculture). In vegetarian as well as in omnivorous diets, unsalted and unfried nuts and seeds are a good alternative for common salty snacks, e.g., potato crisps, due to the lower content of salt and trans-fatty acids.

3.4 Legumes

Legumes from the botanical family *Fabaceae* include beans, peas, peanuts, lentils, and soybeans, whereas pulses exclude peanuts and soybeans (McCrory et al., 2010). Due to their slowly digestible starch and resistant starch properties and their high dietary fiber and protein content, a higher consumption of pulses is suggested as helpful for weight management (McCrory et al., 2010). Whereas in general dietary guidelines as the Optimized Mixed Diet in Germany or MyPlate in the United States where pulses are assigned to vegetables, in guidelines for vegetarian diets, they should be mentioned separately. In such plant-based diets, pulses are important sources for a broad range of potential critical nutrients, e.g., iron and zinc. Due to the high protein content, they are considered as alternatives to meat (United States Department of Agriculture). Soy can be a valuable protein source in vegan diets for children and adolescents as the protein content is higher than in other legumes, and the amino acid pattern is only slightly inferior to that of cow's milk (Singhal et al., 2016). Combining any legumes with cereal results in complementation in amino acid pattern, but such a food selection is uncommon in general dietary habits in children and adolescents in Germany.

 Soy also differs markedly from other legumes due to the higher content of fat and the lower content of carbohydrates (Messina and Messina, 2010). Isoflavones in soybeans may be protective against different types of cancer (Chen et al., 2014; Qu ct al., 2014; van Die et al., 2014), osteoporosis (Wei et al., 2012), and metabolic syndrome (Zhang et al., 2013; Liu et al., 2012). Also, potential harmful effects of high consumption rates especially in early childhood are discussed. A review with meta-analysis on soy-based infant formula, however, showed no strong evidence of adverse effects with regard to growth, mental development, reproductive, endocrine, and immune function (Vandenplas et al., 2014). For adults, an optimal intake of soy would appear to be between two and four servings per day (Messina and Messina, 2010). In our sample menus, consumption of legumes, i.e., pulses plus soy, was much lower and therefore minimized potential for adverse health effects of soy consumption.

3.5 Whole Grains

Whole grain comprises all components of the kernel. Through milling the bran and germ are removed, leaving only the endosperm of the kernel. Those refined grains are character-ized by their fine texture and improved shelf life at the expense of dietary fiber, mineral, and vitamin content. By exchanging refined grain product by the whole grain alternatives, e.g., bread, flakes, pasta, and rice, the nutrient density of diets can be improved signifi-cantly (Table 31.2). Compared to refined grain, especially the content of nutrients that may become critical in vegetarian diets is higher in whole grain products. Therefore, whole grain consumption should be encouraged in omnivorous and vegetarian diets as well. Generally a share of at least half of total grain consumption should be whole grain in the German and US FBDG for children and adolescents (Kersting et al., 2005). However, in dietary practice, this recommendation is often not met (Alexy et al., 2010). Oat flakes are a traditional and easily available whole grain product in child nutrition, but consumption is low at the expense of refined ready-to-eat cereals (RTEC). Muesli made from a mixture of oat flakes and RTEC could increase the acceptance of oats by use of flavor-flavor learning.

3.6 Special Vegetarian Food Products

3.6.1 Dairy and Vegan Dairy Substitutes

In omnivorous and vegetarian diets, dairy is an important source of protein, calcium, vitamin B_2, and vitamin B_{12}. The Optimized Mixed Diet contains only moderate amounts of dairy as a food of animal origin in total. In particular, in young children a high consumption of cow's milk (>500 mL/day) is a risk factor for iron deficiency (Parkin et al., 2016). This applies in par-ticular to vegetarian children, where meat as an important source for iron is lacking.

For vegan diets, there is an increasing supply of plant-based drinks, e.g., of soy, grain, or almonds, which are marketed as cow's milk alternatives. The protein quality of soy is closer to protein of animal origin than the protein quality of the other plant-based ingre-dients. Infant formula and follow-on formula based on soy isolates are suited for vegan diets in children also beyond infancy as their composition is prescribed in EU food law. Otherwise, soy-based drinks fortified with calcium, vitamin B_2, and vitamin B_{12} orientated toward the contents of cow's milk should be used. However, a sound selection of suitable products is hampered because of the different fortification habits in products on the mar-ket as shown by the example of Germany (Table 31.3). Organic products are not allowed to be fortified; therefore the food market offers several unfortified milk substitutes whose regular consumption could hamper a sufficient intake of these dairy specific nutrients.

In ovolactovegetarian diets, dairy and eggs are sources of vitamin B_{12} [one glass of milk: 0.8 µg, one slice of cheese: 0.8 µg, one egg: 1.0 µg (Souci et al., 2008)]. Hence, provided a sufficient consumption of these foods, intake of vitamin B_{12} can reach reference values

Table 31.2 Nutrient Composition of Whole Grain and Refined Grain Products (per 100g)

	Energy (kcal)	Protein (g)	Fat (g)	Carbohydrate (g)	Dietary Fiber (g)	Calcium (mg)	Phosphorus (mg)	Iron (mg)	Zinc (mg)	Folate (µg)	Vitamin B$_1$ (µg)	Vitamin B$_6$ (µg)
Wheat whole meal flour[a]	309	11.4	2.4	59.5	10	32	345	3.4	3.4	n.s.	470	460
Wheat flour type 405[b]	335	10.6	1	71.8	4	15	74	1.4	0.7	10	60	180
Rye flour type 1370[b]	313	8.9	1.4	66.7	9	31	170	2.6	n.s.	n.s.	300	n.s.
Rye flour type 815[b]	319	6.9	1	71	6.5	22	128	2.1	1.5	15	180	110
Oat flakes[b]	348	13.5	7	58.7	10	43	430	5.8	4.3	87	590	160
Rice, unpolished[b]	345	7.8	2.2	74.1	2.2	16	282	3.2	1.6	16	410	275
Rice, polished[b]	344	7.4	0.6	77.7	1.4	6.2	110	0.9	1.1	11	60	150
Millet, raw[b]	350	10.6	3.9	68.8	3.8	9.5	275	6.9	2.9	n.s.	433	519
Buckwheat, raw[b]	336	9.8	1.7	71	3.7	18	320	3.8	2.7	n.s.	240	n.s.
Pasta, whole meal[a]	323	13.4	2.5	60.6	11.5	34	370	3.9	3	40	670	200
Pasta, refined[b]	348	12.5	1.2	70.5	5.1	22	165	1.5	1.5	31	90	170

n.s., not specified.
[a]Bundeslebensmittelschlüssel, https://blsdb.de.
[b]Souci et al. (2008).

Table 31.3 Nutrient Composition of Cow's Milk, Variants of Plant-Based Drinks, and Infant Formula on the Market in Germany (per 100 mL) (Effective July/August 2016)

	Energy (kcal)	Fat (g)	Protein (g)	Carbohydrate (g)	Calcium (mg)	Riboflavin (mg)	Vitamin B$_{12}$ (µg)	Vitamin D (µg)
Cow's milk, 3.5% fat	65	3.6	3.4	4.7	120	0.18	0.4	0.09
Cow's milk, 1.5% fat	48	1.6	3.4	4.8	155	0.18	0.4	0.03
Soy drink, plain	35	2.1	3.7	0.1	n.s	n.s.	n.s	n.s
Soy drink, fortified with Ca	43	2.4	4.1	0.9	120	n.s.	n.s.	n.s.
Soy drink, multifortified	39	1.8	3	2.5	120	0.21	0.38	0.75
Almond drink, plain	31	2.9	0.8	0.2	n.s.	n.s.	n.s.	n.s.
Almond drink, fortified	13	1.1	0.4	0.1	120	0.21	0.38	0.75
Oat drink, plain	47	1.3	0.3	8.1	n.s.	n.s.	n.s.	n.s.
Oat drink, fortified	44	1.5	0.3	6.8	120	0.21	0.38	0.75
Coconut milk, plain	194	19	1.0	4.1	n.s.	n.s.	n.s.	n.s.
Coconut drink, fortified	20	0.9	0.1	2.7	120	n.s.	0.38	0.75
Infant formula based on cow's milk protein	66	3.2	1.4	7.7	59	0.1	0.18	0.9
Infant formula based on soy protein isolates	67	3.3	1.7	7.8	68	0.1	0.14	0.95

n.s., not specified.

[1–3 µg/day (Referenzwerte für die Nährstoffzufuhr, 2015)] easily. However, the EPIC-Oxford study showed a higher prevalence of vitamin B_{12} deficiency in adult ovolactoveg-etarians than in omnivores (Gilsing et al., 2010). The readers may refer to Chapter 43 for a detailed review on B_{12} status. Therefore, vegetarian children and adolescents should be aware of their vitamin B_{12} intake. In particular when consumption of dairy and eggs is low, vitamin B_{12}-fortified foods should be consumed at least occasionally. In vegan diets, however, where vitamin B_{12} is absent, the regular consumption of vitamin B_{12}-fortified food and/or vitamin B_{12} supplementation is mandatory since vitamin B_{12} deficiency in childhood may have lasting neurological impairments (van Dusseldorp et al., 1999). In both fortified food and supplements, vitamin B_{12} is not bound to protein. Due to the limited capacity of intrinsic factor, single doses of vitamin B_{12} reach an absorption maximum of approximately 1–2 µg (National Institutes of Health, 2016). Since with fortified food repeated small doses of vitamin B_{12} are ingested, this application may be of advantage over supplements. Up to now, no adverse effects have been associated with excess B_{12} intake from food or supplements in healthy individuals (Staff, Institute of Medicine, 2000).

3.7 Meat Substitutes

There is a broad range of vegetarian meat substitutes on the market. Meanwhile major super-market chains in Germany offer a selection of products such as vegetarian sausages, spread, or burgers. The vegan variants are usually based on soy or wheat protein or, in case of burgers and patties, on grain, while vegetarian variants often contain egg protein. Meat substitutes are designed to equal the animal alternatives in taste and texture, among them convenience products such as vegetarian Bolognese or Gulasch or "crunchy" sticks. The nutrient composition of the vegetarian products varies to a great extent similar to the correspondent meat products. Products with a low to moderate fat content should be preferred, and the source of fat (plant or animal) should be considered. An advantage of the plant-based substitutes is the usually low amount of saturated fat. In addition, they may contribute to fiber intake depending on the ingredients. Burgers and patties based on grains have a high content of carbohydrates and thus may substitute for both meat and side dishes like rice or pasta in a traditional meal.

In contrast to dairy substitutes, meat substitutes are generally not fortified. Hence, these vegetarian alternatives provide no compensation for vitamin B_{12} from animal products. Like many common meat products, the vegetarian alternatives often contain high amounts of salt (about 2 g/100 g). Furthermore, convenience products often contain additives such as flavoring agents or preservatives. Therefore basic products like soy granules, plain tofu, or seitan should be preferred.

4. Eggs

Eggs provide protein of a high biological value and a high content of specific nutrients, especially in egg yolk, such as vitamin A, niacin, folate, selenium, zinc, and also bioactive compounds like carotenoids. In the omnivorous and ovolactovegetarian menus, the contribution of eggs to daily dietary intake is small (1%). Therefore, there is no obvious risk for nutrient deficiencies by excluding eggs from an overall balanced omnivorous or vegetarian diet in children and adolescents.

5. Sweets and Snacks

Sweet preference is common in children already in infancy and decreases during adolescence (Ventura and Worobey, 2013). In dietary practice, most children and adolescents exceed the current recommendations of the WHO not to consume more than 10% of energy from free sugar (Alexy et al., 2003). In the sample menus presented here, added sugar accounts for 6% of energy, well below the WHO limit, although it would be higher if considering free sugar. The total food group of sweets and snacks, called "tolerated food" in the Optimized Mixed Diet, may contribute up to 10% of total energy intake if the consumption of the recommended food groups is balanced.

6. Supplements and Fortification

Ideally, natural foods should cover all nutrient requirements. However, in the general nutrition of children and adolescents in Germany, this option is not achievable for vitamin D and iodine and in a vegan diet additionally for vitamin B_{12}.

In a vegan diet, vitamin B_{12} needs to be supplemented or supplied by fortified foods. Supplementation provides the advantage of standardization and the disadvantage of limited absorption capacity, whereas absorption is increased in smaller fortified dosage but evaluation of provided amount is difficult for parents due to the variable fortification practice at present.

Foods with high vitamin D content are oily fish, liver, egg yolk, butter, and fortified foods as margarine. However, most children and adolescents dislike foods like oily fish or liver. Fortification of usual milk could be an additional dietary approach but is not in general use in Germany. In contrast, vitamin D is added to some of the plant-based cow's milk alternatives (Table 31.3). Vitamin D can be supplied by endogenous production via sunlight (UVB) exposure. However, in Germany, this is not sufficiently practiced as vitamin D status is insufficient in large parts of children and adolescents. Vitamin D supplementation beyond infancy is suggested by pediatric authority and may be in particular advisable for vegetarian children and adolescents (Wabitsch et al., 2011).

To achieve an adequate iodine supply, the use of iodized salt is needed in omnivorous and vegetarian diets, not only as table salt but also in salted food like bread and convenience food (Johner et al., 2013). In a vegan diet where fish and milk as valuable dietary iodine sources are absent, additional iodine supplementation may be necessary as (iodized) salt should be used only sparingly to prevent high blood pressure. The readers may refer to Chapter 42 for a detailed review of iodine in vegetarian diets.

To assure an adequate supply of preformed n-3 long-chain polyunsaturated fatty acids (LC-PUFA) eicosapentaenoic acid (EPA), and docosahexaenoic acid (DHA) is difficult in vegetarian diets since the primary source of these fatty acids is fish and the conversion of plant-derived n-3 PUFA (fatty acids) to EPA and DHA is low (Harris, 2014). To support such conversion, a lower ratio of n-6 to n-3 fatty acids is considered useful and can be achieved in vegetarian diets by the use of (plant) n-3 rich plant oils, such as rapeseed oil or walnut oil. A novel approach is the consumption of foods such as plant oils enriched with pre-formed EPA and DHA from microalgae sources (Harris, 2014).

7. Conclusion and Perspective

Our sample menus showed that well-planned vegetarian diets including the necessary nutrient supplementation or fortification can meet the nutrient reference values. However, such a nutrient-based approach has been criticized since the emphasis on nutrient intake may not capture important nutritional issues and may inhibit a focus on food (Jacobs et al., 2009). However, the food group recommendations derived from our sample menus are in good accordance with food-based strategies for the prevention of cardiovascular disease, diabetes, and obesity (Mozaffarian, 2016).

The reference food group intakes from the ovolactovegetarian and vegan sample menus for children and adolescents (Table 31.1) are similar to those for omnivorous counterparts in Germany. General critical nutrients in the omnivorous and vegetarian menus are vitamin D and iodine, which need supplementation (vitamin D) or fortification (iodized salt). Following an ovolactovegetarian diet, which avoids meat and fish, energy and nutrient requirements can be fulfilled similar to the omnivorous menus, in particular when not only vegetables and fruits but also whole grain and pulses are consumed regularly (Table 31.4). The latter food groups become increasingly important if a vegan diet is practiced.

Table 31.4   Key Food-Based Messages for the Nutrition of Children and Adolescents

Omnivorous and Vegetarian Diets

- Use water as regular beverage at meals and in between.
- Eat a variety and abundance of plant-based food, i.e., vegetables, fruit, grain (preferably as whole grain), legumes, nuts, and seeds.
- Eat sweets, confectionaries, and cakes sparingly.
- Use iodized salt in the household and prefer ready-to-eat foods (e.g., bread, convenience products) produced with iodized salt.
- Choose rapeseed oil or another oil with a high proportion of n-3 PUFA for food preparation.
- Use vitamin D supplements if sunlight exposure is insufficient.

Vegetarian Diets

- Include moderate amounts of dairy or dairy substitutes fortified with calcium, vitamin B_2, and vitamin B_{12}.
- Combine iron-rich plant-based food with a vitamin C source in a meal.

Vegan Diets

- Care for a sufficient vitamin B_{12} supply by supplementation or fortified food.
- Use regular pediatric check-up to evaluate as a first step besides growth curve and developmental status the child's food consumption and as second step to decide if and which nutrients could be "critical" and for which the nutrient status should be examined.

Modified from Haddad, E.H., Sabaté, J., Whitten, C.G., 1999. Vegetarian food guide pyramid: a conceptual framework. Am. J. Clin. Nutr. 70 (Suppl. 3), 615S–619S.

In this case, the combination of pulses, soy, and whole grains contribute to an adequate intake of protein and amino acids. In addition, the supplementation of vitamin B_{12} is necessary, and the use of cow's milk substitutes enriched with dairy key nutrients would be prudent.

Acknowledgment

The support of Dr. Annett Hilbig and Eva Hohoff in the conception of the sample menus is acknowledged.

References

Alexy, U., Sichert-Hellert, W., Kersting, M., 2003. Associations between intake of added sugars and intakes of nutrients and food groups in the diets of German children and adolescents. Br. J. Nutr. 90 (2), 441–447.

Alexy, U., Zorn, C., Kersting, M., 2010. Whole grain in children's diet: intake, food sources and trends. Eur. J. Clin. Nutr. 64 (7), 745–751.

Birch, L.L., Doub, A.E., 2014. Learning to eat: birth to age 2 y. Am. J. Clin. Nutr. 99 (3) 723S–728S.

Blanchette, L., Brug, J., 2005. Determinants of fruit and vegetable consumption among 6-12-year-old children and effective interventions to increase consumption. J. Hum. Nutr. Diet. 18 (6), 431–443.

Chen, M., Rao, Y., Zheng, Y., Wei, S., Li, Y., Guo, T., Yin, P., 2014. Association between soy isoflavone intake and breast cancer risk for pre- and post-menopausal women: a meta-analysis of epidemiological studies. PLoS One 9 (2), e89288.

Clarys, P., Deliens, T., Huybrechts, I., Deriemaeker, P., Vanaelst, B., Keyzer, W.de, Hebbelinck, M., Mullie, P., 2014. Comparison of nutritional quality of the vegan, vegetarian, semi-vegetarian, pesco-vegetarian and omnivorous diet. Nutrients 6 (3), 1318–1332.

Clarys, P., Deriemaeker, P., Huybrechts, I., Hebbelinck, M., Mullie, P., 2013. Dietary pattern analysis: a comparison between matched vegetarian and omnivorous subjects. Nutr. J. 12, 82.

Domellöf, M., Braegger, C., Campoy, C., Colomb, V., Decsi, T., Fewtrell, M., Hojsak, I., Mihatsch, W., Molgaard, C., Shamir, R., Turck, D., van Goudoever, J., 2014. Iron requirements of infants and toddlers. J. Pediatr. Gastroenterol. Nutr. 58 (1), 119–129.

Elorinne, A.-L., Alfthan, G., Erlund, I., Kivimäki, H., Paju, A., Salminen, I., Turpeinen, U., Voutilainen, S., Laakso, J., 2016. Food and nutrient intake and nutritional status of Finnish vegans and non-vegetarians. PLoS One 11 (2), e0148235.

Epp, A., 2016. Vegan – Risiken durch einen neuen Ernährungsstil? (Online). Available at: www.bfr.bund.de/cm/343/vegan-risiken-durch-einen-neuen-ernaehrungsstil.pdf.

Foterek, K., Hilbig, A., Alexy, U., 2015. Associations between commercial complementary food consumption and fruit and vegetable intake in children. Results of the DONALD study. Appetite 85, 84–90.

Galloway, A.T., Fiorito, L.M., Francis, L.A., Birch, L.L., 2006. Finish your soup': counterproductive effects of pressuring children to eat on intake and affect. Appetite 46 (3), 318–323.

Gilsing, A.M.J., Crowe, F.L., Lloyd-Wright, Z., Sanders, T.A.B., Appleby, P.N., Allen, N.E., Key, T.J., 2010. Serum concentrations of vitamin B_{12} and folate in British male omnivores, vegetarians and vegans: results from a cross-sectional analysis of the EPIC-Oxford cohort study. Eur. J. Clin. Nutr. 64 (9), 933–939.

Haddad, E.H., Sabaté, J., Whitten, C.G., 1999. Vegetarian food guide pyramid: a conceptual framework. Am. J. Clin. Nutr. 70 (Suppl. 3) 615S–619S.

Haddad, E.H., Tanzman, J.S., 2003. What do vegetarians in the United States eat? Am. J. Clin. Nutr. 78 (Suppl. 3) 626S–632S.

Harris, W.S., 2014. Achieving optimal n-3 fatty acid status: the vegetarian's challenge… or not. Am. J. Clin. Nutr. 100 (Suppl. 1) 449S–52S.

Hintzpeter, B., Mensink, G.B.M., Thierfelder, W., Müller, M.J., Scheidt-Nave, C., 2008. Vitamin D status and health correlates among German adults. Eur. J. Clin. Nutr. 62 (9), 1079–1089.

Jacobs, D.R., Haddad, E.H., Lanou, A.J., Messina, M.J., 2009. Food, plant food, and vegetarian diets in the US dietary guidelines: conclusions of an expert panel. Am. J. Clin. Nutr. 89 (5) 1549S–1552S.

Johner, S.A., Thamm, M., Nöthlings, U., Remer, T., 2013. Iodine status in preschool children and evaluation of major dietary iodine sources: a German experience. Eur. J. Nutr. 52 (7), 1711–1719.

Kersting, M., Alexy, U., Clausen, K., 2005. Using the concept of food based dietary guidelines to develop an optimized mixed diet (OMD) for German children and adolescents. J. Pediatr. Gastroenterol. Nutr. 40 (3), 301–308.

Libuda, L., Alexy, U., Sichert-Hellert, W., Stehle, P., Karaolis-Danckert, N., Buyken, A.E., Kersting, M., 2008. Pattern of beverage consumption and long-term association with body-weight status in German adolescents – results from the DONALD study. Br. J. Nutr. 99 (06).

Liu, X.X., Li, S.H., Chen, J.Z., Sun, K., Wang, X.J., Wang, X.G., Hui, R.T., 2012. Effect of soy isoflavones on blood pressure: a meta-analysis of randomized controlled trials. Nutr. Metab. Cardiovasc. Dis. 22 (6), 463–470.

Maier, A., Chabanet, C., Schaal, B., Issanchou, S., Leathwood, P., 2007. Effects of repeated exposure on acceptance of initially disliked vegetables in 7-months old infants. Food Qual. Pref. 18, 1023–1032.

Maier, A.S., Chabanet, C., Schaal, B., Leathwood, P.D., Issanchou, S.N., 2008. Breastfeeding and experience with variety early in weaning increase infants' acceptance of new foods for up to two months. Clin. Nutr. Edinb. Scotl. 27 (6), 849–857.

Manz, F., Wentz, A., Sichert-Hellert, W., 2002. The most essential nutrient: defining the adequate intake of water. J. Pediatr. 141 (4), 587–592.

McCrory, M.A., Hamaker, B.R., Lovejoy, J.C., Eichelsdoerfer, P.E., 2010. Pulse consumption, satiety, and weight management. Adv. Nutr. (Bethesda, MD) 1 (1), 17–30.

Messina, M., Messina, V., 2010. The role of soy in vegetarian diets. Nutrients 2 (8), 855–888.

Messina, V., Mangels, A.R., 2001. Considerations in planning vegan diets: children. J. Am. Diet. Assoc. 101 (6), 661–669.

Mozaffarian, D., 2016. 'Dietary and policy priorities for cardiovascular disease, diabetes, and obesity: a comprehensive review'. Circulation.

Muckelbauer, R., Barbosa, C.L., Mittag, T., Burkhardt, K., Mikelaishvili, N., Müller-Nordhorn, J., 2014. Association between water consumption and body weight outcomes in children and adolescents: a systematic review. Obesity (Silver Spring, MD) 22 (12), 2462–2475.

National Institutes of Health, 2016. Vitamin B_{12}: Dietary Supplement Fact Sheet (Online). Available at: https://ods.od.nih.gov/factsheets/VitaminB12-HealthProfessional/.

Orlich, M.J., Jaceldo-Siegl, K., Sabaté, J., Fan, J., Singh, P.N., Fraser, G.E., 2014. Patterns of food consumption among vegetarians and non-vegetarians. Br. J. Nutr. 112 (10), 1644–1653.

Parkin, P.C., DeGroot, J., Maguire, J.L., Birken, C.S., Zlotkin, S., 2016. Severe iron-deficiency anaemia and feeding practices in young children. Public Health Nutr. 19 (4), 716–722.

Pearson, N., Biddle, S.J.H., Gorely, T., 2009. Family correlates of fruit and vegetable consumption in children and adolescents: a systematic review. Public Health Nutr. 12 (2), 267–283.

Popkin, B.M., D'Anci, K.E., Rosenberg, I.H., 2010. Water, hydration, and health. Nutr. Rev. 68 (8), 439–458.

Qu, X.-L., Fang, Y., Zhang, M., Zhang, Y.-Z., 2014. Phytoestrogen intake and risk of ovarian cancer: a meta-analysis of 10 observational studies. Asian Pac. J. Cancer Prev. 15 (21), 9085–9091.

Referenzwerte für die Nährstoffzufuhr, second ed., 2015. Umschau, Frankfurt.

Richter, A., Vohmann, C., Stahl, A., Heseker, H., Mensink, G., 2008. Der aktuelle Lebensmittelverzehr von Kindern und Jugendlichen in Deutschland. Ernähr Umschau 55, 28–36.

Ros, E., 2009. Nuts and novel biomarkers of cardiovascular disease. Am. J. Clin. Nutr. 89 (5) 1649S–1656S.

Schürmann, S., Kersting, M., Alexy, U., 2017. Vegetarian diets in children: a systematic review. Eur. J. Nutr. (in press).

Scientific opinion on establishing food-based dietary guidelines. EFSA J. 8 (3), 2010, 1460.

Sichert-Hellert, W., Kersting, M., Schöch, G., 1999. Consumption of fortified food between 1985 and 1996 in 2- to 14-year-old German children and adolescents. Int. J. Food Sci. Nutr. 50 (1), 65–72.

Sichert-Hellert, W., Wenz, G., Kersting, M., 2006. Vitamin intakes from supplements and fortified food in German children and adolescents: results from the DONALD study. J. Nutr. 136 (5), 1329–1333.

Singhal, S., Baker, R.D., Baker, S.S., 2016. A comparison of the nutritional value of cow's milk and non-dairy beverages. J. Pediatr. Gastroenterol. Nutr.

Souci, S.W., Fachmann, W., Kraut, H., Kirchhoff, E., 2008. Food composition and nutrition tables: On behalf of the Bundesministerium für Ernährung, Landwirtschaft und Verbraucherschutz, seventh ed. MedPharm Scientific Publishers; CRC Press, Stuttgart, Boca Raton, FL.

Staff, Institute of Medicine, 2000. Dietary Reference Intakes for Thiamin, Riboflavin, Niacin, Vitamin B_6, Folate, Vitamin B_{12}, Pantothenic Acid, Biotin, and Choline (Online). National Academies Press, Washington. Available at: http://gbv.eblib.com/patron/FullRecord.aspx?p=3375613.

United States Department of Agriculture *Choose my plate* (Online). Available at: www.choosemyplate.gov/protein-foods.

van Die, M.D., Bone, K.M., Williams, S.G., Pirotta, M.V., 2014. Soy and soy isoflavones in prostate cancer: a systematic review and meta-analysis of randomized controlled trials. BJU Int. 113 (5b), E119–E130.

van Dusseldorp, M., Schneede, J., Refsum, H., Ueland, P.M., Thomas, C.M., Boer, E.de, van Staveren, W.A., 1999. Risk of persistent cobalamin deficiency in adolescents fed a macrobiotic diet in early life. Am. J. Clin. Nutr. 69 (4), 664–671.

Vandenplas, Y., Castrellon, P.G., Rivas, R., Gutiérrez, C.J., Garcia, L.D., Jimenez, J.E., Anzo, A., Hegar, B., Alarcon, P., 2014. Safety of soya-based infant formulas in children. Br. J. Nutr. 111 (8), 1340–1360.

Ventura, A.K., Worobey, J., 2013. Early influences on the development of food preferences. Curr. Biol. 23 (9), R401–R408.

Wabitsch, M., Koletzko, B., Moß, A., 2011. Vitamin-D-Versorgung im Säuglings-, Kindes- und Jugendalter. Monatsschrift Kinderheilkunde 159 (8), 766–774.

Wei, P., Liu, M., Chen, Y., Chen, D.-C., 2012. Systematic review of soy isoflavone supplements on osteoporosis in women. Asian Pac. J. Trop. Med. 5 (3), 243–248.

Zhang, Y.-B., Chen, W.-H., Guo, J.-J., Fu, Z.-H., Yi, C., Zhang, M., Na, X.-L., 2013. Soy isoflavone supplementation could reduce body weight and improve glucose metabolism in non-Asian postmenopausal women–a meta-analysis. Nutrition (Burbank, Los Angel. Cty. Calif.) 29 (1), 8–14.

32

Vegetarian and Plant-Based Diets in Pregnancy

Giorgina B. Piccoli[1,2], Filomena Leone[1], Rossella Attini[1],
Gianfranca Cabiddu[3], Valentina Loi[3], Stefania Maxia[3], Irene Capizzi[1],
Tullia Todros[1]

[1]UNIVERSITY OF TORINO, TORINO, ITALY; [2]LE MANS HOSPITAL, LE MANS, FRANCE;
[3]BROTZU HOSPITAL, CAGLIARI, ITALY

1. Background

"You are pregnant, you have to eat for two," "You are pregnant, you have to eat meat," "You are pregnant you have to eat rich food." All of us have heard such sentences and indeed the idea that pregnant women have to be preserved from undernutrition (i.e., eat for two) and from nutritional deficiencies (e.g., eat meat, eat rich food) is, generally speaking, quite sensible. Meat and animal derivatives are rich in iron and vitamin B_{12}, the most commonly recognized micronutrients needed in pregnancy, while deficiencies in vitamin D are less frequent in meat eaters than in vegetarians (Kaiser and Campbell, 2014; Kaiser and Allen, 2008; Ramakrishnan et al., 2012a; Procter and Campbell, 2014).

A healthy diet during pregnancy has been recognized for centuries as a key for the health of the mother and the fetus. While this concept would protect mothers from undernutrition in times of limited resources, now it may be challenged by the abundance of food, which characterizes the differing social strata of the Western world and is also increasingly being found in the developing world (Kaiser and Campbell, 2014; Kaiser and Allen, 2008; Ramakrishnan et al., 2012a; Procter and Campbell, 2014; Koletzko et al., 2013; Liu et al., 2015; Lee et al., 2013; Blumfield et al., 2013). This abundance is often associated with lower quality of food, at least in the lower social strata.

In fact, the definition of an ideal diet has progressively switched over the last few decades from a diet at a low risk of nutritional deficiency to a diet that protects from diseases that can be induced or enhanced by overeating. If possible, this should also mean that the diet meets some of the requirements of sustainability (Macdiarmid, 2013; Smith and Gregory, 2013; Macdiarmid et al., 2012).

In this context, the rediscovery of the Mediterranean diet and of vegan or vegetarian diets has gained a growing interest, mainly because they may protect from the most commonly encountered chronic diseases linked to "overeating" in the developed and developing world, including the array of cardiovascular diseases, diabetes, obesity, the related metabolic syndrome, and even several types of cancer (Estruch et al., 2013; Valls-Pedret et al., 2015; Widmer et al., 2015; Ostan et al., 2015).

It is quite obvious that pregnancy is not a disease, but it may be associated with diseases, which can be different according to the setting and the availability of economic resources. In high-resource countries, the increasing age of mothers bears in itself an increased risk of hypertension and kidney disease, and the diffusion of medically assisted conception and the obesity epidemics may increase the risk of the negative effects of overnutrition. On the other hand, in underresourced settings the high metabolic demands of the fetus may create nutrient deficiency, with deleterious short- and long-term effects on both mother and child (Table 32.1) (Jebeile et al., 2016; Gresham et al., 2014; Ruchat et al., 2016; Laopaiboon et al., 2014; Jackson et al., 2015; Waldenström et al., 2014; Paulson et al., 2002; Maness and Buhi, 2016; Aminu et al., 2014).

Table 32.1   Obstetric Definitions for the Main Outcomes and Their Analytical Limits

Term	Definition	Main Problems and Limits
At term	Delivery after 37 completed gestational weeks (GW)	This term is usually agreed. It may be difficult if not impossible to assess pregnancy duration in settings where late referral is common, such as many developing countries
Preterm	Delivery before the 37 GW	These are the most commonly agreed definitions. They may
Late preterm	Delivery after 34 and before 37 GW	not be consistently employed in particular in older studies. Clinical relevance is high (Fig. 32.1). Early preterm and very
Early preterm	Delivery before 34 GW	early preterm babies usually need also NICU (see later). While
Extreme preterm	Delivery before 28 GW	late preterm incidence is also linked to the policy toward caesarean sections, early preterm and extreme preterm babies reflect better the presence of important clinical problems in the mother or severe fetal growth impairment
Small baby	Weight at birth <2500 g	These broad definitions have the advantage of simplicity,
Very small baby	Weight at birth <1500 g	but they do not discriminate babies who grew well and were delivered preterm versus babies with intrauterine growth impairment. These two conditions have different pathogenesis and clinical implications for adult health and should be distinguished as much as possible (see SGA-IUGR)
Small for gestational age (SGA)	Below the 5th or below the 10th centile of weight adjusted for gestational age	A more precise measure of intrauterine growth, it should be interpreted together with weight and timing of delivery. It depends upon the availability of growth curves of the resident population and needs precise assessment of GW. It does not discriminate between "small babies" growing harmoniously on their own growth curve and IUGR. Caution on the definition (5th or 10th centile)
Intrauterine growth restriction (IUGR)	Arrest or impairment of intrauterine growth at the growth curve	This is the only way to discriminate between harmonious growth of a small baby and impairment of intrauterine growth in a previously normal or "large" baby; a precise measure of intrauterine problems, associated with future health problems; possible only when repeated measures are available (not in late referrals)

Table 32.1 Obstetric Definitions for the Main Outcomes and Their Analytical Limits—cont'd

Term	Definition	Main Problems and Limits
Preeclampsia (PE)	Clinical syndrome of poor placentation leading to endothelial damage	Usually defined as new onset of proteinuria above 300 mg and hypertension after the 20th gestational week in a patient who was previously normotensive and without proteinuria or kidney disease. Should resolve within 3 months from delivery. New definitions include plasma creatinine increase, even in the absence of proteinuria. This cannot apply to patients with kidney diseases or on dialysis (see superimposed PE)
Mild PE Severe PE Early PE Late PE Maternal PE Placental PE	Several attempts to define, none agreed Cut-point usually set at 34 GW With/without maternal predisposing disease	PE is a complex syndrome, of various severity, ranging from a mild increase in blood pressure and proteinuria at term to a stormy potentially deadly affection. None of the subsets is presently agreed, but their presence underlines the heterogeneity of the disease. May be considered a continuum with pregnancy induced hypertension and HELLP (hemolysis, increase in liver enzymes and low platelets), the most severe expression of endothelial derangement
Need for neonatal intensive care unit (NICU)	Usually needed for very early preterm and very small babies	This is an indirect marker of the severity of the intrauterine problems or of preterm delivery; however, availability depends upon the health care setting and upon the obstetric policy

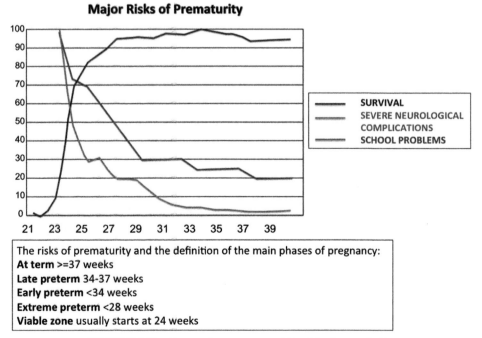

FIGURE 32.1 The phases of pregnancy and the risk of prematurity.

In both cases, well-balanced plant-based diets may theoretically be welcomed: they are rarely "too rich" and may protect from overnutrition in the "rich" countries. Plant-based food is often less expensive than animal-derived food, and thus a well-balanced vegan or vegetarian diet could be more easily affordable in "poor" countries.

While appealing, these are still ungrounded hypotheses, and the literature on vegan, vegetarian, plant-based, and pescetarian diets in pregnancy is still very limited, highly heterogeneous, and not easily analyzed.

In this context, the following narrative review was undertaken to try to answer some of the questions and highlight some of the unsolved problems of what we will call for clarity and simplicity vegetarian diets in pregnancy (encompassing different types of vegetarian diets, including ovolactovegetarian and vegan diets; see Chapter 1 for the definitions), as a complement to a wider discussion on plant-based diets in the prevention of several diseases.

2. Vegetarian Diets in Pregnancy: The Reviews

In 2009, the American Dietetic Association (ADA) provided the following favorable, albeit generic, statement: "appropriately planned vegetarian diets, including total vegetarian or vegan diets, are healthful, nutritionally adequate, and may provide health benefits in the prevention and treatment of certain diseases," followed by an appreciation of its validity across the entire lifecycle: "well-planned vegetarian diets are appropriate for individuals during all stages of the lifecycle, including pregnancy, lactation, infancy, childhood …" (Craig and Mangels, 2009).

However, these highly favorable statements are weakened by the short review available online, which summarized the data, from only seven papers, on fetal outcomes and underlined the limitations of the studies and reported different outcomes and contrasting results (Craig and Mangels, 2009).

Despite the great interest in this issue, when we were reviewing our experience with vegetarian diets in pregnant women with chronic kidney disease, we were unable to find any other reviews apart from the ADA Website, and for this reason, we undertook a systematic review, targeting the studies performed and reported outside of a context of malnutrition and limited resources (Piccoli et al., 2015a).

Our study was able to retrieve and analyze 13 papers on materno-fetal outcomes and 9 papers on vitamin or mineral deficiencies from 2329 references (Piccoli et al., 2015a; Table 32.2). The results underlined a few key points: the first was the difficulty in discriminating between the effects of lifestyle and diet, considering the lack of randomized controlled trials, which are questionable for the general population (as they would be too intrusive in their daily lives) and almost impossible during pregnancy from an ethical perspective.

The second point was the need for more studies on vegan diets in pregnancy, due to the heterogeneity of studies, methods, populations, and results. A common limitation shared by most of the studies was the lack of homogeneous control groups. Furthermore, no large

Table 32.2   Characteristics of the Studies Included in the Previous Systematic Review

References	All Cases (Vegans-Vegetarians)	Main Outcomes Reported in the Papers
Papers Reporting on Materno-Fetal Outcomes in Vegan/Vegetarian Pregnancies		
Wen et al. (2013)	852 w (ns)	Vegetarian diet during second trimester associated with lower fetal (−0.39 [−0.71, −0.08]) and placental weight (−0.40 [−0.79, −0.01]) (abstract)
Robic et al. (2012)	27 w (9)	No significant differences between groups in pregnancy mass gain and birth mass (abstract)
Alwan et al. (2011)	1257 w (114)	Vegetarians most likely to take iron-containing supplements
Stuebe et al. (2009)	1388 w (50)	To identify modifiable risk factors for excessive gestational weight gain
North and Golding (2000)	7928 c (3211)	Vegetarian mothers had an adjusted OR of 4.99 of giving birth to a boy with hypospadias
Lakin et al. (1998)	19 women (4)	Birth weight (g): 3673±485 (omnivores), 3770±500 (vegetarians), 3365±302 (diabetic omnivores) (not statistically significant)
Drake et al. (1998)	25 (ovolacto) 29 (fish) 29 (omnivores)	No significant differences in any pregnancy outcomes between groups
Fonnebo (1994)	7285 (most vegetarians)	Birth weight length (cm): 50.7 (SDA), 50.4 (non-SDA) (difference 0.3, 95% CI 0.1–0.5). RR of death from 28th week onward: 0.87 (95% CI 0.43–0.75)
Reddy et al. (1994)	144 w (48)	Birth weight lower in vegetarians, head circumference shorter No significant differences in length/APGAR index at 1 and 5 min
Ward et al. (1988)	73 Gujerat (53) 92 Harrow (59)	Birth weight equal (in vegetarian and nonvegetarian)
Carter et al. (1987)	775 women (775)	One mother had four small for gestational age babies
Campbell-Brown et al. (1985)	144 women (59)	No differences in Hindu vegetarian and meat eaters; significant difference between Hindus and Europeans ($P<.001$)
Thomas et al. (1977)	32 women (14)	Birth weight (kg): 3.1±0.8 (vegans), 3.3±1.2 (nonvegans). Live births (%): 86 (vegans), 88 (nonvegans). Stillbirths/miscarriages (%): 14 (vegans), 12 (nonvegans)
Papers Reporting on Nutritional Deficiencies in Vegan/Vegetarian Pregnancies		
Koebnick et al. (2005)	108 women (27)	Dietary magnesium intake (mg/day): 508±14 and 504±11 (plant-based diets), 412±9 (controls) ($P<.001$). No significant difference in serum and RBC magnesium between groups. Lower occurrence of calf cramps in plant-based diets versus controls
Koebnick et al. (2004)	109 women (27)	Vitamin B_{12} intake and serum vitamin B_{12} levels: lower in plant-based diets than in controls ($P<.001$). Higher plasma homocysteine versus controls
Sharma et al. (2003)	1150 women (524)	Anemia (%): 96.18 (vegetarians), 95.3 (halal meat eaters), 96.2 (jhatka meat eaters) (ns)

Continued

Table 32.2 Characteristics of the Studies Included in the Previous Systematic Review—cont'd

References	All Cases (Vegans-Vegetarians)	Main Outcomes Reported in the Papers
Koebnick et al. (2001)	109 women (27)	Folate deficiency: OR=0.1 (95% CI=0.01,0.56) in only vegetarians, OR=0.52 (95% CI=0.2,1.34) in low meat eaters versus WD
Sharma et al. (1994)	46 women (21)	Maternal Hb (g/dL): 9.64±0.46 (vegetarians), 10.16±0.35 (nonvegetarians) ($P<.001$). Maternal ferritin (ng/mL): 40.4±18 (vegetarians), 61.6±32.2 (nonvegetarians) ($P<.02$)
Stammers et al. (1989)	47 women (28)	Maternal plasma free fatty acid (mmol/L): 1.110±0.157 (vegetarians), 0.964±0.096 (nonvegetarians) (ns). Umbilical cord plasma free fatty acid: ns
Abraham (1982)	60 women (20)	Zinc intake (mg/day): 7.35±0.42 (vegetarians), 10.2±0.55 (nonvegetarians), 11.5±0.49 (controls) ($P<.001$). Copper intake (mg/day): 1.38±0.07 (vegetarians), 1.93±0.25 (nonvegetarians), 1.72±0.20 (controls)
Jathar and Inamdar-Deshmukh (1981)	60 women (60)	RBC vitamin B_{12} (ng/L): 157±30.4 (nonpregnant), 126±12.5 (pregnant with Hb >10 g/dL), 81±10.7 (pregnant with Hb <10 g/dL) (ns)
King et al. (1981)	23 women (12+5)	Zinc intake (mg/day): 12.6±0.9 (pregnant vegetarians), 14.4±0.6 (pregnant nonvegetarians) ($P\le.01$)

study had adjusted the model for the attainment of biochemical goals, such as ferritin or hemoglobin levels, thus making it impossible to conclude if the differences, when present, were due to the overall dietary pattern or to the lack of attainment of the minimum requirements of specific vitamins and minerals needed in pregnancy.

Within these limits, the third important point was that none of the studies reporting on materno-fetal outcomes demonstrated, or even strongly suggested, a higher risk for severe adverse pregnancy-related events in vegetarian mothers (Piccoli et al., 2015a). Prematurity is one of the most studied outcomes, for its relevance throughout lifetime (Fig. 32.1).

Overall, the data available at that time suggested that vegetarian mothers could have a slightly shorter duration of gestation as compared to omnivorous mothers. However, since the mean and median data were in the "at term" range, this observation was substantially devoid of clinical significance. Also, in keeping with a slightly lower duration of pregnancy, birth weight was significantly lower in some studies. Once more, the clinical relevance is of difficult interpretation, as no study discussed in detail whether the effect was due to protection against large for gestational age (LGA) babies (which would have been favorable), or to the presence of more small for gestational age (SGA) babies (which could be negative), or to a shift toward a lower normal birth weight (probably devoid of clinical relevance) (Piccoli et al., 2015a; Wen et al., 2013; Robic et al., 2012; Alwan et al., 2011; Stuebe et al., 2009; Drake et al., 1998; Fonnebo, 1994; Carter et al., 1987).

Conversely, a positive effect of a well-balanced vegetarian diet was suggested by some studies that supported the idea that plant-based diets protect against "high weight gain" in pregnancy. Likewise, the review did not detect any effect of the diet on the most important outcomes of pregnancy, including preeclampsia, preterm labor, and of caesarean section (Piccoli et al., 2015a; Wen et al., 2013; Robic et al., 2012; Alwan et al., 2011; Stuebe et al., 2009; Drake et al., 1998; Fonnebo, 1994; Carter et al., 1987).

One note of caution was the finding, in one large study, of a higher incidence of hypospadias in children from vegan mothers, which remained both unexplained and unconfirmed at the time of the present review (North and Golding, 2000).

Deficiencies in vitamin B_{12}, iron, zinc, and copper were described as being more frequent in vegetarians, again without clear evidence of the clinical meaning in both the short and long term. Thus, our conclusions were the following: evidence regarding vegetarian diets in pregnancy is heterogeneous and influences lifestyle choices. Within these limits, vegetarian diets are probably safe in pregnancy, provided that attention is given to vitamin and trace elements (mainly vitamin B_{12} and iron) requirements (Reddy et al., 1994; Lakin et al., 1998; Ward et al., 1988; Campbell-Brown et al., 1985; Koebnick et al., 2005, 2001, 2004; Sharma et al., 2003, 1994; Stammers et al., 1989; Abraham, 1982; Jathar and Inamdar-Deshmukh, 1981; King et al., 1981).

Since the conclusion of our previous research strategy, and until the present update of March 2016, no further broad systematic review has been made available on PubMed. Conversely, a systematic review on zinc in vegan pregnancies is now available, together with an in-depth, nonsystematic review on the advantages and drawbacks of vegetarian diets in pregnancy (Foster et al., 2015).

Zinc is an essential trace element and is involved in several biological processes that include enzyme action, stabilization of cell membranes, regulation of gene expression, and cell signaling. Therefore, zinc deficiencies have protean effects, and an extreme deficiency is not compatible with life; severe deficiency may lead to immunologic deficits, bullous dermatitis, alopecia, diarrhea, emotional disorder, weight loss, and hypogonadism (Foster et al., 2015).

The role of zinc in growth is important and a moderate deficiency may lead to growth retardation and delayed puberty together with mental impairment, taste abnormalities, and abnormal dark adaptation in sight. According to the study, based upon six English language observational studies, the zinc intake of vegetarians was lower than that of omnivores. However, overall, neither vegetarian nor omnivorous pregnant patients fully satisfied the recommended dietary allowance for zinc in pregnancy (Drake et al., 1998; Ward et al., 1988; Campbell-Brown et al., 1985; King et al., 1981; Abraham et al., 1985; Abu-Assal and Craig, 1984). In such a context, there is still an open question regarding whether physiological adaptations in zinc metabolism are sufficient to meet maternal and fetal requirements on overall zinc-poor diets in pregnancy (Foster et al., 2015).

The narrative review on diets, broadly defined as "Plant-Based and Plant-Rich," in pregnancy analyzes in-depth their advantages and shortcomings, merging personal experience and specific studies; we will refer to this extensive analysis on specific issues. However, it may be worth mentioning that the conclusions highlighted the need for further observational studies on a larger scale to investigate the relationship between "consolidated diets, gestation, and health," with the ultimate goal of providing targeted counseling for managing nutrition in each individual and for finding tailored interventions in each patient (Pistollato et al., 2015).

3. Vegetarian Diets in Pregnancy: Four Major Categories, According to the Reasons of Choice

Vegetarian and plant-based diets may have a different connotation in richer and poorer countries, often being associated with higher educational levels and income in the former and with poverty in the latter (Pistollato et al., 2015; Dwyer, 1999; Jacobs et al., 2009; Hu, 2003; Albert, 2005; Piccoli et al., 2014; Arora et al., 2011).

Furthermore, particularly in industrialized countries, the frequent association with particular lifestyles, healthy habits, and religious groups makes it difficult to disentangle the dietary effect from other elements, such as cigarette smoke, alcohol consumption, or exercise (Goswmai and Das, 2015; Fraser et al., 2016; Appleby and Key, 2015; Ho-Pham et al., 2009).

Anorexia and eating disorders are also associated with vegetarian diets, and their distinction from a "healthy lifestyle" suggests that these cases should be considered as a specific form of "malnutrition," and that they may share more features with the vegan diets observed in poor countries, even if the baseline trigger is unrelated to poverty (Leitzmann, 2014; O'Connor et al., 1987; Robinson-O'Brien et al., 2009; Bardone-Cone et al., 2012; Klopp et al., 2003).

The increasing use of vegetarian diets in the care of different diseases may raise issues of whether to continue these diets during pregnancy or not. This may be of particular importance in chronic kidney diseases (CKD), affecting up to 3% of women of childbearing age, and in which vegetarian diets may be used in severe cases (Forestell et al., 2012; Barsotti et al., 1996; Piccoli et al., 2015b; Cupisti et al., 2002; Chauveau et al., 2013; Piccoli et al., 2013).

Pregnancy is a peculiar situation in which, more than in other phases of life, socioeconomic and lifestyle (including dietary) choices merge. We will therefore discuss some clinically relevant aspects, advantages, limitations, and risks of vegetarian diets in four major situations: the "healthy and wealthy," the "poor and obliged," the "nutritionally disturbed," and the "sick and controlled."

Their intrinsic characteristics make each of these broad categories prone to display one or more aspects of vegetarian diets. The study of the "healthy and wealthy" may allow for the identification of the specific benefits of plant-based diets in settings in which the lifespan is long, and degenerative chronic diseases are the main causes of morbidity and mortality. The population of the "poor and obliged" highlights the main side effects due to nutritional deficiencies, which are more frequently due to qualitatively poor food even when in sufficient quantity, while the "nutritionally disturbed" individuals on vegan diets may help in understanding the risk of the dangerous combination of vegetarian and quantitatively limited alimentation. Even if obtained in a relatively small niche of cases, the experience of "sick and controlled" patients with CKD, in which a vegetarian diet is prescribed in pregnancy to counteract the negative effect of renal hyperfiltration on damaged nephrons, may highlight the potential of a tailored dietetic approach in the care of specific diseases in the most delicate phase of pregnancy (Garneata et al., 2016; Piccoli et al., 2015c).

4. What Is a "Well-Balanced" Vegetarian Diet in Pregnancy?

There are three major issues in nutritional approaches to vegetarian diets, whose importance is obviously increased in pregnancy: energy, essential amino acids, and trace elements. The first one is easily fulfilled. The second may be more difficult, especially in diets mainly or exclusively based upon vegetable proteins such as in the vegan ones, on which our review is mostly focused. Minerals are the last issue, and they will be extensively reviewed, considering once more the most "difficult" situation: strictly vegan diets.

Many papers on vegetarian or plant-based diets in pregnancy use the term "varied" to identify suitable diets in pregnancy and "unvaried" to refer to vegetarian diets often associated with nutritional deficiencies of quality and quantity proteins, or of trace elements, the most important (and studied in pregnancy) being iron, vitamin B_{12}, and vitamin D. However, zinc, iodine, and even calcium may also be below their required levels during pregnancy, in particular in some settings (Craig and Mangels, 2009; Piccoli et al., 2015a; Pistollato et al., 2015) (Table 32.4).

Vegan and vegetarian diets are, however, completely different with regard to nutritional attention in pregnancy. While milk and dairy products and, where consumed, eggs (and fish, in pescetarian diets) provide many trace elements and complement the vegetable proteins, which are low in some essential amino acids, vegan diets require greater attention, in particular in the final phase of rapid fetal growth. In the latter, from the point of view of integration among the different essential amino acids, a good rule of thumb is to consume together in each meal, whenever possible, at least two different types of grains and at least two different types of legumes, or protein-rich vegetables such as soy or quinoa, amaranth or buckwheat. The enormous quantity of papers published, however, bears witness to how much we still have to discover about these complex issues (Piccoli et al., 2014; Abugoch James, 2009; Alvarez-Jubete et al., 2009; Vega-Gálvez et al., 2010; Jukanti et al., 2012).

Several case reports analyzed the effects of vitamin B_{12} deficiencies in children from vegan and, less often, vegetarian mothers, mainly in those who were breastfed for a long period. While severe deficiencies are rare, the important and disabling neurologic symptoms in early life are relatively well known. The clinical picture of other deficiencies may be subtler and therefore more difficult to diagnose (Table 32.4) (Guez et al., 2012; Idris and Arsyad, 2012; Erdeve et al., 2009; Schlapbach et al., 2007).

In developing countries, nutritional deficiencies are common, and their correction usually requires dedicated programs to improve the outcomes of the pregnancies, in particular in the poorer population groups. The efficacy of such approaches, however, is not always clear, also probably due to the complexity of the underlying problems and to the multifactorial interventions (Nahar et al., 2009; Pérez-Expósito and Klein, 2009).

Indeed, the millenary experience with vegetarian diets and the richness of fruits, vegetables, and plants may allow for safe, nonsupplemented vegan diets in pregnant women in some settings and cultures. However, we also have to be aware that this is a rapidly developing field and that we still know very little on these subjects (Saunders et al., 2014; Grieger et al., 2014; Martin et al., 2015; Englund-Ögge et al., 2014; Hillesund et al., 2014; Brantsaeter et al., 2009; Chatzi et al., 2012).

A further remark may be that, in most Western, industrialized "rich" countries, in which the classical cuisine integrates a plant-based diet with at least small amounts of animal-derived food (such as in the Mediterranean diet, or in the Okinawa diet, both heavily associated with longevity), pregnant vegan patients may face a dilemma. Is it preferable to use specific supplements (for example, vitamin B_{12}, calcium, iron, or vitamin D) that are perceived by some as a medicalization of a natural approach, or is it preferable to stay on this classical diet, which is based on local food (a Zero Kilometer diet), but adjust with some exotic products that often come from thousands of kilometers away.

While vegan and vegetarian diets are overall considered feasible and harmless when well-balanced, controlled, and supplemented as needed, these considerations may warn against "excessively committed" vegan patients in pregnancy, and the usual definition of "varied diets" suggests paying attention to the possible association between vegetarian choices and nutritional disturbances, whose combination may be particularly dangerous in pregnancy (Klopp et al., 2003; Robinson-O'Brien et al., 2009; Neumark-Sztainer et al., 1997; Zuromski et al., 2015; Micali et al., 2012).

5. The "Healthy and Wealthy": The Benefits of the Vegetarian Diet in Preventing Diseases

When vegetarian diets are chosen in a context of having full access to all kinds of food, they may be taken as an example of dietary options that reflect attention and interest toward health-related matters; in other words, we often deal with very committed individuals, with respect to self-care and lifestyle (Piccoli et al., 2015a; Appleby and Key, 2015).

As previously mentioned, however, this favorable situation makes it difficult to disentangle the effects of lifestyle from those of diet, and once more because of the lack of large randomized controlled trials, the studies reporting on these individuals may overestimate the positive effects of vegetarian choices.

Furthermore, some large studies, such as the classic observational studies on the Adventist population, not only merge various types of plant-based diets but are also performed in very particular "cultural islands" (Piccoli et al., 2015a; Fonnebo, 1994; Fraser et al., 2016; Pettersen et al., 2012; Le and Sabaté, 2014).

Due to the high level of heterogeneity of the populations studied, the periods of study, the compared populations, and ethnic backgrounds, the previously mentioned systematic review did not succeed in identifying any clearcut advantages of vegetarian diets in pregnancy (Piccoli et al., 2015a).

However, when we merge the limited experience of vegetarian diets and the growing body of evidence that suggests correcting some potentially negative habits, such as excessive consumption of red meat or insufficient intake of vegetables and fruits, it is possible to highlight some further advantages, including a lower incidence of calf cramps, which is linked to a higher magnesium intake (Koebnick et al., 2005; Pistollato et al., 2015; Shiell et al., 2001; Saito et al., 2010; Jedrychowski et al., 2012).

Furthermore, one of the very few randomized controlled trials, concerning 52 women with gestational diabetes, found that the DASH (Dietary Approach to Stop Hypertension) diet, while not being strictly vegetarian, is however enriched by fruits, vegetables, and grains, and reduced the need for caesarean section and reduced the risk of LGA babies (Asemi et al., 2014). Another interesting indirect suggestion comes from the large Nurses' Health Study, which showed that a higher total intake of fiber (10 g/day) was associated with a lower incidence of gestational diabetes (Gaskins et al., 2014).

The effects of vegetarian diets on fetal growth are very difficult to analyze from the current literature (Table 32.3). In fact, most of the older studies only provide information on the mean and median values, which are unlikely to be significantly affected by well-balanced plant-based diets, particularly in physiological pregnancies. On the other hand, the mean and median values may not reveal information on two clinically relevant outcomes: the incidence of SGA (associated with poor placentation or placental damage) and LGA (associated with maternal diabetes or glucose intolerance) babies. Interestingly, and almost paradoxically, the two conditions are associated with a higher risk of metabolic syndrome and hypertension in adulthood, which in turn are associated with less favorable pregnancy-related outcomes (Table 32.3; Nguyen and Wilcox, 2005; Fleischman et al., 2010).

The attempts to associate maternal diets and diseases in childhood and adulthood have led to conflicting or nonconclusive results, due to the complexity of the diet issue, the heterogeneity of the populations, and the differences in study designs (Gernand et al., 2016; Milman et al., 2016). One exception is the association between high intake of dietary folate (whose content is higher in plant-based diets) and the lower incidence of neural tube defects and cleft palate/lip. Nothing is simple in pregnancy, and excessive folate intake has been associated with epigenetic modification and with a higher probability of twin pregnancies (Wilson et al., 2015).

Moreover, some evidence suggests that diets rich in fruits and vegetables are associated with a lower risk of common allergic diseases, including asthma, and atopic dermatitis for the offspring (Shiell et al., 2001; Saito et al., 2010). Furthermore, diets rich in fish and vegetables may have some effects on the incidence of childhood brain tumors (Jedrychowski et al., 2012; Huncharek and Kupelnick, 2004).

Many pieces of the puzzle are, however, missing, as most of the studies that have been conducted so far focused on macronutrients and vitamins. However the effects of additives, including taste enhancers, preservatives, and contaminants, including pesticides,

Table 32.3   Pregnancy as a "Source" of Future Diseases: Main Risks of Overeating and Undereating in Pregnancy

	Mother	Child
Overeating		
Excessive weight gain	Preeclampsia, hypertensive disorders of pregnancy, linked to a higher risk of developing chronic hypertension, diabetes, CKD later in life	Prematurity, which is not only linked to the known major neurological risks depicted in Fig. 32.1, but also to impaired kidney growth and deranges adipocyte metabolism, increasing the risk of CKD and of obesity-metabolic syndrome later in life
High consumption of refined sugars	Besides increasing the risk of excessive weight gain, diabetes in pregnancy is associated with prematurity and hypertensive disorders of pregnancy	See earlier
High consumption of canned and preserved food	May be deficient in many micronutrients, including vitamin D, whose deficit is associated with an increase in risk of hypertensive disorders of pregnancy Usually rich in sodium, may increase edema, and the risk of hypertensive disorders of pregnancy	As for hypertensive disorders and prematurity, see earlier Little is known on the eventual long-term effect of trace elements, mainly assumed as preservatives or additives, and diseases occurring later in life
High consumption of red meat	Usually rich in sodium, may increase edema, and the risk of hypertensive disorders of pregnancy	Little is known on the long-term effects on the fetus; a pro-cancerogenic effect of high red meat consumption has been described in adults
Undereating		
Low caloric intake	Preeclampsia, hypertensive disorders of pregnancy	Prematurity associated with other deficiencies
Low protein intake	Malnutrition, anemia, or edema	Prematurity, intrauterine growth restriction
Unbalanced protein intake	Malnutrition, anemia, or edema	Prematurity, intrauterine growth restriction
Vitamin B_{12}	Anemia, fatigue, neurological problems	Delayed neurological development, failure to thrive, flaccid paralysis
Vitamin D and calcium	Preeclampsia, hypertensive disorders of pregnancy	Prematurity, intrauterine growth restriction; however, some data suggest that combining vitamin D and calcium may increase the risk of preterm delivery
Vitamin A	Blindness, malabsorption, immunologic deficiencies	Blindness, immunodepression, stunted growth
Iron	Anemia, fatigue, or edema	Intrauterine growth restriction, prematurity
Iodine	Impaired thyroid function, fatigue	Cretinism
Other trace elements (Zn...)	Fatigue, neurological problems, dermatitis	Not completely known
Water soluble vitamins	Fatigue, dermatitis, impaired coagulation	Not completely known

that may be avoided in a meat-free diet, but that may be present, for example, in vegetable canned food, are much less known (Huncharek and Kupelnick, 2004; Genuis, 2009). For instance, the effect on the offspring of contamination of vegetables with pesticides has not been adequately studied so far (Tyagi et al., 2015; Pathak et al., 2010; Yagev and Koren, 2002; Perera et al., 2005; Rappazzo et al., 2016). An interesting paper with a captivating title, "Nowhere to hide: chemical toxicants and the unborn child" warns against the dangers hidden in otherwise healthy food, such as large fish, because of the possible contamination with mercury or other heavy metals, polychlorinated biphenyls, or dioxins (Genuis, 2009).

6. The "Poor and Obliged": The Main Side Effects of Low Quality in Vegetarian Diets

The high incidence of clinical problems related to nutritional deficits in pregnancies in low-resource environments is not surprising, considering the increased nutritional requirements that are often hard to be met by omnivorous individuals even in high-resource settings (Table 32.4).

The definition of a clinically relevant deficiency is, however, quite difficult, and its grading, of high importance in contextualizing the risks, is only rarely available. The case of iron deficiency is emblematic: a subtle iron deficiency is common and widespread all over the world; the "normal" levels of hemoglobin and hematocrit are usually set lower due to the hemodilution of pregnancy, compared to those of nonpregnant individuals. Mild anemia often develops in the final trimester, where it is reported in up to 30% of cases, and its clinical relevance is unclear (American College of Obstetricians and Gynecologists, 2008; Peña-Rosas et al., 2015). However, higher degrees of anemia are associated with an increase in adverse pregnancy-related outcomes, including SGA babies and preterm deliveries (American College of Obstetricians and Gynecologists, 2008; Peña-Rosas et al., 2015; Haider and Bhutta, 2015).

However, iron deficiency may not stand alone, particularly in the context of low food availability, as it could be associated with protein deficiencies (from a qualitative or quantitative view point) as well as calcium, zinc, vitamin B_{12}, or vitamin D deficits. Therefore, interpreting the findings may be difficult, and while pragmatic supporting programs with multiple integrations may be useful in such contexts, these considerations may warn against extrapolating results to "healthy and wealthy" vegetarian pregnancies (Gernand et al., 2016; Peña-Rosas et al., 2015; Haider and Bhutta, 2015; West et al., 2014; Persson et al., 2012; Ramakrishnan et al., 2012b).

Besides iron and vitamin B_{12} deficiencies, whose effects on pregnancy outcomes and on brain development are well known, some evidence is accumulating regarding calcium, phosphate, and vitamin D balance in pregnancy (Jathar and Inamdar-Deshmukh, 1981; Guez et al., 2012; Idris and Arsyad, 2012; Erdeve et al., 2009; Schlapbach et al., 2007; De-Regil et al., 2016; Bärebring et al., 2016; Achkar et al., 2015; Bodnar et al., 2014).

Table 32.4   Nutritional Requirements in Pregnancy [WHO (nutrition)]

	Daily Requirements	Note
Calories (added to the "usual" intake)	85 Kcal/day	First trimester
	285 Kcal/day	Second trimester
	475 Kcal/day	Third trimester
Proteins (added to the "usual" intake)	0.7 g/day	First trimester
	9.6 g/day	Second trimester
	31.2 g/day	Third trimester
Iron	30 mg/day	
Iodine	200 µg/day	
Calcium	1200 mg/day	
Magnesium	220 mg/day	
Zinc	11 mg/day	
Selenium	28 µg/day	Second trimester
	30 µg/day	Third trimester
Vitamin C	55 mg/day	
Thiamine	1.4 mg/day	
Riboflavin	1.4 mg/day	
Niacin	18 mg NE/day	NE = niacin equivalent
Vitamin B_6	1.9 mg/day	
Pantothenate	6.0 mg/day	
Biotin	30 µg/day	
Folate	600 µg DFE/day	DFE = dietary folate equivalent
Vitamin B_{12}	2.6 µg/day	
Vitamin A	800 RE/day	1 µg retinol = 1 RE
Vitamin D	5 µg/day	
Vitamin E	12 mg α-TE/day	No specific recommendation; no evidence of vitamin E requirements different from other adults
Vitamin K	55 µg/day	

A deficit in vitamin D and a low calcium intake have both been associated with an increased risk of hypertensive disorders of pregnancy. However, once more the results are conflicting and nonconsistent, leading to the suggestion of targeting supplementation toward confirmed deficiencies, at least in high-resource settings.

7. The "Nutritionally Disturbed": The Main Side Effects of Low Quantity in Vegetarian Diets

"Too healthy" may not in fact be "too good." An obsessive attitude toward food often merges with evident eating disorders and vegetarian patterns, and plant-based diets are frequently in question when such cases are described (O'Connor et al., 1987; Robinson-O'Brien et al., 2009; Bardone-Cone et al., 2012; Klopp et al., 2003; Forestell et al., 2012). Albeit rarely, pregnancy is also reported in patients with full-blown anorexia, but subtler imbalances may be difficult to identify; this is probably why data on pregnancies in women who have previously suffered from anorexia has led to conflicting results (Langley, 2014; Bulik et al., 2010; Solmi et al., 2014).

In such settings, the problem of low quantity food may add to the lack of variety in the diet, and anorexic patients in high-resource settings may present with the same clinical problems as those induced by poverty in low-resource settings.

From the point of view of research, while a high BMI is only rarely associated with plant-based diets, the association between plant-based diets, low BMI, and eating disorders may suggest the exclusion of individuals with low to very low BMI from the studies, to avoid a carry-over effect of alimentary disturbance in the analysis of the diets.

8. The "Sick and Controlled": The Benefits of the Vegetarian Diets in Counteracting Kidney Diseases

CKD is a heterogeneous condition in which low-protein diets have been a milestone in postponing the onset of end-stage kidney failure, or delaying the need for dialysis (Fouque and Laville, 2009; Mitch and Remuzzi, 2004). Pregnancy is increasingly frequent in advanced CKD, a population in which low-protein diets are increasingly needed in a growing number of settings (Piccoli et al., 2015d; Holley et al., 2015).

While some groups discontinue low-protein diets in pregnant CKD women, others mitigate the restriction or propose specific schemas. This is the case of our group that has adapted the moderately restricted vegetarian low-protein diets for pregnant patients, increasing the protein intake from about 0.6 to 0.8 g/Kg/day and integrating the major nutritional indications on calories, calcium, and oligo-elements prescribed in pregnant patients without CKD (Appleby and Key, 2015; Piccoli et al., 2011). The diet was basically vegan but was defined as vegetarian because it occasionally allowed milk and yogurt, and at least one (and up to three) unrestricted meals per week. Supplementation of essential amino acids and ketoacids was added, as has been described elsewhere in more detail (Appleby and Key, 2015; Piccoli et al., 2011).

A reevaluation of the results obtained over the last 15 years allowed us to compare 36 on-diet CKD pregnancies with 47 CKD control cases on unrestricted diets. In spite of having a similar baseline age, referral week, kidney function, hypertension, and proteinuria, the incidence of SGA (<10th centile) and/or extremely preterm babies (<28th week) was significantly lower in singletons from on-diet mothers than in the control cases (on diet: 12.9% vs. control cases: 33.3). This almost paradoxical finding of better fetal growth in on-diet patients as compared to control cases on unrestricted diets (mostly because of late referral or of milder disease) shifted our attention from the maternal kidneys to the maternal–fetal exchanges, suggesting a potential effect of the diet on the utero–placental axis (Attini et al.).

Once more, at least theoretically, a positive effect of plant-based diets could be due to a decrease in "vaso-toxic" elements or to an increase in "vaso-protective" factors; both are present in the study diet. A growing amount of data suggests that red meat consumption is associated with an increase in cardiovascular risk, while diets that are rich in vegetables, legumes, and grains (especially those with a low glycemic index) may be protective against endothelial dysfunction (Defagó et al., 2014; Nettleton et al., 2006; Lopez-Garcia et al., 2004; Wang and Mitch, 2011; Messina, 2014; Flight and Clifton, 2006; van den Broek et al., 2015). The specific advantage of vegetable proteins (soya) and of supplementation with ketoacids has been suggested in experimental models (Gao et al., 2010, 2011; Cahill et al., 2007; Bonacasa et al., 2011).

With the limitations of a small population, this data may suggest that vegetarian diets are safe during pregnancy even in fragile individuals, such as those with CKD; while a favorable trend was observed for all outcomes, it reached statistical significance for the most robust predictors of future health. Such findings may raise awareness not only of the specific issue of diet, CKD, and pregnancy, but also of the wider aspects of the interface between vegetarian diets and fetal growth.

9. Conclusions

Well-balanced, varied, and controlled vegan and vegetarian diets in pregnancy are nutritionally safe, and they are not associated with clinical problems in either mother nor child. However, the studies are still limited and highly heterogeneous, and the potential advantages of plant-based diets have to be balanced with the risks of protein malnutrition or trace element deficiencies. The favorable experience in patients with CKD may further stress this point. However, the problems described in low-resource settings, in which vegan diets are often the marker of poverty, warn against generalization. In vegetarian and in particular in vegan pregnant mothers, a close attention should be paid to the intake of key nutrients, in particular vitamin B_{12}, with a much varied diet, tailored control policies, and surveillance for even subtle eating disorders that can precipitate clinically relevant problems.

References

Abraham, R., 1982. Trace element intake by Asians during pregnancy. Proc. Nutr. Soc. 41, 261–265.

Abraham, R., Campbell-Brown, M., Haines, A., North, W., Hainsworth, V., McFadyen, I., 1985. Diet during pregnancy in an Asian community in Britain—energy, protein, zinc, copper, fiber and calcium. Hum. Nutr. Appl. Nutr. 39, 23–35.

Abu-Assal, M., Craig, W., 1984. The zinc status of pregnant vegetarian women. Nutr. Rep. Int. 29, 485–494.

Abugoch James, L.E., 2009. Quinoa (*Chenopodium quinoa* Willd.): composition, chemistry, nutritional, and functional properties. Adv. Food Nutr. Res. 58, 1–31.

Achkar, M., Dodds, L., Giguère, Y., Forest, J.C., Armson, B.A., Woolcott, C., Agellon, S., Spencer, A., Weiler, H.A., April 2015. Vitamin D status in early pregnancy and risk of preeclampsia. Am. J. Obstet. Gynecol. 212 (4), 511.e1–511.e7.

Albert, N.M., November-December 2005. We are what we eat: women and diet for cardiovascular health. J. Cardiovasc. Nurs. 20 (6), 451–460.

Alvarez-Jubete, L., Arendt, E.K., Gallagher, E., 2009. Nutritive value and chemical composition of pseudo-cereals as gluten-free ingredients. Int. J. Food Sci. Nutr. 60 (Suppl. 4), 240–257.

Alwan, N.A., Greenwood, D.C., Simpson, N.A.B., McArdle, H.J., Godfrey, K.M., Cade, J.E., 2011. Dietary iron intake during early pregnancy and birth outcomes in a cohort of British women. Hum. Reprod. 26, 911–919.

American College of Obstetricians and Gynecologists, July 2008. ACOG Practice Bulletin No. 95: anemia in pregnancy. Obstet. Gynecol. 112 (1), 201–207.

Aminu, M., Unkels, R., Mdegela, M., Utz, B., Adaji, S., van den Broek, N., September 2014. Causes of and factors associated with stillbirth in low- and middle-income countries: a systematic literature review. BJOG 121 (Suppl. 4), 141–153.

Appleby, P.N., Key, T.J., December 28, 2015. The long-term health of vegetarians and vegans. Proc. Nutr. Soc. 1–7 (Epub ahead of print).

Arora, P., Jha, P., Nagelkerke, N., May 2011. Association between history of tuberculosis and vegetarianism from a nationally representative survey in India. Int. J. Tuberc. Lung Dis. 15 (5), 706–708.

Asemi, Z., Samimi, M., Tabassi, Z., Esmaillzadeh, A., April 2014. The effect of DASH diet on pregnancy outcomes in gestational diabetes: a randomized controlled clinical trial. Eur. J. Clin. Nutr. 68 (4), 490–495.

Attini, R., et al., unpublished data.

Bardone-Cone, A.M., Fitzsimmons-Craft, E.E., Harney, M.B., Maldonado, C.R., Lawson, M.A., Smith, R., Robinson, D.P., August 2012. The inter-relationships between vegetarianism and eating disorders among females. J. Acad. Nutr. Diet. 112 (8), 1247–1252.

Bärebring, L., Bullarbo, M., Glantz, A., Leu Agelii, M., Jagner Å, E.J., Hulthén, L., Schoenmakers, I., Augustin, H., March 29, 2016. Preeclampsia and blood pressure trajectory during pregnancy in relation to vitamin D status. PLoS One 11 (3), e0152198.

Barsotti, G., Morelli, E., Cupisti, A., Meola, M., Dani, L., Giovannetti, S., 1996. A low-nitrogen low-phosphorus vegan diet for patients with chronic renal failure. Nephron 74 (2), 390–394.

Blumfield, M.L., Hure, A.J., Macdonald-Wicks, L., Smith, R., Collins, C.E., February 2013. A systematic review and meta-analysis of micronutrient intakes during pregnancy in developed countries. Nutr. Rev. 71 (2), 118–132.

Bodnar, L.M., Simhan, H.N., Catov, J.M., Roberts, J.M., Platt, R.W., Diesel, J.C., Klebanoff, M.A., March 2014. Maternal vitamin D status and the risk of mild and severe preeclampsia. Epidemiology 25 (2), 207–214.

Bonacasa, B., Siow, R.C., Mann, G.E., May 2011. Impact of dietary soy isoflavones in pregnancy on fetal programming of endothelial function in offspring. Microcirculation 18 (4), 270–285.

Brantsaeter, A.L., Haugen, M., Samuelsen, S.O., Torjusen, H., Trogstad, L., Alexander, J., Magnus, P., Meltzer, H.M., June 2009. A dietary pattern characterized by high intake of vegetables, fruits, and vegetable oils is associated with reduced risk of preeclampsia in nulliparous pregnant Norwegian women. J. Nutr. 139 (6), 1162–1168.

Bulik, C.M., Hoffman, E.R., Von Holle, A., Torgersen, L., Stoltenberg, C., Reichborn-Kjennerud, T., November 2010. Unplanned pregnancy in women with anorexia nervosa. Obstet. Gynecol. 116 (5), 1136–1140.

Cahill, L.E., Peng, C.Y., Bankovic-Calic, N., Sankaran, D., Ogborn, M.R., Aukema, H.M., January 2007. Dietary soya protein during pregnancy and lactation in rats with hereditary kidney disease attenuates disease progression in offspring. Br. J. Nutr. 97 (1), 77–84.

Campbell-Brown, M., Ward, R.J., Haines, A.P., North, W.R.S., Abraham, R., McFadyen, I.R., et al., 1985. Zinc and copper in Asian pregnancies-is there evidence for a nutritional deficiency? Br. J. Obstet. Gynaecol. 92, 875–885.

Carter, J.P., Furman, T., Hutcheson, H.R., 1987. Preeclampsia and reproductive performance in a community of vegans. South. Med. J. 80, 692–697.

34

Nutritional Profiles of Elderly Vegetarians

Stephen Walsh[1], Peter Deriemaeker[1,2], Marcel Hebbelinck[1], Peter Clarys[1,2]

[1]VRIJE UNIVERSITEIT BRUSSEL, BRUSSELS, BELGIUM; [2]ERASMUS UNIVERSITY COLLEGE, BRUSSELS, BELGIUM

1. Introduction

Diet continues to be important for good health even in the oldest old (Fraser and Shavlik, 1997), and meeting nutrient requirements becomes more challenging with increased age as energy requirements decrease with age (Henry, 2005).

This chapter looks at published reports on the nutritional profiles and nutrient status of elderly vegetarians and considers whether the observations presented point to any specific recommendations for elderly vegetarians or for further research. As there is very limited specific data available for elderly vegetarians, we will briefly consider evidence for vegetarians of all ages or for elderly people following all diets where this provides a useful context for the limited direct studies on elderly vegetarians. For details regarding nutritional status for many nutrients in adults and the general population, readers can refer to other chapters of this book (Section 5).

Studies are included on vegetarians with an average age greater than 65 that report on nutrient intakes, nutrient biomarkers, or other outcomes influenced by diet, such as body mass index (BMI), bone mineral density (BMD), blood pressure, and blood cholesterol.

2. Overview of Studies on Elderly Vegetarians

The studies available fall into three clusters: North America (usually Seventh-day Adventists), Western Europe, and Hong Kong and Taiwan Chinese (usually Buddhist or Taoist). Unless otherwise stated, the studies include both men and women.

2.1 North America

Gibson et al. (1983) report on trace metal status in 36 Canadian women (28 ovolactovegetarians and 8 vegans) with an average age of 69. Three-day dietary records were collected along with hair samples.

A series of US reports focused on BMD. Marsh et al. (1980, 1983) presented BMD results on Adventist ovolactovegetarian subjects in southwestern Michigan *by decade of age*. These results included BMD values for 32 female and 18 male vegetarians over the age of 60 compared with age-matched nonvegetarians. Marsh et al. (1988) reviewed these results and presented detailed diet comparisons, using a 7-day weighed diet record, comparing 10 ovolactovegetarians (average age 67) and matched Methodist nonvegetarians (average age 66).

Hunt et al. (1988, 1989) reported on 144 female Adventist vegetarians (average age 67) and matched nonvegetarians. A 24-h diet recall method was used. Tylavsky and Anderson (1988) reported on 88 female Adventist ovolactovegetarians (average age 73) compared with 287 nonvegetarians (average age 79). Reed et al. (1994) reported a 5-year follow-up of 189 participants in this study (average age 81 at end of follow-up). A Food Frequency Questionnaire (FFQ) was used.

Nieman et al. (1989) did not consider BMD but reported on the diet of 23 female Adventist vegetarians (average age 72) compared with 14 female nonvegetarians (average age 71) based on a 7-day food record.

Fraser and Shavlik (1997) reported on the oldest old (85 years or older) within the first Adventist Health Study, exploring links between diet and lifestyle and mortality. More than 1400 people were observed at age 85 or older. Of 603 participants who were 85 or older at baseline, 44% ate meat less than once a month. An FFQ was used.

Sarter et al. (2015) examined blood fatty acids and dietary intake in 165 vegans recruited via the Internet. Results were reported by age group and included those for 23 men and 19 women between 60 and 69 years and for 10 men and 17 women between 70 and 85.

2.2 Western Europe

Brants et al. (1990) and Löwik et al. (1990) reported results from a single study of 44 Dutch ovolactovegetarians or lactovegetarians (average age 82, 18 men and 26 women) living in a "vegetarian community" compared with 108 nonvegetarian elderly in a national survey (average age 72, 54 men and 54 women). Twenty-seven of the 44 vegetarians were institutionalized. Diet was assessed by a 2-week dietary recall. Comparative data for nonvegetarians was given as mean values without stating standard deviations or statistical significance. For this review, statistical significance was estimated approximately by assuming that the observed standard deviations for the omnivores are the same as for the vegetarians and using a two-sided *t*-test for the difference in means.

Davey et al. (2003) presented baseline BMI information by diet group and decade of age from the EPIC-Oxford cohort in the United Kingdom.

Deriemaeker et al. (2011) reported on 29 institutionalized ovolactovegetarians from the Netherlands (average age 83, 7 men and 22 women) and matched institutionalized nonvegetarians from the Dutch-speaking part of Belgium (average age 83, 7 men and 22 women). An FFQ was used to evaluate diet.

2.3 Chinese Vegetarians

Four reports are available on elderly Chinese vegetarian women in Hong Kong. Woo et al. (1998) reported on the nutritional status of 179 Chinese vegetarian women (average age 81) compared with 250 nonvegetarians (average age 71). The vegetarians were either Buddhist or Taoist and included a significant number of vegans. Nutrient intakes were assessed by 24-h recall. Lau et al. (1998) reported on BMD in 76 Buddhist vegetarian women (average age 79) compared with 109 nonvegetarians (average age 77). Kwok et al. (2002) reported in more detail on vitamin B_{12} and hematological status in 119 vegetarian women (average age 78) from the study by Woo et al. (1998). Kwok et al. (2003) focused on blood pressure and sodium and potassium intakes in 111 vegetarian women (average age 78).

Wang et al. (2008) compared BMD in 872 vegetarians and 993 nonvegetarians by sex and decade of age, based on observations in a Buddhist hospital in Taiwan. Two-thirds of the vegetarians drank milk.

Huang et al. (2011) reported on vegetarians compared with nonvegetarians within the Elderly Nutrition and Health Survey in Taiwan (all participants 65 years or older). The classification of vegetarians and vegans in this study was problematic in that it classified people as "vegetarians"/"vegans" ($n=269$) if between a third and all of their meals were vegetarian/vegan. There were also some results on "consistent" vegetarians (10 men and 31 women), who ate at least 90 vegetarian meals a month. Diets were assessed by 24-h recall.

While to a very good approximation the studies of European and North American elderly vegetarians are studies of ovolactovegetarians, the studies of Chinese elderly vegetarians include a significant number of vegans as well as ovolactovegetarians. The studies provide some comparisons between the different types of vegetarians, but in some cases the only result available is for all types of vegetarian combined.

3. Nutritional Profiles of Elderly Vegetarians

Based on studies of all age groups, typical vegetarian diets (Appleby et al., 2016; Clarys et al., 2014; Davey et al., 2003; Elorinne et al., 2016; Orlich et al., 2014; Rizzo et al., 2013) are higher in fruit, fiber, vitamin C, and folate than omnivorous diets but lower in EPA and DHA. They are often lower in saturated fat and in vitamins B_{12} and D, and sometimes lower in zinc, iodine, selenium, protein, or calcium. The bioavailability of iron and zinc may be lower in a vegetarian diet.

Milk makes little contribution to vitamin D intake unless it is fortified, but it makes a significant contribution to calcium, vitamin B_{12}, iodine, zinc, and protein intakes, while full fat dairy products make a major contribution to saturated fat intake (Bates et al., 2014).

Milk intake of lactovegetarians is often lower than that of nonvegetarians, though this is not a consistent pattern. For vegans, calcium intake is sometimes low, and this has been associated with increased risk of fracture (Appleby et al., 2007).

The differences in nutritional profiles and diet-related biomarkers in general studies of vegetarians may have a particular significance in elderly people as food intakes decline and loss of muscle and risk of fracture become significant health issues.

This review starts with general health outcomes and then considers intermediate measures such as BMI and BMD before moving on to macronutrients and micronutrients. Markers of nutrient intake such as hair or blood measurements will be considered alongside estimates of dietary intake. The review will focus on aspects of nutritional profile that are considered potentially significant for health.

3.1 Diet and Death

Fraser and Shavlik (1997) examined diet, lifestyle, and death rates in Adventists aged 85 years or more. Dietary intakes suggested a health-conscious population: 90% of the subjects used whole meal bread rather than white bread, and two-thirds ate two or more servings of fruit a day. Three diet and lifestyle factors were significantly associated with all-cause mortality: one or more doughnuts a week versus none was associated with increased death rates [Relative Risk (RR) 1.24]; nuts 5 or more times a week versus less than once a week was associated with decreased death rates (RR 0.82); moderate and high activity levels were both associated with decreased death rates compared with low activity (RRs of 0.81, 0.80).

These three factors were also found to play a key role in the overall Adventist population (Fraser and Shavlik, 2001). Fraser and Shavlik (2001) also showed a significant advantage for vegetarians over nonvegetarians that was not apparent in the older subgroup considered in Fraser and Shavlik (1997): red meat intake was not associated with all-cause mortality, though it was associated with death from coronary heart disease in men.

There was an increased risk of death in the lowest quartile of BMI versus higher quartiles, but this largely disappeared when the first 6 years of follow-up were excluded. Unintentional weight loss in elderly people is often a marker of ill health.

Fraser and Shavlik (1997) confirm that at least some diet and lifestyle choices continue to predict longevity in the oldest old.

3.2 BMI and Energy Intake

Reported BMI in European and North American studies is usually lower in vegetarians than in nonvegetarians and lowest in vegans (Davey et al., 2003; Rizzo et al., 2013). Such a difference was not apparent in Vietnamese vegans (Ho-Pham et al., 2012) but was seen in South Korean vegetarians (Kim et al., 2007).

Estimated energy intakes are sometimes reported as notably lower in vegetarians than in nonvegetarians (Davey et al., 2003). This may be partly attributed to the limitations of FFQs in measuring diet, particularly portion sizes. The expected differences in required energy intake based on the observed differences in BMI are too small to be reliably measured. Where large differences in estimated energy intakes appear when comparing diet groups, these may point to a limitation in the measurement rather than a real difference.

Woo et al. (1998) found a very similar BMI distribution in vegetarian and nonvegetarian women in Hong Kong, with a median of 22.5 kg/m² for the vegetarians and 22.3 kg/m² for the nonvegetarians.

Tylavsky and Anderson (1988) found significantly *higher* BMI in vegetarians (31.5 vs. 30.1 kg/m$^{1.5}$). Note that they measured BMI as weight divided by height to the power of 1.5. In the usual units the values would be 25 versus 23.9 kg/m². The fact that the nonvegetarians were 6 years older than the vegetarians may have influenced the result.

Other studies reported BMIs in vegetarians that were numerically lower than nonvegetarians but mostly not significant (NS): Nieman et al. (1989), 22.8 versus 24.2[NS] kg/m²; Löwik et al. (1990), 23.5 versus 25.5[NS] kg/m² in men and 24.7 versus 27.1 kg/m² in women; Deriemaeker et al. (2011), 23.5 versus 25.2[NS] kg/m² in men and 26.1 versus 26.8[NS] kg/m² in women. The differences in BMI in Löwik et al. (1990) may be in part due to the vegetarians being 10 years older.

Löwik et al. (1990) reported body fat percentage and skinfold measurements. Body fat followed the same pattern as BMI with vegetarians showing lower values (25.9% vs. 29.5% in men and 34.7% vs. 39.9% in women). Skinfold measurements in vegetarians were also lower than in nonvegetarians. Deriemaeker et al. (2011) reported waist-to-hip ratio and skinfold measurements. Waist-to-hip ratio was consistent with BMI (0.91 vs. 0.94[NS] in men and 0.90 vs. 0.90[NS] in women). The subscapular skinfold was significantly lower in vegetarian women (9.2 vs. 13.5 mm), but other skinfold measurements were similar in vegetarians and nonvegetarians.

Davey et al. (2003) report BMI by diet group and age group for the EPIC-Oxford cohort at baseline (Fig. 34.1). This shows a clear trend toward lower BMI both with age and with increasing exclusion of animal products.

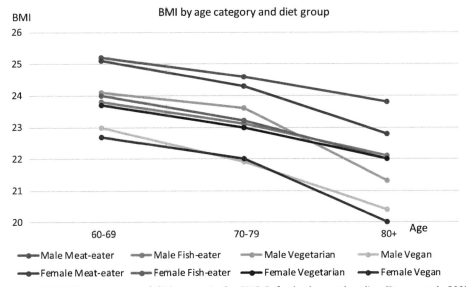

FIGURE 34.1 BMI by sex, age, and diet group, in the EPIC-Oxford cohort at baseline (Davey et al., 2003).

It is noteworthy that the difference in BMI between the various diet groups does not decline with age; instead, it appears to widen. In the EPIC-Oxford cohort, this would translate to a significant prevalence of underweight in vegans in old age. This is less likely to be the case in Adventist cohorts, where the average BMIs are higher in all diet groups, ranging from 28.3 in meat eaters to 24.1 in vegans (Rizzo et al., 2013).

In general, the studies of older vegetarians confirm the finding that BMI decreases with increasing restriction of foods derived from animals at least in Europe and North America. This effect may be conditional on other factors, since it does not appear as consistently in Asian studies as in European and North American studies. While such a decrease is favorable against a background of overweight and obesity, it may not be desirable in all elderly people.

BMI is a crude measure of body composition, and the use of additional and more direct measures of body fat and its distribution is desirable.

3.3 Blood Cholesterol and Related Nutrients (Fats, Cholesterol, Fiber)

Vegans generally have the lowest intakes of saturated fat and the highest intakes of fiber and show lower blood levels of cholesterol than other vegetarians who (usually) show lower blood cholesterol than nonvegetarians (Bradbury et al., 2014).

Most studies of older vegetarians found the cholesterol levels of vegetarians to be lower than those of nonvegetarians: Nieman et al. (1989), 5.62 versus 6.46 mmol/L; Löwik et al. (1990), 4.3 versus 6.0 mmol/L in men and 5.5 versus 6.5 mmol/L in women; Woo et al. (1998), 4.8 versus 5.9 mmol/L. Differences in the ratio of total to HDL cholesterol were less consistent and often NS: Nieman et al. (1989), 3.66 versus 3.80[NS]; and Löwik et al. (1990), 4.83 versus 6.13 for men and 5.66 versus 5.17[NS] for women.

Deriemaeker et al. (2011) found slightly *higher* cholesterol levels in ovolactovegetarians (5.5 mmol/L) than in nonvegetarians (4.9 mmol/L). The vegetarians in this study showed slightly lower intakes of saturated fat (31.4 vs. 33.4[NS] g/day in men and 25.4 vs. 32.2 g/day in women) and monounsaturated fat (28.8 vs. 39.1[NS] g/day in men and 22.8 vs. 37.1 g/day in women) but similar intakes of cholesterol (181 vs. 208[NS] mg/day in men and 161 vs. 205[NS] mg/day in women), fiber (28 vs. 36[NS] g/day in men and 28 vs. 32[NS] in women), and polyunsaturated fat (14.3 vs. 13.8[NS] g/day in men and 13.4 vs. 12.2[NS] g/day in women). Differences in dietary factors influencing cholesterol levels were therefore modest and in conflicting directions. In addition, the use of cholesterol-reducing drugs was not recorded and could significantly affect the results.

Cholesterol intakes are usually lower in vegetarians than in nonvegetarians: Marsh et al. (1988), 194 versus 294 mg/day; Tylavsky and Anderson (1988), 167 versus 305 mg/day; Nieman et al. (1989), 89 versus 183 mg/day; Brants et al. (1990), 200 versus 355 mg/day in men and 215 versus 294 mg/day in women; and Huang et al. (2011), 45 versus 182 mg/day in men and 24 versus 164 mg/day in women.

Saturated fat intakes are usually lower in vegetarians than in nonvegetarians: Nieman et al. (1989), 7.6% versus 10.9% (of energy); Brants et al. (1990), 15.0% versus 17.3% in men and 15.8% versus 17.2%[NS] in women; and Huang et al. (2011), 3.3% versus 7.1%[NS] in men and 4.7% versus 7.7%[NS] in women.

The ratio of polyunsaturated fat to saturated fat (P/S) is usually higher in vegetarians: Marsh et al. (1988), 0.75 versus 0.48; Nieman et al. (1989), 0.85 versus 0.5; Brants et al. (1990), 0.65 versus 0.42 in men and 0.62 versus 0.40 in women; and Huang et al. (2011), 1.9 versus 1[NS] in men and 1.8 versus 1 in women.

Fiber intakes are usually higher in vegetarians than in nonvegetarians. Marsh et al. (1988) found no significant difference in crude fiber intakes for vegetarians versus non-vegetarians (5.2 vs. 4.7[NS] g/day), while Tylavsky and Anderson (1988) found a significant difference (5.6 vs. 4.2 g/day). Other reports refer to total fiber rather than crude fiber. Total dietary fiber intake is approximately five times crude fiber intake. Total fiber intakes were generally higher in vegetarians: Nieman et al. (1989), 21.5 versus 13 g/day; Brants et al. (1990), 34 versus 27 g/day in men and 29 versus 24 g/day in women; and Huang et al. (2011), 29.1 versus 16.6 g/day in men and 25.4 versus 16.6[NS] g/day in women.

Overall, the results on blood cholesterol in elderly populations are consistent with those in younger adults in showing reduced cholesterol levels with restriction of animal products, driven mainly by reduced saturated fat and cholesterol intake along with higher P/S ratio and higher fiber.

3.4 Blood Pressure and Related Nutrients

Vegetarian and plant-based diets have been shown in randomized trials to reduce blood pressure (Margetts et al., 1986; Appel et al., 1997). This effect occurs even if sodium intake does not differ, and it is only partly explained by potassium intake.

There have been few comparisons of blood pressure between elderly vegetarians and nonvegetarians: Löwik et al. (1990), 143/76 versus 151[NS]/85 mm Hg in men and 153/79 versus 156[NS]/88 mm Hg in women (differences in diastolic blood pressure were significant); and Woo et al. (1998), 150/76 versus 143/79.

The vegetarians studied in Woo et al. (1998) were further analyzed by Kwok et al. (2003), who found that hypertensive vegetarians (64% of subjects with blood pressure > 140/90) had higher urinary sodium to creatinine ratios, higher sodium to potassium ratios, and lower calcium intakes than normotensive vegetarians. Comparing vegetarians with both low sodium to potassium ratio and high calcium intake with those with both high sodium to potassium ratio and low calcium intake showed a substantial difference in systolic blood pressure (130 vs. 159) and prevalence of hypertension (78% vs. 25%). The prevalence of hypertension was similar in vegans and lactovegetarians (70% vs. 56%[NS]).

Comparisons of elderly vegetarians and nonvegetarians have found that vegetarians have similar or higher potassium intakes: Tylavsky and Anderson (1988), 2600 versus 2600[NS] mg/day; Nieman et al. (1989), 2600 versus 2300[NS] mg/day; Löwik et al. (1990), 2700 versus 2600[NS] mg/day in men and 2500 versus 2200[NS] mg/day in women (based on 24-h urine samples); Woo et al. (1998), 7.7 versus 4.3 mmol potassium/mmol creatinine; and Deriemaeker et al. (2011), 4000 versus 3100 mg/day in men and 3200 versus 3200[NS] mg/day in women.

Most comparisons of elderly vegetarians and nonvegetarians have found that vegetarians have similar or lower sodium intakes: Tylavsky and Anderson (1988), 1900 versus 1900[NS] mg/day; Nieman et al. (1989), 1900 versus 1900[NS] mg/day; Löwik et al. (1990), 2000 versus 3400 mg/day in men and 1900 versus 2700 mg/day in women (based on 24-h urine samples); and Deriemaeker et al. (2011), 4100 versus 4900[NS] mg/day in men and 2900 versus 4900 mg/day in women. In contrast, Woo et al. (1998) found higher urinary sodium in the vegetarians: 30.3 versus 17.5 mmol sodium/mmol creatinine.

3.5 Bone Mineral Density and Related Nutrients

A meta-analysis by Ho-Pham et al. (2009) concluded that BMD in lactovegetarians was about 2% lower than for nonvegetarians at both the femoral neck and the lumbar spine and about 6% lower for vegans. Readers may refer to Chapter 17 for further review of vegan bone health. Ho-Pham et al. (2009) categorize the vegetarians in most Asian studies as vegans, though this is an oversimplification. In Wang et al. (2008), two-thirds of the vegetarians consumed some animal milk. In Lau et al. (1998) about half the vegetarians were vegan, and separate results were provided for vegans and other vegetarians, but in the meta-analysis all the vegetarians were treated as vegan. Although the meta-analysis indicated statistically significant differences, the magnitude of the estimated effect was small and may be exaggerated slightly due to confounding by age differences, e.g., in Chiu et al. (1997).

Most of the BMD studies discussed subsequently were excluded from the meta-analysis by Ho-Pham et al. (2009), which only considered BMD measurements at the hip or lumbar spine. Most of the studies discussed in Ho-Pham et al. (2009) were excluded from this chapter, as the average age was too low. Lau et al. (1998) and Wang et al. (2008) are included in both the meta-analysis and this review.

BMD declines with age from about 30 years, with a particularly rapid decline in women in the decade after menopause.

Marsh et al. (1980) reported much better BMD for the radius in elderly female vegetarians than in matched elderly nonvegetarians. For example, based on 19 pairs between 60 and 69 years old, the vegetarians showed a BMD of 0.623 versus 0.559 g/cm^2. This large and statistically significant difference was not observed in a later study of men (Marsh et al., 1983), which reported 0.78 versus 0.77[NS] g/cm^2 in the same age range.

Marsh et al. (1988) reported on a 7-day weighed dietary record for 10 vegetarians and matched nonvegetarians. The ratio of calcium to phosphorus was higher for the vegetarians than the nonvegetarians (0.81 vs. 0.66), while calcium (900 vs. 710[NS] mg/day) and protein (56 vs. 68[NS] g/day) intakes were similar.

The work by Marsh et al. was followed by further studies on vegetarian diet and BMD (Tylavsky and Anderson, 1988; Hunt et al., 1989; Reed et al., 1994), which found no significant differences in BMD or rate of change in BMD between vegetarians and nonvegetarians. Tylavsky and Anderson (1988) found BMD for vegetarians compared with nonvegetarians to be 0.32 versus 0.32[NS] g/cm^2 at the distal radius and 0.546 versus 0.563[NS] g/cm^2 at the mid-radius after adjustment for age. Hunt et al. (1989) found 0.570 versus 0.573[NS] g/cm² at the cortical radius after adjustment for age. BMD values by decade of age showed no significant differences. Reed et al. (1994) followed up on Tylavsky and Anderson (1988) and found no impact of vegetarian diet or calcium intake on rate of change of BMD but observed a protective effect of lean body mass.

In contrast, Lau et al. (1998) found lower BMD for elderly female vegetarians in Hong Kong compared with nonvegetarians (0.70 vs. 0.72[NS] g/cm² for the spine, 0.49 vs. 0.53 g/cm² for the neck of the femur, 0.69 vs. 0.73[NS] g/cm² for the intertrochantic area). The vegetarians were on average just 2 years older than the nonvegetarians, so age is unlikely to be a confounding factor. BMD measurements of the 36 vegans were similar to those of the 40 lactovegetarians (0.72 vs. 0.68[NS] g/cm² for the spine, 0.50 vs. 0.48[NS] g/cm² for the neck of the femur, and 0.69 vs. 0.69[NS] g/cm² for the intertrochantic area). Total calcium intakes were similarly low in both vegetarians and nonvegetarians (around 400 mg/day): vegetarians had both a lower energy intake (1142 vs. 1557 kcal) and a higher calcium intake relative to energy intake (338 vs. 221 mg/1000 kcal). The much lower reported energy intake in vegetarians is not explained by age or weight and may well underestimate the actual energy intake. Sodium excretion in urine was 50% higher in vegetarians compared with nonvegetarians, and protein intake was much lower in vegetarians (35 vs. 60 g/day). A regression analysis did not find any significant relationships between nutrient intakes and BMD. Other reports (Woo et al., 1998; Kwok et al., 2002) have indicated low vitamin B_{12} levels in these vegetarians (see Section 6.2).

Wang et al. (2008) studied 872 vegetarians and 993 nonvegetarians who attended a Buddhist hospital. Differences in BMD were NS in either men or women, though in both cases the average BMD in the vegetarians was about 2% lower. Graphs of BMD by decade of age for vegetarians and nonvegetarians tracked each other very closely, with both showing a drop in BMD of about 25% with age. Analyses of the risk of osteopenia or osteoporosis showed no difference in either men or women between the third of the vegetarians who did not drink milk and the milk-drinking vegetarians.

Calcium intakes in elderly US and European ovolactovegetarians are generally similar to those in elderly nonvegetarians: Marsh et al. (1988), 900 versus 710[NS] mg/day; Hunt et al. (1988), both slightly below the RDA; Tylavsky and Anderson (1988), 823 versus 902[NS] mg/day; Nieman et al. (1989), 628 versus 633[NS] mg/day; Brants et al. (1990), 1219 versus 1128[NS] mg/day in men and 1141 versus 1013[NS] mg/day in women; and Deriemaeker et al. (2011), 1096 versus 969[NS] mg/day in men and 894 versus 858[NS] mg/day in women.

Huang et al. (2011) found higher calcium intakes in "consistent" vegetarians (consuming at least 90 vegetarian meals a month) versus nonvegetarians: 745 versus 423 mg/day in men and 749 versus 439 mg/day in women. This result is unusual in showing calcium intakes in Asian vegetarians comparable with those of European and North American vegetarians.

Overall, studies of BMD in elderly vegetarians are consistent with those at younger ages in showing at most a slight disadvantage to vegetarians. The results of Marsh et al. (1980) suggesting a substantial beneficial effect of vegetarianism must be viewed as an outlier, given the results of later studies. Further studies of elderly and very elderly vegetarians who consume little or no milk are needed to establish whether the study by Lau et al. (1998) is an outlier in the other direction or highlights a real concern about certain vegetarian diets, such as low protein or vitamin B_{12} or high sodium.

4. Energy Macronutrients

4.1 Protein Intake

Protein intakes are sometimes but not always lower in vegetarians, particularly in vegans, and intakes of lysine may be particularly low (Schmidt et al., 2016). Low protein levels may lead to low IGF-1 levels in vegans with low soya protein intakes (Allen et al., 2002; Fontana et al., 2008). Some studies find protein intakes to be comparable regardless of the degree of exclusion of animal products (Rizzo et al., 2013).

Most studies of the elderly report ovolactovegetarians to have slightly lower protein intakes than nonvegetarians: Marsh et al. (1988), 56 versus 68[NS] g/day; Tylavsky and Anderson (1988), 55 versus 70 g/day; Nieman et al. (1989), 12.9% versus 16.2% of energy; Brants et al. (1990), 60 versus 82 g/day in men and 54 versus 70 g/day in women; and Deriemaeker et al. (2011), 17.8% versus 21.0%[NS] of energy in men and 17.3% versus 19.5% in women. Huang et al. (2011) report essentially no difference between consistent vegetarians and nonvegetarians: 16.3% versus 16.6%[NS] for men 15.7% versus 16%[NS] in women. Lau et al. (1998) report a particularly large difference between vegetarians and nonvegetarians: 35 versus 60 g/day.

None of these studies indicated any functional consequences of the lower protein intake, though the intakes reported by Lau et al. (1998) would not be expected to be adequate. In general, the studies of elderly vegetarians are consistent with those of younger vegetarians.

4.2 Total Fat

Most studies of the elderly report vegetarians to have lower fat intakes as a percentage of energy intake: Marsh et al. (1988), 36% versus 42%[NS]; Tylavsky and Anderson (1988), 33% versus 39%; Nieman et al. (1989), 32% versus 36%[NS]; Brants et al. (1990), 37% versus 41% in men and 37% versus 40% in women; Woo et al. (1998), 14% versus 19%; and Huang et al. (2011), 16.6% versus 24.9%[NS] for men 21.3% versus 26.4%[NS] in women. Deriemaeker et al. (2011) found no difference: 33% versus 33%[NS] in men and 35% versus 35%[NS] in women.

The differences between countries show a stronger effect than the differences between vegetarians and nonvegetarians: vegetarians in the United States and Europe consume more fat than nonvegetarians in Hong Kong and Taiwan.

4.3 Carbohydrate

Typically, carbohydrate intake as a percentage of energy is increased by 5%–10% in vegetarians at the expense of protein and/or fat: Tylavsky and Anderson (1988), 56% versus 46%; Nieman et al. (1989), 60% versus 50%; Brants et al. (1990), 51% versus 42% in men and

50% versus 43% in women; Woo et al. (1998), 75% versus 64%; Deriemaeker et al. (2011), 48% versus 42%[NS] in men and 48% versus 43% in women; and Huang et al. (2011), 68% versus 57%[NS] in men 61% versus 57%[NS] in women.

4.4 Sugar (Mono- and Di-Saccharides)

Studies on elderly vegetarians report sugar intake to be substantial and slightly greater in vegetarians than nonvegetarians: Nieman et al. (1989), 21.5% versus 18.5%[NS] of energy; Brants et al. (1990), 25.3% versus 21.1% in men and 26.8% versus 22.0% in women; and Deriemaeker et al. (2011), 32.8% versus 26.5%[NS] in men and 33.8% versus 27.9%[NS] in women.

It is not clear how much of this high sugar intake is contributed by free or added sugar, which could be of importance for health. Deriemaeker et al. (2011) observed a considerable intake of added sugar from biscuits and pastries in both vegetarians and nonvegetarians.

4.5 Omega-3 Fatty Acids

Sarter et al. (2015) found that the proportion of eicosapentaenoic acid (EPA, 20:5n-3) plus docosahexaenoic acid (DHA, 22:6n-3) in red blood cells was slightly higher in older vegans (about 4%) than younger vegans (about 3.5%), but this trend disappeared after adjustment for dietary alpha-linolenic acid (ALA, 18:3n-3). This study reported the proportion in a sample of US soldiers to be similar to that of the younger vegans (3.5%).

We found no other results on ALA, EPA, and DHA in elderly vegetarians. This is potentially an important omission as direct dietary intakes of EPA and DHA in vegetarians are low so that vegetarians rely mainly on conversion of ALA. Poor zinc status may impair this conversion (Knez et al., 2016).

Low EPA and DHA are hypothesized to have adverse effects on death rates, dementia, and mood. However, none of these effects have been observed in vegetarians (Giem et al., 1993; Beezhold et al., 2010; Orlich et al., 2013), suggesting that either the actual impact is low or that other factors in vegetarian diets outweigh any adverse effect.

5. Minerals

5.1 Iron

Iron intakes can be higher in vegetarians and vegans than in nonvegetarians, but iron stores (ferritin levels) are consistently lower in vegetarians (Hunt, 2003), as nonheme iron is less absorbable, and its absorption is almost inversely proportional to ferritin levels: as iron stores approach depletion, the absorption of heme and nonheme iron becomes similar (Hallberg et al., 1997; Hallberg and Hulthén, 2000). The lower stores in vegetarians do not seem to translate to increased iron deficiency (Hunt, 2003). The reader may refer to Chapter 39 for a general review.

Guralnik et al. (2004) report that in the general population in the United States, prevalence of anemia increases substantially with age within the elderly population, and only about a third of anemia in people over 65 is explained by nutritional deficiencies. Nieman et al. (1989) found no evidence of differences in iron status between vegetarian and non-vegetarian women. Average hemoglobin levels were above 14 g/dL in both groups, and no participants had hemoglobin levels below 12.

Löwik et al. (1990) found lower hemoglobin levels in vegetarians, but based on a regression model included in this paper, this was accounted for by the vegetarians being about 10 years older. As expected, ferritin levels were much lower in the vegetarians (42 vs. 85 μg/L). Based on the same study, Brants et al. (1990) reported that the percentage of women with ferritin levels below 12 μg/L was similar in vegetarians and nonvegetarians (about 10%), but three out of 17 vegetarian men showed low ferritin compared to one out of 54 nonvegetarian men. The difference for men was statistically significant (P = .04), but the difference for men and women combined was not (P = .3).

Woo et al. (1998) found lower hemoglobin in vegetarian women compared with non-vegetarian women (12.3 vs. 13.4 g/dL), and 30% of vegetarians had levels below 12 compared with 10% of nonvegetarians. However, the prevalence of iron deficiency appeared similar among vegetarians and nonvegetarians, and only 15% of the anemic vegetarians showed confirmed iron deficiency. The vegetarians were about 10 years older than the nonvegetarians, which may partly explain their higher levels of anemia.

Deriemaeker et al. (2011) found very similar hemoglobin levels in vegetarians and non-vegetarians. Average ferritin levels were much lower in vegetarians compared with non-vegetarians (66 vs. 159 μg/L), but incidence of abnormally low ferritin values was similar.

Taken as a whole, the comparisons between elderly vegetarians and nonvegetarians suggest no clear difference in the prevalence of iron deficiency despite a clear difference in ferritin levels. In looking at anemia in the elderly, it is particularly important that comparisons are made between age-matched subjects.

5.2 Zinc

Bioavailability of zinc may be lower in vegetarian diets, particularly if phytate intake is high (Hunt, 2003). Vegetarian zinc intakes are sometimes also reported to be lower than nonvegetarian intakes (Davey et al., 2003). A meta-analysis by Foster et al. (2013) found serum zinc levels in vegetarians to be about 1 μmol/L lower than for nonvegetarians. This is a modest effect set against a normal range of about 10–25 μmol/L but may be significant for some people. Readers may refer to Chapter 38 for a detailed review of the general topic.

The ZINCAGE study, which included over 1000 healthy elderly people from the general population in five European countries, provides a useful picture of trends in fasting plasma zinc with age. Linear regression indicated that levels fall from about 12.5 μmol/L at 65 to about 11.2 μmol/L at 90 (Giacconi et al., 2016). The scatter plot of plasma zinc versus age is consistent with an accelerated decline at ages above 80, and Mariani et al. (2008) note that almost half those over 90 had plasma zinc levels below 10 μmol/L.

The estimated decline in fasting plasma zinc level with age was reduced by a quarter on adjustment for blood albumin and was only slightly further attenuated by adjustment for dietary zinc intake, though zinc intake also declined with age. This suggests that the decline is more related to the physiology of aging than to changes in dietary intakes, though it is also possible that variations in zinc bioavailability obscure the effect of changes in dietary intakes.

Marcellini et al. (2006), in an earlier report on the ZINCAGE study, presented fasting plasma zinc levels by 5-year age band and country, showing a striking difference between countries, ranging from Greece (average of 11.3 µmol/L) to France (average of 14.2 µmol/L). Hotz et al. (2003) reported a median level of 13 µmol/L for 75-year-olds in the United States, and De Paula et al. (2014) reported a median level of 15 µmol/L in people over 80 in Brazil. There seems to be substantial variability in average levels between different populations.

Löwik et al. (1990) found average levels of serum zinc in vegetarians to be much lower than in nonvegetarians (12.4 µmol/L vs. 16.4 µmol/L). Brants et al. (1990) further reported that nine out of 40 vegetarians had zinc levels below 11.5 µmol/L compared with two out of 108 nonvegetarians ($P=.0001$). As previously noted, the vegetarians were about 10 years older than the nonvegetarians in this study, but this is not enough to realistically explain such a large difference. The nonvegetarian average (16.4 µmol/L) seems rather high relative to the ZINCAGE study results discussed earlier, while the vegetarian levels seem unexceptional.

Deriemaeker et al. (2011) found similar levels of serum zinc in vegetarians (9.5 µmol/L) and nonvegetarians (9.9 µmol/L). These levels are strikingly low compared with other reports on elderly people and are lower than the lowest result for 80- to 84-year-olds among the five countries in the ZINCAGE study (11.2 µmol/L in Greece).

Zinc levels are known to decrease after meals (Hotz et al., 2003), but this does not explain the difference between the two studies, as Löwik et al. (1990) used nonfasting samples and Deriemaeker et al. (2011) used fasting samples. Brants et al. (1990) reported zinc intakes of 8 mg/day in vegetarians compared with about 10 mg/day in nonvegetarians. Deriemaeker et al. (2011) reported zinc intakes of 13 versus 12[NS] mg/day. This, again, does not explain the lower plasma levels in Deriemaeker et al. (2011), but the fact that all subjects in Deriemaeker et al. (2011) were institutionalized may be relevant.

Zinc levels in elderly vegetarians deserve further study, as do zinc levels in the oldest old population generally. In the absence of clear reference values for plasma zinc in the oldest old, careful age matching is essential for comparisons between diet groups.

5.3 Selenium

Gibson et al. (1983) found hair selenium levels and dietary intakes of selenium to be similar between vegetarians and nonvegetarians. This study was carried out in Canada, where wheat is a good source of selenium. Selenium is only an issue for vegetarians if most plant foods used are grown in soil low in selenium. The reader may refer to Chapter 40 for a review.

5.4 Iodine

Iodine intakes are best measured based on urinary excretion rather than diet analysis as the iodine content of plant foods varies considerably depending on where they are grown. Iodine intakes are often low in vegans, but can be very high if seaweed is consumed.

The studies of elderly vegetarians are largely silent on this, but Löwik et al. (1990) report much higher iodine excretion in vegetarians both for men (765 vs. 122 µg/day) and for women (660 vs. 101 µg/day), suggesting significant use of seaweed. The reader may refer to Chapter 42 for a review.

6. Vitamins

6.1 Folate

In line with studies on younger vegetarians, most studies on elderly vegetarians report that vegetarians have higher folate intakes and higher blood levels of folate than nonvegetarians: Nieman et al. (1989), 273 versus 215[NS] µg/day; Löwik et al. (1990), 12.7 versus 6.6 µmol/L in men and 14.2 versus 7.3 µmol/L in women; and Deriemaeker et al. (2011), 22 versus 16.5[NS] µmol/L.

6.2 Vitamin B_{12}

Homocysteine levels in vegetarians, and particularly in vegans, are often found to be high as a consequence of low vitamin B_{12} status (Elmadfa and Singer, 2009). Vitamin B_{12} status in vegetarians is improved by use of animal milks, foods fortified with vitamin B_{12}, or vitamin B_{12} supplements.

Nieman et al. (1989) found estimated intakes in US Adventist vegetarians to be similar to nonvegetarians (2.3 vs. 2.6[NS] µg/day).

Löwik et al. (1990) found lower blood levels of vitamin B_{12} in vegetarians than nonvegetarians (205 vs. 278 pmol/L). Mean corpuscular volume (MCV) in the vegetarians studied was higher than in nonvegetarians (95 vs. 91 fL in men and 94 vs. 89 fL in women). The vegetarian MCV levels were close to the top of the reference range (80–96 fL). Brants et al. (1990) reported that 9 out of 40 vegetarians showed blood vitamin $B_{12} < 138$ pmol/L compared with five out of 108 nonvegetarians ($P = .002$). The fact that the vegetarians were 10 years older may play a part in these differences, as poor absorption of vitamin B_{12} becomes more common with increasing age.

In contrast, Deriemaeker et al. (2011) found no disadvantage in blood vitamin B_{12} levels in elderly institutionalized vegetarians compared with nonvegetarians. The vegetarians in this study had similar average vitamin B_{12} levels (430 vs. 340[NS] pmol/L). The prevalence of low vitamin B_{12} values (<160 pmol/L) was also comparable in vegetarians (7 out of 22) and nonvegetarians (7 out of 26, $P = .76$).

Brants et al. (1990) reported that dairy products contributed 87% of the vitamin B_{12} intake of the vegetarians in their study population. Both Brants et al. (1990) and Deriemaeker et al. (2011) found calcium intakes to be fairly high in both vegetarians (1170 and 940 mg/day) and nonvegetarians (1060 and 880 mg/day), suggesting important use of dairy in all groups. Dairy intake as estimated through calcium intake therefore does not explain why blood vitamin B_{12} levels in vegetarians were twice as high in Deriemaeker et al. (2011) as in Löwik et al. (1990).

Woo et al. (1998) and Kwok et al. (2002) found a high prevalence of biochemical vitamin B_{12} deficiency in elderly Chinese vegetarian women and also a high prevalence of anemia.

Woo et al. (1998) reported that low vitamin B_{12} values (<150 pmol/L) were common among the vegetarians, but not notably more common among anemic vegetarians (58%) than among nonanemic vegetarians (52%).

Kwok et al. (2002) analyzed the same population but included an analysis of serum methylmalonic acid (MMA). Elevated serum MMA is a marker of vitamin B_{12} deficiency. Elevated MMA was associated with increased prevalence of anemia. The increase in anemia was statistically significant for serum MMA above 1 µmol/L, though even in this group only a third of the anemia was macrocytic (the form associated with clinical vitamin B_{12} deficiency). Poor renal function can cause both anemia and elevated MMA, but subjects with elevated serum creatinine were excluded to try to minimize this effect.

Subjects showing both vitamin B_{12} greater than 150 pmol/L and serum MMA below 0.4 µmol/L were classified as *not* vitamin B_{12} deficient (24%). Subjects with one indicator of vitamin B_{12} deficiency were classified as possibly deficient (29%), while subjects with both indicators of deficiency were classified as definitely deficient (47%). Hemoglobin levels were higher in those who were not deficient in vitamin B_{12} (13 vs. 12.3 g/dL). Definite vitamin B_{12} deficiency was associated with consuming neither animal milk nor vitamin B_{12} supplements, even though milk consumption by those who did use it was noted to be infrequent. Calcium intake in this population was about 400 mg/day in both vegetarians and nonvegetarians, which is qualitatively lower than in North American and European populations.

In general, the picture for vitamin B_{12} for elderly vegetarians seems similar to that in younger populations: vitamin B_{12} deficiency is more likely in vegetarians than nonvegetarians if and only if the intake from dairy products, fortified foods, and supplements is low. The reasons for the large difference in vegetarian blood vitamin B_{12} levels between the studies of Löwik et al. (1990) and Deriemaeker et al. (2011) are unclear.

6.3 Vitamin C

Vitamin C intakes are typically higher in vegetarians than nonvegetarians, reflecting higher intakes of fruits and vegetables: Marsh et al. (1988), 92 versus 105[NS] mg/day; Tylavsky and Anderson (1988), 184 versus 159 mg/day; Nieman et al. (1989), 155 versus 114[NS] mg/day; Brants et al. (1990), 136 versus 94 mg/day in men and 149 versus 101 mg/day in women; and Deriemaeker et al. (2011), 162 versus 96 mg/day in men and 149 versus 123[NS] mg/day in women.

6.4 Vitamin D

Vitamin D levels are mainly driven by sun exposure, but diet becomes important whenever sun exposure is limited. Vegetarian intakes of vitamin D from diet are generally lower than nonvegetarian intakes.

Löwik et al. (1990) found no difference in 25(OH)D blood levels between vegetarians and nonvegetarians but their survey was carried out in June (and the authors note that it was very sunny), so blood levels would be strongly influenced by sun exposure, and differences due to diet would be minimized.

Vitamin D intakes were reported in a few studies comparing elderly vegetarians with nonvegetarians: Nieman et al. (1989), 2.2 versus 2.7[NS] μg/day; and Deriemaeker et al. (2011), 0.31 versus 0.27[NS] μg/day in men and 0.11 versus 0.23 μg/day in women.

7. Conclusion

7.1 Nutritional Status

In general, vegetarian diets show a healthy profile for most nutrients in the elderly as well as in younger adults. Blood cholesterol levels and BMI values are generally, but not always, favorable. There may be a slight disadvantage in BMD.

Iron deficiency appears to be much less of an issue in practice than in popular perception, though iron *stores* are lower in vegetarians. Protein intakes range from higher than recommended (particularly measured in terms of calorie density) to rather low. The inclusion of sufficient animal or soya milk or legumes avoids low protein intakes.

Sodium intakes are usually slightly lower in vegetarians than in nonvegetarians, but were found to be higher in Hong Kong vegetarians. High sodium intakes should be avoided to reduce risk of hypertension.

Low vitamin B_{12} intakes in those vegetarians with low intakes of milk and fortified foods/supplements are an important concern, albeit one that can be easily addressed.

Low calcium levels can be a concern in those vegetarian diets with low intakes of milk and fortified foods/supplements, and low intakes may impact fracture risk.

Low zinc levels and low EPA/DHA levels may be significant in elderly vegetarians, but more research is needed. Sprouted seeds and legumes and whole meal bread are good sources of zinc, since sprouting or leavening reduces phytate content.

7.2 Research Approach

The use of biomarkers of nutritional status and intermediate diet-related outcomes is very helpful in complementing analyses of nutrient intakes, particularly when multiple factors affect a relevant outcome (as in BMI, blood pressure, cholesterol, and BMD) or when bioavailability plays a critical role but cannot be predicted accurately from diet records (as in iron and zinc).

The limited amount of research on elderly vegetarians is striking, given the aging of populations and the increased interest in vegetarian and plant-based diets. Further research should look at elderly participants in ongoing large studies of vegetarians as well as looking at samples drawn from vegetarian organizations or religious communities. To limit confounding by age, studies should use subjects matched for age and sex whenever possible.

Failing that they should adjust carefully for age, considering the possibility of nonlinear trends.

Conflicts of interest

Stephen Walsh is Chair of The Vegan Society in the United Kingdom.

References

Allen, N.E., Appleby, P.N., Davey, G.K., Kaaks, R., Rinaldi, S., Key, T.J., 2002. The associations of diet with serum insulin-like growth factor I and its main binding proteins in 292 women meat-eaters, vegetarians, and vegans. Cancer Epidemiol. Biomarkers Prev. 11 (11), 1441–1448.

Appel, L.J., Moore, T.J., Obarzanek, E., Vollmer, W.M., Svetkey, L.P., Sacks, F.M., Bray, G.A., Vogt, T.M., Cutler, J.A., Windhauser, M.M., Lin, P.H., 1997. A clinical trial of the effects of dietary patterns on blood pressure. N. Engl. J. Med. 336 (16), 1117–1124.

Appleby, P., Roddam, A., Allen, N., Key, T., 2007. Comparative fracture risk in vegetarians and nonvegetarians in EPIC-Oxford. Eur. J. Clin. Nutr. 61 (12), 1400–1406.

Appleby, P.N., Crowe, F.L., Bradbury, K.E., Travis, R.C., Key, T.J., 2016. Mortality in vegetarians and comparable nonvegetarians in the United Kingdom. Am. J. Clin. Nutr. 103 (1), 218–230.

Bates, B., Lennox, A., Prentice, A., Bates, C., Page, P., Nicholson, S., Swan, G. (Eds.), 2014. National Diet and Nutrition Survey Results from Years 1, 2, 3 and 4 (Combined) of the Rolling Programme (2008/2009–2011/2012): A Survey Carried Out on Behalf of Public Health England and the Food Standards Agency. [Appendices, (Chapter 5) Tables, 5.5, 5.6, 5.11, 5.27, 5.30, 5.40, 5.44, 5.47].

Beezhold, B.L., Johnston, C.S., Daigle, D.R., 2010. Vegetarian diets are associated with healthy mood states: a cross-sectional study in Seventh Day Adventist adults. Nutr. J. 9 (1), 1–7.

Bradbury, K.E., Crowe, F.L., Appleby, P.N., Schmidt, J.A., Travis, R.C., Key, T.J., 2014. Serum concentrations of cholesterol, apolipoprotein AI and apolipoprotein B in a total of 1694 meat-eaters, fish-eaters, vegetarians and vegans. Eur. J. Clin. Nutr. 68 (2), 178–183.

Brants, H.A., Löwik, M.R., Westenbrink, S., Hulshof, K.F., Kistemaker, C., 1990. Adequacy of a vegetarian diet at old age (Dutch Nutrition Surveillance System). J. Am. Coll. Nutr. 9 (4), 292–302.

Chiu, J.F., Lan, S.J., Yang, C.Y., Wang, P.W., Yao, W.J., Su, I.H., Hsieh, C.C., 1997. Long-term vegetarian diet and bone mineral density in postmenopausal Taiwanese women. Calcif. Tissue Int. 60 (3), 245–249.

Clarys, P., Deliens, T., Huybrechts, I., Deriemaeker, P., Vanaelst, B., De Keyzer, W., Hebbelinck, M., Mullie, P., 2014. Comparison of nutritional quality of the vegan, vegetarian, semi-vegetarian, pesco-vegetarian and omnivorous diet. Nutrients 6 (3), 1318–1332.

Davey, G.K., Spencer, E.A., Appleby, P.N., Allen, N.E., Knox, K.H., Key, T.J., 2003. EPIC–Oxford: lifestyle characteristics and nutrient intakes in a cohort of 33 883 meat-eaters and 31 546 non meat-eaters in the UK. Public Health Nutr. 6 (03), 259–268.

De Paula, R.C., Aneni, E.C., Costa, A.P., Figueiredo, V.S.N., Moura, F.A., Freitas, W.M., Quaglia, L.A., Santos, S.N., Soares, A.A., Nadruz Jr., W., Blaha, M., 2014. Low zinc levels is associated with increased inflammatory activity but not with atherosclerosis, arteriosclerosis or endothelial dysfunction among the very elderly. BBA Clin. 2, 1–6.

Deriemaeker, P., Aerenhouts, D., De Ridder, D., Hebbelinck, M., Clarys, P., 2011. Health aspects, nutrition and physical characteristics in matched samples of institutionalized vegetarian and non-vegetarian elderly (> 65 yrs). Nutr. Metab. 8 (1), 1–8.

Elmadfa, I., Singer, I., 2009. Vitamin B-12 and homocysteine status among vegetarians: a global perspective. Am. J. Clin. Nutr. 89 (5), 1693S–1698S.

Elorinne, A.L., Alfthan, G., Erlund, I., Kivimäki, H., Paju, A., Salminen, I., Turpeinen, U., Voutilainen, S., Laakso, J., 2016. Food and nutrient intake and nutritional status of Finnish vegans and non-vegetarians. PLoS One 11 (2), e0148235.

Fontana, L., Weiss, E.P., Villareal, D.T., Klein, S., Holloszy, J.O., 2008. Long-term effects of calorie or protein restriction on serum IGF-1 and IGFBP-3 concentration in humans. Aging Cell 7 (5), 681–687.

Foster, M., Chu, A., Petocz, P., Samman, S., 2013. Effect of vegetarian diets on zinc status: a systematic review and meta-analysis of studies in humans. J. Sci. Food Agric. 93 (10), 2362–2371.

Fraser, G.E., Shavlik, D.J., 1997. Risk factors for all-cause and coronary heart disease mortality in the oldest-old: the Adventist Health Study. Arch. Intern. Med. 157 (19), 2249–2258.

Fraser, G.E., Shavlik, D.J., 2001. Ten years of life: is it a matter of choice? Arch. Intern. Med. 161 (13), 1645–1652.

Giacconi, R., Costarelli, L., Piacenza, F., Basso, A., Rink, L., Mariani, E., Fulop, T., Dedoussis, G., Herbein, G., Provinciali, M., Jajte, J., 2016. Main biomarkers associated with age-related plasma zinc decrease and copper/zinc ratio in healthy elderly from ZincAge study. Eur. J. Nutr. 1–10.

Gibson, R.S., Anderson, B.M., Sabry, J.H., 1983. The trace metal status of a group of post-menopausal vegetarians. J. Am. Dietetic Assoc. 82 (3), 246–250.

Giem, P., Beeson, W.L., Fraser, G.E., 1993. The incidence of dementia and intake of animal products: preliminary findings from the Adventist Health Study. Neuroepidemiology 12 (1), 28–36.

Guralnik, J.M., Eisenstaedt, R.S., Ferrucci, L., Klein, H.G., Woodman, R.C., 2004. Prevalence of anemia in persons 65 years and older in the United States: evidence for a high rate of unexplained anemia. Blood 104 (8), 2263–2268.

Hallberg, L., Hulten, L., Gramatkovski, E., 1997. Iron absorption from the whole diet in men: how effective is the regulation of iron absorption? Am. J. Clin. Nutr. 66 (2), 347–356.

Hallberg, L., Hulthén, L., 2000. Prediction of dietary iron absorption: an algorithm for calculating absorption and bioavailability of dietary iron. Am. J. Clin. Nutr. 71 (5), 1147–1160.

Henry, C.J.K., 2005. Basal metabolic rate studies in humans: measurement and development of new equations. Public Health Nutr. 8 (7a), 1133–1152.

Ho-Pham, L.T., Nguyen, N.D., Nguyen, T.V.S., 2009. Effect of vegetarian diets on bone mineral density: a Bayesian meta-analysis. Am. J. Clin. Nutr. 90 (4), 943–950.

Ho-Pham, L.T., Vu, B.Q., Lai, T.Q., Nguyen, N.D., Nguyen, T.V.S., 2012. Vegetarianism, bone loss, fracture and vitamin D: a longitudinal study in Asian vegans and non-vegans. Eur. J. Clin. Nutr. 66 (1), 75–82.

Hotz, C., Peerson, J.M., Brown, K.H., 2003. Suggested lower cutoffs of serum zinc concentrations for assessing zinc status: reanalysis of the second National Health and Nutrition Examination Survey data (1976–1980). Am. J. Clin. Nutr. 78 (4), 756.

Huang, C.J., Fan, Y.C., Liu, J.F., Tsai, P.S., 2011. Characteristics and nutrient intake of Taiwanese elderly vegetarians: evidence from a national survey. Br. J. Nutr. 106 (03), 451–460.

Hunt, I.F., Murphy, N.J., Henderson, C., 1988. Food and nutrient intake of Seventh-day Adventist women. Am. J. Clin. Nutr. 48 (3), 850–851.

Hunt, I.F., Murphy, N.J., Henderson, C., Clark, V.S.A., Jacobs, R.M., Johnston, P.K., Coulson, A.H., 1989. Bone mineral content in postmenopausal women: comparison of omnivores and vegetarians. Am. J. Clin. Nutr. 50 (3), 517–523.

Hunt, J.R., 2003. Bioavailability of iron, zinc, and other trace minerals from vegetarian diets. Am. J. Clin. Nutr. 78 (3), 633S–639S.

Kim, M.H., Choi, M.K., Sung, C.J., 2007. Bone mineral density of Korean postmenopausal women is similar between vegetarians and nonvegetarians. Nutr. Res. 27 (10), 612–617.

Knez, M., Stangoulis, J.C., Zec, M., Debeljak-Martacic, J., Pavlovic, Z., Gurinovic, M., Glibetic, M., 2016. An initial evaluation of newly proposed biomarker of zinc status in humans-linoleic acid: dihomo-γ-linolenic acid (LA: DGLA) ratio. Clin. Nutr. ESPEN 15, 85–92.

Kwok, T., Cheng, G., Woo, J., Lai, W.K., Pang, C.P., 2002. Independent effect of vitamin B12 deficiency on hematological status in older Chinese vegetarian women. Am. J. Hematol. 70 (3), 186–190.

Kwok, T.C.Y., Chan, T.Y.K., Woo, J., 2003. Relationship of urinary sodium/potassium excretion and calcium intake to blood pressure and prevalence of hypertension among older Chinese vegetarians. Eur. J. Clin. Nutr. 57 (2), 299–304.

Lau, E.M.C., Kwok, T., Woo, J., Ho, S.C., 1998. Bone mineral density in Chinese elderly female vegetarians, vegans, lacto-vegetarians and omnivores. Eur. J. Clin. Nutr. 52 (1), 60–64.

Löwik, M.R., Schrijver, J., Odink, J., Van Den Berg, H., Wedel, M., 1990. Long-term effects of a vegetarian diet on the nutritional status of elderly people (Dutch Nutrition Surveillance System). J. Am. Coll. Nutr. 9 (6), 600–609.

Marcellini, F., Giuli, C., Papa, R., Gagliardi, C., Dedoussis, G., Herbein, G., Fulop, T., Monti, D., Rink, L., Jajte, J., Mocchegiani, E., 2006. Zinc status, psychological and nutritional assessment in old people recruited in five European countries: Zincage study. Biogerontology 7 (5–6), 339–345.

Margetts, B.M., Beilin, L.J., Vandongen, R., Armstrong, B.K., 1986. Vegetarian diet in mild hypertension: a randomised controlled trial. Br. Med. J. Clin. Res. Ed. 293 (6560), 1468–1471.

Mariani, E., Mangialasche, F., Feliziani, F.T., Cecchetti, R., Malavolta, M., Bastiani, P., Baglioni, M., Dedoussis, G., Fulop, T., Herbein, G., Jajte, J., 2008. Effects of zinc supplementation on antioxidant enzyme activities in healthy old subjects. Exp. Gerontol. 43 (5), 445–451.

Marsh, A.G., Sanchez, T.V.S., Midkelsen, O., Keiser, J., Mayor, G., 1980. Cortical bone density of adult lacto-ovo-vegetarian and omnivorous women. J. Am. Dietetic Assoc. 76 (2), 148–151.

Marsh, A.G., Sanchez, T.V.S., Chaffee, F.L., Mayor, G.H., Mickelsen, O., 1983. Bone mineral mass in adult lacto-ovo-vegetarian and omnivorous males. Am. J. Clin. Nutr. 37 (3), 453–456.

Marsh, A.G., Sanchez, T.V.S., Michelsen, O., Chaffee, F.L., Fagal, S.M., 1988. Vegetarian lifestyle and bone mineral density. Am. J. Clin. Nutr. 48 (3), 837–841.

Nieman, D.C., Underwood, B.C., Sherman, K.M., Arabatzis, K., Barbosa, J.C., Johnson, M., Shultz, T.D., 1989. Dietary status of Seventh-Day Adventist vegetarian and non-vegetarian elderly women. J. Am. Dietetic Assoc. 89 (12), 1763–1769.

Orlich, M.J., Singh, P.N., Sabaté, J., Jaceldo-Siegl, K., Fan, J., Knutsen, S., Beeson, W.L., Fraser, G.E., 2013. Vegetarian dietary patterns and mortality in Adventist health study 2. JAMA Intern. Med. 173 (13), 1230–1238.

Orlich, M.J., Jaceldo-Siegl, K., Sabaté, J., Fan, J., Singh, P.N., Fraser, G.E., 2014. Patterns of food consumption among vegetarians and non-vegetarians. Br. J. Nutr. 112 (10), 1644–1653.

Reed, J.A., Anderson, J.J., Tylavsky, F.A., Gallagher, P.N., 1994. Comparative changes in radial-bone density of elderly female lacto-ovovegetarians and omnivores. Am. J. Clin. Nutr. 59 (5), 1197S–1202S.

Rizzo, N.S., Jaceldo-Siegl, K., Sabate, J., Fraser, G.E., 2013. Nutrient profiles of vegetarian and nonvegetarian dietary patterns. J. Acad. Nutr. Dietetics 113 (12), 1610–1619.

Sarter, B., Kelsey, K.S., Schwartz, T.A., Harris, W.S., 2015. Blood docosahexaenoic acid and eicosapentaenoic acid in vegans: associations with age and gender and effects of an algal-derived omega-3 fatty acid supplement. Clin. Nutr. 34 (2), 212–218.

Schmidt, J.A., Rinaldi, S., Scalbert, A., Ferrari, P., Achaintre, D., Gunter, M.J., Appleby, P.N., Key, T.J., Travis, R.C., 2016. Serum concentrations and intakes of amino acids in male meat-eaters, fish-eaters, vegetarians and vegans: a cross-sectional analysis in the EPIC-Oxford cohort. Eur. J. Clin. Nutr. 70 (3), 306–312.

Tylavsky, F.A., Anderson, J.J., 1988. Dietary factors in bone health of elderly lactoovovegetarian and omnivorous women. Am. J. Clin. Nutr. 48 (3), 842–849.

Wang, Y.F., Chiu, J.S., Chuang, M.H., Chiu, J.E., Lin, C.L., 2008. Bone mineral density of vegetarian and non-vegetarian adults in Taiwan. Asia Pac. J. Clin. Nutr. 17 (1), 101–106.

Woo, J., Kwok, T., Ho, S.C., Sham, A., Lau, E., 1998. Nutritional status of elderly Chinese vegetarians. Age Ageing 27 (4), 455–461.

Nutrients and Other Substances Intake and Status

Plant Protein, Animal Protein, and Protein Quality

François Mariotti

UMR PHYSIOLOGIE DE LA NUTRITION ET DU COMPORTEMENT ALIMENTAIRE, AGROPARISTECH, INRA, UNIVERSITÉ PARIS-SACLAY, PARIS, FRANCE

1. Introduction

This first chapter on plant protein will focus on the fundamental role of dietary protein: to supply nitrogen and amino acids that ensure normal growth and the normal renewal of body protein pools. This is the criterion that has always been used to evaluate protein quality. In line with this viewpoint, this chapter will therefore deal with plant and animal proteins as sources of amino acids, and not of the other nutrients and substances with which they are commonly associated. As we shall explain, protein quality as defined here mostly relates to the bioavailability of amino acids from dietary protein, the quantities of individual amino acids and the amino acid profile, the utilization of these amino acids for anabolic purposes, and their overall, final, although often theoretical, impact on body protein pools. The myriad of functions related to specific body proteins are supposed to be assured if protein pools are globally balanced by dietary protein intake. We shall be reviewing these relationships and different sources of information that range from theoretical assessments to experimental results. We shall then turn to the complexity of amino acid metabolism and the uncertainties attached to our understanding of dietary protein and protein metabolism, while attempting to clarify the practical implications of using plants as a major source of protein.

2. Initial Evaluations of Plant and Animal Protein Quality

Nearly 100 years ago, Mitchell described the basic concept used to estimate protein quality as being the fraction of a dietary protein that is lost during digestion plus the fraction that is lost in metabolism, i.e., not retained in the body (the so-called "biological value"), and proposed a method to measure the level of nitrogen losses beyond the obligatory losses that could be accounted for by consumption of the protein (Mitchell, 1923, 1924). Under this principle, the fundamental value of a dietary protein is to supply alpha-amino nitrogen to be used for anabolic purposes, thereby ensuring optimum growth or, in an adult, enabling the normal renewal of body protein with an equilibrated nitrogen balance

(Sherman, 1920). This was judging protein quality on experimental grounds—a highly pragmatic viewpoint—based on the basic criteria of metabolic indispensability, a very fundamental viewpoint.

Much research has been based on this approach in rodents. Numerous studies have measured the "protein efficiency ratio" (PER, weight gain divided by the amount of protein consumed) of different protein sources in rodent diets, or other similar indexes such as the "relative protein efficiency ratio" or "(relative) net protein ratio," to compare weight gain between groups receiving a reference protein, or to compare the weight loss of a group receiving a protein-free diet. For a review, readers can refer to the publication by Boye et al. (2012). Based on these criteria, a series of studies in rodents concluded that plant proteins were of poor quality. For example, protein efficiency ratios were found to lie within the 1.2–2.4 range for plant proteins (including pea flour, soy protein, beans) and could be as low as 0.95 for wheat flour, whereas animal proteins were in the 3.1–3.7 range (Sarwar et al., 1984; Cruz et al., 2003).

These studies were also useful in demonstrating the concept of a limiting amino acid. The protein efficiency ratio of soy flour in a rodent diet increases with the addition of methionine to reach a ratio similar to that of casein, showing that the low level of sulfur amino acid in soy protein limits the utilization of other amino acids for the most quantitatively important pathway, i.e., protein synthesis. Interestingly, while the PER of soy protein and casein increase with the amount of protein in the diet, a difference between the two sources remains whatever the level of protein, provided it is not too low. Therefore, in the case of a single source of protein, the limiting amino acid is the key factor regarding relative protein utilization. From this literature, cereals have been established as being deficient in lysine and legumes deficient in methionine, or more generally speaking in sulfur amino acids (Friedman and Brandon, 2001; Sarwar et al., 1978). In line with this concept, it has also been demonstrated by experiments in rats that proteins can complement each other (Sarwar et al., 1978).

Another key factor demonstrated by these approaches with respect to protein quality is digestibility. The antinutritional factors found in many plant proteins may limit the digestion of protein, resulting in a reduction in its final global efficiency of utilization. This is particularly important regarding the trypsin inhibitors found in many beans, the inhibitory effect of which is markedly decreased by heat treatment or chemical reduction, resulting in a structural change (via the disulphide bonds) (Friedman and Brandon, 2001; Friedman and Gumbmann, 1986; Faris et al., 2008; Sarwar Gilani et al., 2012; Gilani and Sepehr, 2003).

As argued by Mitchell a century ago, and based on series of classic growth experiments in rats, plant protein is more digestible when the protein fraction is purer, and poorer digestibility estimates are limited to legumes, but this depends on previous heat treatment. With respect to legumes, including white bean, lima bean, and velvet beans, he wrote "The value of these proteins in growth experiments on rats in large part depended upon whether or not the proteins were cooked or uncooked" (Mitchell, 1923).

Assessing protein quality by measuring the efficiency of protein utilization in a rat model has some important limitations. Protein requirements for rapid growth in animals are not the same as those in humans, which are mainly driven by maintenance, even in young children (Young, 1991). Furthermore, individual amino acid requirements are not the same in rodents and humans, due to the different metabolic demands of specific tissues. A higher sulfur amino acid requirement in rodents than in humans has long been suspected, and it has been evidenced by the fact that the PER of animal proteins (or a mixture of proteins) is not maximal and increases with the addition of methionine. These initial evaluations based on rat growth had many limitations regarding their application to the human diet, but together with the predominance of plant-based diets in a context of protein-energy malnutrition, they have shaped the lasting view that plant proteins have a very poor quality for human nutrition.

3. Protein Quality Based on the Nitrogen Balance in Humans

Because of the limitations of animal models, it has long been argued that protein quality should be evaluated in humans. Based on the principle of nitrogen balance studies, the utilization of a protein can be assessed in humans by measuring fecal and urinary nitrogen (N) losses. The results of such studies have confirmed that some plant proteins have a lower utilization, in particular certain beans and wheat (FAO/WHO, 1973; Alford and Onley, 1978; Young et al., 1975). When compared to egg protein, the net protein utilization of wheat was estimated at 41% (Young et al., 1975). Lysine was confirmed as being the limiting amino acid in wheat (Bailey and Clark, 1976). However, some plant proteins have produced good results, comparable to those achieved with animal proteins. For instance, it was reported that amaranth had a net protein utilization that was 89% of that of cheese protein, and lupine a net protein utilization that was 77% of that of egg protein, which is comparable to the value found for beef (78%). Likewise, soy protein isolate has the same overall utilization as milk, egg, or beef proteins (Young et al., 1984a,b). Contrary to the results found in rats, the addition of methionine does not improve the utilization of soy protein (Young et al., 1984a). A mixture of plant protein sources, particularly including small amounts of animal protein (such as milk) can result in an equilibrated nitrogen balance at a level of intake similar to that of animal proteins, indicating their good utilization for body protein maintenance.

4. Digestibility

Investigations in animals and humans have also generated much data regarding the digestibility of plant protein, and helped us to understand the main factors at issue. Data in humans have indicated a range of values for plant protein, with most plant sources exhibiting true digestibility within the 80%–90% range, although with some from specific sources being lower (e.g., "rice, cereal": 75% and "rice, polished": 88%), and a few higher (e.g., "wheat, refined": 96%, "soy protein isolate": 95%) (FAO/WHO/UNU, 2007). The digestibility of meat, fish, milk, or eggs reaches ~95%. Digestibility is usually higher for refined products (e.g., soy flour: 86% and soy protein isolate: 95%) (FAO/WHO/UNU, 2007; Boye et al., 2012). The digestibility of protein in the traditional diets of developing countries is considered to be lower than that in Western diets, which is attributed to more unprocessed protein sources and higher levels of antinutritional factors (Sarwar Gilani et al., 2012).

However, true fecal digestibility is not the best measure of the digestibility of dietary protein. The amount of ingested protein nitrogen absorbed in the small intestine better reflects the quantity of amino acids made available for body metabolism before the protein enters the colon, and this measure is referred to as "ileal digestibility." Further, the nitrogen found after the colon or ileum originates from both endogenous and dietary sources, so the digestibility calculation requires that an estimate of endogenous nitrogen losses should be subtracted from the total losses. When basal (endogenous) losses are considered, this constitutes "true digestibility," but when precise endogenous/dietary losses can be estimated directly, this is called "real digestibility." Real ileal digestibility has been assessed in humans during the past 20 years. Using sophisticated methods, these studies reported that the real ileal digestibility of various dietary proteins was within the 89%–95% range. For soy protein isolate, pea protein flour or isolate, wheat flour, and lupine flour, the figures were 89%–92%; these were similar to those found for eggs (91%) or meat (90%–94%), and slightly lower than those reported for milk protein (95%) (Tomé, 2013). It is important to note that most of the plant proteins studied came from raw, untreated (unheated, or minimally heated) sources, and some were ingested in complex food matrices such as (unheated) flour. Data in rats and pigs have shown that moderate heat treatment, which reduces trypsin inhibitor activity in legumes and increases the accessibility of most proteins to proteolytic enzymes, tends to improve digestibility (Van Der Poel et al., 1990; Gilani and Sepehr, 2003; Clemente et al., 2000; Boye et al., 2012). Furthermore, it was shown that pea globulin alone—the major fraction of pea protein—has a high digestibility of 94%, whereas total pea protein (i.e., globulin plus albumin) had a digestibility of 90% (Mariotti et al. 2001). Given that the albumin fraction contains all the trypsin inhibitors, that this protein displays the structure that is the most resistant to hydrolysis, and that the proteins were untreated, this 4% difference is finally very small. In this series of studies reporting a close range of values for different proteins, one exception was rapeseed protein isolate, the digestibility of which was found to be 84%, although there was marked interindividual variability in the results (84±9%) (Bos et al., 2007). Rapeseed contains proteins that are particularly resistant to hydrolysis and whose structure is little affected by heat treatment. For rapeseed, as for other protein sources, intense heat treatment tends to impair digestibility (Eklund et al., 2015). However, the precise effects of different heat treatments on the structure and resulting digestibility of proteins remains little documented (Samadi et al., 2013). Heat treatment may also decrease the availability of some amino acids, and particularly lysine, depending on the conditions and substrates available (Gilani et al., 2005), but the final impact in humans is difficult to determine. The digestibility issue may be more specific to certain plant protein fractions, and the extraction processes and subsequent treatments applied.

Finally, the differences found between the digestibility of plant proteins and animal proteins appear to be small, contrary to historical findings in rats or pigs, or determinations using less precise methods in humans.

For many years, it has been proposed that digestibility should be studied at the level of each individual amino acid rather than the overall total nitrogen level (Gilani and Sepehr, 2003). There are several reasons why the individual digestibility of some amino acids may vary or be poorer than that of others, so overall digestibility is an imperfect proxy for the bioavailability of each amino acid. Although individual amino acid levels may vary between and within protein sources, it remains difficult to delineate a systematic bias in the evaluation of dietary protein quality that could be resolved by means of ileal digestibility (Rutherfurd et al., 2015). One exception to this rule is the reduction in available lysine due to food manufacturing processes such as Maillard reactions (FAO/WHO/UNU, 2007). Indeed, the issue of lysine availability remains unclear, and methodological advances will be necessary to determine clear estimates (Rutherfurd, 2015).

Data on the digestibility of individual amino acids at the ileal level remain rare, and the theoretical rationale for improving the evaluation of amino acid availability is plagued by numerous methodological problems. FAO (2013) has suggested that this could be an important opportunity to improve the evaluation of protein quality, but it is acknowledged that until these data are available, fecal crude protein digestibility should be used as a proxy for individual amino acid bioavailability. This will be further discussed next. In the meantime, data to refine our understanding of the differences between plant and animal proteins are scarce (Rutherfurd et al., 2015). In a study that compared the ileal amino acid digestibility of soy and milk proteins, the average digestibility was 94% for soy, with individual amino acids within the 89%–97% range (89 ± 5%–97 ± 3%), while for milk the average figure was 95%, and values ranged from 92% to 99% regarding the digestibility of individual amino acids (Gaudichon et al., 2002).

5. Amino Acid Profiles and Requirements

Theoretically, the amino acids available are used efficiently if they are supplied in quantities and proportions that are optimal for their incorporation in protein synthesis. In line with the concept of limiting amino acids, when sufficient alpha-amino nitrogen is consumed in the absolute, a protein of good quality should supply enough of each of the nine indispensable amino acids. This is the concept of the amino acid score (AAS). The AAS ascribes to a protein the lowest proportion of each indispensable amino acid relative to the amount in a reference pattern that is optimal for protein utilization. This reference pattern was initially that of a real protein (egg protein), but since 1973 it has been based on an estimate of individual amino acid requirements (FAO/WHO, 1973). Based on the AAS, a dietary protein that is consumed at a level that covers the overall protein requirement (i.e., an average of 0.66 g/kg body weight) and has an AAS of 1, supplies exactly the absolute amounts of individual amino acids that meet metabolic demand, and at a proportion where no amino acid constrains utilization of the others.

6. Amino Acid Scores and Protein Digestibility Corrected Amino Acid Score (PDCAAS) of Plant Proteins

When reviewing the AAS of plant protein, two amino acids often appear as being limiting: lysine in cereals and sulfur amino acids in legumes. A closer look at the data reveals that the amounts of lysine are low or very low in cereals (and pseudocereals) such as wheat, sorghum, triticale (49%, 47%, 62%), and rice (80%), and low in a few other sources (almonds and walnuts: 60%), whereas it is high or very high in other sources and particularly in legumes (e.g., pea: 168%; fava bean: 152%; soybean: 134%) as in animal proteins (milk: 168%; beef: 193%; egg: 160%) (US Department of Agriculture – Agricultural Research Service, 2013). The very low level of lysine in cereals has long been an important aspect of protein quality, and there is an ongoing debate as to the implications of these low levels (see later). Because of the very low lysine level in cereals, there have been major concerns about whether diets mainly composed of cereals can cover protein and amino acid requirements at a marginal level of total protein intake. This will be further discussed subsequently.

As far as sulfur amino acids are concerned, small quantities are found in many legumes, with a few being below the reference value, e.g., fava bean (95% of the reference value) and some lupines (88%), although most have AAS that is >1 (e.g., pea, kidney bean, and soybean at 112%–118%). Most cereals contain very high levels of sulfur amino acids (e.g., wheat: 160%; rice: 190%), similar to those in animal proteins (e.g., milk: 148%; beef: 167%; egg: 235%). Before 1973 (because the reference pattern for the AAS was egg protein, which is very high in sulfur amino acids), the AAS for legumes was dramatically low (FAO/WHO, 1973). Revision of the reference pattern between 1990 and 2007 also resulted in a further lowering of the value for sulfur amino acids (from 25 mg/g to 22 mg/g), and although this was a slight decrease, it resulted in most legumes being no longer "deficient" in sulfur amino acids, with an AAS > 1.

Apart from virtually all cereals and a very few legumes, dietary proteins are not limiting in any amino acids when compared to the most recent reference pattern (FAO/WHO/UNU, 2007); see Fig. 35.1. This figure also shows that the overall average plant protein AAS is superior to one, and protein sources can easily complement each other. This is readily achieved once cereals and legumes are mixed together in the diet, or plant sources are mixed with some animal sources (such as milk and eggs). This has practical implications for ovolactovegetarians and vegans, and for plant-based diets that incorporate small quantities of animal protein. The low levels of lysine in cereals and sulfur amino acids in legumes have long been acknowledged, but it is also known that cereals and legumes can combine to yield a mix that is no longer deficient in these amino acids, as they complement each other. Combining cereals and legumes is also probably one of the oldest features of "cultural nutrition." Numerous traditional dishes that are staples in many cultures in large parts of the world combine cereals with legumes or dairy, such as couscous that combines wheat and chickpeas, diverse bread or pasta with cheese, or the famous rice and beans.

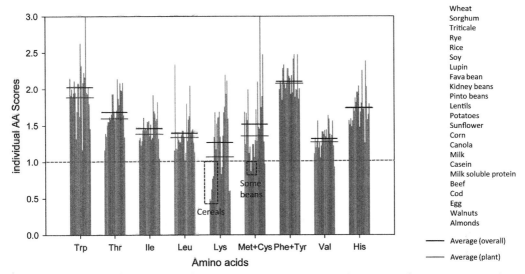

FIGURE 35.1 Individual amino acid scores (calculated as the ratio between the amount of a given amino acid in dietary protein and its value in the FAO/WHO (2007) reference pattern) for a broad range of plant and animal proteins. *Lines* indicate the overall average for all protein sources (black) and the average for plant proteins only. *Data were calculated from the USDA database (USDA National Nutrient Database for Standard Reference, Release 26).*

7. PDCAAS as a Proxy for the Protein Quality of Single Protein Sources

Because it only requires data on amino acid composition, the AAS approach has been widely applied. It has long been combined with estimates of digestibility (such as protein digestibility measured experimentally in rats) to yield the well-known PDCAAS. Interestingly, this score combines estimates of the two main factors for protein utilization: digestibility and the amino acid pattern. It can be applied in the context of marginal protein intake when the overall protein requirement is covered, i.e., when the intake of "good quality" protein is sufficient to secure the nitrogen balance. It has become the official international consensus for the routine evaluation of protein quality. For plant proteins, the PDCAAS is the result of the combination of what has been presented earlier. Briefly, the slightly poorer digestibility of most plant proteins amplifies low or marginally adequate amino acid patterns. A low PDCAAS (i.e., lower than 1) is still mainly found with cereals.

To understand this approach, it is important to note that the PDCAAS was proposed as a method to assess the protein quality of both individual protein food sources AND dietary mixtures. For a given protein, a PDCAAS higher than 1 does not mean that it has an advantage over a protein with a PDCAAS of 1 if it were the only source of protein in the diet. Therefore, when calculated for a diet, the PDCAAS and other indicators should be truncated to 1. If a protein has a PDCAAS higher than 1, this indeed indicates its clear potential to be used to complement other protein sources with a PDCAAS lower than 1. Conversely, the PDCAAS system does not account for the fact that two proteins of "low(er) quality" (PDCAAS < 1) may achieve a mix of adequate quality (PDCAAS = 1) when combined, a typical example being cereals and legumes.

Clearly, the PDCAAS therefore has limitations when it is used to communicate on the protein quality of different foodstuffs, which may be important inasmuch as the PDCAAS (and its current variation the DIAAS) is recommended for regulatory purposes. All approaches that are designed to provide information on diet but are based on fragmented, reductionist information on individual foodstuffs are ultimately subject to such limitations as they may disregard and finally hinder their integration at the dietary level, a classic pitfall in nutrition (Mariotti et al., 2010).

8. PDCAAS of Mixed Protein Diets and Protein Intake in Plant-Based Diets

It is important to understand that the evaluation of protein quality is based on the theoretical situation of a marginal protein intake. For populations in developing countries where the protein intake is low, the issue of protein quality is of acute importance, particularly since the protein source may be insufficiently varied, but the general concern is that of overall protein-energy malnutrition. Again, the problem is most important for diets that are mainly cereal-based, because of the lysine limitation (Nuss and Tanumihardjo, 2011), as we shall discuss later in this chapter. In this context, evaluating the protein quality of diets comprising components from different protein sources could make a valuable contribution to analyzing the specific constraints of different models on the supply of an equilibrated amino acid pattern to meet protein requirements (Suri et al., 2014; Nuss and Tanumihardjo, 2011).

As a corollary, if protein quality is still inadequate when assessed at the level of the diet (and as estimated by the PDCAAS), this means that the total protein intake needs to be higher than the standard requirement (based on good quality protein). It is a matter of opinion whether this will mean compensating for quality by quantity, or simply recognizing that there is no quality issue when the protein intake is high. In Western countries, this option is preferable inasmuch as protein intakes are indeed considerably higher than the needs of the general population, where even vegetarians (including vegans) have protein intakes above the recommended dietary allowance (or population reference intake, to use the EU wording). In an analysis of the nutrient intake of the Adventist cohort of the AHS-2 study, Rizzo et al. reported median protein intakes of 75 g/day for nonvegetarians and 71 g/day for both ovolactovegetarians and vegans, even though the vegetarians were relying on plant protein to meet >83% of their total protein needs. When only considering the groups with the lowest protein intakes (i.e., the 5th percentile of protein intakes), the values were 54 g/day in nonvegetarians, 53 g/day in ovolactovegetarians, and 52 g/day in vegans. These results clearly illustrate the fact that the risk of an inadequate protein intake may little differ as a function of the plant protein content in the diet of communities of Western adults. Based on absolute protein amounts, i.e., without information on body weight, a rigorous estimate of the prevalence of inadequate protein intake in these populations is not possible, and this would be necessary for an in-depth analysis. However, if 54 g is considered as the reference value to comply with the population reference intake (of 0.83 g/kg body weight) with a body weight of 65 kg, the data indicate that this prevalence of inadequate intake, even among those with the lowest intake (5th percentile), is virtually null. The fact that vegans achieve a sufficient protein intake is also corroborated by a protein:energy ratio >10% at the 5th percentile. These conclusions are in line with data from other studies reporting on the protein intakes of vegetarians and nonvegetarians in Western countries (Clarys et al., 2014; Halkjaer et al., 2009; Millward and Garnett, 2010). In these countries, concerns regarding protein nutrition may be limited to older adults because of their lower protein intake, lower energy intake, and possibly higher absolute requirement (Mariotti, 2016; Berner et al., 2013). This situation also involves a peculiar metabolic constraint, linked to their resistance to postprandial anabolism. This will be discussed in further detail subsequently.

9. Limitations of the AAS, PDCAAS, and DIAAS Approaches

The theoretical and practical limitations of AAS-based methods are numerous. The PDCAAS has been widely criticized as being ineffective in predicting the nutritional quality of certain specific sources containing high levels of antinutritional factors (including trypsin inhibitors or growth-depressing factors such as glucosinolates), which have been proved to impair growth in rats. However, these sources are quite specific and tested as raw, and it is thought that these limitations to PDCAAS should only concern novel and single sources of protein (Gilani, 2012). It has also been thought that, depending on the conditions such as high temperatures, processing can reduce the levels of bioavailable amino acids (although this improves their digestibility) by degrading these amino acids (Boye et al., 2012). Lysine is particularly sensitive processing. Finally, AAS-based approaches, including PDCAAS, come in for criticism at two ends of the theoretical spectrum: they are too general to assess the value of highly specific proteins, but they are too specific to reflect the real utilization of complex combinations of broad protein sources.

It should also be remembered that PDCAAS also suffers from the practical limitations of amino acid analysis in terms of how amino acid contents are expressed relative to protein, either as "crude protein" (i.e., using the classic $N \times 6.25$ factor) or as a sum of amino acids (using specific conversion factors or direct comprehensive analysis). We have shown that using crude protein for plant protein (which has a real conversion factor <6.25) underestimates the AAS of plant protein, and it equally overestimates the quantity of protein in the food source (Mariotti et al., 2008); this concern was recently reiterated (Rutherfurd et al., 2015). It is a good example of how, in practice, it is difficult to disentangle protein quantity and quality.

To account for variations in the digestibility of individual amino acids, the DIAAS approach was proposed by the FAO as an improvement to the PDCAAS estimate. However, the DIAAS targets a more specific and individual ileal amino acid balance (as discussed earlier), but for practical reasons it is calculated using the amino acid content of a protein multiplied by the overall protein fecal digestibility, as estimated in rats. In short, where the PDCAAS typically multiplies digestibility by the AAS, the DIAAS directly considers the quantities of amino acids and their overall digestibility to calculate the ratios of digestible indispensable amino acids against the value in the reference pattern, ultimately retaining the lowest. DIAAS values are therefore slightly lower than those of the PDCAAS, but the differences are very similar among protein sources ($4 \pm 2\%$ lower) (Rutherfurd et al., 2015). As discussed later, applying estimates of individual amino acids available at the ileal level also results in lowering the index for all proteins, with some slightly more important differences between protein sources (in the study by Rutherfurd et al., $-4 \pm 3\%$).

Clearly, although the PDCAAS and DIAAS are theoretically sound methods to estimate protein quality, it is doubtful whether the differences in estimates between the indexes and different protein sources are meaningful from a human nutritional standpoint, given all the methodological uncertainties and constraints and the theoretical limitations that affect our understanding of protein requirements, as we shall be discussing next.

10. Uncertainties Affecting Protein Quality Evaluation

The indirect approaches used to assess protein quality are based on a separate accounting of the total protein (i.e., nitrogen) requirement and that of each individual amino acid, and the define quality as the minimum amino acids that will permit the best efficiency of utilization, based on fragmentary information. For example, they do not account for the influence of each amino acid on the metabolism of others, nor their complex influence on background/endogenous metabolism. As can be expected, the metabolic reality is much more complex.

First, it has repeatedly been argued that the dietary protein requirement model is adaptive (Millward and Rivers, 1988), or in other words the metabolic demand for amino acids increases in line with amino acid intake. However, this is not usually taken into account by studies that are too short-term to show any adaptation in the amplitude of the diurnal cycling of fasting losses and postprandial gain according to protein intake (WHO/FAO/UNU, 2007). On this basis, it has been argued that the lysine requirement (the value of which is included in the amino acid reference pattern) has been overestimated, which is a matter of long-standing controversy (Young, 1998). Furthermore, studies in humans have shown that some dietary proteins are better retained/utilized than might be predicted by their AASs. For example, this has been shown for wheat protein (Millward et al., 2002) and pea protein fractions (Mariotti et al., 2001). It is not surprising that the real utilization of dietary proteins, in both the acute and adaptive settings, will not be readily predicted by amino acid scoring that assesses the minimum required based on individual amino acid requirements. Amino acids are both the substrates and signals for protein metabolism. As is well-known for leucine, a higher intake increases its oxidation at the same time as positively regulating the utilization of all amino acids for protein synthesis (Millward et al., 2008). The utilization of a mixture of amino acid is not the same as that of a protein (Daenzer et al., 2001). The numerous ramifications of such questions are beyond the scope of this paper, but in short, neither the utilization of a dietary protein not its metabolic impact can be reduced to just the separate amounts of the individual amino acids they convey, so once again, the whole is more than the sum of its parts.

A final example of the uncertainties that still affect our understanding of nitrogen and amino acid conservation in humans is the existence of nitrogen cycling in the lower gut. It has long been acknowledged that some amino acids are synthesized in the lower gut and then made available to the body, and this includes indispensable amino acids. It is also known that this synthesis may operate de novo, i.e., using nonalpha-amino nitrogen, and the NH_3 used to synthesize amino acids (including lysine) is supplied by the hydrolysis of urea ("urea N salvage") (FAO/WHO/UNU, 2007). The level of urea N salvage seems to vary according to the conditions, and it occurs as early as the postprandial period. It has been reported that the degree of urea hydrolysis increases when urea production increases as a result of a lower efficiency of postprandial utilization, in the case of plant protein (Fouillet et al., 2008). We therefore know that all the mechanisms that might modulate differences in the quantity and quality of protein are present and operational. What remains unknown is the degree of impact, and if this causes a nutritionally important effect.

Uncertainties concerning protein and amino acid requirements in the long term, taking account of the adaptive component, still limit estimates of adequacy based on comparing intakes from a plant-based protein diet and estimated requirements. On the other hand, as we will discuss further, we lack relevant markers for protein status that can be used directly to assess protein adequacy in adults. There is certainly little evidence that a low protein intake from a plant-based diet in well-nourished populations has adverse effects on health. This type of argument has a long history and still persists. In 1950, Mirone argued against the recommended daily allowance for protein (which was set at 70 g/day, with 50% of animal origin) after reporting that a group of vegetarians consuming 50 g total protein plus ~6 g animal protein was in apparent good health, as indicated by normal blood hematology and chemistry markers (including serum albumin); this was taken as an indication that a plant protein combination could substitute for animal protein (Mirone, 1950; Albanese, 2012).

11. When Might Protein Quantity and Quality Be Limiting With Respect to Protein Requirements?

An inadequate protein intake can be estimated in a population by comparing the protein intake and the distribution of requirements. This statistical estimation provides the percentage of individuals in the population whose protein requirements are not met by their protein intake. Another way to address this question is to calculate the protein:energy requirement ratios for different groups of individuals. This approach is based on the fact that when sufficient food is eaten to meet energy needs, those for protein will also be satisfied if the ratio of protein to energy is appropriate (FAO/WHO/UNU, 2007). Accordingly, different population groups are not at the same risk of insufficient intake. The mean and reference protein:energy ratios increase with age, being higher in women than in men, higher in small as opposed to large adults, and markedly lower in active individuals. It is therefore not surprising that the risk of inadequacy is very low in the general population but higher in older and inactive females of small stature. Likewise, in the general population with a high energy intake whose diet contains substantial amounts of protein, the intake of protein is indeed very high. As shown earlier, this has been confirmed in the general population in Western countries, and it is also the case for ovolacto-vegetarians. The protein intake of most vegans is lower than that of other vegetarians, but there are few concerns regarding insufficient intake among adults. Some elderly people with a low animal protein intake may have a marginal protein intake when compared to their requirement, and as predicted by the protein:energy approach, this is probably the case among elderly vegan women of small stature who have an inactive lifestyle (Millward and Garnett, 2010; FAO/WHO/UNU, 2007). It may be considered that the total protein requirement should be indeed be slightly higher with plant-based diets, to "compensate" for the slightly lower digestibility of plant protein sources or an imperfect supplementation in amino acids (mostly lysine) in some mixed protein diets. On this basis, and using the rough estimate of differences in digestibility between plant and animal sources, it may seem reasonable to consider a safety margin of an additional 5%–10% protein intake in diets that are predominantly or exclusively based on plant protein. This could be further increased if the diet is based exclusively on plant protein and is insufficiently varied to supply sufficient lysine. In line with this reasoning, the American Dietetic Association has proposed that "protein needs might be somewhat higher than the recommended dietary allowance in those vegetarians whose dietary protein sources are mainly those that are less well digested, such as some cereals and legumes" (Craig et al., 2009). However, this remains highly theoretical and approximate, and, importantly, it was refuted by a meta-analysis of nitrogen balance data, which did not find any influence of the type of protein (Rand et al., 2003). In their analysis, Rand et al. considered the protein sources in the study diets as being divided into three groups: animal, vegetable, and mixed, and they found no effects on this metaregression (slope and intercept), indicating that the total protein requirement is similar with plant-based or animal-based diets (Rand et al., 2003; FAO/WHO/UNU, 2007). When interpreting this analysis, however, it is important to note that the "vegetable" diets included complementary mixtures of plant proteins (cereals and legumes) or good quality soy protein.

In contrast with the inactive elderly, protein intake is high in well-nourished children, because of their high energy requirements whatever the dietary level of animal protein intake, and there is no risk of insufficiency based on requirements (AFSSA, 2008). In other words, the protein requirement of well-nourished children is high but their energy requirement is even higher, so that energy intake is the most limiting factor for protein adequacy.

That the protein quality of a plant-based diet is insufficient to meet the protein requirement may also be relevant, but only in situations of low total protein intakes and high requirements. In this context, as we have discussed before, consuming a variety of plant proteins is key to ensuring the adequacy of overall amino acid intake, and plant protein sources that are low in lysine (such as cereals) will not make the most important contribution to the protein intake.

Likewise, it is clear that the adequacy of a plant protein-based diet remains an issue in some developing countries: where total energy and protein intakes are low, the diet is based on complex plant sources with poorer digestibility, and these plant sources are insufficiently varied to supply adequate quantities of certain indispensable amino acids. For example, an insufficient intake of tryptophan has typically been shown in cases of pellagra in a population receiving a very monotonous diet of untreated maize that combines a very low protein and energy intake, insufficient niacin, B_2, and B_6 intakes and poor overall health status. The addition of groundnuts, fish, or eggs as sources of tryptophan and niacin can markedly reduce this risk (Seal et al., 2007; Malfait et al., 1993). By contrast, the level of available lysine is a primary concern regarding the quality of plant-based diets in some developing countries. There remain concerns about the amount of available lysine in some cereal-based diets in certain regions because its intake is lower than the estimated requirement; even in a mixed protein source, lysine levels appear to be insufficient when the protein (and energy) intake is low (Nuss and Tanumihardjo, 2011; FAO, 2013). As shown by Heck et al. (2010) in a rural area of Bangladesh, a larger share of animal protein (such as fish) in a mostly rice-based diet enabled an adequate protein and lysine intake, but the low BMI values seen in this population classically indicates a degree of (protein)-energy malnutrition. As we have discussed earlier, there are some very important limitations to our characterization of the risk of inadequacy in many situations of low lysine intake because we lack a specific and objective measure of protein deficiency that is independent of energy intake.

12. Refining With Metabolic Aspects: the Timing of Protein and Amino Acid Intake and Protein Metabolism, Especially Among Older People

It is usually considered that dietary proteins that complete each other do not need be consumed at the same meal, and that an assortment over the course of day may be appropriate. Expressing recommendations on a daily basis, because balances are the result of integrated changes over days, is a classical approach in nutrition, and indeed stems from our lack of information on how the metabolism may be regulated more precisely, particularly during the key window for protein utilization that is the postprandial period. The specificity of protein metabolism, compared to that of other energy nutrients, is that no inactive form of protein exists that can be used to store dietary protein in the postprandial state, so the precise regulation of postprandial metabolism is critical to protein homeostasis (Fouillet et al., 2003; Millward et al., 1996; Waterlow, 1999). Likewise, there is no true reservoir of certain specific amino acids that could be used between meals to smooth the variable intakes of each amino acid. Such buffering operates in a limited manner, and in part, through the total free amino acid pools. It has been suggested that the relatively large free lysine pool (as compared to leucine and other indispensable amino acids) enables lysine recycling during diurnal cycling, which in turn enables the conservation of lysine between meals, to some extent at least (Millward et al., 2000). This falls in line with an earlier study in rats that showed that the utilization of a lysine supplement added to a deficient diet over 24 h was similar to that of lysine given 12 h after feeding with a deficient diet (Yang et al., 1968). However, evidence that this would operate over more than 24 h remains scarce. It has also been suggested that variations in cysteine intake may be buffered because of its involvement in other pathways, and notably the existence of a large pool of cysteine in the form of glutathione (Mariotti et al., 2001). By contrast, tryptophan is known to be tightly regulated and has a small pool that is rapidly turned over, thus impairing its potential to buffer variations in intake (Yang et al., 1968).

However, our knowledge of postprandial metabolism is insufficient to understand how intakes between two meals or 2 days may be integrated. What we do know is that factors other than amino acid composition impact postprandial protein metabolism (such as the speed of amino acid availability), irrespective of this composition (Beaufrere et al., 2000; Dangin et al., 2001; Fouillet et al., 2009), and we suspect that this influence may differ depending on the amino acid studied (e.g., lysine vs. leucine) (Daenzer et al., 2001). Overall, protein turnover in skeletal muscle is highly responsive to amino acid intake in healthy adults (Groen et al., 2015). What is still little studied is how a difference in amino acid composition between two meals may impact the overall nitrogen balance or regional protein metabolism in adults. The influence of the rate of absorption and the specific effect of certain amino acids is different in older adults, a feature that offers an interesting refinement of the question at issue. Our current understanding of dietary protein and amino acids in the context of aging is that older people are resistant to postprandial anabolic stimulation by dietary protein, a resistance which can be overcome by supplying daily protein in the form of protein-rich meals (Paddon-Jones and Leidy, 2014; Rodriguez, 2014; Wall et al., 2015). A higher level of postprandial anabolism has been evidenced in older people (but not in younger adults) following a single large protein meal versus several smaller ones (Arnal et al., 1999, 2000; Mamerow et al., 2014). There is now consensus that a protein-rich meal in this context contains more than 30 g protein, which is considered to be the amount necessary to pass the "anabolic threshold" and to optimize postprandial anabolism (Paddon-Jones and Leidy, 2014; Paddon-Jones and Rasmussen, 2009). Similarly, in older people, proteins that are absorbed and delivered rapidly elicit a better postprandial amino acid balance than those which are absorbed slowly, while the reverse holds true in younger adults (Dangin et al., 2003; Fouillet et al., 2009; Beasley et al., 2013). This argues in favor of an age-related decrease in the ability of available amino acids to stimulate anabolism, lending further credence to the "anabolic threshold" paradigm (Dardevet et al., 2012). However, the rate of absorption is not the only factor involved in postprandial anabolism: the concomitant ingestion of carbohydrates, which delay amino acid absorption, does not reduce postprandial protein anabolism in older adults

(Churchward-Venne et al., 2015; Gorissen et al., 2014). When testing for protein consumed within a mixed meal, the overall daily level of protein in the diet, and not its distribution over the day, was reported to impact postprandial protein synthesis and the net protein balance (Kim et al., 2015). Indispensable amino acids, and particularly branched-chain amino acids, are considered to be key in eliciting the optimum anabolic response in the postprandial state, so a threshold (at 3 g) for peak anabolism has also been proposed for meal leucine (Gryson et al., 2014), triggering a signal for the anabolic utilization of the bulk of amino acids (Magne et al., 2012; Dardevet et al., 2002). In line with this, at a relatively low dose (20 g), whey protein (a leucine-rich, "fast" protein) causes a greater increase in postprandial anabolism in older people than casein (slow and lower in leucine) and casein hydrolysate (fast, but lower in leucine) (Pennings et al., 2011). Note should also be made of the possible long-term benefits of leucine-rich protein and/or high-protein diets in older people, probably because of their lower rates of muscle proteolysis (Mosoni et al., 2014).

These metabolic aspects have implications for protein nutrition in the elderly beyond the basic requirement for amino acids and our consideration of the potential of protein from different sources with respect to protein nutrition. To achieve optimum benefits in the elderly, it is not sufficient that the diet should include enough BCAA (when compared to what is required for a high PDCAAS), but it is important that the protein sources in a meal should be rich in BCAA, i.e., rich in proteins that are rich in BCAA. Indeed, most sources of plant protein are rich in leucine when compared to animal protein (e.g., an average of 8 g/100 g, with a range of 6–14 in a set of 18 plant proteins selected from the USDA database; an average of 9.5 g/100 g, with a range of 8–12 in a set of 6 animal proteins). Mixing different proteins is not expected to be key in this situation. However, it may be beneficial to include large quantities of protein-rich foodstuffs/ingredients to compose a meal that is rich in protein. In the current situation, protein-rich meals in the elderly are clearly associated with a higher intake of animal protein (Tieland et al., 2015; Paddon-Jones et al., 2015).

Alongside the specific case of leucine, it is necessary to define the optimum amino acid profile that will maximize postprandial anabolism in older individuals and could thus be used to refine amino acid requirements and the reference amino acid profile by applying more precise metabolic criteria. The usefulness of plant versus animal proteins in terms of protein nutrition needs to be reassessed using these dynamic metabolic criteria; this could lead to a further characterization of strategies for the enhanced use of plant protein, including optimum mixes of these proteins (van Vliet et al., 2015). However, achieving this goal is still a long way off.

13. Beyond Protein Metabolism? Functional Impacts

There remain numerous uncertainties regarding how different protein sources might impact protein metabolism and even more about how ultimately this may result in changes to muscle mass and function. If global protein homeostasis is considered alone, this may mask the importance of the profound impact of protein and amino acid intakes on protein and amino acid metabolism and their associated functions. Metabolic adaptation and accommodation to changes in the level of protein intake enable the final homeostasis of body nitrogen, with important changes to protein metabolism (changes to protein fluxes or reductions in lean mass) (Millward and Roberts, 1996). Likewise, while ensuring nitrogen homeostasis and muscle mass, the amount and nature of protein intake may impact many aspects of protein and amino acid metabolism. For instance, during adaptation to the protein reference intake, healthy adults experience changes in glutathione kinetics and in the turnover of some specific proteins, suggesting a functional cost (Afolabi et al., 2004; Jackson et al., 2004). In more specific populations such as older people at risk of developing sarcopenia, accommodating to a marginal protein intake may secure the nitrogen balance, but the associated metabolic cost may have implications for the optimum maintenance of muscle function during aging (Campbell et al., 2002).

Finally, the benefits of different levels of protein and amino acid intake have been addressed unsuccessfully using an indirect approach that compares intakes with theoretical requirements. However, we also lack relevant markers of protein status in adults who are not undernourished. In older individuals, where this becomes an important question, it is necessary to generate data to determine whether the quantity and nature (notably plant vs. animal) of dietary protein influences long-term markers of muscle mass and function and ultimately the risk of sarcopenia. Metabolic data alone have indeed proved insufficient to clarify an optimum level (toward the lower end of the range of intakes) to which the body can adapt or accommodate, nor to establish whether a different pattern of amino acids might have real implications for health. We need a more detailed characterization of the metabolic processes involved and their relationships with physiological and pathophysiological impacts.

As well as determining their impact on musculoskeletal health, it is also important to understand how the changes to amino acid metabolism that occur following the intake of plant or animal protein might affect other health-related endpoints. There is evidence that consuming plant or animal proteins does not result in the same configurations in the underlying metabolism (Poupin et al., 2011, 2014), and systems biology should help to improve our knowledge of the influences of dietary amino acids on both the overall metabolism and the precise pathways that might explain their physiological effects (He et al., 2011). This will be dealt with in the next chapter, but the importance of this area of research is well illustrated by the finding that the profile of some amino acids in the plasma is central to the metabolomic profiles that are associated with obesity and cardio-metabolic health (Ho et al., 2016; LeMieux et al., 2013).

14. Conclusion

Many uncertainties remain in terms of how human metabolism can adapt to or accommodate a lower intake of some individual amino acids when compared to the overall set of amino acid and protein requirements, even when considering a theoretically simple criterion such as protein homeostasis. Amino acid metabolism is a much more dynamic and complex process that is still only appreciated from fragmented information. Nonetheless, based on our current knowledge, proteins from plant sources are wholly adequate to ensure protein nutrition in healthy adults, even at the exclusion of animal protein, provided the sources are mixed in a varied, high-quality diet. This might not be the case among elderly people, but this remains a research question that awaits studies to depict the final functional impacts (e.g., on fitness, in the short/medium term, and the long-term risk of sarcopenia). When plant protein sources are not mixed and mostly arise from cereals, in a diet that is associated with low protein and energy intakes (as in some developing regions), a low lysine intake remains a concern whose impact needs to be further characterized. More generally, the effects of plant/animal protein intake on the background metabolism of amino acids remains largely unexplored, although this is expected to be the rationale for studies on the impact of dietary protein sources on numerous functions and health outcomes. In Western countries, the standard view of "protein quality" is now outdated. We need to further study the metabolic impact of plant and animal protein sources with respect to amino acid–related metabolic pathways that have key relationships with functional impact. Last, different proteins (animal vs. plant) are not consumed in isolation but in association with the foodstuffs that contain them, and they will together build the final nutritional characteristics of a diet. This is part of the bigger picture that we shall try to analyze in Chapter 36, as this is important to deciphering the relationships between plant protein, animal protein, and health.

Acknowledgments

I would like to thank Professor Jean-François Huneau for our fruitful discussions.

References

Afolabi, P.R., Jahoor, F., Gibson, N.R., Jackson, A.A., 2004. Response of hepatic proteins to the lowering of habitual dietary protein to the recommended safe level of intake. Am. J. Physiol. Endocrinol. Metab. 287, E327–E330.

AFSSA, 2008. Apport en protéines : consommation, qualité, besoins et recommandations. AFSSA.

Albanese, A., 2012. Protein and Amino Acid Nutrition. Elsevier Science.

Alford, B.B., Onley, K., 1978. The minimum cottonseed protein required for nitrogen balance in women. J. Nutr. 108, 506–513.

Arnal, M.A., Mosoni, L., Boirie, Y., Houlier, M.L., Morin, L., Verdier, E., Ritz, P., Antoine, J.M., Prugnaud, J., Beaufrere, B., Mirand, P.P., 1999. Protein pulse feeding improves protein retention in elderly women. Am. J. Clin. Nutr. 69, 1202–1208.

Arnal, M.A., Mosoni, L., Boirie, Y., Houlier, M.L., Morin, L., Verdier, E., Ritz, P., Antoine, J.M., Prugnaud, J., Beaufrere, B., Mirand, P.P., 2000. Protein feeding pattern does not affect protein retention in young women. J. Nutr. 130, 1700–1704.

Bailey, L.B., Clark, H.E., 1976. Plasma amino acids and nitrogen retention of human subjects who consumed isonitrogenous diets containing rice and wheat or their constituent amino acids with and without additional lysine. Am. J. Clin. Nutr. 29, 1353–1358.

Beasley, J.M., Shikany, J.M., Thomson, C.A., 2013. The role of dietary protein intake in the prevention of sarcopenia of aging. Nutr. Clin. Pract. 28, 684–690.

Beaufrere, B., Dangin, M., Boirie, Y., 2000. The 'fast' and 'slow' protein concept. Nestle Nutr. Workshop Ser. Clin. Perform. Programme 3, 121–131 discussion 131–133.

Berner, L.A., Becker, G., Wise, M., Doi, J., 2013. Characterization of dietary protein among older adults in the United States: amount, animal sources, and meal patterns. J. Acad. Nutr. Diet. 113, 809–815.

Bos, C., Airinei, G., Mariotti, F., Benamouzig, R., Bérot, S., Evrard, J., Fénart, E., Tomé, D., Gaudichon, C., 2007. The poor digestibility of rapeseed protein is balanced by its very high metabolic utilization in humans. J. Nutr. 137, 594–600.

Boye, J., Wijesinha-Bettoni, R., Burlingame, B., 2012. Protein quality evaluation twenty years after the introduction of the protein digestibility corrected amino acid score method. Br. J. Nutr. 108 (Suppl. 2), S183–S211.

Campbell, W.W., Trappe, T.A., Jozsi, A.C., Kruskall, L.J., Wolfe, R.R., Evans, W.J., 2002. Dietary protein adequacy and lower body versus whole body resistive training in older humans. J. Physiol. 542, 631–642.

Churchward-Venne, T.A., Snijders, T., Linkens, A.M., Hamer, H.M., Van Kranenburg, J., Van Loon, L.J., 2015. Ingestion of casein in a milk matrix modulates dietary protein digestion and absorption kinetics but does not modulate postprandial muscle protein synthesis in older men. J. Nutr. 145, 1438–1445.

Clarys, P., Deliens, T., Huybrechts, I., Deriemaeker, P., Vanaelst, B., De Keyzer, W., Hebbelinck, M., Mullie, P., 2014. Comparison of nutritional quality of the vegan, vegetarian, semi-vegetarian, pesco-vegetarian and omnivorous diet. Nutrients 6, 1318–1332.

Clemente, A., Vioque, J., Sanchez-Vioque, R., Pedroche, J., Bautista, J., Millan, F., 2000. Factors affecting the in vitro protein digestibility of chickpea albumins. J. Sci. Food Agric. 80, 79–84.

Craig, W.J., Mangels, A.R., American Dietetic, A, 2009. Position of the American dietetic association: vegetarian diets. J. Am. Diet. Assoc. 109, 1266–1282.

Cruz, G., Oliveira, M., Pires, C., Gomes, M., Costa, N., Brumano, M., Moreira, M., 2003. Protein quality and in vivo digestibility of different varieties of bean (*Phaseolus vulgaris* L.). Braz. J. Food Technol. 6, 157–162.

Daenzer, M., Petzke, K.J., Bequette, B.J., Metges, C.C., 2001. Whole-body nitrogen and splanchnic amino acid metabolism differ in rats fed mixed diets containing casein or its corresponding amino acid mixture. J. Nutr. 131, 1965–1972.

Dangin, M., Boirie, Y., Garcia-Rodenas, C., Gachon, P., Fauquant, J., Callier, P., Ballevre, O., Beaufrere, B., 2001. The digestion rate of protein is an independent regulating factor of postprandial protein retention. Am. J. Physiol. Endocrinol. Metab. 280, E340–E348.

Dangin, M., Guillet, C., Garcia-Rodenas, C., Gachon, P., Bouteloup-Demange, C., Reiffers-Magnani, K., Fauquant, J., Ballevre, O., Beaufrere, B., 2003. The rate of protein digestion affects protein gain differently during aging in humans. J. Physiol. 549, 635–644.

Dardevet, D., Remond, D., Peyron, M.A., Papet, I., Savary-Auzeloux, I., Mosoni, L., 2012. Muscle wasting and resistance of muscle anabolism: the "anabolic threshold concept" for adapted nutritional strategies during sarcopenia. Sci. World J. 2012, 269531.

Dardevet, D., Sornet, C., Bayle, G., Prugnaud, J., Pouyet, C., Grizard, J., 2002. Postprandial stimulation of muscle protein synthesis in old rats can be restored by a leucine-supplemented meal. J. Nutr. 132, 95–100.

Eklund, M., Sauer, N., Schone, F., Messerschmidt, U., Rosenfelder, P., Htoo, J.K., Mosenthin, R., 2015. Effect of processing of rapeseed under defined conditions in a pilot plant on chemical composition and standardized ileal amino acid digestibility in rapeseed meal for pigs. J. Anim. Sci. 93, 2813–2825.

FAO, 2013. Dietary Protein Quality Evaluation in Human Nutrition Report of an FAO Expert Consultation. March 31–April 2, 2011, Auckland, New Zealand. FAO, Rome, Italy. Food and Nutrition Paper 92.

FAO/WHO, 1973. Energy and Protein Requirements. Report of a Joint FAO/WHO Ad Hoc Expert Committee. World Health Organization, Geneva. WHO Technical Report Series, No 522.

FAO/WHO/UNU, 2007. Protein and Amino Acid Requirements in Human Nutrition: Report of a Joint FAO/WHO/UNU Expert Consultation (2002: Geneva, Switzerland). World Health Organization, WHO. Technical Report Series, No 935.

Faris, R.J., Wang, H., Wang, T., 2008. Improving digestibility of soy flour by reducing disulfide bonds with thioredoxin. J. Agric. Food Chem. 56, 7146–7150.

Fouillet, H., Gaudichon, C., Bos, C., Mariotti, F., Tome, D., 2003. Contribution of plasma proteins to splanchnic and total anabolic utilization of dietary nitrogen in humans. Am. J. Physiol. Endocrinol. Metab. 285, E88–E97.

Fouillet, H., Juillet, B., Bos, C., Mariotti, F., Gaudichon, C., Benamouzig, R., Tome, D., 2008. Urea-nitrogen production and salvage are modulated by protein intake in fed humans: results of an oral stable-iso-tope-tracer protocol and compartmental modeling. Am. J. Clin. Nutr. 87, 1702–1714.

Fouillet, H., Juillet, B., Gaudichon, C., Mariotti, F., Tome, D., Bos, C., 2009. Absorption kinetics are a key fac-tor regulating postprandial protein metabolism in response to qualitative and quantitative variations in protein intake. Am. J. Physiol. Regul. Integr. Comp. Physiol. 297, R1691–R1705.

Friedman, M., Brandon, D.L., 2001. Nutritional and health benefits of soy proteins. J. Agric. Food Chem. 49, 1069–1086.

Friedman, M., Gumbmann, M.R., 1986. Nutritional improvement of legume proteins through disulfide interchange. Adv. Exp. Med. Biol. 199, 357–389.

Gaudichon, C., Bos, C., Morens, C., Petzke, K.J., Mariotti, F., Everwand, J., Benamouzig, R., Dare, S., Tome, D., Metges, C.C., 2002. Ileal losses of nitrogen and amino acids in humans and their importance to the assessment of amino acid requirements. Gastroenterology 123, 50–59.

Gilani, G.S., 2012. Background on international activities on protein quality assessment of foods. Br. J. Nutr. 108 (Suppl. 2), S168–S182.

Gilani, G.S., Cockell, K.A., Sepehr, E., 2005. Effects of antinutritional factors on protein digestibility and amino acid availability in foods. J. AOAC Int. 88, 967–987.

Gilani, G.S., Sepehr, E., 2003. Protein digestibility and quality in products containing antinutritional fac-tors are adversely affected by old age in rats. J. Nutr. 133, 220–225.

Gorissen, S.H., Burd, N.A., Hamer, H.M., Gijsen, A.P., Groen, B.B., Van Loon, L.J., 2014. Carbohydrate coingestion delays dietary protein digestion and absorption but does not modulate postprandial mus-cle protein accretion. J. Clin. Endocrinol. Metab. 99, 2250–2258.

Groen, B.B., Horstman, A.M., Hamer, H.M., De Haan, M., Van Kranenburg, J., Bierau, J., Poeze, M., Wodzig, W.K., Rasmussen, B.B., Van Loon, L.J., 2015. Post-prandial protein handling: you are what you just ate. PLoS One 10, e0141582.

Gryson, C., Walrand, S., Giraudet, C., Rousset, P., Migne, C., Bonhomme, C., Le Ruyet, P., Boirie, Y., 2014. "Fast proteins" with a unique essential amino acid content as an optimal nutrition in the elderly: grow-ing evidence. Clin. Nutr. 33, 642–648.

Halkjaer, J., Olsen, A., Bjerregaard, L.J., Deharveng, G., Tjonneland, A., Welch, A.A., Crowe, F.L., Wirfalt, E., Hellstrom, V., Niravong, M., Touvier, M., Linseisen, J., Steffen, A., Ocke, M.C., Peeters, P.H., Chirlaque, M.D., Larranaga, N., Ferrari, P., Contiero, P., Frasca, G., Engeset, D., Lund, E., Misirli, G., Kosti, M., Riboli, E., Slimani, N., Bingham, S., 2009. Intake of total, animal and plant proteins, and their food sources in 10 countries in the European Prospective Investigation into Cancer and Nutrition. Eur. J. Clin. Nutr. 63 (Suppl. 4), S16–S36.

He, Q., Yin, Y., Zhao, F., Kong, X., Wu, G., Ren, P., 2011. Metabonomics and its role in amino acid nutrition research. Front. Biosci. (Landmark Ed.) 16, 2451–2460.

Heck, J.E., Nieves, J.W., Chen, Y., Parvez, F., Brandt-Rauf, P.W., Howe, G.R., Ahsan, H., 2010. Protein and amino acid intakes in a rural area of Bangladesh. Food Nutr. Bull. 31, 206–213.

Ho, J.E., Larson, M.G., Ghorbani, A., Cheng, S., Chen, M.H., Keyes, M., Rhee, E.P., Clish, C.B., Vasan, R.S., Gerszten, R.E., Wang, T.J., 2016. Metabolomic profiles of body mass index in the Framingham heart study reveal distinct cardiometabolic phenotypes. PLoS One 11, e0148361.

Jackson, A.A., Gibson, N.R., Lu, Y., Jahoor, F., 2004. Synthesis of erythrocyte glutathione in healthy adults consuming the safe amount of dietary protein. Am. J. Clin. Nutr. 80, 101–107.

Kim, I.Y., Schutzler, S., Schrader, A., Spencer, H., Kortebein, P., Deutz, N.E., Wolfe, R.R., Ferrando, A.A., 2015. Quantity of dietary protein intake, but not pattern of intake, affects net protein balance primarily through differences in protein synthesis in older adults. Am. J. Physiol. Endocrinol. Metab. 308, E21–E28.

LeMieux, M., Al-Jawadi, A., Wang, S., Moustaid-Moussa, N., 2013. Metabolic profiling in nutrition and metabolic disorders. Adv. Nutr. 4, 548–550.

Magne, H., Savary-Auzeloux, I., Migne, C., Peyron, M.A., Combaret, L., Remond, D., Dardevet, D., 2012. Contrarily to whey and high protein diets, dietary free leucine supplementation cannot reverse the lack of recovery of muscle mass after prolonged immobilization during ageing. J. Physiol. 590, 2035–2049.

Malfait, P., Moren, A., Dillon, J.C., Brodel, A., Begkoyian, G., Etchegorry, M.G., Malenga, G., Hakewill, P., 1993. An outbreak of pellagra related to changes in dietary niacin among Mozambican refugees in Malawi. Int. J. Epidemiol. 22, 504–511.

Mamerow, M.M., Mettler, J.A., English, K.L., Casperson, S.L., Arentson-Lantz, E., Sheffield-Moore, M., Layman, D.K., Paddon-Jones, D., 2014. Dietary protein distribution positively influences 24-h muscle protein synthesis in healthy adults. J. Nutr. 144, 876–880.

Mariotti, F., 2016. Protein intake throughout life and current dietary recommendations. In: Dardevet, D. (Ed.), The Molecular Nutrition of Amino Acids and Proteins. Elsevier.

Mariotti, F., Kalonji, E., Huneau, J.F., Margaritis, I., 2010. Potential pitfalls of health claims from a public health nutrition perspective. Nutr. Rev. 68, 624–638.

Mariotti, F., Pueyo, M.E., Tome, D., Berot, S., Benamouzig, R., Mahe, S., 2001. The influence of the albumin fraction on the bioavailability and postprandial utilization of pea protein given selectively to humans. J. Nutr. 131, 1706–1713.

Mariotti, F., Tomé, D., Patureau-Mirand, P., 2008. Converting nitrogen into protein – beyond 6.25 and Jones' factors. Crit. Rev. Food Sci. Nutr. 48, 177–184.

Millward, D.J., Fereday, A., Gibson, N.R., Cox, M.C., Pacy, P.J., 2002. Efficiency of utilization of wheat and milk protein in healthy adults and apparent lysine requirements determined by a single-meal [1-13C] leucine balance protocol. Am. J. Clin. Nutr. 76, 1326–1334.

Millward, D.J., Fereday, A., Gibson, N.R., Pacy, P.J., 1996. Post-prandial protein metabolism. Baillieres Clin. Endocrinol. Metab. 10, 533–549.

Millward, D.J., Fereday, A., Gibson, N.R., Pacy, P.J., 2000. Human adult amino acid requirements: [1-13C] leucine balance evaluation of the efficiency of utilization and apparent requirements for wheat protein and lysine compared with those for milk protein in healthy adults. Am. J. Clin. Nutr. 72, 112–121.

Millward, D.J., Garnett, T., 2010. Plenary Lecture 3: food and the planet: nutritional dilemmas of greenhouse gas emission reductions through reduced intakes of meat and dairy foods. Proc. Nutr. Soc. 69, 103–118.

Millward, D.J., Layman, D.K., Tome, D., Schaafsma, G., 2008. Protein quality assessment: impact of expanding understanding of protein and amino acid needs for optimal health. Am. J. Clin. Nutr. 87, 1576S–1581S.

Millward, D.J., Rivers, J.P., 1988. The nutritional role of indispensable amino acids and the metabolic basis for their requirements. Eur. J. Clin. Nutr. 42, 367–393.

Millward, D.J., Roberts, S.B., 1996. Protein requirements of older individuals. Nutr. Res. Rev. 9, 67–87.

Mirone, L., 1950. Blood findings in men on a diet devoid of meat and low in animal protein. Science 111, 673.

Mitchell, H.H., 1923. The place of proteins in the diet in the light of the newer knowledge of nutrition. Am. J. Public Health (NY) 13, 17–23.

Mitchell, H.H., 1924. A method of determining the biological value of protein. J. Biol. Chem. 58, 873–903.

Mosoni, L., Gatineau, E., Gatellier, P., Migne, C., Savary-Auzeloux, I., Remond, D., Rocher, E., Dardevet, D., 2014. High whey protein intake delayed the loss of lean body mass in healthy old rats, whereas protein type and polyphenol/antioxidant supplementation had no effects. PLoS One 9, e109098.

Nuss, E.T., Tanumihardjo, S.A., 2011. Quality protein maize for Africa: closing the protein inadequacy gap in vulnerable populations. Adv. Nutr. 2, 217–224.

Paddon-Jones, D., Campbell, W.W., Jacques, P.F., Kritchevsky, S.B., Moore, L.L., Rodriguez, N.R., Van Loon, L.J., 2015. Protein and healthy aging. Am. J. Clin. Nutr.

Paddon-Jones, D., Leidy, H., 2014. Dietary protein and muscle in older persons. Curr. Opin. Clin. Nutr. Metab. Care 17, 5–11.

Paddon-Jones, D., Rasmussen, B.B., 2009. Dietary protein recommendations and the prevention of sarcopenia. Curr. Opin. Clin. Nutr. Metab. Care 12, 86–90.

Pennings, B., Boirie, Y., Senden, J.M., Gijsen, A.P., Kuipers, H., Van Loon, L.J., 2011. Whey protein stimulates postprandial muscle protein accretion more effectively than do casein and casein hydrolysate in older men. Am. J. Clin. Nutr. 93, 997–1005.

Poupin, N., Bos, C., Mariotti, F., Huneau, J.F., Tome, D., Fouillet, H., 2011. The nature of the dietary protein impacts the tissue-to-diet 15N discrimination factors in laboratory rats. PLoS One 6, e28046.

Poupin, N., Mariotti, F., Huneau, J.F., Hermier, D., Fouillet, H., 2014. Natural isotopic signatures of variations in body nitrogen fluxes: a compartmental model analysis. PLoS Comput. Biol. 10, e1003865.

Rand, W.M., Pellett, P.L., Young, V.R., 2003. Meta-analysis of nitrogen balance studies for estimating protein requirements in healthy adults. Am. J. Clin. Nutr. 77, 109–127.

Rodriguez, N.R., 2014. Protein-centric meals for optimal protein utilization: can it be that simple? J. Nutr. 144, 797–798.

Rutherfurd, S.M., 2015. Use of the guanidination reaction for determining reactive lysine, bioavailable lysine and gut endogenous lysine. Amino Acids 47, 1805–1815.

Rutherfurd, S.M., Fanning, A.C., Miller, B.J., Moughan, P.J., 2015. Protein digestibility-corrected amino acid scores and digestible indispensable amino acid scores differentially describe protein quality in growing male rats. J. Nutr. 145, 372–379.

Samadi, Theodoridou, K., Yu, P., 2013. Detect the sensitivity and response of protein molecular structure of whole canola seed (yellow and brown) to different heat processing methods and relation to protein utilization and availability using ATR-FT/IR molecular spectroscopy with chemometrics. Spectrochim. Acta A Mol. Biomol. Spectrosc. 105, 304–313.

Sarwar, G., Blair, R., Friedman, M., Gumbmann, M.R., Hackler, L.R., Pellett, P.L., Smith, T.K., 1984. Inter- and intra-laboratory variability in rat growth assays for estimating protein quality of foods. J. Assoc. Off. Anal. Chem. 67, 976–981.

Sarwar, G., Sosulski, F.W., Bell, J.M., Bowland, J.P., 1978. Nutritional evaluation of oilseeds and legumes as protein supplements to cereals. Adv. Exp. Med. Biol. 105, 415–441.

Sarwar Gilani, G., Wu Xiao, C., Cockell, K.A., 2012. Impact of antinutritional factors in food proteins on the digestibility of protein and the bioavailability of amino acids and on protein quality. Br. J. Nutr. 108 (Suppl. 2), S315–S332.

Seal, A.J., Creeke, P.I., Dibari, F., Cheung, E., Kyroussis, E., Semedo, P., Van Den Briel, T., 2007. Low and deficient niacin status and pellagra are endemic in postwar Angola. Am. J. Clin. Nutr. 85, 218–224.

Sherman, H.C., 1920. The protein requirement of maintenance in man. Proc. Natl. Acad. Sci. U.S.A. 6, 38–40.

Suri, D.J., Tano-Debrah, K., Ghosh, S.A., 2014. Optimization of the nutrient content and protein quality of cereal-legume blends for use as complementary foods in Ghana. Food Nutr. Bull. 35, 372–381.

Tieland, M., Borgonjen-Van Den Berg, K.J., Van Loon, L.J., De Groot, L.C., 2015. Dietary protein intake in Dutch elderly people: a focus on protein sources. Nutrients 7, 9697–9706.

Tomé, D., 2013. Digestibility issues of vegetable versus animal proteins: protein and amino acid requirements – functional aspects. Food Nutr. Bull. 34, 272–274.

U.S. Department of Agriculture – Agricultural Research Service, 2013. USDA National Nutrient Database for Standard Reference, Release 26. Nutrient Data Laboratory. Available at: http://www.ars.usda.gov/ba/bhnrc/ndl.

Van Der Poel, T.F.B., Blonk, J., Van Zuilichem, D.J., Van Oort, M.G., 1990. Thermal inactivation of lectins and trypsin inhibitor activity during steam processing of dry beans (*Phaseolus vulgaris*) and effects on protein quality. J. Sci. Food Agric. 53, 215–228.

van Vliet, S., Burd, N.A., Van Loon, L.J., 2015. The skeletal muscle anabolic response to plant- versus animal-based protein consumption. J. Nutr. 145, 1981–1991.

Wall, B.T., Gorissen, S.H., Pennings, B., Koopman, R., Groen, B.B., Verdijk, L.B., Van Loon, L.J., 2015. Aging is accompanied by a blunted muscle protein synthetic response to protein ingestion. PLoS One 10, e0140903.

Waterlow, J.C., 1999. The mysteries of nitrogen balance. Nutr. Res. Rev. 12, 25–54.

WHO/FAO/UNU, 2007. Protein and Amino Acid Requirements in Human Nutrition. World Health Organ Tech. Rep. Ser. 1–265, back cover.

Yang, S.P., Tilton, K.S., Ryland, L.L., 1968. Utilization of a delayed lysine or tryptophan supplement for protein repletion of rats. J. Nutr. 94, 178–184.

Young, V.R., 1991. Nutrient interactions with reference to amino acid and protein metabolism in nonruminants; particular emphasis on protein-energy relations in man. Z. Ernahrungswiss. 30, 239–267.

Young, V.R., 1998. Human amino acid requirements: counterpoint to Millward and the importance of tentative revised estimates. J. Nutr. 128, 1570–1573.

Young, V.R., Fajardo, L., Murray, E., Rand, W.M., Scrimshaw, N.S., 1975. Protein requirements of man: comparative nitrogen balance response within the submaintenance-to-maintenance range of intakes of wheat and beef proteins. J. Nutr. 105, 534–542.

Young, V.R., Puig, M., Queiroz, E., Scrimshaw, N.S., Rand, W.M., 1984a. Evaluation of the protein quality of an isolated soy protein in young men: relative nitrogen requirements and effect of methionine supplementation. Am. J. Clin. Nutr. 39, 16–24.

Young, V.R., Wayler, A., Garza, C., Steinke, F.H., Murray, E., Rand, W.M., Scrimshaw, N.S., 1984b. A long-term metabolic balance study in young men to assess the nutritional quality of an isolated soy protein and beef proteins. Am. J. Clin. Nutr. 39, 8–15.

36

Plant Protein, Animal Protein, and Cardiometabolic Health

François Mariotti

UMR PHYSIOLOGIE DE LA NUTRITION ET DU COMPORTEMENT ALIMENTAIRE, AGROPARISTECH, INRA, UNIVERSITÉ PARIS-SACLAY, PARIS, FRANCE

1. Introduction

This chapter follows on naturally from the previous chapter dedicated to plant/animal protein and protein quality. The basic role of dietary protein is to ensure adequate growth and the renewal of body proteins, and it has been the focus of protein research for many years. However, as explained in the previous chapter, debate continues on certain unresolved issues. Refining our understanding of the protein nutritional system under different conditions remains an important area of research. In particular, it is necessary to clarify the specific conditions that cause changes to the protein nutritional system with aging, since this has important impact on musculoskeletal health and the risk of sarcopenia. It is also essential to fully characterize the detailed metabolic effects of changes to protein and amino acid intakes that do not apparently affect the classic rough criteria applied for protein quality. It is still largely unknown how the metabolic fluxes concerning virtually all amino acid pathways are affected by changes to protein sources, although it is expected that this will mediate both the physiological and pathophysiological impacts. When broaching this topic, we indeed need to consider the relationship between dietary protein and disease prevention from a metabolic standpoint. The fact that the type of protein may modify disease risk is a long-standing issue that can be dated back to 1908 and the pioneering work by Alexander I. Ignatowski on animal protein, cholesterol, and experimental atherosclerosis in rabbits (Kritchevsky, 1995).

In this chapter, we will be reviewing the broad topic of plant and animal proteins and their relationships with cardiometabolic health from a variety of standpoints, which include basic science such as amino acid metabolism, clinical trials on the intermediary endpoints of cardiovascular health, and nutritional epidemiology to decipher the potential effects of plant/animal protein intakes. These different issues will be addressed at different levels of understanding, from specific amino acids to overall diet adequacy.

Vegetarian and Plant-Based Diets in Health and Disease Prevention. http://dx.doi.org/10.1016/B978-0-12-803968-7.00036-8

2. Plant Protein, Amino Acids, and Underlying Metabolism

2.1 Overall Changes to Background Amino Acid Metabolism

As well as supplying indispensable amino acids to ensure body protein growth/turnover, dietary proteins also affect amino acid metabolism. It has been shown that animal versus plant proteins (milk and soy proteins), which can both meet the requirements for maintenance and growth in rodents, do indeed leave a footprint, as identified from their natural isotopic abundance in tissues, demonstrating that the utilization of these proteins in response to metabolic demand is not assured by the same arrangements in the underlying metabolism (Poupin et al., 2011, 2014). In turn, changes to the underlying metabolism may have a physiological or pathophysiological impact in the longer term. Systems biology should help to increase our knowledge of the influence of dietary amino acids on both the overall metabolism and the precise pathways that are candidates to explain a physiological effect (He et al., 2011). This is important because alterations to the profiles of some amino acids in plasma have been demonstrated to be central to the metabolomic profiles that are associated with obesity, cardiometabolic risk factors, and the risks of cardiovascular disease (CVD) and diabetes (Ho et al., 2016; LeMieux et al., 2013). It remains unclear how these metabolomic characteristics are affected by protein and individual amino acid intakes (Cavallaro et al., 2016; Schmidt et al., 2015). Dietary intakes and plasma concentrations of amino acids were assayed in a subsample of the EPIC cohort, and the differences analyzed across the spectrum of vegetarian diet types (Schmidt et al., 2015). The data showed that plasma methionine, tryptophan, and tyrosine levels were higher in ovolactovegetarians than in meat eaters, but the values were the lowest among vegans. In contrast, plasma glycine concentrations were higher in vegans, followed by ovolactovegetarians and pescetarians, than in meat eaters. Lysine levels were lower in vegans than in ovolactovegetarians, followed by meat eaters. These differences between dietary groups were, in general, little or not explained by differences in dietary intakes, although there was a general correlation between the intakes and concentrations of lysine, methionine, tyrosine, and tryptophan (Schmidt et al., 2015). Currently, the health consequences of the background metabolic changes induced by changes to amino acid intakes remain unknown.

2.2 Could Some Amino Acids in Plant Versus Animal Protein Procure Specific Benefits?

As well as their utilization for protein synthesis or oxidation, amino acids enter specific metabolic pathways that lead to the synthesis of metabolites that play key roles in physiology and pathophysiology. Mention should be made of two amino acids that are present at varying levels in plant and animal proteins and have been widely studied for their probable impact on physiology: arginine and cysteine.

Arginine, a conditionally indispensable amino acid, has attracted attention since the discovery that it provides the substrate for the synthesis of nitric oxide (NO), a mediator involved in a series of pivotal physiological functions (Moncada and Higgs, 2006).

Epidemiological studies have closely related CVD risk with an impairment of endothelial function, and have shown that endothelial dysfunction precedes and predicts atherosclerosis (Juonala et al., 2004; Flammer et al., 2012). Endothelial dysfunction primarily results in alterations to NO metabolism, the critical modulator of vascular homeostasis (Maxwell, 2002; Moncada and Higgs, 2006). Indeed, an impairment of NO production and/or bioactivity is largely reported as a central feature associated with cardiometabolic risk, including that of coronary artery disease, stroke, and diabetes (Reriani et al., 2010). As shown by a meta-analysis, arginine supplementation improves endothelial function when it is low at baseline (Bai et al., 2009). The beneficial effects of arginine supplementation on endothelial function may be achieved with a low intake, such as that seen by modifying the amount or type of protein in the diet, as shown by its ability to blunt postprandial endothelial function after a high-fat meal (Borucki et al., 2009; Deveaux et al., 2016b). The kinetics of arginine bioavailability may also play an important role inasmuch as arginine that is slowly made available—as dietary, protein-bound arginine—is directed more toward NO synthesis than arginine that is rapidly available (for example, in a dietary supplement) (Deveaux et al., 2016a). The potential of arginine-rich proteins to prevent alterations to postprandial endothelial function has been demonstrated (Westphal et al., 2006; Magne et al., 2009). It has also been suggested that arginine has a beneficial impact on many other metabolism systems and functions. For instance, animal data have shown that arginine supplementation can affect body composition (Jobgen et al., 2009; Tan et al., 2009; Wu et al., 2012). In humans, it has been concluded that arginine may mediate some of the beneficial effects of including 25 g/day lupine protein (which is very rich in arginine) in the diet (Bahr et al., 2015). Improvements to metabolic health with arginine may be concomitant with the possible effect of NO modulation of the physiology of adipose tissue (Roberts, 2015). Low plasma arginine levels have been associated with obesity, as well as inflammation and oxidative stress in obese humans (Niu et al., 2012).

The benefits of a high arginine intake have also been studied for many years in connection with lysine levels. Indeed, the early historical relationship between plant and animal proteins, plasma cholesterol, and atherosclerosis in animal models has largely been attributed to varying amounts of arginine and lysine, and the lysine:arginine ratio; a high lysine:arginine ratio has been associated with these adverse effects (Debry, 2004a, 2004b). More recently, in a closely controlled trial, Vega-Lopez et al. found that a low (vs. high) lysine:arginine ratio lowered postprandial plasma levels of triglycerides, VLDL cholesterol, and C-reactive protein (CRP) in moderately hypercholesterolemic subjects. This study did not demonstrate any effects of changes to the lysine:arginine ratio on fasting endothelial function, but postprandial endothelial function was not tested. The addition of 25 g/day lupine protein (which is very rich in arginine) to the diet of hypercholesterolemic subjects also resulted in lower plasma triglyceride and LDL cholesterol levels (Bahr et al., 2014). Overall, the effects of arginine on health and disease is an ongoing topic, but further controlled and longer term studies are necessary to clarify the benefits of different arginine levels in dietary proteins.

Sulfur amino acids, and particularly cysteine, have also been studied for their potential effects on cardiometabolic risk, because of their links with homocysteine (a probable risk factor for CVD) and glutathione (a pivotal molecule in redox homeostasis). The relationship between cysteine intake, glutathione metabolism, and cardiometabolic risk has been widely studied and reviewed elsewhere (Wu, 2009; McPherson and Hardy, 2011). In brief, dietary cysteine supplementation has been reported to reduce diet-induced oxidative stress and insulin resistance in rats (Blouet et al., 2007). This protective effect was notably accompanied by an alteration of glutathione redox status, which has been reported to be an early marker of atherosclerosis in healthy humans (Ashfaq et al., 2006). In humans, variation in sulfur amino acid intakes affect fasting plasma free cysteine concentration and the redox status, as shown by the Cys/CySS redox potential (E(h)CySS) (Jones et al., 2011). The effects of modulating cysteine intake on the synthesis and status of not only glutathione but also hydrogen sulfide and taurine, on redox status and, in turn, on the pathobiology of insulin resistance, inflammation, and atherosclerosis, remain an important area of research (Yin et al., 2016).

Other amino acids have been studied for their links with cardiovascular risk factors and identified as candidates for mediating the effects of protein intakes, based on experimental studies in animal or humans, or associations found in epidemiological studies. For instance, oral glycine was shown to be particularly efficient in potentiating the action of insulin in a series of controlled trials on the effects of adding amino acids to a glucose load (Gannon et al., 2002; Gannon and Nuttall, 2010). Intakes of glutamic acid have been associated with lower systolic blood pressure, independently of other amino acids (Stamler et al., 2009). Other candidates include histidine, tyrosine, or leucine itself (Jennings et al., 2015; Niu et al., 2012). It would be interesting to study the separate and combined effects of amino acid intakes, to identify the most influential amino acids and try to determine how they might account for the effects of plant proteins. In the study by Jenning et al. the association between the intake of several amino acids and blood pressure was found to depend on whether they originated from plant or animal protein sources, which is indicative of the complexity of this issue.

Although it is much too soon, this area of research may eventually have important implications for our evaluation of protein quality based on the level of specific amino acids, and it should stimulate study of the effects of certain plant proteins on cardiovascular/ cardiometabolic health. According to the USDA database (US. Department of Agriculture – Agricultural Research Service, 2013), legumes are generally rich in arginine, with high values being found in soy protein (7.6 g/100 g), lentils (8.4 g/100 g), peas (9.3 g/100 g), fava beans (9.9 g/100 g), and lupine (10.6 g/100 g), as well as in nuts (e.g., almonds: 11.2 g/100 g). High levels are also found in rice (8.3 g/100 g). By contrast, animal proteins contain moderate (beef, fish, and eggs: 6–6.6 g/100 g) or low amounts (milk protein: 3.5 g/100 g). When expressed relative to other amino acids, arginine is that which is the most consumed by vegans when compared to nonvegetarians (Schmidt et al., 2015). Cysteine content also varies considerably between protein sources, in particular in plant versus animal proteins. Sulfur amino acids are mostly cysteine in plant protein but mostly methionine in animal protein.

Cysteine levels are high in cereal protein (wheat: 2.1 g/100 g), moderate in bean protein (peas: 1.6 g/100 g), low in meat and fish (1.1–1.2 g/100 g), and very low in milk protein (0.9 g/100 g). Among animal proteins, the exception is egg protein (2.3 g/100 g). Plant proteins are the main contributor to cysteine intake in an omnivorous population, whereas animal proteins contribute most histidine, tyrosine, and leucine (Jennings et al., 2015). In plant proteins, cereals are rich in glutamic acid (and/or glutamine) (wheat: 35 g/100 g), and much more so than animal protein (average: 16 g/100 g).

Nevertheless, it can be hypothesized that the beneficial effects of plant proteins on cardiovascular risk might not be ascribable to a specific amino acid but rather to a different amino acid pattern. Some effects may result from the combined intake of some of the amino acids we have mentioned as good candidates, such as arginine and cysteine, or of a larger set of amino acids.

This would explain the beneficial effects of some specific proteins, such as rapeseed protein. In rats, adding both cysteine and arginine to a meal was seen to reproduce most of the beneficial effects of replacing milk protein by rapeseed proteins on postprandial endothelial function (Magne et al., 2009). A combined effect of certain amino acids might also explain the beneficial effects of a plant-based diet, as found in vegetarians. Based on the nonvegetarian, ovolactovegetarian, and vegans groups in the study by Schmidt et al. (2016) the more the diet avoids animal protein, the more it is relatively rich in arginine and dispensable amino acids (such as glutamate and aspartate or the amides), and the lower it is in lysine and methionine, the methionine:cysteine ratio, and branched-chain amino acids.

Clearly, there are hypotheses that need to be further tested to delineate the effects of plant proteins and their mediation by different amino acid intakes. However, it remains difficult to specifically ascribe the effect of a protein to that of certain amino acids, or conversely, extrapolate the effect of a specific amino acid to that of a protein. Further studies might interestingly consist in manipulating the dietary amino acid content with different protein sources during controlled trials, as proposed elegantly by Vega-Lopez et al. (2010), or to simulate the addition of amino acids using sustained release forms that mimic slow dietary absorption kinetics and thus synchronize this supplementary supply to the natural dietary intake of all amino acids, as we did (Deveaux et al., 2016a,b). Furthermore, epidemiological studies should try to determine which patterns of amino acid intake are associated with cardiovascular health across different animal protein intakes, adjusting for the usual confounding factors that are associated with consuming a plant versus animal-based diet.

3. Clinical Trials and Interventional Studies With Plant Protein

The literature proposes a large body of studies that have examined the effects of specifically manipulating plant proteins on intermediary endpoints to estimate their benefits in terms of cardiovascular health. This type of study mainly consists in adding a specific protein source, using foodstuffs, to a standard diet, with appropriate controls. The endpoints are either established risk factors, such as plasma cholesterol or blood pressure, or markers that are strongly associated with cardiovascular risk (e.g., hyperhomocysteinemia, low-grade inflammation). A few interesting studies have also proposed an integrative assessment of vascular health using measurement of endothelial function.

3.1 Plant Protein and Plasma Cholesterol

Clearly, the most prominent set of data of this type concerns the effect of soy protein intake on plasma cholesterol. While the dataset that was analyzed at the end of the 1990s concluded that soy protein intake lowered LDL cholesterol levels in humans, the evidence until then had been mixed, leading to less conclusive statements (Sacks et al., 2006). Although they remain controversial (Anderson and Bush, 2011), findings have mainly agreed that a soy protein intake per se (i.e., when compared to other proteins) has little effect on LDL cholesterol except at very high levels (>40–50 g/day, i.e., half the average total protein intake), leading to an estimated reduction in LDL cholesterol of ~3% (Sacks et al., 2006; Reynolds et al., 2006). To judge the practical implications of such levels of intake, it is worth mentioning that the high soy protein intake of Adventist vegans in the United States averages only 13 g (Rizzo et al., 2013). A study found no differences in the plasma cholesterol levels of hypercholesterolemic subjects when testing 25 g/day soy protein versus the wheat protein contained in muffins (Padhi et al., 2015). By contrast, products rich in soy protein may be beneficial to cardiovascular health insofar as their utilization results in a displacement of nutrient intake that results in a higher intake of polyunsaturated fats and fiber and a lower intake of saturated fats (Sacks et al., 2006; Reynolds et al., 2006).

It has always been difficult to ascertain the mechanism underlying the effects of soy protein, which may be linked to its amino acids, bioactive peptides, or other substances tightly associated with the protein fraction, as has been debated with respect to isoflavones, for instance (El Khoury and Anderson, 2013).

Other plant proteins have been investigated in rats and humans, such as lupine, whose cholesterol-lowering potential was reported in rats (Spielmann et al., 2007) and humans (Weisse et al., 2009). Recently, the hypocholesterolemic effect of lupine protein in humans was confirmed in a trial using 25 g lupine protein (vs. milk protein) in a variety of complex food products (Bahr et al., 2015). Interestingly, based on data obtained in rats, it has been suggested that lupine protein, like soy protein, may exert its effect by regulating the metabolism of fatty acids and triglycerides in the liver (Torres et al., 2006; Spielmann et al., 2007; Bettzieche et al., 2008).

It should also be noted that dietary protein may also have effects that are little specific and consist in improving lipid metabolism by slowing lipid absorption and synthesis (El Khoury and Anderson, 2013). This effect may not be more attributable to plant or animal protein per se, but rather depend on several factors that include the food matrix containing them and their specific physicochemical interactions (Mariotti et al., 2015). It may therefore not be surprising that trials using legumes, like those on soy foods, have found reductions in plasma cholesterol. A meta-analysis of these data reported mean net decreases in LDL cholesterol of 8 mg/dL and triglycerides of 0.2 g/L, in subjects receiving a legume-rich diet (from 80 to 440 g/day lentils, beans, lupine, etc.) (Bazzano et al., 2011), which confirmed earlier findings (Anderson and Major, 2002). It is also important to note that these studies equilibrated the amounts of energy nutrients in the legume and control diets, including the levels and types of fatty acids (Bazzano et al., 2011). However, other nutrients differ, such as fiber, associated micronutrients, and other substances, so it is not possible to ascribe the effect to the protein per se.

Many researchers have therefore chosen to focus their trials on more marked changes to the diet, where modulating the protein type is only part of the intervention. The well-known portfolio approach combines several foods with cholesterol-lowering properties. Thus Jenkins et al. (2003, 2011) showed that combining soy protein, plant sterols, viscous fibers, and almonds in an intervention diet, or in dietary guidelines, resulted in an important reduction in LDL cholesterol that was much greater than that seen with the low-fat control diet or guidelines. This intervention diet also benefited other cardiovascular risk factors, such as blood pressure and low-grade inflammation (Jenkins et al., 2005, 2008). Approaches that rely on simultaneous changes to several foods in a diet, like a more food-based and dietary pattern method, are useful to clarify dietary recommendations to achieve a reduction in cardiovascular risk (Kris-Etherton et al., 2002).

3.2 Plant Protein and Other Cardiometabolic Factors

Plant protein sources have been studied for their effects on blood pressure. According to a meta-analysis published in 2011, a soy protein isolate reduces systolic and diastolic blood pressures by 2.2 mm Hg and 1.4 mm Hg, respectively (Dong et al., 2011; Hooper et al., 2008). This could be explained by the isoflavones present in soy protein (Liu et al., 2012; Hooper et al., 2008). However, as with the effect on plasma cholesterol, these trials involved large quantities of soy protein (~35 g/day on average). Furthermore, many of them did not use soy protein isolate but soy-containing foods versus control foods, and those using a protein isolate did not all compare their findings with a reference animal protein (such as casein) but rather with carbohydrates, thus hindering interpretation of the entire dataset. Again, soy-containing foodstuffs have been reported as exerting a clearer effect than soy protein isolates (Hooper et al., 2008). Other plant proteins have also been studied, but the evidence remains inconclusive.

Whether plant protein affects other parameters related to metabolic syndrome remains unknown, but many of them have been reported to be modulated in subjects with metabolic syndrome of type 2 diabetes (Zhang et al., 2016). The favorable effects of soy protein products on insulin sensitivity have also been reported following the replacement of meat in the diet with mixed protein sources (from meat, dairy, and bread, mainly) (van Nielen et al., 2014b). During this meticulous study, the macronutrient intakes (including SFA, MUFA, PUFA, cholesterol, and fiber) were matched, so most of the effect could be ascribed to the protein fraction itself, although the role of subtle differences in the whole-food package could not be ruled out. Products containing lupine protein have been shown to exert protein from fish and low-fat dairy (positively associated with the nutrient cluster related to global nutrient adequacy) and protein from processed meat, cheese, and eggs (negatively associated). Associations also varied according to gender, with a negative association of red meat protein in men only. By contrast, plant proteins, whatever the source (i.e., grains, legumes, seeds, and nuts) and gender were consistently associated with nutrient adequacy (Camilleri et al., 2013).

It is still not certain whether the association between plant protein intake and overall nutrient adequacy should be ascribed to the intrinsic characteristic of the foods in our basic diet, as depicted with the "whole-food package," or if it might also be confounded by the healthy behaviors of people seeking a more plant-based diet. Dietary diversity is an overarching factor of diet quality associated with healthy behaviors that is well known for being associated with dietary quality and nutrient adequacy, and which we proved to be associated with plant protein intake in French adults (Bianchi et al., 2016). However, we also found that the association between plant protein intake and nutrient adequacy was independent of overall dietary diversity (Bianchi et al., 2016). This result further strengthens the view that plant protein intake is a robust marker of the nutritional adequacy of the diet (Camilleri et al., 2013). Satija et al. (2016) found that the negative association between a plant-based diet and a risk of diabetes in three cohorts in the United States was stronger when the plant-based diet was considered to be healthy, as measured using a plant-based diet index that positively counts plant groups that are not fruit juices, sweetened beverages, refined grains, potatoes, and sweets/desserts. When looking more closely at the data, it can be seen that the plant-based diet index is negatively associated with total protein intake, whereas a healthy plant-based diet is positively associated with total protein intake, apparently because of a higher intake of plant protein and a moderately lower intake of animal protein (Satija et al., 2016). Therefore, plant/animal protein intake appears to be associated with diet quality, even across different levels of intake of a plant-based diet in the general population.

We also consider that although these data are still limited and fragmented, they lend credence to the idea that a large part of the association between plant and animal protein intakes and cardiometabolic risk could be ascribed to the large cluster of nutrients and others substances (e.g., phytochemicals) that they directly or indirectly convey (Mariotti and Huneau, 2016; Richter et al., 2015). Nonetheless, we also consider, as we have argued earlier, that the type of a protein per se (i.e., the relative amounts of amino acids that it supplies) may affect CVD risk. One interesting observation that may emerge from reviewing the epidemiological data is that the strength of the association decreases when models include nutrient intakes for the purposes of adjustment. For example, during the INTERMAP study, when further adjusting for calcium, SFA, PUFA, cholesterol, magnesium, and fiber, estimates of the strength of the association between plant protein intake were approximately halved and no longer significant (Elliott et al., 2006). Yet many studies have reported a significant association with health-related outcomes, even when fully adjusted models were used, i.e., including dietary/nutrient intakes, and despite classic confounding factors related to behaviors and socioeconomic status. For example, this was the case for the report on plant/animal protein intake and the risk of diabetes, which used a model that adjusted for a family history of diabetes, smoking, alcohol intake, physical activity, race/ethnicity, total energy intake, use of postmenopausal hormones/oral contraceptives, percentages of energy from trans fats, saturated fats, monounsaturated fats, and polyunsaturated fat, dietary cholesterol, dietary fiber, and the glycemic index (Malik et al., 2016). Song et al. (2016) also found significant relations between CVD mortality and plant versus animal protein intakes when adjusting for dietary intakes (e.g., whole grains, fruits, and vegetables, glycemic index) and the intake of types of fatty acids. Likewise, in the Adventist health study-2 cohort, we analyzed the relation between the contributing factors of patterns of dietary protein intake and cardiovascular mortality, and we found that the strong association between factors of protein intake were not modified when accounting for potential confounders such as the vegetarian diet category and the intake of a series of nutrients considered as relevant to cardiovascular risk (e.g., PUFA, SFA, sodium, and vitamins A, C, E, B_6, B_9, and B_{12}) (Tharrey et al., unpublished results). The relation between animal and plant protein products and CVD mortality seems to be mostly contributed by meat: processed red meat and red meat (compared to plant protein) made the clearest association in the study of Song et al. (2016) and, in our study, animal protein factor weighing on meat products was very strongly associated with risk. Conversely, we identified a protective association with a plant protein factor weighting on nuts and seeds and not with other plant protein components of patterns of dietary protein intakes (Tharrey et al., unpublished results).

Finally, these results make a strong suggestion for a specific effect of protein per se, and they also suggest the effect of more specific protein sources, within a diet consisting of animal and plant proteins that are probably heterogeneously associated with cardiovascular health.

6. Conclusion

There are numerous possible reasons why plant protein, or certain plant proteins, may affect cardiometabolic health, starting with their composition in particular amino acids. Our review has shown that plant protein intake could well be beneficial to cardiovascular health, but the final picture remains very unclear. Because protein is an energy macronutrient, and dietary proteins are intricately embedded in different foodstuffs, the results of controlled trials have some important limitations. Closely controlled trials using supplementation with a specific protein source given as selectively as possible are still little conclusive regarding the true impact of plant protein on intermediary endpoints of cardiometabolic risk such as plasma lipid levels. Although trials using plant protein foodstuffs rather than purified proteins have yielded more conclusive results, it is still difficult to disentangle the effect of protein per se from that of changes to other nutrients and substances associated with the protein. Furthermore, studies have mostly been restricted to specific protein sources, so that any extrapolation to "plant protein" in general, and versus animal protein, remains problematic. Likewise, the effect of interventional protocols comparing diets that differ markedly in many respects cannot be ascribed to the pattern of protein sources. Observational studies have been very useful in revealing an association between plant/animal protein intakes using hard outcomes of cardiovascular health and under real-life conditions, although the risk of residual confounding is important. We have argued that a large part of the association between plant and animal protein intakes and cardiometabolic risk could be ascribed to the large cluster of nutrients and other substances that they directly or indirectly convey. However, plant protein intake has consistently been proven a robust marker of a healthy diet in developed countries, and this appears to be a good basis for recommending the sourcing of more protein from plant foods. As this review has emphasized, plant protein is a key nutritional characteristic of a plant-based diet, which can be advocated as being healthy provided it is well balanced.

We still lack much information to analyze the role of plant proteins versus animal proteins and that of the different types of plant proteins that could be used to optimize diet quality at different levels: foods, foodstuffs, and ingredients. Further research is now necessary to understand the potential benefits of manipulating protein sources in our diet, and thereby provide opportunities to refine dietary recommendations and consider perspectives for development of this agricultural sector and food supply.

Acknowledgments

I would like to thank Flore Duranton and Jean-François Huneau for their input and fruitful discussions.

References

Altorf-van der Kuil, W., Engberink, M.F., Vedder, M.M., Boer, J.M., Verschuren, W.M., Geleijnse, J.M., 2012. Sources of dietary protein in relation to blood pressure in a general Dutch population. PLoS One 7, e30582.

Anderson, J.W., Bush, H.M., 2011. Soy protein effects on serum lipoproteins: a quality assessment and meta-analysis of randomized, controlled studies. J. Am. Coll. Nutr. 30, 79–91.

Anderson, J.W., Major, A.W., 2002. Pulses and lipaemia, short- and long-term effect: potential in the prevention of cardiovascular disease. Br. J. Nutr. 88 (Suppl. 3), S263–S271.

Ashfaq, S., Abramson, J.L., Jones, D.P., Rhodes, S.D., Weintraub, W.S., Hooper, W.C., Vaccarino, V., Harrison, D.G., Quyyumi, A.A., 2006. The relationship between plasma levels of oxidized and reduced thiols and early atherosclerosis in healthy adults. J. Am. Coll. Cardiol. 47, 1005–1011.

Azadbakht, L., Kimiagar, M., Mehrabi, Y., Esmaillzadeh, A., Hu, F.B., Willett, W.C., 2007. Soy consumption, markers of inflammation, and endothelial function: a cross-over study in postmenopausal women with the metabolic syndrome. Diabetes Care 30, 967–973.

Bahr, M., Fechner, A., Kiehntopf, M., Jahreis, G., 2014. Consuming a mixed diet enriched with lupin protein beneficially affects plasma lipids in hypercholesterolemic subjects: a randomized controlled trial. Clin. Nutr. 34 (1), 7–14.

Bahr, M., Fechner, A., Kiehntopf, M., Jahreis, G., 2015. Consuming a mixed diet enriched with lupin protein beneficially affects plasma lipids in hypercholesterolemic subjects: a randomized controlled trial. Clin. Nutr. 34, 7–14.

Bai, Y., Sun, L., Yang, T., Sun, K., Chen, J., Hui, R., 2009. Increase in fasting vascular endothelial function after short-term oral L-arginine is effective when baseline flow-mediated dilation is low: a meta-analysis of randomized controlled trials. Am. J. Clin. Nutr. 89, 77–84.

Bazzano, L.A., Thompson, A.M., Tees, M.T., Nguyen, C.H., Winham, D.M., 2011. Non-soy legume consumption lowers cholesterol levels: a meta-analysis of randomized controlled trials. Nutr. Metab. Cardiovasc. Dis. 21, 94–103.

Beavers, D.P., Beavers, K.M., Miller, M., Stamey, J., Messina, M.J., 2012. Exposure to isoflavone-containing soy products and endothelial function: a Bayesian meta-analysis of randomized controlled trials. Nutr. Metab. Cardiovasc. Dis. 22, 182–191.

Belski, R., Mori, T.A., Puddey, I.B., Sipsas, S., Woodman, R.J., Ackland, T.R., Beilin, L.J., Dove, E.R., Carlyon, N.B., Jayaseena, V., Hodgson, J.M., 2011. Effects of lupin-enriched foods on body composition and cardiovascular disease risk factors: a 12-month randomized controlled weight loss trial. Int. J. Obes. (Lond.) 35, 810–819.

Bettzieche, A., Brandsch, C., Weisse, K., Hirche, F., Eder, K., Stangl, G.I., 2008. Lupin protein influences the expression of hepatic genes involved in fatty acid synthesis and triacylglycerol hydrolysis of adult rats. Br. J. Nutr. 99, 952–962.

Bianchi, C.M., Egnell, M., Huneau, J.F., Mariotti, F., 2016. Plant protein intake and dietary diversity are independently associated with nutrient adequacy in French adults. J. Nutr. 146, 2351–2360.

Blouet, C., Mariotti, F., Azzout-Marniche, D., Mathe, V., Mikogami, T., Tome, D., Huneau, J.F., 2007. Dietary cysteine alleviates sucrose-induced oxidative stress and insulin resistance. Free Radic. Biol. Med. 42, 1089–1097.

Borucki, K., Aronica, S., Starke, I., Luley, C., Westphal, S., 2009. Addition of 2.5 g L-arginine in a fatty meal prevents the lipemia-induced endothelial dysfunction in healthy volunteers. Atherosclerosis 205, 251–254.

Camilleri, G.M., Verger, E.O., Huneau, J.F., Carpentier, F., Dubuisson, C., Mariotti, F., 2013. Plant and animal protein intakes are differently associated with nutrient adequacy of the diet of French adults. J. Nutr. 143, 1466–1473.

Cavallaro, N.L., Garry, J., Shi, X., Gerszten, R.E., Anderson, E.J., Walford, G.A., 2016. A pilot, short-term dietary manipulation of branched chain amino acids has modest influence on fasting levels of branched chain amino acids. Food Nutr. Res. 60, 28592.

Cupisti, A., Ghiadoni, L., D'alessandro, C., Kardasz, I., Morelli, E., Panichi, V., Locati, D., Morandi, S., Saba, A., Barsotti, G., Taddei, S., Arnoldi, A., Salvetti, A., 2007. Soy protein diet improves endothelial dysfunction in renal transplant patients. Nephrol. Dial. Transpl. 22, 229–234.

Debry, G., 2004a. Experimental Data on Animals. Dietary Proteins and Atherosclerosis. CRC Press.

Debry, G., 2004b. Data on Atherosclerosis. Dietary Proteins and Atherosclerosis. CRC Press.

Deibert, P., Konig, D., Schmidt-Trucksaess, A., Zaenker, K.S., Frey, I., Landmann, U., Berg, A., 2004. Weight loss without losing muscle mass in pre-obese and obese subjects induced by a high-soy-protein diet. Int. J. Obes. Relat. Metab. Disord. 28, 1349–1352.

Dettmer, M., Alekel, D.L., Lasrado, J.A., Messina, M., Carriquiry, A., Heiberger, K., Stewart, J.W., Franke, W., 2012. The effect of soy protein beverages on serum cell adhesion molecule concentrations in prehypertensive/stage 1 hypertensive individuals. J. Am. Coll. Nutr. 31, 100–110.

Deveaux, A., Fouillet, H., Petzke, K.J., Hermier, D., Andre, E., Bunouf, P., Lantoine-Adam, F., Benamouzig, R., Mathe, V., Huneau, J.F., Mariotti, F., 2016a. A slow- compared with a fast-release form of oral arginine increases its utilization for no synthesis in overweight adults with cardiometabolic risk factors in a randomized controlled study. J. Nutr.

Deveaux, A., Pham, I., West, S.G., Andre, E., Lantoine-Adam, F., Bunouf, P., Sadi, S., Hermier, D., Mathe, V., Fouillet, H., Huneau, J.F., Benamouzig, R., Mariotti, F., 2016b. l-Arginine supplementation alleviates postprandial endothelial dysfunction when baseline fasting plasma arginine concentration is low: a randomized controlled trial in healthy overweight adults with cardiometabolic risk factors. J. Nutr.

Dong, J.Y., Tong, X., Wu, Z.W., Xun, P.C., He, K., Qin, L.Q., 2011. Effect of soya protein on blood pressure: a meta-analysis of randomised controlled trials. Br. J. Nutr. 106, 317–326.

Liu, Z.M., Ho, S.C., Chen, Y.M., Woo, J., 2013b. Effect of soy protein and isoflavones on blood pressure and endothelial cytokines: a 6-month randomized controlled trial among postmenopausal women. J. Hypertens. 31, 384–392.

Magne, J., Huneau, J.F., Tsikas, D., Delemasure, S., Rochette, L., Tome, D., Mariotti, F., 2009. Rapeseed protein in a high-fat mixed meal alleviates postprandial systemic and vascular oxidative stress and prevents vascular endothelial dysfunction in healthy rats. J. Nutr. 139, 1660–1666.

Malik, V.S., Li, Y., Tobias, D.K., Pan, A., Hu, F.B., 2016. Dietary protein intake and risk of type 2 diabetes in US men and women. Am. J. Epidemiol. 183, 715–728.

Mariotti, F., Huneau, J.F., 2016. Plant and animal protein intakes are differentially associated with large clusters of nutrient intake that may explain part of their complex relation with CVD risk. Adv. Nutr. 7, 559–560.

Mariotti, F., Valette, M., Lopez, C., Fouillet, H., Famelart, M.H., Mathe, V., Airinei, G., Benamouzig, R., Gaudichon, C., Tome, D., Tsikas, D., Huneau, J.F., 2015. Casein compared with whey proteins affects the organization of dietary fat during digestion and attenuates the postprandial triglyceride response to a mixed high-fat meal in healthy, overweight men. J. Nutr. 145, 2657–2664.

Matthan, N.R., Jalbert, S.M., Ausman, L.M., Kuvin, J.T., Karas, R.H., Lichtenstein, A.H., 2007. Effect of soy protein from differently processed products on cardiovascular disease risk factors and vascular endothelial function in hypercholesterolemic subjects. Am. J. Clin. Nutr. 85, 960–966.

Maxwell, A.J., 2002. Mechanisms of dysfunction of the nitric oxide pathway in vascular diseases. Nitric Oxide 6, 101–124.

McEvoy, C.T., Cardwell, C.R., Woodside, J.V., Young, I.S., Hunter, S.J., Mckinley, M.C., 2014. A posteriori dietary patterns are related to risk of type 2 diabetes: findings from a systematic review and meta-analysis. J. Acad. Nutr. Diet. 114 1759–1775.e4.

McPherson, R.A., Hardy, G., 2011. Clinical and nutritional benefits of cysteine-enriched protein supplements. Curr. Opin. Clin. Nutr. Metab. Care 14, 562–568.

Miller 3rd, E.R., Erlinger, T.P., Appel, L.J., 2006. The effects of macronutrients on blood pressure and lipids: an overview of the DASH and OmniHeart trials. Curr. Atheroscler. Rep. 8, 460–465.

Moncada, S., Higgs, E.A., 2006. The discovery of nitric oxide and its role in vascular biology. Br. J. Pharmacol. 147 (Suppl. 1), S193–S201.

Murtaugh, M.A., Herrick, J.S., Sweeney, C., Baumgartner, K.B., Guiliano, A.R., Byers, T., Slattery, M.L., 2007. Diet composition and risk of overweight and obesity in women living in the southwestern United States. J. Am. Diet. Assoc. 107, 1311–1321.

Niu, Y.C., Feng, R.N., Hou, Y., Li, K., Kang, Z., Wang, J., Sun, C.H., Li, Y., 2012. Histidine and arginine are associated with inflammation and oxidative stress in obese women. Br. J. Nutr. 108, 57–61.

Obarzanek, E., Sacks, F.M., Vollmer, W.M., Bray, G.A., Miller 3rd, E.R., Lin, P.H., Karanja, N.M., Most-Windhauser, M.M., Moore, T.J., Swain, J.F., Bales, C.W., Proschan, M.A., Group, D.R., 2001. Effects on blood lipids of a blood pressure-lowering diet: the Dietary Approaches to Stop Hypertension (DASH) Trial. Am. J. Clin. Nutr. 74, 80–89.

Okubo, H., Sasaki, S., Murakami, K., Takahashi, Y., Freshmen in Dietetic Courses Study II Group, 2011. The ratio of fish to meat in the diet is positively associated with favorable intake of food groups and nutrients among young Japanese women. Nutr. Res. 31, 169–177.

Padhi, E.M., Blewett, H.J., Duncan, A.M., Guzman, R.P., Hawke, A., Seetharaman, K., Tsao, R., Wolever, T.M., Ramdath, D.D., 2015. Whole soy flour incorporated into a muffin and consumed at 2 doses of soy protein does not lower LDL cholesterol in a randomized, double-blind controlled trial of hypercholesterolemic adults. J. Nutr. 145, 2665–2674.

Pasiakos, S.M., Agarwal, S., Lieberman, H.R., Fulgoni 3rd, V.L., 2015. Sources and amounts of animal, dairy, and plant protein intake of US adults in 2007–2010. Nutrients 7, 7058–7069.

Phillips, S.M., Fulgoni 3rd, V.L., Heaney, R.P., Nicklas, T.A., Slavin, J.L., Weaver, C.M., 2015. Commonly consumed protein foods contribute to nutrient intake, diet quality, and nutrient adequacy. Am. J. Clin. Nutr.

Pisa, P.T., Pedro, T.M., Kahn, K., Tollman, S.M., Pettifor, J.M., Norris, S.A., 2015. Nutrient patterns and their association with socio-demographic, lifestyle factors and obesity risk in rural South African adolescents. Nutrients 7, 3464–3482.

Poupin, N., Bos, C., Mariotti, F., Huneau, J.F., Tome, D., Fouillet, H., 2011. The nature of the dietary protein impacts the tissue-to-diet ^{15}N discrimination factors in laboratory rats. PLoS One 6, e28046.

Poupin, N., Mariotti, F., Huneau, J.F., Hermier, D., Fouillet, H., 2014. Natural isotopic signatures of variations in body nitrogen fluxes: a compartmental model analysis. PLoS Comput. Biol. 10, e1003865.

Reriani, M.K., Lerman, L.O., Lerman, A., 2010. Endothelial function as a functional expression of cardiovascular risk factors. Biomark. Med. 4, 351–360.

Reynolds, K., Chin, A., Lees, K.A., Nguyen, A., Bujnowski, D., He, J., 2006. A meta-analysis of the effect of soy protein supplementation on serum lipids. Am. J. Cardiol. 98, 633–640.

Richter, C.K., Skulas-Ray, A.C., Champagne, C.M., Kris-Etherton, P.M., 2015. Plant protein and animal proteins: do they differentially affect cardiovascular disease risk? Adv. Nutr. 6, 712–728.

Rizzo, N.S., Jaceldo-Siegl, K., Sabate, J., Fraser, G.E., 2013. Nutrient profiles of vegetarian and nonvegetarian dietary patterns. J. Acad. Nutr. Diet. 113, 1610–1619.

Roberts, L.D., 2015. Does inorganic nitrate say No to obesity by browning white adipose tissue? Adipocyte 4, 311–314.

Rodriguez-Monforte, M., Flores-Mateo, G., Sanchez, E., 2015. Dietary patterns and CVD: a systematic review and meta-analysis of observational studies. Br. J. Nutr. 114, 1341–1359.

Roussell, M.A., Hill, A.M., Gaugler, T.L., West, S.G., Ulbrecht, J.S., Vanden Heuvel, J.P., Gillies, P.J., Kris-Etherton, P.M., 2014. Effects of a DASH-like diet containing lean beef on vascular health. J. Hum. Hypertens. 28, 600–605.

Sacks, F.M., Lichtenstein, A., Van Horn, L., Harris, W., Kris-Etherton, P., Winston, M., American Heart Association Nutrition Committee, 2006. Soy protein, isoflavones, and cardiovascular health: an American Heart Association Science Advisory for professionals from the nutrition Committee. Circulation 113, 1034–1044.

Saneei, P., Salehi-Abargouei, A., Esmaillzadeh, A., Azadbakht, L., 2014. Influence of Dietary Approaches to Stop Hypertension (DASH) diet on blood pressure: a systematic review and meta-analysis on randomized controlled trials. Nutr. Metab. Cardiovasc. Dis. 24, 1253–1261.

Satija, A., Bhupathiraju, S.N., Rimm, E.B., Spiegelman, D., Chiuve, S.E., Borgi, L., Willett, W.C., Manson, J.E., Sun, Q., Hu, F.B., 2016. Plant-based dietary patterns and incidence of type 2 diabetes in US men and women: results from three prospective cohort studies. PLoS Med. 13, e1002039.

Schmidt, J.A., Rinaldi, S., Ferrari, P., Carayol, M., Achaintre, D., Scalbert, A., Cross, A.J., Gunter, M.J., Fensom, G.K., Appleby, P.N., Key, T.J., Travis, R.C., 2015. Metabolic profiles of male meat eaters, fish eaters, vegetarians, and vegans from the EPIC-Oxford cohort. Am. J. Clin. Nutr. 102, 1518–1526.

Schmidt, J.A., Rinaldi, S., Scalbert, A., Ferrari, P., Achaintre, D., Gunter, M.J., Appleby, P.N., Key, T.J., Travis, R.C., 2016. Plasma concentrations and intakes of amino acids in male meat-eaters, fish-eaters, vegetarians and vegans: a cross-sectional analysis in the EPIC-Oxford cohort. Eur. J. Clin. Nutr. 70, 306–312.

Sherzai, A., Heim, L.T., Boothby, C., Sherzai, A.D., 2012. Stroke, food groups, and dietary patterns: a systematic review. Nutr. Rev. 70, 423–435.

Song, M., Fung, T.T., Hu, F.B., Willett, W.C., Longo, V.D., Chan, A.T., Giovannucci, E.L., 2016. Association of animal and plant protein intake with all-cause and cause-specific mortality. JAMA Intern. Med.

Spielmann, J., Shukla, A., Brandsch, C., Hirche, F., Stangl, G.I., Eder, K., 2007. Dietary lupin protein lowers triglyceride concentrations in liver and plasma in rats by reducing hepatic gene expression of sterol regulatory element-binding protein-1c. Ann. Nutr. Metab. 51, 387–392.

Stamler, J., Brown, I.J., Daviglus, M.L., Chan, Q., Kesteloot, H., Ueshima, H., Zhao, L., Elliott, P., 2009. Glutamic acid, the main dietary amino acid, and blood pressure: the INTERMAP study (International Collaborative Study of Macronutrients, Micronutrients and Blood Pressure). Circulation 120, 221–228.

Stamler, J., Liu, K., Ruth, K.J., Pryer, J., Greenland, P., 2002. Eight-year blood pressure change in middle-aged men: relationship to multiple nutrients. Hypertension 39, 1000–1006.

Steinberg, F.M., Guthrie, N.L., Villablanca, A.C., Kumar, K., Murray, M.J., 2003. Soy protein with isoflavones has favorable effects on endothelial function that are independent of lipid and antioxidant effects in healthy postmenopausal women. Am. J. Clin. Nutr. 78, 123–130.

Swain, J.F., Mccarron, P.B., Hamilton, E.F., Sacks, F.M., Appel, L.J., 2008. Characteristics of the diet patterns tested in the optimal macronutrient intake trial to prevent heart disease (OmniHeart): options for a heart-healthy diet. J. Am. Diet. Assoc. 108, 257–265.

Tan, B., Yin, Y., Liu, Z., Li, X., Xu, H., Kong, X., Huang, R., Tang, W., Shinzato, I., Smith, S.B., Wu, G., 2009. Dietary L-arginine supplementation increases muscle gain and reduces body fat mass in growing-finishing pigs. Amino Acids 37, 169–175.

Teede, H.J., Dalais, F.S., Kotsopoulos, D., Liang, Y.L., Davis, S., Mcgrath, B.P., 2001. Dietary soy has both beneficial and potentially adverse cardiovascular effects: a placebo-controlled study in men and post-menopausal women. J. Clin. Endocrinol. Metab. 86, 3053–3060.

Teede, H.J., Dalais, F.S., Mcgrath, B.P., 2004. Dietary soy containing phytoestrogens does not have detectable estrogenic effects on hepatic protein synthesis in postmenopausal women. Am. J. Clin. Nutr. 79, 396–401.

Tielemans, S.M., Altorf-van der Kuil, W., Engberink, M.F., Brink, E.J., Van Baak, M.A., Bakker, S.J., Geleijnse, J.M., 2013. Intake of total protein, plant protein and animal protein in relation to blood pressure: a meta-analysis of observational and intervention studies. J. Hum. Hypertens. 27, 564–571.

Tielemans, S.M., Kromhout, D., Altorf-van der Kuil, W., Geleijnse, J.M., 2014. Associations of plant and animal protein intake with 5-year changes in blood pressure: the Zutphen Elderly Study. Nutr. Metab. Cardiovasc. Dis. 24, 1228–1233.

Torres, N., Torre-Villalvazo, I., Tovar, A.R., 2006. Regulation of lipid metabolism by soy protein and its implication in diseases mediated by lipid disorders. J. Nutr. Biochem. 17, 365–373.

U.S. Department of Agriculture – Agricultural Research Service, 2013. USDA National Nutrient Database for Standard Reference, Release 26. Nutrient Data Laboratory. Available at: http://www.ars.usda.gov/ba/bhnrc/ndl.

Umesawa, M., Sato, S., Imano, H., Kitamura, A., Shimamoto, T., Yamagishi, K., Tanigawa, T., Iso, H., 2009. Relations between protein intake and blood pressure in Japanese men and women: the Circulatory Risk in Communities Study (CIRCS). Am. J. Clin. Nutr. 90, 377–384.

van Nielen, M., Feskens, E.J., Mensink, M., Sluijs, I., Molina, E., Amiano, P., Ardanaz, E., Balkau, B., Beulens, J.W., Boeing, H., Clavel-Chapelon, F., Fagherazzi, G., Franks, P.W., Halkjaer, J., Huerta, J.M., Katzke, V., Key, T.J., Khaw, K.T., Krogh, V., Kuhn, T., Menendez, V.V., Nilsson, P., Overvad, K., Palli, D., Panico, S., Rolandsson, O., Romieu, I., Sacerdote, C., Sanchez, M.J., Schulze, M.B., Spijkerman, A.M., Tjonneland, A., Tumino, R., Van Der, A.D., Wurtz, A.M., Zamora-Ros, R., Langenberg, C., Sharp, S.J., Forouhi, N.G., Riboli, E., Wareham, N.J., Interact, C., 2014a. Dietary protein intake and incidence of type 2 diabetes in Europe: the EPIC-Interact Case-Cohort Study. Diabetes Care 37, 1854–1862.

van Nielen, M., Feskens, E.J., Rietman, A., Siebelink, E., Mensink, M., 2014b. Partly replacing meat protein with soy protein alters insulin resistance and blood lipids in postmenopausal women with abdominal obesity. J. Nutr. 144, 1423–1429.

Vega-Lopez, S., Matthan, N.R., Ausman, L.M., Harding, S.V., Rideout, T.C., Ai, M., Otokozawa, S., Freed, A., Kuvin, J.T., Jones, P.J., Schaefer, E.J., Lichtenstein, A.H., 2010. Altering dietary lysine: arginine ratio has little effect on cardiovascular risk factors and vascular reactivity in moderately hypercholesterolemic adults. Atherosclerosis 210, 555–562.

Wang, Y.F., Yancy Jr., W.S., Yu, D., Champagne, C., Appel, L.J., Lin, P.H., 2008. The relationship between dietary protein intake and blood pressure: results from the PREMIER study. J. Hum. Hypertens. 22, 745–754.

Weisse, K., Brandsch, C., Zernsdorf, B., Nembongwe, G.S.N., Hofmann, K., Eder, K., Stangl, G.I., 2009. Lupin protein compared to casein lowers the LDL cholesterol: HDL cholesterol-ratio of hypercholesterolemic adults. Eur. J. Nutr.

Westphal, S., Taneva, E., Kastner, S., Martens-Lobenhoffer, J., Bode-Boger, S., Kropf, S., Dierkes, J., Luley, C., 2006. Endothelial dysfunction induced by postprandial lipemia is neutralized by addition of proteins to the fatty meal. Atheroscler. Suppl. 185, 313–319.

Willett, W.C., 2007. Low-carbohydrate diets: a place in health promotion? J. Intern. Med. 261, 363–365.

Winham, D.M., Hutchins, A.M., 2007. Baked bean consumption reduces serum cholesterol in hypercholesterolemic adults. 27, 380–386.

Winham, D.M., Hutchins, A.M., Johnston, C.S., 2007. Pinto bean consumption reduces biomarkers for heart disease risk. J. Am. Coll. Nutr. 26, 243–249.

Wu, G., 2009. Amino acids: metabolism, functions, and nutrition. Amino Acids 37, 1–17.

Wu, Z., Satterfield, M.C., Bazer, F.W., Wu, G., 2012. Regulation of brown adipose tissue development and white fat reduction by L-arginine. Curr. Opin. Clin. Nutr. Metab. Care 15, 529–538.

Yang, X., Croft, K.D., Lee, Y.P., Mori, T.A., Puddey, I.B., Sipsas, S., Barden, A., Swinny, E., Hodgson, J.M., 2010. The effects of a lupin-enriched diet on oxidative stress and factors influencing vascular function in overweight subjects. Antioxid. Redox Signal. 13, 1517–1524.

Yin, J., Ren, W., Yang, G., Duan, J., Huang, X., Fang, R., Li, C., Li, T., Yin, Y., Hou, Y., Kim, S.W., Wu, G., 2016. L-Cysteine metabolism and its nutritional implications. Mol. Nutr. Food Res. 60, 134–146.

Zhang, X.M., Zhang, Y.B., Chi, M.H., 2016. Soy protein supplementation reduces clinical indices in type 2 diabetes and metabolic syndrome. Yonsei Med. J. 57, 681–689.

37

Polyunsaturated Fatty Acid Status in Vegetarians

Thomas A.B. Sanders

KING'S COLLEGE LONDON, UNITED KINGDOM

1. Introduction

There are two series (omega-6 and omega-3) of polyunsaturated fatty acids (PUFA) derived from the essential fatty acids linoleic (18:2n-6) and α-linolenic acid (18:3n-3; ALA), respectively. Both linoleic and ALA undergo alternating chain elongation and desaturation to form longer chain derivatives using the same enzyme system (Fig. 37.1). The abundance of the respective omega-6 and omega-3 metabolites is dependent on the relative amounts of dietary linoleic and ALA as well as the absolute intakes. Linoleic acid is an essential nutrient that has a specific role in the maintenance of the water permeability barrier as a component of acylglycosyl ceramides and the transport of cholesterol in blood. However, its major physiological role is as a precursor to arachidonic acid (20:4n-6), which is an important component of structural lipids found in membranes and gives rise to the major active series of eicosanoids (prostaglandins, prostacyclins, thromboxanes, and leukotrienes) and anandamides (compounds involved in sensory regulation). Dose-dependent increases in the proportion of arachidonic acid (20:4n-6) in phospholipids occur with intakes of linoleic acid up to 1%–2% dietary energy, and thereafter levels plateau or even fall with increasing intakes. The minimum requirement for linoleic acid is estimated as being close to 1% of the dietary energy. Usual dietary intakes are well in excess of this amount (WHO/FAO, 2010). Dietary reference values for linoleic acid range from 3% energy to an upper limit of 10% energy.

Docosahexaenoic acid (22:6n-3; DHA) is the major metabolite of omega-3 series found in the phospholipids of mammalian tissues especially in the brain, retina, cardiac muscle, and testis. ALA is regarded as a dietary essential nutrient because it is converted into DHA, which plays an important physiological role in neurotransmission. There has been a debate surrounding how efficiently ALA is converted to DHA in humans. Diets lacking ALA but containing adequate intakes of linoleic acid have the effect of replacing DHA with the omega-6 homologue docosapentaenoic acid (22:5n-6; omega-6 DPA), which results in impaired retinal and cognitive function. In mammals, including primates, the requirements for omega-3 PUFA for visual and neurological development can be met

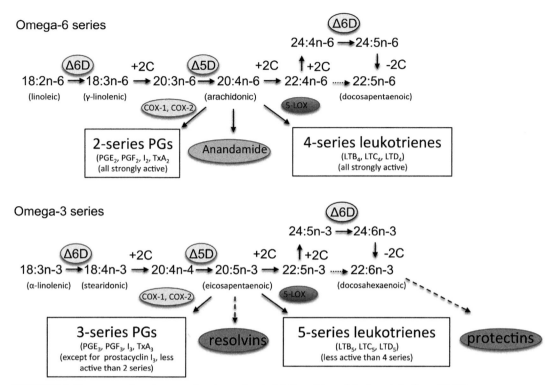

FIGURE 37.1 The omega-6 and omega-3 polyunsaturated fatty acids and their metabolites. *5-LOX,* 5-lipoyxygenase; Δ6D, Δ6 desaturase; Δ5D, Δ5 desaturase; *COX,* cylco-oxygenase; *PG,* prostaglandins. *Taken from Sanders, T.A., 2015. Functional Dietary Lipids. Woodhead Publishing Series in Food Science, Technology and Nutrition: Number 24. Elsevier, Amsterdam.*

by ALA (WHO/FAO, 2010). The estimated human requirement is between 0.2% and 0.5% of the dietary energy intake. High intakes of linoleic acid relative to ALA competitively inhibit the conversion of ALA to DHA and result in its partial replacement with omega-6 DPA. Plasma and erythrocyte lipids are often used as indicators of tissue DHA status but may not always accurately reflect DHA status of brain and retinal tissues, which retain DHA even when intakes of linoleic acid are high (Roshanai and Sanders, 1985). However, dietary DHA is probably required to meet the needs of the preterm infants as rates of synthesis from ALA may be insufficient to meet the needs of the developing brain. Many infant formulas are now supplemented with both arachidonic acid and DHA to provide similar amounts to those present in human breastmilk. Although some studies suggest benefit in terms of increased cognitive function in infants receiving the long-chain PUFA, a meta-analysis shows no overall benefit in infants (Simmer et al., 2011). Human infants can convert linoleic acid to omega-6 DPA and ALA to DHA (Jensen et al., 1997; Makrides et al., 2000), but proportions of DHA are lower in breastmilk, cord blood, and arterial lipids of vegetarians compared to omnivores (Sanders and Reddy, 1992; Reddy et al., 1994) (Figs. 37.2 and 37.3). Studies of DHA supplementation in omnivore pregnancy have failed to demonstrate beneficial effects on cognitive function of the offspring

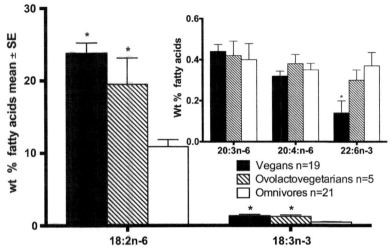

FIGURE 37.2 Proportions of polyunsaturated fatty acid in breast milk lipids of vegans, ovolactovegetarians, and omnivores. *Asterisk* denotes *P*<.01 compared with omnivores using unpaired *t*-test. *Data are from samples collected in 1980 and taken from Sanders, T.A., Reddy, S., 1992. The influence of a vegetarian diet on the fatty acid composition of human milk and the essential fatty acid status of the infant. J. Pediatr. 120, S71–S77.*

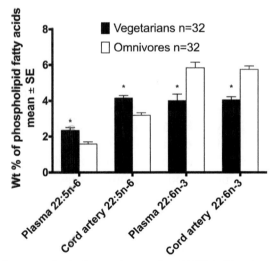

FIGURE 37.3 Differences in the proportions of docosahexaenoic acid (22:6n-3) and omega-6 docosapentaenoic acid (22:5n-6) in cord blood and cord artery phospholipids obtained at delivery from vegetarians compared with omnivores. *Asterisk* denotes *P*<.01 for comparisons between groups using a *t*-test. *Data from Reddy, S., Sanders, T.A., Obeid, O., 1994. The influence of maternal vegetarian diet on essential fatty acid status of the newborn. Eur. J. Clin. Nutr. 48, 358–368.*

(Gould et al., 2013, 2014; Makrides et al., 2014). While the consumption of DHA in pregnancy and lactation augments the supply to the infant, there currently is no evidence of benefit in terms of meaningful clinical outcomes such as cognitive function in vegetarian infants. Furthermore, there is a lack of sound experimental data to support the need for dietary DHA beyond the 6-month age of life.

Many current dietary guidelines advocate the inclusion of oily fish in the diet to supply an intake of long-chain omega-3 PUFA (0.2–0.5 g/day) because of an association of fish intake with a reduced risk of cardiovascular disease (CVD). Long-chain omega-3 PUFA, particularly eicosapentaenoic acid (20:5n-3; EPA), have several pharmacological effects when consumed in relatively high amounts (usually in excess of 3 g/day). Both dietary EPA and DHA displace arachidonic acid from cell membranes and have the effect of reducing the production of active eicosanoids from arachidonic acid and have antiinflammatory effects. They also give rise to some novel compounds termed resolvins and neuroprotectins, but the physiological importance of these is at present uncertain. This chapter discusses the PUFA status in vegetarians compared with omnivores and addresses the issue as to whether vegetarians need to supplement their diets with long-chain omega-3 PUFA.

2. Dietary Sources of Polyunsaturated Fatty Acids

Human diets contain much more linoleic acid than ALA. Linoleic acid accounts for more than half of the fatty acids in cereals and in many nuts and seed oils (Table 37.1). ALA is less widely distributed but found significantly in some of the major oilseed crops such as soybean and rapeseed (which contain about 7% and 10%, respectively, by weight), but most other vegetable oils such as corn, sunflower, olive, and palm oils contain less than 1%. ALA is also found in high proportions in the lipids of flaxseed, hempseed, walnuts, and dark green leafy vegetables. However, the fat content of green leafy vegetables is very low, so the contribution from this source is small. However, it does contribute significantly to the dietary intake of herbivores. Grass-fed ruminants (cows, sheep, and goats) produce milk with a higher content of ALA than those that are stall-fed on cereals (Larsen et al., 2010). Dairy produce also contains small amounts of the longer chain PUFA of the omega-6 and omega-3 series, but significantly higher amounts are found in eggs.

The partial hydrogenation of soybean and rapeseed oil reduces the amount of ALA to make frying oil more stable to high temperatures used in deep frying. Partial hydrogenation was used to increase the melting points of oils, so they could be used to make margarine. However, the practice of partial hydrogenation is being phased out in many countries because industrially produced trans fatty acids increase risk of CVD. Modern margarines are generally virtually free from trans fatty acids. The industry also has new varieties of rapeseed and soybean oil with a reduced content of ALA for deep fat frying. While these oils may have a niche as deep-frying oils, the widespread use of such oils have the potential to have deleterious impact on the intake of ALA particularly for vegetarians. Margarine is currently potentially an important source of ALA for vegans and vegetarians. In the past, many margarines were made from corn or sunflower seed oil and contained very little ALA. Nowadays, most modern margarines/yellow fat spreads contain significant amounts of ALA, especially if they are made using rapeseed and soybean oils or are fortified with richer sources of ALA such as flaxseed. Several supplementary sources of omega-3 fatty acids are also acceptable to vegetarians such as linseed (flaxseed), hempseed, and borage oils, which contain ALA. Research is in progress to develop genetically modified strains of

Table 37.1 Polyunsaturated Fatty Acid Content (g/100 g) of Major Contributors to Fat Intake in Vegetarians

Food	18:2n-6	18:3n-3
Oatmeal, quick cook, raw	3.52	0.19
Brown rice, raw	0.94	0.04
Wheat flour, whole meal	0.83	0.06
Bread, whole meal	1.08	0.08
Muesli	1.69	0.05
Soya flour, full fat	11.68	1.66
Chick peas, hummus	4.55	0.40
Almonds	10.19	0.27
Brazil nuts	25.43	0.00
Peanuts, plain	12.75	0.35
Walnuts	39.29	7.47
Corn snacks	5.11	0.67
Avocado	1.53	0.07
Coconut oil	1.50	0.00
Corn oil	50.40	0.90
Olive oil	7.50	0.70
Palm oil	10.10	0.30
Rapeseed oil	19.70	9.60
Safflower oil	73.90	0.10
Soya oil	51.50	7.30
Sunflower oil	63.20	0.10
Butter	0.95	0.46
Margarine: UK 1998	26.30	0.20
Margarine: UK 2015 (Flora)[a]	19.0	4.60
Whole milk, pasteurized, average	0.07	0.02
Cheddar cheese	0.31	0.23
Chicken eggs	1.60	0.08

[a]Data supplied by Unilever PLC, London.

Data from Royal Society of Chemistry, 1998. Fatty Acids. The Seventh Supplement to McCance and Widdowson's the Composition of Foods. Royal Society of Chemistry, Cambridge.

oilseeds that can make long-chain omega-3 PUFA. However, at present, only single-cell oils provide an acceptable source of DHA for vegans and vegetarians (Table 37.2).

Marine lipids contain high amounts of EPA and DHA, which are derived from synthesis by marine algae not necessarily from ALA but from the polyketide synthase pathway (Metz et al., 2001; Uttaro, 2006). Single-cell oils that are not genetically modified by recombinant DNA technology have been developed for human consumption and are mainly used in breast-milk substitutes, especially oils derived from *Cryptheocodinium cohnii* (DHASCO-C) but are also marketed as dietary supplements for vegetarians. These single-cell oils contain mainly DHA but can be cultured to produce EPA in addition to DHA. The oil from *Schizochytrium* spp. (DHASCO-S, DSM Nutritional, Heerlen, the Netherlands) contains 15% by weight the omega-6 homologue of DHA, n-6 DPA (Sanders et al., 2006a) as well as about 38% DHA.

Table 37.2 Oil Sources of Omega-3 Fatty Acids Acceptable Used in Supplements/Fortified Foods That Are Acceptable to Vegetarians (g/100 g)

	18:2n-6	18:3n-3	20:5n-3	22:6n-3
Hempseed oil[a]	57.7	18.6	–	–
Borage oil[b]	35.3	20.6	–	–
Linseed oil[c]	14.33	53.37	–	–
Microalgae Single-Cell Oils				
Schizochytrium spp.[d]	0.2	–	6.0	41.2
Crypthecodinium cohnii[d]	1.3	–	Trace	43.9

[a]Data from T.A.B. Sanders and F. Lewis (unpublished data).
[b]Data from Royal Society of Chemistry (1998).
[c]Data from the US Nutrient Composition Data base (http://ndb.nal.usda.gov/ndb/nutrients).
[d]Data from DSM Nutritional Products, Heerlen, the Netherlands.

As the diets of most land-based animals contain much higher proportions of linoleic acid than ALA, the major long-chain PUFA metabolites found in eggs, milk, and meat are derived from the omega-6 series with only small amounts from the omega-3 series being present predominantly as DHA. Fish accumulate substantial amounts of EPA, docosapentaenoic acid (22:5n-3; omega-3 DPA), and DHA from marine algae. Thus fish consumption, especially oily fish, can make a substantially contribution to long-chain omega-3 PUFA in omnivores. Consequently, vegan diets are usually devoid of long-chain omega-3 PUFA (Roshanai and Sanders, 1984), and vegetarian diets only supply trace amounts (<0.05 g) from eggs and dairy products (Welch et al., 2010), as shown in Table 37.3. Most omnivore diets contain small amounts of DHA, typically less than 0.2 g/day (Sanders et al., 2006b; Welch et al., 2010; WHO/FAO, 2010). There are no specific recommended daily intakes for long-chain polyunsaturated acids for adults. However, as mentioned earlier, several dietary guidelines advocate the consumption of fish once/twice a week that provide in the range of 0.2–0.4 g of long-chain omega-3 fatty acids daily.

3. Biomarkers of PUFA Intake

Linoleic acid and ALA accumulate in adipose tissue and the levels in these stores are a good indicator of long-term intake. Higher levels of both have been reported in vegans compared with omnivores (Sanders et al., 1978). Adipose tissue stores also make a contribution to the composition of breastmilk and higher proportions of linoleic acid and ALA have been reported in breastmilk from vegans and vegetarians (Finley et al., 1985; Sanders et al., 1978; Sanders and Reddy, 1992). The absence of long-chain omega-3 fatty acids from diet is reflected in the lower proportions of EPA and DHA in blood lipids in vegans and vegetarians compared to omnivores in several populations (Sanders et al., 1978; Sanders and Reddy, 1992; Kornsteiner et al., 2008; Lee et al., 2000; Mann et al., 2006; Melchert et al., 1987; Phinney et al., 1990; Yu et al., 2014; Sanders, 2014), as illustrated in Table 37.4. In the European Prospective Investigation into Cancer (EPIC) study, the proportion of DHA in the plasma lipids of vegans and vegetarians was 59% and 31% lower, respectively, than that in omnivores (Rosell et al., 2005).

Table 37.3 Dietary Intakes in g/day of Polyunsaturated Fatty Acids in Vegans, Vegetarians, and Omnivores

	Method	Gender	n	18:2n-6	18:3n-3	20:5n-3	22:6n-3
Roshanai and Sanders (1984)				Mean (range)			
Vegan	3-d Chemical analysis	M	10	34 (15–50)	1.8 (0.7–3.6)	0	0
Vegan	3-d Chemical analysis	F	10	30 (5–43)	1.2 (0.5–2.3)	0	0
Omnivores	3-d Chemical analysis	M	12	11 (5–26)	1.0 (0.4–2.5)	0.02 (0–0.38)	0.42 (0–2.77)
Omnivores	3-d Chemical analysis	F	12	9 (2–15)	1.1 (0.1, 1.5)	0.09 (0–0.25)	0.04 (0–0.75)
Sanders and Reddy (1992)				Mean±SE			
Vegans, lactating	7-d Weighed intake	F	21	20.4±2.49	1.2±0.28	0	0
White vegetarians	7-d Weighed intake	F	18	14.6±1.69	1.5±0.17	Trace	Trace
Indian vegetarians	7-d Weighed intake	F	21	14.2±1.25	0.9±0.10	Trace	Trace
Omnivores	7-d Weighed intake	F	22	11.8±1.22	1.0±0.08	0.08±0.024	0.10±0.02
Welch et al. (2010)				Mean±SD			
Vegetarians	7-d Food record	M	25	14.78±6.9	1.25±0.57	0.02±0.02	0.0007±0.004
Vegetarians	7-d Food record	F	51	10.96±6.02	0.97±0.45	0.01±0.01	0.0004±0.005
Omnivores	7-d Food record	M	2257	12.41±4.8	1.25±0.41	0.13±0.16	0.19±0.22
Omnivores	7-d Food record	F	1891	9.52±3.75	1.01±0.35	0.11±0.13	0.15±0.19
Sanders (2009)				Mean±SE			
Vegans	7-d Weighed intake	M	57	24.8±1.82	2.2±0.16	0	0
Omnivores	7-d Weighed intake	M	138	12.6±0.31	1.3±0.05	0.2±0.02	0.3±0.03

Table 37.4 Proportions of Docosahexaenoic Acid (22:6n-3) in Red Blood Cell (RBC), Platelet, and Plasma Lipid Fractions in Vegans and Vegetarians Compared With Omnivores (Control)

Study	Country	Gender	Lipid Fraction	n	Vegan Mean ± SEM	n	Vegetarian Mean ± SEM	n	Control Mean ± SEM
Sanders et al. (1978)	UK	M+F	RBC lipids	18	1.9±0.23[a]		–	18	5±0.38
Melchert et al. (1987)	Germany	M	Plasma PC		–	40	0.98±0.15[a]	38	2.85±0.08
Melchert et al. (1987)	Germany	F	Plasma PC		–	62	1.37±0.15[a]	70	2.25±0.11
Miller et al. (1988)	UK	M	Plasma PL		-	18	2.69±0.24[a]	19	4.65±0.28
Phinney et al. (1990)	USA	M+F	Plasma PL		–	25	3.19±0.29	100	3.59±0.11
Sanders and Roshanai (1992)	UK	M+F	Platelet PL	20	0.8±0.07[a]		–	20	2.1±0.10
Reddy et al. (1994)	UK	F	Plasma PL		–	21	1.2±0.09[a]	22	2.26±0.19
Lee et al. (2000)	Hong Kong	M+F	Serum		–	60	1.7±0.32[c]	133	3.4±0.19
Rosell et al. (2005)	UK	M	Serum	232	0.7±0.05[a]	231	1.16±0.05[a]	196	1.69±0.05
Mann et al. (2006)	Australia	M	Plasma	18	2.0±0.09[b]	43	2.2±0.11[b]	60	3.3±0.10
Kornsteiner et al. (2008)	Austria	M+F	RBC PE	37	1.59±0.09[a]	25	2.35±0.15[c]	23	3.18±0.23
Sanders (2014)	UK	M	Plasma	124	0.98±0.09[a]	141	–	141	2.66±0.0.07
Yu et al. (2014)	China	M	Plasma			89	1.59±0.09[a]	106	4.66±0.15

Mean±SD.

PC, phosphatidyl choline; PE, phosphatidyl ethanolamine; PL, phospholipids.

[a] P<.001.

[b] P<.01.

[c] P<.05 compared with control.

3.1 Influence of Omega-3 Supplementation on Biomarkers

Supplementation of vegans (Sanders and Younger, 1981), vegetarians (Li et al., 1999; Wien et al., 2010), and omnivores with ALA results in the synthesis of EPA but does not influence the proportion of DHA in blood lipids. In a dose response study (Sanders et al., 2011) comparing doses of 0.18 g, 0.36, and 0.72 g DHA/day or placebo in omnivore participants who were advised to avoid the consumption of oily fish, the proportion (mean ± SD) of DHA in plasma lipids increased from 2.07 ± 0.52% on placebo to 2.63 ± 0.65%, 3.07 ± 0.48%, and 3.84 ± 0.61%, respectively, after 6 months and in erythrocyte lipids from 6.2 ± 1.3 to 7.3 ± 1.0, 7.8 ± 1.1%, and 8.6 ± 1.2% after 12 months in men and women. Supplementing vegans with 0.2 g DHA/day derived from algae versus placebo significantly increased the concentration of DHA (mean ± SD) in their plasma lipids by 43% from 23 ± 12 to 33 ± 12 mg/L (Sanders, 2009) and in erythrocytes phosphoglycerides by 47% from 1.9 ± 0.6% to 2.8 ± 0.8% (Sanders, unpublished data). However, the values still remained lower than in omnivores from our laboratory. Geppert et al. (2006) reported a 2.9-fold increase in the proportion of DHA in plasma phospholipids in a randomized controlled trial of 0.94 g DHA/day versus placebo in German vegetarians. Burns-Whitmore et al. (2014) compared the effects of supplementing US ovolactovegetarians for 8 weeks with walnuts (28.4 g/day for 6 days/week), a source of ALA or omega-3 enriched eggs (6 eggs/week) on erythrocyte lipids: the enriched eggs increased the percentage of DHA in erythrocyte lipids from 2.72 (95% CI 2.57, 2.87) to 3.15 (3.0, 3.32) in erythrocyte lipids, whereas walnuts decreased DHA from 3.12 (95% CI 2.90, 3.34) to 2.71 (2.55, 2.87). Thus, although there is a basal rate of DHA synthesis from ALA in humans, the proportion in blood lipids is greatly augmented by small amounts of dietary DHA.

4. Differences Between ALA and Long-Chain n-3 PUFA on Cardiovascular Risk

4.1 Serum Lipids and Lipoproteins

Intakes of EPA and DHA in excess of about 1 g/day lower plasma triacylglycerol (TAG) concentrations in a dose-dependent manner (Sanders et al., 2011); ALA does not produce this effect even at high intakes (Pan et al., 2009). This difference is probably related to differences in fatty acid chain length because C20-22 fatty acids are poor substrates for mitochondrial β-oxidation, compared with ALA, which is rapidly oxidized. The process that induces extra-mitochondrial chain shortening and subsequent β-oxidation is induced by the C20-22 fatty acids activating peroxisome proliferator receptor alpha (PPARα) nuclear hormone receptor. Activation of PPARα also has the additional effect of inhibiting hepatic TAG synthesis, which explains why long-chain omega-3 PUFA decreases plasma TAG synthesis and ALA does not.

Pharmacological intakes of EPA and DHA (the dose used in prescription medications is about 3 g/day) decrease very low-density lipoprotein (VLDL) synthesis and secretion

(Harris, 1997). As well as decreasing TAG concentrations, long-chain omega-3 fatty acids reduce postprandial lipemia, probably by reducing competition by VLDL with chylomicrons for lipoprotein lipase. Another consequence of reduced serum TAG concentration is to decrease in exchange of TAG from VLDL to low-density lipoprotein (LDL) and high-density lipoprotein (HDL). This results in the formation of slightly larger LDL and HDL particles, which may be less atherogenic. However, marked increases in LDL apolipoprotein B and LDL cholesterol (LDL-C) occur with long-chain omega-3 supplementation in some individuals, especially those exhibiting the relatively common Fredrickson lipoprotein IV phenotype (raised VLDL triglycerides and low HDL-cholesterol) as well as the less common type V phenotype. This effect is believed to result from less dense VLDL (as a result of a lower TAG content) being converted more efficiently. This potentially adverse effect is relevant to individuals with the metabolic syndrome and people with type 2 diabetes where the type IV phenotype is highly prevalent. However, low intakes of fish oil or oily fish providing mixtures of EPA + DHA generally do not affect total cholesterol (TC) or LDL-C in normolipidemic subjects. In contrast, relatively low intakes of algal DHA, as little as 0.8 g/day, increase LDL-C and apolipoprotein B concentrations in normolipidemic subjects (Theobald et al., 2004). In another study, supplementation of vegetarian diets (Geppert et al., 2006) with algal DHA at 0.9 g/day increased LDL-C by about 0.28 mmol/L. A meta-analysis (Bernstein et al., 2012) confirmed that LDL-C is increased by algal DHA on average by 0.23 mmol/L but showed that HDL-cholesterol (HDL-C) was increased in parallel, so the net effect on TC:HDL-C ratio was null. While this increase in LDL-C caused by DHA may increase risk of cardiovascular risk, it has been argued that this effect may be mitigated by an increase in the lighter LDL particles and HDL-C (Kelley et al., 2007). However, drug trials designed to increase HDL-C do not find risk to be reduced. Furthermore, Mendelian randomization studies comparing individuals with higher HDL-C than average also show no effect on risk. This is in contrast to LDL-C, which is strongly related to risk both in drug trials and Mendelian randomization studies. Although lighter LDL particles may be less atherogenic, the higher proportion of DHA in LDL lipids renders the particles more susceptible to oxidative modification. As the average increase in LDL-C with DHA supplementation is of a similar magnitude to that from increasing the intake of saturated fatty acid by 6% energy, this fact should be considered in any risk/benefit analysis of supplementing vegetarian diets with DHA.

4.2 Blood Pressure, Hemostatic, and Inflammatory Risk Markers

High intakes of EPA + DHA normally in excess of 3 g/day but not ALA (Kestin et al., 1990), lower blood pressure (Appel et al., 1993). However, intakes in the range of a normal diet have no effect on blood pressure (Sanders et al., 2011). Generally, besides their documented effects on blood pressure and fasting and postprandial lipids, they have no influence on clotting factors or fibrinolysis, but they do decrease the production of thromboxane A_2, leukotriene B_4, and interleukin-6 and tumor necrosis factor alpha; thus they have potential antiinflammatory effect at high intakes (WHO/FAO, 2010).

4.3 Effects on Arterial Aging

As it has not been possible to discern effects on blood lipids, blood pressure, and inflammation within the range of intakes normally encountered in Western diets, other mechanisms have been proposed to explain how low intakes of long-chain omega-3 PUFA may influence CVD risk. Arterial stiffness is emerging as a significant predictor of cardiovascular death in older people and is a robust index of arterial aging and correlated with increased carotid intimal media thickness. There have been suggestions that EPA/DHA intake may be associated with decreased arterial stiffness. If this were to be the case, then vegetarians and vegans, in particular, might have stiffer arteries. However, a comparison of arterial stiffness in vegan compared with omnivore men found no evidence to indicate that vegans had stiffer arteries. Indeed, there was a trend for their arteries to be less stiff (Sanders, 2014).

4.4 Results From Prospective Cohort Studies With Clinical Endpoints

Some but not all meta-analysis of prospective cohort studies show risk of CVD to be lower with higher intakes of linoleic acid, ALA, and long-chain n-3 PUFA. Pan et al. (2012) found some evidence for an association of ALA intake with a lower risk of CVD. However, Chowdhury et al. (2014) found no relationship with total omega-6 or omega-3 intake and risk but reported a lower risk to be associated with high proportions of long-chain omega-3 fatty acid in blood. A further meta-analysis (Farvid et al., 2014) including previous unpublished data reported that the replacement of 5% energy as saturated fatty acids with linoleic acid was associated with reductions of 9% in CVD incidence and 11% CVD mortality. Prospective studies, however, only show associations and do not prove causality. A lower rate of deaths and hospital admission for ischemic heart disease (IHD) among vegetarians and vegans compared with omnivores was reported in the UK Oxford cohort of the EPIC study (Crowe et al., 2013). However, Appleby et al. (2016) found no difference in IHD mortality up to the age of 90 in vegans and vegetarians compared to the omnivores.

4.5 Intervention Trials With Clinical Endpoints

Several randomized controlled trials conducted in the 1960–70s compared replacing saturated with PUFA (mainly linoleic acid but also containing omega-3 PUFA) on IHD incidence and mortality. A Cochrane review (Hooper et al., 2012) concluded that there was evidence of reduced IHD incidence but not mortality. The Mediterranean diet study (de Logeril et al., 1999) is often cited as evidence to support recommendations to increase the intake of ALA, but although this dietary intervention trial reduced CVD mortality, it also modified several other dietary components simultaneously. The Indo-Mediterranean diet trial reported that ALA reduced CVD, but it emerged that this claim was fraudulent, so its findings should be ignored (Horton, 2005). Only one sufficiently powered study (the Alpha-Omega trial) has compared EPA/DHA with ALA versus placebo supplementation in secondary prevention, and this showed no difference in the primary or secondary outcomes (Kromhout et al., 2010).

Several other large trials have been conducted with equivocal outcomes, and a meta-analysis (Rizos et al., 2012) concluded there to be no evidence of a reduction in total mortality or CVD events with omega-3 supplementation, although there was a trend for cardiac death to 9% lower (95% CI 15, −2). However, it is important to emphasize that blood pressure and lipids were well controlled by medication in the more recent trials, and this may have obscured any dietary effect. Consequently, the impact of long-chain omega-3 fatty acids on CVD risk may be greater in those with elevated LDL-C and raised blood pressure.

5. Conclusion

Vegetarians generally have higher intakes of linoleic and ALA compared with omnivores but usually have negligible intakes of long-chain omega-3 PUFA compared with omnivores who consume fish. DHA concentrations in plasma and erythrocyte lipids are lower in vegetarians, especially in vegans, than in omnivores, primarily attributable to the absence of DHA from the diet. The regular consumption of eggs or single-cell oils increases DHA levels in blood lipids and breast milk. However, there is a lack of evidence based on meaningful clinical outcomes to support supplementing pregnant and lactating vegetarian women with DHA. Long-chain omega-3 fatty acids have pharmacologic effects different from ALA on CVD risk factors, but these effects are only seen at intakes well above the amounts likely to be consumed in most human diets. Prospective cohort studies find higher intakes of linoleic acid, long-chain omega-3 PUFA, and less consistently ALA are associated with a lower risk of fatal CVD, especially when they replace saturated fatty acids. Randomized controlled trials show that the replacement of saturated fatty acids with PUFAs decreases risk of CVD events but not mortality. However, there appears to be no clear benefit of additional ALA or long-chain omega-3 PUFA in secondary prevention of CVD. Despite the lack of EPA and DHA in their diets, vegetarians are at lower risk of premature CVD compared with omnivores. Further research is needed to ascertain whether any long-term benefits to health might accrue from including DHA in the diets of vegetarians and vegans.

References

Appel, L.J., Miller 3rd, E.R., Seidler, A.J., Whelton, P.K., 1993. Does supplementation of diet with "fish oil" reduce blood pressure? A meta-analysis of controlled clinical trials. Arch. Intern. Med. 153, 1429–1438.

Appleby, P.N., Crowe, F.L., Bradbury, K.E., Travis, R.C., Key, T.J., 2016. Mortality in vegetarians and comparable nonvegetarians in the United Kingdom. Am. J. Clin. Nutr. 103, 218–230. http://dx.doi.org/10.3945/ajcn.115.119461.

Bernstein, A.M., Ding, E.L., Willett, W.C., Rimm, E.B., 2012. A meta-analysis shows that docosahexaenoic acid from algal oil reduces serum triglycerides and increases HDL-cholesterol and LDL-cholesterol in persons without coronary heart disease. J. Nutr. 142, 99–104. http://dx.doi.org/10.3945/jn.111.148973.

Burns-Whitmore, B., Haddad, E., Sabate, J., Rajaram, S., 2014. Effects of supplementing N-3 fatty acid enriched eggs and walnuts on cardiovascular disease risk markers in healthy free-living lacto-ovo-vegetarians: a randomized, crossover, free-living intervention study. Nutr. J. 13, 29. http://dx.doi.org/10.1186/1475-2891-13-29.

Chowdhury, R., Warnakula, S., Kunutsor, S., Crowe, F., Ward, H.A., Johnson, L., Franco, O.H., Butterworth, A.S., Forouhi, N.G., Thompson, S.G., et al., 2014. Association of dietary, circulating, and supplement fatty acids with coronary risk: a systematic review and meta-analysis. Ann. Intern. Med. 160, 398–406. http://dx.doi.org/10.7326/m13-1788.

Crowe, F.L., Appleby, P.N., Travis, R.C., Key, T.J., 2013. Risk of hospitalization or death from ischemic heart disease among British vegetarians and nonvegetarians: results from the EPIC-Oxford cohort study. Am. J. Clin. Nutr. http://dx.doi.org/10.3945/ajcn.112.044073.

de Lorgeril, M., Salen, P., Martin, J.L., Monjaud, I., Delaye, J., Mamelle, N., 1999. Mediterranean diet, traditional risk factors, and the rate of cardiovascular complications after myocardial infarction: final report of the Lyon Diet Heart Study. Circulation 99, 779–785.

Farvid, M.S., Ding, M., Pan, A., Sun, Q., Chiuve, S.E., Steffen, L.M., Willett, W.C., Hu, F.B., 2014. Dietary linoleic acid and risk of coronary heart disease: a systematic review and meta-analysis of prospective cohort studies. Circulation 130, 1568–1578. http://dx.doi.org/10.1161/circulationaha.114.010236.

Finley, D.A., Lonnerdal, B., Dewey, K.G., Grivetti, L.E., 1985. Breast milk composition: fat content and fatty acid composition in vegetarians and non-vegetarians. Am. J. Clin. Nutr. 41, 787–800.

Geppert, J., Kraft, V., Demmelmair, H., Koletzko, B., 2006. Microalgal docosahexaenoic acid decreases plasma triacylglycerol in normolipidaemic vegetarians: a randomised trial. Br. J. Nutr. 95, 779–786.

Gould, J.F., Makrides, M., Colombo, J., Smithers, L.G., 2014. Randomized controlled trial of maternal omega-3 long-chain PUFA supplementation during pregnancy and early childhood development of attention, working memory, and inhibitory control. Am. J. Clin. Nutr. 99, 851–859. http://dx.doi.org/10.3945/ajcn.113.069203.

Gould, J.F., Smithers, L.G., Makrides, M., 2013. The effect of maternal omega-3 (N-3) LCPUFA supplementation during pregnancy on early childhood cognitive and visual development: a systematic review and meta-analysis of randomized controlled trials. Am. J. Clin. Nutr. 97, 531–544. http://dx.doi.org/10.3945/ajcn.112.045781.

Harris, W.S., 1997. N-3 Fatty acids and serum lipoproteins: human studies. Am. J. Clin. Nutr. 65, 1645S–1654S.

Hooper, L., Summerbell, C.D., Thompson, R., Sills, D., Roberts, F.G., Moore, H.J., Davey Smith, G., 2012. Reduced or modified dietary fat for preventing cardiovascular disease. Cochrane Database Syst. Rev. 5, CD002137. http://dx.doi.org/10.1002/14651858.CD002137.pub3.

Horton, R., 2005. Expression of concern: Indo-Mediterranean Diet Heart Study. Lancet 366, 354–356. http://dx.doi.org/10.1016/s0140-6736(05)67006-7.

Jensen, C.L., Prager, T.C., Fraley, J.K., Chen, H., Anderson, R.E., Heird, W.C., 1997. Effect of dietary linoleic/alpha-linolenic acid ratio on growth and visual function of term infants. J. Pediatr. 131, 200–209.

Kelley, D.S., Siegel, D., Vemuri, M., Mackey, B.E., 2007. Docosahexaenoic acid supplementation improves fasting and postprandial lipid profiles in hypertriglyceridemic men. Am. J. Clin. Nutr. 86, 324–333.

Kestin, M., Clifton, P., Belling, G.B., Nestel, P.J., 1990. N-3 Fatty acids of marine origin lower systolic blood pressure and triglycerides but raise LDL cholesterol compared with N-3 and N-6 fatty acids from plants. Am. J. Clin. Nutr. 51, 1028–1034.

Kornsteiner, M., Singer, I., Elmadfa, I., 2008. Very low N-3 long-chain polyunsaturated fatty acid status in Austrian vegetarians and vegans. Ann. Nutr. Metab. 52, 37–47. http://dx.doi.org/10.1159/000118629.

Kromhout, D., Giltay, E.J., Geleijnse, J.M., 2010. N-3 Fatty acids and cardiovascular events after myocardial infarction. N. Engl. J. Med. 363, 2015–2026. http://dx.doi.org/10.1056/NEJMoa1003603.

Larsen, M.K., Nielsen, J.H., Butler, G., Leifert, C., Slots, T., Kristiansen, G.H., Gustafsson, A.H., 2010. Milk quality as affected by feeding regimens in a country with climatic variation. J. Dairy Sci. 93, 2863–2873. http://dx.doi.org/10.3168/jds.2009-2953.

Lee, H.Y., Woo, J., Chen, Z.Y., Leung, S.F., Peng, X.H., 2000. Serum fatty acid, lipid profile and dietary intake of Hong Kong Chinese omnivores and vegetarians. Eur. J. Clin. Nutr. 54, 768–773.

Li, D., Sinclair, A., Wilson, A., Nakkote, S., Kelly, F., Abedin, L., Mann, N., Turner, A., 1999. Effect of dietary alpha-linolenic acid on thrombotic risk factors in vegetarian men. Am. J. Clin. Nutr. 69, 872–882.

Makrides, M., Gould, J.F., Gawlik, N.R., Yelland, L.N., Smithers, L.G., Anderson, P.J., Gibson, R.A., 2014. Four-year follow-up of children born to women in a randomized trial of prenatal DHA supplementation. JAMA 311, 1802–1804. http://dx.doi.org/10.1001/jama.2014.2194.

Makrides, M., Neumann, M.A., Jeffrey, B., Lien, E.L., Gibson, R.A., 2000. A randomized trial of different ratios of linoleic to alpha-linolenic acid in the diet of term infants: effects on visual function and growth. Am. J. Clin. Nutr. 71, 120–129.

Mann, N., Pirotta, Y., O'Connell, S., Li, D., Kelly, F., Sinclair, A., 2006. Fatty acid composition of habitual omnivore and vegetarian diets. Lipids 41, 637–646.

Melchert, H.U., Limsathayourat, N., Mihajlovic, H., Eichberg, J., Thefeld, W., Rottka, H., 1987. Fatty acid patterns in triglycerides, diglycerides, free fatty acids, cholesteryl esters and phosphatidylcholine in serum from vegetarians and non-vegetarians. Atherosclerosis 65, 159–166.

Metz, J.G., Roessler, P., Facciotti, D., Levering, C., Dittrich, F., Lassner, M., Valentine, R., Lardizabal, K., Domergue, F., Yamada, A., et al., 2001. Production of polyunsaturated fatty acids by polyketide synthases in both prokaryotes and eukaryotes. Science 293, 290–293. http://dx.doi.org/10.1126/science.1059593.

Miller, G.J., Kotecha, S., Wilkinson, W.H., Wilkes, H., Stirling, Y., Sanders, T.A., Broadhurst, A., Allison, J., Meade, T.W., 1988. Dietary and other characteristics relevant for coronary heart disease in men of Indian, West Indian and European descent in London. Atherosclerosis 70, 63–72.

Pan, A., Chen, M., Chowdhury, R., Wu, J.H., Sun, Q., Campos, H., Mozaffarian, D., Hu, F.B., 2012. Alpha-linolenic acid and risk of cardiovascular disease: a systematic review and meta-analysis. Am. J. Clin. Nutr. 96, 1262–1273. http://dx.doi.org/10.3945/ajcn.112.044040.

Pan, A., Yu, D., Demark-Wahnefried, W., Franco, O.H., Lin, X., 2009. Meta-analysis of the effects of flaxseed interventions on blood lipids. Am. J. Clin. Nutr. 90, 288–297. http://dx.doi.org/10.3945/ajcn.2009.27469.

Phinney, S.D., Odin, R.S., Johnson, S.B., Holman, R.T., 1990. Reduced arachidonate in serum phospholipids and cholesteryl esters associated with vegetarian diets in humans. Am. J. Clin. Nutr. 51, 385–392.

Reddy, S., Sanders, T.A., Obeid, O., 1994. The influence of maternal vegetarian diet on essential fatty acid status of the newborn. Eur. J. Clin. Nutr. 48, 358–368.

Rizos, E.C., Ntzani, E.E., Bika, E., Kostapanos, M.S., Elisaf, M.S., 2012. Association between omega-3 fatty acid supplementation and risk of major cardiovascular disease events: a systematic review and meta-analysis. JAMA 308, 1024–1033. http://dx.doi.org/10.1001/2012.jama.11374.

Rosell, M.S., Lloyd-Wright, Z., Appleby, P.N., Sanders, T.A., Allen, N.E., Key, T.J., 2005. Long-chain N-3 polyunsaturated fatty acids in plasma in British meat-eating, vegetarian, and vegan men. Am. J. Clin. Nutr. 82, 327–334.

Roshanai, F., Sanders, T.A., 1984. Assessment of fatty acid intakes in vegans and omnivores. Hum. Nutr. Appl. Nutr. 38, 345–354.

Roshanai, F., Sanders, T.A., 1985. Influence of different supplements of N-3 polyunsaturated fatty acids on blood and tissue lipids in rats receiving high intakes of linoleic acid. Ann. Nutr. Metab. 29, 189–196.

Royal Society of Chemistry, 1998. Fatty Acids. The Seventh Supplement to McCance and Widdowson's the Composition of Foods. Royal Society of Chemistry, Cambridge.

Sanders, T.A., 2009. DHA status of vegetarians. Prostagl. Leukot. Essent. Fat. Acids 81, 137–141. http://dx.doi.org/10.1016/j.plefa.2009.05.013.

Sanders, T.A., 2014. Plant compared with marine N-3 fatty acid effects on cardiovascular risk factors and outcomes: what is the verdict? Am. J. Clin. Nutr. 100 (Suppl. 1), 453S–458S. http://dx.doi.org/10.3945/ajcn.113.071555.

Sanders, T.A., 2015. Functional Dietary Lipids. Woodhead Publishing Series in Food Science, Technology and Nutrition: Number 24. Elsevier, Amsterdam.

Sanders, T.A., Ellis, F.R., Dickerson, J.W., 1978. Studies of vegans: the fatty acid composition of plasma choline phosphoglycerides, erythrocytes, adipose tissue, and breast milk, and some indicators of susceptibility to ischemic heart disease in vegans and omnivore controls. Am. J. Clin. Nutr. 31, 805–813.

Sanders, T.A., Gleason, K., Griffin, B., Miller, G.J., 2006a. Influence of an algal triacylglycerol containing docosahexaenoic acid (22 : 6n-3) and docosapentaenoic acid (22 : 5n-6) on cardiovascular risk factors in healthy men and women. Br. J. Nutr. 95, 525–531.

Sanders, T.A., Hall, W.L., Maniou, Z., Lewis, F., Seed, P.T., Chowienczyk, P.J., 2011. Effect of low doses of long-chain N-3 PUFAs on endothelial function and arterial stiffness: a randomized controlled trial. Am. J. Clin. Nutr. 94, 973–980. http://dx.doi.org/10.3945/ajcn.111.018036.

Sanders, T.A., Lewis, F., Slaughter, S., Griffin, B.A., Griffin, M., Davies, I., Millward, D.J., Cooper, J.A., Miller, G.J., 2006b. Effect of varying the ratio of N-6 to N-3 fatty acids by increasing the dietary intake of alpha-linolenic acid, eicosapentaenoic and docosahexaenoic acid, or both on fibrinogen and clotting factors VII and XII in persons aged 45-70 Y: the OPTILIP study. Am. J. Clin. Nutr. 84, 513–522.

Sanders, T.A., Reddy, S., 1992. The influence of a vegetarian diet on the fatty acid composition of human milk and the essential fatty acid status of the infant. J. Pediatr. 120, S71–S77.

Sanders, T.A., Roshanai, F., 1992. Platelet phospholipid fatty acid composition and function in vegans compared with age- and sex-matched omnivore controls. Eur. J. Clin. Nutr. 46, 823–831.

Sanders, T.A., Younger, K.M., 1981. The effect of dietary supplements of omega 3 polyunsaturated fatty acids on the fatty acid composition of platelets and plasma choline phosphoglycerides. Br. J. Nutr. 45, 613–616.

Simmer, K., Patole, S.K., Rao, S.C., 2011. Long-chain polyunsaturated fatty acid supplementation in infants born at term. Cochrane Database Syst. Rev. http://dx.doi.org/10.1002/14651858.CD000376.

Theobald, H.E., Chowienczyk, P.J., Whittall, R., Humphries, S.E., Sanders, T.A., 2004. LDL cholesterol-raising effect of low-dose docosahexaenoic acid in middle-aged men and women. Am. J. Clin. Nutr. 79, 558–563.

Uttaro, A.D., 2006. Biosynthesis of polyunsaturated fatty acids in lower eukaryotes. IUBMB Life 58, 563–571. http://dx.doi.org/10.1080/15216540600920899.

Welch, A.A., Shakya-Shrestha, S., Lentjes, M.A., Wareham, N.J., Khaw, K.T., 2010. Dietary intake and status of N-3 polyunsaturated fatty acids in a population of fish-eating and non-fish-eating meat-eaters, vegetarians, and vegans and the product-precursor ratio [corrected] of alpha-linolenic acid to long-chain N-3 polyunsaturated fatty acids: results from the EPIC-Norfolk cohort. Am. J. Clin. Nutr. 92, 1040–1051. http://dx.doi.org/10.3945/ajcn.2010.29457.

WHO/FAO, 2010. Fats and Fatty Acids in Human Nutrition. Report of an Expert Consultation. Food and Agricultural Organisation, Rome, Italy. Available from: http://www.fao.org.

Wien, M., Rajaram, S., Oda, K., Sabate, J., 2010. Decreasing the linoleic acid to alpha-linolenic acid diet ratio increases eicosapentaenoic acid in erythrocytes in adults. Lipids 45, 683–692. http://dx.doi.org/10.1007/s11745-010-3430-3.

Yu, X., Huang, T., Weng, X., Shou, T., Wang, Q., Zhou, X., Hu, Q., Li, D., 2014. Plasma N-3 and N-6 fatty acids and inflammatory markers in Chinese vegetarians. Lipids Health Dis. 13, 151. http://dx.doi.org/10.1186/1476-511x-13-151.

38

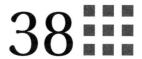

Implications of a Plant-Based Diet on Zinc Requirements and Nutritional Status

Meika Foster[1], Samir Samman[1,2]

[1]UNIVERSITY OF OTAGO, DUNEDIN, NEW ZEALAND; [2]UNIVERSITY OF SYDNEY, SYDNEY, NSW, AUSTRALIA

1. Introduction

Zinc is the second most abundant trace metal (after iron) in the human body. It performs diverse structural, catalytic, and regulatory roles in numerous biological processes (Table 38.1). The ubiquitous nature of zinc highlights its importance in human health and contributes to the recognition of zinc deficiency as a global public health concern (Wuehler et al., 2005).

Human zinc deficiency was first discovered in the Middle East in young men consuming predominantly plant-based diets that were high in wheat and low in animal protein (Prasad et al., 1961, 1963). Populations in low- and middle-income countries (LMIC) who follow predominantly plant-based diets continue to be at risk of diet-induced overt zinc deficiency, which is characterized by severe growth retardation, delayed sexual and bone maturation, impaired immunity, and diarrhea (Samman, 2012). In high-income countries (HIC), severe zinc deficiency is rare; however, based on population estimates of zinc intake, zinc deficiency in a less obvious form is believed to be highly prevalent (Wuehler et al., 2005). The scientific literature suggests that in HIC vegetarians are one of the populations that are most at risk of subclinical zinc deficiency. Although plant-based diets are reported to provide a variety of health benefits (Craig and Mangels, 2009), zinc is less bioavailable when obtained from plant-derived compared with animal food sources.

The present chapter aims to (1) explore dietary zinc requirements, zinc intake, and the factors that complicate the determination of zinc status and deficiency in vegetarian populations across the life cycle and (2) identify areas that require further investigation to support the translation of zinc research in vegetarians into clinical and public health applications.

Table 38.1   Select Structural and Biochemical Roles of Zinc

	Zinc Functions	Examples
Structural roles	Stabilization of cell membranes	Erythrocytes
	Structural component of various proteins and protein complexes, including >3000 transcription factors	Copper, zinc superoxide dismutase; zinc fingers (i.e., retinoic acid and calcitriol receptors)
Catalytic roles	Enzyme cofactor in >50 types of enzymes across all six enzyme classes	Carbonic anhydrases; angiotensin converting enzymes; nucleotide polymerases
Regulatory roles	Modulates numerous zinc-responsive genes and proteins	ZnT and Zip family zinc transporters; metallothionein; NF-κβ
	Endogenous signaling ion	Modulator of neuronal excitability

2. Plant-Based Diets

A diversity of dietary patterns can be described broadly as "plant-based." However, the term is used commonly in scientific literature to refer to semivegetarian and vegetarian diets. In classic terms, vegetarians abstain from eating all flesh foods, including meat, poultry, fish, and shellfish, whereas semivegetarians occasionally include meat and/or fish. Vegetarian populations are categorized as ovolactovegetarians, ovovegetarians, or lactovegetarians, depending on whether their dietary pattern includes egg (ovo) and/or dairy (lacto) products, or vegans for those who exclude all foods of animal origin. Within these patterns, considerable variation may exist in the extent to which animal products are excluded. Chapter 1 of the book explains vegetarian dietary practices in detail.

The composition of plant-based diets is influenced by numerous factors, including food choice motivations, product availability, produce growing conditions, and economic considerations. Particular care must be taken when comparing the composition of LMIC and HIC diets. Due to the limited availability or accessibility of animal foods, vegetarian diets in LMIC are often more similar in zinc content and bioavailability to their nonvegetarian counterparts than to HIC vegetarian diets. On the other hand, as sectors of an LMIC population increase in wealth, their dietary patterns are subject to change in a direction that aligns more closely with HIC diets (Gerbens-Leenes et al., 2010).

3. Food Sources and Bioavailability of Zinc

3.1 Zinc in Foods

Zinc is widely distributed in foods (Table 38.2). In HIC, meat, fish, and poultry are the major contributors of zinc in the adult omnivorous diet (Lim et al., 2013); however, dairy products and many vegetable foods provide amounts of zinc similar to those found in animal tissues. Vegetarians, to varying degrees depending on their dietary pattern, obtain a substantial amount of zinc from dairy foods, cereals, grains, legumes, pulses, nuts, and

Table 38.2   Zinc and Phytate Content and Phytate:Zinc Ratio of Selected Foods

Food	Zinc[a] (mg/100 g, EP on FW Basis)	Phytate[b] (mg/100 g, FW)	Phytate:Zn Molar Ratio
Beef, ground, raw	4.55	0	0
Chicken meat, raw	1.54	0	0
Oysters, Pacific, raw	16.62	0	0
Egg, whole, raw	1.29	0	0
Cheese, cheddar	3.64	0	0
Milk	0.37	0	0
Tofu, raw	0.83	171.6	20.4
Tempeh, raw	1.57	122.5	7.7
Breakfast cereal			
Kellog's All Bran, original[c]	12.40	2158.6	17.1
Kellog's Cornflakes	1.00	9.8	1.0
Quaker Instant Oatmeal	3.07	776.2	24.9
Quaker Puffed Rice	1.10	9.1	0.8
General Mills Wheaties[c]	27.80	551.2	2.0
Oat, whole meal flour	3.20	726.0	22.3
Rye, whole meal flour	2.17	712.8	32.4
Wheat bran	7.27	3161.4	42.8
Lentils, raw	3.27	588.7	17.7
Split peas, green, raw	3.55	471.1	13.1
Chickpeas, raw	2.76	458.2	16.3
Beans			
Baby lima, raw	0.78	718.4	90.7
Red kidney, raw	2.79	888.0	31.3
Pinto, raw	2.28	802.0	34.6
Peanuts, raw	3.27	771.5	23.2
Sesame seeds, whole	7.75	1525.0	19.4

EP, edible portion; *FW*, fresh weight.

[a]US Department of Agriculture, Agricultural Research Service, Nutrient Data Laboratory, 2015. USDA National Nutrient Database for Standard Reference, Release 27 (revised).

[b]IP5 + IP6 content, calculated using HPLC method (Lehrfeld, 1989; Sandberg and Ahderinne, 1986). Note: phytate data is derived from a range of countries [Ethiopia (Abebe et al., 2007), Indonesia (Chan et al., 2007), Sweden (Sandberg and Svanberg, 1991), and United States (Morris and Hill, 1995, 1996)] due to the limited availability of quality phytate data for US foods.

[c]US product fortified with zinc; fortification levels differ depending on country of production (Lim et al., 2013).

seeds. In the plant-based diets of numerous LMIC populations around the world, staple foods such as wheat, maize, rice, and lentils are the primary sources of dietary zinc (Wessells and Brown, 2012).

3.1.1 Zinc Fortification

The zinc content of the diet can be augmented by the fortification of foods with zinc. Food fortification is defined as "the addition of nutrients to commonly eaten foods, beverages, or condiments at levels higher than those originally found in food, with the goal of improving the quality of the overall diet" (Ruel, 2007). Voluntary zinc fortification is widespread in HIC, with variation across countries in the types of foods that are permitted to be vectors for fortificant zinc and the allowable levels of fortification. Cereals and cereal products (such as breakfast cereals, bread, pasta, biscuits, and cereal flours) and meat analogues (such as textured vegetable protein and quorn) are common vehicles for zinc fortification (Food Standards Australia New Zealand, 2013). Fortified foods may make an important zinc contribution to the diets of vegetarians generally, and vegans in particular, given that the latter group do not consume any animal products including dairy and eggs.

In the predominantly plant-based diets of LMIC, fortification increasingly is recognized as an important strategy for reducing the risk of zinc deficiency; efficacy trials indicate that zinc fortification can increase both total daily zinc consumption and the amount of absorbed zinc in children and adults (Brown et al., 2007). Widespread fortification of staple foods (commonly wheat or maize flour) with zinc has been mandatory for at least a decade in Mexico, Indonesia, Jordan, and South Africa (Brown et al., 2010; Food Fortification Initiative, 2015). As of November 2015, the practice of zinc fortification of one or more types of wheat or maize flour or rice is occurring in 39 LMIC (Personal Communication, Food Fortification Initiative, November 4, 2015).

3.2 Zinc Bioavailability

There is no standardized definition of the term "bioavailability" in the context of nutrition. A broad definition refers to the proportion of an ingested nutrient that is absorbed and utilized (Forbes and Erdman, 1983; Wood, 2005): in other words, the accessibility of a nutrient to normal metabolic and physiologic processes (Institute of Medicine (IOM), 2001). Accordingly, factors that may affect the bioavailability of a nutrient include dietary factors, such as the presence or absence in the food matrix of promoters or inhibitors of absorption; and host factors, including age, gender, nutritional status and health. A broad concept of bioavailability is often used also to encompass factors that appear to affect bioavailability but which, more accurately, trigger or result from regulatory responses designed to maintain optimal homeostasis, such as changes in absorption and/or excretion (Hambidge, 2010; Hambidge et al., 2010). The two principal factors that influence zinc bioavailability, in a broad sense, are the quantity of zinc ingested and the dietary level of inositol phosphate (IP), also known as phytic acid, or phytate when in salt form (Oberleas, 1983; Sandberg et al., 1982).

3.2.1 Phytate
Phytate is the principal storage form of phosphorus in cereals, legumes, and oleaginous seeds. It is therefore abundant in the plant-based diets of numerous populations around the world due to its presence in staple foods, such as cereals, beans, and lentils. Phytate in food is composed of a mixture of different phosphorylated forms of IP, with inositol hexaphosphate (IP6) usually the major form. IP6 and inositol pentaphosphate (IP5) form poorly soluble complexes with zinc in the gastrointestinal tract, resulting in reduced zinc

absorption or reabsorption (Oberleas, 1983; Sandberg et al., 1982). Mathematical modeling of zinc absorption suggests that phytate and the total intake of dietary zinc together account for more than 80% of the variability in the quantity of zinc absorbed (Hunt et al., 2008; Miller et al., 2007).

Food groups vary in their phytate content, which is undetectable in animal foods, high in grains and legumes (Table 38.2), and very low in roots and tubers (~0.1% dry weight) (Phillippy et al., 2003). The phytate content of a specific food may vary depending on the location from which it is sourced, due to inherent differences in soil composition, climatic or environmental conditions, crop plant cultivars, and agricultural management practices; the different stages of seed maturation and the use of food processing techniques, such as milling and flour extraction, are additional factors that influence the phytate concentration (Schlemmer et al., 2009). Further, the hydrolysis of phytate by microbial phytases during certain food preparation practices, including germination and fermentation, results in the formation of tetra- and lower phosphate derivatives, which have little influence on zinc availability (Sandström and Sandberg, 1992). A study of major foods consumed in central Iran reported that the IP6 concentration was significantly lower in polished rice compared to rice samples that were abrasively ground but unpolished, and the concentration of IP6 was decreased in all rice varieties after cooking (Roohani et al., 2012). In cereals, phytate is located predominantly in the aleurone layer and the germ, whereas in legume seeds it largely occurs in the protein bodies of the endosperm or cotyledon (Schlemmer et al., 2009); removal of the hull or seed coat therefore could result in a higher phytate concentration in legumes.

There is wide variation in estimates of the daily phytate intakes of different populations, depending on gender, age, dietary patterns, country of origin, and the methods that are used to determine the phytate content of the diet. In adults, phytate intakes have been reported to range from approximately 200–5000 mg/day (Schlemmer et al., 2009). Vegetarian adults in India reportedly ingest phytate in amounts that are comparable to healthy women consuming a mixed diet in Australia (1290 ± 300 mg/day vs. 1316 ± 708 mg/day, mean ± SD, respectively) (Foster et al., 2012; Khokhar and Fenwick, 1994). Similar mean phytate intakes of 1487 ± 791 were observed in ovolactovegetarian Asian immigrants residing in Canada (Bindra et al., 1986). In Sweden, the median phytate intake of vegetarian adults was estimated to be 1146 mg/day compared to 369 mg/day in adults consuming nonvegetarian diets (Brune et al., 1989). Differences between the mean phytate intake in rural (1342 mg/day/reference man) and urban (781 mg/day/reference man) populations are evident in China, which is likely to reflect an evolution from traditional toward more Western-type dietary patterns in metropolitan areas (Ma et al., 2007).

The distribution of phytate in the diet also differs among populations. Breads and breakfast cereals appear to contribute a substantial proportion (40%–61%) of the dietary phytate in HIC (Amirabdollahian and Ash, 2010; Foster et al., 2012; Prynne et al., 2010), suggesting that a large amount of the daily phytate intake is consumed at the morning meal. In contrast, 39% of the phytate intake in a South Korean population was derived from rice (Kwun and Kwon, 2000), while 84% was derived from grain products in the diets of Guatemalan women, of which 48% was from tortillas (Fitzgerald et al., 1993).

3.2.2 Phytate:Zinc Molar Ratio

The inhibitory effect of phytate on zinc absorption can be estimated by the molar ratio of phytate to zinc in the adult diet. Examples of the phytate:zinc ratios of specific foods are provided in Table 38.2.

Based on data mainly from single meal studies, the World Health Organization (WHO) determined that dietary phytate:zinc ratios less than 5 correspond to 50% zinc absorption (described as "high" bioavailability), ratios in the range 5–15 are consistent with 30% zinc absorption (moderate bioavailability), and ratios greater than 15 correspond to 15% absorption (low bioavailability) (WHO, 1996). Vegetarian and vegan diets are described as being of moderate zinc bioavailability provided they are not based primarily on unrefined, unfermented, and ungerminated cereal grains or high extraction rate flours or, if more than 50% of the energy intake is derived from such cereal grains and flours, the phytate:zinc molar ratio of the total diet does not exceed 10 (WHO/Food and Agriculture Organisation of the United Nations (FAO), 2004). The findings of a meta-analysis conducted as part of the European Micronutrient Recommendations Aligned (EURRECA) program of work concur with the WHO's adjustments for diets of moderate and low bioavailability; compared to control meals with phytate:zinc ratios <15, test meals with phytate:zinc ratios >15 resulted in a reduction of fractional zinc absorption (FZA) by a mean of 0.14, representing a fall in FZA of almost half (45%) from the mean for the control meals of 0.31 (Bel-Serrat et al., 2014).

The International Zinc Nutrition Consultative Group (IZiNCG) notes that the effect of phytate on zinc absorption may be exaggerated when measured from single test meals compared to typical total diets (Brown et al., 2004). Preferring to follow a total diet methodology (excluding data from semipurified formula diets), IZiNCG classified diets into two types: mixed diets or refined vegetarian diets characterized by phytate:zinc molar ratios of 4–18 (corresponding to 31% zinc absorption); and unrefined cereal-based diets with phytate:zinc molar ratios greater than 18 (23% zinc absorption) (Brown et al., 2004).

The inhibitory effect of phytate on zinc absorption is a key consideration in dietary zinc intake assessment and planning for individuals and in estimating population requirements for dietary zinc.

4. Dietary Zinc Recommendations

Due to differences in expert opinions, types and availability of evidence, and assumptions employed in establishing requirements, the daily amounts of dietary zinc that are recommended to meet the physiological requirements of practically all healthy people at each stage of the life cycle vary throughout the world (Table 38.3). While it is generally agreed that vegetarians require higher amounts of zinc than nonvegetarians due to the

Table 38.3 Examples of Differences Worldwide in Recommendations for Dietary Zinc Intake (mg/day) by Life Stage and Gender

Region/Organization		Infants	Children	Adolescents Male	Adolescents Female	Adults Male	Adults Female	Pregnancy	Lactation	References
Australia/New Zealand	RDI (age)	2 (0–6 months)e 3 (7–12 months)	3 (1–3 years) 4 (4–8 years)	6 (9–13 years) 13 (14–18 years)	6 (9–13 years) 7 (14–18 years)	14 (≥19 years)	8 (≥19 years)	10 (14–18 years) 11 (≥19 years)	11 (14–18 years) 12 (≥19 years)	NHMRC (2006)l
India	RDA (age)	– –	5 (1–3 years) 7 (4–6 years) 8 (7–9 years)	9 (10–12 years) 11 (13–15 years) 12 (16–17 years)	9 (10–12 years) 11 (13–15 years) 12 (16–17 years)	12 (≥18 years)	10 (≥18 years)	12	12 (0–12 months PP)	ICMR (2010)
Nordic countries	RI (age)	– 5 (6 months–<2 years)	6 (2–5 years) 7 (6–9 years)	11 (10–13 years) 12 (14–17 years)	8 (10–13 years) 9 (14–17 years)	9 (≥18 years)	7 (≥18 years)	9	11	EFSA (2014)
United Kingdom	RNIa (age)	– 5 (7–12 months)	5 (1–3 years) 6.5 (4–6 years) 7 (7–10 years)	9 (11–14 years) 9.5 (15–18 years)	9 (11–14 years) 7 (15–18 years)	9.5 (≥19 years)	7 (≥19 years)	7	+6 (0–4 months PP) +2.5 (>4 months PP)	COMA (1991)
United States/Canada	RDA (age)	2 (0–6 months)g 3 (7–12 months)	3 (1–3 years) 5 (4–8 years)	8 (9–13 years) 11 (14–18 years)	8 (9–13 years) 9 (14–18 years)	11 (≥19 years)	8 (≥19 years)	12 (≤18 years) 11 (≥19 years)	13 (≤18 years) 12 (≥19 years)	IOM (2001)m
IZiNCG (refined vegetarian or mixed diets)a	RDA (age)	– 4 (6–11 months)	3 (1–3 years) 4 (4–8 years)	6 (9–13 years) 10 (14–18 years)	6 (9–13 years) 9 (14–18 years)	13 (≥19 years)	8 (≥19 years)	11 (14–18 years) 10 (≥19 years)	10 (14–18 years) 9 (≥19 years)	Brown et al. (2004)
IZiNCG (unrefined, cereal-based diets)b		– 5 (6–11 months)	3 (1–3 years) 5 (4–8 years)	9 (9–13 years) 14 (14–18 years)	9 (9–13 years) 11 (14–18 years)	19 (≥19 years)	9 (≥19 years)	15 (14–18 years) 13 (≥19 years)	11 (14–18 years) 10 (≥19 years)	

Continued

Table 38.3 Examples of Differences Worldwide in Recommendations for Dietary Zinc Intake (mg/day) by Life Stage and Gender—cont'd

Region/Organization		Infants	Children	Adolescents		Adults		Pregnancy	Lactation	References
				Male	Female	Male	Female			
WHO/FAO (high BA)[c]	RNI[f] (age)	1.1 (0–6 months)[h] 2.5 (7–12 months)[i]	2.4 (1–3 years) 2.9 (4–6 years) 3.3 (7–9 years)	5.1 (10–18 years)	4.3 (10–18 years)	4.2 (≥19 years)	3.0 (≥19 years)	3.4 (T1) 4.2 (T2) 6.0 (T3)	5.8 (0–3 months PP) 5.3 (3–6 months PP) 4.3 (6–12 months PP)	WHO/FAO (2004)
WHO/FAO (moderate BA)[d]		2.8 (0–6 months)[j] 4.1 (7–12 months)	4.1 (1–3 years) 4.8 (4–6 years) 5.6 (7–9 years)	8.6 (10–18 years)	7.2 (10–18 years)	7.0 (≥19 years)	4.9 (≥19 years)	5.5 (T1) 7.0 (T2) 10.0 (T3)	9.5 (0–3 months PP) 8.8 (3–6 months PP) 7.2 (6–12 months PP)	
WHO/FAO (low BA)[e]		6.6 (0–6 months)[k] 8.4 (7–12 months)	8.3 (1–3 years) 9.6 (4–6 years) 11.2 (7–9 years)	17.1 (10–18 years)	14.4 (10–18 years)	14 (≥19 years)	9.8 (≥19 years)	11.0 (T1) 14.0 (T2) 20.0 (T3)	19.0 (0–3 months PP) 17.5 (3–6 months PP) 14.4 (6–12 months PP)	

BA, bioavailability; COMA, Committee on Medical Aspects of Food Policy; EFSA, European Food Safety Authority; ICMR, Indian Council of Medical Research; IOM, Institute of Medicine; NHMRC, National Health and Medical Research Council; PP, postpartum; RDA, recommended dietary allowance; RDI, recommended dietary intake; RI, recommended dietary intake; RNI, recommended nutrient intake; RNIa, reference nutrient intake; T, Trimester; WHO/FAO, World Health Organisation/Food and Agriculture Organisation of the United Nations.

[a]Assumed bioavailability of dietary zinc, 31%.
[b]Assumed bioavailability of dietary zinc, 23%.
[c]Assumed bioavailability of dietary zinc, 50%.
[d]Assumed bioavailability of dietary zinc, 30%.
[e]Assumed bioavailability of dietary zinc, 15%.
[f]Assuming body weights (kg) of 6 kg for infants 0–6 months, 9 kg for infants 7–12 months, 12 kg for children 1–3 years, 17 kg for children 4–6 years, 25 kg for children 7–9 years, 49 kg for adolescent boys, 47 kg for adolescent girls, 65 kg for adult males, 55 kg for adult females.
[g]Adequate intake (AI; used when an RDI cannot be determined).
[h]Exclusively human milk–fed infants (bioavailability of zinc from human milk assumed to be 80%).
[i]With the exception of exclusively human milk–fed infants (7–12 months), who require 0.8 mg/day.
[j]Formula-fed infants fed whey-adjusted milk formula and infants partly human milk fed.
[k]Formula-fed infants fed a phytate-rich vegetable protein-based formula with or without whole grain cereals.
[l]The NHMRC suggests that vegetarians, particularly vegans, may require zinc intakes that are 50% higher than those set.
[m]The IOM notes that the dietary zinc requirement may be as much as 50% greater for vegetarians and particularly vegans whose major food staples are grains and legumes and whose dietary phytate:zinc molar ratio exceeds 15:1. In later summary dietary reference intake tables, the IOM of the National Academies (2015) documents that the zinc requirement for those consuming a vegetarian diet is approximately twofold greater than for those consuming a nonvegetarian diet; however, this incongruity in the summary tables appears to be in error as the tables are adapted from the original IOM recommendations published in 2001.

lower bioavailability of zinc from plant compared to animal foods, the recommendations of expert committees as to the extent of the increase are inconsistent due in part to heterogeneity in the definitions and categorization of vegetarian diets.

IOM (2001) suggests that vegetarians may need to consume as much as 50% more zinc to maintain health than amounts recommended for the general population, which equates to a recommended nutrient intake for zinc in the United States and Canada of 16.5 mg/day for males and 12 mg/day for females. The IOM notes that the higher recommendation is relevant particularly for vegans whose major food staples are grains and legumes and whose dietary phytate:zinc molar ratio exceeds 15:1. In line with the IOM, in Australia and New Zealand it is likewise suggested that vegetarians, particularly vegans, will need intakes that are approximately 50% higher than those set (NHMRC, 2006); this results in recommendations of 21 mg/day and 12 mg/day for male and female vegetarians, respectively. In contrast, two levels of recommended intakes have been set in France, depending on the dietary content of products of animal origin. A daily intake of 9 mg/day for men and 7 mg/day for women is recommended for balanced diets rich in animal products, including meat products (estimated intestinal zinc absorption, 30%). For predominantly plant-based diets (estimated intestinal absorption, 20%), an increased daily intake of 14 mg/day for men and 12 mg/day for women is proposed (Agence française de sécurité sanitaire des aliments (AFSSA), 2001; European Food Safety Authority (EFSA), 2014).

The zinc intake recommendations of the international agencies WHO and IZiNCG are set according to the phytate:zinc ratio of the diet; however, inconsistencies in the categorization and estimated zinc absorption efficiencies of diets with varied phytate:zinc ratios have resulted in varied recommendations (Table 38.3). For example, the WHO recommends a zinc intake of 14 mg/day for men and 9.8 mg/day for women who consume diets of low zinc bioavailability, such as those that are high in unrefined, unfermented, and ungerminated cereal grain and contain negligible amounts of animal protein (WHO/FAO, 2004). In contrast, IZiNCG recommends 19 mg/day for men and 9 mg/day for women consuming unrefined, cereal-based diets (Brown et al., 2004).

Indian Council of Medical Research (ICMR, 2010) has suggested that, at least in India, the adjustments for plant-based diets that are proposed internationally by many expert committees result in higher recommended dietary zinc intakes than those indicated from actual observations. According to the ICMR, data from the National Nutrition Monitoring Bureau show a habitual zinc intake of 9–11 mg/day from the typical cereal- and lentil-based Indian diet, with local zinc balance studies indicating an expected absorption of approximately 25% and marginal risk of zinc inadequacy. After considering the available evidence, the ICMR recommended a daily zinc allowance of 12 mg/day for men and 10 mg/day for women consuming traditional Indian diets. The observations of the ICMR highlight one of the primary challenges in estimating zinc requirements for humans: the strong homeostatic regulation of zinc in the body complicates our understanding of the effects of diet on zinc nutriture.

5. Whole-Body Zinc Homeostasis

Adaptations in zinc absorption, resorption, and excretion along the gastrointestinal tract are the primary means of maintaining a constant zinc state. FZA is dependent on dietary zinc content; a number of studies have shown that when zinc intakes are decreased, fractional absorption increases (King et al., 2001; Taylor et al., 1991; Wada et al., 1985). Superimposed on the relationship between intake and fractional absorption is the effect of enhancing and inhibiting components in the diet. Beyond the immediate influence of a low zinc dose, fractional absorption has been shown to be upregulated further (from 49% to 70%) after several weeks of equilibration to a diet low in zinc and of high bioavailability but not to a diet low in zinc and of low bioavailability (Hunt et al., 2008).

Despite adaptive increases in fractional absorption, the absolute amount of zinc absorbed on a low-zinc diet has been shown to be lower than the amount absorbed when zinc intake is adequate (Wada et al., 1985): the reason being that the largest increases in fractional absorption are applied to the lowest intakes of bioavailable zinc. In isolation, this finding suggests that zinc balance will not be sustained in the presence of chronic exposure to diets that are low in zinc. However, compared to adjustments in absorption, changes in gastrointestinal zinc excretion have the potential to conserve substantially greater quantities of endogenous zinc for tissue use and are sustained in the presence of habitually low zinc intakes (Hambidge and Krebs, 2001; Jackson et al., 1982). Shifts in endogenous fecal zinc excretion occur in concomitant response to changes in zinc absorption and reflect both a reduction in the amount of zinc secreted into the intestinal lumen and increased distal reabsorption of endogenous zinc.

A study of healthy participants who switched from a mixed to a lactovegetarian diet for 12 months illustrates the occurrence of physiological adjustments to a plant-based diet; although the plasma zinc concentration decreased in response to the lower zinc bioavailability of the lactovegetarian diet, the zinc excretion demonstrated a compensatory decrease (Srikumar, 1992). Whether homeostatic adaptations to a habitual vegetarian diet are sufficient to maintain an adequate zinc status throughout the life cycle, particularly during times of increased requirement, is an important subject of debate.

6. Zinc Status Throughout the Life Cycle

The plasma (or serum) zinc concentration and the dietary zinc intake are used, ideally in combination, to indicate the zinc status of populations and to identify subgroups at risk of zinc deficiency.

6.1 Zinc Status in Healthy Vegetarian Adults

It is estimated that approximately 3% of adults in the United Kingdom, Australia, and the United States are vegetarian (Foster and Samman, 2015), with prevalence rates as high as 40% in India (Yadav and Kumar, 2006). A meta-analysis explored the association between habitual vegetarian diets and dietary zinc intake and/or serum zinc concentration in vegetarian compared to nonvegetarian healthy adult populations (Foster et al., 2013a). The dietary zinc intake of vegetarians overall was found to be 0.9 mg/day lower than that of nonvegetarians, which represents a difference of approximately 8% of the RDA (IOM, 2001) for men and 11% for women. Similarly, the serum zinc concentration was 0.9 µmol/L lower in vegetarians compared to nonvegetarian control populations. Combined analyses of the dietary zinc intake and serum zinc concentration support the possibility of a gender difference in zinc status, with the difference in values between vegetarians and nonvegetarians being wider in females than in males. Secondary analyses suggest that not all vegetarian diets impact zinc status to the same extent. Vegans showed the largest differences in dietary zinc intake and serum zinc concentration compared to nonvegetarians (Foster et al., 2013a), although it has been demonstrated that well-planned vegan diets can be higher in dietary zinc than typical omnivorous diets (Abdulla et al., 1981). Differences in the impact on zinc status of plant-based diets from HIC compared to LMIC are also likely to exist.

6.1.1 High-Income Countries

Fig. 38.1 depicts the mean dietary zinc intakes of (A) male and (B) female ovolactovegetarians (defined as excluding all flesh foods and including dairy and eggs), vegans, and nonvegetarians in studies conducted in HIC that were included in the meta-analysis (Foster et al., 2013a). It is noteworthy that, regardless of gender, few vegetarian groups had a mean zinc intake that met the increased requirements recommended for vegetarians by the IOM (16.5 mg/day for men, 12 mg/day for women) (IOM, 2001), even accounting for variability of the data. Although the RDA is not intended to be used to evaluate the adequacy of population intakes, a mean nutrient intake of a group below the RDA likely indicates a nonnegligible prevalence of insufficient intakes as compared to estimated requirements (Gibson, 2005).

In combination, the findings of the meta-analysis and the relationship in vegetarian populations between recommended and mean zinc intakes suggest that vegetarians are at greater risk of zinc deficiency than their nonvegetarian counterparts. However, there do not appear to be any adverse health consequences in HIC adult vegetarians that are attributable to a lower zinc status (Gibson, 1994), supporting suggestions that there is an increase in the efficiency with which zinc is utilized in healthy individuals following plant-based diets. Consistent with this conclusion, zinc balance has been shown to be maintained in healthy men after exposure to a diet that supplied zinc of only 5.5 mg/day (Wada et al., 1985); and in women following an ovolactovegetarian diet during an 8-week crossover intervention study, despite decreases in zinc intake, absorptive efficiency, and the plasma zinc concentration compared to the nonvegetarian diet (Hunt et al., 1998).

6.1.2 Low- and Middle-Income Countries

Three studies (Faber et al., 1986; Pohit and Pal, 1985; Raghunath et al., 2006) that compared the dietary zinc intake of vegetarian and nonvegetarian populations in LMIC were included in the meta-analysis, but none that measured the serum zinc concentration.

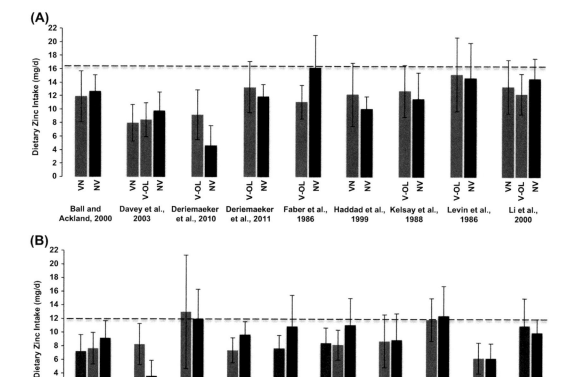

FIGURE 38.1 Comparison of dietary zinc intake in ovolactovegetarians, vegans, and nonvegetarians in high-income countries (define as World Bank Income Group 1) in (A) men; and (B) women. The *dashed line* represents the RDA for vegetarians suggested by the Institute of Medicine (2001). Results are expressed as mean±SD. *NV*, nonvegetarian, *VN*, vegan; *V-OL*, ovolactovegetarian.

One study was conducted in South Africa and reported significantly lower intakes of zinc in ovolactovegetarians compared to controls in both males (11.1 and 16.2 mg/day, respectively) and females (7.4 and 9.7 mg/day, respectively); however, these findings may not have been representative of the wider population as the study participants included vegetarians from a college for Seventh-day Adventists and nonvegetarians that were recruited exclusively from students and staff of a National Research Institute (Faber et al., 1986). The remaining two studies were conducted in India. The mean zinc intake was reported in 1985 to be 6.1 mg/day for Bengalee male vegetarians compared to 5.3 mg/day for nonvegetarians (Pohit and Pal, 1985). In a combined analysis of males and females in 2006, vegetarian adults in Mumbai were reported to have a mean zinc intake of 6.1 mg/day compared to 6.9 mg/day for nonvegetarians (Raghunath et al., 2006). It was noted in both instances that the vegetarian and nonvegetarian dietary patterns in these Indian populations are similar, with cereals and legumes being the primary contributors of zinc to both diets and the latter diet differing only by the inclusion of small amounts of animal protein (Pohit and Pal, 1985; Raghunath et al., 2006). Both the vegetarian and nonvegetarian Indian diets reported in these studies therefore typify the low-zinc, high-phytate dietary composition that is believed to convey the highest risk of zinc deficiency. However, the extent of homeostatic adaptation to the predominantly plant-based diets in LMIC that are low in zinc and high in phytate remains to be established. Further, it is not the case that all plant-based Indian diets are low in zinc. It has been reported that the customary zinc intakes of Indian adults consuming regional diets can be as high as 25 mg/day and that zinc balance is maintained on these diets despite estimated zinc absorption of 6%–8% (ICMR, 2010). It is likely that the higher zinc content of some high-phytate foods compared to products lower in phytate may compensate for the less efficient absorption of zinc, resulting in a greater absolute amount of zinc absorbed (Hunt, 2003).

6.2 Zinc Status in Pregnancy and Lactation

Pregnant and lactating women are vulnerable to a low zinc status due to the additional zinc demands associated with pregnancy and infant growth and development. Estimates of dietary zinc requirements in pregnancy take into account zinc accumulation in late pregnancy, the period of greatest need (NHMRC, 2006). The recommendation for zinc intake in lactation considers the additional needs for milk production counterbalanced with estimates of zinc released for use as a consequence of decreasing maternal blood volume after parturition (NHMRC, 2006). As with vegetarians generally, it is suggested that pregnant and lactating vegetarians need to consume higher amounts of zinc than their nonvegetarian counterparts, although recommendations of the extent of the increase vary throughout the world (Table 38.3).

6.2.1 Pregnancy

To strictly conclude that a particular dietary pattern provides insufficient zinc to meet the additional zinc demands of pregnancy, evidence of adverse effects either to the mother or the fetus as a consequence of low zinc status is needed. Early prospective studies investigating maternal zinc status and pregnancy outcome in healthy primigravidae (Jameson, 1976b) and women with a history of pregnancy complications (Jameson, 1976a) reported a significantly lower serum zinc concentration in women who had complications at delivery and/or gave birth to abnormally formed infants compared to women with normal deliveries. The findings of later observational studies, including numerous surveys of the association between maternal zinc status and the birth weight of infants, have been mixed (King, 2000). There is some research that suggests altered zinc status in pregnancy is associated with the occurrence of anencephaly in infants (Cavdar et al., 1988); however, further investigation is required to elucidate the role of zinc deficiency in the etiology of neural tube defects. Overall, the relationship between zinc status and maternal or fetal health outcomes in pregnancy is unclear.

Limited evidence explores the relationship between zinc status and health outcomes in pregnant vegetarian women. In a systematic review (Foster et al., 2015), the dietary zinc intake of pregnant vegetarians (defined as excluding all flesh foods) was found, using meta-analysis techniques, to be 1.5 mg/day lower than that of nonvegetarians, which represents a difference of approximately 14% of the RDA (IOM, 2001). Despite this, the balance of available evidence evaluated in the systematic review suggests that there is no difference between vegetarian and nonvegetarian groups in the serum zinc concentration or in functional outcomes associated with pregnancy (period of gestation, birth weight) (Foster et al., 2015). It is therefore plausible that adaptations in zinc metabolism to a vegetarian diet occur also in pregnant women, despite the increased zinc requirements of pregnancy.

The studies included in the systematic review (Foster et al., 2015) were too few to allow comparison of HIC and LMIC data by meta-analysis; only three studies explored the relationship between dietary zinc intake, zinc status, and pregnancy outcome in pregnant women consuming vegetarian dietary patterns that are typical in LMIC compared to their nonvegetarian counterparts. In an investigation of the zinc status of Hindu vegetarian pregnant women compared to nonvegetarian controls (Campbell-Brown et al., 1985), no differences were found over time between vegetarians and nonvegetarians in plasma zinc measurements. The amount of zinc excreted in the urine and the increase in urinary zinc excretion during pregnancy were both lower in the pregnant Hindu vegetarian compared to nonvegetarian women; taken together with the lower zinc intake in vegetarians (7.5 vs. 10.2 mg/day) that was reported at the first antenatal visit, this finding may represent a constraint dependent on the lower availability of zinc from the vegetarian diet (Campbell-Brown et al., 1985). Alternatively, it has been suggested that a degree of renal zinc conservation may occur in pregnant women consuming 9 mg or less zinc per day who do not demonstrate the significant increase in urinary zinc during pregnancy that is observed in women consuming higher amounts of zinc (Donangelo et al., 2005). A second study included in the systematic review supports the possibility that homeostatic adaptations occur in pregnant women from LMIC who consume low-zinc diets, whether or not they are vegetarian; it was observed that birth weights were similar between the infants of UK immigrant and indigenous Indian women, regardless of dietary pattern and notwithstanding zinc intakes in the Indian women that, at less than 6 mg/day, were almost half those of the immigrant group (Ward et al., 1988).

As alluded to previously, the predominantly plant-based diets of many LMIC nonvegetarian populations are likely to be closer in composition to traditional vegetarian dietary patterns compared to the omnivorous diets of HIC populations (Abraham et al., 1985). A number of observational studies have explored zinc status during pregnancy in LMIC without differentiating between vegetarian and nonvegetarian eating patterns. Populations who consume predominantly plant-based traditional diets during pregnancy are reported consistently to have a high prevalence of dietary zinc intakes below estimated requirements, phytate:zinc ratios greater than 15, and plasma zinc levels below the cutoff values specific for gestational age (Abebe et al., 2008; Fitzgerald et al., 1993; Huddle et al., 1998; Pathak et al., 2004, 2008), suggesting that zinc is a limiting nutrient in the predominantly plant-based diets that are typical in LMIC populations. However, the relationship between zinc status and birth outcome is rarely studied in LMIC, due in part to difficulties in obtaining data from customary village births (Huddle et al., 1998). The effects of a low zinc status in pregnancy on health outcomes therefore remain controversial. In addition, studies that investigate zinc status in pregnancy need to take into account the well-documented physiological adjustments in zinc metabolism during gestation, which include a decline in the plasma zinc concentration, perhaps as early as the first trimester (Hambridge and Droegemueller, 1974), and an increase in the concentration of urinary zinc (King, 2000).

6.2.2 Lactation

The concentration of zinc in breast milk is highest in colostrum and progressively declines with the duration of lactation (IOM, 1991). The effects of a vegetarian diet on zinc status during lactation are little studied (Foster and Samman, 2015); however, the zinc concentration of human milk is relatively resistant to changes in maternal zinc intake (Krebs, 2000), even in women with intakes that are chronically inadequate (Simmer et al., 1990), suggesting that homeostatic mechanisms rather than an increase in ingested zinc compensate for the maternal contribution of zinc that is secreted into breast milk.

6.3 Zinc Status in Infants, Young Children, and Adolescents

Adequate zinc nutrition is necessary for child growth, immune function, and neurobehavioral development (Brown et al., 2004). Infants, young children, and adolescents are particularly vulnerable to suboptimal zinc status during periods of rapid growth that increase requirements for zinc. As with adults, higher zinc intakes are recommended for vegetarian compared to nonvegetarian children to account for differences in bioavailability between plant and meat sources of zinc (NHMRC, 2006).

6.3.1 High-Income Countries

A narrative review (Foster and Samman, 2015) identified a number of observational studies that compared the effects of vegetarian compared to nonvegetarian diets on dietary zinc intake and serum zinc concentration in HIC populations of children (Table 38.4). The studies canvass populations of children from infancy to adolescence.

   In healthy term infants, zinc requirements to support the very rapid growth of early infancy generally are met by exclusive feeding of human milk; however, after the first 5 or 6 months of life, it becomes necessary to introduce complementary foods to meet infant zinc requirements. A longitudinal observational study (Taylor et al., 2004) that investigated the zinc status of infants consuming no meat with those consuming varying amounts of mixed red and white meat reported no differences among groups in zinc intake, which was assessed at four monthly intervals between the ages of 4 months and 2 years. Zinc bioavailability was not considered; however, no differences were observed at any time point in serum zinc concentrations between nonmeat and meat-eating infant groups, suggesting that zinc status is maintained in vegetarian and nonvegetarian infants to a similar degree. No measurements were taken of zinc-related functional outcomes, such as growth,

Table 38.4 Characteristics of Observational Studies Comparing the Effects of Vegetarian Compared to Nonvegetarian Diets on Dietary Zinc Intake and Serum/Plasma Zinc Concentration in Infants, Children, and Adolescents

Study (Author, Year)	Country	Diet Groups (V-OL, VU, LoM, NV)	Age[a] (years)	Gender (F/M)	N[b]	Dietary Zinc Intake (mg/day)[c]	SD	Serum/Plasma Zinc (μmol/L)	SD
Donovan and Gibson (1995, 1996)	United States	LoM	17.7±1.4	F	78	6.7	2.1	11.6	1.7
		NV	18.2±1.4	F	29	7.8	3.0	12.0	1.6
Gorczyca et al. (2013)	Poland	VU	1–17.6	F and M	22	4.02 (1.93–7.15)[d]			
		NV	2.3–17.8	F and M	18	5.44 (4.68–6.98)[d]			
Nathan et al. (1996)	United Kingdom	LoM	9.1±1.5	F and M	50	5.9[i]	1.4		
		NV	9.4±1.4	F and M	50	6.8	1.6		
Taylor et al. (2004)[e]	United Kingdom	V-OL[f]	24 months[g]	F and M	13	5.0	1.6	14.1	2.2
		NV(low)[f]	24 months[g]	F and M	33	4.1	1.2	14.2	2.5
		NV(medium)[f]	24 months[g]	F and M	40	4.4	1.1	14.3	2.3
		NV(high)[f]	24 months[g]	F and M	45	4.9	1.5	14.5	2.3
Thane and Bates (2000)	United Kingdom	LoM	2.3±0.4[h]	F and M	25	3.6/4.18MJ	1.0	13.1	
		NV	2.3±0.4[h]	F and M	668	4.0/4.18MJ	0.9	13.0	
		LoM	3.7±0.4[h]	F and M	19	3.5/4.18MJ	0.6	13.1	
		NV	3.7±0.4[h]	F and M	639	3.7/4.18MJ	0.9	13.0	
Treuherz (1982)	United Kingdom	VU	10–16	F and M	15	9.31[j]	2.1		
		NV	Age-matched	F and M	12	7.57	2.4		
Yen et al. (2008)	Taiwan, China	V-OL	5.2±1.5	F and M	21	6.2	1.0		
		NV	5.0±1.1	F and M	28	6.6	1.1		

F, female; LoM, low meat (populations that the study defined as vegetarian but who consumed meat, fish, or poultry on limited occasions, such as once per month); M, male; NV, nonvegetarian; V-OL, ovolactovegetarian; VU, vegetarian undefined.

[a]Mean±SD where available, otherwise range unless otherwise stated.
[b]n-Values for dietary zinc intake.
[c]Mean±SD unless otherwise stated.
[d]Median (range).
[e]Longitudinal study.
[f]Diet groups correspond to study definitions, as follows: V-OL (nonmeat eaters), NV (low, middle, and upper tertile meat eaters).
[g]Participants were recruited before they were 4months of age and were followed up until 24months of age (n-values differ at each timepoint).
[h]LoM and NV combined in determination of each age group.
[i]P=.001 (dietary zinc intake lower in LoM compared to NV).
[j]P<.05 (dietary zinc intake higher in VU compared to NV when expressed per 4.18MJ).

neurocognitive development, and infectious morbidity, so it is not possible to comment on whether any of the vegetarian and nonvegetarian dietary patterns contributed to zinc deficiency in the population of infants under study.

In older age groups, one study reported a lower zinc intake in vegetarian compared to nonvegetarian children in the United Kingdom with a mean age of 9 years (Nathan et al., 1996). In contrast, the remaining studies suggest that zinc status is maintained to the same extent in vegetarians and omnivores. No differences in energy-adjusted zinc intake or plasma zinc concentrations were identified using the British National Diet and Nutrition Survey 1992–93 in younger (1.5 to <3 years) or older (3–4.5 years) participants who consumed no meat during the 4-day period of dietary record keeping compared to those who ate meat. Neither were differences observed in the percentages of omnivores and vegetarians with clearly insufficient intakes (below the lower RNI threshold) (Thane and Bates, 2000). Similarly, no differences between vegetarians and omnivores were found in zinc intake or in weight, height, or the weight-for-height index of preschool children in Taiwan (Yen et al., 2008). A trend in the United Kingdom toward a higher zinc intake was observed in a small number of vegetarian children aged 10–16 years compared to age- and sex-matched omnivores (Treuherz, 1982). In a study in Poland (Gorczyca et al., 2013), zinc intakes were reported to be lower but not significantly different in male and female vegetarians aged between 1 and 18 years compared to omnivores, and no differences in height, weight, infectious disease morbidity, or serum immunoglobulin levels were observed between groups. In a Canadian study, no differences in zinc intake, serum zinc, or hair zinc concentrations were found in young vegetarian and nonvegetarian women aged 14–19 years (Donovan and Gibson, 1995); despite a median phytate:zinc molar ratio that was higher in vegetarians, with a higher proportion of vegetarians than omnivores having ratios above 15, similar proportions of each group were observed to have serum zinc concentrations below lower threshold levels.

Further studies are needed to confirm whether zinc status is similar in vegetarian and nonvegetarian children. Regardless of dietary pattern, children and adolescents with measures of zinc intake or status below critical thresholds may benefit from strategies that increase the amount of bioavailable zinc (Gibson et al., 1997; Harland et al., 1988). Targeted zinc supplementation studies have demonstrated increases in height-for-age Z score and height velocity in boys from the United States with low height percentiles (Gibson et al., 1989; Walravens et al., 1983).

6.3.2 Low- and Middle-Income Countries

Children from LMIC who consume predominantly plant-based monotonous diets that include limited intakes of flesh food and high phytate:zinc molar ratios are likely to be at greater risk of suboptimal zinc nutriture than HIC children consuming a more varied diet. Indian girls (10–16 years) with high intakes of cereals (199 g/day) and legumes/pulses (43 g/day) and low intakes of meat, fish, and poultry (13 g/day) were found to have a mean zinc intake of 3.6 mg/day, with almost all (99.5%) consuming zinc in amounts lower than WHO recommended intakes (Tupe and Chiplonkar, 2010). A mean phytate:zinc molar ratio greater than 25 has been reported in India for children aged 4–9 years and adolescents aged 10–19 years (Khokhar and Fenwick, 1994). Elsewhere, 75% and 43% of children in Papua New Guinea (aged 6–10 years) and Malawi (aged 4–6 years), respectively, were reported to have zinc intakes below 80% of the WHO estimated requirements (Gibson et al., 1991). Children (4–6 years) living in low socioeconomic areas in Mexico were reported to consume predominantly plant-based diets that did not meet energy requirements and provided mean zinc intake of 5.1 mg/day, which was significantly lower than the zinc intake of 14.9 mg/day in children from high socioeconomic areas who consumed a greater amount of animal protein (Wyatt and Triana Tejas, 2000). The increasingly widespread practice of zinc fortification in LMIC has the potential to improve the zinc intake of children who consume predominantly plant-based diets; while it appears that meals high in phytate depress zinc absorption from zinc-fortified foods, the absolute amount of zinc absorbed is still likely to be greater than if the foods were not fortified with zinc (Brown et al., 2007). The success of such intervention programs in improving health outcomes is yet to be determined and will depend on the population's access to and consumption of zinc-fortified foods (Brown et al., 2007).

The results of randomized controlled zinc intervention trials in children and adolescents illuminate the influence of zinc intake on zinc status indicators and on health. A recent meta-analysis of 18 randomized controlled zinc intervention trials (13 of which were conducted in LMIC) in apparently healthy children aged 1–17 years indicated that for every doubling in zinc intake, the difference in serum or plasma zinc concentration is 9% (Moran et al., 2012). The primary functional outcome that is most often associated with serum zinc is growth (Raiten et al., 2011). Studies of preventive zinc supplementation have found that increasing zinc intake in at-risk populations increases children's weight gain (Brown et al., 2009) and linear growth (Abdollahi et al., 2014; Brown et al., 2009), thereby reducing the prevalence of stunting. Based on the results of randomized controlled zinc supplementation trials conducted in pediatric populations in LMIC, a recent systematic investigation concluded that zinc deficiency in children younger than 5 years of age increases the risk of incidence for diarrheal disease by 28%, pneumonia by 52%, and malaria by 56%. While it is estimated that the burden of disease due to zinc deficiency is borne most heavily by countries in Africa, the Eastern Mediterranean, and Southeast Asia, epidemiological evidence regarding the contribution of zinc deficiency to morbidity and mortality is limited for all age groups other than children aged 0–4 years (Caulfield and Black, 2004).

6.4 Summary

In studying zinc nutrition in any population, it is important to consider the relationships between intake, status, and health (Fig. 38.2). While concurrent measurement of dietary zinc intake and the plasma zinc concentration may indicate a low zinc status, a true determination of dietary-induced zinc deficiency requires adverse health effects to be established. To conclude that adverse health consequences are attributable to a diet

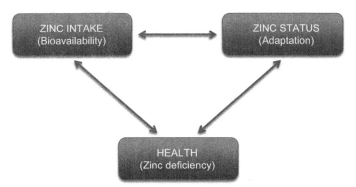

FIGURE 38.2 Triad of considerations in the determination of zinc nutriture. To assess the zinc nutriture of populations following habitual plant-based diets, it is important to consider the interrelationship among the intake of bioavailable zinc (with reference to the dietary phytate:zinc ratio), zinc status (and the extent of homeostatic adaptation to a plant-based diet), and health outcomes; to conclude strictly that the zinc intake from a plant-based diet is inadequate (such that zinc deficiency is present), it is necessary to demonstrate an adverse health outcome or disease that is consequent upon the level of zinc intake provided by the diet.

low in bioavailable zinc, confounding factors need to be considered, such as the potential concomitant prevalence of multiple other nutrient deficiencies and nonnutritional factors that affect zinc status.

Compared to nonvegetarians, adult male and female vegetarians, particularly vegans, tend to have lower dietary zinc intakes and serum zinc concentrations (Foster et al., 2013a); however, there do not appear to be any adverse health consequences in adult vegetarians that are attributable to a lower zinc status, presumably because of homeostatic mechanisms that allow adults to adapt to a vegetarian diet. In pregnant and lactating women, infants, young children, and adolescents, further research is needed to determine the effects of a plant-based diet on status and health. Research findings should take into particular account the differences inherent in the various categories of vegetarian diets and between the plant-based diets of HIC compared to LMIC populations.

7. Translating Research Into Practice

The ultimate aim of nutritional science is to translate nutrition research findings into clinical and public health applications. A range of strategies are available that promote zinc nutrition in individuals and populations following plant-based diets; however, a number of key areas require further investigation to maximize the ability of zinc research to impact positively on health.

7.1 Meeting Zinc Recommendations in Individuals

RDI (or equivalent) values are intended to be used as intake goals (assessed over a period of 3–4 days) for individuals; however, there is concern that the higher amounts of zinc currently recommended for vegetarians at each stage of the life cycle may not be achievable through diet alone without exceeding energy requirements. The Harvard Women's Health Watch (2009) has published online a 1-day menu devised by a clinical dietitian to meet all of the dietary reference intake recommendations for healthy postmenopausal omnivorous women consuming 1500 kcal (6276 kJ) or less per day. Table 38.5 depicts estimated dietary zinc and phytate contents and the phytate:zinc molar ratio of the Harvard Women's Health Watch sample menu in its original form, and with an example adaptation for ovolactovegetarians. At 8.9 and 10 mg of zinc for the nonvegetarian and vegetarian versions of the 1-day meal plan, respectively, both eating patterns exceed the dietary zinc amount of 8 mg/day that is recommended in the United States for the general female adult population. Although the latter sample menu does not meet the 50% higher dietary zinc recommendation of 12 mg/day for vegetarian women (IOM, 2001), a greater zinc intake does not appear to be required in this instance; the estimated phytate:zinc ratio is less than 10 (moderate zinc absorption) for both the nonvegetarian and vegetarian versions of the menu and both 1-day plans exceed the recommendations set by the WHO and IZiNCG for diets of moderate bioavailability (Table 38.3). It is of interest to note that the sample nonvegetarian menu includes only one meal that contains flesh food (salmon). This may be increasingly representative of a typical nonvegetarian diet in women; it appears in HIC that there is a trend toward a reduction in meat consumption, particularly in women (Fayet et al., 2014; Foster and Samman, 2015), and an increase in the consumption of exclusively plant-based meals in recognition that eating less meat (WHO, 2015) and more plant foods improves health.

The sample menu of the Harvard Women's Health Watch contains only one serving of grain-based foods. An Australian study demonstrated that it is possible with careful planning to design 7-day isoenergetic meal plans for ovolactovegetarians that meet both nutrient reference values and food group recommendations, including the guideline to consume at least four grain-based food servings daily (Probst and Tapsell, 2012). Three meal plans were devised based on the type of grain (whole grain, refined grain, and a 50:50 mix of whole and refined grain) for males and females aged 9 years and older (excluding pregnant and lactating women). The RDIs for the general population were used as the targets for zinc content, rather than the 150% RDI recommendations for vegetarians (Table 38.3); nonetheless, the daily zinc values for the ovolactovegetarian meal plans achieved %RDI values that ranged from 233 to 260 for boys and girls aged 9–13 years, 136 to 155 and 217 to 233 for adolescent (14–18 years) males and females, respectively, and 125 to 133 and 185 to 200 for men and women, respectively. Phytate content and the phytate:zinc ratio of the meal plans were not assessed, so it is difficult to evaluate whether the higher recommended zinc intakes for vegetarians would be warranted for the proposed meal plans. It seems likely, however, that zinc requirements would differ between the whole grain and refined grain dietary patterns; the former meal plan contained 30% more fiber than the refined grain meal plan (Probst and Tapsell, 2012), indicating that it has a higher phytate content (Foster et al., 2012). Further, it was noted in the study that the greatest contributors to zinc content were dairy products (cheese, milk, yogurt). Whether similar meal plans could be devised for vegan diets is unclear.

Table 38.5 Estimated Zinc and Phytate Contents and Phytate:Zinc Molar Ratio of a Sample 1-Day Menu Devised to Meet the DRI for All Nutrients, Including Zinc, in Healthy Postmenopausal Nonvegetarian Women Consuming 1500 Calories or Less per Day (Harvard Women's Health Watch 2009)[a] (in Its Original Form and Adapted for Ovolactovegetarians)

	Amount (EP) (g)[b]	Zinc[c] (mg)	Phytate[d] (mg)	Phytate References
Breakfast				
Nonfat yogurt, 8 oz.	226.8	1.9	0	Brown et al. (2004)
Sliced papaya[e], ½ cup	75	0.1	9.8	Umeta et al. (2005)
Sliced kiwifruit, ½ cup	75	0.1	0	Brown et al. (2004)
Walnuts, 14 halves	28.3	0.9	215.1	Harland and Oberleas (1987)
Skim milk, 4 oz.	113.4	0.5	0	Brown et al. (2004)
Lunch				
Whole wheat pita bread, 1 small with green salad:	28	0.4	47.3	Mameesh and Tomar (1993)
• dark green lettuce, 1 cup	75	0.1	0.5	Frossard et al. (2000)
• red capsicum, 1 small	74	0.1	26.3	Joung et al. (2004)
• grape tomatoes[f], 1 cup	85	0.1	3.2	Joung et al. (2004)
• edamame beans[g], ½ cup	78	1.1	227.8	Kamchan et al. (2004)
• sunflower seeds, 1 tbsp	8	0.4	128.5	Harland and Oberleas
• olive oil, 1 tbsp	13.7	0	0	(1987)
• balsamic vinegar	16.2	0	0	
• ground black pepper	0.3	0	0	
Dinner				
Broiled wild salmon, 4 oz with yogurt sauce:	113.4	0.9	0	Brown et al. (2004)
• greek nonfat yogurt, 1 tbsp	17.8	0.1	0	Brown et al. (2004)
• lemon juice, 1 tsp	5.2	0	0	Brown et al. (2004)
• chopped garlic, 1 clove	6	0.1	19.2	Joung et al. (2004)
or				
Cheese omelet[h]				
• scrambled whole egg, 2 large	90.7	1.2	0	Brown et al. (2004)
• grated cheddar cheese, ¼ cup	28.8	1.0	0	Brown et al. (2004)
• olive oil, 1 tbsp	13.7	0	0	
• iodized salt	0.8	0	0	
• ground black pepper	0.3	0	0	
Cooked barley[i] (added spices), ¼ cup	39	0.3	63.96	Harland and Oberleas (1987)
Cooked lentils[j] (added spices), ¼ cup	50	1.6	27.2	Davies and Warrington (1986)
Steamed baby bok choy[k], 1 cup	70	0.1	7.5	Kamchan et al. (2004)
		Total zinc[l] (mg/day)	**Total phytate[l] (mg/day)**	**Phytate:Zn molar ratio[m]**
	Nonvegetarian	8.8[n]	776	8.7
	Vegetarian	10.0	757	7.5

Continued

Table 38.5 Estimated Zinc and Phytate Contents and Phytate:Zinc Molar Ratio of a Sample 1-Day Menu Devised to Meet the DRI for All Nutrients, Including Zinc, in Healthy Postmenopausal Nonvegetarian Women Consuming 1500 Calories or Less Per Day (Harvard Women's Health Watch 2009)[a] (in Its Original Form and Adapted for Ovolactovegetarians)—cont'd

DRI, dietary reference intake; *EP*, edible portion.

[a]Although the "percent daily values" featured on food labels in the United States are based on a diet of 2000 kcal/day, the Harvard Women's Health Watch (2009) recognizes that not all adults require this much energy to remain in energy balance, and others may be wishing to achieve a healthy weight loss. The sample menu achieves all of the nutrient recommendations within a 1200 kcal mixed diet; the inclusion of healthy drinks and snacks would allow the 1500 kcal target to be met.

[b]Weights are estimated based on the provided descriptions of foods.

[c]US Department of Agriculture, Agricultural Research Service, Nutrient Data Laboratory, 2015. USDA National Nutrient Database for Standard Reference, Release 27 (revised).

[d]In all cases, the method used for measuring phytate either was not HPLC or was not described; Nb. phytate data is derived from a range of countries [Ethiopia (Umeta et al., 2005), United Kingdom (Harland and Oberleas, 1987; Davies and Warrington, 1986), Kuwait (Mameesh and Tomar), Korea (Joung et al., 2004), Thailand (Kamchan et al., 2004), United States (Harland and Oberleas, 1987)] due to the limited availability of phytate data for US foods.

[e]Phytate content estimated using values for fresh guava.

[f]Phytate content estimated using values for standard tomatoes.

[g]Phytate content estimated using values for young soy beans, cooked.

[h]Ovolactovegetarian option (not provided in original menu; Nb. cheese omelet option adds approximately 150 kcal to the 1-day menu and removal of salmon will reduce long-chain omega-3 fatty acid content of the diet; the conversion in humans of short-chain omega-3 fatty acids is inefficient, so vegetarians may benefit from consuming microalgae-derived DHA supplements).

[i]Cooking reduced phytate content from 739.2 g/100 g FW (McKenzie-Parnell and Guthrie, 1986) to 164 g/100 g FW (Harland and Oberleas, 1987).

[j]Cooking reduced phytate content from 588.7 g/100 g FW (Morris and Hill, 1996) to 54.4 g/100 g FW (Davies and Warrington, 1986).

[k]Phytate content estimated using values for Chinese cabbage, blanched.

[l]Sum of values before rounding.

[m]Calculated using the following formula: [phytate (mg)/660]/[zinc (mg)/65.4].

[n]Original source (Harvard Women's Health Watch, 2009) calculated zinc as 8.6 mg/day.

A second Australian dietary planning study succeeded in designing isoenergetic ovolactovegetarian meal plans for all age groups and both sexes that meet the nutrient reference value recommendations, including the 150% RDI recommendation for zinc in vegetarians (Reid et al., 2013). The study reports that the best vegetarian sources of zinc in the meal plans included muesli, pumpkin seeds, sunflower seeds, wheat germ, tofu, and brown rice. These foods are known to be high in phytate; however, the study did not assess the phytate content or the phytate:zinc ratio of the meal plans. Although the authors comment that phytate in food is minimized by modern food processing methods, little data is available to confirm this assumption in foods commonly available in HIC. Even assuming a higher zinc intake recommendation is justified in vegetarians and despite it being possible to achieve the greater zinc content in a carefully planned diet, a related issue is how to ensure adequate zinc intakes in individuals who may have decreased or selective appetites, such as children, pregnant women, and the elderly.

In summary, an assessment of the phytate:zinc ratio is necessary to determine whether higher zinc intake recommendations are justified in vegetarian compared to nonvegetarian individuals. It is possible to design an ovolactovegetarian meal plan that is similar in zinc content and bioavailability to well-planned nonvegetarian diets. Dietary assessment and planning is needed to determine the typical zinc and phytate content and phytate:zinc ratio of vegan diets and their ability (in both HIC and LMIC) to meet dietary zinc intake recommendations, with or without the need to incorporate foods fortified with zinc. When assessing the zinc status of individuals following plant-based diets, it is important for health professionals to bear in mind that RDIs are not synonymous with requirements; rather, they reflect the average daily dietary intake level of a particular nutrient that is sufficient to meet the nutrient requirements of nearly all (97%–98%) of the healthy individuals in a particular life stage and gender group, such that the majority of the group will require less than the stipulated amount. In addition, at least in healthy adults, homeostatic mechanisms appear to allow individuals to adapt to a vegetarian diet.

7.2 Research in Populations: Translational Implications

The ability to develop evidence-based and effective programs and policies to achieve global health goals depends on the availability of valid and reliable data. To promote the study of zinc nutrition across the life cycle in populations who consume plant-based diets, further research of consistent design is needed at each level of the intake–status–health triad (Fig. 38.2) in both HIC and LMIC.

In general, revised investigations of the zinc intake, bioavailability, and status of population groups throughout the life cycle are warranted; an increase in the availability and/or use of supplements and fortified foods is likely to have affected positively the zinc status of some groups and modern methods of food processing are likely to have altered the dietary phytate content of plant-based zinc sources. Plasma zinc concentration and dietary zinc intake, which are the recommended biochemical and dietary indicators, respectively, of zinc status in populations should be measured as part of nationally representative surveys, bearing in mind that the types of food consumed and the adequacy of food intakes by young children may differ substantially from those of adults in the same population. In addition, randomized controlled trials are needed to assess the relationship between plant-based diets and health outcome measures in both HIC and LMIC populations.

To support these objectives, when designing studies research groups need to ensure that definitions ascribed to vegetarian populations for research purposes are applied carefully and in a consistent manner; methodologies used to measure dietary zinc and phytate intake are robust; the zinc supplementation practices of vegetarians and their nonvegetarian counterparts are taken into account; and laboratory assessment methods are appropriate and consistent. In relation to the last point, the International Zinc Consultative Group protocols (Brown et al., 2004) are recommended for the measurement of serum/plasma zinc, and methods of PA analysis need to quantify individual IP as only IP5 and IP6 appear to affect zinc absorption (Sandberg and Ahderinne, 1986; Sandström and Sandberg, 1992).

In a related vein, a need exists for further development of accurate food composition tables that include updated and country-specific measurements of the zinc and phytate content of readily available local foods, ideally expressed as an index of zinc bioavailability. To compare results on a common basis, international standardization is essential to ensure that phytate data in food tables are comparable. Currently, food tables that include phytate information often do not describe which IP have been measured, nor do they appear to differentiate between the phytic acid and phytate contents of food items. All analytical procedures determine phytic acid following acidic extraction from food, which eliminates information on the phytate cations; it therefore has been suggested that results should be given correctly as phytic acid even though it is not present in plants (Schlemmer et al., 2009).

As with all zinc research, the identification of specific and reliable biomarkers of zinc exposure, status, and function would be invaluable in the assessment of zinc nutriture in vegetarian populations. Recent improvements in zinc-imaging techniques have afforded a deeper understanding of the maintenance of zinc homeostasis at the cellular level, which involves complex interactions between zinc sensors, such as metal responsive element-binding transcription factor-1 (MTF-1), and cell signaling machinery; the transcriptional and/or posttranslational regulation of two recently discovered classes of zinc transporters, the ZnT (SLC30) and Zip (SLC39) transporter families; and the trafficking of zinc through the cell by metallothionein. The coordinated control of zinc transporters in humans (Foster et al., 2011, 2013b) represents one promising direction in biomarker research that should continue to be explored. In addition to biomarkers that show cellular response to short-term zinc depletion or supplementation, the identification of biomarkers of zinc function across the life course and biomarkers that reflect short-term changes in zinc function with marginal intakes would also be invaluable (Raiten et al., 2011).

As new evidence becomes available that deepens our understanding of zinc nutrition, future revisions of population reference intakes will be enhanced and refined to more closely reflect the needs of specific groups. In the meantime, a cautious interpretation of the amount of dietary zinc required in vegetarian populations throughout the life cycle is merited, with the possible exception of healthy adults who appear to adapt to a wide range of zinc intakes.

7.3 Strategies for Improving the Zinc Bioavailability of Plant-Based Diets

A number of potential strategies are available for improving the zinc bioavailability of plant-based diets. Examples include these:

1. Increasing the zinc content of the diet through supplementation. Low-dose supplements are the most appropriate for children and during pregnancy and lactation until further information is available regarding safe and effective dose ranges in populations with increased zinc requirements. Total zinc intake in excess of the upper limit [40 mg/day (IOM, 2001; NHMRC, 2006)] may induce adverse consequences, such as an interference with copper absorption (Samman and Roberts, 1987). An understanding of patterns of phytate consumption in particular populations may increase the effectiveness of low-dose zinc supplementation regimes; for example, in HIC, given that the morning meal often has a high content of dietary phytate, it may be appropriate to recommend that zinc supplements be taken away from breakfast.

2. Increasing the zinc content of the diet through zinc fortification of widely consumed foods, as discussed earlier. Monitoring and evaluation of the effectiveness of zinc fortification programs are required.

3. Reducing the intake of antagonists of zinc absorption. Phytase can be used either during food processing to degrade phytate in foods that are important sources of zinc or as an active food ingredient to degrade dietary phytate during stomach transit time (Troesch et al., 2013). Further information is needed to determine phytase concentrations that are optimal in improving zinc bioavailability from phytate-rich foods.

4. Promoting the intake of enhancers of zinc absorption. For LMIC populations following predominantly plant-based dietary patterns, the addition of milk or yogurt to the diet has been reported to increase zinc bioavailability (Rosado et al., 2005).

As zinc research progresses, novel solutions are likely to become available that further assist policy-makers and nutritional science practitioners in improving the zinc status and health of populations consuming plant-based diets.

8. Conclusions

To determine the prevalence of zinc deficiency across the life cycle in populations consuming plant-based diets, a more complete understanding is required of the relationships among zinc nutriture, physiological adaptations in zinc metabolism during periods of increased requirement, and health outcomes. Due to fundamental differences in dietary composition, meeting zinc requirements is likely to be more difficult and require more careful planning in vegans compared to ovolactovegetarians and in LMIC populations that consume plant-based diets compared to HIC vegetarians. It is important that studies investigating zinc nutrition in vegetarians consistently assess the bioavailability of dietary zinc, particularly given the absence of reliable zinc biomarkers; however, to support this objective, further development of accurate food composition tables that include the zinc and phytate contents of locally available foods is required.

References

Abdollahi, M., et al., 2014. Oral zinc supplementation positively affects linear growth, but not weight, in children 6-24 months of age. Int. J. Prev. Med. 5 (3), 280–286.

Abdulla, M., et al., 1981. Nutrient intake and health status of vegans. Chemical analyses of diets using the duplicate portion sampling technique. Am. J. Clin. Nutr. 34 (11), 2464–2477.

Abebe, Y., et al., 2008. Inadequate intakes of dietary zinc among pregnant women from subsistence households in Sidama, Southern Ethiopia. Public Health Nutr. 11 (4), 379–386.

Abebe, Y., et al., 2007. Phytate, zinc, iron and calcium content of selected raw and prepared foods consumed in rural Sidama, Southern Ethiopia, and implications for bioavailability. J. Food Compos. Anal. 20 (3–4), 161–168.

Abraham, R., et al., 1985. Diet during pregnancy in an asian community in britain – energy, protein, zinc, copper, fiber and calcium. Hum. Nutr. – Appl. Nutr. 39A (1), 23–35.

Agence française de sécurité sanitaire des aliments (AFSSA), 2001. Apports nutritionnels conseillés pour la population française. Editions Tech & Doc, Paris, France.

Amirabdollahian, F., Ash, R., 2010. An estimate of phytate intake and molar ratio of phytate to zinc in the diet of the people in the United Kingdom. Public Health Nutr. 13 (9), 1380–1388.

Ball, M.J., Ackland, M.L., 2000. Zinc intake and status in Australian vegetarians. Br. J. Nutr. 83 (1), 27–33.

Bel-Serrat, S., et al., 2014. Factors that affect zinc bioavailability and losses in adult and elderly populations. Nutr. Rev. 72 (5), 334–352.

Bindra, G.S., Gibson, R.S., Thompson, L.U., 1986. [Phytate][calcium]/[zinc] ratios in Asian immigrant lacto-ovo vegetarian diets and their relationship to zinc nutriture. Nutr. Res. 6 (5), 475–483.

Brown, K.H., et al., 2004. International Zinc Nutrition Consultative Group (IZiNCG) technical document #1. Assessment of the risk of zinc deficiency in populations and options for its control. Food Nutr. Bull. 25 (1 Suppl. 2), S99–S203.

Brown, K.H., et al., 2009. Preventive zinc supplementation among infants, preschoolers, and older prepubertal children. Food Nutr. Bull. 30 (Suppl. 1), S12–S40.

Brown, K.H., Hambidge, K.M., Ranum, P., 2010. Zinc fortification of cereal flours: current recommendations and research needs. Food Nutr. Bull. 31 (Suppl. 1), S62–S74.

Brown, K.H., Wessells, K.R., Hess, S.Y., 2007. Zinc bioavailability from zinc-fortified foods. Int. J. Vitam. Nutr. Res. 77 (3), 174–181.

Brune, M., Rossander, L., Hallberg, L., 1989. Iron absorption: no intestinal adaptation to a high-phytate diet. Am. J. Clin. Nutr. 49 (3), 542–545.

Campbell-Brown, M., et al., 1985. Zinc and copper in Asian pregnancies–is there evidence for a nutritional deficiency? Br. J. Obstet. Gynaecol. 92 (9), 875–885.

Caulfield, L.E., Black, R.E., 2004. Zinc deficiency. In: Ezzati, M., et al. (Ed.), Comparative Quantification of Health Risks: Global and Regional Burden of Disease Attributable to Selected Major Risk Factors. World Health Organization, Geneva.

Cavdar, A.O., et al., 1988. Zinc status in pregnancy and the occurrence of anencephaly in Turkey. J. Trace Elem. Electrolytes Health Dis. 2 (1), 9–14.

Chan, S.S.L., et al., 2007. The concentrations of iron, calcium, zinc and phytate in cereals and legumes habitually consumed by infants living in East Lombok, Indonesia. J. Food Compos. Anal. 20 (7), 609–617.

Committee on Medical Aspects of Food Policy (COMA), 1991. Dietary Reference Values for Food Energy and Nutrients for the United Kingdom: Report of the Panel on Dietary Reference Values of the Committee on Medical Aspects of Food Policy. H.M. Stationery Office, London.

Craig, W.J., Mangels, A.R., 2009. Position of the American dietetic association: vegetarian diets. J. Am. Diet. Assoc. 109 (7), 1266–1282.

Davey, G.K., et al., 2003. EPIC-Oxford: lifestyle characteristics and nutrient intakes in a cohort of 33 883 meat-eaters and 31 546 non meat-eaters in the UK. Public Health Nutr. 6 (3), 259–269.

Davies, N.T., Warrington, S., 1986. The phytic acid mineral, trace element, protein and moisture content of UK Asian immigrant foods. Hum. Nutr. Appl. Nutr. 40 (1), 49–59.

Deriemaeker, P., et al., 2010. Nutritional status of Flemish vegetarians compared with non-vegetarians: a matched samples study. Nutrients 2 (7), 770–780.

Deriemaeker, P., et al., 2011. Health aspects, nutrition and physical characteristics in matched samples of institutionalized vegetarian and non-vegetarian elderly (>65 yrs). Nutr. Metab 8 (1), 37.

Donangelo, C.M., et al., 2005. Zinc absorption and kinetics during pregnancy and lactation in Brazilian women. Am. J. Clin. Nutr. 82 (1), 118–124.

Donovan, U.M., Gibson, R.S., 1995. Iron and zinc status of young women aged 14 to 19 years consuming vegetarian and omnivorous diets. J. Am. Coll. Nutr. 14 (5), 463–472.

Donovan, U.M., Gibson, R.S., 1996. Dietary intakes of adolescent females consuming vegetarian, semi-vegetarian, and omnivorous diets. J. Adolesc. Health 18 (4), 292–300.

European Food and Safety Authority (EFSA) Panel on Dietetic Products, Nutrition and Allergies, 2014. Scientific opinion on dietary reference values for zinc. EFSA J. 12 (10), 3844.

Faber, M., et al., 1986. Anthropometric measurements, dietary intake and biochemical data of South African lacto-ovovegetarians. South Afr. Med. J. Suid-Afrikaanse tydskrif vir geneeskunde 69 (12), 733–738.

Fayet, F., et al., 2014. Avoidance of meat and poultry decreases intakes of omega-3 fatty acids, vitamin B_{12}, selenium and zinc in young women. J. Hum. Nutr. Diet. 27 (Suppl. 2), 135–142.

Fitzgerald, S.L., et al., 1993. Trace element intakes and dietary phytate/Zn and Ca x phytate/Zn millimolar ratios of periurban Guatemalan women during the third trimester of pregnancy. Am. J. Clin. Nutr. 57 (2), 195–201.

Food Fortification Initiative, 2015. Country Profiles. Available at: http://www.ffinetwork.org/country_profiles/index.php.

Food Standards Australia New Zealand, 2013. Australia New Zealand Food Standards Code – Standard 1.3.2: Vitamins and Minerals. Available at: https://www.comlaw.gov.au/details/F2013C00099.

Forbes, R.M., Erdman, J.W., 1983. Bioavailability of trace mineral elements. Annu. Rev. Nutr. 3, 213–221.

Foster, M., et al., 2012. Dietary fiber intake increases the risk of zinc deficiency in healthy and diabetic women. Biol. Trace Elem. Res. 149 (2), 135–142.

Foster, M., Chu, A., et al., 2013a. Effect of vegetarian diets on zinc status: a systematic review and meta-analysis of studies in humans. J. Sci. Food Agric. 93 (10), 2362–2371.

Foster, M., et al., 2015. Zinc status of vegetarians during pregnancy: a systematic review of observational studies and meta-analysis of zinc intake. Nutrients 7 (6), 4512–4525.

Foster, M., et al., 2011. Zinc transporter genes are coordinately expressed in men and women independently of dietary or plasma zinc. J. Nutr. 141 (6), 1195–1201.

Foster, M., Petocz, P., Samman, S., 2013b. Inflammation markers predict zinc transporter gene expression in women with type 2 diabetes mellitus. J. Nutr. Biochem. 24 (9), 1655–1661.

Foster, M., Samman, S., 2015. Vegetarian diets across the lifecycle: impact on zinc intake and status. Adv. Food Nutr. Res. 74, 93–131.

Frossard, E., et al., 2000. Potential for increasing the content and bioavailability of Fe, Zn and Ca in plants for human nutrition. J. Sci. Food Agric. 80 (7), 861–879.

Gerbens-Leenes, P.W., Nonhebel, S., Krol, M.S., 2010. Food consumption patterns and economic growth. Increasing affluence and the use of natural resources. Appetite 55 (3), 597–608.

Gibson, R., 1994. Content and bioavailability of trace elements in vegetarian diets. Am. J. Clin. Nutr. 59 (Suppl. 5), 1223S–1232S.

Gibson, R.S., et al., 1989. A growth-limiting, mild zinc-deficiency syndrome in some southern Ontario boys with low height percentiles. Am. J. Clin. Nutr. 49 (6), 1266–1273.

Gibson, R.S., et al., 1991. Dietary induced zinc deficiency in children from Papua New Guinea (PNG) and Malawi consuming plant-based diets. In: Momcilovic, B. (Ed.), Trace Elements in Man and Animals (TEMA) 7. Institute for Medical Research and Occupational Health (IMI), Zagreb, pp. 166–168.

Gibson, R.S., 2005. Principles of Nutritional Assessment, second ed. Oxford University Press, New York.

Gibson, R.S., Donovan, U.M., Heath, A.L., 1997. Dietary strategies to improve the iron and zinc nutriture of young women following a vegetarian diet. Plant Foods Hum. Nutr. 51 (1), 1–16.

Gorczyca, D., Prescha, A., Szeremeta, K., 2013. Impact of vegetarian diet on serum immunoglobulin levels in children. Clin. Pediatr. 52 (3), 241–246.

Haddad, E.H., et al., 1999. Dietary intake and biochemical, hematologic, and immune status of vegans compared with nonvegetarians. Am. J. Clin. Nutr. 70 (Suppl. 3), 586S–593S.

Hambidge, M., 2010. Micronutrient bioavailability: dietary reference intakes and a future perspective. Am. J. Clin. Nutr. 91 (Suppl. 5), 1430S–1432S.

Hambidge, M., Krebs, N.F., 2001. Interrelationships of key variables of human zinc homeostasis: relevance to dietary zinc requirements. Annu. Rev. Nutr. 21, 429–452.

Hambidge, M., et al., 2010. Zinc bioavailability and homeostasis. Am. J. Clin. Nutr. 91 (Suppl. 5), 1478S–1483S.

Hambridge, K.M., Droegemueller, W., 1974. Changes in plasma and hair concentrations of zinc, copper, chromium, and manganese during pregnancy. Obstet. Gynecol. 44 (5), 666–672.

Harland, B.F., et al., 1988. Nutritional status and phytate:zinc and phytate x calcium:zinc dietary molar ratios of lacto-ovo vegetarian Trappist monks: 10 years later. J. Am. Diet. Assoc. 88 (12), 1562–1566.

Harland, B.F., Oberleas, D., 1987. Phytate in foods. World Rev. Nutr. Diet. 52, 235–259.

Harvard Women's Health Watch, 2009. Getting Your Vitamins and Minerals through Diet (July 01 2009). Available at: Available at: http://www.health.harvard.edu/womens-health/getting-your-vitamins-and-minerals-through-diet.

Huddle, J.M., Gibson, R.S., Cullinan, T.R., 1998. Is zinc a limiting nutrient in the diets of rural pregnant Malawian women? Br. J. Nutr. 79 (3), 257–265.

Hunt, J.R., 2003. Bioavailability of iron, zinc, and other trace minerals from vegetarian diets. Am. J. Clin. Nutr. 78 (Suppl. 3), 633S–639S.

Hunt, J.R., Beiseigel, J.M., Johnson, L.K., 2008. Adaptation in human zinc absorption as influenced by dietary zinc and bioavailability. Am. J. Clin. Nutr. 87 (5), 1336–1345.

Hunt, J.R., Matthys, L.A., Johnson, L.K., 1998. Zinc absorption, mineral balance, and blood lipids in women consuming controlled lactoovovegetarian and omnivorous diets for 8 wk. Am. J. Clin. Nutr. 67 (3), 421–430.

Indian Council of Medical Research (ICMR), 2010. Nutrient Requirements and Recommended Dietary Allowances for Indians: A Report of the Expert Group of the Indian Council of Medical Research. Indian Council of Medical Research, New Delhi.

Institute of Medicine (IOM), 1991. Nutrition During Lactation. National Academies Press, Washington, D.C.

Institute of Medicine (IOM), 2001. Dietary Reference Intakes for Vitamin a, Vitamin K, Arsenic, Boron, Chromium, Copper, Iodine, Iron, Manganese, Molybdenum, Nickel, Silicon, Vanadium, and Zinc, Washington, DC.

Institute of Medicine of the National Academies, August 19, 2015. Dietary Reference Intakes: Elements Summary Table. Available at: https://iom.nationalacademies.org/~/media/Files/ActivityFiles/Nutrition/DRIs/DRI_Elements.pdf.

Jackson, M.J., Jones, D.A., Edwards, R.H., 1982. Tissue zinc levels as an index of body zinc status. Clin. Physiol. Oxf. Engl. 2 (4), 333–343.

Jameson, S., 1976a. Variations in maternal serum zinc during pregnancy and correlation to congenital malformations, dysmaturity, and abnormal parturition. Acta Medica Scand. Suppl. 593, 21–37.

Jameson, S., 1976b. Zinc and copper in pregnancy, correlations to fetal and maternal complications. Acta Medica Scand. Suppl. 593, 5–20.

Janelle, K.C., Barr, S.I., 1995. Nutrient intakes and eating behavior scores of vegetarian and nonvegetarian women. J. Am. Diet. Assoc. 95 (2), 180–186 189, quiz 187–8.

Joung, H., et al., 2004. Bioavailable zinc intake of Korean adults in relation to the phytate content of Korean foods. J. Food Compos. Anal. 17 (6), 713–724.

Kamchan, A., et al., 2004. In vitro calcium bioavailability of vegetables, legumes and seeds. J. Food Compos. Anal. 17 (3–4), 311–320.

Kelsay, J.L., et al., 1988. Impact of variation in carbohydrate intake on mineral utilization by vegetarians. Am. J. Clin. Nutr. 48 (Suppl. 3), 875–879.

Khokhar, S., Fenwick, G.R., 1994. Phytate content of indian foods and intakes by vegetarian Indians of hisar region, Haryana state. J. Agric. Food Chem. 42 (11), 2440–2444.

King, J.C., 2000. Determinants of maternal zinc status during pregnancy. Am. J. Clin. Nutr. 71 (Suppl. 5), 1334S–1343S.

King, J.C., et al., 2001. Effect of acute zinc depletion on zinc homeostasis and plasma zinc kinetics in men. Am. J. Clin. Nutr. 74 (1), 116–124.

Krebs, N.F., 2000. Dietary zinc and iron sources, physical growth and cognitive development of breastfed infants. J. Nutr. 130 (Suppl. 2S), 358S–360S.

Kwun, I.S., Kwon, C.S., 2000. Dietary molar ratios of phytate:zinc and millimolar ratios of phytate × calcium:zinc in South Koreans. Biol. Trace Elem. Res. 75 (1–3), 29–41.

Lehrfeld, J., 1989. High-performance liquid chromatography analysis of phytic acid on a pH-stable, macroporous polymer column. Cereal Chem. 66, 510–515.

Levin, N., Rattan, J., Gilat, T., 1986. Mineral intake and blood levels in vegetarians. Israel J. Med. Sci. 22 (2), 105–108.

Li, D., et al., 2000. Selected micronutrient intake and status in men with differing meat intakes, vegetarians and vegans. Asia Pac. J. Clin. Nutr. 9 (1), 18–23.

Lim, K., et al., 2013. Iron and zinc nutrition in the economically-developed world: a review. Nutrients 5 (8), 3184–3211.

Ma, G., et al., 2007. Phytate intake and molar ratios of phytate to zinc, iron and calcium in the diets of people in China. Eur. J. Clin. Nutr. 61 (3), 368–374.

Mameesh, M., Tomar, M., 1993. Phytate content of some popular kuwaiti foods. Cereal Chem. 70 (5), 502–503.

McKenzie-Parnell, J.M., Guthrie, B.E., 1986. The phytate and mineral content of some cereals, cereal products, legumes, legume products, snack bars, and nuts available in New Zealand. Biol. Trace Elem. Res. 10 (2), 107–121.

Miller, L.V., Krebs, N.F., Hambidge, K.M., 2007. A mathematical model of zinc absorption in humans as a function of dietary zinc and phytate. J. Nutr. 137 (1), 135–141.

Moran, V.H., et al., 2012. The relationship between zinc intake and serum/plasma zinc concentration in children: a systematic review and dose-response meta-analysis. Nutrients 4 (8), 841–858.

Morris, E.R., Hill, A.D., 1996. Inositol phosphate content of selected dry beans, peas, and lentils, raw and cooked. J. Food Compos. Anal. 9 (1), 2–12.

Morris, E.R., Hill, A.D., 1995. Inositol phosphate, calcium, magnesium, and zinc contents of selected breakfast cereals. J. Food Compos. Anal. 8 (1), 3–11.

Nathan, I., Hackett, A.F., Kirby, S., 1996. The dietary intake of a group of vegetarian children aged 7-11 years compared with matched omnivores. Br. J. Nutr. 75 (4), 533–544.

National Health and Medical Research Council, 2006. Nutrient Reference Values for Australia and New Zealand: Including Recommended Dietary Intakes, Canberra, Australia.

Nieman, D.C., et al., 1989. Dietary status of seventh-day adventist vegetarian and non-vegetarian elderly women. J. Am. Diet. Assoc. 89 (12), 1763–1769.

Oberleas, D., 1983. The role of phytate in zinc bioavailability and homeostasis. ACS Symp. Ser. 210, 145–158.

Pathak, P., et al., 2004. Prevalence of multiple micronutrient deficiencies amongst pregnant women in a rural area of Haryana. Indian J. Pediatr. 71 (11), 1007–1014.

Pathak, P., et al., 2008. Serum zinc levels amongst pregnant women in a rural block of Haryana state, India. Asia Pac. J. Clin. Nutr. 17 (2), 276–279.

Phillippy, B.Q., Bland, J.M., Evens, T.J., 2003. Ion chromatography of phytate in roots and tubers. J. Agric. Food Chem. 51 (2), 350–353.

Pohit, J., Pal, B., 1985. Zinc content of the diets of the sedentary Bengalees. Int. J. Vitam. Nutr. Res. 55 (2), 223–225.

Prasad, A.S., et al., 1963. Zinc metabolism in patients with the syndrome of iron deficiency anemia, hepatosplenomegaly, dwarfism, and hypognadism. J. Lab. Clin. Med. 61, 537–549.

Prasad, A.S., Halsted, J.A., Nadimi, M., 1961. Syndrome of iron deficiency anemia, hepatosplenomegaly, hypogonadism, dwarfism and geophagia. Am. J. Med. 31 (4), 532–546.

Probst, Y., Tapsell, L., 2012. Meeting recommended dietary intakes in meal plans with ≥4 servings of grain-based foods daily. Public Health Nutr. 16 (05), 803–814.

Prynne, C.J., et al., 2010. Dietary fibre and phytate–a balancing act: results from three time points in a British birth cohort. Br. J. Nutr. 103 (2), 274–280.

Raghunath, R., et al., 2006. Dietary intake of metals by Mumbai adult population. Sci. Total Environ. 356 (1–3), 62–68.

Raiten, D.J., et al., 2011. Executive summary–biomarkers of nutrition for development: building a consensus. Am. J. Clin. Nutr. 94 (2), 633S–650S.

Rauma, A.L., et al., 1995. Antioxidant status in long-term adherents to a strict uncooked vegan diet. Am. J. Clin. Nutr. 62 (6), 1221–1227.

Reid, M.A., et al., 2013. Meeting the nutrient reference values on a vegetarian diet. Med. J. Aust. 199 (Suppl. 4), S33–S40.

Roohani, N., et al., 2012. Zinc and phytic acid in major foods consumed by a rural and a suburban population in central Iran. J. Food Compos. Anal. 28 (1), 8–15.

Rosado, J.L., et al., 2005. The addition of milk or yogurt to a plant-based diet increases zinc bioavailability but does not affect iron bioavailability in women. J. Nutr. 135 (3), 465–468.

Ruel, M., 2007. Zinc Fortification. IZiNCG Technical Brief No. 04, Davis, CA.

Samman, S., 2012. Zinc. In: Mann, J., Truswell, S. (Eds.), Essentials of Human Nutrition. Oxford University Press, Oxford.

Samman, S., Roberts, D.C., 1987. The effect of zinc supplements on plasma zinc and copper levels and the reported symptoms in healthy volunteers. Med. J. Aust. 146 (5), 246–249.

Sandberg, A., Hasselblad, C., Hasselblad, K., 1982. The effect of wheat bran on the absorption of minerals in the small-intestine. Br. J. Nutr. 48 (2), 185–191.

Sandberg, A.-S., Ahderinne, R., 1986. HPLC method for determination of inositol tri-, tetra-, penta-, and hexaphosphates in foods and intestinal contents. J. Food Sci. 51 (3), 547–550.

Sandberg, A.-S., Svanberg, U., 1991. Phytate hydrolysis by phytase in cereals; effects on in vitro estimation of iron availability. J. Food Sci. 56 (5), 1330–1333.

Sandström, B., Sandberg, A.S., 1992. Inhibitory effects of isolated inositol phosphates on zinc absorption in humans. J. Trace Elem. Electrolytes Health Dis. 6 (2), 99–103.

Schlemmer, U., et al., 2009. Phytate in foods and significance for humans: food sources, intake, processing, bioavailability, protective role and analysis. Mol. Nutr. Food Res. 53 (S2), S330–S375.

Simmer, K., et al., 1990. Breast milk zinc and copper concentrations in Bangladesh. Br. J. Nutr. 63 (1), 91–96.

Srikumar, T.S., 1992. Trace element status in healthy subjects switching a mixed to a lactovegetarian diet for 12 mo. Am. J. Clin. Nutr. 55 (4), 885–890.

Taylor, A., Redworth, E.W., Morgan, J.B., 2004. Influence of diet on iron, copper, and zinc status in children under 24 months of age. Biol. Trace Elem. Res. 97 (3), 197–214.

Taylor, C.M., et al., 1991. Homeostatic regulation of zinc absorption and endogenous losses in zinc-deprived men. Am. J. Clin. Nutr. 53 (3), 755–763.

Thane, C.W., Bates, C.J., 2000. Dietary intakes and nutrient status of vegetarian preschool children from a British national survey. J. Hum. Nutr. Diet. 13 (3), 149–162.

Treuherz, J., 1982. Possible inter-relationship between zinc and dietary fibre in a group of lacto-ovo vegetarian adolescents. J. Plant Foods 4, 89–93.

Troesch, B., et al., 2013. Absorption studies show that phytase from *Aspergillus niger* significantly increases iron and zinc bioavailability from phytate-rich foods. Food Nutr. Bull. 34 (Suppl. 2), S90–S101.

Tupe, R., Chiplonkar, S.A., 2010. Diet patterns of lactovegetarian adolescent girls: need for devising recipes with high zinc bioavailability. Nutrition 26 (4), 390–398.

Umeta, M., West, C.E., Fufa, H., 2005. Content of zinc, iron, calcium and their absorption inhibitors in foods commonly consumed in Ethiopia. J. Food Compos. Anal. 18 (8), 803–817.

Wada, L., Turnlund, J.R., King, J.C., 1985. Zinc utilization in young men fed adequate and low zinc intakes. J. Nutr. 115 (10), 1345–1354.

Walravens, P.A., Krebs, N.F., Hambidge, K.M., 1983. Linear growth of low income preschool children receiving a zinc supplement. Am. J. Clin. Nutr. 38 (2), 195–201.

Ward, R.J., et al., 1988. Assessment of trace metal intake and status in a Gujerati pregnant Asian population and their influence on the outcome of pregnancy. Br. J. Obstet. Gynaecol. 95 (7), 676–682.

Wessells, K.R., Brown, K.H., 2012. Estimating the global prevalence of zinc deficiency: results based on zinc availability in national food supplies and the prevalence of stunting. PLoS One 7 (11), e50568.

Wood, R.J., 2005. Bioavailability. In: Caballero, B., Allen, L., Prentice, A. (Eds.), Encyclopedia of Human Nutrition, second ed. Elsevier Academic Press, Oxford.

World Health Organization (WHO), 1996. Trace Elements in Human Nutrition and Health. WHO, Geneva.

World Health Organization (WHO)/Food and Agriculture Organization of the United Nations (FAO), 2004. Vitamin and Mineral Requirements in Human Nutrition. Report of a Joint FAO/WHO Expert Consultation, Bangkok, Thailand, 21–30 September 1998, second ed. WHO, Geneva.

World Health Organization (WHO), October 26, 2015. International Agency for Research on Cancer (IARC). IARC Monographs Evaluate Consumption of Red Meat and Processed Meat. Press Release No. 240. Available at: http://www.iarc.fr/en/media-centre/pr/2015/pdfs/pr240_E.pdf.

Wuehler, S.E., Peerson, J.M., Brown, K.H., 2005. Use of national food balance data to estimate the adequacy of zinc in national food supplies: methodology and regional estimates. Public Health Nutr. 8 (7), 812–819.

Wyatt, C.J., Triana Tejas, M.A., 2000. Nutrient intake and growth of preschool children from different socioeconomic regions in the city of Oaxaca, México. Ann. Nutr. Metab. 44 (1), 14–20.

Yadav, Y., Kumar, S., August 14, 2006. The Food Habits of a Nation. The Hindu CNN-IBN State of the Nation Survey. The Hindu. Available at: http://www.thehindu.com/todays-paper/article3089973.ece.

Yen, C.-E., et al., 2008. Dietary intake and nutritional status of vegetarian and omnivorous preschool children and their parents in Taiwan. Nutr. Res. 28 (7), 430–436.

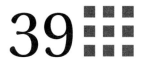

39

Plant-Based Diets and Iron Status

Diego Moretti

ETH ZÜRICH, ZÜRICH, SWITZERLAND

1. Introduction

Iron is abundant in the geosphere, being the fourth most abundant element in the Earth's crust. Despite this, iron deficiency is estimated to affect up to 1.5–2 billion people worldwide (Kassebaum et al., 2014; WHO, 2008). Anemia is estimated to contribute to 8.8% of the total global disability arising from health conditions (Kassebaum et al., 2014), and while the causes of anemia are multifactorial and depend on the geographical setting, iron deficiency is estimated to account to ≈40% of the global prevalence of anemia.

Iron deficiency anemia (IDA) during pregnancy is associated with higher risk of preterm delivery, predicts iron deficiency in 4-month-old children, and may cause deficits in neurocognitive development in infancy and childhood. Further, it generally increases susceptibility to infections (Zimmermann and Hurrell, 2007). In adults, manual laborers afflicted by IDA are more productive if they are given iron (Zimmermann and Hurrell, 2007), and it has been suggested that iron deficiency, even without anemia, can reduce work (Haas and Brownlie, 2001) and athletic performance (Brownlie et al., 2002). In a case study in 2015, the economic and social costs of IDA in 6- to 59-month-old Indian infants and preschool children were estimated to account for 1.3% of gross domestic product (Plessow et al., 2015).

The reasons for the persisting high prevalence of iron deficiency worldwide are complex (Lynch, 2011b), and they include poverty as a limiting factor for dietary diversity but also technical and programmatic challenges in addressing possible solutions, linked to the lack of recognition of its economical and societal impact (Lynch, 2011b).

2. Iron Sources in the Diet, Iron Metabolism, and Assessment of Iron Status

Iron deficiency arises when body iron needs cannot be met by iron absorption from the diet (Zimmermann and Hurrell, 2007). Iron balance is achieved by compensating obligatory iron losses through the gastrointestinal tract, airways, skin, and sweat, which account for approximately ≈1 mg of absorbed Fe/day in an adult 75-kg man (Institute of Medicine, 2001). Women of childbearing age need to compensate for additional losses due

Vegetarian and Plant-Based Diets in Health and Disease Prevention. http://dx.doi.org/10.1016/B978-0-12-803968-7.00039-3

to menstruation, which can vary strongly between individuals but have been estimated to account for an additional ≈0.5 mg Fe/day (Hallberg and Rossander-Hulten, 1991). Increased needs for growth are required in infancy, childhood, adolescence, and during pregnancy, and life stages with increased tissue growth correspond to the phases of highest risk for development of iron deficiency (Institute of Medicine, 2001).

Two main forms of iron can be found in foods: (1) nonheme iron and (2) heme iron. Nonheme iron is present in significant amounts in plant-based foods, while animal foods contain both nonheme as well as heme iron in dietary relevant amounts. In biological systems, nonheme iron has two main oxidation states: ferrous (Fe^{2+}) and ferric (Fe^{3+}) iron. Free iron is highly reactive (as in oxidoreduction reactions and as a catalyst in free radical reactions), and it shows limited solubility at neutral pH, in particular in its ferric form. For this reason, in biological systems, iron is typically associated with proteins and other ligands to prevent reactivity and precipitation in biological fluids. This reactivity is likely also the cause explaining why iron absorption is naturally restricted.

2.1 Iron Metabolism

The particular biological and molecular mechanisms required for iron absorption, transport, and storage are highly conserved across the biological kingdoms (Frazer and Anderson, 2014). The main site of heme and nonheme absorption is the duodenum, where nonheme iron can be reduced to ferrous iron by apical duodenal cytochrome B reductase and absorbed by the dimetal transporter 1 (DMT1). Heme iron, in contrast, is absorbed intact by a distinct transport pathway, but the identification of a dedicated heme receptor has remained elusive (Frazer and Anderson, 2014). Absorption in the distal gut (ileum and colon) has been assessed in early studies and is considered to be quantitatively limited (Wheby, 1970), both due to the lower presence of DMT1 receptors as well as due to the limited solubility of iron at the neutral pH in the distal GI tract. Once absorbed into enterocytes, iron is exported via a unique trans-membrane protein, ferroportin, the only known cellular iron exporter (Drakesmith et al., 2015), which presents iron to the transferrin molecule for systemic iron transport. Ferroportin can be targeted for degradation by hepcidin, a small peptide that is currently considered the main regulator of systemic iron balance. Hepcidin is synthesized and released in the liver, responding to systemic iron needs dictated by iron status (iron stores), erythropoiesis (iron demand for the production of red blood cells), and hypoxia (tissue and systemic local low oxygen partial pressure), as well as infection and inflammation (IL-6). Hepcidin is thought to integrate these various systemic stimuli and in this way match iron absorption with physiologic iron demand (Muckenthaler et al., 2008). While hepcidin is the systemic regulator of iron metabolism, local iron uptake can be regulated at the cellular level via special iron sensing proteins and RNA elements (IRP/IRE) that modulate the translation iron transport and storage proteins (such as the mentioned DMT1, ferritin, and ferroportin). Iron absorption and metabolism is therefore regulated by two tier system: at the systemic-hormonal level and at the cellular level.

Iron solubility and release from the food matrix is a prerequisite for absorption, as adequate gastric acid secretion has been shown to be essential to maintain adequate iron balance (Betesh et al., 2015). As there is no evidence for an excretion mechanism for iron, balance is controlled at the site of absorption in the duodenum, making bioavailability crucial for establishing and maintaining iron balance throughout life.

2.2 Assessment of Iron Status

An individual with a normal iron status can become progressively iron deficient when requirements cannot be met by the amount of absorbed iron. The process can be considered to progress through three stages: (1) storage iron depletion (decreased serum ferritin, <15 µg/L), (2) early functional iron deficiency (or iron-deficient erythropoiesis, increased soluble transferrin receptor), and (3) established functional iron deficiency (IDA, decreased hemoglobin) (Lynch, 2011a).

In healthy individuals, serum ferritin (SF) is linearly proportional with iron stores: 1 µg/L is indicative of 8–10 mg of body storage iron in an adult (Lynch, 2011a). Low SF is diagnostic for storage iron depletion and iron deficiency. However, SF is also increased during infection and inflammation, as well as liver disease, which can cloud its interpretation. The main iron compartment in the body is composed of erythrocytes transporting hemoglobin, by macrophages that capture senescent erythrocytes and recycle iron back to the transferrin molecule, and by the bone marrow where transferrin iron is used to produce new red blood cells. With the exception of SF, iron status measures the adequacy of this iron transport cycle (Lynch, 2011a), typically accounting for 80% of body iron. As ferroportin transports iron from cells (duodenal enterocytes or macrophages, for example) iron is rapidly bound to the transferrin molecule and transported to transferrin receptors, which are expressed on the cell's surface and are proportional to cellular iron needs. Soluble serum transferrin receptors are a sensitive marker and when elevated in plasma are indicative of early functional iron deficiency and increased unmet tissue iron need.

Hemoglobin concentration, proportional to the oxygen carrying capacity in the blood, is associated with the severe consequences when diminished in anemia. It is, however, not a specific nor sensitive marker for iron deficiency: several factors other than iron deficiency can cause a decreased concentration (hemolysis, chronic infection and inflammation, folate and vitamin B_{12} vitamin deficiencies), and a relative important iron deficit is required before hemoglobin is decreased.

3. Iron Bioavailability in Different Dietary Components and Composite Diets

Heme iron typically contributes only to 10%–15% of total iron intake, but because of its higher and generally less variable bioavailability, its contribution to absorbed iron requirements could be much higher and has been estimated to be >40% in meat-eating populations (Hurrell and Egli, 2010; Hunt, 2002). As a naturally chelated form of iron, heme iron absorption is less affected by dietary constituents and has generally lower variability than nonheme iron absorption (Hallberg et al., 1991).

Even in omnivores, nonheme iron constitutes the largest share of dietary iron, and after ingestion, it typically enters a common pool in the digestive tract, and all nonheme iron is absorbed to the same extent (Cook et al., 1972; Bjornrasmussen et al., 1976). Bioavailability from the common pool is dependent on luminal dietary factors being either enhancer or inhibitors of absorption (Hurrell and Egli, 2010) influencing Fe^{3+} and Fe^{2+} redox equilibrium, complex formation by various food ligands, solubility, and gastric and luminal pH. While subjects with low iron status effectively upregulated iron absorption (Moretti et al., 2006), enhancement and inhibition of iron absorption via luminal factors is independent from iron status and anemia (Thankachan et al., 2008).

3.1 Enhancers of Iron Absorption

3.1.1 Ascorbic Acid
The effect of ascorbic acid on iron absorption has been repeatedly established in single meal studies, and its function is likely related to its capacity of forming soluble complexes with iron and reducing ferric to ferrous iron (Conrad and Schade, 1968). Iron absorption from vegetarian diets can be increased by including ascorbic acid–containing foods (Hallberg and Rossander, 1982), and an ascorbic acid to iron molar ratio of 2:1 has been suggested to increase iron absorption between 2-fold and 12-fold from iron-fortified cereals. However, in meals rich in phytic acid and phenolics the ascorbic acid to iron molar ration should be increased beyond 2:1 (Hurrell, 2002) and up 4:1 to guarantee dietary meaningful iron bioavailability (Hurrell, 2002). Ascorbic acid can counteract the inhibitory effect of phytic acid, polyphenols, and calcium (Hurrell and Egli, 2010). Organic acid such as citric acid has been reported to potentially enhance iron absorption, even if the levels required are likely to exceed what would be commonly consumed in a diet (Teucher et al., 2004).

3.1.2 Muscle Protein
Muscle protein has been repeatedly and consistently shown to enhance nonheme iron absorption (Lynch et al., 1989), and 30 g of muscle is considered to be equivalent in its enhancing proprieties on iron absorption to 25 mg ascorbic acid (Monsen et al., 1978). The mechanism or the component by which muscle protein enhances iron absorption has not been directly established (Hurrell and Egli, 2010).

3.2 Inhibitors of Iron Absorption

3.2.1 Phytic Acid
Myo-inositol hexakisphosphate or phytic acid is the phosphate storage form in plants and has been repeatedly shown to inhibit iron absorption in a dose-dependent manner (Hurrell and Egli, 2010). Cereals such as wheat, barley, and rye contain intrinsic phytase,

able to degrade phytic acid, but the conditions required for the degradation to take place are not easily met in common food preparation methods (Koreissi-Dembele et al., 2013). It has been shown in earlier studies that bread making, in particular sourdough bread making, can significantly activate phytase and degrade phytic acid, enhancing iron bioavailability (Brune et al., 1992). The addition of dietary phytase has been shown to enhance iron bioavailability when added to a meal prior consumption (Troesch et al., 2009), a fact that demonstrates that phytase remains active in the stomach for a certain period, thus degrading phytic acid prior its own degradation by digestive enzymes. It is generally considered that a phytic acid to iron molar ratio of <1:1 should be aimed at, preferably <0.4:1, as already minor amounts of phytic acid can have strong inhibitory effects on iron absorption in the absence of ascorbic acid and muscle protein (Hurrell and Egli, 2010).

3.2.2 Polyphenols and Tannins

Polyphenols, similarly to phytic acid, can bind iron in the duodenum and make it unavailable for absorption by inducing its precipitation or reducing its solubility. As polyphenols are a complex and diverse class of chemical compounds, it can be expected that different polyphenols from different foods affect iron absorption differently. Black tea polyphenols, for instance, have been shown to be highly inhibiting (Thankachan et al., 2008) and generally more inhibiting than polyphenols in herbal tea and red wine (Hurrell and Egli, 2010), from cowpeas (Abizari et al., 2012) or beans (Beiseigel et al., 2007; Petry et al., 2013). Nonetheless, the effect of dephytinization on iron bioavailability from beans was only marginal when polyphenols were present, indicating a relevant inhibiting effect of polyphenols from beans on iron absorption (Petry et al., 2010). Similar results were found with sorghum, where phytic acid degradation did not improve iron absorption from high-polyphenol-containing sorghum (Hurrell et al., 2003).

3.2.3 Calcium

Calcium has been shown to be the only dietary component to inhibit both nonheme as well as heme iron absorption (Hallberg et al., 1991), in particular in simple meal matrixes such as bread rolls or milk. In a study in children using a whey drink as fortification medium, calcium inhibited iron absorption modestly (18%–27%), and ascorbic acid greatly overcompensated the inhibitory effect by calcium (Walczyk et al., 2014). In a study where iron was provided as NaFeEDTA, no effect of calcium could be detected (Troesch et al., 2009), suggesting perhaps that the calcium-dependent effect on iron absorption may be small in presence of absorption enhancers and a complex diet (Lynch, 2000).

3.3 Complete Diets and Iron Bioavailability

Data from single-meal studies can overestimate the effect of enhancers and inhibitors of iron absorption. This is likely because, for methodological reasons, meals to be compared are served in a fasting state, a condition that may not always be realized in a real-life situation. This notion has been translated in an alternative algorithm developed using bioavailability data obtained from a complete diet (Armah et al., 2013). The algorithm consisted of the following factors: vitamin C, iron status as SF, meat, fish, and poultry, phytic acid, amount of tea, and calcium.

Hallberg and Rossander-Hultén (1991) have estimated dietary iron bioavailability in a Western type diet (omnivorous) to range between 14% and 17%, while a vegetarian or vegan diet would have a lower bioavailability of 5%–12% for individuals with estimated depleted iron stores, as reflected in an SF value of $15\,\mu g/L$. Similar estimates have been proposed by the WHO/FAO (Table 39.1). Intakes in vegetarians are recommended to be higher to compensate for the overall lower iron bioavailability, as a plant-based diet would contain no heme iron, no muscle protein, and generally higher phytic acid. Iron intakes in vegetarians have been recommended to be increased by 80% compared to omnivores, which would correspond to an increase in women of childbearing age from 15 to 27 mg Fe/day (Gibson et al., 2014). While vegetarians may typically consume more iron in their diet than omnivores, the recommended increase may not be easy to meet when assuming a low-bioavailability diet. Vegetarians are therefore recommended to plan their diet choosing appropriate methods to reduce phytic acid content from whole meal foods (such as with sprouting, fermentation, sourdough preparation, soaking, and discarding soaking water), consuming ample amounts of foods as sources of ascorbic acid into their diet (citrus fruits, juices, vegetables, fresh produce), and avoid consuming polyphenol- and tannin-rich foods and beverages in concomitance with the main meals.

Table 39.1   Recommended Intakes Necessary to Fullfill Iron Requirements for Varying Levels of Bioavailability in Subjects With Negligible Iron Stores [SF< $15\,\mu g/L$ (WHO, 2005)]

		Fe Intake for Bioavailability (mg/day)			
Group	Age	15%[a]	12%[b]	10%[c]	5%[d]
Infants and children	0.5–1	6.2	7.7	9.3	18.6
	1–3	3.9	4.8	5.8	11.6
	4–6	4.2	5.3	6.3	12.6
	7–10	5.9	7.4	8.9	17.8
Males	11–14	9.7	12.2	14.6	29.2
	15–17	12.5	15.7	18.8	37.6
	18+	9.1	11.4	13.7	27.4
Females	11–14[e]	9.3	11.7	14.0	28.0
	11–14	21.8	27.7	32.7	65.4
	15–17	20.7	25.8	31.0	62.0
	18+	19.6	24.5	29.4	58.8
Postmenopausal		7.5	9.4	11.3	22.6
Lactating		10	12.5	15.0	30.0

[a]Moderate meat/fish in two main meals daily; low phytate and calcium; high ascorbic acid.
[b]Meat/fish in 60% of two main meals daily; high phytate and calcium; with ascorbic acid.
[c]Low meat intake; high phytate; with ascorbic acid.
[d]Meat/fish negligible; high phytate; high tannin; and low ascorbic acid.
[e]Premenarche.

3.4 Iron Fortification and Biofortification

When achieving a varied diet with ample amounts of absorption enhancers cannot be met in the short term, mass iron fortification of staple foods, as practiced in a number of countries worldwide (FFI, 2016), is considered a viable and sustainable approach to improve iron status of a population (WHO, 2001; Gera et al., 2012). In several countries, in addition to government mandating food fortification, the private sector is actively fortifying cereals (breakfast cereals, complementary foods). An alternative approach is biofortification, where the required nutrients are expressed in edible parts of plants either through classical plant breeding, via agronomic approaches, or via genetic engineering (Nestel et al., 2006). Biofortification is considered a sustainable approach suitable in reaching vulnerable populations not having access to industrially processed foods in the developing world. Substantial increases in bioavailable iron content have been reported in pearl millet (Cercamondi et al., 2013) and beans (Petry et al., 2015), and it is to be expected that broad adoption of these cultivars can contribute to the global effort in decreasing the prevalence of IDA. In contrast, efforts to biofortify rice, one of the leading staple crops worldwide, have obtained mixed success: while increases of a factor of 2 to 6 have been reported in transgenically transformed polished rice grains (Masuda et al., 2013; Wirth et al., 2009), further increases in iron level in polished grains are likely needed for rice to become a nutritionally meaningful source of iron (Bhullar and Gruissem, 2013).

4. Iron Status and Plant-Based Diets

4.1 Predictors of Iron Status in Epidemiological Studies

While the type and amounts of dietary factors that affect iron absorption are well known, epidemiological studies have not always found strong relationships between dietary determinants and iron status. This is likely related to the fact that iron absorption is directly regulated by iron stores (Hallberg and Rossander-Hultén, 1991), and differences in bioavailability may be effectively detected only in deficient population subgroups who physiologically upregulate iron absorption. Furthermore, accurate dietary assessment of iron intake may require up to 11 days of complete dietary record (Lyle et al., 1992), as a small number of foods can have a strong influence on overall iron dietary adequacy. In a study in the United Kingdom among 90 premenopausal women who underwent 7-day duplicate diet assessment, appurtenance to a dietary pattern group as ovolactovegetarian, poultry/fish, and red meat was a predictor of iron status, with poultry/fish consumers having higher iron status than red meat and the ovolactovegetarian groups. Total iron intake was not a predictor, while appurtenance to either group explained 6.7% of the variance in iron status. An additional significant determinant of iron status in this population group was menstrual loss, which explained 11.5% of the variability. Generally, only a small number of studies have found evidence that total iron intake is related to iron status (Beck et al., 2014; Galan et al., 1998). In contrast, associations between iron status and heme iron or meat intake have been reported in a large number of studies (Pynaert et al., 2009; Cade et al., 2005; Heath et al., 2001; Leonard et al., 2014; Galan et al., 1998; Rigas et al., 2014).

Many known factors affecting iron bioavailability such as ascorbic acid, fiber, and phytic acid have shown conflicting associations with iron status (Galan et al., 1998; Cade et al., 2005; Peneau et al., 2008; Rigas et al., 2014), with some studies suggesting a positive association between SF and ascorbic acid–containing low-fiber drinks (Peneau et al., 2008), as well as a negative association with fiber intake (Cade et al., 2005), but several other studies reporting no association (Beck et al., 2014). This may be due to the fact that the concomitant intake with iron may be important for an effect on iron absorption to take place, information that would be difficult to assess in population dietary assessment studies. Other study approaches using prospective, longitudinal design have, in contrast, shown the effect of a 16-week consumption of ascorbic acid–rich fruits on iron status (Beck et al., 2011). Similarly, a prospective study investigating the effect of consuming the recommended intake of dietary fiber in form of whole bread as a substitute for normal cereals found a decrease in SF in women with replete iron stores (Bach Kristensen et al., 2005).

In preschool children aged between 1.5 and 4.5 years, iron status was directly associated with meat and fruit consumption and inversely with milk products; however, consuming a vegetarian diet was not associated with iron status (Thane et al., 2000), and the authors concluded that over-dependence on milk (with intakes >400 mL/day) may be associated with lower iron status, as this would imply displacing iron-rich or iron absorption-enhancing foods (such as fortified cereals, meat, and fruits). In older children and adolescents between the ages of 4 and 18 years, intake in fruit juices, heme iron and meat, cereals, and breakfast cereals were associated with SF (Thane et al., 2003). In a different setting, a prospective study in school children in northern Morocco, consuming a self-selected diet relying on limited animal sources and fresh foods, a 15-month observation period following a controlled iron fortification intervention led to a drop in body iron stores reflected in a deficit in body iron of 142 mg Fe and an estimated iron bioavailability from the diet of only 2% (Zimmermann et al., 2005). The diet had refined and unrefined cereals (at a ≈0.45:0.55 ratio, respectively) that covered 58% of energy, fat, and oils (18% of energy), legumes (4% of energy), and meat, fish, and poultry (in the form of sardines mainly, covering 5% of energy).

4.2 Iron Status in Vegetarians

Hunt reviewed studies investigating iron status in omnivores and vegetarians until the year 2002, and concluded that from 15 studies investigating iron status and hematological indices in vegetarians and omnivores, only 3 studies out of 11 found small differences in hematological status and IDA, while a higher number of reports indicate that vegetarians have lower body iron stores than meat-eating counterparts (Hunt, 2002). A similar finding was also reported in a study in Australia in women aged between 18 and 35 years (Leonard et al., 2014), where a lower SF level was found in vegetarians compared to omnivores (26 vs. 42 µg/L). In a recent study in 75 german vegans, 40% were defined as iron deficient, but only 4% had IDA (Waldmann et al., 2004). In a further small study in Swedish vegans, no difference in prevalence of low iron stores was reported when compared to omnivores (Larsson and Johansson, 2002), and while there are several indications that vegetarians including vegans do have lower iron status and iron stores, there are no indications that this population group has a higher prevalence of IDA (Hunt, 2002). However, generally, the size of the studies is limited and does not allow a firm conclusion. Furthermore, several of the studies are dated and may not fully reflect current dietary habits.

4.2.1 Pregnancy

Pregnant women have distinctively and substantially higher iron requirements than prior to pregnancy (Bothwell, 2000), and it is generally accepted that these cannot be covered solely by dietary iron intakes (irrespective whether the diet would contain meat). For this reason, in several countries, iron supplements are recommended (Bothwell, 2000; Cook, 2005). The additional net iron requirement that a pregnancy imposes to the becoming mother is of approximatively 1 g, and most of this iron is required and utilized in the second and third trimester (Bothwell, 2000). Without iron supplementation, a becoming mother should approximatively have a level of iron stores equivalent to this expected additional requirement, which would correspond to a SF level of 100–120 µg/L (Cook, 2005). As iron deficiency without anemia is likely more prevalent in vegetarian women, pregnancy generally poses a challenge for covering iron requirements without the use of supplements (Cook, 2005; Bothwell, 2000). Readers can also refer to Chapter 32 for more detail regarding vegetarian diets in pregnancy.

4.2.2 Children

Until 6 months of age, exclusively breastfed infants born at term are able to cover their iron requirement through their stores and via breastmilk. After that age, additional sources of bioavailable iron are required (Institute of Medicine, 2001). IDA is high in infants in rural areas in developing countries (Jaeggi et al., 2013). Data from industrialized countries on iron status in infants is more scanty, but it has been suggested that the increase in use of iron-fortified complementary foods had the effect of substantially decreasing the prevalence of IDA in infancy and early childhood (Fomon, 2001; Lynch, 2011b).

Iron intakes in the United States and the United Kingdom in infants and children up to the age of 4.5 years do not appear to differ between vegetarian children and omnivores (Gibson et al., 2014); this may reflect the high proportion of iron intake coming from fortified foods. Intake of meat, even among omnivores, is usually small in childhood. Nonetheless, the lower bioavailability of iron in plant-based diets is likely to increase the risk of inadequate absorbable iron intakes (Gibson et al., 2014). In a nationally representative sample in the United Kingdom, prevalence of anemia was not different between vegetarians and omnivores, while the prevalence of iron deficiency defined with an SF < 12 µg/L was 73% versus 34% between ages of 1.5 and 3 years, and 40% versus 0.3% between the ages of 3 and 4.5 years in vegetarian children and omnivores, respectively (Thane et al., 2000).

5. Conclusions

A well-planned plant-based diet can provide ample iron to match requirements for absorbed iron (Gibson et al., 2014). However, consuming a plant-based diet is likely to increase the risk for low iron stores, which can expose vegetarian pregnant women to a higher risk for developing iron deficiency if they do not use supplements. However, current data in industrialized countries does not support the notion that a plant-based or vegetarian diet increases the risk for IDA. In contrast, in unprivileged settings in the developing world, monotonous plant diets are considered an etiological risk factor for IDA. Increasing diet diversity within a plant-based diet, coupled with fortification in the short term and biofortification in the medium term are considered viable and sustainable approaches to attempt curbing the high worldwide prevalence of IDA.

References

Abizari, A.R., Moretti, D., Schuth, S., Zimmermann, M.B., Armar-Klemesu, M., Brouwer, I.D., 2012. Phytic acid-to-iron molar ratio rather than polyphenol concentration determines iron bioavailability in whole-cowpea meal among young women. J. Nutr. 142.

Armah, S.M., Carriquiry, A., Sullivan, D., Cook, J.D., Reddy, M.B., 2013. A complete diet-based algorithm for predicting nonheme iron absorption in adults. J. Nutr. 143, 1136–1140.

Bach Kristensen, M., Tetens, I., Alstrup Jorgensen, A.B., Dal Thomsen, A., Milman, N., Hels, O., Sandstrom, B., Hansen, M., 2005. A decrease in iron status in young healthy women after long-term daily consumption of the recommended intake of fibre-rich wheat bread. Eur. J. Nutr. 44, 334–340.

Beck, K., Conlon, C.A., Kruger, R., Coad, J., Stonehouse, W., 2011. Gold kiwifruit consumed with an iron-fortified breakfast cereal meal improves iron status in women with low iron stores: a 16-week randomised controlled trial. Br. J. Nutr. 105, 101–109.

Beck, K.L., Conlon, C.A., Kruger, R., Coad, J., 2014. Dietary determinants of and possible solutions to iron deficiency for young women living in industrialized countries: a review. Nutrients 6, 3747–3776.

Beiseigel, J.M., Hunt, J.R., Glahn, R.P., Welch, R.M., Menkir, A., Maziya-Dixon, B.B., 2007. Iron bioavailability from maize and beans: a comparison of human measurements with Caco-2 cell and algorithm predictions. Am. J. Clin. Nutr. 86, 388–396.

Betesh, A.L., Santa Ana, C.A., Cole, J.A., Fordtran, J.S., 2015. Is achlorhydria a cause of iron deficiency anemia? Am. J. Clin. Nutr. 102, 9–19.

Bhullar, N.K., Gruissem, W., 2013. Nutritional enhancement of rice for human health: the contribution of biotechnology. Biotechnol. Adv. 31, 50–57.

Bjornrasmussen, E., Hallberg, L., Magnusson, B., Rossander, L., Svanberg, B., Arvidsson, B., 1976. Measurement of iron-absorption from composite meals. Am. J. Clin. Nutr. 29, 772–778.

Bothwell, T.H., 2000. Iron requirements in pregnancy and strategies to meet them. Am. J. Clin. Nutr. 72, 257s–264s.

Brownlie, T.T., Utermohlen, V., Hinton, P.S., Giordano, C., Haas, J.D., 2002. Marginal iron deficiency without anemia impairs aerobic adaptation among previously untrained women. Am. J. Clin. Nutr. 75, 734–742.

Brune, M., Rossander-Hulten, L., Hallberg, L., Gleerup, A., Sandberg, A.S., 1992. Iron absorption from bread in humans: inhibiting effects of cereal fiber, phytate and inositol phosphates with different numbers of phosphate groups. J. Nutr. 122, 442–449.

Cade, J.E., Moreton, J.A., O'hara, B., Greenwood, D.C., Moor, J., Burley, V.J., Kukalizch, K., Bishop, D.T., Worwood, M., 2005. Diet and genetic factors associated with iron status in middle-aged women. Am. J. Clin. Nutr. 82, 813–820.

Cercamondi, C.I., Egli, I.M., Mitchikpe, E., Tossou, F., Zeder, C., Hounhouigan, J.D., Hurrell, R.F., 2013. Total iron absorption by young women from iron-biofortified pearl millet composite meals is double that from regular millet meals but less than that from post-harvest iron-fortified millet meals. J. Nutr. 143, 1376–1382.

Conrad, M.E., Schade, S.G., 1968. Ascorbic acid chelates in iron absorption: a role for hydrochloric acid and bile. Gastroenterology 55, 35–45.

Cook, J.D., Finch, C.A., Walker, R., Martinez, C., Layrisse, M., Monsen, E., 1972. Food iron-absorption measured by an extrinsic tag. J. Clin. Invest. 51, 805–815.

Cook, J.D., 2005. Diagnosis and management of iron-deficiency anaemia. Best Pract. Res. Clin. Haematol. 18, 319–332.

Drakesmith, H., Nemeth, E., Ganz, T., 2015. Ironing out ferroportin. Cell Metab. 22, 777–787.

FFI, 2016. Food Fortification Initiative. (Online). Atlanta. Available: http://www.ffinetwork.org/index.html.

Fomon, S., 2001. Infant feeding in the 20th century: formula and beikost. J. Nutr. 131, 409S–420S.

Frazer, D.M., Anderson, G.J., 2014. The regulation of iron transport. Biofactors 40, 206–214.

Galan, P., Yoon, H.C., Preziosi, P., Viteri, F., Valeix, P., Fieux, B., Briancon, S., Malvy, D., Roussel, A.M., Favier, A., Hercberg, S., 1998. Determining factors in the iron status of adult women in the SU.VI.MAX study. SUpplementation en VItamines et Mineraux AntioXydants. Eur. J. Clin. Nutr. 52, 383–388.

Gera, T., Sachdev, H.S., Boy, E., 2012. Effect of iron-fortified foods on hematologic and biological outcomes: systematic review of randomized controlled trials. Am. J. Clin. Nutr. 96.

Gibson, R.S., Heath, A.L., Szymlek-Gay, E.A., 2014. Is iron and zinc nutrition a concern for vegetarian infants and young children in industrialized countries? Am. J. Clin. Nutr. 100 (Suppl. 1), 459s–468s.

Haas, J.D., Brownlie, T.T., 2001. Iron deficiency and reduced work capacity: a critical review of the research to determine a causal relationship. J. Nutr. 131, 676S–688S discussion 688S–690S.

Hallberg, L., Rossander, L., 1982. Absorption of iron from Western-type lunch and dinner meals. Am. J. Clin. Nutr. 35, 502–509.

Hallberg, L., Rossander-Hultén, L., 1991. Iron requirements in menstruating women. Am. J. Clin. Nutr. 54, 1047–1058.

Hallberg, L., Brune, M., Erlandsson, M., Sandberg, A.S., Rossander-Hulten, L., 1991. Calcium: effect of different amounts on nonheme- and heme-iron absorption in humans. Am. J. Clin. Nutr. 53, 112–119.

Heath, A.L., Skeaff, C.M., Williams, S., Gibson, R.S., 2001. The role of blood loss and diet in the aetiology of mild iron deficiency in premenopausal adult New Zealand women. Public Health Nutr. 4, 197–206.

Hunt, J.R., 2002. Moving toward a plant-based diet: are iron and zinc at risk? Nutr. Rev. 60, 127–134.

Hurrell, R., Egli, I., 2010. Iron bioavailability and dietary reference values. Am. J. Clin. Nutr. 91, 1461S–1467S.

Hurrell, R.F., Reddy, M.B., Juillerat, M.A., Cook, J.D., 2003. Degradation of phytic acid in cereal porridges improves iron absorption by human subjects. Am. J. Clin. Nutr. 77, 1213–1219.

Hurrell, R.F., 2002. Fortification: overcoming technical and practical barriers. J. Nutr. 132, 806S–812S.

Institute of Medicine, 2001. Iron. In: (US), N. A. P. (Ed.), Dietary Reference Intakes for Vitamin A, Vitamin K, Arsenic, Boron, Chromium, Copper, Iodine, Iron, Manganese, Molybdenum, Nickel, Silicon, Vanadium, and Zinc Washington, DC.

Jaeggi, T., Moretti, D., Kvalsvig, J., Holding, P.A., Tjalsma, H., Kortman, G.A., Joosten, I., Mwangi, A., Zimmermann, M.B., 2013. Iron status and systemic inflammation, but not gut inflammation, strongly predict gender-specific concentrations of serum hepcidin in infants in rural Kenya. PLoS One 8, e57513.

Kassebaum, N.J., Jasrasaria, R., Naghavi, M., Wulf, S.K., Johns, N., Lozano, R., Regan, M., Weatherall, D., Chou, D.P., Eisele, T.P., Flaxman, S.R., Pullan, R.L., Brooker, S.J., Murray, C.J., 2014. A systematic analysis of global anemia burden from 1990 to 2010. Blood 123, 615–624.

Koreissi-Dembele, Y., Fanou-Fogny, N., Moretti, D., Schuth, S., Dossa, R.A., Egli, I., Zimmermann, M.B., Brouwer, I.D., 2013. Dephytinisation with intrinsic wheat phytase and iron fortification significantly increase iron absorption from fonio (*Digitaria exilis*) meals in West African women. PLoS One 8, e70613.

Larsson, C.L., Johansson, G.K., 2002. Dietary intake and nutritional status of young vegans and omnivores in Sweden. Am. J. Clin. Nutr. 76, 100–106.

Leonard, A.J., Chalmers, K.A., Collins, C.E., Patterson, A.J., 2014. The effect of nutrition knowledge and dietary iron intake on iron status in young women. Appetite 81, 225–231.

Lyle, R.M., Weaver, C.M., Sedlock, D.A., Rajaram, S., Martin, B., Melby, C.L., 1992. Iron status in exercising women: the effect of oral iron therapy vs increased consumption of muscle foods. Am. J. Clin. Nutr. 56, 1049–1055.

Lynch, S.R., Hurrell, R.F., Dassenko, S.A., Cook, J.D., 1989. The effect of dietary proteins on iron bioavailability in man. Adv. Exp. Med. Biol. 249, 117–132.

Lynch, S.R., 2000. The effect of calcium on iron absorption. Nutr. Res. Rev. 13, 141–158.

Lynch, S., 2011a. Case studies: iron. Am. J. Clin. Nutr. 94, 673s–678s.

Lynch, S.R., 2011b. Why nutritional iron deficiency persists as a worldwide problem. J. Nutr. 141, 763s–768s.

Masuda, H., Kobayashi, T., Ishimaru, Y., Takahashi, M., Aung, M.S., Nakanishi, H., Mori, S., Nishizawa, N.K., 2013. Iron-biofortification in rice by the introduction of three barley genes participated in mugineic acid biosynthesis with soybean ferritin gene. Front. Plant Sci. 4, 132.

Monsen, E.R., Hallberg, L., Layrisse, M., Hegsted, D.M., Cook, J.D., Mertz, W., Finch, C.A., 1978. Estimation of available dietary iron. Am. J. Clin. Nutr. 31, 134–141.

Moretti, D., Zimmermann, M.B., Wegmuller, R., Walczyk, T., Zeder, C., Hurrell, R.F., 2006. Iron status and food matrix strongly affect the relative bioavailability of ferric pyrophosphate in humans. Am. J. Clin. Nutr. 83, 632–638.

Muckenthaler, M.U., Galy, B., Hentze, M.W., 2008. Systemic iron homeostasis and the iron-responsive element/iron-regulatory protein (IRE/IRP) regulatory network. Annu. Rev. Nutr. 28, 197–213.

Nestel, P., Bouis, H.E., Meenakshi, J.V., Pfeiffer, W., 2006. Biofortification of staple food crops. J. Nutr. 136, 1064–1067.

Peneau, S., Dauchet, L., Vergnaud, A.C., Estaquio, C., Kesse-Guyot, E., Bertrais, S., Latino-Martel, P., Hercberg, S., Galan, P., 2008. Relationship between iron status and dietary fruit and vegetables based on their vitamin C and fiber content. Am. J. Clin. Nutr. 87, 1298–1305.

Petry, N., Egli, I., Zeder, C., Walczyk, T., Hurrell, R., 2010. Polyphenols and phytic acid contribute to the low iron bioavailability from common beans in young women. J. Nutr. 140, 1977–1982.

Petry, N., Egli, I., Campion, B., Nielsen, E., Hurrell, R., 2013. Genetic reduction of phytate in common bean (*Phaseolus vulgaris* L.) seeds increases iron absorption in young women. J. Nutr. 143, 1219–1224.

Petry, N., Boy, E., Wirth, J.P., Hurrell, R.F., 2015. Review: the potential of the common bean (*Phaseolus vulgaris*) as a vehicle for iron biofortification. Nutrients 7, 1144–1173.

Plessow, R., Arora, N.K., Brunner, B., Tzogiou, C., Eichler, K., Brugger, U., Wieser, S., 2015. Social costs of iron deficiency anemia in 6-59-month-old children in India. PLoS One 10, e0136581.

Pynaert, I., De Bacquer, D., Matthys, C., Delanghe, J., Temmerman, M., De Backer, G., De Henauw, S., 2009. Determinants of ferritin and soluble transferrin receptors as iron status parameters in young adult women. Public Health Nutr. 12, 1775–1782.

Rigas, A.S., Sorensen, C.J., Pedersen, O.B., Petersen, M.S., Thorner, L.W., Kotze, S., Sorensen, E., Magnussen, K., Rostgaard, K., Erikstrup, C., Ullum, H., 2014. Predictors of iron levels in 14,737 Danish blood donors: results from the Danish Blood Donor Study. Transfusion 54, 789–796.

Teucher, B., Olivares, M., Cori, H., 2004. Enhancers of iron absorption: ascorbic acid and other organic acids. Int. J. Vitam. Nutr. Res. 74, 403–419.

Thane, C.W., Walmsley, C.M., Bates, C.J., Prentice, A., Cole, T.J., 2000. Risk factors for poor iron status in British toddlers: further analysis of data from the National Diet and Nutrition Survey of children aged 1.5–4.5 years. Public Health Nutr. 3, 433–440.

Thane, C.W., Bates, C.J., Prentice, A., 2003. Risk factors for low iron intake and poor iron status in a national sample of British young people aged 4–18 years. Public Health Nutr. 6, 485–496.

Thankachan, P., Walczyk, T., Muthayya, S., Kurpad, A.V., Hurrell, R.F., 2008. Iron absorption in young Indian women: the interaction of iron status with the influence of tea and ascorbic acid. Am. J. Clin. Nutr. 87, 881–886.

Troesch, B., Egli, I., Zeder, C., Hurrell, R.F., De Pee, S., Zimmermann, M.B., 2009. Optimization of a phytase-containing micronutrient powder with low amounts of highly bioavailable iron for in-home fortification of complementary foods. Am. J. Clin. Nutr. 89, 539–544.

Walczyk, T., Muthayya, S., Wegmuller, R., Thankachan, P., Sierksma, A., Frenken, L.G., Thomas, T., Kurpad, A., Hurrell, R.F., 2014. Inhibition of iron absorption by calcium is modest in an iron-fortified, casein- and whey-based drink in Indian children and is easily compensated for by addition of ascorbic acid. J. Nutr. 144, 1703–1709.

Waldmann, A., Koschizke, J.W., Leitzmann, C., Hahn, A., 2004. Dietary iron intake and iron status of German female vegans: results of the German vegan study. Ann. Nutr. Metab. 48, 103–108.

Wheby, M.S., 1970. Site of iron absorption in man. Scand. J. Haematol. 7, 56–62.

WHO, 2001. Iron Deficiency Anemia, Assessement, Prevention and Control: A Guide for Programme Managers. WHO, Geneva.

WHO, 2005. Vitamin and Mineral Requirements in Human Nutrition, second ed. Joint FAO/WHO Expert Consultation on Human Vitamin and Mineral Requirements.

WHO, 2008. In: De Benoist, B., Mclean, E., Egli, I., Cogswell, M. (Eds.), Worldwide Prevalence of Anaemia 1993–2005: WHO Global Database on Anaemia. WHO, Geneva.

Wirth, J., Poletti, S., Aeschlimann, B., Yakandawala, N., Drosse, B., Osorio, S., Tohge, T., Fernie, A.R., Gunther, D., Gruissem, W., Sautter, C., 2009. Rice endosperm iron biofortification by targeted and synergistic action of nicotianamine synthase and ferritin. Plant Biotechnol. J. 7, 631–644.

Zimmermann, M.B., Hurrell, R.F., 2007. Nutritional iron deficiency. Lancet 370, 511–520.

Zimmermann, M.B., Chaouki, N., Hurrell, R.F., 2005. Iron deficiency due to consumption of a habitual diet low in bioavailable iron: a longitudinal cohort study in Moroccan children. Am. J. Clin. Nutr. 81, 115–121.

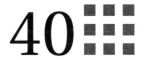
Plant-Based Diets and Selenium Intake and Status

Lutz Schomburg

CHARITÉ - UNIVERSITÄTSMEDIZIN BERLIN, BERLIN, GERMANY

1. Introduction

The mammalian organism needs selenium (Se) as an essential trace element for development, growth, and well-being. This has most convincingly been demonstrated already in the middle of the last century by the pioneering work of Schwarz and Foltz (1957). These researchers worked with rats on a vitamin E–deficient diet, and they showed that some minimal supply of Se (the so-called "Factor 3") was essential and sufficient to prevent vitamin E deficiency–dependent necrotic liver degeneration. Some years later, Leopold Flohé and colleagues identified the first eukaryotic Se-containing protein, the glutathione peroxidase (GPX) from bovine blood, and characterized its importance for the catalytic decomposition of peroxides, realizing that the active enzyme contains Se in stoichiometric amounts, i.e., it represents a true selenoenzyme (Flohé et al., 1973).

With the introduction of transgenic mouse models into basic research, it became possible to directly inactivate certain genes involved in Se metabolism, to address genes implicated in selenoprotein biosynthesis, or to directly delete selenoprotein encoding genes (Schweizer and Schomburg, 2005). These elegant techniques proved the original notion on the essentiality of Se for mammalian development, survival, and certain physiological processes. Deletion of the gene encoding the transfer RNA needed for selenoprotein biosynthesis (gene symbol *TRNAU1*) or of the gene encoding the GPX isozyme that specifically degrades phospholipid hydroperoxides (gene symbol *GPX4*) or of one of the two ubiquitously expressed thioredoxin reductases (gene symbol *TXNRD1*, *TXNRD2*) each caused a lethal phenotype in mice. Other mouse models highlighted the relevance of certain selenoproteins for tumorigenesis, cardiovascular diseases, fertility, brain development, the immune system, or other developmental and degenerative processes (Kasaikina et al., 2012).

2. Importance of Selenoproteins for Human Health

These pioneering experiments along with focused studies with animal models soon became supported by the identification of rare cases of inherited diseases in humans (Schweizer et al., 2011). These case reports highlight the different functions and roles of

Table 40.1   Inherited Defects in Genes Encoding Selenoproteins or Biosynthesis Factors According to (Schweizer et al., 2011)

Gene/Gene Product	Affected Pathway/Process	Phenotype/Symptom
SELN/selenoprotein N	Muscle/myogenesis	Muscular dystrophy
SECISBP2/SECIS binding protein 2	Selenoprotein biosynthesis	Growth impairment, infertility
SEPSECS/selenocysteine synthase	Selenoprotein biosynthesis	Progressive neuronal loss
TXNRD2/thioredoxin reductase 2	Mitochondrial redox control	Failure to thrive, hypoglycemia
TRNAU1/tRNA for selenocysteine	Selenoprotein biosynthesis	Fatigue, hypotonia, pain
GPX4/glutathione peroxidase 4	Arachidonate metabolism	Spondylometaphyseal dysplasia

selenoproteins in humans. Selenoprotein N (gene symbol *SELN*) is a muscle-specific protein. Mutations in *SELN* can cause a rare form of muscular dystrophy (Ferreiro et al., 2002). In 2005, the first subjects with an inherited defect in the biosynthesis machinery of selenoproteins were characterized (Dumitrescu et al., 2005). The phenotype was not lethal, but it was dependent on the remaining biological activity of the mutated gene product. In contrast, a very severe cause of brain atrophy was identified in 2010 and linked to mutations in the gene encoding the selenocysteine synthase gene (gene symbol *SEPSECS*). The affected children develop a progressive loss of brain tissue and neuronal mass, and they have a poor prognosis (Agamy et al., 2010). The strong brain phenotype is reminiscent of selected cases of children with Se-dependent epilepsy and seizures (Ramaekers et al., 1994). Notably, dietary Se supplements were able to improve the health and reduce the symptoms of the children. Recently, mutations in the mitochondrial thioredoxin reductase gene (gene symbol *TXNRD2*) have been identified as responsible for a form of familial glucocorticoid deficiency, characterized by a failure to thrive, hyperpigmentation, high infection rate, hypoglycemia, and neurological symptoms (Prasad et al., 2014). Finally, children with mutations in the gene encoding the selenocysteine tRNA (gene symbol *TRNAU1*) display a spectrum of symptoms, including fatigue, abdominal pain, hypotonia, and low Se concentrations in blood (Schoenmakers et al., 2016).

Collectively, these rare diseases observed in human patients support the conviction that life without Se is not possible and that the personal genotype in selenoprotein genes along with the daily Se intake are important modulators of growth and development, as well as impacting mood, disease risks, aging, and overall quality of life (Table 40.1).

3. Selenium Metabolism and Selenium Transport in Humans

The average daily intake of Se differs around the world (Table 40.2), both in the sheer quantity and partly also in the chemical form of the selenocompounds consumed (Rayman, 2008). This is mainly due to the food choice, soil quality, food availability, and eating habits. However, the range of daily Se intake between different populations is restricted within a certain limit that roughly indicates the thresholds defining deficiency risk and potentially toxic doses. In China, where both very low and very high intakes coexist, minimal levels of around 7 or 14 μg/day are

Table 40.2   Average Se Intake per Person per Day in Different Countries (According to Rayman, 2008)

Country	Se Intake (µg/day)
Australia	57–87
Brazil	28–37
Canada	98–224
China	7–4990
France	29–43
Germany	35
India	27–48
Japan	104–199
Saudi Arabia	15
Switzerland	70
United Kingdom	29–39
United States	106
Venezuela	200–350

reported from the Se-deficient area in the Sichuan Province (Xia et al., 2010), while maximal intakes are reported from the Se-rich area around Enshi, where average daily supplies add up to >500 µg Se (Huang et al., 2013). The reference values in Europe are in between these extremes, and the recommendation in Germany is currently given at about 50–75 µg Se/day for adults (Kipp et al., 2015). The European Food Safety Authority (EFSA) issued in 2014 a "Scientific Opinion on Dietary Reference Values for Selenium" and suggested an adequate daily intake of 15 µg/day for children (1–3 years of age), 70 µg/day for adolescents, and higher intakes in adults (up to 85 µg/day), especially during pregnancy, lactation, or in face of increased health risks (EFSA Journal 2014 12 (10), 3846). The recommendations of the Food and Nutrition Board of the US Institute of Medicine are slightly lower, but do in general conform with these recommendations, according to which 99% of US participants in the third National Health and Nutrition Examination Survey (NHANES III) meet these adequate daily intakes.

In general, all the major selenocompounds in the human diet are well absorbed in the gastrointestinal tract (Fairweather-Tait et al., 2010), with selenomethionine (SeMet) probably showing the most efficient uptake (Thomson et al., 1993). It can be assumed that the current Se status may affect uptake efficiencies of selenocompounds, even though this has formally not been proven, yet. One experimental finding supporting this notion has been obtained in bone Se metabolism, where Se-deficient mice showed an increased expression of the Se uptake receptors in Se deficiency (Pietschmann et al., 2014). The Se-containing amino acids SeMet and selenocysteine (SeCys) are taken up by respective amino acid or peptide transporters. Selenate $\left(SeO_4{}^{2-}\right)$ is mainly transported, like sulfate, by a sodium cotransporter (Wolffram et al., 1988), whereas selenite $\left(SeO_3{}^{2-}\right)$ may be accumulated from the intestinal lumen by sulfate transporters. The passage of the different Se forms from the intestine to liver is only poorly characterized. Liver is the central organ for taking up Se from the diet and for converting it into selenoproteins (Suzuki and Ogra, 2002). There are a number of intracellular selenoproteins in hepatocytes, some of which are highly expressed, e.g., GPX1. However, in terms of Se status, the most important hepatic seleno-protein for Se transport and storage is selenoprotein P (SePP, gene symbol *SEPP1*) (Burk and Hill, 2009). The biosynthesis of SePP is stringently regulated by the available Se pool in hepatocytes. Increased dietary intakes result in increased hepatic SePP biosynthesis and secretion. Likely as a safeguard mechanism to limit Se transport within physiological tolerable limits, SePP biosynthesis reaches a maximal expression level once a sufficiently high saturating Se intake level has been reached (Xia et al., 2010).

Consequently, the SePP concentrations in blood are used as a useful biomarker of Se intake, Se status, and Se transport (Hurst et al., 2010). According to this biomarker, a replete Se status is reached when no further increase in circulating SePP concentrations can be observed despite an increasing nutritional or supplemental intake. Conversely, a Se defi-cit is defined as a state in which SePP biosynthesis and circulating SePP concentrations have not been sufficiently saturated yet and the maximal possible level of serum SePP con-centrations have not yet been reached due to limiting Se availability in hepatocytes. The maximal expression level of the second actively secreted selenoprotein, i.e., GPX3 from the kidneys, is reached at lower Se intake levels than are needed for maximal expression of SePP; hence SePP is considered the more meaningful biomarker (Xia et al., 2010). An average daily intake resulting in circulating Se concentrations of around 70 µg/L would be required for saturating GPX3 expression, while Se concentrations of around 125 µg/L are needed in plasma for a full saturation of SePP expression (Hurst et al., 2010). Target cells for SePP-dependent Se uptake are found in the brain, kidney, muscle, bone, etc. These cells are characterized by lipoprotein receptor–related receptors (LRP). Megalin (gene symbol *LRP2*) was identified as the first SePP receptor in kidney, recognizing SePP in the primary filtrate and likely involved in SePP reuptake to limit Se loss via urinary SePP excre-tion (Olson et al., 2008). Impaired megalin expression is thus associated with a declining Se status (Chiu-Ugalde et al., 2010).

Besides megalin, a second receptor capable of SePP uptake has been identified in the central nervous system, muscle, and in testes, i.e., apolipoprotein E receptor 2 (gene sym-bol *APOER2* or *LRP8*) (Olson et al., 2007). Notably, the phenotype of *ApoER2* knockout mice strongly resembles the one known from SePP-knockout mice, including central nervous defects and low Se status. These findings improve our understanding of the Se transport function of SePP from liver to target tissues, and they highlight that a targeted receptor-mediated uptake of SePP at the site of requirement underlies a preferential supply of Se to certain target tissues and contributes to a selective retention of Se in times of poor supply (Schomburg et al., 2004). Notably, this concept of a hierarchical distribution of dietary Se to those organs most dependent on a sufficiently high Se status is well established in Se biology.

The excretion of Se from the human organism is not fully characterized yet. Some Se inevitably gets lost via cells and blood loss through the fecal excretion, which appears not to constitute a regulated process; a more controlled loss is taking place via the urine in form of selenosugars (Kobayashi et al., 2002). Upon very high or toxic intakes, Se may also become excreted in poorly regulated ways, exhaled in the form of dimethyl-selenide (causing an unpleasant odor) or in soluble charged form in urine as trimethyl-selenonium ions (Suzuki et al., 2005). In general, excretion increases with increasing Se intake, as can be expected from a biologically active micronutrient. However, the relative retention rates differ, with deficient subjects retaining relatively more of the valuable trace element as compared to well-supplied subjects. And moreover, some particular differences between women and men are described (Combs et al., 2011). The underlying molecular mechanisms safeguarding the Se status in a tissue-specific way are partially characterized as the important aim of the hierarchical principles governing Se transport and storage in relation to its current availability, and this well-controlled distribution system is centrally dependent on the preferential uptake of SePP into Se-sensitive target tissues (see later) (Schomburg and Schweizer, 2009).

4. Biomarkers of Selenium Status

The "Se status" is a term that is intuitively well understood but still lacks a precise biochemical definition. In principle, whole body Se content, or even better, whole body Se concentration per body weight or volume and Se availability to the tissues in need, would probably best correspond to the real meaning of Se status. As this parameter is difficult to be determined from living subjects, surrogate biomarkers are needed. A useful biomarker should reliably reflect the corresponding parameter in question. In case of Se status, measuring the Se content per volume or weight unit of a biosample fulfills this requirement. Considering the choice of human biosamples available for analysis, hair or nail clippings, tissue biopsies as well as blood cells, full blood and serum, or plasma samples are available, with the latter two being most widely used in clinical research and routine diagnostics (Fig. 40.1).

Tissue biopsies pose ethical concerns as their acquirement involves a potentially harmful and stressful invasive procedure. Hair and nail may be well suited; however, there are problems with reproducibility, standards for normalization, and cosmetic manipulations by shampoo or nail polish that may interfere with reliable quantitative trace element analyses. Measurements from blood cells or serum and plasma are the most common procedures for assessing biomarkers of Se status (Combs, 2015). The ideal biomarker should correlate to the Se intake over a wide concentration range. The determination of total Se itself from blood, serum, or plasma represents a valid and useful reference, for an increasing intake should nicely be reflected in increasing circulating concentrations of Se. Accordingly, in the majority of human studies, total Se in blood, serum, or plasma is analyzed and used as marker of Se status when trying to elucidate its importance for health issues. However, total Se measurements reflect a mixture of components and not a precise and specific selenocompound (Combs, 2015). For this reason, single selenoproteins may offer an advantage, as their expression can be precisely determined by enzymatic, immunological, or other analytical techniques (Xia et al., 2010).

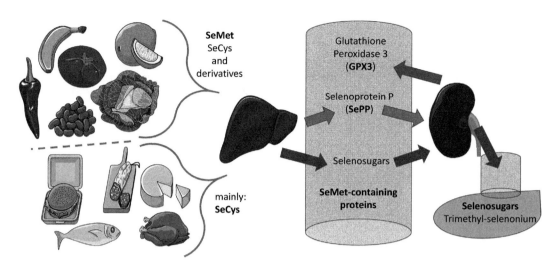

FIGURE 40.1 Overview on Se intake and metabolism in humans. The dietary-derived Se in human nutrition mainly derives from solid food items, and not from drinks. Selenomethionine (SeMet), some selenocysteine (SeCys), and different derivatives of these Se-containing amino acids are the major selenocompounds in plants and plant parts. In contrast, animal-derived nutrients mainly contain SeCys as part of selenoproteins and a variable amount of SeMet-containing proteins and smaller selenocompounds. The liver is the first target for organification of dietary Se, converting the trace element in SeCys-containing selenoproteins, especially selenoprotein P (SePP), to serve as transporter of Se to the other tissues. Besides, some selenosugars as excretory products are synthesized for urinary secretion via the kidney. SePP has also been shown to supply the kidney with Se for the biosynthesis of the circulating glutathione peroxidase 3 (GPX3). SeMet from nutrition can directly be incorporated into newly synthesized proteins; hence, depending on SeMet intake in comparison to Met intake and basal Se status, a considerable fraction of circulating Se-containing proteins harbor SeMet at random positions instead of Met, contributing to the total fraction of circulating Se-containing proteins. Collectively, the total Se concentration in blood, serum, or plasma, consisting of SePP, GPX3, SeMet-containing proteins, and some smaller selenocompounds, is used as a surrogate marker for whole body Se status, as blood is generally well available both for clinical diagnostics as well as for clinical research. Illustration generated with help of Servier Medical Art (Les Laboratoires Servier, Normandy, France).

Among the different selenoproteins, the isozymes of the glutathione peroxidase (GPX) family can reliably be quantified by a coupled enzymatic optic test procedure, both from blood cells and from serum or plasma (Gunzler et al., 1974). However, enzymatic test results stringently depend on the quality of the enzyme source, i.e., on the treatment of the sample prior to analysis. Especially in epidemiological research, serum or plasma samples often have a certain preanalytical history with two or more rounds of freezing and thawing in the process of obtaining the blood samples and aliquoting. Moreover, the time of storage at room temperature often is only poorly controlled and standardized. This may lead to different degrees of proteolysis, hamper a reliable enzymatic determination, and render quantitative comparisons across studies by enzymatic tests almost impossible.

Hence, immunological methods may be a better choice. And in comparison to full blood or blood cells, serum and plasma samples are more stable and most widely used for epidemiological research and clinical diagnostics. There are only two selenoproteins being soluble in blood and becoming actively secreted into the circulation, i.e., GPX3, mainly derived from kidney, and SePP, mainly derived from liver (Burk and Hill, 2015). Animal experiments have shown that renal GPX3 biosynthesis relies on SePP-mediated Se transport from liver to kidney, and thus it depends on SePP for full expression (Renko et al., 2008). These findings argue for measuring SePP instead of GPX3 from serum as the primary and functional biomarker of Se status. This conclusion is further supported by respective supplementation trials in which SePP responded over a larger intake range to the supplemented Se than GPX3 (Xia et al., 2010; Hurst et al., 2010). Moreover, SePP is known to carry up to 10 selenocysteine residues per protein, thereby accounting for the majority of Se in serum and plasma (Persson-Moschos et al., 1995), even in severe disease (Forceville et al., 2009). And finally, the differential dependence of the Se biomarkers including GPX3, SePP, and total serum Se on the Se intake and a sufficiently high Se status was impressively reflected when comparing German omnivores, ovolactovegetarians, and vegans; SePP turned out as the most sensitive parameter suitable for identifying a Se deficit in subjects expressing similar GPX3 activity levels (Hoeflich et al., 2010). In this comparison, both ovolactovegetarians and vegans showed relatively low Se concentrations (Hoeflich et al., 2010). Similarly, in the large European Prospective Investigation into Cancer and Nutrition–Oxford (EPIC) study, the prevalence of insufficient Se intake was two to four times higher in both ovolactovegetarians and vegans as compared to meat or fish eaters (Sobiecki et al., 2016). These findings highlight that, despite the additional Se in milk and eggs, even the ovolactovegetarian diet is usually not sufficient to cover the recommended daily Se intakes.

5. Selenium Content in Food Items

Most contemporary humans consume both plant- and animal-derived food items; yet, an increasing number of subjects is deciding to avoid animal-derived products for reasons of religion, ethics, health, responsibility for the environment, and because of a high respect for living creatures. The specific health impact of different plant-based diets in the large spectrum from low-meat eaters, semivegetarians, ovolactovegetarians, and vegans is a matter of scientific debate, as the readers can appreciate from the other sections and chapters in this book.

Fish and animal products are generally rich sources of Se (Sigrist et al., 2012). This finding is based on two major reasons. First, Se tends to naturally drain from soil into the sea where it is taken up by biological material and accumulates along the food chain, causing fish to contain significant amounts of Se. Second, farm animals normally receive supportive vitamins and trace elements to avoid deficiencies and improve their overall growth, health, fertility, and meat quality. This measure of agricultural fortification ensures relatively high Se concentrations in meat, eggs, milk, and other animal-derived products (Table 40.3). Consequently, human subjects consuming animal-derived food items do not normally develop substantial Se deficiencies. But many contemporary humans do live by choice, religion, or for reasons of availability on a mainly or solely plant-dominated food basis.

Table 40.3 Average Se Content of Selected Animal- and Plant-Based Nutrients (According to Mehdi et al., 2013; Tinggi, 2003; Fairweather-Tait et al., 2010)

Food Item	Se Content (µg/kg)
Cereal (FM)	10–310
White rice (FM)	50–80
Pasta (FM)	10–100
Bread (FM)	60–150
Onions (DM)	<500
Lentils (DM)	240–360
Potatoes (DM)	120
Chicken (FM)	81–142
Pork (FM)	32–198
Crustaceans (DM)	360–1330
Cod (DM)	1500
Tuna (DM)	5600

DM, dry matter; *FM*, fresh matter.

6. Selenium Status of Ovolactovegetarians and Vegans

In comparison to omnivores consuming animal-derived food items that are produced under fortified agricultural production conditions, the Se supply of ovolactovegetarians and vegans is less well predictable and more variable. In general, both undernourished subjects as well as vegans and ovolactovegetarians are at greater risk for micronutrient deficiencies (Kristensen et al., 2015). Plants do not stringently depend on Se for growth, development, and survival, making most plants relatively independent from Se status in soil. This characteristic complicates the assessment of the nutritional value of a certain plant with respect to its Se content. Nevertheless, within the plant kingdom, there are nonaccumulator, Se-accumulator, and Se-indicator plant species that are capable of growing Se independently or on highly seleniferous soils and that may even be used for phytoremediation by accumulation and volatilization of Se (Banuelos et al., 1997). This implies that plants are in general suitable sources of the essential trace element Se in the human diet, given that sufficient Se is supplied during plant growth in a bioavailable form. And indeed, several attempts are currently under way trying to increase Se content in eatable plants by classic breeding and selection, foliar Se spraying, or increasing the Se in soil by enriched fertilizers or even via genetic manipulation of plant species to increase Se uptake and content (Brown and Shrift, 1982; Zhu et al., 2009).

However, at present the consumer is unaware of the Se content of a certain plant-derived dietary component. Even worse, the Se content of the same plant can vary considerably, e.g., as shown in the potentially Se-rich Brazil nuts that may vary in terms of Se concentration from 0.03 µg/g to 512 µg/g (Chang et al., 1995). A vegetarian subject may indeed cover his/her Se requirement by the consumption of a fraction of a single Brazil nut (0.1 g), or the Brazil nuts would practically be a null contributor to Se intake. Similarly, rice or wheat Se concentrations

Table 40.4 Comparison of Selenium Intake (µg/day) or Selenium Status (µg/L or µM) in Vegetarians Including Vegans as Compared to Omnivores From the Same Population

Country, Year	Vegetarians	Omnivores	References
United States, 1983	96–104 µg/L	69–112 µg/L	Shultz and Leklem (1983)
Finland, 1995	27 µg/day	73 µg/day	Rauma et al. (1995)
Sweden, 1985	0.80 ± 0.18 µM (63.2 ± 14.2 µg/L)	0.98 ± 0.15 µM (77.4 ± 11.8 µg/L)	Akesson and Ockerman (1985)
Slovakia, 1995	48.3 ± 1.2 µg/L	57.8 ± 1.4 µg/L	Kadrabova et al. (1995)
Sweden, 2002	10–12 µg/day	27–40 µg/day	Larsson and Johansson (2002)
Brazil, 2009	73.5–77.3 µg/L	–	de Bortoli and Cozzolino (2009)
Germany, 2010	68–81 µg/L	91–94 µg/L	Hoeflich et al. (2010)
Denmark, 2015	25–33 µg/day	39–52 µg/day	Kristensen et al. (2015)
Finland, 2016	79 ± 65 µg/day 1.1 µM (86.9 µg/L)	149 ± 108 µg/day 1.5 µM (118.4 µg/L)	Elorinne et al. (2016)

differ grossly depending on their production site; e.g., wheat Se concentrations vary from as low as a few ng/g when produced in Scandinavia to as high as almost 1 µg/g when produced in Canada (Zhu et al., 2009). Consequently, the Se intake and the status of vegans and ovolactovegetarians may differ considerably from omnivores, especially in those areas where soil Se is low, mainly regional food is consumed, and no supplementation of fertilizers is in place (Table 40.4).

As clearly depicted in Table 40.4, the differences in Se concentrations of vegans, ovolactovegetarians, and omnivores depend on the region of residency. Notably, the very poor Se status of Finnish vegetarians of 27 µg/day only (Rauma et al., 1995) has improved impressively over the recent decades to a current intake of around 79 µg/day (Elorinne et al., 2016); this increase can be attributed to the consequent and systematic supplementation of fertilizers in Finland with selenate, as a safe and very meaningful way of increasing the daily Se intake in a population formerly known to be severely Se deficient (Aro et al., 1995).

These examples nicely highlight the problem ovolactovegetarians and vegans are facing; the Se concentration of plants or plant-derived products varies in an unpredictable manner, as plants do not need Se as an essential micronutrient and thereby do not actively control their Se concentrations within a tight range as animals do, but nevertheless they are capable of accumulating very high Se concentrations, depending on soil quality, Se availability, and plant species or genotype. This is in sharp contrast to animal-derived nutrients, as animals need a certain minimal supply of Se as an essential micronutrient in order not to develop deficiency symptoms, and they are thus a more predictable and uniform source of Se in a quantity comparable to the human need. Se concentrations in human serum, which mirror tissue Se concentrations to a certain degree, may range from a minimal value of around 20 µg/L to a maximal value of around 400 µg/L, i.e., display an interindividual difference of maximal 20-fold. Farm animals, meat, milk, eggs, etc., from controlled agricultural production tend to even contain a more constant and higher Se content, thereby providing a guaranteed Se supply in a concentration range that is likely nontoxic, as too high a concentration would have already harmed the animal. For all of these reasons, vegans and obviously also ovolactovegetarians are at risk of Se deficiency, as reported in several clinical studies (Elorinne et al., 2016; Letsiou et al., 2009; Hoeflich et al., 2010; Kadrabova et al., 1995).

The question thus emerges on how a vegetarian subject can safely and reliably obtain a sufficiently high Se supply to avoid Se deficiency, which clearly constitutes a health risk. The most straightforward strategy would be to consume well-defined dietary supplements containing a specified amount of Se either as SeMet, selenite, or Se-rich yeast preparations (Fagan et al., 2015). Hereby, a reliable and steady supply can be ensured at reasonable costs. However, the supplier should be chosen wisely, as there have been cases of misformulation of Se-containing supplements, containing even up to >100-fold the stated Se content, causing overt endemic selenosis with hair and nail loss as well as other systemic and neurological symptoms (Morris and Crane, 2013).

An alternative approach would be to select foods presumably rich in Se. Here, as mentioned earlier, the geographic origin may help in identifying foods with likely high Se content, however, without guarantee as the specific soil the plant has been grown in together with a number of plant-specific and biogeochemical characteristics determine the ultimate Se concentration in plants. South American Brazil nuts or paranuts may be a good choice as their Se content can be relatively high, but they may also be very low, as mentioned earlier (Chang et al., 1995). An alternative choice would be nutrients derived from areas with naturally high soil Se concentrations, e.g., from North, Middle, or South America, from the Se-rich areas in China, or from along the coastlines as these areas often profit from Se-rich rainfalls if the clouds had passed over ocean areas containing increased biomass highly active in Se volatilization (Winkel et al., 2015).

But again, without a prior analysis and a specified information about the specific Se content of such foods, there is no guarantee on the Se contents. Another potentially Se-rich dietary source would be marine plants and algae (Bottino et al., 1984) or seagrass (Baldwin et al., 1996); however a systematic analysis of these marine products is missing. Finally, Se supplementation of soil, fertilizers, or by foliar spraying may constitute an effective and straightforward way for increasing the Se content of plants in culture. The authorities in Finland together with Finish researchers were the first to decide on a nationwide supplementation effort for increasing the low Se content of their food products by a systematic measure in adding selenite to all mineral fertilizers used in Finland. Hereby, Se intake could be successfully increased in the Finish population from a level being among the lowest in Europe in the 1980s to a daily intake in the recommended range of around 80 µg/day (Alfthan et al., 2015). It is hoped that other countries are learning from this safe, highly desirable, and successful Finish experience, including the most developed countries in Europe.

In the meantime, a number of attempts are ongoing trying to specify the most efficient ways of increasing Se content of plants by breeding and selection, supplementation, or genetic manipulations (Lyons et al., 2004). Certain Se-enriched plants are already available in different parts of the world, especially in China (Wu et al., 2015b) or the United

States (Banuelos and Hanson, 2010), and they have reached a developmental stage close to regular commercial distribution. It can thus be safely assumed that in the very near future, Se-enriched nutrients with specified Se concentrations will become commercially available as a safe, cost-effective, and reliable source of this precious micronutrient.

7. Health Risks of Insufficient Se Intake

Mammals depend on nutritional Se intake mainly for one reason, i.e., for the biosynthesis of selenocysteine-containing selenoproteins. There are 25 genes encoding selenoproteins in humans, some of which have been proven essential for development as observed in respective mouse models with genetic deletion (so-called knockout mice) (Moustafa et al., 2003). Using this strategy, the genes encoding the tRNA (*Trsp*) specifying selenocysteine incorporation into selenoproteins, the two thioredoxin reductases (*Txnrd1, -2*), and the phospholipid hydroperoxide glutathione peroxidase (*Gpx4*) proved to be essential for mammalian development and life (Conrad and Schweizer, 2010).

But besides such a drastic phenotype as developmental failure or premature death, Se deficiency in humans is rather linked to no obvious phenotype but an increased disease predisposition for a number of widespread human diseases. A large body of evidence links a subclinical Se deficit to an increased risk of cancer at several sites (Combs, 2005). Highly significant interactions of Se intake and cancer risk have been obtained for lung, colon, and prostate cancer, in a large randomized controlled supplementation trial (Clark et al., 1996). Notably, the interaction was most significant in those participants who entered into the supplementation trial with lowest baseline Se status (Duffield-Lillico et al., 2002). This notion also likely explains why the large follow-up study failed to replicate the chemopreventive effect of Se supplementation on prostate cancer risk (Lippman et al., 2009). Because of the overwhelming positive findings in the seminal NPC study, there was obviously a trend for an increased Se intake among the US participants of the follow-up trial, resulting in a study population with relatively high baseline Se status, unresponsive to further Se intake (Hatfield and Gladyshev, 2009; Schrauzer, 2009). This is unfortunate, as the study was sufficiently powered, well designed, and sufficiently funded to study the effects of Se supplementation over a time period of 7 years. Now, the negative results from this study on a chemopreventive effect of Se supplementation dominate respective meta-analyses and hinders the attempts to conduct similar supplementation studies in populations with lower baseline Se status, e.g., in the European Union. Here, recent research focuses on observational studies, e.g., associating polymorphisms in selenoprotein genes with increased cancer risks (Meplan and Hesketh, 2014), or associating low serum Se concentrations in healthy subjects with increased cancer incidences in the next decades of life (Hughes et al., 2015).

Besides cancer, also the infectious and inflammatory diseases are closely related to Se status, as a Se deficit increases infection risks and disease progression (Stone et al., 2010), and in turn, infections and inflammation negatively affect Se status in blood and tissues (Nichol et al., 1998; Renko et al., 2009). Even more striking, the mortality risk in different infectious diseases appears to correlate to Se deficiency, as observed in HIV-infected subjects (Baum et al., 1997), in critical disease (Angstwurm et al., 2007), and sepsis (Forceville et al., 1998). Accordingly, Se supplementation trials have been conducted on the intensive care units, with some very positive findings and some null results, collectively yielding an ambiguous picture (Allingstrup and Afshari, 2015). A similar inconclusive situation is given for autoimmune diseases and Se status or Se supplementation. Several trials have reported on positive effects of supplemental Se, especially in autoimmune thyroid disease of the Hashimoto (Toulis et al., 2010) or Graves disease type (Marcocci et al., 2011). However, taking into account all of the published studies, the full picture is rather ambiguous in nature as a number of well-controlled supplementation trials did not observe any positive effects on the thyroid gland or the autoimmune disease parameters (Schomburg, 2012). Despite this inconclusive situation with respect to Se supplementation as an intervention strategy, avoiding a Se deficit has consistently proven as a beneficial health measure for reducing autoimmune thyroid disease risks and other health threats. This has convincingly been shown with respect to goiter development (Derumeaux et al., 2003), thyroid nodules (Rasmussen et al., 2011), or thyroiditis (Wu et al., 2015a).

The interactions of Se status and cardiovascular diseases are less well understood, as both positive and beneficial associations and intervention studies contrast with null results or even negative supplementation effects (Alissa et al., 2003; Brigo et al., 2014; Benstoem et al., 2015). A similar inconclusive picture is given when analyzing the published data concerning Se status, Se supplementation effects, and risk of diabetes mellitus (Bleys et al., 2007; Ogawa-Wong et al., 2016; Rayman and Stranges, 2013; Steinbrenner et al., 2011). Collectively, the studies indicate that there might be an upper limit of Se intake until which an increasing Se supply is rather health promoting, while by surpassing this threshold the effect may be the contrary, and health problems become induced, i.e., the general Se intake and the risk for common diseases display a U-curved interaction (Rayman, 2012).

8. Conclusions

Plants and mammals differ in their relation and dependence to the trace element Se. While the Se concentrations in plants, depending on species, genotype, and supporting soil, may vary over several orders of magnitude, mammals tend to maintain a rather well-controlled and specific Se status, to ensure a sufficiently high rate of biosynthesis of essential selenoproteins while trying to avoid surplus intake eventually causing increased health risks and symptoms of selenosis. For this reason, it is not possible to predict the Se status of a given plant food, while farm animals raised under some form of controlled agricultural production strategy tend to display a Se concentration that is restricted within a limited and predictable range, thereby constituting rich sources of Se.

Consequently, it is challenging to cover the daily Se requirement by a vegetarian diet, as the right nutrients containing a sufficiently high Se content need to be identified and consumed in the necessary amount. South American paranuts and Brazil nuts are typical examples of potentially Se-rich nutrients, even though their Se content strongly depends on the soil used for their production and can thus not safely be predicted. There is a clear lack of labeling and control of these kind of potentially health-promoting nutrients, as the Se content of a single nut can range from a marginal to a potentially toxic source. For these reasons, a number of well-controlled and specified nutrients enriched in Se by different technologies are currently developed and are expected to become commercialized and widely available in the future. By now, suitable supplements containing the inorganic Se-compounds selenite or selenate or the amino acid SeMet or a mixture of selenocompounds as found in Se-enriched yeast constitute efficient supplements for avoiding a Se deficit, which would constitute a health risk for a large number of widespread human diseases.

In addition to trying to find foods rich in Se or suitable supplements, it will always be helpful to get an analysis of the personal Se status from a blood sample. Especially in challenging situations, such as pregnancy, lactation, chronic disease, or in face of infection risks because of traveling or work exposure, the organism will clearly profit from a sufficiently high Se status to strengthen the immune system and the antioxidative defense. On the other hand, too high a chronic Se intake may cause selenosis and disease symptoms; but this oversupply is hardly possible by regular nutrition alone, except for the areas with a history of endemic selenosis when the residents were living on locally produced food only, e.g., as in the Enshi region in China. Other reports on Se oversupply-dependent health risks are all from supplementation studies in populations already well supplied with Se, i.e., from the United States. These findings seem to be of little relevance for subjects residing in large parts of Europe, Africa, or Asia, as their environment must be considered as Se deficient, and beneficial health effects of supplemental Se intake are likely to be observed instead of adverse effects. Large-scale analyses on these notions are currently underway and will provide the necessary scientific database needed for a better understanding of the interaction of Se, Se intake and Se status, and personal health risks and potential health benefits. At present, aiming for a diet with sufficiently high Se content appears as a priority, especially for subjects choosing a purely or predominantly plant-based diet, which clearly increases the risk of an insufficient daily intake of Se.

References

Agamy, O., Ben Zeev, B., Lev, D., Marcus, B., Fine, D., Su, D., Narkis, G., Ofir, R., Hoffmann, C., Leshinsky-Silver, E., Flusser, H., Sivan, S., Soll, D., Lerman-Sagie, T., Birk, O.S., 2010. Mutations disrupting selenocysteine formation cause progressive cerebello-cerebral atrophy. Am. J. Hum. Genet. 87, 538–544.

Akesson, B., Ockerman, P.A., 1985. Selenium status in vegans and lactovegetarians. Br. J. Nutr. 53, 199–205.

Alfthan, G., Eurola, M., Ekholm, P., Venalainen, E.R., Root, T., Korkalainen, K., Hartikainen, H., Salminen, P., Hietaniemi, V., Aspila, P., Aro, A., Selenium Working Group, 2015. Effects of nationwide addition of selenium to fertilizers on foods, and animal and human health in Finland: from deficiency to optimal selenium status of the population. J. Trace Elem. Med. Biol. 31, 142–147.

Alissa, E.M., Bahijri, S.M., Ferns, G.A., 2003. The controversy surrounding selenium and cardiovascular disease: a review of the evidence. Med. Sci. Monit. 9, RA9–18.

Allingstrup, M., Afshari, A., 2015. Selenium supplementation for critically ill adults. Cochrane Database Syst. Rev. 7, CD003703.

Angstwurm, M.W., Engelmann, L., Zimmermann, T., Lehmann, C., Spes, C.H., Abel, P., Strauss, R., Meier-Hellmann, A., Insel, R., Radke, J., Schüttler, J., Gärtner, R., 2007. Selenium in Intensive Care (SIC): results of a prospective randomized, placebo-controlled, multiple-center study in patients with severe systemic inflammatory response syndrome, sepsis, and septic shock. Crit. Care Med. 35, 118–126.

Aro, A., Alfthan, G., Varo, P., 1995. Effects of supplementation of fertilizers on human selenium status in Finland. Analyst 120, 841–843.

Baldwin, S., Maher, W., Kleber, E., Krikowa, F., 1996. Selenium in marine organisms of seagrass habitats (*Posidonia australis*) of Jervis Bay, Australia. Mar. Pollut. Bull. 32, 310–316.

Banuelos, G.S., Hanson, B.D., 2010. Use of selenium-enriched mustard and canola seed meals as potential bioherbicides and green fertilizer in strawberry production. Hortscience 45, 1567–1572.

Banuelos, G.S., Ajwa, H.A., Mackey, B., Wu, L., Cook, C., Akohoue, S., Zambruzuski, S., 1997. Evaluation of different plant species used for phytoremediation of high soil selenium. J. Environ. Qual. 26, 639–646.

Baum, M.K., Shorposner, G., Lai, S.H., Zhang, G.Y., Fletcher, M.A., Sauberlich, H., Page, J.B., 1997. High risk of HIV-related mortality is associated with selenium deficiency. J. Acquir. Immune Defic. Syndr. Hum. Retrovirol. 15, 370–374.

Benstoem, C., Goetzenich, A., Kraemer, S., Borosch, S., Manzanares, W., Hardy, G., Stoppe, C., 2015. Selenium and its supplementation in cardiovascular disease—what do we know? Nutrients 7, 3094–3118.

Bleys, J., Navas-Acien, A., Guallar, E., 2007. Serum selenium and diabetes in U.S. adults. Diabetes Care 30, 829–834.

de Bortoli, M.C., Cozzolino, S.M., 2009. Zinc and selenium nutritional status in vegetarians. Biol. Trace Elem. Res. 127, 228–233.

Bottino, N.R., Banks, C.H., Irgolic, K.J., Micks, P., Wheeler, A.E., Zingaro, R.A., 1984. Selenium containing amino-acids and proteins in marine-algae. Phytochemistry 23, 2445–2452.

Brigo, F., Storti, M., Lochner, P., Tezzon, F., Nardone, R., 2014. Selenium supplementation for primary prevention of cardiovascular disease: proof of no effectiveness. Nutr. Metab. Cardiovasc. Dis. 24, e2–e3.

Brown, T.A., Shrift, A., 1982. Selenium – toxicity and tolerance in higher-plants. Biol. Rev. Camb. Philos. Soc. 57, 59–84.

Burk, R.F., Hill, K.E., 2009. Selenoprotein P-expression, functions, and roles in mammals. Biochim. Biophys. Acta 1790, 1441–1447.

Burk, R.F., Hill, K.E., 2015. Regulation of selenium metabolism and transport. Annu. Rev. Nutr. 35, 109–134.

Chang, J.C., Gutenmann, W.H., Reid, C.M., Lisk, D.J., 1995. Selenium content of Brazil nuts from two geographic locations in Brazil. Chemosphere 30, 801–802.

Chiu-Ugalde, J., Theilig, F., Behrends, T., Drebes, J., Sieland, C., Subbarayal, P., Kohrle, J., Hammes, A., Schomburg, L., Schweizer, U., 2010. Mutation of megalin leads to urinary loss of selenoprotein P and selenium deficiency in serum, liver, kidneys and brain. Biochem. J. 431, 103–111.

Clark, L.C., Combs Jr., G.F., Turnbull, B.W., Slate, E.H., Chalker, D.K., Chow, J., Davis, L.S., Glover, R.A., Graham, G.F., Gross, E.G., Krongrad, A., Lesher Jr., J.L., Park, H.K., Sanders Jr., B.B., Smith, C.L., Taylor, J.R., 1996. Effects of selenium supplementation for cancer prevention in patients with carcinoma of the skin. A randomized controlled trial. Nutritional Prevention of Cancer Study Group. JAMA 276, 1957–1963.

Combs Jr., G.F., Watts, J.C., Jackson, M.I., Johnson, L.K., Zeng, H., Scheett, A.J., Uthus, E.O., Schomburg, L., Hoeg, A., Hoefig, C.S., Davis, C.D., Milner, J.A., 2011. Determinants of selenium status in healthy adults. Nutr. J. 10, 75.

Combs Jr., G.F., 2005. Current evidence and research needs to support a health claim for selenium and cancer prevention. J. Nutr. 135, 343–347.

Combs Jr., G.F., 2015. Biomarkers of selenium status. Nutrients 7, 2209–2236.

Conrad, M., Schweizer, U., 2010. Unveiling the molecular mechanisms behind selenium-related diseases through knockout mouse studies. Antioxid. Redox Signal. 12, 851–865.

Derumeaux, H., Valeix, P., Castetbon, K., Bensimon, M., Boutron-Ruault, M.C., Arnaud, J., Hercberg, S., 2003. Association of selenium with thyroid volume and echostructure in 35-to 60-year-old French adults. Eur. J. Endocrinol. 148, 309–315.

Duffield-Lillico, A.J., Reid, M.E., Turnbull, B.W., Combs Jr., G.F., Slate, E.H., Fischbach, L.A., Marshall, J.R., Clark, L.C., 2002. Baseline characteristics and the effect of selenium supplementation on cancer incidence in a randomized clinical trial: a summary report of the Nutritional Prevention of Cancer Trial. Cancer Epidemiol. Biomarkers Prev. 11, 630–639.

Dumitrescu, A.M., Liao, X.H., Abdullah, M.S., Lado-Abeal, J., Majed, F.A., Moeller, L.C., Boran, G., Schomburg, L., Weiss, R.E., Refetoff, S., 2005. Mutations in *SECISBP2* result in abnormal thyroid hormone metabolism. Nat. Genet. 37, 1247–1252.

Elorinne, A.L., Alfthan, G., Erlund, I., Kivimaki, H., Paju, A., Salminen, I., Turpeinen, U., Voutilainen, S., Laakso, J., 2016. Food and nutrient intake and nutritional status of Finnish vegans and nonvegetarians. PLoS One 11, e0148235.

Fagan, S., Owens, R., Ward, P., Connolly, C., Doyle, S., Murphy, R., 2015. Biochemical comparison of commercial selenium yeast preparations. Biol. Trace Elem. Res. 166, 245–259.

Fairweather-Tait, S.J., Collings, R., Hurst, R., 2010. Selenium bioavailability: current knowledge and future research requirements. Am. J. Clin. Nutr. 91, 1484S–1491S.

Ferreiro, A., Quijano-Roy, S., Pichereau, C., Moghadaszadeh, B., Goemans, N., Bonnemann, C., Jungbluth, H., Straub, V., Villanova, M., Leroy, J.P., Romero, N.B., Martin, J.J., Muntoni, F., Voit, T., Estournet, B., Richard, P., Fardeau, M., Guicheney, P., 2002. Mutations of the selenoprotein N gene, which is implicated in rigid spine muscular dystrophy, cause the classical phenotype of multiminicore disease: reassessing the nosology of early-onset myopathies. Am. J. Hum. Genet. 71, 739–749.

Flohé, L., Günzler, W.A., Schock, H.H., 1973. Glutathione peroxidase: a selenoenzyme. FEBS Lett. 32, 132–134.

Forceville, X., Vitoux, D., Gauzit, R., Combes, A., Lahilaire, P., Chappuis, P., 1998. Selenium, systemic immune response syndrome, sepsis, and outcome in critically ill patients. Crit. Care Med. 26, 1536–1544.

Forceville, X., Mostert, V., Pierantoni, A., Vitoux, D., Le Toumelin, P., Plouvier, E., Dehoux, M., Thuillier, F., Combes, A., 2009. Selenoprotein P, rather than glutathione peroxidase, as a potential marker of septic shock and related syndromes. Eur. Surg. Res. 43, 338–347.

Gunzler, W.A., Kremers, H., Flohe, L., 1974. An improved coupled test procedure for glutathione peroxidase (EC 1-11-1-9-) in blood. Z. Klin. Chem. Klin. Biochem. 12, 444–448.

Hatfield, D.L., Gladyshev, V.N., 2009. The Outcome of Selenium and Vitamin E Cancer Prevention Trial (SELECT) reveals the need for better understanding of selenium biology. Mol. Interv. 9, 18–21.

Hoeflich, J., Hollenbach, B., Behrends, T., Hoeg, A., Stosnach, H., Schomburg, L., 2010. The choice of biomarkers determines the selenium status in young German vegans and vegetarians. Br. J. Nutr. 104, 1601–1604.

Huang, Y., Wang, Q., Gao, J., Lin, Z., Banuelos, G.S., Yuan, L., Yin, X., 2013. Daily dietary selenium intake in a high selenium area of Enshi, China. Nutrients 5, 700–710.

Hughes, D.J., Fedirko, V., Jenab, M., Schomburg, L., Meplan, C., Freisling, H., Bueno-de-Mesquita, H.B., Hybsier, S., Becker, N.P., Czuban, M., Tjonneland, A., Outzen, M., Boutron-Ruault, M.C., Racine, A., Bastide, N., Kuhn, T., Kaaks, R., Trichopoulos, D., Trichopoulou, A., Lagiou, P., Panico, S., Peeters, P.H., Weiderpass, E., Skeie, G., Dagrun, E., Chirlaque, M.D., Sanchez, M.J., Ardanaz, E., Ljuslinder, I., Wennberg, M., Bradbury, K.E., Vineis, P., Naccarati, A., Palli, D., Boeing, H., Overvad, K., Dorronsoro, M., Jakszyn, P., Cross, A.J., Quiros, J.R., Stepien, M., Kong, S.Y., Duarte-Salles, T., Riboli, E., Hesketh, J.E., 2015. Selenium status is associated with colorectal cancer risk in the European prospective investigation of cancer and nutrition cohort. Int. J. Cancer 136, 1149–1161.

Hurst, R., Armah, C.N., Dainty, J.R., Hart, D.J., Teucher, B., Goldson, A.J., Broadley, M.R., Motley, A.K., Fairweather-Tait, S.J., 2010. Establishing optimal selenium status: results of a randomized, double-blind, placebo-controlled trial. Am. J. Clin. Nutr. 91, 923–931.

Kadrabova, J., Madaric, A., Kovacikova, Z., Ginter, E., 1995. Selenium status, plasma zinc, copper, and magnesium in vegetarians. Biol. Trace Elem. Res. 50, 13–24.

Kasaikina, M.V., Hatfield, D.L., Gladyshev, V.N., 2012. Understanding selenoprotein function and regulation through the use of rodent models. Biochim. Biophys. Acta 1823, 1633–1642.

Kipp, A.P., Strohm, D., Brigelius-Flohe, R., Schomburg, L., Bechthold, A., Leschik-Bonnet, E., Heseker, H., German Nutrition, S., 2015. Revised reference values for selenium intake. J. Trace Elem. Med. Biol. 32, 195–199.

Kobayashi, Y., Ogra, Y., Ishiwata, K., Takayama, H., Aimi, N., Suzuki, K.T., 2002. Selenosugars are key and urinary metabolites for selenium excretion within the required to low-toxic range. Proc. Natl. Acad. Sci. U. S. A. 99, 15932–15936.

Kristensen, N.B., Madsen, M.L., Hansen, T.H., Allin, K.H., Hoppe, C., Fagt, S., Lausten, M.S., Gobel, R.J., Vestergaard, H., Hansen, T., Pedersen, O., 2015. Intake of macro- and micronutrients in Danish vegans. Nutr. J. 14, 115.

Larsson, C.L., Johansson, G.K., 2002. Dietary intake and nutritional status of young vegans and omnivores in Sweden. Am. J. Clin. Nutr. 76, 100–106.

Letsiou, S., Nomikos, T., Panagiotakos, D., Pergantis, S.A., Fragopoulou, E., Antonopoulou, S., Pitsavos, C., Stefanadis, C., 2009. Serum total selenium status in Greek adults and its relation to age. The ATTICA study cohort. Biol. Trace Elem. Res. 128, 8–17.

Lippman, S.M., Klein, E.A., Goodman, P.J., Lucia, M.S., Thompson, I.M., Ford, L.G., Parnes, H.L., Minasian, L.M., Gaziano, J.M., Hartline, J.A., Parsons, J.K., Bearden 3rd, J.D., Crawford, E.D., Goodman, G.E., Claudio, J., Winquist, E., Cook, E.D., Karp, D.D., Walther, P., Lieber, M.M., Kristal, A.R., Darke, A.K., Arnold, K.B., Ganz, P.A., Santella, R.M., Albanes, D., Taylor, P.R., Probstfield, J.L., Jagpal, T.J., Crowley, J.J., Meyskens Jr., F.L., Baker, L.H., Coltman Jr., C.A., 2009. Effect of selenium and vitamin E on risk of prostate cancer and other cancers: the Selenium and Vitamin E Cancer Prevention Trial (SELECT). JAMA 301, 39–51.

Lyons, G.H., Stangoulis, J.C.R., Graham, R.D., 2004. Exploiting micronutrient interaction to optimize bio-fortification programs: the case for inclusion of selenium and iodine in the HarvestPlus program. Nutr. Rev. 62, 247–252.

Marcocci, C., Kahaly, G.J., Krassas, G.E., Bartalena, L., Prummel, M., Stahl, M., Altea, M.A., Nardi, M., Pitz, S., Boboridis, K., Sivelli, P., von Arx, G., Mourits, M.P., Baldeschi, L., Bencivelli, W., Wiersinga, W., Orbitopathy, E.G.G., 2011. Selenium and the course of mild graves' orbitopathy. N. Engl. J. Med. 364, 1920–1931.

Mehdi, Y., Hornick, J.L., Istasse, L., Dufrasne, I., 2013. Selenium in the environment, metabolism and involvement in body functions. Molecules 18, 3292–3311.

Meplan, C., Hesketh, J., 2014. Selenium and cancer: a story that should not be forgotten-insights from genomics. Cancer Treat. Res. 159, 145–166.

Morris, J.S., Crane, S.B., 2013. Selenium toxicity from a misformulated dietary supplement, adverse health effects, and the temporal response in the nail biologic monitor. Nutrients 5, 1024–1057.

Moustafa, M.E., Kumaraswamy, E., Zhong, N., Rao, M., Carlson, B.A., Hatfield, D.L., 2003. Models for assessing the role of selenoproteins in health. J. Nutr. 133, 2494S–2496S.

Nichol, C., Herdman, J., Sattar, N., O'Dwyer, P.J., O'Reilly, D.St.J., Littlejohn, D., Fell, G., 1998. Changes in the concentrations of plasma selenium and selenoproteins after minor elective surgery: further evidence for a negative acute phase response? Clin. Chem. 44, 1764–1766.

Ogawa-Wong, A.N., Berry, M.J., Seale, L.A., 2016. Selenium and metabolic disorders: an emphasis on type 2 diabetes risk. Nutrients 8.

Olson, G.E., Winfrey, V.P., Nagdas, S.K., Hill, K.E., Burk, R.F., 2007. Apolipoprotein E receptor-2 (ApoER2) mediates selenium uptake from selenoprotein P by the mouse testis. J. Biol. Chem. 282, 12290–12297.

Olson, G.E., Winfrey, V.P., Hill, K.E., Burk, R.F., 2008. Megalin mediates selenoprotein P uptake by kidney proximal tubule epithelial cells. J. Biol. Chem. 283, 6854–6860.

Persson-Moschos, M., Huang, W., Srikumar, T.S., Akesson, B., Lindeberg, S., 1995. Selenoprotein P in serum as a biochemical marker of selenium status. Analyst 120, 833–836.

Pietschmann, N., Rijntjes, E., Hoeg, A., Stoedter, M., Schweizer, U., Seemann, P., Schomburg, L., 2014. Selenoprotein P is the essential selenium transporter for bones. Metallomics 6, 1043–1049.

Prasad, R., Chan, L.F., Hughes, C.R., Kaski, J.P., Kowalczyk, J.C., Savage, M.O., Peters, C.J., Nathwani, N., Clark, A.J., Storr, H.L., Metherell, L.A., 2014. Thioredoxin Reductase 2 (*TXNRD2*) mutation associated with familial glucocorticoid deficiency (FGD). J. Clin. Endocrinol. Metab. 99, E1556–E1563.

Ramaekers, V.T., Calomme, M., Vanden Berghe, D., Makropoulos, W., 1994. Selenium deficiency triggering intractable seizures. Neuropediatrics 25, 217–223.

Rasmussen, L.B., Schomburg, L., Kohrle, J., Pedersen, I.B., Hollenbach, B., Hog, A., Ovesen, L., Perrild, H., Laurberg, P., 2011. Selenium status, thyroid volume, and multiple nodule formation in an area with mild iodine deficiency. Eur. J. Endocrinol. 164, 585–590.

Rauma, A.L., Torronen, R., Hanninen, O., Verhagen, H., Mykkanen, H., 1995. Antioxidant status in long-term adherents to a strict uncooked vegan diet. Am. J. Clin. Nutr. 62, 1221–1227.

Rayman, M.P., Stranges, S., 2013. Epidemiology of selenium and type 2 diabetes: can we make sense of it? Free Radic. Biol. Med. 65, 1557–1564.

Rayman, M.P., 2008. Food-chain selenium and human health: emphasis on intake. Br. J. Nutr. 100, 254–268.

Rayman, M.P., 2012. Selenium and human health. Lancet 379, 1256–1268.

Renko, K., Werner, M., Renner-Muller, I., Cooper, T.G., Yeung, C.H., Hollenbach, B., Scharpf, M., Kohrle, J., Schomburg, L., Schweizer, U., 2008. Hepatic selenoprotein P (SePP) expression restores selenium transport and prevents infertility and motor-incoordination in *Sepp*-knockout mice. Biochem. J. 409, 741–749.

Renko, K., Hofmann, P.J., Stoedter, M., Hollenbach, B., Behrends, T., Kohrle, J., Schweizer, U., Schomburg, L., 2009. Down-regulation of the hepatic selenoprotein biosynthesis machinery impairs selenium metabolism during the acute phase response in mice. FASEB J. 23, 1758–1765.

Schoenmakers, E., Carlson, B., Agostini, M., Moran, C., Rajanayagam, O., Bochukova, E., Tobe, R., Peat, R., Gevers, E., Muntoni, F., Guicheney, P., Schoenmakers, N., Farooqi, S., Lyons, G., Hatfield, D., Chatterjee, K., 2016. Mutation in human selenocysteine transfer RNA selectively disrupts selenoprotein synthesis. J. Clin. Invest. 126, 992–996.

Schomburg, L., Schweizer, U., 2009. Hierarchical regulation of selenoprotein expression and sex-specific effects of selenium. Biochim. Biophys. Acta 1790, 1453–1462.

Schomburg, L., Schweizer, U., Kohrle, J., 2004. Selenium and selenoproteins in mammals: extraordinary, essential, enigmatic. Cell. Mol. Life Sci. 61, 1988–1995.

Schomburg, L., 2012. Selenium, selenoproteins and the thyroid gland: interactions in health and disease. Nat. Rev. Endocrinol. 8, 160–171.

Schrauzer, G.N., 2009. RE: Lessons from the selenium and vitamin E cancer prevention trial (SELECT). Crit. Rev. Biotechnol. 29, 81.

Schwarz, K., Foltz, C.M., 1957. Selenium as an integral part of factor 3 against dietary necrotic liver degeneration. J. Am. Chem. Soc. 79, 3292.

Schweizer, U., Schomburg, L., 2005. New insights into the physiological actions of selenoproteins from genetically modified mice. IUBMB Life 57, 737–744.

Schweizer, U., Dehina, N., Schomburg, L., 2011. Disorders of selenium metabolism and selenoprotein function. Curr. Opin. Pediatr. 23, 429–435.

Shultz, T.D., Leklem, J.E., 1983. Selenium status of vegetarians, nonvegetarians, and hormone-dependent cancer subjects. Am. J. Clin. Nutr. 37, 114–118.

Sigrist, M., Brusa, L., Campagnoli, D., Beldomenico, H., 2012. Determination of selenium in selected food samples from Argentina and estimation of their contribution to the Se dietary intake. Food Chem. 134, 1932–1937.

Sobiecki, J.G., Appleby, P.N., Bradbury, K.E., Key, T.J., 2016. High compliance with dietary recommendations in a cohort of meat eaters, fish eaters, vegetarians, and vegans: results from the European Prospective Investigation into Cancer and Nutrition-Oxford study. Nutr. Res. 36, 464–477.

Steinbrenner, H., Speckmann, B., Pinto, A., Sies, H., 2011. High selenium intake and increased diabetes risk: experimental evidence for interplay between selenium and carbohydrate metabolism. J. Clin. Biochem. Nutr. 48, 40–45.

Stone, C.A., Kawai, K., Kupka, R., Fawzi, W.W., 2010. Role of selenium in HIV infection. Nutr. Rev. 68, 671–681.

Suzuki, K.T., Ogra, Y., 2002. Metabolic pathway for selenium in the body: speciation by HPLC-ICP MS with enriched Se. Food Addit. Contam. 19, 974–983.

Suzuki, K.T., Kurasaki, K., Okazaki, N., Ogra, Y., 2005. Selenosugar and trimethylselenonium among urinary Se metabolites: dose- and age-related changes. Toxicol. Appl. Pharmacol. 206, 1–8.

Thomson, C.D., Robinson, M.F., Butler, J.A., Whanger, P.D., 1993. Long-term supplementation with selenate and selenomethionine: selenium and glutathione peroxidase (EC 1.11.1.9) in blood components of New Zealand women. Br. J. Nutr. 69, 577–588.

Tinggi, U., 2003. Essentiality and toxicity of selenium and its status in Australia: a review. Toxicol. Lett. 137, 103–110.

Toulis, K.A., Anastasilakis, A.D., Tzellos, T.G., Goulis, D.G., Kouvelas, D., 2010. Selenium supplementation in the treatment of Hashimoto's thyroiditis: a systematic review and a meta-analysis. Thyroid 20, 1163–1173.

Winkel, L.H.E., Vriens, B., Jones, G.D., Schneider, L.S., Pilon-Smits, E., Banuelos, G.S., 2015. Selenium cycling across soil-plant-atmosphere interfaces: a critical review. Nutrients 7, 4199–4239.

Wolffram, S., Grenacher, B., Scharrer, E., 1988. Transport of selenate and sulphate across the intestinal brush-border membrane of pig jejunum by two common mechanism. Q. J. Exp. Physiol. 73, 103–111.

Wu, Q., Rayman, M.P., Lv, H., Schomburg, L., Cui, B., Gao, C., Chen, P., Zhuang, G., Zhang, Z., Peng, X., Li, H., Zhao, Y., He, X., Zeng, G., Qin, F., Hou, P., Shi, B., 2015a. Low population selenium status is associated with increased prevalence of thyroid disease. J. Clin. Endocrinol. Metab. 100, 4037–4047.

Wu, Z., Banuelos, G.S., Lin, Z.Q., Liu, Y., Yuan, L., Yin, X., Li, M., 2015b. Biofortification and phytoremediation of selenium in China. Front. Plant Sci. 6, 136.

Xia, Y., Hill, K.E., Li, P., Xu, J., Zhou, D., Motley, A.K., Wang, L., Byrne, D.W., Burk, R.F., 2010. Optimization of selenoprotein P and other plasma selenium biomarkers for the assessment of the selenium nutritional requirement: a placebo-controlled, double-blind study of selenomethionine supplementation in selenium-deficient Chinese subjects. Am. J. Clin. Nutr. 92, 525–531.

Zhu, Y.G., Pilon-Smits, E.A.H., Zhao, F.J., Williams, P.N., Meharg, A.A., 2009. Selenium in higher plants: understanding mechanisms for biofortification and phytoremediation. Trends Plant Sci. 14, 436–442.

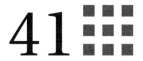

41

B Vitamins Intake and Plasma Homocysteine in Vegetarians

Amalia Tsiami, Derek Obersby

UNIVERSITY OF WEST LONDON, LONDON, UNITED KINGDOM

1. Introduction

Worldwide, there are 75 million vegetarians by choice and 1.45 billion by necessity (The Economic and Social Research Institute, 2011). This is consistent with the approximation of 25% of the world's population consuming a largely vegetarian diet (Foods Standards Agency, 2010).

Lactovegetarians (LVs), ovolactovegetarians (OLVs), and vegan groups of the population are potentially at greater risk of vitamin B_{12} deficiency than omnivores. (The readers may refer to Chapter 43 for a detailed review.) Hence, they are more susceptible to developing elevated homocysteine that may result in developing primary cardiovascular disease (CVD).

2. Vegetarianism

2.1 Classification of Vegetarians

As presented in Chapter 1 of this book, vegetarian diets cover a spectrum of diets.

The most common types of vegetarians are vegan, LV, OLV, and semivegetarian.

Until recently, vegetarian literature claimed that certain plant foods could provide vitamin B_{12}, such as seaweed, fermented soybeans, spirulina, and even unwashed vegetables that have been fertilized with manure. Proponents of vegetarianism pointed to inhabitants of India, who did not seem to exhibit signs of vitamin B_{12} deficiency in spite of very low levels of animal foods in the diet (Dong and Scott, 1982). It is also now known that a source of vitamin B_{12} in the vegetarian diet in India was insect excrement and parts in stored grains and legumes (Dong and Scott, 1982). There is very little nonscientific literature that warns about the real possibility and risk of vitamin B_{12} depletion of vegetarians (Pawiak et al., 2014).

2.2 Homocysteine Status of Vegetarians Compared to Omnivores

A systematic review and meta-analysis, comprising eight Cohort Case Studies and 11 cross-sectional studies involving 3230 participants (Obersby et al., 2013a), demonstrated that an inverse relationship exists between plasma tHcy and serum vitamin B_{12}. The results are

Table 41.1 Calculated Mean, Standard Deviation, and Significant Difference Value P of Lactovegetarians or Ovolactovegetarians (LV-OLVs) and Vegans From Omnivores for Plasma tHcy and Serum Vitamin B_{12} Levels

	Plasma tHcy				Serum Vitamin B_{12}			
Diet	Mean (µmol/L)	SD (µmol/L)	n	P	Mean (pmol/L)	SD (pmol/L)	n	P
Omnivores	11.03	2.89	14		303	72	14	
LV-OLVs	13.91	3.15	15	<0.025	209	47	15	<0.005
Vegans	16.40	4.80	9	<0.005	172	59	9	<0.005

presented in Table 41.1. This supports previous research conducted by Elmadfa and Singer (2009). The same systematic review and meta-analysis conducted by Obersby et al. (2013a) presents in Fig. 41.1 the correlation between plasma tHcy and serum vitamin B_{12} for omnivores, LV-OLVs, and vegans.

3. What Is Homocysteine?

Homocysteine was discovered approximately 83 years ago by Butz and du Vigneaud (1932) at the University of Illinois. These researchers heated methionine in sulfuric acid and isolated a substance with similar features as cysteine and cystine; they had, in fact, synthesized "bis-(Y-amino-Y-carboxypropyl) disulphide." They called it "Homocysteine" since it had the structure of the next higher symmetrical homologue of cysteine (Butz and du Vigneaud, 1932). Structurally, it closely resembles methionine and cysteine.

Homocysteine belongs to a group of molecules known as cellular thiols (Lu, 1999); it is a sulfur-containing potentially injurious amino acid with the molecular formula $C_4H_9NO_2S$. Homocysteine does not occur naturally within proteins and is thought to be a "bad thiol," due to its association with disease states such as CVD (Refsum et al., 1998) and cognitive dysfunctions including Alzheimer disease (Lehmann et al., 1999). Conversely, glutathione and cysteine are considered to be "good thiols" because their functions include maintaining intracellular and extracellular redox homeostasis and facilitating the removal of toxic compounds, and they are also part of the cellular antioxidant defense system (Lu, 1999). Homocysteine stands at the biochemical intersection of two metabolic pathways and converts to glutathione, a powerful antioxidant, and into the important chemical S-adenosylmethionine (SAM). Methionine is the precursor of homocysteine (Finkelstein and Martin, 2000).

Thiols contain a free sulfhydryl group. Other low-molecular weight biological thiols include glutathione, coenzyme A, and dihydrolipoic acid. A general property of thiols is their ability to oxidize in the presence of an electron receptor such as molecular oxygen to form disulfides (-S-S-). Homocysteine can oxidize with other thiols such as

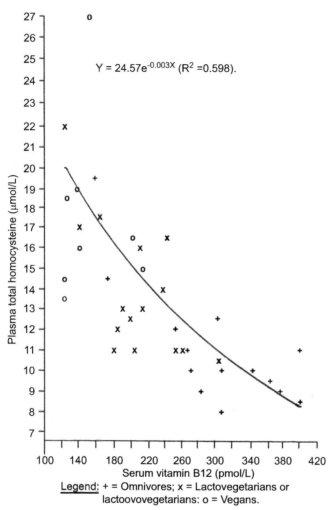

$$Y = 24.57e^{-0.003X} \ (R^2 = 0.598).$$

FIGURE 41.1 Association between plasma tHcy and serum vitamin B_{12} for omnivores, lactovegetarians–ovolactovegetarians, and vegans reported in studies as systematically reviewed by Obersby et al. (2013a).

cysteine and glutathione to form mixed disulfides, which are referred to as "homocysteine–cysteine–mixed disulfide" and "homocysteine–glutathione–mixed disulfide" (Jacobsen, 2001).

The other major class of thiols and disulfides consist of those found in the peptide and proteins that contain cysteine. The intermolecular disulfide bond formed by the oxidation of cysteine resides in peptide, and proteins are primary structural elements that contribute to the final three-dimensional conformations. Peptides and proteins may also contain "free-cysteine residues" that can autooxidize or can react with low-molecular thiols to form stable disulfide bond complexes (Jacobsen, 2001).

Therefore, homocysteine exists as either "free homocysteine" or "protein-bound homocysteine."

Free homocysteine comprises three distinct fractions, namely:

1. reduced homocysteine
2. homocysteine–homocysteine disulfide (homocystine)
3. cysteine–homocysteine (Cys-Hcy)–mixed disulfide

Note that 2 and 3 are commonly referred to as the oxidized homocysteine equivalents. These oxidized forms of homocysteine account for approximately 30% of the body's total homocysteine pool. A small percentage $<3\mu mol/L$ is found as reduced homocysteine 1. The remaining 70% of circulating homocysteine is bound to albumin as a free sulfhydryl moiety.

The sum of the free and protein-bound homocysteine is referred to as "total homocysteine" (tHcy) (Stamm and Reynolds, 1999; Amores-Sanchez and Medina, 2000; Refsum et al., 2004). Homocysteine is a normal metabolite of the amino acid methionine (Jacobsen, 2001). Since homocysteine is virtually nonexistent in food (Sakamoto et al., 2002), all homocysteine in the body is derived from methionine from consumed animal and plant protein, as shown in Fig. 41.2 (methionine cycle).

3.1 The Metabolism of Homocysteine

Homocysteine is an intermediate product of the one-carbon metabolism whose transformation stands at the intersection of two remethylation pathways, namely the "transsulfuration pathway" and the "remethylation pathway or folate cycle."

Remethylation of homocysteine to generate methionine requires folate and vitamin B_{12} of the methylcobalamin form (or TMG or choline in an alternative reaction), and transsulfuration to cystathionine, which requires vitamin B_6 of the pyridoxal-5-phosphate (P-5-P) form, as illustrated in Fig. 41.2 (Verhoef et al., 1996; Selhub, 1999; Obersby et al., 2013b).

The two pathways are coordinated by SAM, which acts as an allosteric inhibitor of the enzyme methylenetetrahydrofolate reductase (MTHFR) reaction and as an activator of the enzyme cystathionine β-synthase (CBS).

3.1.1 Methionine Cycle in Its Role in Homocysteine Formation

A considerable proportion of the essential amino acid methionine obtained from the diet is activated by adenosine triphosphate and used either for protein synthesis or the formation of SAM, in a reaction catalyzed by methionine adenosyltransferases.

The high-energy compound, SAM, serves primarily as a methyl donor via reactions catalyzed by a variety of methyltransferases and involving a variety of acceptors. These SAM-dependent methylations are essential for biosynthesis of a variety of cellular components including creatine, epinephrine, carnitine, phospholipids, proteins, DNA, and RNA. In fact, SAM serves as the methyl donor for essentially all known biological methylation

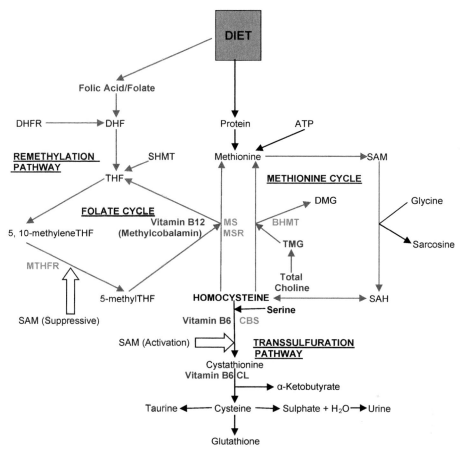

FIGURE 41.2 The methionine cycle, remethylation pathway of homocysteine to methionine via the folate cycle, the transsulfuration pathway, the TMG reaction, and the regulation of methionine methyl group synthesis. *APT*, adenosine triphosphate; *BHMT*, betaine homocysteine methyltransferase; *CBS*, cystathionine β-synthase; *CL*, cystathionine γ-lyase; *DHF*, dihydrofolic acid; *DHFR*, dihydrofolate reductase; *DMG*, dimethylglycine; *MS*, methionine synthase; *MSR*, methionine synthase reductase; *MTHFR*, methylenetetrahydrofolate reductase; *SAH*, s-adenosylhomocysteine; *SAM*, s-adenosylmethionine; *SHMT*, serine hydroxymethyltransferase; *THF*, tetrahydrofolate; *TMG*, trimethylglycine. *Adapted from Verhoef et al. (1996), Selhub (1999), and Obersby et al. (2013b).*

reactions, with the notable exception of those involved in the methylation of homocysteine, the coproduct of transmethylation.

S-adenosylhomocysteine (SAH) is hydrolyzed to yield adenosine and homocysteine, which can be remethylated to methionine or condensed with serine to form cystathionine (see Fig. 41.2). It should be noted that this hydrolysis is a reversible reaction that favors the synthesis of SAH, and elevated cellular concentrations of this metabolite are likely to precede and accompany all forms of hyperhomocysteinemia (Selhub, 1999).

Every tissue in the human body performs the methionine cycle.

3.1.2 Folate Cycle

Homocysteine can be remethylated through the folate cycle (see Fig. 41.2): it is recycled to methionine in a reaction catalyzed by the enzyme methionine synthase (MS) and is dependent on the essential vitamin B_{12} (Dudman et al., 1996), but only in its methylcobalamin form as this is the only type of vitamin B_{12} that contains a methyl group (Herrmann et al., 2005), together with another enzyme methionine synthase reductase (MSR). Homocysteine acquires a methyl group from 5-methyl tetrahydrofolate (THF) that is catalyzed from 5, 10-methyleneTHF by the enzyme methylenetetrahydrofolate reductase (MTHFR) and folic acid/folate from the diet (Selhub, 1999). Folic acid/folate enters the folate cycle as THF via dihydrofolic acid (DHF), which has been reduced to THF by the enzyme dihydrofolate reductase (DHFR). This is the major route for the remethylation of homocysteine to methionine. According to Selhub (1999) homocysteine concentrations may be substantially increased by the deficiency of folate and/or vitamin B_{12}.

Metabolism of folate to different forms can take place in different cell compartments including the cytoplasm, mitochondria, and the nucleus (Thorn, 2010).

3.1.3 Transsulfuration Pathway

Homocysteine is degraded in the transsulfuration pathway to other substances.

Referring to Fig. 41.2, homocysteine condenses with serine to form cystathionine in an irreversible reaction utilizing vitamin B_6 and the enzyme cystathionine β-synthase (CBS). Cystathionine is hydrolyzed a second time by the vitamin B_6-dependent enzyme cystathionine γ-lyase (CL) to form cysteine and α-ketobutyrate.

However, prior to this occurring, if vitamin B_6 in the form of pyridoxine is present, it must be converted into P-5-P, the activated form of vitamin B_6. This conversion is dependent on zinc and vitamin B_2 (Robinson et al., 1995; Leblanc, 2000; Bates, 1999; Dalery, 1995). Excess cysteine is oxidized to taurine or inorganic sulfate or excreted in the urine.

Transsulfuration occurs only in the liver, small intestine, and pancreas (Finkelstein, 1998). This pathway catabolizes excess homocysteine, which would otherwise be required for remethylation (Selhub, 1999).

Homocysteine levels can be regulated, up to a point, by SAM acting in various roles in the remethylation and transsulfuration pathways. Referring to Fig. 41.2, the following are seen:

1. When the diet is rich in methionine, the incoming methionine is rapidly converted to SAM, resulting in the inhibition of MTHFR, which suppresses 5-methylTHF synthesis. The increased level of SAM also increases activation of CBS enzyme, thus increasing the rate of homocysteine catabolism. In this way, homocysteine transsulfuration is promoted over remethylation, consistent with the reduced need for de novo methionine synthesis due to the higher dietary supply of methionine.
2. Conversely, when the diet is low in methionine, SAM concentration is insufficient for the inhibition of MTHFR, resulting in an elevated rate of 5-methylTHF production. The result is a rise in intracellular 5-methylTHF concentration, thereby

conservation of SAM and increase in the availability of substrate for homocysteine remethylation. Thus, remethylation will be favored over transsulfuration because the concentration of SAM is too low to activate the CBS enzyme. This process is consistent with the increased need for de novo methionine synthesis attributed to the low dietary input of methionine.

3.1.4 The Trimethylglycine Reaction

In the methionine cycle, Fig. 41.2, homocysteine is converted to methionine, and the enzyme involved is betaine homocysteine methyltransferase (BHMT). This reaction is independent of the one that is mediated by MS and independent of vitamin B_{12} or the folate cycle. In this case, methionine is regenerated from homocysteine by the transfer of a methyl group from trimethylglycine (TMG) to homocysteine (Brouwer et al., 2000). Once TMG loses a methyl group to homocysteine, it converts to dimethylglycine (DMG). In turn, homocysteine gains a methyl group and becomes methionine. BHMT is a zinc metalloenzyme (Breksa and Garrow, 1999; Bella et al., 2002; Evans et al., 2002) that uses preformed methyl groups from dietary TMG (Sakamoto et al., 2002) or from TMG derived from either dietary choline (Zeisel et al., 2003) or choline synthesized through successive SAM-dependent methylations of phosphatidylethanolamine. TMG may be an important methylating agent when the folate-dependent methylating pathway is impaired by ethanol ingestion, drugs, nutritional imbalances, or when TMG or choline levels are high (Finkelstein et al., 1982, 1983; Townsend et al., 2004; Stipanuk et al., 2004). The TMG reaction is considered to be a minor route since it can only take place in the liver and kidney of humans, as the enzyme involved, BHMT, has only been identified to be present in these organs (Finkelstein et al., 1994). TMG is obtainable from foods such as wheat bran, wheat germ, spinach, and beets. It can also be synthesized in the body from choline (Millian and Garrow, 1998). Total choline can be obtained from food such as beef liver, eggs, and soybeans in the form of choline phosphocholine, glycerophosphocholine, sphingomyelin, and phosphatidylcholine. When total choline is taken up by tissues, it is either converted to TMG and then employed as an osmolyte and methyl donor, or it is phosphorylated and used for the synthesis of phospholipids (Zeisel et al., 2003). The conversion of total choline to TMG is irreversible (Zeisel and Blvsztajn, 1994).

3.1.5 Impact of Methionine on Status of Plasma tHcy of Vegetarians

Obersby (2015) demonstrated from the results of a clinical pilot study involving LVs, OLVs, and vegans with concentrations of plasma tHcy ≥10 μmol/L that there exists a positive relationship between baseline plasma tHcy and mean dietary methionine intake of the form $Y = A \cdot \ln(X) - C$ (see Fig. 41.3). This dispersed following methylcobalamin intervention, with coefficients of determination (R^2) reducing from a very strong statistical significance of 0.79 to a very weak statistical significance of 0.03 (not shown).

Since methionine is a unique precursor of homocysteine, it is reasonable to deduce that concentrations of plasma tHcy can be exacerbated by the consumption of high

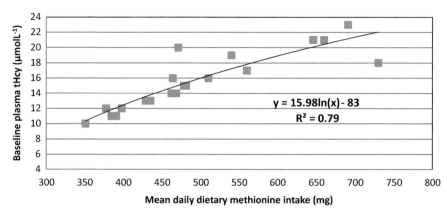

FIGURE 41.3 Correlation between baseline plasma tHcy and mean dietary methionine intake, for vitamin B_{12}-deficient lactovegetarians, ovolactovegetarians, and vegans from the intervention group.

methionine-containing foods, for example, muesli, soy products, nuts, wheat germ, chickpeas, beans, and rice, which are rich in LV, OLV, and vegan low-status vitamin B_{12} diets, as well as cheese for LV and OLV diets.

4. Homocysteine-Related Nutrients

4.1 Recommended Dietary Allowances and Adequate Intakes

By definition the OLV diet differs from the LV diet by the addition of eggs. However, for the purposes of this chapter, it will be assumed that these diets will be nutritionally equal since the vitamin B_{12} content from eggs is generally poorly absorbed due to the presence of vitamin B_{12} analogues (cobamides) that inhibit absorption of actual vitamin B_{12} (Doscherholmen et al., 1976).

The recommended dietary allowances (RDAs) and adequate intakes (AIs) for adults of the main cofactor and associated nutrients connected with the enzymes for normal conversion of homocysteine to other substances, as illustrated in Fig. 41.2, are outlined in Table 41.2. Table 41.2 also presents the results of a study of the diets of LV, OLV, and vegan participants taken over a 14-day period (Obersby, 2015). The participants of this study all had baseline plasma tHcy levels of ≥10 μmol/L, which was normalized for a vast majority of subjects by the intervention of methylcobalamin. The results indicate that apart from vitamin B_{12} for vegans, choline, and TMG, all other nutrients met the RDA or AI requirements.

The findings are what one would expect from these types of diet with high intake of folate and low intake of vitamin B_{12} resulting in elevated plasma tHcy.

The manner in which vitamin B_{12} deficiency produces its effects in humans has not been fully verified. The methyl folate trap hypothesis (Herbert and Zalusky, 1962; Noronha and Silverman, 1962; Scot and Weir, 1981) has been widely accepted over decades despite the difficulty in testing the hypothesis in any meaningful way. The methyl folate trap proposes that

Table 41.2 Results of a Clinical Pilot Study Involving lactovegetarian (LV), ovolactovegetarian (OLV), and Vegan Participant Dietary Intake of the Main Cofactor and Associated Nutrients Connected With the Enzymes for the Normal Remethylation of Homocysteine to Methionine, via the Folate Cycle and the TMG Reaction, and the Degrading of Homocysteine to Glutathione in the Transsulfuration Pathway, Taken Over 14 Days

	LV and OLV		Vegan		Adult RDA or AI/Day	
	Male	Female	Male	Female		
	(n = 11)	(n = 14)	(n = 2)	(n = 12)		
Nutrient	Mean/Day	Mean/Day	Mean/Day	Mean/Day	Male	Female
Vitamin B12 (µg)	2.5	3.2	1.3	1.2	2.4	2.4
Folate (µg)	511	407	425	434	400	400
Vitamin B6 (mg)	1.8	1.4	1.8	1.8	1.3	1.3
Vitamin B2 (mg)	2.1	1.3	1.3	1.3	1.3	1.1
Zinc (mg)	11.7	10.4	12.5	15.3	11	8
Choline (mg)	197	214	205	183	550	425
TMG (mg)	136	238	148	223	500–1000	500–1000

Adapted from National Institute of Health (2012), Linus Pauling Institute (2013), Food and Nutritional Board and Institute of Medicine (2011), USDA Agricultural Research Service (2014), and Foods Standards Agency (2002).

folate can be trapped as methylfolate as a consequence of vitamin B_{12} deficiency. This is due to the fact that vitamin B_{12} is required for the generation of folate from its methylated form. Since methylfolate cannot return to the tetrahydrofolate pool for conversion to 5, 10-methyleneTHF (Fig. 41.2), the transfer of the methyl group of 5-methylTHF to homocysteine is held up, and homocysteine levels rise as a result (Chanarin et al., 1985; Butensky et al., 2008).

The most important nutrients are folate and vitamin B_{12}, as they are required for remethylation of homocysteine back to methionine in the major folic cycle pathway, and they have the largest impact on regulating homocysteine. Low intake of these nutrients causes a very significant rise in plasma tHcy levels.

Vitamins B_6 and B_2 together with zinc are required in the more minor transsulfuration pathway, and TMG and choline play a role in the minor TMG reaction. It should be noted that according to Huang et al. (2003), vitamin B_6 and folate, which are rich in vegetarian diets, have little or no effect on plasma tHcy concentrations when individuals have an adequate dietary supply of these nutrients.

The findings of this study indicate that vegetarians would benefit from supplementation of vitamin B_{12} of the methylcobalamin type. Furthermore, the results imply that the RDA of 2.4 µg for vitamin B_{12} maybe too low, and both genders of LV and OLV diets meet the present RDA but had elevated plasma tHcy. This supports previous research (Bor et al., 2006), which demonstrated that doses of vitamin B_{12} of ≥6 µg/day appear to be sufficient to maintain a steady-state concentration of serum vitamin B_{12}. Furthermore, it is considered by the European Food Safety Authority (2015) that the 2.4-µg/day RDA for vitamin B_{12} for the total population is low.

Table 41.3 Summary of the Effects of Folate, Vitamin B_{12}, and Vitamin B_6 on Fasting Plasma Homocysteine Levels

	Vitamin B_{12} Deficiency	Control	Folate Deficiency	Control	Vitamin B_6 Deficiency	Control
Homocysteine (μmol/L)	25	10	60	6	12	12

Adapted from Selhub (1999).

4.2 Supporting Evidence for Nutritional Causes of Elevated Homocysteine

Table 41.3 summarizes the findings of Selhub (1999), who found that using rats as models established that fasting plasma homocysteine concentrations increased 10-fold in folate-deficient rats and 2.5-fold in vitamin B_{12}-deficient rats. In vitamin B_6-deficient rats, fasting plasma homocysteine concentrations were not elevated.

Obersby (2015) demonstrated that during the analysis of the confidential questionnaires of 49 LV, OLV, and vegans who were participating in a clinical pilot study, 53.13% were oblivious to the potential detrimental effect to health of elevated plasma tHcy, largely due to a deficiency of vitamin B_{12} in their vegetarian diets.

Methylcobalamin is the only form of vitamin B_{12} that contains a methyl group, and as a consequence, it is the only form of vitamin B_{12} that can directly reduce homocysteine (Herrmann et al., 2005).

The other forms of vitamin B_{12} (i.e., cyanocobalamin, artificially synthesized and widely used in supplements and fortification of food and beverages, hydroxocobalamin, and adenosylcobalamin) on entry to the bloodstream must be converted in the body to methylcobalamin before they can be utilized in the folate cycle for remethylation of homocysteine to methionine (Cooper and Rosenblatt, 1987; Pezacka et al., 1990). This conversion process is necessary to regulate plasma tHcy, and in the case of cyanocobalamin, it may take from 4–9 weeks for the synthesis of methylcobalamin to occur (Kelly, 1997), assuming there is no disruption by genetic factors, age-related issues, and metabolic problems (Obersby et al., 2013a). Despite the relative low intake of vitamin B_{12} by vegetarians, vitamin B_{12} deficiency may take years to realize since ~75% of the body's pool of vitamin B_{12} is reabsorbed by the enterohepatic circulation (Green and Mille, 2007) and stored in the liver.

Malabsorption of vitamin B_{12} is by far the most common cause of vitamin B_{12} deficiency, which can lead to pernicious anemia or Biermer disease.

5. Cobalamin

5.1 Origins

Cobalamin is a very complex molecule because, unlike other vitamins, it can be configured to form different forms of vitamin B_{12} (see Fig. 41.4A–D). It is only synthesized by microorganisms, and all mammalian cells can convert it into the coenzyme forms of methylcobalamin and adenosylcobalamin.

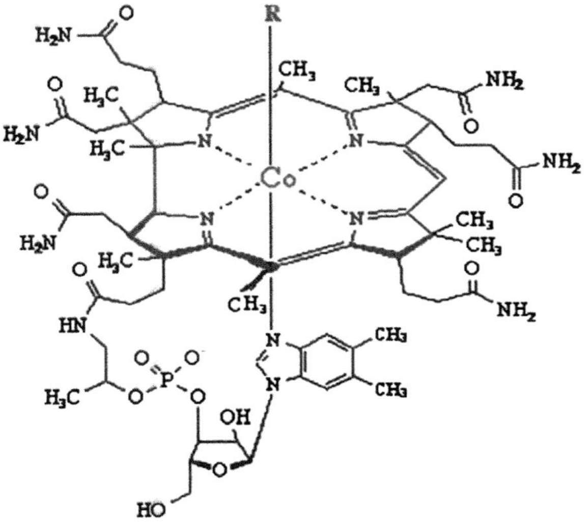

FIGURE 41.4 Chemical structure of cobalamin. *Adapted from Warren et al. (2002) and The European Food Safety Authority (2008).*

A CN

FIGURE 41.4A R=cyano group. *Adapted from Warren et al. (2002).*

B CH_3

FIGURE 41.4B R=methyl group. *Adapted from Warren et al. (2002).*

C OH

FIGURE 41.4C R=hydroxo group. *Adapted from Warren et al. (2002).*

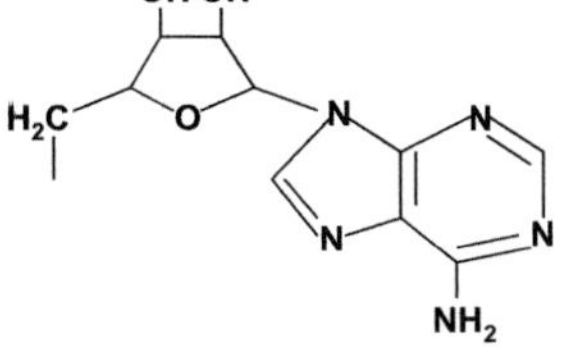

FIGURE 41.4D R=adenosyl group. *Adapted from Warren et al. (2002).*

Vitamin B_{12} is found abundantly mainly in animal products where it is ubiquitous and where it is ultimately derived from bacteria. Certain types of fungi and algae provide the only natural source of this vitamin (Herbert et al., 1984; Herbert, 1987; Herbert and Colman, 1988; Expert Group on Vitamins and Minerals, 2002). Animal products provide the vast majority of dietary vitamin B_{12}. The principal forms found in food are methylcobalamin, adenosylcobalamin, and hydroxocobalamin. The richest source of vitamin B_{12} is edible chlorella algae;

other foods such as ox liver, clams, lambs liver, lambs kidney, oysters, and liver sausage contain good levels of vitamin B_{12}. It has long been assumed that vitamin B_{12} is produced by bacteria in the human colon, but it has now been established that vitamin B_{12} is produced in the caecum below the ileum where vitamin B_{12} is absorbed by the microvilli of the ileum, so it is not available for absorption (Herbert, 1985, 1987; Herbert and Colman, 1988). This is supported by the fact that many animals, which are primarily vegetarian or near vegetarian, obtain their vitamin B_{12} from eating their feces (Herbert, 1988).

5.1.1 Summary of Types of Cobalamin (Vitamin B_{12})

Vitamin B_{12} or cobalamin is a water-soluble vitamin. It has the largest and most complex chemical structure of all the vitamins. It is a member of a family of related molecules known as corrinoids that contain a corrin nucleus made up of a tetrapyrrolic ring structure. The center of the tetrapyrrolic ring nucleus contains a cobalt ion that can be coordinated to a methyl, adenosyl, hydroxo, or cyano group to form the different types of vitamin B_{12}, which have similar effects and are mostly associated with human interaction (Expert Group on Vitamins and Minerals, 2002). Cobalamin is illustrated in Fig. 41.4.

There is also another form of vitamin B_{12}, which is present in edible cyanobacteria and is often mistaken for the normal vitamin B_{12}. It is designated as pseudovitamin B_{12} and is known to be biologically inactive in humans (Watanabe et al., 1999; Watanabe, 2007). Its structural formula is shown in Fig. 41.4E.

The chemical structures for R=cyano, R=methyl, R=hydroxo, and R=adenosyl to structure the vitamin B_{12} form of cyanocobalamin, methylcobalamin, hydroxocobalamin,

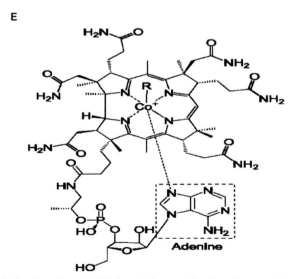

FIGURE 41.4E Pseudovitamin B_{12}. Note that the 5, 6-dimethylbenzimidazole as the α-axial ligand in Fig. 41.4 is replaced by an adenine nucleobase (a purine derivative) (Hoffmann et al., 2000). *Adapted from Watanabe et al. (2014).*

and adenosylcobalamin are shown in Figs. 41.4A–D, respectively, where R represents the β-axial ligand position.

5.1.1.1 CYANOCOBALAMIN

It has a structural formula shown in Fig. 41.4 where R is per Fig. 41.4A. It has a molecular formula of $C_{63}H_{88}C_ON_{14}O_{14}P$ with a molecular weight of 1355.4 g/mol.

It is an especially common vitamin of the vitamin B_{12} family because it is, in chemical terms, the most air stable. It is the easiest to crystallize and, therefore, easiest to purify following its production. Cyanocobalamin does not occur in nature (Qureshi et al., 1994); it is artificially synthesized by the introduction of the cyanide group into hydroxocobalamin, which has been sourced from bacteria. This was accidentally discovered when vitamin B_{12} was first isolated in the eluate from charcoal columns (Herbert and Colman, 1988). It is the most widespread in supplements and in the food industry and can be used as an injectable solution (Herbert, 1988). Cyanocobalamin is highly water soluble and heat stable and has a long shelf life (Expert Group on Vitamins and Minerals, 2002). Cyanocobalamin is very cheap to manufacture and can be classified as a drug.

5.1.1.2 METHYLCOBALAMIN

It has a structural formula shown in Fig. 41.4 where R is per Fig. 41.4B. It has a molecular formula of $C_{63}H_{91}C_ON_{13}O_{14}P$ with a molecular weight of 1344.8 g/mol (The European Food Safety Authority, 2008). This form of vitamin is one of two active coenzymes in the body. It is specifically the cofactor vitamin B_{12} form required by 5-methyTHF to recycle homocysteine back to methionine. Methylcobalamin is found in food and can also be artificially produced by bacteria. It predominates in blood plasma and certain other body fluids, such as cerebrospinal fluid, and in cellular cytosol (Cooper and Rosenblatt, 1987). Its biological function in humans is as a cofactor for the enzyme MS and participates in the transfer of methyl groups from 5-methyltetrahydrofolate to homocysteine, resulting in the subsequent regeneration/remethylation of methionine from homocysteine (see Fig. 41.2) (Kelly, 1997). In addition, methylcobalamin enhances synaptic transmission in learning and memory.

Methylcobalamin is less stable than cyanocobalamin, and it is particularly susceptible to photodecomposition. However, in terms of dietary supplementation, the efficiency of methylcobalamin in tablet or liquid form is usually improved by increasing the dose size.

It is found in foods such as meat, dairy, produce, and seafood, and it is relatively expensive to manufacture in supplementary form.

5.1.1.3 HYDROXOCOBALAMIN

It has a structural formula shown in Fig. 41.4 where R is per Fig. 41.4C. It has a molecular formula of $C_{62}H_{89}C_ON_{13}O_{15}P$ with a molecular weight of 1346.4 g/mol. It is synthesized in the human body by commensal organisms, including a number of specific bacterial species including *Streptomyces olivaceus* (Hall et al., 1953), *Streptomyces griseus*, and *Bacillus megatherium* (Basu and Dickerson, 1996), which can be used to manufacture the vitamin commercially. It is also found in some food such as meat and fish. Pharmaceutically, hydroxocobalamin is usually produced as a sterile injectable solution, and it is used for treatment of vitamin deficiency and because of its affinity for cyanide ions as a treatment for cyanide poisoning (Dart, 2006; Hall et al., 2007; Shepherd and Velez, 2006). It is encountered also in supplementary form.

5.1.1.4 ADENOSYLCOBALAMIN

Known also as 5-deoxyadenosylcobalamin, adenosylcobalamin has a structural formula as shown in Fig. 41.4 where R is per Fig. 41.4D. It has a molecular formula of $C_{72}H_{100}C_0N_{18}O_{17}P$ with a molecular weight of 1579.6 g/mol (The European Food Safety Authority, 2008). It occurs naturally in animal-derived food types such as fish, meat, eggs, and milk. Adenosylcobalamin functions in reactions in which hydrogen atoms are exchanged for organic groups. In humans, adenosylcobalamin is required for the enzyme methylmalonyl-CoA mutase, which is used in the catabolic isomerization of methylmalonyl-CoA to succinyl-CoA (used in the synthesis of porphyrin) and as an intermediate in the degradative pathway for valine, isoleucine, threonine, methionine, thymine, odd-chain fatty acids, and cholesterol (Qureshi et al., 1994). It plays an essential role in the production of blood and the maintenance of normal cerebral and nervous function in the human body. It is involved in the synthesis of thymidylate, a substance necessary for DNA synthesis.

5.1.1.5 PSEUDOVITAMIN B$_{12}$

It has a structural formula shown in Fig. 41.4E. It has a molecular formula of $C_{59}H_{83}C_0N_{17}O_{14}P$ with a molecular weight of 1344.3 g/mol. Pseudovitamin B$_{12}$ was shown not to function in humans and therefore has received less attention than cobalamin (Fig. 41.4). The 500-fold-lower binding affinity of pseudovitamin B$_{12}$ for the human receptor, intrinsic factor, largely contributes to the inability of humans to use pseudovitamin B$_{12}$ (Stupperich and Nexo, 1991).

6. Impact of Elevated Plasma tHcy

The normal range of plasma tHcy level has been defined as 5–15 μmol/L. Hyperhomocysteinemia (HHCY) has been defined as a plasma tHcy level of >15 μmol/L (Ravaglia et al., 2006). HHCY has been linked to the risk level of developing a homocysteine-related medical condition. The classification of HHCY is summarized in Table 41.4.

However, other studies on targeted segments of the population have shown that the upper limit of 15 μmol/L is too high for the normal upper range of plasma tHcy in well-nourished populations without obvious vitamin deficiency (Ubbink, 1995; Nygard et al., 1998).

Table 41.4 Classification of Hyperhomocysteinemia (HHCY)

Homocysteine (μmol/L) Classification	Level HHCY
15–30	Moderate
30–100	Intermediate
>100	Severe

Adapted from Refsum et al. (1998, 2004).

There are numerous health-related risk factors associated with HHCY; in particular, the risk of cancer (Weinstein et al., 2001; Wu and Wu, 2002), hip fracture with Parkinson disease (Sato et al., 2005), diabetes (Buysschaert, 2001), hypothyroidism (Bicikova, 2001; Toft and Toft, 2001), pregnancy miscarriages (Nelen, 2000), Alzheimer disease, and other forms of dementia (Seshadri et al., 2002) and CVD (Wald et al., 2002).

Ueland et al. (2000) and Humphrey et al. (2008) have demonstrated that each increase in 5 μmol/L in plasma tHcy increases the risk of coronary heart disease (CHD) by approximately 20%, independently of the traditional CHD risk factors. Additionally, it is well documented that the risk for CHD is represented by a continuum of homocysteine concentrations with a substantial risk occurring between 10 and 15 μmol/L (Duthie, 1999). Robinson et al. (1995) reports that any plasma tHcy level over 6.3 μmol/L represents an increased risk of CHD.

Malinow et al. (1999) and Ubbink (2001) have shown that the optimum level of plasma tHcy is <10 μmol/L. The odds ratio for the risk of developing a CHD event increases with increasing plasma tHcy. The relationship between the odds ratio and CHD is presented in Fig. 41.5.

A systematic review and meta-analysis (Obersby et al., 2013b) demonstrated that there is strong evidence indicating that elevated plasma tHcy levels are a major independent biomarker and/or risk factor to chronic conditions, such as CVD. It indicated that elevated plasma tHcy is a risk factor in 82.8% of the CVD conditions examined. From these studies, 71.4% of the reported CVD conditions showed that plasma tHcy levels can be employed as a biomarker for the risk of developing CVD (Obersby et al., 2013b).

Obersby et al. (2013b) have suggested that normal levels of plasma tHcy need to be maintained, as a precaution to avoid increasing the risk of developing or exacerbating CVD.

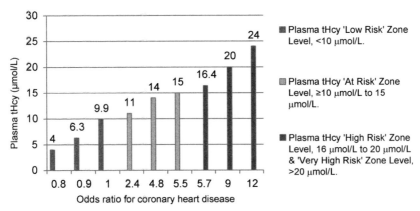

FIGURE 41.5 The odds ratio for coronary heart disease compared to plasma total homocysteine. *Adapted from Robinson et al. (1995), Boushey et al. (1995), Ueland et al. (2000), Ubbink (2001), Stanger et al. (2003), and Obersby et al. (2013b).*

7. Main Conclusions

The following conclusions can be deduced from the aforementioned data:

1. An inverse relationship exists between plasma tHcy and serum B_{12}, from which it can be concluded that the normal source is from animal products, and those who omit this from their diet are destined to show that feature of vitamin B_{12} deficiency.

2. Vegans have the highest mean plasma tHcy of 16.4 μmol/L and the lowest mean serum vitamin B_{12} of 172 pmol/L, which theoretically corresponds to an odds ratio of developing CHD of 5.7, while according to some estimates in LVs and OLVs, mean plasma tHcy is 13.9 μmol/L with a mean serum vitamin B_{12} of 209 pmol/L, which theoretically corresponds to an odds ratio of developing CHD of 4.8. Omnivores have the lowest mean plasma tHcy of 11 μmol/L and the highest mean serum vitamin B_{12} of 303 pmol/L, which theoretically corresponds to an odds ratio of developing CHD of 2.4 according to some estimates. It is noted, however, that this slightly high mean plasma tHcy may be due to a deficiency of folate and not vitamin B_{12} as omnivore diets are notoriously low in folate.

3. Vegetarian diets generally provide adequate amounts of nutrients that concur in the regulation of Hcy, with the exception of vitamin B_{12}, TMG, and choline. However, TMG and choline only play a minor role in reducing homocysteine.

4. In vegetarians with mild hyperhomocysteinemia, plasma tHcy are strongly affected by methionine intake, in a quasilinear way. This indicates that concentrations of plasma tHcy can be exacerbated by the consumption of high methionine-containing foods.

5. LVs and OLVs and particularly vegans should consider supplementing their diet with methylcobalamin, the only form of vitamin B_{12} that can directly reduce plasma tHcy to reduce the risk of developing homocysteine-related primary CVD.

Methylcobalamin would also avoid the potential conversion problems associated with other forms of vitamin B_{12} that are more commonly employed in supplementation.

References

Amores-Sanchez, M.I., Medina, M.A., 2000. Methods for the determination of plasma total homocysteine: a review. Clin. Chem. Lab. Med. 38 (3), 199–204.

Basu, T.K., Dickerson, J.W.T., 1996. Vitamins in Human Health and Disease. CAB International, Oxford.

Bates, C.J., 1999. Plasma pyridoxal phosphate (P-5-P) and pyridoxic acid their relationship to plasma homocysteine in a representative sample of British men and women aged 65 years and over. Br. J. Nutr. 81, 191–201.

Bella, D.L., Hirschberger, L.L., Kwon, Y.H., Stipanuk, M.H., 2002. Cysteine metabolism in periportal and perivenous hepatocytes: cells have greater capacity for glutathione production and taurine bit not for cysteine catabolism. Amino Acids 23, 454–458.

Bicikova, M., 2001. Effect of treatment of hypothyroidism on plasma concentrations of neuroactive steroids and homocysteine. Clin. Chem. Lab. Med. 39 (8), 753–757.

Bor, M.V., Lydeking-Olsen, E., Meller, J., Nexe, E., 2006. A daily intake of approximately 6 µg vitamin B_{12} appears to saturate all vitamin B_{12} related variables in Danish post-menopausal women. Am. J. Clin. Nutr. 83, 52–58.

Boushey, C.J., Beresford, S.A., Omenn, G.S., Motulsky, A.G., 1995. A quantitative assessment of plasma homocysteine as a risk factor for vascular disease: probable benefits of increasing folic acid intakes. J. Am. Med. Assoc. 274, 1049–1057.

Breksa, A.P., Garrow, T.A., 1999. Recombinant human liver betaine-homocysteine S-methyltransferase: identification of three cysteine residues critical for zinc binding. Biochemistry 38, 13991–13998.

Brouwer, I.A., Verhoef, P., Urgent, R., 2000. Betaine supplementation and plasma homocysteine in healthy volunteers. Archiv. Intern. Med. 160, 2546–2547.

Butensky, E., Harmatz, P., Lubin, B., 2008. Nutritional Anemias. Nutrition in Paediatrics, fourth ed. BC Decker Inc., Hamilton (Chapter 62).

Butz, L.W., du Vigneaud, V., 1932. The formation of a homologue of cysteine by the decomposition of methionine with sulphuric acid. J. Biol. Chem. 99, 135–142.

Buysschaert, M., 2001. Micro and macrovascular complications and hyperhomocysteinemia in type 1 diabetic patients. Diabetics Metab. 6, 655–659.

Chanarin, I., Deacon, R., Lumb, M., Muir, M., Perry, J., 1985. Cobalamin-folate interrelations: a critical review. Blood 66 (3), 478–489.

Cooper, B.A., Rosenblatt, D.S., 1987. Inherited defects of vitamin B_{12} metabolism. Annu. Rev. Nutr. 7, 291–320.

Dalery, K., 1995. Homocysteine and coronary artery disease in Canadian subjects: relation with vitamins B_{12}, B_6, pyridoxal phosphate and folate. Am. J. Cardiol. 75, 1107–1111.

Dart, R.C., 2006. Hydroxocobalamin for acute cyanide poisoning. Clin. Toxicol. 44, 1–3.

Dong, A., Scott, S.C., 1982. Serum vitamin B_{12} and blood cell values in vegetarians. Ann. Nutr. Metab. 26 (4), 209–216.

Doscherholmen, A., McMahon, J., Ripley, D., 1976. Inhibitory effect of eggs on vitamin B_{12} absorption: description of a simple ovalbumin co-vitamin B_{12} absorption test. Br. J. Haematol. 33, 261–272.

Dudman, N.P.B., Guo, X., Gordon, R.B., Dawson, P.A., Wilcken, D.E.L., 1996. Human homocysteine catabolism: 3 major pathways and their relevance to the development of arterial occlusive disease. J. Nutr. 126 (Suppl.), 1295S–1300S.

Duthie, S., 1999. Folic acid deficiency and cancer: mechanisms of DNA instability. Br. Med. Bull. 55, 578–592.

Elmadfa, I., Singer, I., 2009. Vitamin B_{12} and homocysteine status among vegetarians: a global perspective. Am. J. Clin. Nutr. 1693s–1698s.

European Food Safety Authority, 2015. Scientific opinion on dietary reference values for cobalamin (vitamin B_{12}). EFSA J. 13 (7), 4150.

Evens, J.C., Huddler, D.P., Jiracek, J., Castro, C., Millian, N.S., 2002. Betaine-homocysteine methyltransferase: zinc in a distorted barrel. Structure 10, 1159–1171.

Expert Group on Vitamins and Minerals, 2002. Revised Review of Vitamin B_{12}. (Online) Available from: https://cot.food.gov.uk/sites/default/files/vitmin2003.pdf.

Finkelstein, J.D., Martin, J.J., 2000. Homocysteine. Int. J. Biochem. Cell Biol. 32 (4), 385–389.

Finkelstein, J.D., Harris, B.J., Martin, J.J., Kyle, W.E., 1982. Regulation of hepatic betaine-homocysteine methyltransferase by dietary methionine. Biochem. Biophys. Res. Commun. 108, 344–348.

Finkelstein, J.D., Martin, J.J., Harris, B.J., Kyle, W.E., 1983. Regulation of hepatic betaine-homocysteine methyltransferase by dietary betaine. J. Nutr. 113, 519–521.

Finkelstein, J.D., Kyle, W.E., Harris, B., 1994. Methionine metabolism in mammals: regulatory effects of s-adenosylhomocysteine. Archiv. Biochem. 165, 77–79.

Finkelstein, J.D., 1998. The metabolism of homocysteine: pathways and regulation. Eur. J. Paediatr. 157 (2), S40–S44.

Food and Nutritional Board, Institute of Medicine, 2011. Reference Intakes: Recommended Dietary Allowances and Adequate Intakes. National Academy Press, Washington, DC.

Foods Standards Agency: McCance and Widdowson's, 2002. The Composition of Foods, Sixth Summary Edition. Royal Society of Chemistry, Cambridge.

Foods Standards Agency, 2010. Vegetarian and Vegan Diets. (Online) Available from: http://www.food.gov.uk/northernireland/nutritionni/nigourypeople/survivorform/brea.

Green, R., Miller, J.W., 2007. Vitamin B_{12}. In: Zemplent, J., Rucker, R.B., McCormick, D.B., Suttle, J.W. (Eds.), Handbook of Vitamins. CRC Press, Boca Raton, Florida, pp. 413–457.

Hall, H.H., Benedict, R.G., Wiesen, C.F., Smith, C.E., Jackson, R.W., 1953. Studies on vitamin B_{12} production with *Streptomyces olivaceus*. Appl. Microbiol. 1, 124.

Hall, A.H., Dart, R., Bogdan, G., 2007. Sodium thiosulfate or hydroxocobalamin for the empiric treatment of cyanide poisoning. Ann. Emerg. Med. 49 (6), 806–813.

Herbert, V., Colman, N., 1988. Folic acid and vitamin B_{12}. In: Shils, M., Young, V. (Eds.), Modern Nutrition in Health and Disease, seventh ed. Lea and Febiger, Philadelphia, pp. 388–416.

Herbert, V., Zalusky, R., 1962. Interrelationship of vitamin B_{12} and folic acid metabolism: folic acid clearance studies. J. Clin. Investig. 41, 1263.

Herbert, V., Drivas, G., Manusselis, C., Mackler, B., Eng, J., Schwartz, E., 1984. Are colon bacteria a major source of cobalamin analogues in human tissue? 24 hour human stool contains only about 5 mcg of cobalamin but about 100 mcg of apparent analogue and 200 mcg of folate. Trans. Assoc. Am. Physicians 97, 161–171.

Herbert, V., 1985. Biology of disease: megaloblastic anemias. Lab. Investig. 52, 3–19.

Herbert, V., 1987. Recommended dietary intakes (RDI) of vitamin B_{12} in humans. Am. J. Clin. Nutr. 45, 671–678.

Herbert, V., 1988. Vitamin B_{12}: plant sources, requirements, and assay. Am. J. Clin. Nutr. 48 (3), 852–858.

Herrmann, W., Obeid, R., Schorr, H., et al., 2005. The usefulness of holotranscobalamin in predicting vitamin B_{12} status in different clinical settings. Curr. Drug Metab. 6 (1), 47–53.

Hoffmann, B., Oberhuber, M., Stupperich, E., et al., 2000. Native corrinoids from *Clostridium cochlearium* and adeninylcobamides: spectroscopic analysis and identification of pseudovitamin B_{12} and factor A. J. Bacteriol. 182, 4773–4782.

Huang, Y.C., Chang, S.J., Chiu, C.T., et al., 2003. The status of plasma homocysteine related to B-vitamins in healthy young vegetarians and non-vegetarians. Eur. J. Nutr. 42 (2), 84–90.

Humphrey, L.L., Fu, R., Rogers, K., Freeman, M., Helfand, M., 2008. Homocysteine level and coronary heart disease: a systematic review and meta-analysis. Mayo Clin. Proc. 83 (11), 1203–1212.

Jacobsen, D.W., 2001. Practical chemistry of homocysteine and other thiols. In: Carmel, R., Jacobsen, D.W. (Eds.), Homocysteine in Health and Disease. Cambridge University Press, pp. 63–78.

Kelly, G., 1997. The coenzyme forms of vitamin B_{12}: towards an understanding of their therapeutic potential. Altern. Med. Rev. 2 (6), 459–471.

Leblanc, M., 2000. Folate and pyridoxal-5-phosphate losses during high efficiency hemodialysis in patients without hydrosoluble vitamin supplementation. J. Ren. Nutr. 10, 196–201.

Lehmann, M., Gottfries, C.G., Regland, B., 1999. Identification of cognitive impairment in the elderly: homocysteine is an early marker. Dementia 10, 12–20.

Linus Pauling Institute, 2013. Recommended Dietary Allowances. (Online) Available from: http://lpi.oregonstate.edu/infocenter/choline/ribotlavin/.

Lu, S.C., 1999. Regulation of hepatic glutathione synthesis: current concepts and controversies. FASEB J. 13, 1169–1183.

Malinow, M.R., Boston, A.G., Krauss, R.M., 1999. Homocyst(e)ine, diet, and cardiovascular diseases. Circulation 99, 178–182.

Millian, N.S., Garrow, T.A., 1998. Human betaine-homocysteine methyltransferase is a zinc metalloenzyme. Arch. Biochem. Biophys. 356, 93–98.

National Institute of Health, 2012. Factsheets, Vitamin B_{12}, B_6, Folate, Zinc. (Online) Available from: http://ods.nih.gov/factsheets/Vitamin.B12/Vitamin B6/Folate/Zinc-HealthProfessonal/.

Nelen, W.L., 2000. Homocysteine and folate levels as risk factors for recurrent early pregnancy loss. Obstet. Gynaecol. 95 (4), 136–143.

Noronha, J.M., Silverman, M., 1962. On folic acid, vitamin B_{12}, methionine and formiminoglutamic acid. In: Heinrich, H.C. (Ed.), Vitamin B_{12} and Intrinsic Factor 2 Europasches Symposion, Hamburg, p. 72.

Nygard, O., Refsum, H., Ueland, P.M., Vollset, S.E., 1998. Major lifestyle determinants of plasma total homocysteine distribution: 'The Hordaland Homocysteine Study'. Am. J. Clin. Nutr. 67, 263–270.

Obersby, D., Chappell, D.C., Dunnett, A., Tsiami, A.A., 2013a. Plasma total homocysteine status of vegetarians compared with omnivores: a systematic review and meta-analysis. Br. J. Nutr. 109, 785–794.

Obersby, D., Chappell, D.C., Tsiami, A.A., 2013b. Plasma total homocysteine and its relationship with cardiovascular disease. J. Nutr. Ther. 2 (4), 182–193.

Obersby, D., 2015. To Critically Investigate and Evaluate Supplementary Vitamin B_{12} Effects on Elevated Homocysteine Levels of Vegetarians, Who May Have a Resultant Susceptibility to Hyperhomocysteinemia Related Diseases (Ph.D. thesis). University of West London.

Pawiak, R., Lester, S.E., Babatunde, T., 2014. The prevalence of cobalamin deficiency among vegetarians assessed by serum vitamin B_{12}: a review of literature. Eur. J. Clin. Nutr. 88 (5), 541–548.

Pezacka, E., Green, R., Jacobsen, D.W., 1990. Glutathionylcobalamin as an intermediate in the formation of cobalamin coenzymes. Arch. Biochem. Biophys. 2, 443–450.

Qureshi, A.A., Rosenblant, D.S., Cooper, B.A., 1994. Inherited disorders of cobalamin metabolism. Crit. Rev. Oncol. Haematol. 17, 133–151.

Ravaglia, G., Forti, P., Maioli, F., Chiappelli, M., Montesi, F., Bianchin, M., et al., 2006. Apolipoprotein E e4 allele affects risk of hyperhomocysteinemia in the elderly. Am. J. Clin. Nutr. 84, 1473–1480.

Refsum, H., Smith, A.D., Ueland, P.M., Nexo, E., Clarke, R., McPartlin, J., Johnston, C., Engback, F., Schneede, J., McPartlin, C., Scott, J.M., 2004. Facts and recommendations about total homocysteine determinations: 'an expert opinion'. Clin. Chem. 50, 3–32.

Refsum, H., Ueland, P., Nygard, O., Vollset, S.E., 1998. Homocysteine and cardiovascular disease. Annu. Rev. Med. 49, 31–62.

Robinson, K., Miller, D.P., van Lente, F., Green, R., Gupta, A., Kottke-Marchant, K., Savon, S.R., Selhub, J., Nissen, E., Kutner, M., Topol, E.T., Jacobsen, D.W., 1995. Hyperhomocysteinemia and low pyridoxal phosphate. Common and independent reversible risk factors for coronary artery disease. Circulation 92, 2825–2830.

Sakamoto, A., Nishimora, Y., Ono, H., Sakura, I.V., 2002. Betaine and homocysteine concentrations in foods. Paediatr. Int. 44, 409–413.

Sato, Y., Iwamoto, J., Kanoko, T., Satoh, K., 2005. Homocysteine as a predictive factor for hip fracture in elderly women with Parkinson's disease. Am. J. Med. 118 (11), 1250–1255.

Scott, J.M., Weir, D.G., August 15, 1981. The methyl folate trap. A physiological response in man to prevent methyl group deficiency in kwashiorkor (methionine deficiency) and an explanation for folic-acid induced exacerbation of subacute combined degeneration in pernicious anaemia. Lancet 2 (8242), 337–340.

Selhub, J., 1999. Homocysteine metabolism. Annu. Rev. Nutr. 19, 217–246.

Seshadri, S., Beiser, A., Selhub, J., Jacques, P.F., Rosenberg, I.H., D'Agostino, R.B., Wilson, P.W., Wolf, P.A., 2002. Plasma homocysteine as a risk factor for dementia and Alzheimer's disease. N. Engl. J. Med. 346 (7), 476–483.

Shepherd, G., Velez, L.I., 2006. Role of hydroxocobalamin in active cyanide poisoning. Ann. Pharmacother. 42 (5), 661–669.

Stamm, E.B., Reynolds, R.D., 1999. Plasma total homocystein(e)ine may not be the most appropriate index for cardiovascular disease risk. J. Nutr. 129, 1927–1930.

Stanger, O., Herrmann, W., Pietrzik, K., Fowler, B., Geisel, J., Dierkes, J., Weger, M., 2003. Homocysteine [German, Austrian and Swiss Homocysteine Society]: consensus paper on the rational clinical use of homocysteine, folic acid and B vitamins in cardiovascular and thrombotic disease: guidelines and recommendations. Clin. Chem. Lab. Med. 41 (11), 1392–1403.

Stipanuk, M.H., Londono, M., Hirschberger, L.L., Hickey, C., Thiel, D.J., Wang, L., 2004. Evidence for expression of a single distinct form of mammalian cysteine dioxygenase. Amino Acids 26, 99–106.

Stupperich, E., Nexo, E., 1991. Effect of the cobalt-N coordination on the cobamide recognition by the human vitamin B_{12} binding proteins intrinsic factor, transcobalamin and haptocorrin. Eur. J. Biochem. 199, 299–303.

The Economic and Social Research Institute, 2011. World Population of Vegetarians. (Online) Available from: http://www.answers.com/worldpopulationofvegetarians.

The European Food Safety Authority, 2008. Scientific opinion on 5-deoxyadenosylcobalamin and methylcobalamin as sources of vitamin B_{12} added as a nutritional substance in food supplements. Eur. Food Saf. Auth. 815, 1–21.

Thorn, C.F., 2010. Folate Cycle Pathway. (Online) Available from: https://www.pharmgkb.org/search/pathway/folate-cycle/folate-cycle.jsp.

Toft, J.C., Toft, H., 2001. Hyperhomocysteinemia and hypothyroidism. Ugeskr. Laeg. 163 (34), 4593–4594.

Townsend, J.H., Davis, S.R., Mackey, A.D., Gregory, J.F., 2004. Folate deprivation reduces homocysteine remethylation in a human intestinal epithelial cell culture model: role of serine in one-carbon donation. Am. J. Physiol. Gastrointest. Liver Physiol. 286, G588–G595.

Ubbink, J.B., 1995. Results of B-vitamin supplementation study used in a prediction model to define a reference range for plasma homocysteine. Clin. Chem. 41, 1033–1037.

Ubbink, J.B., 2001. What is a desirable homocysteine level? In: Carmel, R., Jacobsen, D.W. (Eds.), Homocysteine in Health and Disease. CamUp, pp. 485–490.

Ueland, P.M., Refsum, H., Beresford, M., Vollset, S.E., 2000. The controversy over homocysteine and cardiovascular risk. Am. J. Clin. Nutr. 72, 324–332.

USDA Agricultural Research Service, 2014. National Database for Standard Reference Release 26. Available from: ndb.nal.usda.gov/ndb/search/list.

Verhoef, P., Stampfer, M.J., Buring, J.E., Gazianio, J.M., Allen, R.H., Stabler, S.P., Reynolds, R.D., Kok, F.J., Hennekens, C.H., Willett, W.C., 1996. Homocysteine metabolism and risk of myocardial infarction: relation with vitamins B_6, B_{12}, and folate. Am. J. Epidemiol. 143 (9), 845–859.

Wald, D.S., Law, M., Morris, J.K., 2002. Homocysteine and cardiovascular disease: evidence on causality from a meta-analysis. Br. Med. J. 325 (7374), 1202.

Warren, M.J., Raux, E., Schubert, H.L., Escalante-Semerena, J.C., 2002. The biosynthesis of adenosylcobalamin (vitamin B_{12}). J. R. Soc. Chem. 19, 390–412.

Watanabe, F., Yabuta, Y., Bito, T., Teng, F., 2014. Vitamin B_{12}-containing plant food sources for vegetarians. Nutrients 6 (5), 1861–1873.

Watanabe, F., Katsura, H., Takenaka, S., Fujita, T., Abe, K., Tamura, Y., Nakatsuka, T., Nakano, Y., 1999. Pseudovitamin B_{12} is the predominate cobamide of an algal health food, spirulina tablets. J. Agric. Food Chem. 47, 4736–4741.

Watanabe, F., 2007. Vitamin B_{12} sources and bioavailability. Exp. Biol. Med. 232, 1266–1274.

Weinstein, S.J., Ziegler, R.G., Selhub, J., Fears, T.R., Strickler, H.D., Brinton, L.A., Hamman, R.F., Levine, R.S., Mallin, K., Stolley, P.D., 2001. Elevated serum homocysteine levels and increased risk of invasive cervical cancer in US women. Cancer Causes Control 12 (4), 317–324.

Wu, L.L., Wu, J.T., 2002. Hyperhomocysteinemia is a risk factor for cancer and a new potential tumour marker. Clin. Chim. 322 (1–2), 21–28.

Zeisel, S.H., Blvsztajn, J.K., 1994. Choline and human nutrition. Annu. Rev. Nutr. 14, 269–296.

Zeisel, S.H., Mar, M.H., Howe, J.C., Holden, J.M., 2003. Concentrations of choline-containing compounds and betaine in common foods. J. Nutr. 133, 1302–1307.

Further Reading

Antony, A.C., 2003. Vegetarianism and vitamin B_{12} (cobalamin) deficiency. Am. J. Clin. Nutr. 78 (1), 3–6.

Craig, W.J., 2009. Position of the American Dietetic Association: vegetarian diets. J. Am. Diet. Assoc. 109 (7), 1266–1282.

Egekeze, J.O., Oehme, F.W., 1980. Cyanides and their toxicity. Vet. Q. 2 (2), 104–114.

Key, T.J., Appleby, P.N., Rosell, S., 2006. Health effects of vegetarian and vegan diets. Proc. Nutr. Soc. 65, 35–41.

Watanabe, F., Miyamoto, E., Fujita, T., Takenaka, H., Tanioka, Y., Nakano, Y., 2007. Purification and characterization of a corrinoid compounds from the dried powder of an edible cyanobacterium, *Nostoc commune* (ishikurage). J. Nutr. Sci. Vitaminol. 53, 183–186.

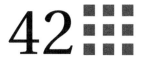

42

Iodine Status, Thyroid Function, and Vegetarianism

Emilie Combet

UNIVERSITY OF GLASGOW, GLASGOW, UNITED KINGDOM

Vegetarian diets, when well planned, have the potential to be balanced and provide the full range of nutrients essential to sustain health. In some instances, especially for the more restrictive diets excluding all animal products, i.e., vegan diets, there is a need to use supplemented foods or dietary supplements to meet reference values. While those following vegetarian diets in developed countries, who are usually well-educated, health conscious, and likely to adhere to published recommendations and guidelines (Sobiecki et al., 2016), some groups may be more vulnerable to nutrient deficiencies. These groups include vegetarians following a vegan diet, women of child-bearing age (peri-conception and during pregnancy), as well as teenagers and those who have recently adopted a vegetarian dietary pattern (Craig et al., 2009). This chapter focuses in particular on iodine nutrition and its role for thyroid function in the context of the vegetarian diets.

1. The Thyroid and Iodine

The thyroid is a gland located in the neck, responsible for the production of the thyroid hormones. Iodine, a trace element obtained from the diet, is an essential component of the two thyroid hormones: thyroxine (tetra-iodo-thyronine, or T_4) and its active metabolite tri-iodo-thyronine (T_3). These thyroid hormones consist of two coupled tyrosine molecules to which four (T_4) or three (T_3) iodine atoms are attached. T_3 and T_4 are critical for normal early neurodevelopment (especially in utero and during lactation) and metabolism throughout life, with implications for cardiovascular health later in life.

Iodide is effectively taken up from the gut lumen (from our food) into the blood and from the blood to the thyroid (via sodium/iodine symporters) (Glinoer, 2001). Depending on iodine stores in the thyroid gland, the anterior pituitary gland secretes thyroid stimulating hormone (TSH) to stimulate this transfer. After entering the thyroid gland, the iodide is oxidized to iodine and bound to the tyrosine residues of thyroglobulin (by the heme-dependent thyroid peroxidase), to form monoiodotyrosines and diiodotyrosines. These are then coupled into T_3 and T_4 by thyroperoxidase and proteases. Under the action of TSH, T_3 and T_4 are then released in the bloodstream.

Vegetarian and Plant-Based Diets in Health and Disease Prevention. http://dx.doi.org/10.1016/B978-0-12-803968-7.00042-3

The iodine-replete body excretes most of the iodine ingested in urine and feces (~9:1 ratio, unchanged in pregnancy) (Jahreis et al., 2001). The excreted iodine, referred to as urinary iodine (UI, expressed as a concentration in microgram per liter of urine or, less often, per gram of creatinine), is therefore a direct reflection of what has been consumed in the preceding hours, and not necessarily a reflection of the true background iodine status. When iodine intake is not meeting demand, thyroid–iodine stores diminish. The first hormone to decrease is T_4, accompanied by an increase in TSH. An early manifestation of this is adaptation to increase uptake of iodide from the blood (and possibly the intestine) accompanied by decreased urinary excretion (Zimmermann and Andersson, 2012).

Given that iodine is extensively stored in the thyroid, it can safely be consumed intermittently, which makes use of iodine-rich ingredients, in a range of foods, attractive, with occasional intake enough to ensure iodine sufficiency.

2. Thyroid Health and Nutrition in Pregnancy

A particular vulnerable period is the time of peri-conception and pregnancy, as maternal iodine requirements increase to meet the needs of the fetus. Although few people have frank iodine deficiency and dietary hypothyroidism, a low or marginal intake will present a potential hazard in pregnancy because of the increased demand placed on maternal thyroid function (Glinoer, 2004).

While hypothyroidism complicates some pregnancies (Abalovich et al., 2002), it does not preclude hypothyroid women to become pregnant (Montoro et al., 1981), making iodine intake crucial during the period surrounding childbearing. When the iodine intake is below the recommended intake (250 μg/day in pregnancy; World Health Organization, 2007; although a new threshold value of 200 μg/day has been proposed; EFSA NDA Panel, 2014), adequate secretion of the thyroid hormones may still be achieved by physiological adaptation. Modifications of thyroid and pituitary activities increase TSH secretion, which enhances production of T_3 relative to T_4 and rapid iodine turnover (Delange and Lecomte, 2000), but fetal supply and placental transfer remain low, as it is primarily maternal T_4, and not T_3 that crosses the placenta.

Since the fetal thyroid is not functional in the first trimester, transfer of iodine to the fetus only becomes essential after about week 16 of gestation, when the fetal thyroid starts to function. During the first trimester especially, severe disruption of thyroid hormone delivery to the fetus through maternal iodine deficiency has been shown to be associated with adverse pregnancy outcomes including spontaneous miscarriage, fetal death, preterm delivery, fetal distress, small head circumference, low birth weight, and impaired neuropsychological development (Glinoer, 2007). Mild iodine deficiency (ID) can also result in a range of developmental impairments including poor visual-motor performance and motor skills, decreased neuromotor and perceptual ability, and lower developmental and intelligence quotients associated with ID (Delange, 2001). There have been cases of transient neonatal hypothyroidism attributed to very low maternal iodine status (and thyroid function) linked with veganism. In this case, the child had a goiter at 10 days of life and elevated TSH. Thyroxine prescription and feeding with an iodine-rich formula reversed the symptoms. However, the long-term impact of the ID on the infant cognition will not be clear until later (Shaikh et al., 2003).

Low maternal iodine status in pregnancy (individual iodine-to-creatinine ratios below 150 μg/g in spot urine samples) was associated with decreased cognitive functions in the ALSPAC cohort (*n*=1040 children) from the south of England (Bath et al., 2013) and the Tasmanian Gestational Iodine Cohort (*n*=228) (Hynes et al., 2013). While the dietary iodine is not scarce in these regions (Mian et al., 2009), the explanation may be that many of the young female population commonly exclude fish and/or dairy products from their diets, for social or other reasons, leading to either low or marginal iodine intakes (Olsen, 2003).

3. Nutrients and Dietary Compounds Affecting Thyroid Function

Other nutrients, beside iodine, are important to sustain thyroid function. They include selenium and iron. Selenium is an essential component of the selenoproteins. These selenoproteins are ubiquitous in the thyroid cells, and they include the iodothyronine deiodinases (which scavenge iodide and produce active thyroid hormone), thioredoxinreductase, and glutathione peroxidase, which are essential to protect the cells against free radical damage otherwise generated by hydrogen peroxide (itself essential to the thyroid hormone production) (De Fusco et al., 2013; Zimmermann and Köhrle, 2002; Rayman, 2012). In individuals deficient in both selenium and iodine, it is likely that selenium deficiency mitigates hypothyroidism; supplementation with selenium is therefore not recommended until iodine levels are corrected (since selenium supplementation can stimulate thyroxin metabolism via iodothyronine deiodinase) (Contempre et al., 1991).

The contribution of iron to thyroid function may also take place via heme-containing enzymes. In the early stages of thyroid hormone formation, iodide is incorporated to the tyrosine residues of thyroglobulin by the heme-dependent thyroid peroxidase. As such, both selenium and iron deficiency can influence thyroid function and may influence the response to iodine prophylaxis (Zimmermann and Köhrle, 2002).

Vitamin A and zinc are also important, although mechanisms are less clear. Zinc may be an important component of the thyroid hormone receptor (Olivieri et al., 1996). Vitamin A may play a role in the activation of the pituitary receptor, with deficiency increasing TSH secretion (Zimmermann et al., 2004).

It is important to consider the impact of supplementing with selenium and vitamin A in iodine-deficient populations, as supplementations could otherwise precipitate or aggravate hypothyroidism (Olivieri et al., 1996; Zimmermann, 2007).

Another class of dietary compounds commonly classified as "goitrogens" have been reported to influence thyroid function. This evidence has, however, been mostly collected in animals. Goitrogenic substances include soy isoflavones (genistein and daidzein, via inhibition of thyroid peroxidase activity in rats), perchlorate (an environmental contaminant, competitively inhibiting the sodium/iodine symporter), thiocyanate (from cigarettes, another competitive inhibitor of sodium/iodine symporter), and thiocyanate (found in Brassica vegetables including broccoli, sprouts, cabbages) (Cao et al., 2010; Gaitan, 1990).

4. Iodine Nutrition, Food Sources

4.1 Dairy, Fish

Dairy and seafood are the main dietary sources of iodine in Europe (Haldimann et al., 2005). In areas with historical endemic goiter (in the United Kingdom, endemic goitre was referred to as the "Derbyshire neck") clinical dietary hypothyroidism was eliminated, in what was termed an accidental public health success, following change to farming practice and supplementation of dairy herds (Phillips, 1997). Dairy/milk intake was the major contributor to the decreased occurrence of goiter (a visible symptom of iodine insufficiency) in the United Kingdom.

Further changes in farming practice, including the decreased use of iodophores for milking (to sanitize the udder, resulting in leaching of iodine in the milk), organic farming, and formulation of fortified cattle feeds, mean that less iodine is now present in milk (Bath et al., 2012), with dairy intake and especially milk intake steadily decreasing since 1975 (Elwood, 2005). Milk, however, remains a good source of iodine, contributing to 22%–47% of the total iodine intake in the United Kingdom (Chambers, 2015). A substantial proportion of the young female population excludes at least one of the iodine-rich food groups (dairy/fish) from their diets, leading to either low or marginal iodine intake (Mian et al., 2009). Indeed, we have shown that women struggle to reach the recommended iodine daily intake (140 µg/day for non-pregnant adults, the reference nutrient intake (RNI), which would provide an amount sufficient to meet the needs of the majority of the population) (Combet et al., 2015; Lampropoulou et al., 2012). This will be the case for vegetarians. Meanwhile, 70 µg/day, the lower RNI (LRNI) for adults, was defined as the minimum intake necessary to avoid goiter in a population (Scientific Advisory Committee on Nutrition, 2014).

4.2 Salt

While iodine fortification of common foods (salt, bread) is widespread, it is not enacted in all countries. There is no requirement for iodine fortification of foods in the United Kingdom, and iodine fortification is therefore unusual. With growing concern that subclinical ID may be emerging in post-industrial countries previously assumed to be iodine sufficient, there is currently very little evidence about the need for specific dietary advice or for iodine fortification/supplementation targeted toward these two key vulnerable groups: young women and their infants. In the absence (or in the case of poor uptake) of universal salt iodization (USI), iodine is mostly secured via consumption of seafood and dairy products. This is a particular challenge for those following a vegetarian or vegan diet. In the United Kingdom, where there is no prophylaxis, consumption of iodine supplements is virtually nonexistent, with iodized salt used by less than 5% (Lazarus, 2007).

In contrast to mandatory fortification (a national public health measure, usually monitored), voluntary fortification is a commercial choice to add nutritional value to a food product (Casala et al., 2014), and it has been monitored since 2007 by the European Union (EC Regulation, 1925, 2006) to protect consumers. USI is the main method of iodine prophylaxis worldwide (World Health Organization, 2014), with USI adopted in over 120 countries. Iodine deficiency disorders have been successfully eliminated or controlled in many countries as a result of this public health strategy in combination with diet diversification. However, studies in numerous countries, including Italy (Marchioni et al., 2008), Turkey (Kut et al., 2010), Tasmania (Burgess et al., 2007), France (Raverot et al., 2012), and Belgium (Vandevijvere et al., 2013), showed that ID in pregnant women persisted even after the application of USI. Despite recent implementation of mandatory fortification of bread with iodized salt, a large proportion of Australian pregnant women also remain iodine deficient unless they take iodine-containing supplements (Charlton et al., 2010, 2013).

To date, there is no mandatory or voluntary measure for salt iodization in the United Kingdom. There is still a concern, among some clinical and public health professionals, that attributing a positive, health-promoting characteristic to salt may blunt the public health effort toward salt reduction in relation to the prevention of cardiovascular diseases. This is despite a recent joint WHO/ICCIDD meeting highlighting that it is possible to synergize salt reduction and iodine fortification agendas, assuming the appropriate level of coordination (World Health Organisation, 2014).

4.3 Seaweed

Seaweed or edible algae, a food produced on the coast of many countries, is a rich source of micronutrients. Data on seaweed consumption are lacking, despite the fact that it is a rich source of iodine. A key issue is the wide variation in the iodine content between species (from 16 to 8165 µg/g) (Teas et al., 2004; Bouga and Combet, 2015). Seaweed consumption, mainly when seaweed is kelp, can lead to very high iodine intake, and excretion in the urine. Indeed, Leung et al. measured urinary excretion of iodine at 9437 µg/L in a kelp-consuming vegan, likely to denote an excessive intake (the reference range being 100–300 µg/L; Leung et al., 2011).

Due to the large variations in the iodine content of seaweed, consumption is usually not recommended. High iodine intake has potential health consequences, which are discussed further on in this chapter.

4.4 Supplements

The iodine content of dietary supplements varies a lot, and intakes are generally poorly reported in the literature. From the point of view of the most restrictive vegetarian diets (vegan), certain nutrients, including B_{12} and iodine, should be obtained from supplements. Kelp tablets containing very high amounts of iodine are not recommended.

5. Assessing Iodine Sufficiency and Iodine Intake

For epidemiological purposes, iodine insufficiency is defined as a population, or subgroup, with a median urinary concentration (UIC) less than 100 µg/L for non-pregnant adults, and below 150 µg/L for groups of pregnant women (World Health Organization, 2007). The WHO criteria for iodine sufficiency in non-pregnant adult populations is based on UI concentration of 100–200 µg/L. Mild ID at population level is defined as a median UI < 100 µg/L, moderate deficiency as UI < 50 µg/L, and severe deficiency as UI < 20 µg/L (WHO/UNICEF/ICCIDD, 2007).

It is also possible to measure the dietary iodine intake, using dietary assessment techniques. These will typically rely on weighed or estimated food diaries or food frequency questionnaires (Combet and Lean, 2014; Rasmussen et al., 2001). A limitation for both of these methods is the reliance on national food composition tables, which are often inadequate or incomplete to provide a sufficiently accurate picture for this nutrient. In populations where iodine is secured mostly via iodized salt, dietary assessment might be less useful and able to derive meaningful values, because of error in the estimation of salt intake (Schüpbach et al., 2015). Lightowler and Davies (1998, 2002) have used the duplicate diet method, where participants set aside the equivalent foods that they have eaten for chemical analysis. While more precise and accurate, the method is also burdensome and costly.

ID is a global threat affecting 2 billion individuals worldwide. In Europe, despite commitment to eradicate ID, 21 countries (out of 35) declared no mandatory iodine fortification, leaving 24.2 million children (34% of the age groups) exposed to ID (Lazarus, 2014; Zimmermann and Boelaert, 2015). While ID is not necessarily "visible," it has lifelong consequences and a financial cost, estimated to short of 1 billion Euros for health care in Germany alone (Kahaly and Dietlein, 2002). ID is highlighted by the World Health Organization as a major public health issue and the most preventable cause of mental retardation and brain damage (Zimmermann and Andersson, 2012).

Previously, the United Kingdom has been assumed to be iodine replete; however, a survey of British school girls aged 14–15 years in 2011 (Vanderpump et al., 2011) demonstrated otherwise, with a median UIC of 80 µg/L. While young children aged 8–10 years old are sufficient (median 144 µg/L) (Bath et al., 2015), females of childbearing age (median 75–85 µg/L) (Lampropoulou et al., 2012; Bath et al., 2014) and breast-feeding women (median 79 µg/L) (Bouga et al., 2014) are iodine insufficient. This scenario remains true for numbers of other developed countries that, contrary to the United Kingdom, have implemented an iodization strategy. It also highlights entry in adolescence as a key point for changed dietary behaviors related to iodine nutrition.

6. Iodine Intake and Status in Ovolactovegetarians and Vegans

There are few comprehensive cross-sectional studies assessing the iodine status of individuals following a vegetarian or vegan diet, and the usefulness of the data will be highly dependent on the dietary assessment tool used. Dietary assessment is not the preferred method to estimate sufficiency for iodine, with urinary excretion the more widely used method. Indeed, while a RNI (140 μg/day) and LRNI (70 μg/day) are used in the United Kingdom, there are no estimated average requirements (EAR). The Institute of Medicine states an EAR of 95 μg/day (approximating the mean turnover of iodine by the thyroid in healthy adults).

Dietary iodine intake, reported by Sobiecki et al. (2016), Kristensen et al. (2015), Waldmann et al. (2003), Lightowler and Davies (1998, 2002), Rauma et al. (1994) and Draper et al. (1993), for vegetarian diets varied a lot, depending on dietary assessment methods and country of evaluation. Vegetarian iodine intakes were close or above the RNI of 140 μg/day (and EAR of 95 μg/day) for the EPIC-Oxford study (mean 141–146 μg/day) (Sobiecki et al., 2016), and the study by Draper (126 and 167 μg/day) (Draper et al., 1993), but not in the German Vegan Study (intake of 88 and 78 μg/day) (Waldmann et al., 2003). The iodine intake for the vegan groups was consistently below recommendation, with values ranging from 42 μg/day to 98 μg/day (Table 42.1), except in the studies of Lightowler and Davies, where a higher mean intake was reported (Lightowler and Davies, 1998, 2002). This higher intake is potentially skewed by seaweed consumption by one of the volunteers, compounded by the use of the mean to describe central tendency, when the median would be more appropriate given the distribution of intake data. The duplicate diet methods also led to a much higher assessment of iodine intake. This is an important observation, since it is recognized that food composition tables may not be appropriate to estimate iodine intake in individuals following non-conventional diets. Krajcovicova-Kudlackova mentions that, for the same sample of Finnish vegans, using regional Finnish food tables, led to the estimation of a daily intake of 29 μg/day, threefold higher than when British food composition tables were used (Krajcovicova-Kudlackova et al., 2003).

Sobiecki highlights that while only 58% of the vegan group meet the recommended UK intake, all other (United Kingdom) groups, including omnivores, all nonvegan vegetarians, and pescetarians, exceed it (Sobiecki et al., 2016); however, the RNI is not the adequate reference value to estimate adequacy of intake for a population based on the number of individuals with intake below or above this value. In the German Vegan Study, only 1.3% of German vegans reached the recommended national intake of 200 μg, with no difference between vegans and ovolactovegetarians (Waldmann et al., 2003). A potential limitation of studies assessing iodine intake with FFQ, including the EPIC-Oxford study, is the lack of information on iodized salt intake and seaweed foods captured: indeed the iodine intake in vegans may have been underestimated (Sobiecki et al., 2016). This finding is echoed by all the other studies, except that of Lightowler, with both diaries and duplicate plates.

Table 42.1 Dietary Intake in Vegetarian Diets Compared to Omnivorous Diets

Author	Region		Sample Size				Dietary Method	Iodine Reference Intake: 140 (UK DRV) or 150 µg/day (WHO)				Comment
			OV	VG	VN	Others[a]		OV	VG	VN	Others[a]	
Sobiecki et al. (2016)	Oxfordshire, Buckinghamshire, and Greater Manchester, UK	M	3798	1516	269	782	FFQ	214 (85.6)	141 (77)	55 (40)	197 (85)	Mean (SD); others are fish eaters; for iodine, the value developed by the Food and Nutrition Board of the Institute of Medicine (IOM) was used as surrogate EAR
		F	14,446	5157	534	3749		214 (85)	146 (79)	54 (40)	195 (86)	
Kristensen et al. (2015)	Denmark	M	566		33		4-day weighed food diary	213 (180–269)[a]		64 (43–91)[b]		Median (IQR)
		F	691		37			178 (146–215)		65 (54–86)		
Waldmann et al. (2003)	Germany	M		48	19		2 × 9-day FFQ		88 (31)	94 (28)		Mean (SD)
		F		50	37				78 (26)	82 (34)		
Lightowler and Davies (1998)	UK	M			11		4-day duplicate diets			137 (149) (25–521)		Mean (SD) (range)
		F			19					187 (346) (25–1467)		
Lightowler and Davies (2002)	UK	M			11		4-day diaries			42 (46) (5–173)		
		F			15					1448 (3878) (12–13256)		
		M			11		4-day duplicate plate			137 (147) (25–521)		
		F			15					216 (386) (25–1467)		
Rauma et al. (1994)	Finland	M and F	12		12		7-day food records	222 (93)		29 (18)		Mean (SD); vegans following "living food diet" or raw; some with illnesses
Draper et al. (1993)	London, UK	M	16	18	13		3-day weighed diaries	244	216 (73)	98 (42)	253 (164)	Mean (SD)
		F	36	20	24			190	167 (59)	66 (22)	172 (91)	

OV, omnivores, or meat eaters; VG, vegetarians, including ovolactovegetarians; VN, vegans.
[a]Others: Sobiesk, fish eater (those who do not eat meat, but eat fish); Draper, semivegetarians who usually avoid meat.

Lightowler reported 64% males and 67% females not meeting the UK recommended intake using the duplicate plate method, and 91% and 87% using the diet diaries (Lightowler and Davies, 1998, 2002). The women's results in these studies were skewed by two participants consuming seaweed, bringing the average up significantly; moreover, the iodine content of seaweed on food composition tables was significantly higher than that measured by duplicate diet (Lightowler and Davies, 1998, 2002). Again, it is worth noting that the fact that any individual intake lower than the reference intake does not mean that this individual has an insufficient intake, and the proportion of individuals not meeting the reference intake, when this is an "adequate intake," is not a proxy for the prevalence of insufficient intake in the population.

In contrast, the prevalence of insufficient intake has been more precisely estimated in the EPIC-Oxford study (using the EAR cut-point method with the Institute of Medicine surrogate EAR of 95 µg/day), and figures for vegans were high, at 94%–93% (male/females), versus 33% for male ovolactovegetarians and 29% for female ovolactovegetarians. Of further concern, a very high proportion of female vegans had intake below the LRNI of 70 µg/day using the duplicate plate method and diet diaries (67%, 87%, respectively). The proportion of vegan males with intake below 70 µg/day remained at 91% with diet diaries, but it was 27% with the duplicate plate method (Lightowler and Davies, 1998, 2002).

All dietary assessment exercises rely on the representativeness of the diet period assessed, and the methods to quantitatively derive a nutrient intake. The findings of Lightowler identify an important issue with the adequacy of food composition tables. However, regardless which method is used, a high proportion of vegans do not apparently cover the iodine requirement.

There is very little evidence relative to the dietary behaviors of women following vegetarian diets during pregnancy. The nutrient was not part of the outcome measures in a systematic review of pregnancy outcomes for vegetarian diets (Piccoli et al., 2015). Omnivorous UK pregnant women ($n=893$) have a median daily iodine intake (including supplemental iodine) of 236 µg/day (IQR 164–320) in the first trimester of pregnancy, versus 241 µg/day (IQR 178–309) for vegetarian women ($n=75$) and 104 µg/day (IQR 38–721) for vegan women ($n=5$). While 62% of omnivorous and 73% of vegetarian women met the lower (EU) recommendation of 200 µg/day, only 20% of the vegan pregnant mothers did. The proportions meeting the higher (WHO) recommendation of 250 µg/day were slightly lower for omnivores (46%) and vegetarians (43%) with only 20% of vegan mothers meeting the WHO recommendation (Combet, unpublished data).

7. Iodine Status

Iodine status has been measured via UI excretion in five studies (Table 42.2). The studies use a range of samples, from single spot samples to repeat 24-h urine collections. The use of single spot samples are usually not adequate to define the iodine status of an individual, and repeated samples, ideally 10, are required (König et al., 2011). The use of mean, median to describe central tendency, as well as range, standard deviation, or

Table 42.2 Urinary Iodine Excretion in Vegan, Vegetarian, and Omnivorous Populations

Author	Region	Sample	Method	(n=)			Iodine µg/L			% <100 µg/L Iodine			Comments
				OV	VG	VN	OV	VG	VN	OV	VG	VN	
Leung et al. (2011, p. 67)	Boston, US	M and F	Urinary spot		78	62	164[a]	78 (7–965)a	147 (9–779)b				Median (range)
Elorinne et al. (2016)	Finland	M and F	24-h urine×1	18		21	37 (18–86)		(5–22)	91		100	Median (IQR)
Krajcovicova-Kudlackova et al. (2003)	Slovakia	M and F	24-h urine×2	35	31	15	210 (76–423)	177 (44–273)	71 (9–204)	9	26	80	Median (range)
Schüpbach et al. (2015)	Switzerland	M and F	4×spot urine	100	53	53	83 (22–228)a	75 (1–610)a	56 (27–586)b	64	66	79	Median (min–max)

A different letter (a, b) indicates significant difference between groups.
[a]US (NHANES) adult median urinary iodine concentrations 2007–08.

interquartile range to describe dispersion renders interpretation difficult. However, again, the iodine status of vegans appears inadequate. In a cross-sectional study in Boston, the median UI was found to be significantly lower in vegans (78.5 µg/L) than ovolactovegetarians (147 µg/L) and that observed for the northeastern US population (134 µg/L) (Leung et al., 2011). Similarly, in Slovakia, the urinary excretion of iodine was significantly lower in vegans (78 µg/L) compared to ovolactovegetarians (172 µg/L) or omnivorous participants (216 µg/L). Additionally, 80% of vegan respondents were found to be below the sufficiency threshold of 100 µg/L UI excretion compared to just 9% of omnivores (Krajcovicova-Kudlackova et al., 2003). Despite iodine prophylaxis, a large majority of the Swiss omnivorous, vegetarian, and vegan samples displayed iodine concentrations below the threshold (64% for omnivores to 79% for vegans; Schüpbach et al., 2015). In Finland, UI excretion was lower than the threshold for all vegans and most omnivorous controls (91%) (Elorinne et al., 2016). In the United Kingdom, Lightowler measured iodine concentration over 4 days (with complete urine collections), with very low excretion (mean 24 µg/L and 34 µg/L for male and females, respectively) (Lightowler and Davies, 1998). These concentrations were not in line with the iodine intake determined via the duplicate plate method. Potential explanations may reside in the reduced bioavailability of iodine from certain food sources (especially seaweed) (Aquaron et al., 2002; Combet et al., 2014).

8. Supplement Usage

Information on the type of supplement usage in vegetarian diets was not always well reported or focused on iodine-containing supplements (Table 42.3). Only Lightowler and Davies and Leung identified iodine-specific supplement usage, with 17% and 40%, respectively, reporting regular consumption. According to Draper, dietary supplement contributed to only 11% of the iodine RNI, lower than the 39% reported by Lightowler using the duplicate plate method (Draper et al., 1993; Lightowler and Davies, 1998; Leung et al., 2011, p. 67). All other reports (Elorinne et al., 2016; Sobiecki et al., 2016; Schüpbach et al., 2015) point toward a minority making regular use of dietary supplements, with the exception of Draper, reporting 54% of the (small) UK sample taking (any) dietary supplements, and Kristensen et al. (2015) in Denmark, reporting 66% of vegans supplementing their diet. The larger EPIC-Oxford study reports a third of ovolactovegetarians and vegans taking dietary supplements regularly, with about half consuming multimineral-enriched multivitamins (Sobiecki et al., 2016). While ovolactovegetarians have the potential to meet their iodine requirements via consumption of milk and dairy products, fortified foods, and occasionally through seaweed consumption, vegans are restricted to seaweed or iodine-fortified foods to meet their requirement. The use of a supplement is therefore likely to be warranted, especially when considering the intake and excretion data presented.

During pregnancy, in the United Kingdom, 37% of the omnivorous pregnant women used an iodized supplement, versus 63% of vegetarian women and only 20% of the vegan women (Combet, unpublished data). This is a particular concern for vegan diets, at a time when iodine requirements are increased.

Table 42.3 Supplement Usage in Vegetarian Diets

Author	Region	Sample	n				Regular/Daily Supplement (%)				Comments
			OV	VG	VN	Others[a]	OV	VG	VN	Others[a]	
Sobiecki et al. (2016)	Oxfordshire, Buckinghamshire, and Greater Manchester, UK	M	3798	1516	269	782	19	29	35	28	Any multivitamin (iodine not specifically mentioned), multivitamin with multimineral typically represented 50% of the multivitamin supplements
		F	14,446	5157	534	3749	26	35	37	33	
Elorinne et al. (2016)	Finland	M and F	18		21		71		32		Multivitamin/multiminerals
Schüpbach et al. (2015)	Switzerland	M and F	100	53	53				43		Estimated as B12-containing supplements
Leung et al. (2011)	Boston, US	M and F		78	62			23	39		Iodine-containing supplements
Lightowler and Davies (1998)	UK	M and F			30				17		Iodine-containing supplement
Draper et al. (1993)	London, UK	M and F		52	38	37		41	54	49	Any dietary supplement

OV, omnivores, or meat eaters; VG, vegetarians, including ovolactovegetarians; VN, vegans.

[a]Others: Sobieski, fish eater (those who do not eat meat, but eat fish); Draper, semivegetarians who usually avoid meat.

9. Selenium and Iron Intake and Status

As outlined previously, iron and selenium are important for thyroid function. These two nutrients are covered in detail in dedicated chapters in this book.

Selenium intake was generally low in the vegetarian groups, which could affect thyroid function. In the EPIC-Oxford study, only 55% of the selenium reference intake was met for vegans and 47% for ovolactovegetarians (Sobiecki et al., 2016). This was also the case in Denmark, where only 34% of the vegans reached the recommended intake of selenium (Kristensen et al., 2015). However, dietary intake is not the preferred method to establish selenium status. In Finland, Elorinne reported lower selenium concentrations in vegans than in nonvegans, with those values similar to those in countries that do not add selenium to fertilizers (Finland is the only country where this happens) and above reference for both vegans and ovolactovegetarians (Elorinne et al., 2016). The readers may report to Chapter 40 for a full review of selenium intake and status in plant-based and vegetarian diets.

A plant-based diet with no supplementation can increase the risk for low iron stores, which may possibly lead to subsequent iron deficiency, especially in women. However, there is no clear evidence that such a diet, in industrialized countries, increases the risk for iron deficiency anemia. The readers may report to Chapter 39 for a full review of iron intake and status in plant-based and vegetarian diets.

In terms of iron intake, Sobiecki showed a slightly higher iron intake in vegans (18 mg) compared to ovolactovegetarians and omnivorous participants (16 mg) (Sobiecki et al., 2016). Prevalence of inadequate intake was assessed only for men and women aged over 51 in the EPIC-Oxford study (due to distribution of the data for the younger female age groups); after bioavailability adjustment, with 11%–13% of vegans (male, female, respectively) and 11%–19% of ovolactovegetarians (male, female, respectively) had inadequate intakes, versus 0.4%–0.8% of omnivorous subjects. These figures are likely to be compounded, since younger females were not included, and do not necessarily reflect iron stores. In Switzerland, there was no difference in the proportion of individuals with plasma ferritin lower than the reference range (11% of vegetarians, 13% of vegans, and 14% of omnivores) (Schüpbach et al., 2015). In Denmark, all male vegans reached the iron recommendation, but only 60% of the female vegans did (Kristensen et al., 2015).

Meanwhile, in pregnancy, a systematic review identified a risk of iron deficiency in vegan and vegetarian diets (Piccoli et al., 2015). The readers may report to Chapter 32 for a full review of vegetarian diet in pregnancy.

10. Iodine Toxicity: Prevalence in General and Links to Thyroid Health

The upper tolerable limit of iodine intake have been defined as 1.1 mg/day by the IOM in the United States and 600 µg/day by the European Food Safety Authority for healthy individuals (Goldhaber, 2003; Flynn et al., 2003; Food and Board, 2001). These thresholds are designed for the general (euthyroid) population, rather than groups with thyroid pathologies, who may have an increased sensitivity to iodine (EFSA NDA Panel, 2014). For vegan diets, a natural source of iodine is seaweed. A small daily dose of seaweed (0.5 g, equivalent to 356 μg iodine) can increase the iodine status of women (Combet et al., 2014). Moreover, a 2-week iodine supplementation with up to 500 μg/day had no impact on thyroid function tests in euthyroid subjects (Combet et al., 2014). However, regular seaweed consumption is not recommended, as consumption has been associated with concerns over both iodine toxicity (the seaweed may contain toxic levels of iodine, especially if belonging to the kelps) and ingestion of contaminants and heavy metals. In the United Kingdom, a study identified a substantial ($n=26$) range of retailed food products that, if consumed, could lead to an iodine intake higher than the TUL of 600 μg/day (Bouga and Combet, 2015). Large (excessive) iodine intake can inhibit the formation of thyroid hormones and increase plasma TSH, a phenomenon known as the Wolff-Chaikoff effect, which is transient and uncommon in Western countries. Restricting seaweed intake postacute exposure can reverse the iodine-induced goiter and transient hypothyroidism (Zava and Zava, 2011).

11. Thyroid Diseases and Vegetarianism

Chronic iodine insufficiency may lead to hypothyroidism (an elevated TSH level, accompanied with a decreased free T_4 level in overt hypothyroidism, or normal free T_4 in subclinical hypothyroidism). Several studies reported that iodine-insufficient populations were diagnosed with iodine-induced hyper- or hypothyroidism following high iodine intake (Roti and Degli Uberti, 2001; Leung and Braverman, 2012; Emder and Jack, 2011; Camargo et al., 2008).

Smaller studies, such as that of Leung, found no significant difference in the TSH levels between vegans (median 1.1 mUI/L) and vegetarians (median 1.38 mUI/L) (Leung et al., 2011). In this study, only one vegan participant had a TSH value over 5.5 mUI/L. In the study of Key et al. (1992), vegans had a slightly elevated TSH compared to omnivorous participants (geometric mean thyroid stimulating hormone concentrations 2.4 mUI/L; 95% CI 2.0–2.8) and 1.7 mUI/L (1.5–2.0), respectively). Five of the 48 vegans but none of the 53 omnivores had a TSH concentration above 5 mUI/L. Only one vegan was hypothyroxinemic. The three who took kelp were hypothyroid (two subclinical and one overt).

The Adventist Health Study-2 is a large cohort study of a religious group where the consumption of a plant-based diet is advocated (over 96,000 church members). In this group, there was no association between vegan diets and the prevalence of incidence of hypothyroidism (OR 0.89, CI 95% 0.78–1.01, and OR 0.78, 95% CI 0.59–1.03, respectively) (Tonstad et al., 2013). However, an ovolactovegetarian diet was associated with slightly elevated odds for the prevalence of hypothyroidism (1.09, 95% CI 1.01–1.18), but not the incidence. While iodized salt use was not determined per se, salt use more than once a day was associated with elevated odds of prevalent hypothyroidism (OR 1.15 1.05–1.25) (Tonstad et al., 2013). However, in a more recent report focusing on a subsample of the Adventist Health Study-2 ($n=843$), Tonstad found that those with elevated TSH (>5 mUI/L) were more likely to be women following a vegan or vegetarian diet. High

TSH was not always correlated with hypothyroidism diagnosis, with 13 out of 43 women and 2 out of 23 men with high TSH having received a hypothyroidism diagnosis. This may be confounded partly by attitudes to health management of this group (Tonstad et al., 2015a).

The cause of hyperthyroidism (low to undetectable TSH, with high T_3 and T_4) is most often thyroid autoimmunity (Graves' disease). While dietary causes of hyperthyroidism are rare, excess dietary iodine is a potential cause of hyperthyroidism. In the same Adventist Health Study-2, the prevalence of hyperthyroidism was 0.9% (compared to general US population 1.2%–1.3%; NHANES III). Vegan and vegetarian diets were both associated with a lower incidence of hyperthyroidism in the previous 12 months (OR 0.49, 95% CI 0.33–0.72 and 0.65, 95% CI 0.53–0.81, respectively). This was only the case for ovolactovegetarian diets (OR 0.77, 95% CI 0.66–0.89), not vegan diets, when the diagnosis or treatment of hyperthyroidism any time prior to the assessment was taken in consideration. This may be linked to the length of time the diet pattern was adopted (Tonstad et al., 2015b). Predictors of hypothyroidism and hyperthyroidism include age and being female and overweight or obese. As such, vegan and ovolactovegetarian diets may be protective via the lower BMI of these diet groups (Rosell et al., 2006). In an iodine-sufficient pregnant population in India, Jaiswal showed that vegetarian women did not have lower iodine intakes or higher risk of hypothyroidism than their omnivorous counterparts; however, overweight/obesity and anemia predicted thyroid insufficiency (Jaiswal et al., 2014).

No studies, to date, have looked at the specific incidence of thyroid cancer in those following a vegetarian or vegan diet. There are two major histological subtypes of differentiated thyroid cancer: papillary carcinoma and follicular carcinoma. Genetic susceptibility is an important risk factor; however, dietary causes have also been examined (Dal Maso et al., 2009). Iodine-rich and iodine-deficient diets have both been linked to the incidence of these cancers, and a small increase in the risk of thyroid cancer has been reported when iodine was supplemented in areas of previous deficiency (Szybiński et al., 2002; Zimmermann et al., 2004; Zimmermann and Galetti, 2015). The mechanism is, however, not clear. ID is a clear risk factor for goiter and thyroid nodules (Knudsen et al., 2002), and goiter and nodules are themselves a clear risk factor for thyroid cancer (risk ratio 3.4 to 5.9, 30 with history of benign nodules/adenoma). Epidemiological evidence has linked high consumption of seaweed/iodine with higher thyroid cancer risk in Japan (Michikawa et al., 2012); however, this observation was not supported by experimental studies in rats with chronic high iodine intake (up to 1 g/L in drinking water) (Takegawa et al., 2000). In a 2015 meta-analysis, there was, however, no association found between dietary iodine intake and thyroid cancer risk (RR: 0.83; 95% CI: 0.49–1.42) (Cho and Kim, 2015).

12. Goitrogens and Thyroid Function

Certain dietary factors, the goitrogens, are believed to limit the ability of the body to utilize iodine. Goitrogenic foods include (1) cruciferous vegetables (i.e., broccoli, kale, and cabbage) that contain thioglucosides, which are metabolized to thiocyanates and inhibit iodine uptake from the thyroid gland, (2) sweet potatoes, cassava, and lima beans, which contain cyanogenic glucosides that may be metabolized into thiocyanates as well, and (3) soy products and millet, which contain flavonoids, believed to have "antithyroid" activity via thyroperoxidase inhibition (it is not clear whether it is soy/millet flavonoids that exert this activity or all flavonoids), contributing to the genesis of endemic goiter (Gaitan, 1990, 1996). Drinking water and eating foods that contain perchlorate may inhibit of iodine uptake by the thyroid. Some of these factors will be relevant to the vegetarian diets.

In a cross-sectional study of ovolactovegetarians and vegans in Boston, no significant association between UI, perchlorate, and thiocyanate concentrations and thyroid function were found (Leung et al., 2011). In a cross-over study in the United Kingdom, short term high goitrogenic food intake in a population with marginal iodine intake did not impact thyroid function (Bouga et al., 2015). More recently, an association was demonstrated in a subsample of the Adventist Health Study (AHS-2), between soya isoflavone intakes and higher odds of high TSH concentrations in women only (OR 4·17, 95% CI 1·73, 10·06) but not in men (OR 1·05, 95% CI 0·27, 4·07) (Tonstad et al., 2015a). As just over half of the sample had UI concentration below 100 μg/L, it is possible that soy isoflavones exert an effect on thyroid function when iodine status is insufficient. Genistein aglycone, a soy-derived isoflavone, did not affect thyroid function (TSH, free T_3, free T_4) after 3 years of treatment in postmenopausal women (Bitto et al., 2010), in accordance with the results of a 6-month study that used isoflavone supplements (Bruce et al., 2003). It is perhaps important to point out that the iodine intake or excretion of these populations was not evaluated, and the outcomes may be a function of the iodine status.

The relationship between cruciferous vegetables (goitrogenic, and enriched in vegetarian diets) is not clear. Dal Maso points to a nonsignificant relationship between cruciferous vegetable intake and thyroid cancer (RR = 0.9, 95% CI: 0.8–1.1) (Dal Maso et al., 2009). Meanwhile, a case–control study in New Caledonia found an increased association between consumption of cruciferous vegetables and odds of thyroid cancer, but again only in women with low iodine intake (Truong et al., 2010). There are studies, though, that have focused on goitrogens intake from the diet.

13. Final Considerations: Nutritional Knowledge of Ovolactovegetarians and Vegans

Awareness of iodine and thyroid function is generally low among the population and health-care professionals (Williamson et al., 2012). In developed countries, those following vegetarian diets tend to be older, well educated, and health conscious. However, the low iodine intake of vegans and low supplementation demonstrates that there is a gap between knowledge and intentions. Draper showed that 57% of vegetarians and 67% of vegans believed they secured all the required nutrients from foods only. Assuming a deep knowledge of nutrition, this is of course achievable. However, in this sample, while the reference intake value was met by ovolactovegetarians, it was not met by vegans. In young Swedish and Norwegian adolescents, only 24% perceived their diet as adequate (33% for vegans), but 86% of both ovolactovegetarians and vegans felt informed sufficiently about eating for health. While 54% of ovolactovegetarians reported taking dietary supplements to prevent or treat a nutritional deficiency, 75% of vegans reported taking a dietary supplement (Larsson et al., 2001). Most ovolactovegetarians (84%) and vegans (80%) were unaware of the role of iodine in pregnancy, for the neurodevelopment of the unborn child, similar to their omnivorous counterparts (82%) (Combet, unpublished data). The role of professional and charitable organizations is important to disseminate core knowledge regarding diet and nutrition; however, Draper reported that only 56% of vegans and 28% of ovolactovegetarians belonged to such an organization. In the light of the poor iodine status and poor supplement uptake (especially in pregnancy), it is important that those following vegetarian diets (especially vegan) can make informed choices. Retail availability and intake of iodine-rich foods are essential for individuals to meet their daily iodine requirements. When table salt is available, it can contribute to the iodine status of these groups. Given that iodine is extensively stored in the thyroid, it can safely be consumed intermittently, which makes seaweed use in a range of foods attractive and occasional seaweed intake enough to ensure iodine sufficiency. However, it should be used with caution due to its high iodine content. With table salt usage falling in the United Kingdom and Europe following successful public health campaigns, it may be contradictory to portray salt as a vehicle for iodine. However, the WHO highlights that sodium reduction and salt iodization are not incompatible, and they are mostly affected by a public perception problem (World Health Organisation, 2014). Viable alternatives to increase iodine status include fortification of staple foods suitable for vegetarian diets, such as bread, with mandatory fortification already in place in Australia, New Zealand, and Denmark (Edmonds et al., 2016; Rasmussen et al., 2014; Clifton et al., 2013). The use of naturally iodine-rich seaweed as an ingredient for reformulation also offers opportunities, with dried seaweed successfully incorporated in a nutritionally balanced pizza, designed in the context of health-by-stealth improvement of ready meals (Combet et al., 2013). While these modifications to the food supply are implemented with the consumer in mind, they, however, render the process of dietary assessment even more challenging, as food composition tables do not dynamically reflect these changes.

References

Abalovich, M., Gutierrez, S., Alcaraz, G., Maccallini, G., Garcia, A., Levalle, O., 2002. Overt and subclinical hypothyroidism complicating pregnancy. Thyroid 12, 63–68.

Andersson, M., Karumbunathan, V., Zimmermann, M.B., 2012. Global iodine status in 2011 and trends over the past decade. J. Nutr. 142, 744–750.

Aquaron, R., Delange, F., Marchal, P., Lognone, V., Ninane, L., 2002. Bioavailability of seaweed iodine in human beings. Cell. Mol. Biol. 48, 563–569.

Bath, S.C., Button, S., Rayman, M.P., 2012. Iodine concentration of organic and conventional milk: implications for iodine intake. Br. J. Nutr. 107, 935–940.

Bath, S.C., Steer, C.D., Golding, J., Emmett, P., Rayman, M.P., 2013. Effect of inadequate iodine status in UK pregnant women on cognitive outcomes in their children: results from the Avon Longitudinal Study of Parents and Children (ALSPAC). Lancet 382, 331–337.

Bath, S.C., Walter, A., Taylor, A., Wright, J., Rayman, M.P., 2014. Iodine deficiency in pregnant women living in the South East of the UK: the influence of diet and nutritional supplements on iodine status. Br. J. Nutr. 111, 1622–1631.

Bath, S.C., Combet, E., Scully, P., Zimmermann, M.B., Hampshire-Jones, K.H., Rayman, M.P., 2015. A multi-centre pilot study of iodine status in UK schoolchildren, aged 8–10 years. Eur. J. Nutr. 1–9.

Bitto, A., Polito, F., Atteritano, M., Altavilla, D., Mazzaferro, S., Marini, H., Adamo, E.B., D'anna, R., Granese, R., Corrado, F., Russo, S., Minutoli, L., Squadrito, F., 2010. Genistein aglycone does not affect thyroid function: results from a three-year, randomized, double-blind, placebo-controlled trial. J. Clin. Endocrinol. Metab. 95, 3067–3072.

Bouga, M., Combet, E., 2015. Emergence of seaweed and seaweed-containing foods in the UK: focus on labeling, iodine content, toxicity and nutrition. Foods 4, 240–253.

Bouga, M., Layman, S., Mullaly, S., Lean, M.E.J., Combet, E., 2014. Iodine intake and excretion are low in British breastfeeding mothers. Nutr. Soc. Summer Meet.

Bouga, M., Cousins, F., Lean, M., Combet, E., 2015. Influence of goitrogenic foods intake on thyroid functions in healthy females of childbearing age with low habitual iodine intake. Proc. Nutr. Soc. 74, E39.

Bruce, B., Messina, M., Spiller, G.A., 2003. Isoflavone supplements do not affect thyroid function in iodine-replete postmenopausal women. J. Med. Food 6, 309–316.

Burgess, J.R., Seal, J.A., Stilwell, G.M., Reynolds, P.J., Taylor, E.R., Parameswaran, V., 2007. A case for universal salt iodisation to correct iodine deficiency in pregnancy: another salutary lesson from Tasmania. Med. J. Aust. 186, 574–576.

Camargo, R.Y.A., Tomimori, E.K., Neves, S.C., Rubio, I.G.S., Galrao, A.L., Knobel, M., Mcdeiros-Neto, G., 2008. Thyroid and the environment: exposure to excessive nutritional iodine increases the prevalence of thyroid disorders in Sao Paulo, Brazil. Eur. J. Endocrinol. 159, 293–299.

Cao, Y., Blount, B.C., Valentin-Blasini, L., Bernbaum, J.C., Phillips, T.M., Rogan, W.J., 2010. Goitrogenic anions, thyroid-stimulating hormone, and thyroid hormone in infants. Environ. Health Perspect. 118, 1332–1337.

Casala, E., Matthys, C., Péter, S., Baka, A., Kettler, S., Mcnulty, B., Stephen, A., Verkaik-Kloosterman, J., Wollgast, J., Berry, R., 2014. Monitoring and addressing trends in dietary exposure to micronutrients through voluntarily fortified foods in the European Union. Trends Food Sci. Technol. 37, 152–161.

Chambers, L., 2015. Iodine in milk–implications for nutrition? Nutr. Bull. 40, 199–202.

Charlton, K.E., Gemming, L., Yeatman, H., Ma, G., 2010. Suboptimal iodine status of Australian pregnant women reflects poor knowledge and practices related to iodine nutrition. Nutrition 26, 963–968.

Charlton, K.E., Yeatman, H., Brock, E., Lucas, C., Gemming, L., Goodfellow, A., Ma, G., 2013. Improvement in iodine status of pregnant Australian women 3 years after introduction of a mandatory iodine fortification programme. Prev. Med. 57, 26–30.

Cho, Y.A., Kim, J., 2015. Dietary factors affecting thyroid cancer risk: a meta-analysis. Nutr. Cancer 67, 811–817.

Clifton, V.L., Hodyl, N.A., Fogarty, P.A., Torpy, D.J., Roberts, R., Nettelbeck, T., Ma, G., Hetzel, B., 2013. The impact of iodine supplementation and bread fortification on urinary iodine concentrations in a mildly iodine deficient population of pregnant women in South Australia. Nutr. J. 12, 1.

Combet, E., Lean, M.E., 2014. Validation of a short food frequency questionnaire specific for iodine in UK females of childbearing age. J. Hum. Nutr. Diet.

Combet, E., Jarlot, A., Aidoo, K.E., Lean, M.E., 2013. Development of a nutritionally balanced pizza as a functional meal designed to meet published dietary guidelines. Public Health Nutr. 1–10.

Combet, E., Ma, Z.F., Cousins, F., Thompson, B., Lean, M.E., 2014. Low-level seaweed supplementation improves iodine status in iodine-insufficient women. Br. J. Nutr. 112, 753–761.

Combet, E., Bouga, M., Pan, B., Lean, M.E.J., Christopher, C.O., 2015. Iodine and pregnancy – a cross-sectional survey of maternal awareness, knowledge and practice. Br. J. Nutr. 114, 108–117.

Combet, E., Dietary Pattern and Iodine Status in the UK, (unpublished data).

Contempre, B., Bebe, N., Vanderpas, J., 1991. Effect of selenium supplementation in hypothyroid subjects of an iodine and selenium deficient area: the possible danger of indiscriminate supplementation of iodine-deficient subjects with selenium. J. Clin. Endocrinol. Metab. 73, 213–215.

Craig, W.J., Mangels, A.R., Ada, 2009. Position of the American Dietetic Association: vegetarian diets. J. Am. Diet. Assoc. 109, 1266–1282.

Dal Maso, L., Bosetti, C., La Vecchia, C., Franceschi, S., 2009. Risk factors for thyroid cancer: an epidemiological review focused on nutritional factors. Cancer Causes Control 20, 75–86.

De Fusco, C., Nettore, I.C., Colao, A., Macchia, P.E., 2013. Selenium in the thyroid: physiology and pathology. Rev. Endocrinol. Metab. 1, 34–40.

Delange, F., Lecomte, P., 2000. Iodine supplementation – benefits outweigh risks. Drug Saf. 22, 89–95.

Delange, F., 2001. Iodine deficiency as a cause of brain damage. Postgrad. Med. J. 77, 217–220.

Draper, A., Lewis, J., Malhotra, N., Wheeler, E., 1993. The energy and nutrient intakes of different types of vegetarian – a case for supplements. Br. J. Nutr. 69, 3–19.

Edmonds, J.C., Mclean, R.M., Williams, S.M., Skeaff, S.A., 2016. Urinary iodine concentration of New Zealand adults improves with mandatory fortification of bread with iodised salt but not to predicted levels. Eur. J. Nutr. 55, 1201–1212.

EFSA NDA PANEL, 2014. Scientific opinion on dietary reference values for iodine. EFSA J. 12, 57 3660.

Elorinne, A.-L., Alfthan, G., Erlund, I., Kivimaki, H., Paju, A., Salminen, I., Turpeinen, U., Voutilainen, S., Laakso, J., 2016. Food and nutrient intake and nutritional status of Finnish vegans and non-vegetarians. PLoS One 11.

Elwood, P.C., 2005. Time to value milk. Int. J. Epidemiol. 34, 1160–1162.

Emder, P.J., Jack, M.M., 2011. Iodine-induced neonatal hypothyroidism secondary to maternal seaweed consumption: a common practice in some Asian cultures to promote breast milk supply. J. Paediatr. Child Health 47, 750–752.

Flynn, A., Moreiras, O., Stehle, P., Fletcher, R.J., Muller, D.J.G., Rolland, V., 2003. Vitamins and minerals: a model for safe addition to foods. Eur. J. Nutr. 42, 118–130.

Food, I.O.M., Board, N., 2001. DRI, Dietary Reference Intakes for Vitamin A, Vitamin K, Arsenic, Boron, Chromium, Copper, Iodine, Iron, Manganese, Molybdenum, Nickel, Silicon, Vanadium, and Zinc: A Report of the Panel on Micronutrients and of Interpretation and Uses of Dietary Reference Intakes, and the Standing Committee on the Scientific Evaluation of Dietary Reference Intakes. National Academy Press.

Gaitan, E., 1990. Goitrogens in food and water. Annu. Rev. Nutr. 10, 21–39.

Gaitan, E., 1996. Flavonoids and the thyroid. Nutrition 12, 127–129.

Glinoer, D., 2001. Pregnancy and iodine. Thyroid 11, 471–481.

Glinoer, D., 2004. The regulation of thyroid function during normal pregnancy: importance of the iodine nutrition status. Best Pract. Res. Clin. Endocrinol. Metab. 18, 133–152.

Glinoer, D., 2007. The importance of iodine nutrition during pregnancy. Public Health Nutr. 10, 1542–1546.

Goldhaber, S.B., 2003. Trace element risk assessment: essentiality vs. toxicity. Regul. Toxicol. Pharmacol. 38, 232–242.

Haldimann, M., Alt, A., Blanc, A., Blondeau, K., 2005. Iodine content of food groups. J. Food Compos. Anal. 18, 461–471.

Hynes, K.L., Otahal, P., Hay, I., Burgess, J.R., 2013. Mild iodine deficiency during pregnancy is associated with reduced educational outcomes in the offspring: 9-year follow-up of the gestational iodine cohort. J. Clin. Endocrinol. Metab. 98, 1954–1962.

Jahreis, G., Hausmann, W., Kiessling, G., Franke, K., Leiterer, M., 2001. Bioavailability of iodine from normal diets rich in dairy products-results of balance studies in women. Exp. Clin. Endocrinol. Diabetes 109, 163–167.

Jaiswal, N., Melse-Boonstra, A., Thomas, T., Basavaraj, C., Sharma, S.K., Srinivasan, K., Zimmermann, M.B., 2014. High prevalence of maternal hypothyroidism despite adequate iodine status in Indian pregnant women in the first trimester. Thyroid 24, 1419–1429.

Kahaly, G.J., Dietlein, M., 2002. Cost estimation of thyroid disorders in Germany. Thyroid 12, 909–914.

Key, T., Thorogood, M., Keenan, J., Long, A., 1992. Raised thyroid stimulating hormone associated with kelp intake in British vegan men. J. Hum. Nutr. Diet. 5, 323–326.

Knudsen, N., Laurberg, P., Perrild, H., Bülow, I., Ovesen, L., Jørgensen, T., 2002. Risk factors for goiter and thyroid nodules. Thyroid 12, 879–888.

König, F., Andersson, M., Hotz, K., Aeberli, I., Zimmermann, M.B., 2011. Ten repeat collections for urinary iodine from spot samples or 24-hour samples are needed to reliably estimate individual iodine status in women. J. Nutr. 141, 2049–2054.

Krajcovicova-Kudlackova, M., Buckova, K., Klimes, I., Sebokova, E., 2003. Iodine deficiency in vegetarians and vegans. Ann. Nutr. Metab. 47, 183–185.

Kristensen, N.B., Madsen, M.L., Hansen, T.H., Allin, K.H., Hoppe, C., Fagt, S., Lausten, M.S., Gobel, R.J., Vestergaard, H., Hansen, T., Pedersen, O., 2015. Intake of macro- and micronutrients in Danish vegans. Nutr. J. 14.

Kut, A., Gursoy, A., Senbayram, S., Bayraktar, N., Budakoglu, I., Akgun, H.S., 2010. Iodine intake is still inadequate among pregnant women eight years after mandatory iodination of salt in Turkey. J. Endocrinol. Invest. 33, 461–464.

Lampropoulou, M., Lean, M., Combet, E., 2012. Iodine status of women of childbearing age in Scotland. Proc. Nutr. Soc. 71.

Larsson, C.L., Klock, K.S., Åstrøm, A.N., Haugejorden, O., Johansson, G., 2001. Food habits of young Swedish and Norwegian vegetarians and omnivores. Public Health Nutr. 4, 1005–1014.

Lazarus, J.H., 2007. Evaluating iodine deficiency in pregnant women and young infants-complex physiology with a risk of misinterpretation – comments. Public Health Nutr. 10, 1553.

Lazarus, J.H., 2014. Iodine status in Europe in 2014. Eur. Thyroid J. 3, 3–6.

Leung, A.M., Braverman, L.E., 2012. Iodine-induced thyroid dysfunction. Curr. Opin. Endocrinol. Diabetes Obes. 19, 414–419.

Leung, A.M., Lamar, A., He, X., Braverman, L.E., Pearce, E.N., 2011. Iodine status and thyroid function of Boston-area vegetarians and vegans. J. Clin. Endocrinol. Metab. 96, E1303–E1307.

Lightowler, H.J., Davies, G.J., 1998. Iodine intake and iodine deficiency in vegans as assessed by the duplicate-portion technique and urinary iodine excretion. Br. J. Nutr. 80, 529–535.

Lightowler, H.J., Davies, G.J., 2002. Assessment of iodine intake in vegans: weighed dietary record vs duplicate portion technique. Eur. J. Clin. Nutr. 56, 765–770.

Marchioni, E., Fumarola, A., Calvanese, A., Piccirilli, F., Tommasi, V., Cugini, P., Ulisse, S., Rossi Fanelli, F., D'armiento, M., 2008. Iodine deficiency in pregnant women residing in an area with adequate iodine intake. Nutrition 24, 458–461.

Mian, C., Vitaliano, P., Pozza, D., Barollo, S., Pitton, M., Callegari, G., Di Gianantonio, E., Casaro, A., Nacamulli, D., Busnardo, B., Mantero, F., Girelli, M.E., 2009. Iodine status in pregnancy: role of dietary habits and geographical origin. Clin. Endocrinol. 70, 776–780.

Michikawa, T., Inoue, M., Shimazu, T., Sawada, N., Iwasaki, M., Sasazuki, S., Yamaji, T., Tsugane, S., Japan Public Health Center Based Prospective Study Group, 2012. Seaweed consumption and the risk of thyroid cancer in women: the Japan public health center-based prospective study. Eur. J. Cancer Prev. 21, 254–260.

Montoro, M., Collea, J.V., Frasier, S.D., Mestman, J.H., 1981. Successful outcome of pregnancy in women with hypothyroidism. Ann. Intern. Med. 94, 31–34.

Olivieri, O., Girelli, D., Stanzial, A.M., Rossi, L., Bassi, A., Corrocher, R., 1996. Selenium, zinc, and thyroid hormones in healthy subjects. Biol. Trace Elem. Res. 51, 31–41.

Olsen, S.O., 2003. Understanding the relationship between age and seafood consumption: the mediating role of attitude, health involvement and convenience. Food Qual. Prefer. 14, 199–209.

Phillips, D., 1997. Iodine, milk, and the elimination of endemic goitre in Britain: the story of an accidental public health triumph. J. Epidemiol. Community Health 51, 391–393.

Piccoli, G., Clari, R., Vigotti, F., Leone, F., Attini, R., Cabiddu, G., Mauro, G., Castelluccia, N., Colombi, N., Capizzi, I., 2015. Vegan–vegetarian diets in pregnancy: danger or panacea? A systematic narrative review. BJOG 122, 623–633.

Rasmussen, L.B., Ovesen, L., Bulow, I., Jorgensen, T., Knudsen, N., Laurberg, P., Perrild, H., 2001. Evaluation of a semi-quantitative food frequency questionnaire to estimate iodine intake. Eur. J. Clin. Nutr. 55, 287–292.

Rasmussen, L.B., Jørgensen, T., Perrild, H., Knudsen, N., Krejbjerg, A., Laurberg, P., Pedersen, I.B., Bjergved, L., Ovesen, L., 2014. Mandatory iodine fortification of bread and salt increases iodine excretion in adults in Denmark–a 11-year follow-up study. Clin. Nutr. 33, 1033–1040.

Rauma, A., Törmälä, M., Nenonen, M., Hänninen, O., 1994. Iodine status in vegans consuming a living food diet. Nutr. Res. 14, 1789–1795.

Raverot, V., Bournaud, C., Sassolas, G., Orgiazzi, J., Claustrat, F., Gaucherand, P., Mellier, G., Claustrat, B., Borson-Chazot, F., Zimmermann, M., 2012. Pregnant French women living in the Lyon area are iodine deficient and have elevated serum thyroglobulin concentrations. Thyroid 22, 522–528.

Rayman, M.P., 2012. Selenium and human health. Lancet 379, 1256–1268.

Rosell, M., Appleby, P., Spencer, E., Key, T., 2006. Weight gain over 5 years in 21 966 meat-eating, fish-eating, vegetarian, and vegan men and women in EPIC-Oxford. Int. J. Obes. 30, 1389–1396.

Roti, E., Degli Uberti, E., 2001. Iodine excess and hyperthyroidism. Thyroid 11, 493–500.

Schüpbach, R., Wegmüller, R., Berguerand, C., Bui, M., Herter-Aeberli, I., 2015. Micronutrient status and intake in omnivores, vegetarians and vegans in Switzerland. Eur. J. Nutr. 1–11.

Scientific Advisory Committee on Nutrition, 2014. Statement on Iodine and Health. (Online). Available from: https://www.gov.uk/government/uploads/system/uploads/attachment_data/file/339439/SACN_Iodine_and_Health_2014.pdf.

Shaikh, M.G., Anderson, J.M., Hall, S.K., Jackson, M.A., 2003. Transient neonatal hypothyroidism due to a maternal vegan diet. J. Pediatr. Endocrinol. Metab 16, 111–113.

Sobiecki, J.G., Appleby, P.N., Bradbury, K.E., Key, T.J., 2016. High compliance with dietary recommendations in a cohort of meat eaters, fish eaters, vegetarians, and vegans: results from the European Prospective Investigation into Cancer and Nutrition-Oxford study. Nutr. Res. 36, 464–477.

Szybiński, Z., Huszno, B., Zemla, B., Bandurska-Stankiewicz, E., Przybylik-Mazurek, E., Nowak, W., Cichon, S., Buziak-Bereza, M., Trofimiuk, M., Szybiński, P., 2002. Incidence of thyroid cancer in the selected areas of iodine deficiency in Poland. J. Endocrinol. Invest. 26, 63–70.

Takegawa, K., Mitsumori, K., Onodera, H., Shimo, T., Kitaura, K., Yasuhara, K., Hirose, M., Takahashi, M., 2000. Studies on the carcinogenicity of potassium iodide in F344 rats. Food Chem. Toxicol. 38, 773–781.

Teas, J., Pino, S., Critchley, A., Braverman, L.E., 2004. Variability of iodine content in common commercially available edible seaweeds. Thyroid 14, 836–841.

Tonstad, S., Nathan, E., Oda, K., Fraser, G., 2013. Vegan diets and hypothyroidism. Nutrients 5, 4642–4652.

Tonstad, S., Jaceldo-Siegl, K., Messina, M., Haddad, E., Fraser, G.E., 2015a. The association between soya consumption and serum thyroid-stimulating hormone concentrations in the Adventist Health Study-2. Public Health Nutr. 1–7.

Tonstad, S., Nathan, E., Oda, K., Fraser, G.E., 2015b. Prevalence of hyperthyroidism according to type of vegetarian diet. Public Health Nutr. 18, 1482–1487.

Truong, T., Baron-Dubourdieu, D., Rougier, Y., Guenel, P., 2010. Role of dietary iodine and cruciferous vegetables in thyroid cancer: a countrywide case-control study in New Caledonia. Cancer Causes Control 21, 1183–1192.

Vanderpump, M.PJ., Lazarus, J.H., Smyth, P.P., Laurberg, P., Holder, R.L., Boelaert, K., Franklyn, J.A., British Thyroid Association, U.K. Iodine Survey Group, 2011. Iodine status of UK schoolgirls: a cross-sectional survey. Lancet 377, 2007–2012.

Vandevijvere, S., Amsalkhir, S., Mourri, A.B., Van Oyen, H., Moreno-Reyes, R., 2013. Iodine deficiency among Belgian pregnant women not fully corrected by iodine-containing multivitamins: a national cross-sectional survey. Br. J. Nutr. 109, 2276–2284.

Waldmann, A., Koschizke, J., Leitzmann, C., Hahn, A., 2003. Dietary intakes and lifestyle factors of a vegan population in Germany: results from the German Vegan Study. Eur. J. Clin. Nutr. 57, 947–955.

WHO/UNICEF/ICCIDD, 2007. Assessment of Iodine Deficiency Disorders and Monitoring Their Elimination. A Guide for Programme Managers, third ed. WHO, Geneva.

Williamson, C., Lean, M.E., Combet, E., 2012. Dietary iodine: awareness, knowledge and current practice among midwives. Proc. Nutr. Soc. 71, E142.

World Health Organisation, 2014. Salt Reduction and Iodine Fortification Strategies in Public Health: Report of a Joint Technical Meeting Convened by the World Health Organization and the George Institute for Global Health in Collaboration with the International Council for the Control of Iodine Deficiency Disorders Global Network, Sydney, Australia. World Health Organisation, Switzerland. March 2013.

World Health Organization, 2007. Assessment of Iodine Deficiency Disorders and Monitoring Their Elimination. A Guide for Programme Managers, third ed. United Nations Children's Fund, International Council for the Control of Iodine Deficiency Disorders, Geneva, Switzerland.

World Health Organization, 2014. Guideline: Fortification of Food-Grade Salt with Iodine for the Prevention and Control of Iodine Deficiency Disorders.

Zava, T.T., Zava, D.T., 2011. Assessment of Japanese iodine intake based on seaweed consumption in Japan: a literature-based analysis. Thyroid Res. 4, 14.

Zimmermann, M.B., Andersson, M., 2012. Assessment of iodine nutrition in populations: past, present, and future. Nutr. Rev. 70.

Zimmermann, M.B., Boelaert, K., 2015. Iodine deficiency and thyroid disorders. Lancet Diabetes Endocrinol. 3, 286–295.

Zimmermann, M.B., Galetti, V., 2015. Iodine intake as a risk factor for thyroid cancer: a comprehensive review of animal and human studies. Thyroid Res. 8, 1.

Zimmermann, M.B., Köhrle, J., 2002. The impact of iron and selenium deficiencies on iodine and thyroid metabolism: biochemistry and relevance to public health. Thyroid 12, 867–878.

Zimmermann, M.B., Wegmu¨Ller, R., Zeder, C., Chaouki, N., Torresani, T., 2004. The effects of vitamin A deficiency and vitamin A supplementation on thyroid function in goitrous children. J. Clin. Endocrinol. Metab. 89, 5441–5447.

Zimmermann, 2007. Interactions of vitamin A and iodine deficiencies: effects on the pituitary-thyroid axis. Int. J. Vitam. Nutr. Res. 77, 236–240.

Further Reading

Andersson, M., Karumbunathan, V., Zimmermann, M.B., 2012. Global iodine status in 2011 and trendsover the past decade. J. Nutr. 142, 744–750.

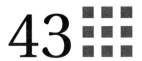

43

Vitamin B$_{12}$ Deficiency in Vegetarians

Wolfgang Herrmann

SAARLAND UNIVERSITY HOSPITAL, HOMBURG, GERMANY

1. Vitamin B$_{12}$ and Its Metabolism

Vitamin B$_{12}$ [cobalamin (Cbl)] had been discovered after several years of intensive investigation on the previously fatal disease pernicious anemia. In the early 1920s, Minot and Murphy demonstrated that pernicious anemia was treatable by whole liver extract, which is rich in vitamin B$_{12}$. Later, vitamin B$_{12}$ was then isolated, and the crystallized molecule was identified. Vitamin B$_{12}$ belongs to a group of compounds of similar chemical structure but displays completely different biological functions. The vitamin B$_{12}$ structure consists of a corrinoid molecule with cobalt in the center. The synthetic forms of vitamin B$_{12}$ are cyanocobalamin and hydroxycobalamin. In humans, there are only two forms of vitamin B$_{12}$ that have biological activity as cofactors in enzyme reactions, adenosylcobalamin (AdoCbl) and methylcobalamin (MeCbl) (Herzlich and Herbert, 1988) (Fig. 43.1). Vitamin B$_{12}$ is required by all cells for its role in one-carbon metabolism and in DNA synthesis and maintenance.

Only two vitamin B$_{12}$–dependent enzymes are known in humans, methionine synthase and L-methylmalonyl-CoA mutase. Methionine synthase mediates the formation of methionine from homocysteine, which requires MeCbl as a cofactor. This reaction occurs in the cytosol. The second pathway takes place in the mitochondria and involves isomerization of methylmalonyl-CoA to succinyl-CoA. This reaction is catalyzed by methylmalonyl-CoA mutase and requires AdoCbl as a cofactor (Stroinsky and Schneider, 1987). That pathway is part of the catabolism of odd-chained fatty acids, cholesterol, and several amino acids. The excess of methylmalonyl-CoA is converted into methylmalonic acid (MMA). Therefore, vitamin B$_{12}$ deficiency leads to MMA elevation, which is considered a sensitive marker for this deficiency. A reduced flux through the methylmalonyl-CoA mutase reaction is discussed to contribute to subsequent neurological tissue damage. Serum concentrations of MMA and homocysteine (Hcy) are, therefore, accepted as metabolic indicators of vitamin B$_{12}$ status. Of these, only MMA is specific for vitamin B$_{12}$ deficiency, whereas homocysteine concentrations also increase in case of folate deficiency or disturbed transsulfuration pathway. Hcy is constituent of the methionine cycle and becomes remethylated to methionine by takeover of a methyl group from 5-methyl-tetrahydrofolate.

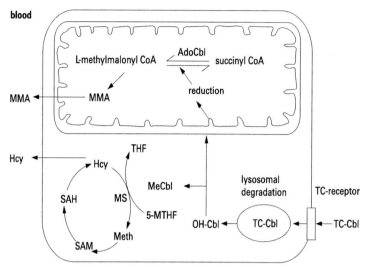

FIGURE 43.1 The metabolic pathways enhanced by cobalamin. *AdoCbl*, adenosylcobalamin; *Cbl*, cobalamin; *Hcy*, homocysteine; *MeCbl*, methylcobalamin; *Meth*, methionine; *MMA*, methylmalonic acid; *MS*, methionine synthase; *MTHF*, methyltetrahydrofolate; *SAH*, S-adenosylhomocysteine; *SAM*, S-adenosylmethionine; *TC*, transcobalamin; *THF*, tetrahydrofolate. (Herrmann and Obeid, 2011).

2. Vitamin B$_{12}$ Sources and Hemostasis

Neither humans nor animals are able to synthesize the vitamin B$_{12}$ molecule. Vitamin B$_{12}$ synthesis is very complex and restricted to a certain strain of bacteria. As well, plants and fungi do not synthesize vitamin B$_{12}$ or use this vitamin. Animals can get vitamin B$_{12}$ by consuming foods contaminated with synthesizing bacteria and then incorporate the vitamin into their body organs. Foods of animal source are the only natural source of vitamin B$_{12}$ in the human diet (Scott, 1997). Vitamin B$_{12}$ is essential for normal maturation and development of all DNA synthesizing cells, including blood cells and cells of the central nervous system. The ultimate source of vitamin B$_{12}$ in the human diet is from foods contaminated with vitamin B$_{12}$–synthesizing bacteria. Not all forms of vitamin B$_{12}$ synthesized by bacteria are metabolically active for mammalian cells. Some naturally occurring forms of corrinoids have similar structure but no biological role in humans. These are produced by some algae (spirulina) and are termed analogues. Cobalamin-analogues may even block the normal metabolism of the vitamin (Herbert and Drivas, 1982; Dagnelie et al., 1991).

Dietary vitamin B$_{12}$ is bound to food proteins and must be released before the vitamin can be absorbed. The release of vitamin B$_{12}$ from its food-binding proteins is achieved by the action of gastric acid and proteolytic enzymes in the stomach. In the stomach, vitamin B$_{12}$ is captured by haptocorrin (transcobalamin I), an R-binder protein made in the saliva and stomach. In the upper small intestine, pancreatic enzymes and an alkaline pH degrade the haptocorrin–vitamin B$_{12}$ complex (Markle, 1996; Herrmann and Geisel, 2002). The free vitamin is then captured by intrinsic factor (IF), another vitamin B$_{12}$–binding protein. The IF–vitamin B$_{12}$ complex is transported to the terminal ileum where the complex is recognized and internalized by specific membrane receptors of the enterocytes (intrinsic factor receptor). The receptor-mediated absorption of vitamin B$_{12}$ is a saturable process, and a maximal amount of 3 µg of the vitamin per meal is capable of being internalized by this pathway.

After absorption of vitamin B$_{12}$–IF complex into the enterocytes, the complex is degraded, and vitamin B$_{12}$ is transferred to a third binding protein, transcobalamin (transcobalamin II, TCII). TCII is synthesized within the enterocytes and is the only binder that can deliver vitamin B$_{12}$ into cells via TCII-receptor. The TCII–vitamin B$_{12}$ complex is released into the portal circulation and is subsequently recognized by TCII-receptors that are expressed by all cell types. The part of vitamin B$_{12}$ that is bound to TCII is named holotranscobalamin II (holoTCII) (Carmel, 1985). Only 6%–20% of total plasma vitamin B$_{12}$ is present as holoTCII (Hall, 1977). HoloTCII is a modern biomarker in detecting vitamin B$_{12}$ deficiency and is seen to be the earliest marker for a low vitamin B$_{12}$ status because it is more sensitive and specific compared with total vitamin B$_{12}$ (Herrmann et al., 2005). The remaining part of vitamin B$_{12}$ is bound to haptocorrin and is called holohaptocorrin (holoHC), which amounts for almost 80% of total vitamin B$_{12}$ (England et al., 1976).

A considerable amount of vitamin B$_{12}$ is secreted into the bile. Two-thirds of the secreted vitamin B$_{12}$ in the bile is reabsorbed in the ileum. The liver stores most of the vitamin B$_{12}$ in the body (2–3 mg) (Markle, 1996). The kidney and the brain are also two important organs that accumulate vitamin B$_{12}$. The kidney can release vitamin B$_{12}$ in case of short-term depletion of the vitamin. Vitamin B$_{12}$ is excreted into urine, and this can be reabsorbed in the proximal tubules via a specific receptor (megalin/cubilin) (Moestrup et al., 1996). The major route by which vitamin B$_{12}$ is lost from the body is through the feces.

The bioavailability of vitamin B$_{12}$ from vitamin preparations is greater than that from foods. In contrast to the receptor-mediated absorption, about 1% of free vitamin B$_{12}$ is absorbed by passive diffusion even in the absence of intrinsic factor (Herrmann and Obeid, 2012). Therefore, even patients with pernicious anemia, or those with disturbed gastrointestinal pH or atrophic gastritis, benefit from relatively high doses (100–1000 µg/day) of oral vitamin B$_{12}$ treatment.

3. Vitamin B$_{12}$ Deficiency

Vitamin B$_{12}$ deficiency is common worldwide (Sipponen et al., 2003; Clarke et al., 2004; Morris et al., 2002; Obeid et al., 2002a,b). In developed countries, it is restricted to patients with malabsorption, intestinal resection, or those who do not ingest a sufficient amount of the vitamin or who practice a vegetarian lifestyle (Herrmann et al., 2003b; Carmel, 1997). Besides in individuals using a vegetarian diet, vitamin B$_{12}$ deficiency is also common in elderly people. Furthermore, low vitamin B$_{12}$ status has been reported in children, and in adults in developing countries. Vitamin B$_{12}$ deficiency takes years to develop, even when one stops ingesting the vitamin. This is due to the relatively large body stores of vitamin B$_{12}$ and to the effective enterohepatic circulation that ensures reabsorption of the vitamin. Natural vitamin B_{12} sources in the human diet are restricted to foods of animal origin (Herbert, 1988). Subjects who practice a long-term vegetarian diet are at high risk to develop vitamin B_{12} deficiency (Herbert, 1994; Herrmann et al., 2003b). Despite milk and eggs containing some vitamin B_{12}, the intake of this vitamin by means of a lacto-/ovolactovegetarian diet is limited. Studies have shown that vitamin B_{12} status (indicated by MMA, holoTCII, and homocysteine) was lower in lacto-/ovolactovegetarians compared with omnivorous subjects (Herrmann et al., 2003b). In addition, metabolic signs of vitamin B_{12} deficiency were more common in vegans compared with lacto-/ovolactovegetarians (Herrmann et al., 2003b). Chronic low intake of vitamin B_{12} and its deficiency can be endemic in developing countries and is related to poverty and malnutrition in this case (Refsum et al., 2001; Rogers et al., 2003; Herrmann et al., 2003a, 2009).

Preclinical or asymptomatic vitamin B_{12} deficiency is the state of metabolic evidence of insufficiency, without symptoms of anemia or neurological complications. The measurement of serum concentrations of metabolic markers allows detection of a large number of asymptomatic subjects who are depleted from vitamin B_{12}. The classification of vitamin B_{12} deficiency introduced by Herbert (1994) suggests that vitamin B_{12} deficiency develops through different stages. In the early stages of vitamin B_{12} deficiency, the plasma and cell stores become depleted, which is indicated by low plasma level of holoTCII while MMA and homocysteine are still normal (Herbert et al., 1990; Lindgren et al., 1999). In the second stage where the body stores are exhausted, functional dysbalances occur. Beside lowered holoTCII, increased plasma levels of MMA and homocysteine are observed. The third stage, according to Herbert et al. (1990), is characterized by clinical signs of vitamin B_{12} deficiency like macroovalocytosis, elevated mean corpuscular volume (MCV) of erythrocytes, or lowered hemoglobin. However, in practice, neurological symptoms of deficiency may already develop before hematological symptoms occur. An early diagnosis of vitamin B_{12} deficiency is therefore of great clinical relevance because neurological damage can be irreversible even at an early stage, while this damage can easily be prevented by early diagnosis followed by vitamin B_{12} substitution (Weir and Scott, 1999).

Symptoms of subclinical vitamin B_{12} deficiency are subtle and often overlooked. The long-term consequences of subclinical deficiency are not fully known but may include adverse effects on pregnancy outcomes and vascular, cognitive, bone, and eye health (O'Leary and Samman, 2010). Abnormal biomarkers, which precede clinical signs of vitamin B_{12} deficiency, are early indicators and display the metabolic consequence of vitamin B_{12} deficiency (Hultberg et al., 2001).

3.1 Vitamin B_{12} Status and Vegetarian Diet

In a systematic review using multiple search engines including PubMed, Medline, CINAHL plus, ERIC, Nursing and Allied Health Collection, and Nursing/Academic Edition, Pawlak et al. (2014) reported the prevalence of vitamin B_{12} deficiency among vegetarians assessed by serum vitamin B_{12}. The deficiency prevalence among infants reached 45%; among children and adolescents it ranged from 0% to 33%; the deficiency among pregnant women

Table 43.1   Cobalamin Status and Metabolites in Vegetarian and Nonvegetarian Subjects

	Omnivores	LV/OLV	Vegans
Number	109	114	50
Age, years	41 (24–61)	50 (35–71)[a]	44 (20–66)[b]
Vitamin B$_{12}$, pmol/L	280 (191–416)	190 (130–320)[a]	146 (98–294)[a,b]
MMA, nmol/L	160 (113–253)	308 (155–1014)[a]	698 (180–2728)[a,b]
HoloTC, pmol/L	55 (33–91)	31 (7–64)[a]	13 (2–110)[a,b]
Hcy, µmol/L	9.3 (6.5–14.4)	10.9 (7.2–21.5)[a]	13.0 (6.4–35.6)[a,b]
Folic acid, nmol/L	25.7 (16.2–45.6)	21.2 (13.2–39.8)[a]	28.9 (19.0–65.9)[a]
Vitamin B$_6$, nmol/L	50.3 (25.3–122.2)	52.1 (27.6–99.3)	46.0 (19.8–116.6)

Data are median (10th–90th) percentiles. $P < .05$. *LV/OLV*, lacto-/ovolactovegetarians (Herrmann et al., 2005).
[a]Compared to the omnivores.
[b]Compared to the LV/LOV subjects (ANOVA and Bonferroni tests).

ranged from 17% to 39%, dependent on the trimester. Adults and elderly individuals had a deficiency range of 0%–86%. Higher deficiency prevalence was reported in vegans than in other vegetarians. The review also documented a rather high prevalence of vitamin B$_{12}$ deficiency among vegetarians adhering to different types of vegetarian diets. Vegans who do not ingest vitamin B$_{12}$ supplements were found to be at especially high risk. All vegetarians and especially vegans should, therefore, give strong consideration to the use of vitamin B$_{12}$ supplements to ensure adequate vitamin B$_{12}$ intake.

Vitamin B$_{12}$ status is directly correlated with dietary intake and length of time following a vegetarian diet (Chanarin et al., 1985). It has been suggested that, depending on the strictness of the diet, 30%–60% of all vegetarian and vegan subjects might have metabolic evidence of vitamin B$_{12}$ deficiency (Donaldson, 2000; Rauma et al., 1995). Serum concentrations of MMA, holoTCII, homocysteine, and total vitamin B$_{12}$ are related to the type of the diet (Table 43.1; Fig. 43.2). Lowered holoTCII as well as raised MMA and homocysteine are common in vegetarians and vegans and are in agreement with functional B$_{12}$ deficiency. Vegan subjects have the lowest vitamin B$_{12}$ status. This is expected because a vegan diet includes no kind of animal foods. Although lacto-/ovolactovegetarians consume some animal foods (egg, milk, and milk products), metabolic signs of vitamin B$_{12}$ deficiency were also common in this group (Table 43.1). The lactovegetarian and ovolactovegetarian group displays intermediate vitamin B$_{12}$ status compared with vegans and omnivorous (Fig. 43.2).

3.2 Vitamin B$_{12}$ Deficiency in Early Life

The requirements for B vitamins (folate, vitamin B$_{12}$, and vitamin B$_6$) are exceptionally high during pregnancy as a result of increased maternal metabolic rate and fetal demands (Heller et al., 1973). Maternal nutritional status before and during pregnancy is the main determinant of the nutritional status of the offspring (Bjorke Monsen et al., 2001; Murphy

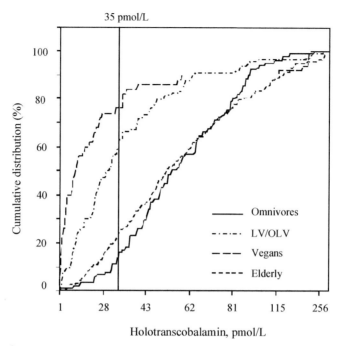

FIGURE 43.2 The cumulative distribution of holotranscobalamin II (holoTCII) in subjects with different diets in addition to the distribution in elderly people. The lower cutoff of holoTCII = 35 pmol/L is indicated. *LV/OLV*, lacto-/ovolactovegetarians (Herrmann et al., 2005).

et al., 2004). Vitamin B_{12}, folate, and vitamin B_6 function as cofactors in one-carbon metabolism, DNA synthesis, and numerous methylation reactions. These metabolic pathways are particularly active in developing embryos. Therefore, vitamin B_{12} deficiency in developing embryos can occur in women on vegetarian diets who do not ingest a sufficient amount of this vitamin. During the fetal period, the liver of the fetus stores vitamin B_{12}, so normally the newborn child has a considerable reserve of vitamin B_{12} (Allen, 2004; Doyle et al., 1989). In vegetarian or vegan mothers, however, this prenatal store is less or not built, giving the newborn an additional high risk of deficiency (Weiss et al., 1989), especially since the breast milk of the same mother contains little or no B_{12} (Weiss et al., 1989; Grange and Finlay, 1994).

Metabolic and clinical signs of vitamin B_{12} deficiency have also been reported in newborn babies from vegetarian mothers or in breastfed infants from deficient mothers (Dagnelie et al., 1989; Graham et al., 1992; Schneede et al., 1994; Bjorke Monsen et al., 2001). These conditions were partly reversible after vitamin B_{12} supplementation. The content of vitamin B_{12} in breast milk is related to markers of vitamin B_{12} deficiency in the infants (Bjorke Monsen et al., 2001). This explains the finding that exclusively breastfed babies from deficient mothers are at increased risk for developing metabolic and clinical signs of deficiency.

It has been reported that the most common cause of vitamin B_{12} deficiency at early childhood is being born from or lactated by a vitamin-deficient mother. A serious neurological syndrome and developmental disorders have been described in case reports of exclusively breastfed infants of strict vegetarian mothers who were vitamin B$_{12}$ deficient (Higginbottom et al., 1978; Kuhne et al., 1991). Vitamin B$_{12}$ deficiency in infants is associated with a marked developmental regression, poor brain growth, or a poor intellectual outcome. Other signs include impaired communicative reactions and fine and gross motor functions. Low vitamin B$_{12}$ status had also negative influence on school achievement. Adolescents who previously consumed a macrobiotic diet had lower scores in some measures of cognitive performance as compared with adolescents who consumed an omnivorous diet from birth onward (Louwman et al., 2000). Furthermore, attention should be paid to familial factors (maternal vitamin status) and predisposing environmental factors (vegetarian diet or poverty). Vitamin B$_{12}$ deficiency should be suspected in children with unexplained neurological symptoms, failure to thrive, or poor intellectual performance.

3.3 Diagnosis of Vitamin B$_{12}$ Deficiency

There is no single parameter that can be reliably used to diagnose vitamin B$_{12}$ deficiency. Megaloblastic anemia and neurological symptoms are neither sensitive nor they are specific for vitamin B$_{12}$ deficiency. Metabolic signs of deficiency (elevated MMA and homocysteine) were observed in the absence of hematological or clinical manifestations. Concentrations of total vitamin B$_{12}$ in serum are too insensitive to be used for diagnosing a vitamin-deficient state with high sensitivity and specificity (Herrmann et al., 2000, 2001). Measurement of serum concentration of MMA alone or in conjunction with homocysteine has partly resolved the demand for a sensitive and a specific test, especially for studies on vitamin B$_{12}$ status in otherwise healthy populations. For the purpose of individual diagnosis, however, the results of the metabolites should be interpreted with some caution because it is difficult to determine to which extent an impaired kidney function may participate in MMA and homocysteine elevation. Subjects with serum vitamin B$_{12}$ concentrations in the normal range up to 400 pmol/L may have increased MMA and low holoTCII indicating functional vitamin B$_{12}$ deficiency. Therefore, the measurement of holoTCII has been introduced with promising results. Studies in vegetarian subjects have shown that the majority of them had low holoTCII in addition to abnormal metabolic signs like elevated MMA and homocysteine (Herrmann et al., 2003b, 2005).

3.4 Modern and Traditional Biomarkers for Metabolic Vitamin B$_{12}$ Deficiency

As a biomarker of vitamin B$_{12}$ status, total vitamin B$_{12}$ measurement is often used cost effectively as the parameter of choice, but it has limited sensitivity and specificity, especially in persons with vitamin B$_{12}$ concentrations <400 pmol/L (Herrmann et al., 2003b; Loikas et al., 2003). If the total vitamin B$_{12}$ concentration is in the lower reference range, 156–400 pmol/L, vitamin B$_{12}$ deficiency cannot be ruled out. Furthermore, clinical signs of vitamin B$_{12}$ deficiency can be seen in persons with vitamin B$_{12}$ concentrations within

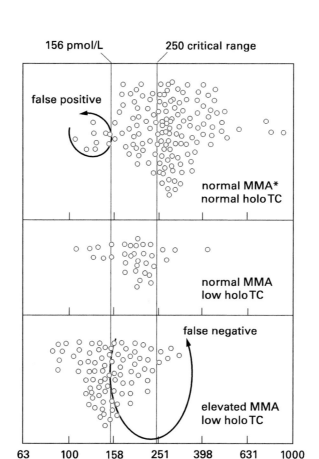

FIGURE 43.3 Serum concentrations of cobalamin in subjects (omnivorous, lacto-/ovolactovegetarians, vegans) with normal holoTCII and normal MMA and in those with at least one abnormal test. Only subjects with normal concentration of serum creatinine are included in this figure. *Normal cobalamin status defined as MMA ≤271 nmol/L/holo TCII >35 pmol/L. *MMA*, methylmalonic acid; *holoTCII*, holotranscobalamin II (Herrmann et al., 2005).

the lower reference range (>156 pmol/L) (Lesho and Hyder, 1999). Persons with normal concentrations of vitamin B_{12} may have raised concentrations of MMA (>300 nmol/L) and lowered concentrations of holoTCII (<35 pmol/L), owing to intracellular, metabolically manifest (functional) vitamin B_{12} deficiency (Herrmann et al., 2003b). By contrast, lowered concentrations of vitamin B_{12} and normal MMA as well as normal holoTCII indicate a false positive finding (Fig. 43.3). On the other hand, a decreased serum holoTCII concentration only is the earliest marker of vitamin B_{12} deficiency and signals that the body does not have sufficient available vitamin B_{12} within the cells and that the B_{12} stores are being exhausted as a result of the negative balance of vitamin B_{12} (Herrmann and Obeid 2012, 2011). At this stage, clinical or hematological symptoms might not yet be present. Lowered holoTCII combined with raised MMA and homocysteine levels are indicative of metabolically manifest vitamin B_{12} deficiency. Clinical signs may already be present but can still be missing; the patient may therefore still be clinically inconspicuous. Metabolically manifest B$_{12}$ deficiency can affect bone metabolism, for example, and stimulate osteoclasts (Herrmann et al., 2007). The exact prevalence of clinically significant B$_{12}$ deficiency is not known; the range of symptoms is wide, and the new markers enable the detection of vitamin deficiency notably more often.

In studies in mixed groups of vegetarians, lowered holoTCII concentrations (<35 pmol/L) were found in 8%–11% of omnivores, in 61%–77% of lacto-/ovolactovegetarians, and in 76%–92% of vegans; raised MMA (>271 nmol/L) was detected in 5%–7% of omnivores, in 57%–68% of lacto-/ovolactovegetarians, and in 74%–83% of vegan subjects (Herrmann et al., 2005; 2003b). Low vitamin B$_{12}$ status in lacto-/ovolactovegetarians and vegan subjects was associated with hyperhomocysteinemia (Hcy > 12 μmol/L). Hyperhomocysteinemia was present in 16% of the omnivores, in 38% of the lacto-/ovolactovegetarians, and in 67% of the vegan subjects. The combination of low holoTCII and high MMA was detected in 43% of the lacto-/ovolactovegetarians and 64% of the vegan subjects, respectively (Herrmann et al., 2003b, 2005). Therefore, the prevalence of subclinical functional vitamin B$_{12}$ deficiency is dramatically higher than previously assumed, if sensitive and relatively specific markers are used, such as MMA, holoTCII, and homocysteine (Sipponen et al., 2003; Clarke et al., 2004; Herrmann et al., 2005; Herrmann and Obeid, 2008).

Fig. 43.2 illustrates the cumulative distribution of holoTCII concentrations in the three groups with different diets. The values found in vegans were notably shifted toward the lower end of the distribution. On the other hand, the distribution of holoTCII concentrations in lacto-/ovolactovegetarians subjects showed an intermediate pattern between that found in the vegans and the omnivores. Fig. 43.3 shows the concentrations of total B$_{12}$ in subjects (omnivorous, lacto-/ovolactovegetarians, vegans) with one or two abnormal results concerning MMA and holoTCII compared to those having combined normal holoTCII and normal MMA (Herrmann et al., 2005). Some cases with normal holoTCII and MMA had low concentrations of total B$_{12}$ in serum, indicating a false positive result. More importantly, about 45% of subjects with low holoTCII and elevated MMA had normal serum B$_{12}$, which should be categorized as false negative results (Herrmann and Obeid, 2011). The high prevalence of some biochemical dysfunction in subjects who adhere to any type of vegetarian diet should be emphasized. In vegetarians, the low vitamin B$_{12}$ may cause the so-called "folate trap" because the remethylation of homocysteine to methionine is inhibited (methionine synthase is vitamin B$_{12}$ dependent). Therefore, a concentration of folate of ~40 nmol/L is required to metabolize sufficient folate and to keep homocysteine in a normal range, as compared to only ~10 nmol/L in omnivores (Herrmann et al., 2003b) (Fig. 43.4). This gives additional emphasis that vegetarians are at high risk of vitamin B$_{12}$ deficiency and should therefore ensure adequacy of vitamin B$_{12}$ intake since this is of great importance for them, especially for vegans. Nonanimal sources of vitamin B$_{12}$ include cobalamin supplements, fortified breakfast cereals, and vitamin B$_{12}$–fortified soy products (Tucker, 2014).

Measuring MMA is expensive and requires special equipment, such as mass spectrometers. The holoTCII immunoassay is now available as an automated test. The costs for holoTCII test are higher than for vitamin B$_{12}$. With regard to the cost-benefit effect of early detection of vitamin B$_{12}$ deficiency by using holoTCII, this test will become established as

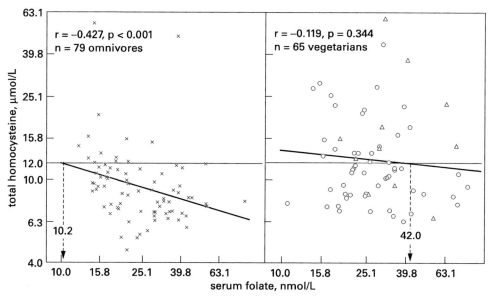

FIGURE 43.4 Scatterplot showing concentrations of total homocysteine in relation to serum folate in omnivores (left plot) and vegetarians (right plot). Numbers on the axis are anti-Log (Herrmann et al., 2003b).

the laboratory parameter of choice to measure vitamin B_{12} status. Currently, no consensus exists with regard to screening for vitamin B_{12} deficiency. Nevertheless, regular monitoring of vitamin B_{12} status is essential for early detection and treatment of metabolic vitamin B_{12} deficiency both in vegans and lactovegetarians, and possibly for prevention of related diseases, like osteoporosis, stroke, or neurodegenerative diseases (Tucker, 2014; Woo et al., 2014; Spence, 2015).

Screening and monitoring would especially make sense if it is possible to detect first signs of subclinical vitamin B_{12} deficiency before neurological or hematological anomalies develop. Although holoTCII is a very early marker and MMA a functional biomarker for vitamin B_{12} deficiency, there is no universal marker for vitamin B_{12} status because limitations exist with regard to their diagnostic informative value. An optimal monitoring of vitamin B_{12} status in vegetarians should include the measurement of holoTCII, MMA, and homocysteine. Additionally, the levels of folate and vitamin B_6 should be controlled. Despite the superior role of holoTCII compared with total B_{12} in diagnosing vitamin B_{12} deficiency, the diagnostic power of holoTCII seems not sufficient to distinguish deficient from nondeficient individuals with high diagnostic correctness. This is related to the fact that normal holoTCII is common in individuals with elevated MMA, especially those with a decline in renal function. Therefore, the implementation of a gray range of holoTCII has been suggested that is defined as the range of the diagnostic uncertainty between 90% sensitivity and 90% specificity, which covers the serum holoTCII concentration range between 23 and 75 pM. In this case, additional MMA testing is recommended (Herrmann and Obeid, 2012). The suggested diagnostic algorithm may significantly improve classification of vitamin B_{12} status.

4. Clinical Manifestations of Vitamin B_{12} Deficiency

4.1 Hematological Symptoms

Megaloblastic anemia is the classical finding of vitamin B_{12} deficiency. The underlying mechanism of anemia in vitamin B_{12} deficiency is a slowed DNA synthesis in rapidly dividing blood cell. This will lead to large red cells with increased MCV. Nevertheless, megaloblastic anemia is neither sensitive, nor it is specific for vitamin B_{12} deficiency. As already mentioned, recent studies have shown that many vitamin B_{12} deficient subjects may develop neurological disorders without macrocytosis of red blood cells. Furthermore, because vitamin B_{12} and iron deficiencies might coincide in many cases, MCV to diagnose vitamin B_{12} deficiency is not valid since microcytic anemia due to iron deficiency can mask the macrocytic anemia of vitamin B_{12} deficiency (Obeid et al., 2002a,b). The result is hypochromic red blood cells with, on average, a normal size. However, since the "normal average" is caused by the sum of microcytic and macrocytic cells, this could be solved by replacing MCV by red cell distribution width, which can be routinely determined in any hematological laboratory nowadays along with other hematological characteristics (Hb, Ht, MCV, MCH, etc.).

It should also be mentioned that hematological manifestation of vitamin B_{12} deficiency can be mistaken by that of folate deficiency. Hypersegmented neutrophils are also common in vitamin B_{12}–deficient subjects. Nevertheless, in general, hematological indices are not valid in diagnosing early stages of vitamin B_{12} deficiency.

4.2 Neurological Complications

Concentrations of homocysteine >12.0 μmol/L and that of MMA >300 nmol/L are common in neuropsychiatric population even in the absence of hematological manifestations (Lindenbaum et al., 1988; Obeid et al., 2007). Vitamin B_{12} deficiency can cause lesions in spinal cord, peripheral nerves, and cerebrum, and it can cause neurological and psychiatric disorders (Maktouf et al., 2007; Andrès et al., 2003; Teplitsky et al., 2003). The most common symptoms are sensory disturbances in the extremities, memory loss, dementia, and psychosis. Improvements have been reported after initiation of vitamin B_{12} treatment (Masalha et al., 2001; Lorenzl et al., 2003). In infants, these improvements can occur within days.

The association between vitamin B_{12} deficiency and depression has also been documented in elderly subjects (Penninx et al., 2000). Metabolically significant vitamin B_{12} deficiency was present in approximately 15% of nondepressed women, 17% of mildly depressed women, and in 27% of the severely depressed women (Penninx et al., 2000). Women with vitamin B_{12} deficiency were 2.05 times as likely to be suffering from severe depression as were nondeficient women. Moreover, peripheral neuropathy occurred in 40% of vitamin B_{12}–deficient subjects (Shorvon et al., 1980). As an example, vitamin B_{12} deficiency in India is often overlooked, but it is very common and connected with varied religious, ethnic, and socioeconomic reasons. It increases the load of cognitive decline and accentuates vascular risk factors in neuropsychiatric illnesses (Issac et al., 2015).

Therefore, prevention, early detection, and management of this reversible vitamin B_{12} deficiency state are of profound importance.

Vitamin B_{12} deficiency may cause serious neurological symptoms in infants, especially in breastfed babies from strictly vegetarian mothers (Graham et al., 1992; Kuhne et al., 1991; Higginbottom et al., 1978). Significant developmental regression, reduced brain growth, and low intellectual outcome has been observed. Furthermore, impaired communicative reactions and impaired fine as well as gross motor functions have been noticed (Dagnelie et al., 1989). In school children, a low vitamin B_{12} status may also be associated with lower school achievement, and in a study on adolescents who were previously fed a macrobiotic diet, they had lower cognitive performance (Louwman et al., 2000). Prolonged insufficient intake of vitamin B_{12} is seen as a common cause of vitamin B_{12} deficiency in children. Therefore, available studies emphasize the need for early recognition and prevention or treatment of B vitamins deficiency in children. Although large-scale screening programs in the general population are currently not recommended (Refsum et al., 2004), a regular checking of vitamin B_{12} status in all lacto-/ovolactovegetarians and vegans and in other cases at risk of vitamin B_{12} deficiency is recommended (Doyle et al., 1989; Weiss et al., 1989; Grange and Finlay, 1994). Children with unexplained neurological symptoms, failure to thrive, or poor intellectual performance should be tested for vitamin B_{12} deficiency.

4.3 Vitamin B_{12} Deficiency and Osteoporosis

Considering the potential association between vitamin B_{12} and bone health, it can be suggested that vegetarians may be particularly prone to disturbances in bone metabolism (Chiu et al., 1997). There is evidence that vegetarians, and particularly vegans, may be at greater risk of lower bone mineral density (BMD) and fracture (Tucker, 2014). First evidence for the relationship between a vegetarian lifestyle, low vitamin B_{12} status, and low BMD was derived from a cross-sectional study of adolescents who were fed a macrobiotic diet up to the age of 6 years, followed by a lacto-/ovolactovegetarian or omnivorous diet (Dhonukshe-Rutten et al., 2005). Total vitamin B_{12}, BMD, and bone mineral content were lower, and MMA was higher in the formerly macrobiotic-fed individuals compared with controls. Consistent with this, the Longitudinal Aging Study Amsterdam (LASA) study reported a significant relationship between vitamin B_{12} and BMD, measured by calcaneal broadband ultrasound attenuation (BUA) in women (Dhonukshe-Rutten et al., 2005). The strongest evidence for accelerated bone loss in vegetarians comes from the EPIC-Norfolk study, which included over 11,000 men and women (Welch et al., 2005). Male vegetarians exhibited a 6%–15% reduction in BUA, indicating a significant deterioration in bone composition in vegetarians. Previous studies suggested lower body weight as well as lower intake of protein, calcium, vitamin D, and acid substances as potential causative factors for reduced BMD and an increased fracture rate in vegetarians and vegans (Fontana et al., 2005; Chiu et al., 1997; Appleby et al., 2007; Welch et al., 2005). However, in the LASA and the EPIC studies the relationship between BMD/BUA and vegetarian lifestyle, as well as vitamin B_{12} status, remained significant after adjusting for body weight, food intake, and nutrients.

Data regarding BMD in vegetarians are not always consistent with data on bone turnover markers (BTMs). In one study, individuals consuming a raw food vegetarian diet had lower BMD at the hip and lumbar spine, compared to controls ingesting an omnivorous diet (Fontana et al., 2005). However, the bone turnover as measured by C-terminal telopeptides of collagen I (CTx) and by bone alkaline phosphatase (BAP) did not differ. Furthermore, in vegetarian children, reduced serum concentrations of bone formation markers [BAP, osteocalcin (OC)] by 10%–20% and of the bone resorption marker CTx by 15% have been reported (Ambroszkiewicz et al., 2007). Since animal products are a good source of vitamin D and vitamin B$_{12}$, a vegetarian diet might be associated with depletion of both vitamin B$_{12}$ and vitamin D stores, the latter being of major importance for bone health. While the association between a vegetarian lifestyle and BMD and fracture risk has been addressed in several studies (Fontana et al., 2005; Dhonukshe-Rutten et al., 2005; Ambroszkiewicz et al., 2007), there is limited information regarding the association between vitamin B$_{12}$ status and bone metabolism in vegetarians. A 2009 study (Herrmann et al., 2009) reported that German vegetarians had higher circulating activities of BAP as well as higher CTx, OC, and procollagen type I N-terminal peptide compared with omnivorous controls. HoloTCII and MMA were correlated with OC, CTx, and BAP (Fig. 43.5). Subjects with low vitamin B$_{12}$ status (holoTCII <35 pmol/L and MMA >271 nmol/L) had significantly lower serum concentrations of 25(OH)-vitamin D but higher homocysteine, and the BTMs (P1NP,

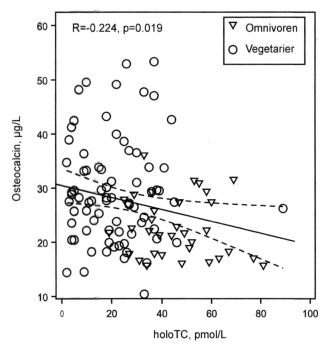

FIGURE 43.5 Scatter plot showing the inverse correlation between osteocalcin and holotranscobalamin II (holoTCII) concentrations according to diet.

BAP, OC, and CTx) compared with subjects having normal vitamin B_{12} status. Multiple regression analysis showed, however, that the association between BTMs and markers of vitamin B_{12} status was independent from the association with 25(OH)-vitamin D. Approximately 12%–14% of the variation in the concentration of BTMs was explained by a regression model including holoTCII, MMA, and 25(OH)-vitamin D.

5. Conclusion

A vegetarian lifestyle, especially a vegan lifestyle, increases the risk of developing deficiencies of several essential nutrients such as vitamins and trace elements. Investigations in populations with different types of vegetarian diets revealed a high prevalence of vitamin B_{12} deficiency, which was over 60% in vegans but also over 40% in lacto-/ovolactovegetarians. Thus, the prevalence of deficiency in lactovegetarians is considerably higher than was previously assumed. The degree of animal foods deprivation and the length of time following this lifestyle are important determinants of the vitamin B_{12} status in vegetarians. Total serum vitamin B_{12} concentrations are widely used when investigating vitamin B_{12} status, but they are too insensitive and unspecific to correctly diagnose vitamin B_{12} deficiency. Modern metabolic markers, especially holoTCII and MMA, allow a far more sensitive and specific detection of vitamin B_{12} deficiency. Thus, the prevalence of vitamin B_{12} deficiency is much higher than till now assumed. HoloTCII represents the metabolically active vitamin B_{12} fraction, and a decreased level is considered as the earliest marker of vitamin B_{12} deficiency; it signals the fact that the body does not have sufficient vitamin B_{12} available and that the B_{12} stores are being exhausted. At this stage, clinical or hematological symptoms, which are late markers of deficiency, might not yet be present. Lowered holoTCII combined with raised MMA (and homocysteine) are indicative of metabolically manifest vitamin B_{12} deficiency. In vegetarians with vitamin B_{12} deficiency, the delivery of active methyl groups may be reduced, leading to hypomethylation of DNA, RNA, proteins, myelin, or neurotransmitters. As a clinical consequence, this may contribute to the development of psychiatric and neurological disorders, like cognitive dysfunction, depression, dementia, or Alzheimer disease. Regarding the potential association between vitamin B_{12} and bone health, vegetarians might be particularly prone to disturbances in bone metabolism resulting in reduced BMD and increased fracture risk. Vegetarians, especially vegans, should, therefore, give strong consideration to the use of vitamin B_{12} supplements to ensure sufficient vitamin B_{12} intake. Furthermore, regular monitoring is urgent to assure an early diagnosis of biochemical vitamin B_{12} deficiency, using holoTCII and MMA, to prevent later clinical vitamin B_{12} deficiency.

References

Allen, L.H., 2004. Multiple micronutrients in pregnancy and lactation: an overview (2005). Am. J. Clin. Nutr. 81 (Suppl.), 1206S–1212S.

Ambroszkiewicz, J., Klemarczyk, W., Gajewska, J., Chel-chowska, M., Laskowska-Klita, T., 2007. Serum concentration of biochemical bone turnover markers in vegetarian children. Adv. Med. Sci. 52, 279–282.

Andrès, E., Perrin, A.E., Demangeat, C., Kurtz, J.E., Vinzio, S., Grunenberger, F., Goichot, B., Schlienger, J.L., 2003. The syndrome of food-cobalamin malabsorption revisited in a department of internal medicine. A monocentric cohort study of 80 patients. Eur. J. Intern. Med. 14 (4), 221–226.

Appleby, P., Roddam, A., Allen, N., Key, T., 2007. Comparative fracture risk in vegetarians and nonvegetarians in EPIC-Oxford. Eur. J. Clin. Nutr. 61, 1400–1406.

Bjorke Monsen, A.L., Ueland, P.M., Vollset, S.E., Guttormsen, A.B., Markestad, T., Solheim, E., Refsum, H., 2001. Determinants of cobalamin status in newborns. Pediatrics 108, 624–630.

Carmel, R., 1985. The distribution of endogenous cobalamin among cobalamin-binding proteins in the blood in normal and abnormal states. Am. J. Clin. Nutr. 41, 713–719.

Carmel, R., 1997. Cobalamin, the stomach, and aging. Am. J. Clin. Nutr. 66, 750–759.

Chanarin, I., Malkowska, V., O'Hea, A.M., Rinsler, M.G., Price, A.B., 1985. Megaloblastic anaemia in a vegetarian Hindu community. Lancet 2, 1168–1172.

Chiu, J.F., Lan, S.J., Yang, C.Y., Wang, P.W., Yao, W.J., Su, L.H., Hsieh, C.C., 1997. Long-term vegetarian diet and bone mineral density in postmenopausal Taiwanese women. Calcif. Tissue Int. 60, 245–249.

Clarke, R., Grimley, E.J., Schneede, J., Nexo, E., Bates, C., Fletcher, A., Prentice, A., Johnston, C., Ueland, P.M., Refsum, H., Sherliker, P., Birks, J., Whitlock, G., Breeze, E., Scott, J.M., 2004. Vitamin B$_{12}$ and folate deficiency in later life. Age Ageing 33, 34–41.

Dagnelie, P.C., van Staveren, W.A., Vergote, F.J., Dingjan, P.G., van den, B.H., Hautvast, J.G., 1989. Increased risk of vitamin B-12 and iron deficiency in infants on macrobiotic diets. Am. J. Clin. Nutr. 50, 818–824.

Dagnelie, P.C., van Staveren, W.A., van den Berg, H., 1991. Vitamin B-12 from algae appears not to be bioavailable. Am. J. Clin. Nutr. 53, 695–697.

Dhonukshe-Rutten, R.A., Van, D.M., Schneede, J., de Groot, L.C., van Staveren, W.A., 2005. Low bone mineral density and bone mineral content are associated with low cobalamin status in adolescents. Eur. J. Nutr. 44, 341–347.

Donaldson, M.S., 2000. Metabolic vitamin B$_{12}$ status on a mostly raw vegan diet with follow-up using tablets, nutritional yeast, or probiotic supplements. Ann. Nutr. Metab. 44, 229–234.

Doyle, J.J., Langevin, A.M., Zipursky, A., 1989. Nutritional vitamin B$_{12}$ deficiency in infancy: three case reports and a review of the literature. Pediatr. Hematol. Oncol. 6 (2), 161–172.

England, J.M., Down, M.C., Wise, I.J., Linnell, J.C., 1976. The transport of endogenous vitamin B$_{12}$ in normal human serum. Clin. Sci. Mol. Med. 51, 47–52.

Fontana, L., Shew, J.L., Holloszy, J.O., Villareal, D.T., March 28, 2005. Low bone mass in subjects on a long-term raw vegetarian diet. Arch. Intern. Med. 165 (6), 684–689.

Graham, S.M., Arvela, O.M., Wise, G.A., 1992. Long-term neurologic consequences of nutritional vitamin B$_{12}$ deficiency in infants. J. Pediatr. 121, 710–714.

Grange, D.K., Finlay, J.L., 1994. Vitamin B$_{12}$ deficiency in a breastfed infant following maternal gastric bypass. Pediatr. Hematol. Oncol. 11 (3), 311–318.

Hall, C.A., 1977. The carriers of native vitamin B$_{12}$ in normal human serum. Clin. Sci. Mol. Med. 53, 453–457.

Heller, S., Salkeld, R.M., Korner, W.F., 1973. Vitamin B$_6$ status in pregnancy. Am. J. Clin. Nutr. 26, 1339–1348.

Herbert, V., Drivas, G., 1982. Spirulina and vitamin B$_{12}$. JAMA 248, 3096–3097.

Herbert, V., Fong, W., Gulle, V., Stopler, T., 1990. Low holotranscobalamin II is the earliest serum marker for subnormal vitamin B$_{12}$ (cobalamin) absorption in patients with AIDS. Am. J. Hematol. 34, 132–139.

Herbert, V., 1988. Vitamin B-12: plant sources, requirements, and assay. Am. J. Clin. Nutr. 48, 852–858.

Herbert, V., 1994. Staging vitamin B-12 (cobalamin) status in vegetarians. Am. J. Clin. Nutr. 59, 1213S–1222S.

Herrmann, W., Geisel, J., 2002. Vegetarian lifestyle and monitoring of vitamin B-12 status. Clin. Chim. Acta 326, 47–59.

Herrmann, W., Obeid, R., 2008. Cause and early diagnosis of vitamin B_{12} deficiency. Dtsch. Arztebl. Int. 105 (40), 680–685.

Herrmann, W., Obeid, R., 2011. Cobalamin deficiency. In: Herrmann, W., Obeid, R. (Eds.), Vitamins in the Prevention of Human Diseases. De Gruyter, Berlin, pp. 213–242.

Herrmann, W., Obeid, R., 2012. Cobalamin and its metabolism. In: Stanger, O. (Ed.), Water Soluble Vitamins. Springer, Heidelberg, pp. 301–322.

Herrmann, W., Schorr, H., Bodis, M., Knapp, J.P., Muller, A., Stein, G., Geisel, J., 2000. Role of homocysteine, cystathionine and methylmalonic acid measurement for diagnosis of vitamin deficiency in high-aged subjects. Eur. J. Clin. Invest. 30, 1083–1089.

Herrmann, W., Schorr, H., Purschwitz, K., Rassoul, F., Richter, V., 2001. Total homocysteine, vitamin B-12, and total antioxidant status in vegetarians. Clin. Chem. 47, 1094–1101.

Herrmann, W., Obeid, R., Jouma, M., 2003a. Hyperhomocysteinemia and vitamin B-12 deficiency are more striking in Syrians than in Germans – causes and implications. Atherosclerosis 166, 143–150.

Herrmann, W., Schorr, H., Obeid, R., Geisel, J., 2003b. Vitamin B-12 status, particularly holotranscobalamin II and methylmalonic acid concentrations, and hyperhomocysteinemia in vegetarians. Am. J. Clin. Nutr. 78, 131–136.

Herrmann, W., Obeid, R., Schorr, H., Geisel, J., 2005. The usefulness of holotranscobalamin in predicting vitamin B_{12} status in different clinical settings. Curr. Drug Metab. 6, 47–53.

Herrmann, M., Schmidt, J., Umanskaya, N., et al., 2007. Stimulation of osteoclast activity by low B-vitamin concentrations. Bone 41, 584–591.

Herrmann, W., Obeid, R., Schorr, H., Hübner, U., Geisel, J., Sand-Hill, M., Nayyar, A., Herrmann, M., 2009. Enhanced bone metabolism in vegetarians – the role of vitamin B_{12} deficiency. Clin. Chem. Lab. Med. 47, 1381–1387.

Herzlich, B., Herbert, V., 1988. Depletion of serum holotranscobal-amin II. An early sign of negative vitamin B_{12} balance. Lab. Invest. 58 (3), 332–337.

Higginbottom, M.C., Sweetman, L., Nyhan, W.L., 1978. A syndrome of methylmalonic aciduria, homo-cystin-uria, megaloblastic anemia and neurologic abnormalities in a vitamin B_{12}-deficient breast-fed infant of a strict vegetarian. N. Engl. J. Med. 299, 317–323.

Hultberg, B., Isaksson, A., Nilsson, K., Gustafson, L., 2001. Markers for the functional availability of cobalamin/folate and their association with neuropsychiatric symptoms in the elderly. Int. J. Geriatr. Psychiatry 16, 873–878.

Issac, T.G., Soundarya, S., Christopher, R., Chandra, S.R., 2015. Vitamin B_{12} deficiency: an important reversible co-morbidity in neuropsychiatric manifestations. Indian J. Psychol. Med. 37 (1), 26–29.

Kuhne, T., Bubl, R., Baumgartner, R., 1991. Maternal vegan diet causing a serious infantile neurological disorder due to vitamin B_{12} deficiency. Eur. J. Pediatr. 150, 205–208.

Lesho, E.P., Hyder, A., 1999. Prevalence of subtle cobalamin deficiency. Arch. Intern. Med. 159, 407.

Lindenbaum, J., Healton, E.B., Savage, D.G., Brust, J.C., Garrett, T.J., Podell, E.R., Marcell, P.D., Stabler, S.P., Allen, R.H., 1988. Neuropsychiatric disorders caused by cobalamin deficiency in the absence of anemia or macrocytosis. N. Engl. J. Med. 318, 1720–1728.

Lindgren, A., Kilander, A., Bagge, E., Nexo, E., 1999. Holotranscobalamin – a sensitive marker of cobalamin malabsorption. Eur. J. Clin. Invest. 29, 321–329.

Loikas, S., Löppönen, M., Suominen, P., Møller, J., Irjala, K., Isoaho, R., Kivelä, S.L., Koskinen, P., Pelliniemi, T.T., 2003. RIA for serum holo-transcobalamin: method evaluation in the clinical laboratory and reference interval. Clin. Chem. 49, 455–462.

Lorenzl, S., Vogeser, M., Muller-Schunk, S., Pfister, H.W., 2003. Clinically and MRI documented funicular myelosis in a patient with metabolical vitamin B_{12} deficiency but normal vitamin B_{12} serum level. J. Neurol. 250 (8), 1010–1011.

Louwman, M.W., Van Dusseldorp, M., van der Vijver, F.J., Thomas, C.M., Schneede, J., Ueland, P.M., Refsum, H., van Staveren, W.A., 2000. Signs of impaired cognitive function in adolescents with marginal cobalamin status. Am. J. Clin. Nutr. 72, 762–769.

Maktouf, C., Bchir, F., Louzir, H., Elloumi, M., Ben Abid, H., Mdhaffer, M., Elleuch, N., Meddeb, B., Mhiri, C., Hassen, Z., Makni, F., Abid, M., Cherif, O., Rokbani, L., Souissi, T., Hafsia, A., Dellagi, K., 2007. Clinical spectrum of cobalamin deficiency in Tunisia. Ann. Biol. Clin. (Paris) 65 (2), 135–142.

Markle, H.V., 1996. Cobalamin. Crit. Rev. Clin. Lab. Sci. 33, 247–356.

Masalha, R., Chudakov, B., Muhamad, M., Rudoy, I., Volkov, I., Wirguin, I., 2001. Cobalamin-responsive psychosis as the sole manifestation of vitamin B$_{12}$ deficiency. Isr. Med. Assoc. J. 3, 701–703.

Moestrup, S.K., Birn, H., Fischer, P.B., Petersen, C.M., Verroust, P.J., Sim, R.B., et al., 1996. Megalin-mediated endocytosis of transcobalamin-vitamin-B$_{12}$ complexes suggests a role of the receptor in vitamin-B$_{12}$ homeostasis. Proc. Natl. Acad. Sci. U.S.A. 93, 8612–8617.

Morris, M.S., Jacques, P.F., Rosenberg, I.H., Selhub, J., 2002. Elevated serum methylmalonic acid concentrations are common among elderly Americans. J. Nutr. 132, 2799–2803.

Murphy, M.M., Scott, J.M., Arija, V., Molloy, A.M., Fernandez-Ballart, J.D., 2004. Maternal homocysteine before conception and throughout pregnancy predicts fetal homocysteine and birth weight. Clin. Chem. 50, 1406–1412.

Obeid, R., Geisel, J., Schorr, H., Hübner, U., Herrmann, W., 2002a. The impact of vegetarianism on some haematological parameters. Eur. J. Haematol. 69 (5–6), 275–279.

Obeid, R., Jouma, M., Herrmann, W., 2002b. Cobalamin status (holo-transcobalamin, methylmalonic acid) and folate as determinants of homocysteine concentration. Clin. Chem. 48, 2064–2065.

Obeid, R., McCaddon, A., Herrmann, W., 2007. The role of hyperhomocysteinemia and B-vitamin deficiency in neurological and neuropsychiatric diseases. Clin. Chem. Lab. Med. 45, 1590–1606.

O'Leary, F., Samman, S., 2010. Vitamin B$_{12}$ in health and disease. Nutrients 2 (3), 299–316.

Pawlak, R., Lester, S.E., Babatunde, T., 2014. The prevalence of cobalamin deficiency among vegetarians assessed by serum vitamin B$_{12}$: a review of literature. Eur. J. Clin. Nutr. 68 (5), 541–548.

Penninx, B.W., Guralnik, J.M., Ferrucci, L., Fried, L.P., Allen, R.H., Stabler, S.P., 2000. Vitamin B(12) deficiency and depression in physically disabled older women: epidemiologic evidence from the Women's Health and Aging Study. Am. J. Psychiatry 157, 715–721.

Rauma, A.L., Torronen, R., Hanninen, O., Mykkanen, H., 1995. Vitamin B-12 status of long-term adherents of a strict uncooked vegan diet ("living food diet") is compromised. J. Nutr. 125, 2511–2515.

Refsum, H., Yajnik, C.S., Gadkari, M., Schneede, J., Vollset, S.E., Orning, L., Guttormsen, A.B., Joglekar, A., Sayyad, M.G., Ulvik, A., Ueland, P.M., 2001. Hyperhomocysteinemia and elevated methylmalonic acid indicate a high prevalence of cobalamin deficiency in Asian Indians. Am. J. Clin. Nutr. 74, 233–241.

Refsum, H., Grindflek, A.W., Ueland, P.M., Fredriksen, A., Meyer, K., Ulvik, A., Guttormsen, A.B., Iversen, O.E., Schneede, J., Kase, B.F., 2004. Screening for serum total homocysteine in newborn children. Clin. Chem. 50, 1769–1784.

Rogers, L.M., Boy, E., Miller, J.W., Green, R., Sabel, J.C., Allen, L.H., 2003. High prevalence of cobalamin deficiency in Guatemalan schoolchildren: associations with low plasma holotranscobalamin II and elevated serum methylmalonic acid and plasma homocysteine concentrations. Am. J. Clin. Nutr. 77, 433–440.

Schneede, J., Dagnelie, P.C., van Staveren, W.A., Vollset, S.E., Refsum, H., Ueland, P.M., 1994. Methylmalonic acid and homocysteine in plasma as indicators of functional cobalamin deficiency in infants on macrobiotic diets. Pediatr. Res. 36, 194–201.

Scott, J.M., 1997. Bioavailability of vitamin B$_{12}$. Eur. J. Clin. Nutr. 51 (Suppl. 1), S49–S53.

Shorvon, S.D., Carney, M.W., Chanarin, I., Reynolds, E.H., 1980. The neuropsychiatry of megaloblastic anaemia. Br. Med. J. 281, 1036–1038.

Sipponen, P., Laxen, F., Huotari, K., Harkonen, M., 2003. Prevalence of low vitamin B_{12} and high homocysteine in serum in an elderly male population: association with atrophic gastritis and *Helicobacter pylori* infection. Scand. J. Gastroenterol. 38, 1209–1216.

Spence, J.D., October 21, 2015. Metabolic B_{12} deficiency: a missed opportunity to prevent dementia and stroke. Nutr. Res. 36 (Epub ahead of print).

Stroinsky, A., Schneider, Z., 1987. Cobamide dependant enzymes. In: Schneider, Z., Stroinsky, A. (Eds.), Comprehensive B-12. De Gruyter, Berlin, pp. 225–266.

Teplitsky, V., Huminer, D., Zoldan, J., Pitlik, S., Shohat, M., Mittelman, M., 2003. Hereditary partial transcobalamin II deficiency with neurologic, mental and hematologic abnormalities in children and adults. Isr. Med. Assoc. J. 5, 868–872.

Tucker, K.L., 2014. Vegetarian diets and bone status. Am. J. Clin. Nutr. 100 (Suppl.), 329S–335S.

Weir, D.G., Scott, J.M., 1999. Brain function in the elderly: role of vitamin B_{12} and folate. Br. Med. Bull. 55, 669–682.

Weiss, R., Fogelman, Y., Bennett, M., 1989. Severe vitamin B_{12} deficiency in an infant associated with a maternal deficiency and a strict vegetarian diet. J. Pediatr. Hematol. Oncol. 26 (4), 270–271.

Welch, A., Bingham, S., Camus, J., Dalzell, N., Reeve, J., Day, N., Khaw, T.T., 2005. Calcaneum broadband ultrasound attenuation relates to vegetarian and omnivorous diets differently in men and women: an observation from the European Prospective Investigation into Cancer in Norfolk (EPIC-Norfolk) population study. Osteoporos. Int. 16, 590–596.

Woo, K.S., Kwok, T.C., Celermajer, D.S., 2014. Vegan diet, subnormal vitamin B-12 status and cardiovascular health. Nutrients 6 (8), 3259–3273.

Further Reading

Herrmann, W., Obeid, R., 2013. Utility and limitations of biochemical markers of vitamin B_{12} deficiency. Eur. J. Clin. Invest. 43 (3), 231–237.

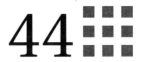

44

Probiotics in Nondairy Products

Gabriel Vinderola, Patricia Burns, Jorge Reinheimer

INSTITUTO DE LACTOLOGÍA INDUSTRIAL (CONICET-UNL), FACULTAD DE INGENIERÍA QUÍMICA, UNIVERSIDAD NACIONAL DEL LITORAL, SANTA FE, ARGENTINA

1. Introduction

The World Health Organization recognized in 2002 that some microorganisms, when orally administered, can confer health benefits on the host. They were named probiotics. The majority of probiotic microorganisms developed until now belong to the genera *Lactobacillus* and *Bifidobacterium*. The latter are natural inhabitants of the large intestine and only health benefits have been ascribed to them; the former might naturally occur in traditional or artisanal fermented foods and belong to the group of lactic acid bacteria (LAB). There is an ancient connection between traditional fermented foods, LAB, bifidobacteria, and intestinal health. The immune and molecular mechanisms that support that connection are being described today by metagenomic studies on the effects of specific probiotic strains on the gut microbiota and the impact on health and diseases. The industrialization and the transition from rural to modern life in cities led people to a lesser intake of the beneficial LAB present in traditional or artisanal fermented foods. The production of fermented dairy products, especially yogurt and fresh cheeses, fortified with probiotic bacteria is an option for the reintroduction of these benefic microorganisms into the diet. In this chapter, a brief description of the gut microbiota and its importance in the host health are depicted. A brief description of the incorporation of probiotic bacteria into fermented dairy products and their health benefits are provided. The importance of the food matrix in the functionality of probiotic bacteria and the reasons for developing nondairy plant-based probiotic products are also described. Finally, different technologies for the development of this kind of product are shown, but in a different way from the majority of the reviews on this topic, where probiotic products are presented and classified on the basis of the substrate used (cereals, legumes, fruits, or vegetables). In the approach used in this chapter, nondairy plant-based probiotic products were classified into three types: (1) products obtained by spontaneous (uncontrolled) fermentation of botanical species by resident fermentative microbiota, (2) products manufactured using controlled fermentation of vegetable substrates by the addition of selected probiotic strains displaying fermentation capacity, or (3) a probiotic plant-based product developed by the addition of the probiotic culture as an adjunct culture to the food matrix (unfermented products). Uncontrolled fermented products (traditional or artisanal fermented foods) display a complex and variable microbial population, dominated by yeasts and LAB, which renders it difficult to standardize and fully characterize them from a microbiological point of view, a condition required by the regulatory authorities for the approval of a health claim for the marketing of the food product. Fermentation of plant-based material with specific strains of probiotics might render a stable product (as the probiotic culture would be adapted to the food matrix); however, care must be taken as fermentation might change the sensorial properties in a negative way from what a consumer expects. Masking of unpleasant flavors is a technological possibility to cope with this issue. Finally, the use of plant material as carrier (i.e., without fermentation) requires a probiotic strain with great stability during storage. There are opportunities and challenges for probiotics in nondairy plant-based food products. The vast experience already achieved with probiotics in dairy products might be of help to overcome those challenges and to finally take advantage of the present opportunities.

2. The Gut Microbiota–Probiotic Axis

The largest microbial community of the human microbiome is located in the digestive tract, more precisely in the large intestine (Matamoros et al., 2013), and it is normally referred to as gut or intestinal microbiota. The massive use in the last decade of molecular biology techniques for mass sequencing of total DNA of complete bacterial communities has contributed to the increasing knowledge about the role of the gut microbiota in health and disease (Toh and Allen-Vercoe, 2015), as only approximately 10% of the gut bacteria are culturable on traditional agar plates (Eckburg et al., 2005). Strong and increasing evidence shows that the early acquisition, development, and maintenance of specific bacterial populations within the gut are critical to human health, and a better understanding of these offers great opportunities for intervention (Saavedra and Dattilo, 2012). In this regard, the use of probiotics is an option that we will discuss later. Throughout the human lifetime, the intestinal microbiota performs vital functions, such as barrier function, metabolic reactions, trophic effects, and maturation of the host's innate and adaptive immune responses. Development of the intestinal microbiota in infants is characterized by rapid and large changes in microbial abundance, diversity, and composition. These changes are influenced by medical, cultural, and environmental factors such as mode of delivery, diet, familial environment, diseases, and therapies used (Matamoros et al., 2013). The intestine of the human baby is sterile at birth, and the composition of the intestinal microbiota is relatively simple in infants but becomes more complex (and stable) in adults. The intestinal microbiota is thought to derive from the microbiota its own mother (vagina, skin, and mother's breastmilk) and from the environment where the infant is born. With regard to bacterial diversity, there is a high degree of variability among individuals, even among those living under the same conditions. This variability depends on age, diet, immune status, stress factors, and many other factors not yet completely known (Isolauri et al., 2004). Briefly, vaginal delivery, breastfeeding, and interaction of the infant with the environment were pointed out as factors that favor a proper microbial gut colonization and maturation of the gut-associated immune system, whereas C-section delivery, pre-term delivery, intake of antibiotics, formula feeding, indoor living, excessive sanitation, and chemical preservation of food are on the list of factors that might impair natural colonization (Moreau and Gaboriau-Routhiau, 2000; Toh and Allen-Vercoe, 2015). The total population of the large intestine has been estimated in approximately 10^{11}–10^{12} CFU/g of intestinal content, to harbor around 500–1000 different bacterial species in a given individual (Zhu et al., 2010) and to represent approximately 10^{12} cells/g dry weight feces. Then, a lot of metabolic activity is carried out by the intestinal microbiota to support the constant elimination through feces. Not only bacteria are present in the gut, the viral micro-biome (the "virome") load is estimated to be higher than that of the bacterial load, the majority being viruses that infect bacteria and Archaea (bacteriophage). Yeasts and other eukaryotes (e.g., protists) are estimated to make up only a small fraction of the colonic microbiota (Schulze and Sonnenborn, 2009; Reyes et al., 2010; Mills et al., 2013; Parfrey et al., 2014). Common genera or species found within the gut intestinal microbiota include *Bacteroides, Eubacterium, Ruminococcus, Clostridium,* and *Bifidobacterium,* and as sub-dominant microbiota, *Escherichia coli, Veillonella, Staphylococcus, Proteus, Streptococcus,* and *Lactobacillus* (Tannock, 2003; Krych et al., 2013). These microorganisms exert vari-ous metabolic activities, such as formation of short-chain fatty acids, upon dietary fiber breakdown and fermentation, that act as a carbon source for colonocytes, the synthesis of vitamins, and the activation or inactivation of bioactive food components. As it was said, their normal functioning is essential for the development of the host gut anatomy and for a proper education of the mucosal immune system. Regarding the functions carried out by the members of the intestinal microbiota, it is possible to categorize the gut microbiota species on the basis of whether they exert potentially pathogenic activities, potentially pathogenic and health-promoting activities at the same time, or exclusively potentially health-promoting aspects (Gibson et al., 2003). Species from the genera *Bifidobacterium* and *Lactobacillus,* commonly found within the gut microbiota in healthy subjects, have a long tradition of being considered health-promoting bacteria, and only health posi-tive effects have been ascribed to them. It seems, however, that the increasing amount of studies of intestinal microbiota components and their function will reveal in the near future that many other members of the intestinal microbiota might display only health positive effects for the host, converting them into potential candidates for probiotic inter-vention. The joint FAO/WHO working group adopted the definition that establishes that probiotics are "live microorganisms which when administered in adequate amounts con-fer a health benefit on the host" (FAO/WHO, 2002). This joint commission also released a series of guidelines for the evaluation of probiotics in foods.

The probiotic capacity of a microorganism is strain dependent. A strain can be referred to as a probiotic culture only once a health effect has been properly dem-onstrated on the host, following its consumption. Some species from which spe-cific strains have been isolated, characterized and proposed as probiotics include *Lactobacillus acidophilus, Lactobacillus gasseri, Lactobacillus johnsonii, Lactobacillus casei, Lactobacillus paracasei, Lactobacillus rhamnosus, Lactobacillus plantarum,*

Lactobacillus reuteri, Lactobacillus crispatus, Lactobacillus fermentum, Bifidobacterium animalis, Bifidobacterium bifidum, Bifidobacterium adolescentis, Bifidobacterium lactis, Bifidobacterium breve, Bifidobacterium infantis, Bifidobacterium longum, Saccharomyces boulardii, Saccharomyces cerevisiae, Enterococcus faecium, and *Escherichia coli*, among others. LAB constitute a broad heterogeneous group of generally food-grade microorganisms historically used in food preservation, composed of genera such as *Lactobacillus, Leuconostoc, Pediococcus, Lactococcus*, and *Streptococcus* (Mozzi, 2016). LAB is by far the most used group for the development of probiotic cultures. Interestingly, in the case of *E. coli* species, only the commercial probiotic strain *E. coli* Nissle has been reported so far. Although some strains of the genera *Enterococcus* were studied for their probiotic capacity and there are even some well-known examples of probiotic enterococci in European markets, their participation in diseases and their role as vectors for antibiotic resistance transmission still raise concerns on their safety for use as a probiotic for humans and also because these bacteria are still often viewed as problematic since many strains belonging to specific genetic subsets are known to be involved in nosocomial infections (Franz et al., 2011, 2014).

The definition of "probiotics" requires the term to be only applied to live microbes having a substantiated beneficial effect, as evidenced by a randomized double-blind, placebo-controlled, human clinical study. Nevertheless, in some cases, health benefits were also observed, to a certain degree, followed the administration of nonviable cells (Lahtinen, 2012). Recent studies have raised the question of whether nonviable probiotic strains can confer health benefits on the host by influencing the immune system. As the potential health effect of these nonviable bacteria depends on whether the mechanism of this effect is dependent on viability, future research needs to consider each probiotic strain on a case-by-case basis (Power et al., 2014). Some probiotic bacteria strains may release bioactive peptides by the breakdown of proteins (Pessione and Cirrincione, 2016) during the fermentation of a vegetal matrix and can also produce metabolites that can also confer health benefits, such as exopolysaccharides (Patten and Laws, 2015) or neuroactive substances such as gamma-aminobutyric acid and serotonin, which act on the brain-gut axis by displaying antidepressant or anxiolytic activity. This new generation of probiotics were called "psychobiotics" (Dinan et al., 2013). Starters commonly used in the fermentative dairy industry that belong to the species *Streptococcus thermophilus, Lactobacillus delbrueckii* subsp. *bulgaricus* or *Lactococcus lactis* are consumed alive on the food products manufactured with them (fermented dairy products mainly), but they do not survive the gastric and intestinal transit. Anyway, they (or their food products) can be considered probiotics according to Reid et al. (2003) and Guarner et al. (2005).

Different species from the genera *Bifidobacterium* and *Lactobacillus* can be normally found as members of the intestinal microbiota of healthy individuals. They can be recovered from feces, breastmilk, and grown in laboratory culture media (so they can be further industrialized), and only health-promoting effects have been ascribed to them. These facts make these genera the main chosen ones for the development of probiotic strains for use in food products or supplements. The human gut microbiota is getting a lot of attention today, and research has already demonstrated that alteration of its population may have far-reaching consequences. One of the possible routes for correcting intestinal dysbiosis is consuming probiotics (Fijan, 2014). Then, the strategy behind probiotic intervention would be to reinforce the intestinal microbiota diversity with "naturally occurring beneficial bacteria," at least as a transient intestinal colonization (as probiotics do not permanently colonize the gut), using a health-promoting candidate with credibility of specific health claims established through science-based clinical studies.

Probiotics do not derive exclusively from breastmilk (Martín et al., 2003) or from the intestinal environment or feces of healthy individuals. Beyond the human microbiota, strains for probiotic use, mainly from the genus *Lactobacillus*, can be isolated from certain food products, as they naturally occur in artisanal fermented foods such as fermented milks, cheeses, sausages, or cereal-based fermented foods (Farnworth, 2008). Considering the species-specific criterion, largely and historically used in the research of new probiotic strains, one might think that a probiotic candidate isolated from the human intestinal microbiota would perform better in humans compared to a strain isolated from another source (food, for instance) or from another species (pigs, for example), as it could be supposed that it would be ecologically better adapted to the human intestinal environment if it comes from that place. Nevertheless, probiotic properties were found in strains derived from the intestinal environment as well as in strains derived from fermented foods. For example, many commercial probiotic strains of intestinal origin performed well in the, sometimes harsh, acidic conditions found in fermented milks (Lourens-Hattingh and Viljoen, 2001; Vinderola et al., 2002). Haller et al. (2001) and Ren et al. (2014) found interesting metabolic and functional properties in lactobacilli derived from the gut as well as in strains isolated from food. Commensal and noncommensal strains of *L. fermentum* and *L. acidophilus* were both able to activate the gut mucosal immune response in mice (Dogi and Perdigón, 2006), a feature of interest for probiotic bacteria. The criterion of human origin still holds true, but more for "historical reasons" and "common sense," rather than for scientifically based reasons, which are still not evident (Morelli, 2000). It is the specificity of the action, not the source of the microorganism that is important for a strain to be considered a probiotic (FAO/WHO, 2002).

3. Probiotic Bacteria in Fermented Dairy Products: What Was Lost After the Industrial Revolution Is Being Recovered Today

The association between man and fermented milks stretches back thousands of years before the Christian era. The main geographical areas in which the traditional use of fermented milk dates back to ancient times include North and North Eastern Europe, South Eastern Europe including the Caucasus, Transcaucasia, and North East Asia in the

Soviet Union, the Near East, and the Indian subcontinent (Kanbe, 1992). The idea that LAB prevent intestinal disorders and diseases is nearly as old as the science of microbiology and due to the work of a disciple of Louis Pasteur, the father of microbiology. At the beginning of the 20th century, the Russian bacteriologist Eli Metchnikoff gave the first scientific explanation for the beneficial effects of LAB present in fermented milks. The good health and longevity observed in the Bulgarian population by Metchnikoff was attributed to the large amounts of fermented milks consumed. In 1908 he postulated his "longevity-without-aging" theory considering that the LAB resulted in the displacement of toxin-producing bacteria normally present in the intestine, resulting in a healthier environment (Lourens-Hattingh and Viljoen, 2001). Lactic acid–fermented (artisanal) foods have constituted a significant portion of the human diet for a long time and still constitute it in many countries, mainly in Africa and Asia. Lactic acid fermentation is the simplest and often the safest way of preserving food, and before the Industrial Revolution, this process was used just as much in Europe as it still is in Africa. In this way, humans consumed large numbers of live LAB, and presumably those associated with plant material were consumed before those associated with milk (Molin, 2001). The microbiological composition of traditional (artisanal) fermented products from Africa and Asia, mainly fermented milks, is composed of species such as *L. casei, L. acidophilus, L. rhamnosus, L. fermentum, L. delbrueckii* subsp. *bulgaricus, S. thermophilus, L. lactis,* or *L. plantarum*, among others (Watanabe et al., 2009; Schoustra et al., 2013; Franz et al., 2014). Many artisanal fermented foods may contain potential probiotic strains that will become important in the future (Farnworth, 2004). One of the first industrial productions of yogurt in Europe was undertaken by Danone in 1922 in Madrid, Spain (Rasic and Kurmann, 1978). After World War II, the technology of yogurt production, its consumption, and the understanding of its properties have increased rapidly (Prajapati and Nair, 2003). In the 1960s, the first concentrated deep-frozen/freeze bulk set starter cultures for yogurt manufacture were released into the market. From then on, commercial yogurt became more and more popular and it was massively produced by dairy companies around the world. Then, the natural supply of a variety of LAB through artisanal fermented milks ceased in industrialized countries during the 20th century, which may have contributed to the increasing occurrence of gastrointestinal problems, perhaps even immunologically dependent ones (Molin, 2001). If not completely ceased, the ingested diversity of LAB might have been reduced when commercial yogurt replaced artisanal fermented milks as part of the human diet. Yogurt is impressively old: it dates back to the third millennium BC, when Turkish goatherds fermented milk in sheep-skin bags to conserve it. Today, commercial yogurt is perhaps the fermented milk most consumed worldwide. Yogurt is the product of milk fermentation by only two species: *S. thermophilus* and *L. delbrueckii* subsp. *bulgaricus*. Although many beneficial health effects (metabolic, cardiovascular, gastrointestinal, and bone health as well as weight, cancer, or diabetes management and nutrition-related health outcomes) were linked to consumption of yogurt along with these two species (Adolfsson et al., 2004; McKinley, 2005; Glanville et al., 2015), the use of specific strains of other *Lactobacillus* species and bifidobacteria as adjuncts probiotics in commercial yogurt may be a way for consumers to take back some of those beneficial microorganisms lost by the transition from artisanal fermented milks to commercial (microbiologically simplified) yogurt or to incorporate, in the case of bifidobacteria, benefic microorganisms derived from the gut environment to reinforce the intestinal health through diet. In this sense, application of LAB has changed from traditionally fermented foods and beverages to rationally controlled food fermentation (Mozzi, 2016). Other facts that justify the incorporation of probiotic cultures to traditional yogurts are the following: microorganisms used for yogurt production (*S. thermophilus* and *L. delbrueckii* subsp. *bulgaricus*) are not common members of the human intestinal microbiota, and they hardly survive the harsh conditions found in the stomach (Reid et al., 2003). For probiotics, a criterion for strain selection is their capacity to survive along the gastrointestinal tract (Sanders, 2008), which means to withstand the low pH of the stomach and the inhibitory compounds found during the intestinal transit (bile salts mainly) (Russell et al., 2005; Lehrer et al., 2005). Viability in the intestine confers probiotics the possibility to have desirable metabolic activity during their passage through the gut (Bron et al., 2004) and to interact with gut-associated immune cells (Vinderola et al., 2005), launching desirable immune responses. Finally, numerous studies have demonstrated the importance of cell viability for the accomplishment of many health-promoting effects (Ouwehand and Salminen, 1998; Galdeano and Perdigón, 2004; Lahtinen, 2012). Although there is still debate on whether yogurt starters should be regarded as probiotics (Senok et al., 2005), sound evidence supports the idea that these cultures fulfill the current concept of probiotics (Guarner et al., 2005). The presence of probiotic bacteria able to survive the gastrointestinal transit will also assure many other health benefits for which cell viability and cell integrity in the intestinal lumen is required. However, it is worth to mention that the European Food Safety Authority (EFSA) has acknowledged, in 2010, a probiotic role to live yogurt cultures in relation to their capacity to improve lactose digestion in a nonstrain-dependent manner. The first commercial foods with probiotic bacteria were yogurt and fermented milks and are still the most important food vehicle for the delivery of probiotic bacteria in terms of worldwide diversity and sales (Farnworth and Champagne, 2016). Some facts made yogurt the main food vehicle for the delivery of probiotics. Yogurts are perceived by consumers as healthy food. From the point of view of the manufacture of yogurt in the dairy industry, and the feasibility of probiotic bacteria addition, probiotics can be aseptically added, after milk pasteurization, before (in set or firm yogurts) or after (in drinking or liquid yogurts) milk fermentation, depending on the type of product. The methods used to manufacture stirred and drinking yogurt, in particular, are well suited to the addition of probiotics after milk fermentation (Stanton et al., 2003). Additionally, yogurts are kept at refrigeration temperatures for up to more or less 1 month, which helps probiotic cell viability along storage. The commercial stability of the fermented milks allows the expansion and coverage of the needs of different consumer categories (Prado et al., 2008). Finally, yogurts are consumed, in general, on a regular basis. This might warrant the efficacy of probiotics in the intestine, as an eventual or sporadic probiotic intake is not likely to induce any health benefit.

4. Health Benefits of Probiotic Bacteria

In vitro investigations on adhesion properties, pathogen inhibition, and stimulation of immune parameters in cell culture, for example, are not sufficient to call a strain probiotic (Franz et al., 2014). Therefore, although in vitro (eukaryotic cell cultures) and animal studies are key steps to estimate the potential health effects of probiotic bacteria, the ultimate evidence of probiotic action must be provided by well-designed randomized double-blind placebo-controlled human clinical trials. The most popular food matrix used up to now for delivery of probiotics, yogurt, has health benefits itself derived from its multiple bioactive components. Typical dairy starters such as *L. lactis, S. thermophilus,* and *L. delbrueckii* subsp. *lactis* or *bulgaricus* have only rarely been used in animal or human in vivo studies, because they are not considered to exert health benefits comparable to those of probiotic strains (Lick et al., 2001), although there are some reports indicating that yogurt starters might arrive viable to the intestine (Lick et al., 2001; Elli et al., 2006; Vázquez et al., 2013). There is a large body of evidence that conventional yogurts containing *S. thermophilus* and *L. delbrueckii* subsp. *bulgaricus* do exert many health-promoting effects (Adolfsson et al., 2004; Guarner et al., 2005) due to their content of lactase released in the gut from the starters that are sensitive to the detergent action of bile salts (Lin et al., 1998), to the release of bioactive peptides from milk proteins (Vinderola, 2008), to the production of soluble immunomodulatory exopolysaccharides (Vinderola et al., 2006) or antimicrobial components (Ouwehand and Vesterlund, 2004), or to health effects related to the immunomodulation of the gut-associated lymphoid tissue by cell-wall debris (Morata de Ambrosini et al., 1996; Tejada-Simon and Pestka, 1999) derived from cells of *S. thermophilus* and *L. delbrueckii* subsp. *bulgaricus* that are inactivated by gastric acidity and disrupted by bile salts and lysozyme during the intestinal transit.

A detailed discussion of the health benefits of different probiotic strains and their mechanisms of action is far beyond the scope of this chapter. Some of the health benefits of the consumption of probiotic bacteria as pure cultures (as found in dietary supplements) or included in fermented dairy products or other foods are the beneficial modulation of the gut microbiota activity by the reduction of the risk associated with mutagenicity and carcinogenicity (Druart et al., 2014), alleviation of lactose intolerance (Shaukat et al., 2010), reinforcement of gut mucosal immunity (Ganesh and Versalovic, 2015), acceleration of intestinal mobility (Miller and Ouwehand, 2013) or reduction of constipation (Dimidi et al., 2014), lowering of blood cholesterol (Kumar et al., 2012), prevention or shortening of the duration of different diarrheas (Ahmadi et al., 2015; Guarino et al., 2015; Szajewska et al., 2015; Wong et al., 2015), prevention of urinary tract infections (Schwenger et al., 2015) or human diarrhea infections associated with domestic animal husbandry (Zambrano et al., 2014), prevention of inflammatory bowel disease (IBD) and pouchitis (Saez-Lara et al., 2015; Wasilewski et al., 2015) prevention of colon cancer (Wang et al., 2015), inhibition of *Helicobacter pylori* and intestinal pathogens, or treatment and prevention of allergies such as atopic dermatitis (Zuccotti et al., 2015) or celiac disease (de Sousa Moraes et al., 2014). Positive results after probiotic intervention were also observed at distant sites from the gut such as the skin (Vaughn and Sivamani, 2015). Additionally, probiotics were also positively involved in emotions (Slyepchenko et al.,

2014) and weight loss (Park and Bae, 2015). It is unlikely that a probiotic strain might accomplish all the different health benefits attributed to probiotics in general. The health effects of a given strain are limited to those demonstrated by the human clinical trials in which it was used and in the concentration, format (pure culture or included in a food matrix), and period of administration reported. Some commercially available probiotic strains with well-documented health effects are *L. acidophilus* LA1, *L. paracasei* CRL 431, *B. animalis* subsp. *lactis* Bb-12 and *L. rhamnosus* GR1 from Chr. Hansen, *L. acidophilus* NCFM from Dupont, *L. acidophilus* DDS-1 from Nebraska Cultures, *L. acidophilus* NCFB 1748 and *L. paracasei* F19 from Arla, *L. paracasei* Shirota and *B. breve* Yakult from Yakult, *L. casei* Immunitas (DN 114-001) and *B. animalis* subsp. *lactis* (DN 173-010) from Danone, *L. johnsonii* LA-1 from Nestec, *L. plantarum* 299v and *L. rhamnosus* 271 from Probi AB, *L. reuteri* SD2112 from Biogaia, *L. rhamnosus* GG from Valio Dairy, *L. salivarius* UCC118 from University College Cork, *B. longum* BB536 from Morinaga, or *B. animalis* subsp. *lactis* DR10 from Fonterra (Franz et al., 2014). For some of them, their health effects have been reviewed. One example is *L. rhamnosus* GG (Szajewska et al., 2011; Liu et al., 2013; Szajewska and Kołodziej, 2015), which accounts for more than 760 scientific publications and more than 260 clinical studies; *L. rhamnosus* GG (trademark LGG) is the world's best documented lactobacilli probiotic strain (http://www.chr-hansen.com). Other well-documented probiotic strains are *L. casei* Shirota (Matsuzaki, 1998), included in the popular Japanese product Yakult, *L. acidophilus* NCFM, or *B. animalis* subsp. *lactis* BB12 (Szajewska and Chmielewska, 2013; Jungersen et al., 2014), backed by 360 scientific publications out of which more than 165 are clinical studies; BB-12 is the world's best documented probiotic bifidobacteria (http://www.chr-hansen.com). It must be taken into account that effects observed for a strain administered as pure culture will not necessarily be the same if the strain is administered within a product matrix, as the food matrix might highly determine the functionality of probiotic bacteria. This is worth mentioning since the majority of the clinical trials for probiotics were carried out with the strain as pure cultures (supplements) or within a dairy matrix, so much less information has been available up to now about the effects of probiotics when administered in nondairy foods.

Perturbations in the composition or functions of the microbiota are linked to inflammatory and metabolic disorders (e.g., IBD, irritable bowel syndrome, and obesity); however, it is not clear yet whether these changes are symptoms of the disease or a contributing factor for disease development. While evidence of the preventive and therapeutic effects of probiotic strains on various intestinal conditions is promising, the exact mechanisms of the beneficial effects are not fully understood (Power et al., 2014).

5. Functionality of Probiotic Bacteria: The Food Matrix Matters

According to the definition of probiotic bacteria, cells must be viable. The determination of probiotic viability (assessment of the concentration of viable cells on agar plates as the simplest method to monitor cell viability) along the manufacture chain of probiotic cultures and foods containing probiotic bacteria has been the gold standard to claim for the probiotic capacity of the strain or the product containing it. Although plate counting on agar media can assess bacterial viability, it actually only indicates how many cells can replicate under the conditions provided for growth (Ben Amor et al., 2007). Noncultivable or dead cells, which may be still functional, are not considered. Then, "viable cells" is, for the moment, a sign of a "functional culture." Nonetheless, evidence suggests that the level of viable cells would no longer be a definite parameter that indicates the real probiotic capacity or functionality of the strain. Some examples where functional traits changed without changes in cell viability will be briefly commented on now and were further discussed in previous works (Sanders and Marco, 2010). Adhesion of probiotics to the surface of intestinal epithelial cells is important for, at least a transient, gut colonization. Additionally, cell adhesion was linked to several beneficial effects such as shortening of duration of diarrhea, immunogenic effects, and competitive exclusion (Isolauri et al., 1991; Saavedra et al., 1994; Salminen et al., 1996; Malin et al., 1997; Van Tassell and Miller, 2011). Tuomola et al. (2001) reported a reduction in the adhesion capacity of *L. acidophilus* when this parameter was compared in the strain isolated from a dairy product at the beginning and at the end of the production line of manufacture of the product. If the adhesion capacity of the probiotic is altered during the manufacture of the food product due to technological issues (shear stress when pumping liquids trough pipes), then its functionality (persistence in the gut) might be also altered without noticeable changes in cell viability. Saarela et al. (2003) reported that resistance to acidic conditions found in the stomach, a desirable feature of probiotic candidates, depended on the carbon source used as substrate for the production of biomass of probiotic bacteria. Similar levels of viable cells were obtained with different substrates, but cultures differed on their capacity to withstand low pH. Acid tolerance in a probiotic strain of *B. animalis* was influenced by the processing and storage conditions, whereas the level of viable cells in the product was not affected during storage (Matto et al., 2006). The immunomodulatory capacity of *L. gasseri* OLL2809 was dependent on the pH at which cells were grown as well as on the time at which cells were harvested (Sashihara et al., 2007). The resistance to gastric acidity of the breastmilk-derived probiotic candidate *B. animalis* subsp. *lactis* INL1 also depends on the pH at which biomass was produced, and also on the food matrix where the strain is included (Vinderola et al., 2012). It was reported that *L. casei* BL23 was more effective for the attenuation of colitis in a murine model when administered in milk compared to the administration of the strain as a pure culture in a buffered solution (Lee et al., 2015). A key study showing the impact of the food matrix on the functionality of the probiotic strain is the one performed by Grześkowiak et al. (2011). In the aforementioned study, the commercial probiotic strain *L. rhamnosus* GG was reisolated from different foods and dietary supplements obtained in different parts of the world. All *L. rhamnosus* GG isolates showed similar tolerance to acid and were able to bind to human colonic mucus. However, pathogen exclusion by inhibition and competition varied significantly among the different isolates and pathogens tested. The results suggest that different sources of the same probiotic may have significantly altered strain properties. A comprehensive revision on the importance of the food matrix on probiotic viability efficacy was reported (Ranadheera et al., 2010; do Espírito Santo et al., 2011). As already mentioned, when considering nondairy foods it must be taken into account that the majority of the clinical trials for probiotics were carried out with the strain as pure cultures (supplements) or within a dairy matrix. So, we must be aware of the fact that efficacy of probiotics might change when a probiotic strain supported by clinical studies performed as single culture or within a dairy matrix is incorporated in a vegetable, cereal, or fruit matrix.

6. Opportunities and Challenges for Probiotic Bacteria in Nondairy Foods

Beyond artisanal milk-based fermented products, LAB are present in other traditional fermented foods, such as brined olives, salted gherkins, or sauerkraut, but for one reason or another, these plant-based foods are rarely considered carriers for probiotic bacteria (Molin, 2001). With an increase in the number of vegetarians in developing countries, there is also a demand for vegetarian probiotic products. Concomitantly, lactose intolerance, allergy to milk proteins, and the cholesterol content of dairy products are major drawbacks related to fermented dairy products as attractive carriers for probiotic bacteria (Prado et al., 2008; Granato et al., 2010). Anyway, it is fair to mention that there are also allergies to soy, gluten, and vegetables, which means that milk-based products are not the only ones that may confer allergenicity on consumers (Granato et al., 2010). Additionally, some people may reject consuming dairy products for economic, cultural, or religious reasons. Yet, milk products are hardly accessible to consumers in some parts of the world (Rivera-Espinoza and Gallardo-Navarro, 2010), thus creating opportunities for the development of nondairy probiotic products. For instance, the Asian diets are relatively low in meat and dairy food, whereas plant-based foods constitute the core of the daily intake (Vasudha and Mishra, 2013). At the same time, lactose intolerance in East Asia may have up to a 90% of incidence in the population (Kumar et al., 2015). In economic terms, the only hope for business survival is the ability to continue innovating (Granato et al., 2010). Therefore, permanent seeking of innovation by the food industry is another factor that fuels the diversification of the food matrices where probiotics might be included, to satisfy the growing demand for new foods. Nondairy foods that might be a potential vehicle for probiotic bacteria include meat, fish, cereals, legumes, vegetables, or fruits; however, due to the characteristics of this book, we will focus on plant materials. Plant materials, as carriers for probiotic bacteria, may have the same positive perception by consumers of being as good for health as dairy products. They are a source of fibers, nutrients, and minerals, and they are intended for consumption by all individuals and widely accepted among consumers (Furtado Martins et al., 2013). A particular and possible advantage of the incorporation of probiotics to fruit juices is that they stay much less time in the stomach compared to dairy products; thus probiotic strains could find their way to the gut more quickly, and in higher amounts of viable cells, evading faster the harsh acidic conditions of the stomach (Kumar et al., 2015). However, it must be acknowledged that dairy products may have more buffering capacity compared to fruit juices and seem to better neutralize the acid in the stomach (Tompkins et al., 2011). However, contradictory results were reported by Elizaquível et al. (2011) as well. In the referenced work, survival of certain probiotic strains to simulated gastrointestinal digestion was higher in orange juice than in yogurt. These results indicate the strain-matrix dependency of survival in food.

There are opportunities, but there are also challenges. Fruit or vegetable juices contain important nutrients (minerals, vitamins, dietary fibers), but there are also some factors that could limit probiotic survival, mainly low acidity related to the high level of organic acids (Perricone et al., 2015) and dissolved oxygen (Shori, 2016). However, these same hurdles had to be overcome previously by probiotic bacteria in fermented milks (and indeed they succeed due to proper strain selection). Dairy products are stored at temperatures close to 5°C in commercial retailers, so probiotic cell viability is presumably warranted along the shelf life of the product if low temperatures are maintained. Storage at room temperature, which is common for many types of nondairy products such as cereal products, fruit juices, drinks, confectionary, and so on, can create an overwhelming challenge for probiotic stability (Matilla-Sandholm et al., 2002). Yogurt-type products when not consumed immediately require refrigeration to ensure stability of both the product and the probiotics, but the high ambient temperatures of many regions around the globe, the great distribution distances within some countries, and potential problems with maintaining the cold chain in rural areas present logistical problems for probiotic dairy products (Franz et al., 2014).

Marketing a strain, food, or a dietary supplement or pharmaceutical product containing a strain as probiotic and bearing a health claim requires the approval of the specific health claim by the local or regional health authority. This authority will determine which health or nutritional claims can be advertised or not on the label of the product (packaging) or in the messages delivered through audiovisual media (Arora and Baldi, 2015). In Europe, probiotic health claims must be evaluated and approved by an ad hoc committee named by the EFSA before being authorized by the European Commission (Salminen and van Loveren, 2012). While hundreds of human trials are published, the term is in danger of falling into disrepute as a result of negative publicity associated with the lack of support of numerous health claims by agencies such as EFSA, who are demanding quasi-medical standards of proof in a bid to "protect the consumer" (Hill and Sanders, 2013). This controversy makes the European probiotics industry fear that regulations will scuttle the market for health-promoting or disease-preventing foods (Vogel, 2010), making substantiation of their health effects a present challenge for probiotics.

7. Plant Material and Technological Strategies for the Development of Nondairy Probiotic Products

Fermented dairy products, such as fermented milks and fresh cheeses, have been the food vehicles with the biggest technological and commercial success for the incorporation of

Table 44.1 Technological Strategies for the Development of Nondairy Plant-Based Probiotic Products

Fermentation	Characteristics	Advantages	Disadvantages
Uncontrolled	Raw material fermented with indigenous microorganisms	No need for inoculation	Difficulty for product standardization
Controlled	Inoculation and growth of a specific probiotic strain	Use of a smaller inoculum	Possible negative impact on flavor
Unfermented	Use of a specific probiotic strain as adjunct (no growth on the substrate)	No negative impact on flavor	Need for a higher inoculum

probiotic bacteria (Figueroa-González et al., 2011). The technological process for the manufacture of yogurt is rather simple. In most cases, milk is fermented by a mixed starter culture composed of *S. thermophilus* and *L. delbrueckii* subsp. *bulgaricus*, and the probiotic cultures are added along with the starters (for set or firm yogurts) or after milk fermentation (in stirred or drinking yogurts). The most common probiotic microorganisms used and marketed in food worldwide belong to the genera *Lactobacillus* and *Bifidobacterium* (Champagne et al., 2011). They are generally fastidious bacteria and require rich media for propagation. They grow poorly in milk (Robitaille and Champagne, 2014), or their growth in milk-based media, even with an added nitrogen source, is very slow (Burns et al., 2008) when compared to the starter cultures. The protocooperation established between *S. thermophilus* and *L. delbrueckii* subsp. *bulgaricus* can lower milk pH from 6.5 to 4.5 in less than 6 h, whereas the majority of probiotic strains need more than 10 h to reach that pH (Østlie et al., 2003). As probiotic bacteria generally do not grow rapidly in cows' milk, in yogurt manufacture, they do not attain as high numbers as the starter cultures (Champagne et al., 2005). So, probiotics in yogurts are mostly used as adjuncts or ingredients (Granato et al., 2010); they are not expected to significantly grow during milk fermentation if inoculated prior to fermentation. For plant-based probiotic products, there is a wider range of possible growth substrates (vegetables, fruits, cereals, legumes), and probiotics might act as starters or as adjuncts (Table 44.1).

7.1 Nondairy Plant-Based Probiotic Beverages Derived From Uncontrolled Fermentations

Over centuries, fermentations have been used to preserve, improve the quality, or modify the flavor of cereals, fruits, vegetables, legumes, meat, or fish. As the spontaneous fermentation process involves mixed cultures such as yeast, LAB, and fungi, traditional fermented foods are a plentiful source of microorganisms, and some strains were studied for their probiotic characteristics (Rivera-Espinoza and Gallardo-Navarro, 2010). Boza is a beverage consumed in Bulgaria, Albania, Turkey, and Romania that is derived from the spontaneous fermentation of wheat, rye, millet, maize, and other cereals mixed with sugar. Yeasts and LAB were isolated from Bulgarian boza, including *L. plantarum*, *L. acidophilus*, *L. fermentum*, *Lactobacillus coprophilus*, *Leuconostoc reffinolactis*,

Leuconostoc mesenteroides, L. brevis, S. cerevisiae, Candida tropicalis, Candida glabrata, Geotrichum penicillatum, and *Geotrichum candidum.* Bushera is the most common traditional beverage prepared in Uganda from sorghum or millet flour from the germinated sorghum and millet grains mixed with boiling water and left to cool to ambient temperature to ferment for 1–6 days. The LAB isolated from Bushera comprised *Lactobacillus,* mainly *L. brevis,* but also *Lactococcus, Leuconostoc, Enterococcus,* and *Streptococcus.* In line with this kind of spontaneously fermented beverages, where a plethora of yeasts and LAB species were reported to be naturally present, also mentioned can be Mahewu, consumed in Africa and in some Arabian Gulf countries (made from corn meal), Pozol in Mexico (made from maize), Togwa in Africa (obtained from maize flour and finger millet malt), or Hardaliye in Turkey, a lactic acid–fermented beverage produced from the natural fermentation of red grape, or grape juice with the addition of the crushed mustard seeds and benzoic acid (Prado et al., 2008). A multitude of nondairy fermented cereal products has been created throughout history for human nutrition, but only recently probiotic characteristics of microorganisms involved in traditional fermented cereal foods have been reported. Although LAB are the principal microorganisms responsible for the natural fermentation of these products, the indigenous LAB microbiota varies as a function of the quality of the raw material, temperature, harvesting, and fermentation conditions, which make difficult the complete characterization of the LAB strains involved and the standardization of the product required to be regarded and marketed as a probiotic food. Although there is a large quantity of traditional fermented food produced from different substrates, we still lack information about the identity of the potential probiotic strains naturally present in those foods (Rivera-Espinoza and Gallardo-Navarro, 2010). However, they constitute an important source for the isolation, characterization, and marketing of new probiotic strains, as the information available on these matrices as raw material for probiotic microorganisms is still significantly less compared to their dairy counterparts (Kumar et al., 2015). The possibility of obtaining an accepted health claim for a traditional fermented food from the local authority is of interest for the promotion of probiotic foods; as local populations in developing countries may prefer a "local" solution to nourishment, health maintenance, and restoration rather than purchasing a foreign company's product on a regular basis, especially if that traditional food is part of their normal diet (Franz et al., 2014) or of their cultural identity.

7.2 Nondairy Plant-Based Probiotic Beverages Derived From Controlled Fermentation

L. plantarum 299v is to the plant-based food industry perhaps what *L. rhamnosus* GG is to the dairy products industry. The first probiotic food that did not contain milk or milk constituents was launched in Sweden in 1994 and was named ProViva (Skane Dairy, Malmö, Sweden). The active component is oatmeal gruel fermented by *L. plantarum* 299v where malted barley is added to enhance the liquefaction of the product. This formula is used as the active ingredient in the food product in which 5% of the oatmeal gruel is mixed with a fruit drink (rose hip, strawberry, blueberry, black currant, or tropical fruits). The drink contains approximately 5×10^7 CFU/mL of *L. plantarum* 299v. The product was effective in a human clinical trial with patients with irritable bowel syndrome (Molin, 2001), among other clinical conditions that will be discussed later. Another *L. plantarum* strain (*L. plantarum* B28) was used for the controlled fermentation (8 h) of whole-grain oat. The shelf life of this functional drink was 21 days (Angelov et al., 2006).

Probiotic products developed with soy extract mixed with fruit juices are a new generation of foods on the market, which is a convenient way to include soy protein in the basic diet (Champagne and Gardner, 2008). Soymilk is a suitable substrate for the growth of LAB and bifidobacteria in a controlled fermentation (Prado et al., 2008). One technological benefit of soy fermentation is the reduction of its "beany" flavor and chalkiness. Fermentation by probiotics has also the potential to reduce the content of carbohydrates possibly responsible for gas production in the gut, such as raffinose and stachyose, to increase free isoflavone levels, and to favor desirable changes in the intestinal microbiota (Champagne et al., 2009). Fermentation has been a traditional option to increase digestibility of soy products and make them more flavored (Han et al., 2001). Even antioxidant activity of phenolic compounds might be enhanced by fermentation (Sheih et al., 2000; Wang et al., 2006). Some examples of fermented soy products are a water-soluble soy extract fermented beverage with *B. breve* Yakult (Shimakama et al., 2003) or a soy yogurt product fermented with *L. casei* and supplemented with oligofructose and inulin that presented an acceptance index above 70% (Hauly et al., 2005). Potential probiotic strains of *L. plantarum* and *L. fermentum*, isolated from cocoa fermentation in Southern Bahia (Brazil), adequately fermented soymilk, rendering a product with sensorial acceptance. Strains also displayed good survival in refrigerated storage (Saito et al., 2014).

In the dairy industry, cheeses were the second massive successful food matrix for the delivery of probiotic bacteria (Vinderola et al., 2009). The preparation of cheese-like products from soymilk coagulated with LAB is also an option. Liu et al. (2006) developed a soy cheese based on the Chinese sufu, including a probiotic strain of *L. rhamnosus*, without negative effects on sensory properties and satisfactory viability of the strain in storage at 10°C.

Fruit and vegetable juices as a food matrix for the development of probiotic drinks display a number of attractive advantages (inherent content of beneficial nutrients, tasteful and pleasant to all age groups, perceived as being healthy and refreshing), but there are also potential sensory challenges when lactic acid fermentation takes place, especially if bifidobacteria are used as they produce acetic acid that may impart a vinegar taste. Yoon et al. determined the suitability of tomato (Yoon et al., 2004), beet juice (Yoon et al., 2005), and cabbage juice (Yoon et al., 2006) using four strains of probiotic LAB. Fermentation took from 48 to 72 h until pH reached 4.1–4.5. However, not all LAB strains used remained viable in storage for 4 weeks at 4°C. Rakin et al. (2007) fermented beetroot and carrot juices with a strain of *L. acidophilus*. Fermentation was faster in the presence of yeast autolysate. Other commercially available products that fall into this category of plant-based drinks fermented with probiotic microorganisms are Grainfields Wholegrain Liquid, a drink made from oat, maize, rice, alfalfa seed, pearl barley, linseed, mung beans, rye grain, wheat, and millet fermented with *L. acidophilus, L. delbrueckii, S. cerevisiae,* and *S. boulardii* and Vita Biosa, a mixture of aromatic herbs and other plants fermented with LAB and yeasts, aimed at improving intestinal conditions (Prado et al., 2008). As fermentation with LAB or bifidobacteria may produce unpleasant flavors, masking can be used to reduce the sensations of unpleasant odors and flavors through the addition of new substances or flavors to juices (Reineccius, 2000). Addition of 10% (v/v) of tropical fruit juices was reported to be enough for masking the perceptible off-flavors caused by probiotics that often contribute to consumer dissatisfaction (Luckow et al., 2006). Fruit purees were also assessed as a substrate for fermentation with LAB strains. Kim et al. (2010) and Tsen et al. (2004), reported a successful pear puree and banana puree fermentation with *Leuconostoc mesenteroides* and *L. acidophilus,* respectively; however, the probiotic capacity of the strains used remains unknown.

7.3 Nondairy Plant-Based Beverages Added With Probiotic Cultures

Application of probiotic cultures in nondairy products represents a great challenge. Since the probiotic cultures are included as ingredients to these products, they do not usually multiply, as there will be no fermentation, which sets great demands for the probiotic survival. Stability is conditioned by factors such as pH, storage temperature, dissolved oxygen levels, and presence of chemical inhibitors (Granato et al., 2010). Storage at room temperature, which is common for many types of nondairy products, can be detrimental for probiotic stability (Matilla-Sandholm et al., 2002). For example, unsatisfactory probiotic cell viability was observed when two probiotic strains of *L. casei,* commonly used in dairy products, were added to commercial fruit and soya drinks and stored at 5°C for 4 weeks. Yet, negative sensorial characteristics appeared in those juices due to the growth of *L. casei* in the food product during storage at room temperature (Céspedes et al., 2013). Storage under refrigeration, as for probiotics in dairy products, is mandatory for this kind of product. Fortunately, successful cases were reported as well, but success is dependent on the probiotic strain used and on the fruit juice used. Sheehan et al. (2007) assessed the acid tolerance and the technological robustness of probiotic cultures for fortification of fruit juices. A variable survival capacity of *L. rhamnosus, L. casei,* and *L. paracasei* in orange, pineapple, and cranberry juices was observed. Champagne and Gardner (2008) studied the effect of storage on a commercial fruit drink on subsequent survival to gastrointestinal stresses. Nine probiotic lactobacilli strains were evaluated for their ability to survive in a commercial fruit drink stored at 4°C for up to 80 days. Authors found that *L. rhamnosus* seemed more stable than *L. acidophilus.* The famous *L. rhamnosus* GG, largely used in dairy products, has also been present since 1996 in nondairy drinks developed by Valio Ltd., in products such as Gefilus fruit drinks. Another series of fruit juices containing the same probiotic strain is Biola, manufactured by Tine BA in Norway. Rela is a fruit juice with added *L. reuteri* MM53 manufactured by BioGaia in Sweden (Prado et al., 2008). The awareness of consumers about the presence of a functional ingredient might condition the acceptance of the product. Luckow and Delahunty (2004a) evaluated the consumer's acceptance of black currant juices containing probiotic cultures. Consumers were told that one of the juices contained a healthy ingredient. In general, the consumers selected their most preferred product as the "healthiest" sample. However, in another trial (Luckow and Delahunty, 2004b), consumer's preference was directed toward conventional orange juice instead of a probiotic one, as consumers detected "dairy" and "medicinal" flavors. Sometimes, in fact, consumers are influenced to associate "healthy" foods with unacceptable flavors, assuming in their minds that sensory pleasure must be sacrificed to achieve a healthy diet (Tuorila and Cardello, 2002). The issue of the presence of perceptible dairy flavors may be due to the presence of traces of dairy ingredients (skim milk, milk proteins) commonly used as protectants by manufacturers of probiotic bulk cultures. This may happen when probiotic cultures developed for the dairy food industry are used as adjuncts for the development of nondairy products. In this sense, it is still needed the development of probiotic cultures where nondairy ingredients are used as protectants for freeze-dried or deep-frozen cultures intended for direct inoculation. For example, *L. paracasei* 431, a probiotic strain isolated in the middle 1980s at CERELA (Tucumán, Argentina) and marketed by Chr. Hansen, has been largely used in fermented dairy products. This strain was reengineered for use in juice drinks (Céspedes et al., 2013). The key for the direct inoculation of probiotics into the final food product is a special direct liquid inoculation system. It allows food producers to add the probiotic bacteria directly to the finished food product, which can lead to a higher number of viable microorganisms (Prado et al., 2008), without the need (and the possible negative impact on sensorial properties) of product fermentation. Another strategy reported for the delivery of probiotics is their immobilization on minimally processed pieces of apple and quince (Kourkoutas et al., 2005) or on wheat grains (Loulouda et al., 2009).

8. Human Clinical Trials Supporting the Health Benefits of Probiotics in Nondairy Plant-Based Foods

As it was mentioned before, the health claims of probiotics in the food matrix used must be supported by sound evidence derived from well-designed randomized placebo-controlled double-blind human clinical trials. Clinical trials of probiotic bacteria in plant-based food are still low in number compared to their dairy counterparts. The commercial product ProViva (rose hip fruit drink supplemented with oatmeal gruel fermented by *L. plantarum* 299v) was administrated to patients with irritable bowel syndrome in a double-blind, placebo-controlled study for 4 weeks. Abdominal bloating was significantly lower in the treatment group than in the placebo group, and pain decrease was more rapid in the treated group. Twelve months after treatment, the treatment group was still experiencing better overall gastrointestinal function than the placebo group (Nobaek et al., 2000). The same fruit drink was effective in reducing fibrinogen and LDL cholesterol concentrations in serum of Polish men with moderately elevated cholesterol after 6 week of administration (Bukowska et al., 1998) and gastrointestinal symptoms during treatment with antibiotics (Lönnermark et al., 2010), and the product proved to be effective in increasing iron absorption in women of reproductive age (Hoppe et al., 2015). Ouwehand et al. (2004) reported the detection in feces of *B. lactis* BB-12 when administered in an oat cereal bar, whereas Valerio et al. (2006) demonstrated the presence in feces of *L. paracasei* IMPC2 when orally administered to humans in artichokes. The presence of probiotic bacteria in feces following oral administration is a desirable attribute for a probiotic candidate; however, it says little about the probiotic effect, which should be demonstrated. Pitkala et al. (2007) reported that fermented cereal with two bifidobacteria strains normalized bowel movements in elderly nursing home residents in a randomized controlled trial. The administration of *L. paracasei* F19 in cereals to infants had a positive effect on the serum lipid profile and plasma metabolome in infants (Chorell et al., 2013). Nevertheless, the same product seemed not to be effective either on the prevention of dental caries (Hasslöf et al., 2013) nor for primary prevention of allergic disease (West et al., 2013). In the latter study, the authors hypothesized that the lack of differences between the control and treated group might have been due to the small size of the population involved in the clinical trial. Lee et al. (2013) reported a reduced medication use and improved pulmonary function in asthmatic school children aged 10–12 years that received for 16 weeks supplements containing vegetable and fruit concentrate, fish oil, and probiotics. However, the concomitant administration of several potential functional products does not permit establishing the real contribution of the probiotics used to the health effects observed.

9. Concluding Remarks

The popular positive and ancient connection between ingestion of fermented foods and the proliferation of friendly bacteria in the gut has been gradually more and more supported by the knowledge emerging from the metagenomics studies concerning intestinal microbiota and its modulation through the diet, and the consequences on health and disease. The most typical food matrices for probiotic bacteria have been fermented dairy products, mainly yogurts and fresh cheeses. Yet it is possible to obtain probiotic foods from several plant-based matrices (cereals, legumes, fruits, and vegetables), including both fermented (spontaneously or controlled) and nonfermented products. Among the factors that fueled the development of nondairy plant-based probiotic products are increasing numbers of vegetarians (including vegans), lactose intolerance, allergy to milk proteins, cholesterol content of dairy products, and the permanent need for innovation of the food industry. Although there is a large quantity of traditional fermented food produced from different substrates, where a plethora of LAB and yeast occurs naturally, we still lack information about the identity and stability of those complex ecosystems to apply for a health claim for those products to the regulatory authority. Food products obtained by controlled fermentation with specific probiotic strains or those where the food is used as a carrier for probiotic microorganisms delivery (unfermented products) seem to be more likely to successfully pass the rigorous exams about functionality required by the regulatory authorities today. Most probiotic strains has been developed for the dairy industry where dairy ingredients are used as protectants for the concentrated commercial cultures. Considering that the food matrix might exert a key role on the functionality of the products, further studies are needed to evaluate the impact of the plant-based matrix on the functionality of traditional probiotics or newly isolated ones. Even with all these challenges, the future of nondairy plant-based probiotic products is promising, considering the vast variety of fruits, vegetables, herbs, cereals, legumes, and all their possible combinations to manufacture innovative and attractive healthy food products for a growing world population looking for non-dairy functional products.

References

Adolfsson, O., Meydani, S.N., Russell, R.M., 2004. Yogurt and gut function. Am. J. Clin. Nutr. 80, 245–256.

Ahmadi, E., Alizadeh-Navaei, R., Rezai, M.S., 2015. Efficacy of probiotic use in acute rotavirus diarrhea in children: a systematic review and meta-analysis. Caspian J. Intern. Med. 6 (4), 187–195.

Angelov, A., Gotcheva, V., Kuncheva, R., Hristozova, T., 2006. Development of a new oat-based probiotic drink. Int. J. Food Microbiol. 112 (1), 75–80.

Arora, M., Baldi, A., 2015. Regulatory categories of probiotics across the globe: a review representing existing and recommended categorization. Indian J. Med. Microbiol. 33 (5), 2–10.

Ben Amor, K., Vaughan, E.E., de Vos, W.M., 2007. Advanced molecular tools for the identification of lactic acid bacteria. J. Nutr. 137, 741S–747S.

Bron, P.A., Grangette, C., Mercenier, A., de Vos, W.M., Kleerebezem, M., 2004. Identification of *Lactobacillus plantarum* genes that are induced in the gastrointestinal tract of mice. J. Bacteriol. 186, 5721–5729.

Bukowska, H., Pieczul-Mróz, J., Jastrzebsk, K., Chelstowski, K., Naruszewicz, M., 1998. Significant decrease in fibrinogen and LDL cholesterol levels upon supplementation of the diet with *Lactobacillus plantarum* (ProViva) in subjects with moderately elevated cholesterol concentrations. Atherosclerosis 137, 437–438.

Burns, P., Vinderola, G., Molinari, F., Reinheimer, J., 2008. Suitability of whey and buttermilk for the growth and frozen storage of probiotic lactobacilli. Int. J. Dairy Technol. 61 (2), 156–164.

Céspedes, M., Cárdenas, P., Staffolani, M., Ciappini, M.C., Vinderola, G., 2013. Performance in nondairy drinks of probiotic *L. casei* strains usually employed in dairy products. J. Food Sci. 78 (5), 756–762.

Champagne, C.P., Gardner, N.J., 2008. Effects of storage in a fruit drink on subsequent survival of probiotic lactobacilli to gastro-intestinal stresses. Food Res. Int. 41, 539–543.

Champagne, C.P., Green-Johnson, J., Raymond, Y., Barrete, J., Buckley, N., 2009. Selection of probiotic bacteria for the fermentation of a soy beverage in combination with *Streptococcus thermophilus*. Food Res. Int. 42, 612–621.

Champagne, C.P., Ross, R.P., Saarela, M., Hansen, K.F., Charalampopoulos, D., 2011. Recommendations for the viability assessment of probiotics as concentrated cultures and in food matrices. Int. J. Food Microbiol. 149, 185–193.

Champagne, C.P., Roy, D., Gardner, N., 2005. Challenges in addition of probiotic cultures to foods. Crit. Rev. Food Sci. Nutr. 45, 61–84.

Chorell, E., Karlsson Videhult, F., Hernell, O., Antti, H., West, C.E., 2013. Impact of probiotic feeding during weaning on the serum lipid profile and plasma metabolome in infants. Br. J. Nutr. 110 (1), 116–126.

de Sousa Moraes, L.F., Grzeskowiak, L.M., de Sales Teixeira, T.F., Gouveia Peluzio Mdo, C., 2014. Intestinal microbiota and probiotics in celiac disease. Clin. Microbiol. Rev. 27 (3), 482–489.

Dinan, T.G., Stanton, C., Cryan, J.F., 2013. Psychobiotics: a novel class of psychotropic. Biol. Psychiatry 74, 720–726.

Dimidi, E., Christodoulides, S., Fragkos, K.C., Scott, S.M., Whelan, K., 2014. The effect of probiotics on functional constipation in adults: a systematic review and meta-analysis of randomized controlled trials. Am. J. Clin. Nutr. 100, 1075–1084.

do Espírito Santo, A.P., Perego, P., Converti, A., Oliveira, M.N., 2011. Influence of food matrices on probiotic viability: a review focusing on the fruity bases. Trends Food Sci. Technol. 22, 377–385.

Dogi, C., Perdigón, G., 2006. Importance of the host specificity in the selection of probiotic bacteria. J. Dairy Res. 73, 357–366.

Druart, C., Alligier, M., Salazar, N., Neyrinck, A.M., Delzenne, N.M., 2014. Modulation of the gut microbiota by nutrients with prebiotic and probiotic properties. Adv. Nutr. 5 (5), 624S–633S.

Eckburg, P., Bik, E., Bernstein, C., Purdom, E., Dethlefsen, L., Sargent, M., et al., 2005. Diversity of the human intestinal microbial flora. Science 308, 1635–1638.

Elli, M., Callegari, M.L., Ferrari, S., Bessi, E., Cattivelli, D., Soldi, S., et al., 2006. Survival of yogurt bacteria in the human gut. Appl. Environ. Microbiol. 72 (7), 5113–5117.

Elizaquível, P., Sánchez, G., Salvador, A., Fiszman, S., Dueñas, M.T., López, P., Fernández de Palencia, P., Aznar, R., 2011. Evaluation of yogurt and various beverages as carriers of lactic acid bacteria producing 2-branched (1-3)-B-D-glucan. J. Dairy Sci. 94, 3271–3278.

FAO/WHO, 2002. In: Guidelines for the Evaluation of Probiotics in Food. Food and Agriculture Organization of the United Nations and World Health Organization Working Group Report. http://www.who.int/foodsafety/fs_management/en/probiotic_guidelines.pdf.

Farnworth, E. (Ed.), 2008. Handbook of Fermented Functional Foods, second ed. CRC Press, Boca Raton.

Farnworth, E.R., 2004. The beneficial health effects of fermented foods – potential probiotics around the world. J. Nutraceuticals Funct. Med. Foods 4, 93–117.

Farnworth, E.R., Champagne, C.P., 2016. Production of probiotic cultures and their incorporation into foods. In: Watson, R.R., Preedy, V.R. (Eds.), Probiotics, Prebiotics, and Synbiotics. Bioactive Foods in Health Promotion. Academic Press, London, pp. 303–317.

Figueroa-González, I., Quijano, G., Ramírez, G., Cruz-Guerrero, A., 2011. Probiotics and prebiotics. Perspectives and challenges. J. Sci. Food Agric. 91, 1341–1348.

Fijan, S., 2014. Microorganisms with claimed probiotic properties: an overview of recent literature. Int. J. Environ. Res. Public Health 11 (5), 4745–4767.

Franz, C.M., Huch, M., Abriouel, H., Holzapfel, W., Gálvez, A., 2011. Enterococci as probiotics and their implications in food safety. Int. J. Food Microbiol. 151 (2), 125–140.

Franz, C.M., Huch, M., Mathara, J.M., Abriouel, H., Benomar, N., Reid, G., et al., 2014. African fermented foods and probiotics. Int. J. Food Microbiol. 190, 84–96.

Furtado Martins, E.M., Mota Ramos, A., Lago Vanzela, E.S., Stringheta, P.C., de Oliveira Pinto, C.L., Martins, J.M., 2013. Products of vegetable origin: a new alternative for the consumption of probiotic bacteria. Food Res. Int. 51, 764–770.

Galdeano, C.M., Perdigón, G., 2004. Role of viability of probiotic strains in their persistence in the gut and in mucosal immune stimulation. J. Appl. Microbiol. 97, 673–681.

Ganesh, B.P., Versalovic, J., 2015. Luminal conversion and immunoregulation by probiotics. Front. Pharmacol. 6, 269. http://dx.doi.org/10.3389/fphar.2015.00269.

Gibson, G.R., Rastall, R.A., Fuller, R., 2003. The health benefits of probiotics and prebiotics. In: Fuller, R., Perdigón, G. (Eds.), Gut Flora, Nutrition, Immunity and Health. Balckwell Publishing, Oxford, pp. 52–76.

Glanville, J.M., Brown, S., Shamir, R., Szajewska, H., Eales, J.F., 2015. The scale of the evidence base on the health effects of conventional yogurt consumption: findings of a scoping review. Front. Pharmacol. 6, 246. http://dx.doi.org/10.3389/fphar.2015.00246.

Granato, D., Branco, G.F., Nazzaro, F., Cruz, A.G., Faria, J.A.F., 2010. Functional foods and nondairy probiotic food development: trends, concepts, and products. Compr. Rev. Food Sci. Food Saf. 9, 292–302.

Grześkowiak, Ł., Isolauri, E., Salminen, S., Gueimonde, M., 2011. Manufacturing process influences properties of probiotic bacteria. Br. J. Nutr. 105 (6), 887–894.

Guarino, A., Guandalini, S., Lo Vecchio, A., 2015. Probiotics for prevention and treatment of diarrhea. J. Clin. Gastroenterol. 49 (1), S37–S45.

Guarner, F., Perdigón, G., Corthier, G., Salminen, S., Koletzko, B., Morelli, L., 2005. Should yoghurt cultures be considered probiotics? Br. J. Nutr. 93, 783–786.

Haller, D., Colbus, H., Ganzle, M.G., Scherenbacher, P., Bode, C., Hammes, W.P., 2001. Metabolic and functional properties of lactic acid bacteria in the gastro-intestinal ecosystem: a comparative in vitro study between bacteria of intestinal and fermented food origin. Syst. Appl. Microbiol. 24, 218–226.

Han, B.Z., Rombouts, F.M., Nout, J.M.J.R., 2001. A Chinese fermented soybean food. Int. J. Food Microbiol. 65, 1–10.

Hasslöf, P., West, C.E., Videhult, F.K., Brandelius, C., Stecksén-Blicks, C., 2013. Early intervention with probiotic *Lactobacillus paracasei* F19 has no long-term effect on caries experience. Caries Res. 47 (6), 559–565.

Hauly, M.C.O., Fuchs, R.H.B., Prudencio-Ferreira, S.H., 2005. Soymilk yoghurt supplemented with fructooligosaccharides: probiotic properties and acceptance. Braz. J. Nutr. 18, 613–622.

Hill, C., Sanders, M.E., 2013. Rethinking probiotics. Gut Microbes 4 (4), 269–270.

Hoppe, M., Önning, G., Berggren, A., Hulthén, L., 2015. Probiotic strain *Lactobacillus plantarum* 299v increases iron absorption from an iron-supplemented fruit drink: a double-isotope cross-over single-blind study in women of reproductive age. Br. J. Nutr. 114 (8), 1195–1202.

Isolauri, E., Juntunen, M., Rautanen, T., Sillanaukee, P., Koivula, T., 1991. A human *Lactobacillus* strain (*Lactobacillus* GG) promotes recovery from acute diarrhea in children. Pediatrics 88, 90–97.

Isolauri, E., Salminen, S., Ouwehand, A.C., 2004. Probiotics. Best Pract. Res. Clin. Gastroenterol. 18, 299–313.

Jungersen, M., Wind, A., Johansen, E., Christensen, J.E., Stuer-Lauridsen, B., Eskesen, D., 2014. The science behind the probiotic strain *Bifidobacterium animalis* subsp. *lactis* BB-12®. Microorganisms 2 (2), 92–110.

Kanbe, M., 1992. Traditional fermented milks of the world. In: Nakazawa, Y., Hosono, A. (Eds.), Functions of Fermented Milk. Elsevier Science Publishers Ltd., Cambridge, pp. 41–60.

Kim, D.C., Chae, H.J., In, M.J., 2010. Fermentation characteristics of Korean pear (*Pyrus pyrifolia* Nakai) puree by the *Leuconostoc mesenteroides* 51-3 strain isolated from kimchi. Afr. J. Biotechnol. 9, 5735–5738.

Kourkoutas, Y., Xolias, V., Kallis, M., Bezirtzoglou, E., Kanellaki, M., 2005. *Lactobacillus casei* cell immobilization on fruit pieces for probiotic additive, fermented milk and lactic acid production. Process Biochem. 40, 411–416.

Krych, L., Hansen, C.H., Hansen, A.K., van den Berg, F.W., Nielsen, D.S., 2013. Quantitatively different, yet qualitatively alike: a meta-analysis of the mouse core gut microbiome with a view towards the human gut microbiome. PLoS One 8 (5), e62578. http://dx.doi.org/10.1371/journal.pone.0062578.

Kumar, B.V., Vijayendra, S.V.N., Reddi, O.V.S., 2015. Trends in dairy and non-dairy products- a review. J. Food Sci. Technol. http://dx.doi.org/10.1007/s13197-015-1795-2.

Kumar, M., Nagpal, R., Kumar, R., Hemalatha, R., Verma, V., Kumar, A., et al., 2012. Cholesterol-lowering probiotics as potential biotherapeutics for metabolic diseases. Exp. Diabetes Res. http://dx.doi.org/10.1155/2012/902917. ID 902917, 14 pages.

Lahtinen, S.J., 2012. Probiotic viability – does it matter? Microb. Ecol. Health Dis. 23, 18567. http://dx.doi.org/10.3402/mehd.v23i0.18567.

Lee, B., Yin, X., Griffey, S.M., Marco, M.L., 2015. Attenuation of colitis by *Lactobacillus casei* BL23 is dependent on the dairy delivery matrix. Appl. Environ. Microbiol. 81 (18), 6425–6435.

Lee, S.C., Yang, Y.H., Chuang, S.Y., Huang, S.Y., Pan, W.H., 2013. Reduced medication use and improved pulmonary function with supplements containing vegetable and fruit concentrate, fish oil and probiotics in asthmatic school children: a randomised controlled trial. Br. J. Nutr. 110 (1), 145–155.

Lehrer, R.I., Bevins, C.L., Ganz, T., 2005. Defensins and other antimicrobial peptides and proteins. In: Mestecky, J., Lamm, M.E., Strober, W., Bienenstock, J., McGhee, J.R., Mayer, L. (Eds.), Mucosal Immunology, third ed. Academic Press, San Diego, pp. 94–110.

Lick, S., Drescher, K., Heller, K.J., 2001. Survival of *Lactobacillus delbrueckii* subsp. *bulgaricus* and *Streptococcus thermophilus* in the terminal ileum of fistulated Göttingen minipigs. Appl. Environ. Microbiol. 67 (9), 4137–4143.

Lin, M.-Y., Yen, C.-L., Chen, S.-H., 1998. Management of lactose maldigestion by consuming milk containing lactobacilli. Dig. Dis. Sci. 43 (1), 133–137.

Liu, S., Hu, P., Du, X., Zhou, T., Pei, X., 2013. *Lactobacillus rhamnosus* GG supplementation for preventing respiratory infections in children: a meta-analysis of randomized, placebo-controlled trials. Indian Pediatr. 50 (4), 377–381.

Liu, D.M., Li, L., Yang, X.Q., Liang, S.Z., Wang, J.S., 2006. Survivability of *Lactobacillus rhamnosus* during the preparation of soy cheese. Food Technol. Biotechnol. 44, 417–422.

Lönnermark, E., Friman, V., Lappas, G., Sandberg, T., Berggren, A., Adlerberth, I., 2010. Intake of *Lactobacillus plantarum* reduces certain gastrointestinal symptoms during treatment with antibiotics. J. Clin. Gastroenterol. 44 (2), 106–112.

Loulouda, A.B., Kourkoutas, Y., Albantaki, N., Tzia, C., Koutinas, A.A., Kanellaki, M., 2009. Functionality of freeze-dried *L. casei* cells immobilized on wheat grains. LWT-Food Sci. Technol. 42, 1696–1702.

Lourens-Hattingh, A., Viljoen, B.C., 2001. Yogurt as probiotic carrier food. Int. Dairy J. 11 (1–2), 1–17.

Luckow, T., Delahunty, C., 2004a. Which juice is 'healthier'? A consumer study of probiotic non-dairy juice drinks. Food Qual. Prefer. 15, 751–759.

Luckow, T., Delahunty, C., 2004b. Consumer acceptance of orange juice containing functional ingredients. Food Res. Int. 37, 805–814.

Luckow, T., Sheehan, V., Fitzgerald, G., Delahunty, C., 2006. Exposure, health information and flavor-masking strategies for improving the sensory quality of probiotic juice. Apetite 47, 315–325.

Malin, M., Verronen, P., Korhonen, H., Syväoja, E.L., Salminen, S., Mykkänen, H., et al., 1997. Dietary therapy with *Lactobacillus* GG, bovine colostrum or bovine immune colostrum in patients with juvenile chronic arthritis: evaluation of effect on gut defence mechanisms. Inflammopharmacology 5, 219–236.

Martín, R., Langa, S., Reviriego, C., Jimínez, E., Marín, M.L., Xaus, J., et al., 2003. Human milk is a source of lactic acid bacteria for the infant gut. J. Pediatr. 6, 754–758.

Matamoros, S., Gras-Leguen, C., Le Vacon, F., Potel, G., de La Cochetiere, M.F., 2013. Development of intestinal microbiota in infants and its impact on health. Trends Microbiol. 21 (4), 167–173.

Matilla-Sandholm, T., Myllarinen, P., Crittenden, R., Mogensen, G., Fonden, R., Saarela, M., 2002. Technological challenges for future probiotic foods. Int. Dairy J. 12, 173–182.

Matsuzaki, T., 1998. Immunomodulation by treatment with *Lactobacillus casei* strain Shirota. Int. J. Food Microbiol. 41 (2), 133–140.

Matto, J., Alakomi, H.L., Vaari, A., Virkajarvi, I., Saarela, M., 2006. Influence of processing conditions on *Bifidobacterium animalis* subsp. *lactis* functionality with a special focus on acid tolerance and factors affecting it. Int. Dairy J. 16, 1029–1037.

McKinley, M.C., 2005. The nutrition and health benefits of yoghurt. Int. J. Dairy Technol. 58 (1), 1–12.

Miller, L.E., Ouwehand, A.C., 2013. Probiotic supplementation decreases intestinal transit time: meta-analysis of randomized controlled trials. World J. Gastroenterol. 19 (29), 4718–4725.

Mills, S., Shanahan, F., Stanton, C., Hill, C., Coffey, A., Ross, R.P., 2013. Movers and shakers: influence of bacteriophages in shaping the mammalian gut microbiota. Gut Microbes 4 (1), 4–16.

Molin, G., 2001. Probiotics in foods not containing milk or milk constituents, with special reference to *Lactobacillus plantarum* 299v. Am. J. Clin. Nutr. 73 (2), 380S–385S.

Morata de Ambrosini, V., Gonzalez, S., Perdigón, G., Pesce de Ruiz Holgado, A., Oliver, G., 1996. Chemical composition of the cell wall of lactic acid bacteria and related species. Chem. Pharm. Bull. 44, 2263–2267.

Moreau, M.C., Gaboriau-Routhiau, V., 2000. Influence of resident intestinal microflora on the development and functions of the intestinal-associated lymphoid tissue. In: Fuller, R., Perdigón, G. (Eds.), Probiotics 3: Immunomodulation by the Gut Flora and Probiotics. Kluwer Academic Publishers, Dordrecht, pp. 69–114.

Morelli, L., 2000. In vitro selection of probiotic lactobacilli: a critical appraisal. Curr. Issues Intest. Microbiol. 1 (2), 59–67.

Mozzi, F., 2016. Lactic acid bacteria reference module in food science encyclopedia of food and health, 501–508. http://dx.doi.org/10.1016/B978-0-12-384947-2.00414-1.

Nobaek, S., Johansson, M.L., Molin, G., Ahrné, S., Jeppsson, B., 2000. Alternation of intestinal microflora is associated with reduction in abdominal bloating and pain in patients with irritable bowel syndrome. Am. J. Gastroenterol. 95, 1231–1238.

Østlie, H.M., Helland, M.H., Narvhus, J.A., 2003. Growth and metabolism of selected strains of probiotic bacteria in milk. Int. J. Food Microbiol. 87 (1–2), 17–27.

Ouwehand, A.C., Kurvinen, T., Rissanen, P., 2004. Use of a probiotic *Bifidobacterium* in a dry food matrix, an in vivo study. Int. J. Food Microbiol. 95, 103–106.

Ouwehand, A.C., Salminen, S.J., 1998. The health effects of cultured milk products with viable and non-viable bacteria. Int. Dairy J. 8, 749–758.

Ouwehand, A.C., Vesterlund, S., 2004. Antimicrobial components from lactic acid bacteria. In: Salminen, S., von Wright, A., Ouwehand, A. (Eds.), Lactic Acid Bacteria: Microbiological and Functional Aspects: Third Edition, Revised and Expanded, Edition. Marcel Dekker, Inc., New York, pp. 375–396.

Patten, D.A., Laws, A.P., 2015. *Lactobacillus*-produced exopolysaccharides and their potential health benefits: a review. Benef. Microbes 6, 457–471.

Parfrey, L.W., Walters, W.A., Lauber, C.L., Clemente, J.C., Berg-Lyons, D., Teiling, C., et al., 2014. Communities of microbial eukaryotes in the mammalian gut within the context of environmental eukaryotic diversity. Front. Microbiol. 5 (298), 1–13.

Park, S., Bae, J.H., 2015. Probiotics for weight loss: a systematic review and meta-analysis. Nutr. Res. 35, 566–575.

Perricone, M., Bevilacqua, A., Altieri, C., Sinigaglia, M., Corbo, M.R., 2015. Challenges for the production of probiotic fruit juices. Beverages 1, 95–103.

Pessione, E., Cirrincione, S., 2016. Bioactive molecules released in food by lactic acid bacteria: encrypted peptides and biogenic amines. Front. Microbiol. 7, 876.

Pitkala, K.H., Strandberg, T.E., Finne Soveri, U.H., Ouwehand, A.C., Poussa, T., Salminen, S., 2007. Fermented cereal with specific bifidobacteria normalizes bowel movements in elderly nursing home residents. A randomized, controlled trial. J. Nutr. Health Aging 11 (4), 305–311.

Power, S.E., O'Toole, P.W., Stanton, C., Ross, R.P., Fitzgerald, G.F., 2014. Intestinal microbiota, diet and health. Br. J. Nutr. 111 (3), 387–402.

Prado, F.C., Parada, J.L., Pandey, A., Soccol, C.R., 2008. Trends in non-dairy probiotic beverages. Food Res. Int. 41 (2), 111–123.

Prajapati, J.B., Nair, B.M., 2003. The history of fermented foods. In: Farnworth, E.R. (Ed.), Handbook of Fermented Functional Foods. CRC Press, Boca Raton, pp. 1–26.

Rakin, M., Vukasinovic, M., Siler-Marinkovic, S., Maksimovic, M., 2007. Contribution of lactic acid fermentation to improved nutritive quality vegetable juices enriched with brewer's yeast autolysate. Food Chem. 100, 599–602.

Ranadheera, R.D.C.S., Baines, S.K., Adams, M.C., 2010. Importance of food in probiotic efficacy. Food Res. Int. 43 (1), 1–7.

Rasic, J.L.J., Kurmann, J.A. (Eds.), 1978. Yoghurt-Scientific Grounds, Technology, Manufacture and Preparations. Technical Dairy Pub. House, Copenhagen.

Reid, G., Sanders, M.E., Gaskins, H.R., Gibson, G.R., Mercenier, A., Rastall, R., et al., 2003. New scientific paradigms for probiotics and prebiotics. J. Clin. Gastroenterol. 37, 105–118.

Reineccius, G.A., 2000. Flavouring systems for functional foods. In: KSchmidl, M., Labuza, T.B. (Eds.), Essentials in Functional Foods. Aspen Publishing, Gaithersburgh, MD, pp. 89–97.

Ren, D., Li, C., Qin, Y., Yin, R., Du, S., Ye, F., et al., 2014. In vitro evaluation of the probiotic and functional potential of *Lactobacillus* strains isolated from fermented food and human intestine. Anaerobe 30, 1–10.

Reyes, A., Haynes, M., Hanson, N., Angly, F.E., Heath, A.C., Rohwer, F., et al., 2010. Viruses in the faecal microbiota of monozygotic twins and their mothers. Nature 466, 334–338.

Rivera-Espinoza, Y., Gallardo-Navarro, Y., 2010. Non-dairy probiotic products. Food Microbiol. 27, 1–11.

Robitaille, G., Champagne, C.P., 2014. Growth-promoting effects of pepsin- and trypsin-treated caseinomacropeptide from bovine milk on probiotics. J. Dairy Res. 81 (3), 319–324.

Russell, M.W., Bobek, L.A., Brock, J.H., Hajishengallis, G., Tenuovo, J., 2005. Innate humoral defense factors. In: Mestecky, J., Lamm, M.E., Strober, W., Bienenstock, J., McGhee, J.R., Mayer, L. (Eds.), Mucosal Immunology, third ed. Academic Press, San Diego, pp. 73–93.

Saarela, M., Hallamaa, K., Mattila-Sandholm, T., Matto, J., 2003. The effect of lactose derivatives lactulose, lactitol and lactobionic acid on the functional and technological properties of potentially probiotic *Lactobacillus* strains. Int. Dairy J. 13, 291–302.

Saavedra, J.M., Dattilo, A.M., 2012. Early development of intestinal microbiota: implications for future health. Gastroenterol. Clin. North Am. 41 (4), 717–731.

Saavedra, J.M., Bauman, N., Oung, I., Perman, J., Yolken, R., 1994. Feeding of *Bifidobacterium bifidum* and *Streptococcus thermophilus* to infants in hospital for prevention of diarrhea and shedding of rotavirus. Lancet 344, 1046–1049.

Saez-Lara, M.J., Gomez-Llorente, C., Plaza-Diaz, J., Gil, A., 2015. The role of probiotic lactic acid bacteria and bifidobacteria in the prevention and treatment of inflammatory bowel disease and other related diseases: a systematic review of randomized human clinical trials. Biomed Res. Int.. ID 505878, 15 pages http://dx.doi.org/10.1155/2015/505878.

Saito, V.S., Dos Santos, T.F., Vinderola, C.G., Romano, C., Nicoli, J.R., Araújo, L.S., Costa, M.M., Andrioli, J.L., Uetanabaro, A.P., 2014. Viability and resistance of lactobacilli isolated from cocoa fermentation to simulated gastrointestinal digestive steps in soy yogurt. J. Food Sci. 79 (2), M 208–213.

Salminen, S., van Loveren, H., 2012. Probiotics and prebiotics: health claim substantiation. Microb. Ecol. Health Dis. 23, 18568. http://dx.doi.org/10.3402/mehd.v23i0.18568.

Salminen, S., Isolauri, E., Salminen, E., 1996. Clinical uses of probiotics for stabilizing the gut mucosal barrier: successful strains and future challenges. Antonie Van Leeuwenhoek 70, 347–358.

Sanders, M.E., 2008. Probiotics: definition, sources, selection, and uses. Clin. Infect. Dis. 46 (2), S58–S61.

Sanders, M.E., Marco, M.L., 2010. Food formats for effective delivery of probiotics. Annu. Rev. Food Sci. Technol. 1, 65–85.

Sashihara, T., Sueki, N., Furuichi, K., Ikegami, S., 2007. Effect of growth conditions of *Lactobacillus gasseri* OLL2809 on the immunostimulatory activity for production of interleukin-12 (p70) by murine spleno-cytes. Int. J. Food Microbiol. 120 (3), 274–281.

Schoustra, S.E., Kasase, C., Toarta, C., Kassen, R., Poulain, A.J., 2013. Microbial community structure of three traditional zambian fermented products: mabisi, chibwantu and munkoyo. PLoS One 8 (5), e63948. http://dx.doi.org/10.1371/journal.pone.0063948.

Schulze, J., Sonnenborn, U., 2009. Yeasts in the gut: from commensals to infectious agents. Dtsch. Ärztebl. Int. 106 (51–52), 837–842.

Schwenger, E.M., Tejani, A.M., Loewen, P.S., 2015. Probiotics for preventing urinary tract infections in adults and children. Cochrane Database Syst. Rev. 12, CD008772. http://dx.doi.org/10.1002/14651858.CD008772.pub2.

Senok, A.C., Ismaeel, A.Y., Botta, G.A., 2005. Probiotics: facts and myths. Clin. Microbiol. Infect. 11, 958–966.

Shaukat, A., Levitt, M.D., Taylor, B.C., MacDonald, R., Shamliyan, T.A., Kane, R.L., et al., 2010. Systematic review: effective management strategies for lactose intolerance. Ann. Intern. Med. 152 (12), 797–803.

Sheehan, V.M., Ross, P., Fitzgerald, G.F., 2007. Assessing the acid tolerance and the technological robustness of probiotic cultures for fortification in fruit juices. Innovative Food Sci. Emerg Technol. 8, 279–284.

Sheih, I., Wu, H.Y., Lai, Y.J., Lin, C.F., 2000. Preparation of high free radical scavenging tempeh by a newly isolated *Rhizopus* sp. R-69 from Indonesia. J. Food Sci. Agric. Chem. 2 (1), 35–40.

Shimakama, Y., Matsubara, S., Yuki, N., Ikeda, M., Ishikawa, F., 2003. Evaluation of *Bifidobacterium breves* strain Yakult-fermented soymilk as a probiotic food. Int. J. Food Microbiol. 81, 131–136.

Shori, A.B., 2016. Influence of food matrix on the viability of probiotic bacteria: a review based on dairy and non-dairy beverages. Food Biosci. 13, 1–8.

Slyepchenko, A., Carvalho, A.F., Cha, D.S., Kasper, S., McIntyre, R.S., 2014. Gut emotions – mechanisms of action of probiotics as novel therapeutic targets for depression and anxiety disorder's. CNS Neurol. Disord. Drug Targets 13 (10), 1770–1786.

Stanton, C., Desmond, C., Coakley, M., Collins, J.K., Fitzgerald, G., Ross, R.P., 2003. Challenges facing development of probiotic-containing functional foods. In: Farnworth, E.R. (Ed.), Handbook of Fermented Functional Foods. CRC Press, Boca Raton, pp. 27–58.

Szajewska, H., Chmielewska, A., 2013. Growth of infants fed formula supplemented with *Bifidobacterium lactis* Bb12 or *Lactobacillus* GG: a systematic review of randomized controlled trials. BMC Pediatr. 13, 185. http://dx.doi.org/10.1186/1471-2431-13-185.

Szajewska, H., Kołodziej, M., 2015. Systematic review with meta-analysis: *Lactobacillus rhamnosus* GG in the prevention of antibiotic-associated diarrhoea in children and adults. Aliment. Pharmacol. Ther. 42 (10), 1149–1157.

Szajewska, H., Canani, R.B., Guarino, A., Hojsak, I., Indrio, F., Kolacek, et al., 2015. Probiotics for the prevention of antibiotic-associated diarrhea in children. J. Pediatr. Gastroenterol. Nutr. (Epub ahead of print).

Szajewska, H., Wanke, M., Patro, B., 2011. Meta-analysis: the effects of *Lactobacillus rhamnosus* GG supplementation for the prevention of healthcare-associated diarrhoea in children. Aliment. Pharmacol. Ther. 34 (9), 1079–1087.

Tannock, G.W., 2003. The intestinal microflora. In: Fuller, R., Perdigón, G. (Eds.), Gut Flora, Nutrition, Immunity and Health. Balckwell Publishing, Oxford, pp. 1–23.

Tejada-Simon, M.V., Pestka, J.J., 1999. Proinflammatory cytokine and nitric oxide induction in murine macrophages by cell wall and cytoplasmic extracts of lactic acid bacteria. J. Food Prot. 62, 1435–1444.

Toh, M.C., Allen-Vercoe, E., 2015. The human gut microbiota with reference to autism spectrum disorder: considering the whole as more than a sum of its parts. Microb. Ecol. Health Dis. 26, 26309. http://dx.doi.org/10.3402/mehd.v26.26309.

Tompkins, T.A., Mainville, I., Arcand, Y., 2011. The impact of meals on a probiotic during transit through a model of the human upper gastrointestinal tract. Benef. Microbes 2, 295–303.

Tsen, J.H., Lin, Y.P., King, E., 2004. Fermentation of banana media by using k-carrageenan immobilized *Lactobacillus acidophilus*. Int. J. Food Microbiol. 91, 215–220.

Tuomola, E., Crittenden, R., Playne, M., Isolauri, E., Salminen, S., 2001. Quality assurance criteria for probiotic bacteria. Am. J. Clin. Nutr. 73 (2), 393S–398S.

Tuorila, H., Cardello, A.V., 2002. Consumer responses to an off flavour in juice in the presence of specific health claims. Food Qual. Prefer. 13, 561–569.

Valerio, F., de Bellis, P., Lonigro, S.L., Morelli, L., Visconti, A., Lavermicocca, P., 2006. In vitro and in vivo survival and transit tolerance of potentially probiotic strains carried by artichokes in the gastrointestinal tract. Appl. Environ. Microbiol. 72, 3042–3045.

Van Tassell, M.L., Miller, M.J., 2011. *Lactobacillus* adhesion to mucus. Nutrients 3 (5), 613–636.

Vasudha, S., Mishra, H.N., 2013. Non dairy probiotic beverages. Int. Food Res. J. 20 (1), 7–15.

Vaughn, A.R., Sivamani, R.K., 2015. Effects of fermented dairy products on skin: a systematic review. J. Altern. Complement. Med. 21 (7), 380–385.

Vázquez, C., Botella-Carretero, J.I., García-Albiach, R., Pozuelo, M.J., Rodríguez-Baños, M., Baquero, F., et al., 2013. Screening in a *Lactobacillus delbrueckii* subsp. *bulgaricus* collection to select a strain able to survive to the human intestinal tract. Nutr. Hosp. 4, 1227–1235.

Vinderola, C.G., Costa, G.A., Regenhardt, S., Reinheimer, J.A., 2002. Influence of compounds associated with fermented dairy products on the growth of lactic acid starter and probiotic bacteria. Int. Dairy J. 12, 579–589.

Vinderola, C.G., Matar, C., Perdigón, G., 2005. Role of intestinal epithelial cells in the immune effects mediated by Gram-positive probiotic bacteria. Involvement of toll-like receptors. Clin. Diagn. Lab. Immunol. 12, 1075–1084.

Vinderola, C.G., Perdigón, G., Duarte, J., Farnworth, E., Matar, C., 2006. Modulation of the gut immune response by the exopolysaccharide produced by *Lactobacillus kefiranofaciens*. Cytokine 36, 254–260.

Vinderola, G., 2008. Dried cell-free fraction of fermented milks: new functional additives for the food industry. Trends Food Sci. Technol. 19, 40–46.

Vinderola, G., de los Reyes-Gavilán, C., Reinheimer, J., 2009. Probiotics and prebiotics in fermented dairy products. In: Ribeiro, C.P., Passos, M.L. (Eds.), Contemporary Food Engineering, vol. 20. CRC Press, Taylor & Francis Group, Boca Raton, FL, USA, pp. 601–634.

Vinderola, G., Zacarías, M.F., Bockelmann, W., Neve, H., Reinheimer, J., Heller, K.J., 2012. Preservation of functionality of *Bifidobacterium animalis* subsp. *lactis* INL1 after incorporation of freeze-dried cells into different food matrices. Food Microbiol. 30 (1), 274–280.

Vogel, L., 2010. European probiotics industry fears regulations will scuttle market for health-promoting or disease-preventing foods. Can. Med. Assoc. J. 182 (11), E493–E494.

Wang, S., Zhang, L., Shan, Y., 2015. Lactobacilli and colon carcinoma-a review. Wei Sheng Wu Xue Bao 55 (6), 667–674.

Wang, Y.C., Yu, R.C., Yang, H.Y., Chou, C.C., 2006. Antioxidatives activities of soymilk fermented with acid lactic bacteria and bifidobacterias. Food Microbiol. 23, 128–135.

Wasilewski, A., Zielińska, M., Storr, M., Fichna, J., 2015. Beneficial effects of probiotics, prebiotics, synbiotics, and psychobiotics in inflammatory bowel disease. Inflamm. Bowel Dis. 21 (7), 1674–1682.

Watanabe, T., Hamada, K., Tategaki, A., Kishida, H., Tanaka, H., Kitano, M., et al., 2009. Oral administration of lactic acid bacteria isolated from traditional South Asian fermented milk 'dahi' inhibits the development of atopic dermatitis in NC/Nga mice. J. Nutr. Sci. Vitaminol. 55 (3), 271–278.

West, C.E., Hammarström, M.L., Hernell, O., 2013. Probiotics in primary prevention of allergic disease–follow-up at 8-9 years of age. Allergy 68 (8), 1015–1020.

Wong, S., Jamous, A., O'Driscoll, J., Sekhar, R., Saif, M., O'Driscoll, S., et al., 2015. Effectiveness of probiotic in preventing and treating antibiotic-associated diarrhoea and/or *Clostridium difficile*-associated diarrhoea in patients with spinal cord injury: a protocol of systematic review of randomised controlled trials. Syst. Rev. 4, 170. http://dx.doi.org/10.1186/s13643-015-0159-3.

Yoon, K.Y., Woodams, E.E., Hang, Y.D., 2004. Probiotication of tomato juice by lactic acid bacteria. J. Microbiol. 42, 315–318.

Yoon, K.Y., Woodams, E.E., Hang, Y.D., 2005. Fermentation of beet juice by beneficial lactic acid bacteria. Lebensm. Wiss. Technol. 38, 73–75.

Yoon, K.Y., Woodams, E.E., Hang, Y.D., 2006. Production of probiotic cabbage juice by lactic acid bacteria. Bioresour. Technol. 97, 1427–1430.

Zambrano, L.D., Levy, K., Menezes, N.P., Freeman, M.C., 2014. Human diarrhea infections associated with domestic animal husbandry: a systematic review and meta-analysis. Trans. R. Soc. Trop. Med. Hyg. 108, 313–325.

Zhu, B., Wang, X., Li, L., 2010. Human gut microbiome: the second genome of human body. Protein Cell 1 (8), 718–725.

Zuccotti, G., Meneghin, F., Aceti, A., Barone, G., Callegari, M.L., Di Mauro, A., et al., 2015. Probiotics for prevention of atopic diseases in infants: systematic review and meta-analysis. Allergy 70 (11), 1356–1371.

45

Exposure to Pesticide Residues and Contaminants of the Vegetarian Population—French data

Ségolène Fleury[1], Nawel Bemrah[1], Alexandre Nougadère[1], Benjamin Alles[2], Mathilde Touvier[2], Gilles Rivière[1]

[1]RISK ASSESSMENT UNIT – FRENCH AGENCY FOR FOOD, ENVIRONMENTAL AND OCCUPATIONAL HEALTH & SAFETY (ANSES), MAISONS-ALFORT, FRANCE; [2]SORBONNE PARIS CITÉ EPIDEMIOLOGY AND STATISTICS RESEARCH CENTER (CRESS), NUTRITIONAL EPIDEMIOLOGY RESEARCH TEAM (EREN), INSERM U1153, INRA U1125, CONSERVATOIRE NATIONAL DES ARTS ET MÉTIERS (CNAM), PARIS 5, 7, 13 UNIVERSITIES, BOBIGNY, FRANCE

1. Introduction

People choose vegetarianism for several reasons: preservation of natural resources, protection of animal welfare, or health benefits, as it has been described in other chapters of this book (the readers may refer to Section 1). Avoiding meat and resorting to a plant-based diet lead to a variety of diets. As described in Chapter 1, the pescetarian diet includes the consumption of fish, seafood, eggs, and milk. The ovolactovegetarian diet (OLV) includes the consumption of eggs and milk, whereas the vegan diet excludes the consumption or the use of any products of animal origin.

The American Dietetic Association stated that well-planned vegetarian diets are healthy and nutritionally adequate and might be beneficial in the prevention and treatment of some diseases (Craig et al., 2009), as it has been reviewed in many chapters of this book (see Section 3). For instance, Kahleova and Pelikanova (2015) showed that type 2 diabetes is 1.6–2 times lower in vegetarians than in the general population. However, a vegetarian diet can also be deleterious to health (Dwyer, 1988). It has been reported that eliminating all animal products from the diet increases the risk of certain nutritional deficiencies; there are concerns for some vitamins and minerals in vegans.

With regard to the consequences of vegetarianism on the exposure to environmental contaminants, few data exist as of today in the literature, except Clarke et al. (2003), who reported the exposure of vegetarians to some trace elements and phytoestrogens in the UK population. With regard to pesticide residues (PRs), a screening French study including 421 PR and the whole diet of each subgroup of consumers showed that, except for organochlorine compounds and particularly PR classified as persistent organic pollutants (POPs), the vegetarian population may be globally more exposed to PR than the general population, even if differences exist from one population subgroup to another and depending on the pesticide considered (Van Audenhaege et al., 2009). The study showed that dietary habits have a significant impact on PR exposure in terms of intake levels, number, and type of pesticides.

With regard to environmental contaminants, our group calculated the exposure of the French vegetarian population to environmental contaminants (Fleury et al., to be submitted). This was made possible using the consumption data from the Nutrinet-Santé study previously published and launched in France in May 2009 (Hercberg et al., 2010) and the contamination data generated in the context of the second total diet study run in France for which food items were collected between 2007 and 2009 (Sirot et al., 2009). With regard to the consumption data, the survey was performed using the Internet only. To participate, an initial set of questionnaires was first fully completed. During 3 days (randomly selected), participants had to describe their diet (both liquid and solid). It relied on a meal-based approach, recording all foods and beverages consumed. Participants had to list all consumed food items and directly record the quantity consumed, when known, or estimated portion sizes for each food and beverage previously listed based on photographs of portion sizes. A second questionnaire focused on physical activity and, finally, the third with anthropometry, lifestyle, socioeconomic conditions, and health status. The participants were requested to fill out this set of questionnaires every year. Monthly, an email was sent to participants inviting them to complete a new questionnaire (Hercberg et al., 2010). With regard to the contamination data, the second total diet study run in France did not specifically take into account organic products, whereas the vegetarian population of the Nutrinet-Santé study seemed to consume a large part of organic food (Baudry et al., 2015, 2016) for which the concentration of contaminants can be different than that in conventional food. Because the concentration data used to perform exposure calculation did not take into account this type of product, the estimate of dietary exposure to chemicals in the present study could be biased. Further studies using complementary data about chemical composition of organic food could overcome this limitation.

Due to the different diets in the vegetarian spectrum (including pescetarian,[1] ovolactovegetarian, or vegan), one can expect exposure to contaminants to be substantially different. For instance, the consumption of fish in the pescetarian diet can significantly increase the exposure to POPs. The consequences of these different diets on the exposure of contaminants were investigated.

2. Dietary Exposure to Pesticide Residues

Long-term exposure to phytopharmaceutical products (pesticides) and their residues is increasingly suspected of being linked to a broad spectrum of medical problems such as cancer, neurotoxic effects, reproductive health concerns, and endocrine disruption,

---

[1] For sake of simplicity, in this chapter, people consuming a pescetarian diet will be considered belonging to the large populations of vegetarians (i.e., together with ovolactovegetarians and vegans).

particularly for specific populations such as farmers and their children (Kesavachandran et al., 2009; Bailey et al., 2011; Baldi et al., 2011; Koutros et al., 2011; Naidoo et al., 2011; INSERM, 2013). Therefore, although plant protection products are subject to a rigorous safety evaluation, improving knowledge on the human health impact of environmental and dietary exposure to pesticides remains a central concern in public health. For the general population, dietary intake is considered to be a major potential route of exposure to most pesticides (Lu et al., 2006; Luo and Zhang, 2009; Panuwet et al., 2009; Cao et al., 2011).

In the European Union (EU), the evaluation of plant protection products and the monitoring of PR in food are harmonized (Regulation (EC) No 396/2005; Regulation (EC) No 1107/2009). To ensure that residue levels in food do not present a risk to consumers, an assessment of the dietary intake of pesticides is carried out by national safety agencies and the European Food Safety Authority (EFSA) at the pre- and postregulation level. Each year, EFSA publishes a report on the results of the EU Member States' monitoring of PR in food commodities (EFSA, 2014, 2015). Some countries also releases an equivalent national report on dietary risk to consumers (Anses, 2014; Nougadère et al., 2014) or multiannual studies such as total diet studies (TDS) (Rawn et al., 2004; Gimou et al., 2008; MAF, 2009; ANSES, 2011; Caldas et al., 2011; Wong et al., 2014; Chen et al., 2015). These dietary exposure assessments are based on international guidelines for predicting dietary intake of PR, and on indicators calculated by combining consumption and occurrence data (e.g., results from national monitoring programs or TDS) for the diet representative of the general population, therefore not specifically for vegetarians (WHO, 1997; EFSA, 2011, 2012; EFSA et al., 2011).

The results of these studies showed that the toxicological reference values such as the acceptable daily intake (ADI) is exceeded for few substances, and foods of plant origin (fruits, vegetables, and cereals) are the main contributors to the dietary exposure of the majority of PR in the general population aged more than 3 years old. For PR classified as POPs, i.e., old pesticides prohibited by Stockholm Convention, foods of animal origin are the main contributors to the dietary intake (ANSES, 2011; Nougadère et al., 2012, 2014; EFSA, 2014).

Numerous studies have shown several important health benefits for vegetarians or underlined the importance of monitoring and ensuring an appropriate energy intake and an adequate protein intake and sources of essential fatty acids, iron, zinc, calcium, and vitamins (Renda and Fischer, 2009; Amit et al., 2010). But few studies have investigated the dietary exposure of vegetarians to chemicals such as PR or studied the benefit–risk ratio. The majority of the publications on vegetarians only included some substances or chemical families, not the whole diet. However, thousands of PRs can be potentially found in the diet of the general population or vegetarians (European Commission, 2015).

Van Audenhaege et al. (2009) reported exposures calculated by combining EU maximum residue levels (MRLs) and French consumption data from 1999 for the general population (Volatier, 2000) and 1997 for the vegetarian subjects (Leblanc et al., 2000). The vegetarian population was separated into five specific diets: pseudo-vegetarian omnivorous (OMN), lactovegetarian (LV), ovolactovegetarian (OLV), pesco-lactovegetarian (PLV), and vegan (VG). Among the 421 PRs studied, 48 had a theoretical maximum daily intake (TMDI) above ADI for at least one population subgroup. An excessive exposure was found for 44, 43, 42, 41, and 30 pesticides in the OLV, VG, OMN, LV, and PLV groups, respectively, versus 29 in the general population. The exposure of the PLV group was extremely close to those of the general population, but the lack of MRL for fish certainly distorts the evaluation of PR intake, particularly for PR classified as POPs. As the limited consumption of foods of animal origin was largely offset by a higher fruit, vegetable, and cereal intake in the vegetarian diets, vegetarians appeared to be preferentially exposed to pesticides, for which these plant foods are the main contributors: chlorpyrifos, dimethoate, imazalil, and phosmet for fruits, dithiocarbamates and chlorpropham for vegetables, and chlorpyrifos-methyl and pirimiphos-methyl for cereals. However, meat and egg products consumption were responsible for higher intakes of PRs classified as POPs, e.g., dieldrin or hexachloro-cyclohexane (HCH) in the general population than in the vegetarian population.

Although dietary exposure to these substances was confirmed by analyses in food prepared as consumed (Nougadère et al., 2012), it would be necessary to reassess the vegetarian exposure using more recent consumption data and actual levels in food (from monitoring programs or TDS) instead of MRLs. Indeed, the TMDI approach is very conservative and usually leads to an overestimation of exposure levels. The authors concluded that "even if this study shows a higher risk for vegetarians regarding some PR, such a diet (or lifestyle) presents better health advantages. Thus, it is important to develop a methodology to simultaneously consider the benefits and risks associated with this particular diet/lifestyle" (Van Audenhaege et al., 2009).

These results on a likely lower exposure to PRs classified as POPs for vegetarians seems to be confirmed by some biomonitoring studies, and particularly a study evaluating the potential of some nutritional approaches to prevent or reduce the body load of organo-chlorines (OCs) in humans (Arguin et al., 2010). This study compared plasma OC concentrations (hexachlorobenzene, aldrin, oxychlordane, beta-HCH, p,p'-DDT, p,p'-DDE, etc.) between vegans and omnivores and concluded that except for p,p'-DDT and beta-HCH, there was a trend toward lesser contamination by OCs in vegans than in omnivores. The authors underlined that "the present results are the outcome of preliminary work and that due to evident lack of statistical power, they cannot be generalised to the entire population and should be interpreted with caution. Indeed, nonsignificant results should be interpreted as trends."

This study confirmed older conclusions about the low levels of contaminants—including PR classified as POPs such as dieldrin, heptachlor epoxide, and oxychlordane—in breastmilk of women that eliminated all animal products from the diet and used soybeans and grains for protein source. In particular, levels of OCs in breastmilk of US vegetarian women were much lower than that in the breastmilk from the US nonvegetarian women. The highest vegetarian value was lower than the lowest value obtained in the nonvegetarian population (Rogan et al., 1980; Hergenrather et al., 1981).

Nevertheless, some authors noted that the vegetarians may have been breastfed as infants, and might thus have been exposed to OC accumulated by the mother and transferred to them during pregnancy and lactation (Anderson and Wolff, 2000). Some studies stated that dietary intake is not the unique source of exposure and that the contamination might not only come from food sources. Some countries still use OCs that can be transported by air and contaminate the environment in a different country (Ma et al., 2003). Therefore, OCs may contaminate the water that vegetarians drink, the air that they breathe, and the plant food from contaminated fields. Therefore, even if an individual eats exclusively organically certified plant food, exposure to OCs cannot be excluded (Arguin et al., 2010).

In another study from India, 28 samples of vegetarian meals (table-ready) were collected at home and in hotels, and analyzed for 31 PRs OCs (including POPs), organophosphates, carbamates, and pyrethroids. All 28 samples were found contaminated by one or several PRs, particularly HCH, DDT/DDE, and endosulfan (Kathpal and Kumari, 2009).

3. Dietary Exposure to Environmental Contaminants

3.1 Trace Elements

Table 45.1 summarizes the exposure of the vegetarian population to some trace elements. The results are presented considering two hypotheses due to the nondetected concentrations: the lower and the upper bound hypotheses. For the purpose of exposure calculations, the lower bound hypothesis, nondetected values were considered to be equal to 0, whereas for the upper bound hypothesis, these values were considered as being equal to the limit of detection.

The average exposure to total As in the Nutrinet-Santé vegetarian population (including pescetarians, ovolactovegetarians, and vegans) was approximately 0.60 µg kg/bw day, and 2.1 at the 95th percentile. Main arsenic contributors were similar to those of the general population (i.e., fish, crustaceans, and mollusks). These results showed that the average exposure of the vegetarian population was lower than that of the general French population. Highest exposure values were close to values of the two benchmark dose lower limits[2] (BMDL) that the JECFA established for inorganic arsenic ($BMDL_{01}$ set at 0.3

Table 45.1 Dietary Exposure to Trace Elements of the Vegetarian Population

	Lower Bound Hypothesis			Upper Bound Hypothesis		
	Mean	SD	95th Percentile	Mean	SD	95th Percentile
As (µg/kg bw day)	0.56	0.81	2.08	0.64	0.82	2.17
Pb (µg/kg bw day)	0.18	0.08	0.33	0.23	0.09	0.40
Cd (µg/kg bw day)	1.12	0.06	1.96	1.19	0.07	2.03
Al (mg/kg bw day)	0.39	0.03	0.74	0.40	0.03	0.76
Hg (µg/kg bw day)	0.02	0.03	0.07	0.16	0.07	0.28
Ni (µg/kg bw day)	2.95	1.34	5.45	3.36	1.44	6.16

Dietary exposures were calculated for the vegetarian population (including pescetarians) using contamination data of food items collected between 2007 and 2009.

[2] BMDL are set after modeling of dose-toxicological response curve and allowed to set a dose corresponding to a quantified effect (1% increase of lung cancer, for instance).

and 8 μg/kg bw day depending of the considered toxicological endpoint), and they indicate that this observed level of exposure is of health concern for the vegetarian population as well as for the general French population. These levels are higher than the UK estimates from Clarke et al. (2003) in the vegetarian population (mean dietary exposure: 0.018 mg/day resulting in 0.3 μg/kg bw day for a 60 kg bw adult).

With regard to lead, mean exposure of the vegetarian population was estimated at 0.20 μg/kg bw day. At the 95th percentile, exposure was 0.36 μg/kg bw day. Main contributors to lead exposure were vegetables (excluding potatoes), bread, and dry baking products. These exposure values were similar to those observed in the general French population. Considering the BMDLs established by EFSA (0.5 μg/kg bw day for central nervous system effects, 0.63 μg/kg bw day for nephrotoxic effects, and 1.5 μg/kg bw day for cardiovascular effects), the margin of exposure was lower than 10 for all toxicological endpoints, indicating that the risk related to lead dietary exposure cannot be excluded for the vegetarian population. These results are lower than those estimated for the UK vegetarian population: 0.016 mg/day resulting in 0.26 μg/kg bw day for an adult of 60 kg bw (Clarke et al., 2003).

The mean cadmium exposure for the French vegetarian population was estimated at 1.15 μg/kg bw week. Main contributors were vegetables (excluding potatoes), bread, and dried bread products. These exposure values were very close to those reported for the general French population. However, the highest contributor was potatoes for the general population compared to vegetables for the vegetarian population. Some exceedances of the health-based guidance value established by EFSA in 2009 (EFSA, 2009) were still observed for 1.3% of the vegetarian population. French estimates for the vegetarian population were close to that estimated for the vegetarian in the United Kingdom (1.75 μg/kg bw week; Clarke et al., 2003).

The mean aluminum exposure was estimated at 0.40 and 0.75 mg/kg bw week at the 95th percentile. Main aluminum contributors were hot beverages and vegetables (excluding potatoes). Exposure to aluminum of the vegetarian population was 1.5 times higher than that observed for the general French population. However, the exposure at the 95th percentile in the present study was below the provisional weekly tolerable intake value offset at 1 mg/kg bw week (EFSA, 2013). Clarke et al. (2003) calculated the same dietary exposures for the UK vegetarian population.

The mean exposure of vegetarians to mercury in the French population ranged from 0.02 to 0.16 μg/kg bw week. At the 95th percentile, exposure ranged from 0.07 to 0.28 μg/kg bw week. These wide ranges were due to different vegetarian populations and the pescetarian diet including fish (which are known to be the main contributor to Hg exposure), contrary to the other vegetarian diets. UK figures for the vegetarian population (Clarke et al., 2003) were close to the French upper bound estimate (0.15 μg/kg bw day for a 60 kg bw adult).

For nickel, mean exposure of French vegetarians was estimated at 3.1 μg/kg bw day and around 6 μg/kg bw day at the 95th percentile. Main nickel contributors were dried fruits, nuts and seeds, and fruits. Nickel exposures were between 1.2 and 1.6 times higher than those for the general French population. Sixty percent of the population had nickel exposure exceeding the health-based guidance value established by EFSA (2015) at 2.8 µg/kg bw day based on perinatal toxicity endpoints. Consequently, with regard to nickel, the risk cannot be excluded for the vegetarian population. The UK results from Clarke et al. (2003) were in the same range of magnitude as those estimated for the French general population (3 µg/kg bw day).

3.1.1 Summary for Trace Elements

The risk cannot be excluded for several trace elements; this includes cadmium, aluminum, and nickel. The studied vegetarian population was more exposed to cadmium and aluminum than the general French population. In the French vegetarian population, exceedances of the respective health-based guidance values for Cd, Al, and Ni were higher than that of the general population. For arsenic and lead, margin of exposures indicated that the risk could not be excluded for both contaminants. Compared to the general population, it appeared that some exceedances of the health-based guidance values were for the same substances.

3.2 Persistent Organic Pollutants

3.2.1 Exposure to PCB, Dioxins, and Furans

As one of the main contributors to PCB, dioxins, and furans exposure are fish, vegan and nonvegan (including pescetarian) exposure have been calculated for these two specific populations separately. PCDD/F + PCB-DL exposures were calculated using the toxicological equivalent factors (regulation (UE) n°1259/2011) known as $TEF_{WHO2005}$. The selected health-based guidance value was the monthly tolerable intake set by JECFA (2001a,b), 70 pg/TEQ_{WHO} kg bw month, i.e., 2.33 pg/$TEQ_{WHO2005}$ kg bw day. With regard to nondioxin-like PCB, the health-based guidance value set by Afssa at 10 ng/kg bw day was selected (Sirot et al., 2012a,b). Table 45.2 summarizes the exposures of the vegetarian populations to PCDD/F and PCB-NDL.

3.2.1.1 EXPOSURES OF THE VEGETARIAN POPULATION

For the total vegetarian population, the mean exposure to PCDD/F + PCB-DL was estimated at 0.4 and 1.5 pg/$TEQ_{WHO2005}$ kg bw day at the 95th percentile. Main PCDD/F + PCB-DL contributors were fish (22%) and cheese (17%). In the case of PCB-NDL, vegetarians had a

Table 45.2 Exposure of Different French Populations to PCDD/F and PCB-NDL

	PCDD/F (pg/$TEQ_{WHO2005}$ kg bw day)		PCB-NDL (ng/kg bw day)	
	Mean	95th Percentile	Mean	95th Percentile
Vegetarian	0.44	1.56	0.97	4.64
Vegan	0.073	0.23	0.068	0.284
Nonvegan	0.480	1.61	1.08	4.45
General population	0.4	0.83	1.83	5.05

The vegetarian population includes all people consuming vegetarian diets as categorized in this study (i.e., pescetarians, ovolactovegetarians, and vegan). The nonvegan population refers to all vegetarian populations (including pescetarians) except vegans. Dietary exposures were calculated using contamination data of food items collected between 2007 and 2009.

mean exposure of 0.97 ng/kg bw day. At the 95th percentile, exposure was 4.6 ng/kg bw day. Main PCB-NDL contributors were fish (47%) and mixed dishes (12%). Vegetarian exposures to PCB-NDL and PCDD/F + PCB-DL were all below their respective health-based guidance value.

3.2.1.2 EXPOSURES OF THE VEGAN POPULATION

Mean exposure to PCDD/F + PCB-DL in vegans was estimated at 0.06 pg/TEQ$_{WHO2005}$ kg bw day. Exposure at the 95th percentile, was estimated at 0.2 pg/TEQ$_{WHO2005}$ kg bw day. Main PCDD/F + PCB-DL contributors were oil and pizzas, quiches, savory pastries, and cakes. Mean exposure to PCB-NDL was estimated at 0.07 ng/kg bw day for both hypotheses. At the 95th percentile, exposure was 0.28 ng/kg bw day. Main PCB-NDL contributors were oil (42.6%) and pizzas, quiches, savory pastries, and cakes (28%). Vegan mean exposure to PCDD/F + PCB-DL was 15–30 times lower than that of the general population.

3.2.1.3 EXPOSURES OF THE NONVEGAN POPULATION

The nonvegan population (i.e., vegetarians including pescetarians but not vegans) had a mean exposure to PCDD/F + PCB-DL of 0.45 pg/TEQ$_{WHO2005}$ kg bw day. At the 95th percentile, exposure was 1.6 pg/TEQ$_{WHO2005}$ kg bw day. Main PCDD/F + PCB-DL contributors were fish (22%, at the lower bound evaluation) and cheese (LB: 17%). The mean exposure to PCB-NDL was estimated at 1.08 and 5.5 ng/kg bw day at the 95th percentile. Main PCB-NDL contributors were fish (48%) and mixed dishes.

It appeared that due to the consumption of fish, the nonvegan population had PCB and PCDD/F exposures much lower than those of the general French population. For all the vegetarian population, health-based guidance values were not exceeded at the 95th percentile.

3.2.2 Perfluoalkyl Acids

Mean exposures of the vegetarian population in France to Perfluorooctanesulfonic acid (PFOS) ranged from 0.031 to 0.447 ng/kg bw day depending on the calculation hypotheses. Perfluorooctanoic acid (PFOA) mean exposure ranged from 0.005 to 0.429 ng/kg bw day. These wide ranges were due to a high number of samples for which the concentration was below the limit of detection. Main contributors to PFOS and PFOA were fish and cheese. Mean vegetarian exposures to perfluoalkyl acids were lower than those described for the general French population (Rivière et al., 2014). Exposure values were below the respective health-based guidance values (PFOS: 0.15 µg/kg bw day and PFOA: 1.5 µg/kg bw day; EFSA, 2008).

3.2.3 Brominated Flame Retardants (BFR)

Table 45.3 summarizes the exposure of the vegetarian population in France to several brominated flame retardants.

Mean vegetarian exposure to HBCDD was estimated at 0.04 ng/kg bw day. At the 95th percentile, exposure was 0.20 ng/kg bw day. Main HBCDD contributors were fish and oil. Mean and 95th percentile exposure values to HBCDD are half of those of the general French population.

Table 45.3 Exposure to Brominated Flame Retardants of the Vegetarian Population

	Lower Bound Hypothesis			Upper Bound Hypothesis		
	Mean	SD	95th Percentile	Mean	SD	95th Percentile
HBCDD (ng/kg bw day)	0.04	0.09	0.19	0.05	0.97	0.21
7-PBDE (ng/kg bw day)	0.11	0.29	0.57	0.12	0.29	0.57
7-PBDE + PBDE209 (ng/kg bw day)	0.25	0.37	0.90	0.27	0.38	0.93

Dietary exposures were calculated for the vegetarian population (including pescetarians) using contamination data of food items collected between 2007 and 2009.

The mean exposure to polybromodiphenylether in vegetarians was estimated at 0.1 and 0.57 ng/kg bw day at the 95th percentile. Main contributors to the exposure of PBDE were fish and mixed dishes.

3.2.4 Summary for Persistent Organic Pollutants

All exposure results to POPs in vegetarians were below those of the general population. Exposure to furans, dioxins, and PCB are lower in vegans (compared to nonvegans) by one order of magnitude. This was due to the strong contribution of fish and mollusks to the exposures of these compounds that are not consumed by the vegan population. No exceedance has been identified in the vegan subpopulation in contrast to the general population.

3.3 Mycotoxins

Mean exposure to ochratoxin A (OTA) ranged from 0.21 to 3.5 ng/kg bw day at the 95th percentile. Main contributors to ochratoxin A exposure were bread and dry baking products and fruits. Considering the health-based guidance value established by EFSA in 2010, the exposure of the vegetarian population to ochratoxin A was considered to be of concern.

Mean exposure of vegetarians to patulin was estimated between 1.03 to 72 ng/kg bw day. Exposure to patulin in vegetarians was slightly higher than that in the general population. Main patulin contributors were fruits (especially apples), cooked fruits, and compotes. The Scientific Committee for Food in 2000 set a health-based guidance value at 400 ng/kg bw day. Consequently, the exposure of the vegetarian population calculated in the present study is considered of no concern.

Table 45.4 summarizes the exposure of the French vegetarian population to various additional mycotoxins. Due to the uncertainties associated with these results (especially due to the analytical limits that did not allow drawing a robust estimate of exposure), details were not discussed here.

Table 45.4 Exposure to Mycotoxins of the Vegetarian Population

| | Lower Bound Hypothesis | | | Upper Bound Hypothesis | | |
	Mean	SD	95th Percentile	SD	Mean	95th Percentile
Aflatoxins (ng/kg bw day)	0.00	0.00	0.00	0.78	0.38	1.49
Fumonisin B1 (ng/kg bw day)	8.9	16.0	31.4	25.7	24.2	63.8
Fumonisin B2 (ng/kg bw day)	2.39	7.82	12.5	12.7	11.7	32.6
Zearalenone (ng/kg bw day)	5.7	3.0	11.2	26.0	10.5	45.3
Ochratoxin A (ng/kg bw day)	0.21	0.17	0.54	1.91	0.86	3.48
Patulin (ng/kg bw day)	1.03	1.60	4.17	29.2	24.7	71.7
Trichothecen						
T2 and HT-2 toxins (ng/kg bw day)	9.3	6.5	21.5	50.4	26.7	99.6
Deoxynivalenol (ng/kg bw day)	285	179	60.9	321	193	670
Nivalenol (ng/kg bw day)	16.8	17.9	51.3	31.2	21.1	70.6

Dietary exposures were calculated for the vegetarian population (including pescetarians) using contamination data of food items collected between 2007 and 2009.

3.3.1 Summary for Mycotoxins

For most of the mycotoxins, the vegetarian population had exposures close to those previously reported for the general population except for T2/HT2 toxins, which mean exposures values were 1.2- to 2.5-fold higher than in the general population. Percentage of the population exceeding the respective health-based guidance values of DON and T2/HT2 toxins were in the same order of magnitude for both the vegetarian and the general populations. The risk could not be excluded for these two substances, but additional data are needed to confirm these results. On the other hand, the risk could be excluded for all other mycotoxins studied.

3.4 Phytoestrogens

Main phytoestrogens belong to the classes of isoflavones, coumestans, and lignans:

- Isoflavones include genistein and biochanin A, daidzein, formononetin, and glycitein.
- Lignans include matairesinol and secoisolariciresinol.
- Coumestans primarily include coumestrol.

Table 45.5   Exposure to Phytoestrogens of the Vegetarian Population

	Lower Bound Hypothesis			Upper Bound Hypothesis		
	Mean	SD	95th Percentile	Mean	SD	95th Percentile
Isoflavones (µg/kg bw day)	199.1	306.4	794.1	199.7	306.6	795.0
Lignans (µg/kg bw day)	2.64	3.79	9.38	3.24	3.71	10.1
Coumestans (ng/kg bw day)	123.0	398.3	775.2	594.5	559.5	1630.5

Isoflavones include genistein, biochanin A, daidzein, formononetion, and glycitein. Lignans include matairesinol and secoisolariciresinol.

For phytoestrogens, exposures of the vegetarian population were far above those reported for the general population (10–300 times higher). Overall exposure was mainly due to isoflavone, and there was a smaller contribution of coumestrol and equol. Consumption rate of "food for particular nutritional uses" was 50% instead of 12% in the general French population. The quantity of food consumed from that category was six times higher in the vegetarian population. "Food for particular nutritional uses" category was the main contributor of phytoestrogens exposure in vegetarian population.

Table 45.5 summarizes the exposure of the French vegetarian population to various phytoestrogens.

4. Conclusion

Based on theoretical exposure calculation, we showed that vegetarians had excessive exposure for many pesticides (48 out of 421), the pescetarian population being very close to the situation observed for the general population. On the other hand, some biomonitoring studies demonstrated that there was a trend toward lower organochlorine contamination in the vegan population compared to that of the general population.

As a conclusion, it appears that there are some differences in exposures to some contaminants between the vegetarian and the general population in France.

Exposure to phytoestrogens or some trace elements (Cd, Al, Ni) was higher for the vegetarian population compared to that of the general population. Among the vegetarian population, the main contributor to phytoestrogens appeared to be "foods for particular nutritional uses" in France. These products are consumed by a larger part of the vegetarian population (50% instead of 12% within the general population) and in a higher amount: six times more than the mean consumption of the general French population.

In vegetarians, exposure to patulin was mostly due to fruits, cooked fruits, and compotes and nonalcoholic flavored drinks. Consumption rates and consequently their contribution to the overall patulin exposure were seen to be higher in the vegetarian population than in the general population. Higher exposure to tin, nickel, cadmium, as well as aluminum was demonstrated in the vegetarian population compared to the general population. High consumption of fruits and vegetables (cooked, raw, and dry) in the vegetarian population appeared to be the reason for this observation.

The vegetarian population studied in the present study was, however, less exposed than the general population to some contaminants. This was true for POPs, some mycotoxins (NIV, DON, and aflatoxins), and some trace elements (As for instance). Primary contributors to the exposure of POP were "fish" and "crustaceans and mollusks." These categories were consumed by 30% of the vegetarian population compared to 80% in the French general population. Bread and dried bread products were the main contributors to certain mycotoxins (DON and Niv) exposures. Foods in this category were consumed by fewer vegetarians and in smaller amounts than that in the general population. This explained the existing differences in exposure between the vegetarian and the general populations. The lower consumption of coffee, cheese, and fish contributed to lower arsenic exposures. Last, exposure to some substances did not appear to be dramatically different between vegetarian and nonvegetarian populations. This is the case for lead, mercury, and some mycotoxins (fumonisin, for instance) that showed similar exposure to those previously reported for the general population.

Overall, it appears that despite the fact that the vegetarian population is not an insignificant part of the general population and the development of plant-based diet is of growing interest, little is known about the consequences of these diets on the exposure to contaminants or PRs. The study we conducted tried to fill gaps, but it suffers some limitations. For instance, as mentioned earlier, vegetarians are prone to consume more organic food that the general population, whereas organic food was not specifically considered in the total diet study that generated the contamination data that we used for estimating the exposure. Similarly, contamination data were not available for some very specific vegetarian dishes. For both contaminants and PRs, it appears that further studies specifically dedicated to vegetarian diets are needed.

References

Amit, M., Cummings, C., Grueger, B., Feldman, M., Lang, M., Grabowski, J., Wong, D., Greig, A., Patel, H., 2010. Vegetarian diets in children and adolescents. Paediatr. Child Health 15, 303–314.

Anderson, H.A., Wolff, M.S., 2000. Environmental contaminants in human milk. J. Expo. Anal. Environ. Epidemiol. 10.

ANSES, 2011. The Second Total Diet Study – Part 2: pesticide residues, additives, acrylamide, polycyclic aromatic hydrocarbons. In: scientifique, E. (Ed.), Rapport D'expertise. ANSES, Maisons-Alfort, p. 405.

Anses, 2014. Avis de l'Anses relatif à l'actualisation des indicateurs de risque alimentaire lié aux résidus de pesticides. Réponse à la saisine n°2013-SA-0138. Opinion on the Update of Dietary Exposure Indicators for Pesticide Residues. Request No 2013-SA-0138. ANSES, Maisons-Alfort, p. 36.

Arguin, H., Sánchez, M., Bray, G.A., Lovejoy, J.C., Peters, J.C., Jandacek, R.J., Chaput, J.P., Tremblay, A., 2010. Impact of adopting a vegan diet or an olestra supplementation on plasma organochlorine concentrations: results from two pilot studies. Br. J. Nutr. 103, 1433–1441.

Bailey, H.D., Armstrong, B.K., De Klerk, N.H., Fritschi, L., Attia, J., Scott, R.J., Smibert, E., Milne, E., 2011. Exposure to professional pest control treatments and the risk of childhood acute lymphoblastic leukemia. Int. J. Cancer 129, 1678–1688.

Baldi, I., Gruber, A., Rondeau, V., Lebailly, P., Brochard, P., Fabrigoule, C., 2011. Neurobehavioral effects of long-term exposure to pesticides: results from the 4-year follow-up of the PHYTONER Study. Occup. Environ. Med. 68, 108–115.

Baudry, J., Méjean, C., Allès, B., et al., 2015. Contribution of organic food to the diet in a large sample of French adults (the NutriNet-santé cohort study). Nutrients. 7 (10), 8615–8632. http://dx.doi.org/10.3390/nu7105417. http://www.mdpi.com.gate2.inist.fr/2072-6643/7/10/5417.

Baudry, J., Touvier, M., Allès, B., et al., June 2016. Typology of eaters based on conventional and organic food consumption: results from the NutriNet-Santé cohort study. Br. J. Nutr. 1–10. http://dx.doi.org/10.1017/S0007114516002427.

Caldas, E.D., de Souza, M.V., Jardim, A.N.O., 2011. Dietary risk assessment of organophosphorus and dithiocarbamate pesticides in a total diet study at a Brazilian university restaurant. Food addit. contam. Part A Chem. Anal. Control Expo. Risk Assess. 28, 71–79.

Cao, L.L., Yan, C.H., Yu, X.D., Tian, Y., Zhao, L., Liu, J.X., Shen, X.M., 2011. Relationship between serum concentrations of polychlorinated biphenyls and organochlorine pesticides and dietary habits of pregnant women in Shanghai. Sci. Total Environ. 409, 2997–3002.

Chen, M.Y.Y., Wong, W.W.K., Chen, B.L.S., Lam, C.H., Chung, S.W.C., Ho, Y.Y., Xiao, Y., 2015. Dietary exposure to organochlorine pesticide residues of the Hong Kong adult population from a total diet study. Food addit. contam. Part A Chem. Anal. Control Expo. Risk Assess. 32, 342–351.

Clarke, D.B., Barnes, K.A., Castle, L., Rose, M., Wilson, L.A., Baxter, M.J., Price, K.R., DuPont, M.S., 2003. Levels of phytoestrogens, inorganic trace-elements, natural toxicants and nitrate in vegetarian duplicate diets. Food Chem. 81, 287–300.

Craig, W.J., Mangels, A.R., American Dietetic, A., 2009. Position of the American Dietetic Association: vegetarian diets. J. Am. Diet. Assoc. 109, 1266–1282.

Dwyer, J.T., 1988. Health aspects of vegetarian diets. Am. J. Clin. Nutr. 48 (3), 712–738.

EFSA, 2008. Scientific Opinion of the Panel on Contaminants in the Food Chain. Perfluorooctane sulfonate (PFOS), perfluorooctanoic acid (PFOA) and their Salts (Question No EFSA-Q-2004-163). EFSA, Parma, Italy.

EFSA, 2009. Cadmium in food. Scientific opinion of the panel on contaminants in the food chain. EFSA 980 Parma, Italy.

EFSA, 2013. Technical Report: Dietary Exposure to Aluminium-Containing Food Additives. EFSA, Parma, Italy.

EFSA, 2011. Overview of the procedures currently used at EFSA for the assessment of dietary exposure to different chemical substances. EFSA J. 9, 2490.

EFSA, 2012. Guidance on the use of probabilistic methodology for modelling dietary exposure to pesticide residues. EFSA J. 10, 2839.

EFSA, 2014. The 2011 European union report on pesticide residues in food. EFSA J. EFSA, Parma, Italy.

EFSA, 2015. The 2013 European Union report on pesticide residues in food. Scientific Report of EFSA. EFSA J. 13, 4038.

EFSA, FAO, WHO, 2011. Towards a harmonised Total Diet Study approach: a guidance document. EFSA J. 9, 2450.

European Commission, 2015. EU Pesticides Database. European Commission, DG-SANCO. http://ec.europa.eu/food/plant/pesticides/eu-pesticides-database/public/?event=homepage&language=EN.

Gimou, M.M., Charrondiere, U.R., Leblanc, J.C., Pouillot, R., 2008. Dietary exposure to pesticide residues in Yaoundé: the Cameroonian total diet study. Food Addit. Contam. Part A Chem. Anal. Control Expo. Risk Assess. 25, 458–471.

JECFA, June 2001a. Joint FAO/WHO expert committee on food additives. In: Summary and Conclusions of the Fifty-Seventh Meeting, Rome, pp. 5–14.

JECFA, 2001b. Safety evaluation of certain mycotoxins in food prepared by the fifty-sixth meeting of the Joint FAO/WHO Expert Committee on Food Additives. WHO Food Addit. Ser. 47.

Hercberg, S., Castetbon, K., Czernichow, S., Malon, A., Mejean, C., Kesse, E., Touvier, M., Galan, P., 2010. Nutrinet-Santé Study: a web-based prospective study on the relationship between nutrition and health and determinants of dietary patterns and nutritional status. BMC Public Health.

Hergenrather, J., Hlady, G., Wallace, B., Savage, E., 1981. Pollutants in breast milk of vegetarians. N. Engl. J. Med. 304, 792.

INSERM, 2013. Pesticides, Effets sur la santé. In: Collection Expertise Collective Inserm, Paris. http://www.inserm.fr.

Kahleova, H., Pelikanova, T., 2015. Vegetarian diets in the prevention and treatment of type 2 diabetes. J. Am. Coll. Nutr.

Kathpal, T.S., Kumari, B., 2009. Monitoring of pesticide residues in vegetarian diet. Environ. Monit. Assess. 151, 19–26.

Kesavachandran, C.N., Fareed, M., Pathak, M.K., Bihari, V., Mathur, N., Srivastava, A.K., 2009. Adverse health effects of pesticides in Agrarian populations of developing countries. In: Whitacre, M.D. (Ed.). Whitacre, M.D. (Ed.), Reviews of Environmental Contamination and Toxicology, vol. 200. Springer US, Boston, MA, pp. 33–52.

Koutros, S., Andreotti, G., Berndt, S.I., Hughes Barry, K., Lubin, J.H., Hoppin, J.A., Kamel, F., Sandler, D.P., Burdette, L.A., Yuenger, J., Yeager, M., Alavanja, M.C.R., Freeman, L.E.B., 2011. Xenobiotic-metabolizing gene variants, pesticide use, and the risk of prostate cancer. Pharmacogenet. Genomics 21, 615–623.

Leblanc, J.-C., Yoon, H., Kombadjian, A., Verger, P., 2000. Nutritional intakes of vegetarian populations in France. Eur. J. Clin. Nutr.

Lu, C., Toepel, K., Irish, R., Fenske, R.A., Barr, D.B., Bravo, R., 2006. Organic diets significantly lower children's dietary exposure to organophosphorus pesticides. Environ. Health Perspect. 114, 260–263.

Luo, Y., Zhang, M., 2009. Multimedia transport and risk assessment of organophosphate pesticides and a case study in the northern San Joaquin Valley of California. Chemosphere 75, 969–978.

Ma, J., Daggupaty, S., Harner, T., Li, Y., 2003. Impacts of lindane usage in the Canadian prairies on the Great Lakes ecosystem. 1. Coupled atmospheric transport model and modeled concentrations in air and soil. Environ. Sci. Technol. 37, 3774–3781.

MAF, 2009. New Zealand Total Diet Study – Agricultural compound residues, selected contaminant and nutrient elements. Ministry Agric. For. 178 Crown Copyright November 2011.

Naidoo, S., London, L., Burdorf, A., Naidoo, R., Kromhout, H., 2011. Spontaneous miscarriages and infant deaths among female farmers in rural South Africa. Scand. J. Work Environ. Health 37, 227–236.

Nougadère, A., Merlo, M., Héraud, F., Réty, J., Truchot, E., Vial, G., Cravedi, J.P., Leblanc, J.C., 2014. How dietary risk assessment can guide risk management and food monitoring programmes: the approach and results of the French Observatory on Pesticide Residues (ANSES/ORP). Food Control. 41, 32–48.

Nougadère, A., Sirot, V., Kadar, A., Fastier, A., Truchot, E., Vergnet, C., Hommet, F., Baylé, J., Gros, P., Leblanc, J.C., 2012. Total diet study on pesticide residues in France: Levels in food as consumed and chronic dietary risk to consumers. Environ. Int. 45, 135–150.

Panuwet, P., Prapamontol, T., Chantara, S., Barr, D.B., 2009. Urinary pesticide metabolites in school students from northern Thailand. Int. J. Hyg. Environ. Health 212, 288–297.

Rawn, D.F.K., Cao, X.L., Doucet, J., Davies, D.J., Sun, W.F., Dabeka, R.W., Newsome, W.H., 2004. Canadian total diet study in 1998: pesticide levels in foods from Whitehorse, Yukon, Canada, and corresponding dietary intake estimates. Food Addit. Contam. 21, 232–250.

Regulation (EC) No 396/2005, of the European Parliament and of the Council on Maximum Residue Levels of Pesticides in or on Food and Feed of Plant and Animal Origin and Amending Council Directive 91/414/EEC (OJEU, 16/03/2005) and Regulations Modifying Its Annexes II, III and IV on Maximum Levels Applicable to Residues of Products Appearing in Its Annex I.

Regulation (EC) No 1107/2009, of the European Parliament and of the Council of 21 October 2009 Concerning the Placing of Plant Protection Products on the Market and Repealing Council Directives 79/117/EEC and 91/414/EEC.

Renda, M., Fischer, P., 2009. Vegetarian diets in children and adolescents. Pediatr. Rev. 30, e1–e8.

Rivière, G., Sirot, V., Tard, A., Jean, J., Marchand, P., Veyrand, B., Le Bizec, B., Leblanc, J.C., 2014. Food risk assessment for perfluoroalkyl acids and brominated flame retardants in the French population: results from the second French total diet study. Sci. Total Environ. 491–492.

Rogan, W.J., Bagniewska, A., Damstra, T., 1980. Pollutants in breast milk. N. Engl. J. Med. 302, 1450–1453.

Sirot, V., Volatier, J.L., Calamassi-Tran, G., Dubuisson, C., Ménard, C., Dufour, A., Leblanc, J.C., 2009. Core food of the French food supply: second total diet study. Food Addit. Contam. Part A.

Sirot, V., Tard, A., Venisseau, A., Brosseaud, A., Marchand, P., Le Bizec, B., Leblanc, J.C., 2012a. Dietary exposure to polychlorinated dibenzo-p-dioxins, polychlorinated dibenzofurans and polychlorinated biphenyls of the French population: results of the second French Total Diet Study. Chemosphere 88, 492–500.

Sirot, V., Hommet, F., Tard, A., Leblanc, J.C., 2012b. Dietary acrylamide exposure of the French population: results of the second French total diet study. Food Chem. Toxicol. 50, 889–894.

Van Audenhaege, M., Héraud, F., Menard, C., Bouyrie, J., Morois, S., Calamassi-Tran, G., Lesterle, S., Volatier, J.L., Leblanc, J.C., 2009. Impact of food consumption habits on the pesticide dietary intake: comparison between a French vegetarian and the general population. Food Addit. Contam. Part A Chem. Anal. Control Expo. Risk Assess. 26, 1372–1388.

Volatier, J.L., 2000. Enquête INCA individuelle et nationale des consommations alimentaires. Tech & Doc, Paris.

WHO, 1997. Guidelines for Predicting Dietary Intake of Pesticides Residues (Revised). Prepared by the Global Environment Monitoring System – Food Contamination Monitoring and Assessment Programme (GEMS/Food) in Collaboration With the Codex Committee on Pesticide Residues. WHO Publications. WHO/FSF/FOS/97.7, WHO, Geneva, p. 31. CH (1997).

Wong, W.W.K., Yau, A.T.C., Chung, S.W.C., Lam, C.H., Ma, S., Ho, Y.Y., Xiao, Y., 2014. Dietary exposure of Hong Kong adults to pesticide residues: results of the first Hong Kong total diet study. Food Addit. Contam. Part A Chem. Anal. Control Expo. Risk Assess. 31, 852–871.

Index

'*Note*: Page numbers followed by "f" indicate figures, "t" indicate tables.'

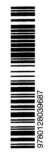